ESPNIC Children's Intensive Care Textbook

Joe Brierley • Pierre Tissieres • Akash Deep
Editors

ESPNIC Children's Intensive Care Textbook

Springer

Editors
Joe Brierley
Paediatric and Neonatal Intensive Care
Great Ormond Street Hospital
London, UK

Akash Deep
Paediatric Intensive Care Unit
King's College Hospital NHS Foundation Trust
London, UK

Pierre Tissieres
Pediatric and Neonatal ICU
University of Paris-Sud
Le Kremlin-Bicêtre Cedex
France

ISBN 978-3-031-64761-1   ISBN 978-3-031-64762-8 (eBook)
https://doi.org/10.1007/978-3-031-64762-8

This Springer imprint is published by the registered company Springer Nature Switzerland AG
The registered company address is: Gewerbestrasse 11, 6330 Cham, Switzerland

Introduction

In its mission to promote the highest quality care to critically ill children throughout Europe, the European Society of Paediatric and Neonatal Intensive Care recognises that education and the ongoing dissemination of best practices to intensive care professionals across Europe and beyond are crucial.

Why another textbook? We seek no forgiveness for wanting to provide the first European textbook covering all aspects of Paediatric and Neonatal Intensive Care.

The previous seismic shift in our speciality, with increased numbers of children with complexity living with life-limiting diseases and dependent on technological support, transformed the ICU environment over recent decades and has been a driving force. But now, in a less-stable post-pandemic world, with war in Europe once again after many years of peace, with near-vanquished infectious diseases returning due to vaccine hesitancy, and with core-PIC diseases likely to reduce due to novel vaccines, critical care is changing again.

Congenital interventions have become safe and standardised, led by experts in European centres in paediatric cardiac surgery and general surgery—the ICU team's role in this ever-safer environment is a core feature of this book. Safer, yet clearly more aggressive organ support with RRT and increasingly ECMO have become standard in most European centres. Knowledge of such organ support and transplants, rapidly developing oncology treatments and patient safety governance standards are now core knowledge for the intensivist. Working with colleagues to support children and their families during and after periods of critical illness, including delivering excellent end-of-life care within the ICU for children and their families, is a clear duty—all feature in this book.

This first ESPNIC paediatric and neonatal intensive care textbook provides the core knowledge of the speciality for clinicians in Europe and further afield from European experts. It is an offering from a European society with increasingly global reach and collaborations. The textbook links into other ESPNIC educational developments, includes sections on all contemporary critical care support for children, and features chapters from leading experts in the field.

It is suitable for those training in paediatric and neonatal intensive care, whether physicians, nurses or allied health professionals. It will also provide a resource for those seeking continuing professional development in this relatively young and developing speciality.

At a time when the Society has recently launched its own journal, Intensive Care Medicine Paediatric and Neonatal, the launch of this new textbook is another step in ESPNIC's goal to help educate PIC/NIC professionals throughout Europe. In this, it joins the now annual ESPNIC conference, standalone workshops and frequent online training offerings.

We are grateful to those authors who have taken the time to provide chapters. While we must acknowledge the interruption of the COVID pandemic to the genesis of this book, one of the few benefits has been the spotlight on critical care in health.

We encourage all members of the intensive care community throughout Europe to seize the zeitgeist and join ESPNIC in its journey to improve the care of critically ill children, wherever they are.

Joe Brierley
Great Ormond Street Hospital
London, UK

Akash Deep
King's College Hospital NHS Foundation Trust
London, UK

Contents

V The Lung and Mechanical Ventilation in ICU

IX Neurocritical Care

X Hematological Issues in PICU

XI Specific Situations

XIII Looking After People

XV Research Needed in the ICU

XVI Education

Contributors

Susana Abreu Hospital Santa Marta, Centro Hospitalar Universitário Lisboa Central, Lisbon, Portugal

Shruti Agrawal Paediatric Intensive Care, Cambridge University Hospitals NHS Foundation Trust, Cambridge, UK

Department of Paediatrics, University of Cambridge, Cambridge, UK

Emma C. Alexander Paediatric Intensive Care Unit, King's College Hospital NHS Foundation Trust, London, UK

Nadirah El-Amin, DO, MPH Division of Pediatric Haematology and Oncology, Department of Pediatrics, Children's Hospital of Richmond, Richmond, VA, USA

John van den Anker Intensive Care and Department of Paediatric Surgery, Erasmus MC-Sophia Children's Hospital, Rotterdam, the Netherlands

Division of Clinical Pharmacology, Children's National Hospital, Washington, D.C., USA

Division of Paediatric Pharmacology and Pharmacometrics, University Children's Hospital Basel, University of Basel, Basel, Switzerland

Angela Aramburo Paediatric Intensive Care Unit, Royal Brompton & Harefield NHS Foundation Trust, London, UK

Roelie Wösten-van Asperen PICU, UMC Utrecht, Utrecht, The Netherlands

Omer Aziz Paediatric Intensive Care Unit, Bristol Royal Hospital for Children, Bristol, UK

Julien Baleine PICU, Hospital Arnaud de Villeneuve, Montpellier, France

Harish Bangalore Great Ormond Street Hospital for Children, London & St Andrews Burns Centre, Chelmsford, UK

Mehak Bansal Pediatric Intensive Care Unit, Clio Mother and Child Institute, Ludhiana, India

Aurélie Bardaji Division of Neonatal and Paediatric Intensive Care, Geneva University Hospitals and Faculty of Medicine, Geneva, Switzerland

Hanaa Benjeddi Amsterdam UMC, Amsterdam, The Netherlands

Jonas Berner Paediatric Perioperative Medicine and Intensive Care, Astrid Lindgren Children's Hospital, Karolinska University Hospital, Stockholm, Sweden

Division of Clinical Pharmacology, Karolinska Institutet and Karolinska University Hospital, Stockholm, Sweden

Robert G. T. Blokpoel Division of Paediatric Critical Care Medicine, Department of Paediatrics, Beatrix Children's Hospital, University Medical Center Groningen, University of Groningen, Groningen, The Netherlands

Tom Breen St Georges' Hospital, London, UK

Joe Brierley Paediatric Intensive Care and Paediatric Bioethics, Great Ormond Street Hospital, London, UK

PICU and Bioethics, Great Ormond Street Hospital, London, UK

Great Ormond St Hospital, London, PIC, London, UK

Katherine L. Brown Paediatric Intensive Care, Heart and Lung Division, Great Ormond Street Hospital NHS Foundation Trust, London, UK

Institute Cardiovascular Science, University College London, London, UK

Ashleigh E. Butler School of Nursing and Midwifery, La Trobe University, Melbourne, VIC, Australia

Corinne Buysse Department of Neonatal and Pediatric Intensive Care, Division of Pediatric Intensive Care, Erasmus MC Sophia Children's Hospital, Rotterdam, The Netherlands

Gilles Cambonie PICU, Hospital Arnaud de Villeneuve, Montpellier, France

Michael J. Carter Centre for Human Genetics, University of Oxford, Oxford, UK

Paediatric Intensive Care Unit, Oxford University Hospitals NHS Foundation Trust, Oxford, UK

Roberta Centorino Division of Pediatrics and Neonatal Critical Care, "A. Beclere" Medical Center, Paris Saclay University Hospitals, APHP, Paris, France

Physiopathology and Therapeutic Innovation Unit-INSERM U999, Paris Saclay University, Paris, France

Maria Chalia Neonatal Intensive Care Unit, Great Ormond Street Hospital for Children, London, UK

Corinne Jotterand Chaparro Department of Nutrition and Dietetics, Geneva School of Health Sciences, HES-SO University of Applied Sciences and Arts Western Switzerland, Geneva, Switzerland

Susan M. Chapman Great Ormond Street Hospital for Children NHS Foundation Trust, London, UK

Teresa Chila' Newcastle upon Tyne Hospitals Foundation Trust, Newcastle upon Tyne, UK

Gillian Colville St George's University Hospitals NHS Foundation Trust, London, UK

Population Health Research Institute, City St George's, University of London, London, UK

Pam D'Silva King's College Hospital, London, UK

Yemi Jegede Paediatric Critical Care, King's College Hospital London, London, UK

Dennis Daniel Department of Anesthesiology, Critical Care and Pain Medicine, Boston Children's Hospital, Boston, MA, USA

Theodore Dassios Faculty of Life Science and Medicine, Department of Women and Children's Health, School of Life Course Sciences, King's College London, London, UK

Neonatal Intensive Care Centre, King's College Hospital NHS Foundation Trust, London, UK

Akash Deep Pediatric Intensive Care Unit, King's College Hospital NHS Foundation Trust, London, UK

Stéphanie Delangue Univ. Lille, CHU Lille, Lille, France

Sandeep Dhingra Department of Pediatrics, Army Hospital (Research & Referral), New Delhi, India

Karolijn Dulfer Department of Neonatal and Pediatric Intensive Care, Division of Pediatric Intensive Care, Erasmus MC Sophia Children's Hospital, Rotterdam, The Netherlands

Caroline Duracher, MD University Paris Cité, Paris, France

Iria Duran Cardiac Intensive Care Unit, Great Ormond Street Hospital, London, UK

Matt Edwards King's College Hospital, London, UK

Y. Feinstein, MD Pediatric Cardiac Intensive Care Unit, Schneider Children's Medical Center, Petach Tikva, Israel

Analía Fernández Paediatric Critical Care Unit, Hospital General de Agudos "C. Durand", Ciudad Autónoma de Buenos Aires, Buenos Aires, Argentina

Serge Grazioli Division of Neonatal and Paediatric Intensive Care, Geneva University Hospitals and Faculty of Medicine, Geneva, Switzerland

Anne Greenough Faculty of Life Science and Medicine, Department of Women and Children's Health, School of Life Course Sciences, King's College London, London, UK

Neonatal Intensive Care Centre, King's College Hospital NHS Foundation Trust, London, UK

Asthma UK Centre for Allergic Mechanisms in Asthma, King's College London, London, UK

NIHR Biomedical Research Centre based at Guy's and St Thomas' NHS Foundation Trust and King's College London, London, UK

Dhiren Gupta Division of Pediatric Emergency and Critical Care, Institute of Child Health, Sir Ganga Ram Hospital, New Delhi, India

Francesco Guzzi Nephrology and Dialysis Unit, Santo Stefano Hospital, Prato, Italy

Simon Hannam Neonatal Intensive Care Unit, Great Ormond Street Hospital for Children, London, UK

Lotte Haverman Amsterdam UMC, University of Amsterdam, Emma Children's Hospital, Department of Child and Adolescent Psychiatry and Psychosocial Care, Amsterdam Reproduction and Development, Amsterdam Public Health, Amsterdam, The Netherlands

Géraldine Hery Pediatric Surgery, Hopital Bicetre, APHP, Paris, France

Aparna Hoskote, MBBS, DCH, MD, MRCP Cardiac Intensive Care Unit, Great Ormond Street Hospital For Children NHS Foundation Trust, London, UK

Maayke Hunfeld Department of Neonatal and Pediatric Intensive Care, Division of Pediatric Intensive Care, Erasmus MC Sophia Children's Hospital, Rotterdam, The Netherlands

David Philip Inwald Paediatric Intensive Care Unit, Cambridge University Hospitals NHS Foundation Trust, Cambridge, UK

Pauline de Jager Division of Paediatric Critical Care Medicine, Department of Paediatrics, Beatrix Children's Hospital, University Medical Center Groningen, University of Groningen, Groningen, The Netherlands

Yemi Jegede Paediatric Critical Care, King's College Hospital, London, UK

Oliver Karam, MD, PhD Pediatric Critical Care, Department of Pediatrics, Yale School of Medicine, New Haven, CT, USA

Pediatric Critical Care Medicine, Yale, New Haven, CT, USA

Sonia Khamis Paediatric Neurology Department, Evelina London Children's Hospital, London, UK

Martin C. J. Kneyber Division of Paediatric Critical Care Medicine, Department of Paediatrics, Beatrix Children's Hospital, University Medical Center Groningen, University of Groningen, Groningen, The Netherlands

Critical Care, Anaesthesiology, Peri-operative and Emergency Medicine (CAPE), University of Groningen, Groningen, The Netherlands

Alette Koopman Division of Paediatric Critical Care Medicine, Department of Paediatrics, Beatrix Children's Hospital, University Medical Center Groningen, University of Groningen, Groningen, The Netherlands

Hari Krishnan Birmingham Children's Hospital, Birmingham, UK

Sonia Labarinas, MD Division of Pediatric Critical Care Medicine, Memorial Hermann Texas Medical Center, University of Texas Health, Houston, TX, USA

Lynne Latten Alder Hey Children's Hospital NHS Foundation Trust, Liverpool, UK

Joris Lemson Department of Intensive Care Medicine, Radboud University Medical Center/Amalia Children's Hospital, Nijmegen, The Netherlands

Stéphane Leteurtre Univ. Lille, CHU Lille, Lille, France

Service de réanimation et de surveillance continue pédiatrique, Hopital Jeanne de Flandre, CHRU de Lille, Lille Cedex, France

Jim Linthicum Chaplaincy and Paediatric Bioethics, Great Ormond Street, Chaplaincy, London, UK

Barbara Loi Division of Pediatrics and Neonatal Critical Care, "A. Beclere" Medical Center, Paris Saclay University Hospitals, APHP, Paris, France

Yolanda M. López-Fernandez PICU, Cruces University Hospital, BioBizkaia Health Research Institute, Barakaldo, Bizkaia, Spain

Daniele De Luca Division of Pediatrics and Neonatal Critical Care, "A. Beclere" Medical Center, Paris Saclay University Hospitals, APHP, Paris, France

Physiopathology and Therapeutic Innovation Unit INSERM U999, Paris Saclay University, Paris, France

Mona Mahyub Paediatric Intensive Care, Great Ormond Street Hospital, London, UK

Joseph C. Manning Nottingham Children's Hospital, Nottingham University Hospitals NHS Trust and Children and Young People's Health Research, School of Health Sciences, The University of Nottingham, Nottingham, UK

Sundaram Manu PICU, San Juan de Deu Hospital, Barcelona, Spain

Luise V. Marino Southampton Children's Hospital, University Hospital Southampton NHS Foundation Trust, Southampton, UK

Faculty of Health and Wellbeing, University of Winchester, Winchester, UK

Jordi Miatello Department of Paediatric and Neonatal Intensive Care, Hôpital Bicêtre, Assistance-Publique Hôpitaux de Paris, Le Kremlin-Bicêtre, Paris, France

Université Paris Saclay, Le Kremlin Bicêtre, Paris, France

Christophe Milési PICU, Hospital Arnaud de Villeneuve, Montpellier, France

Simon Nadel Paediatric Intensive Care, Imperial College London, London, UK

Matteo Di Nardo Pediatric Intensive Care Unit, Bambino Gesù Children's Hospital, IRCCS, Rome, Italy

Rufaro Ndokera Great Ormond Street Hospital, London, UK

Marti Pons Odena PICU, San Juan de Deu Hospital, Barcelona, Spain

Helen Ord Birmingham Children's Hospital, Birmingham, UK

Gilles Orliaguet, MD, PhD University Paris Cité, Paris, France

UMR 1343 Pharmacologie et évaluation des thérapeutiques chez l'enfant et la femme enceinte, Université Paris Cité, INSERM, Paris, France

Aarti Pandit Paediatric Intensive Care, Great Ormond Street Hospital, London, UK

Niha Peshimam Imperial College Healthcare NHS Trust, London, UK

Lucilla Pezza Division of Pediatrics and Neonatal Critical Care, "A. Beclere" Medical Center, Paris Saclay University Hospitals, APHP, Paris, France

C. M. Pierce Great Ormond Street Hospital NHS Trust, London, UK

Pavla Pokorná First Faculty of Medicine, Department of Paediatrics and Inherited Metabolic Disorders, Charles University and General University Hospital, Prague, Czech Republic

First Faculty of Medicine, Institute of Pharmacology, Charles University and General University Hospital, Prague, Czech Republic

Intensive Care and Department of Paediatric Surgery, Erasmus MC-Sophia Children's Hospital, Rotterdam, the Netherlands

Division of Clinical Pharmacology, Karolinska Institutet and Karolinska University Hospital, Stockholm, Sweden

Angelo Polito Geneva, Switzerland

Uri Pollak, MD Department of Pediatric Critical Care, Hadassah University Medical Center, The Hebrew University of Jerusalem, Jerusalem, Israel

Suresh Pujar Paediatric Neurology Department, Great Ormond Street Hospital for Children, London, UK

Institute of Child Health, University College London, London, UK

Lucas Rabaux Pediatric Surgery, Hopital Bicetre, APHP, Paris, France

Padmanabhan Ramnarayan Children's Acute Transport Service, Great Ormond Street Hospital, London, UK

Paediatric Intensive Care Unit, St Mary's Hospital, London, UK

Samiran Ray Paediatric Intensive Care Unit, Great Ormond Street Hospital, London, UK

Morgan Recher Univ. Lille, CHU Lille, Lille, France

Service de réanimation et de surveillance continue pédiatrique, Hopital Jeanne de Flandre, CHRU de Lille, Lille Cedex, France

Karl Reiter Dr. von Hauner Children's Hospital, Ludwig Maximilians University, Munich, Germany

Zaccaria Ricci Pediatric Cardiac Intensive Care Unit, Department of Pediatrics, Meyer Children's Hospital, IRCCS, Florence, Italy

Pediatric Intensive Care Unit, Meyer Children's Hospital, Florence, Italy

Peter Rimensberger Division of Neonatology and Paediatric Intensive Care, University Hospital of Geneva, University of Geneva, Geneva, Switzerland

Alessandra Rizza Rome, Italy

Isadora Rodriguez Paediatric Intensive Care Unit, King's College Hospital NHS Foundation Trust, London, UK

Peter Paul Roeleveld Leiden University Medical Center, Leiden, The Netherlands

Nwanneka N. Sargant Bristol Royal Hospital for Children, Bristol, UK

Emma Simpson Freeman Hospital, Newcastle Hospitals NHS Trust, Newcastle-upon-Tyne, UK

Rahul Raman Singh Paediatric Neurology Department, Evelina London Children's Hospital, London, UK

Yogen Singh Department of Pediatrics—Neonatology and Pediatric Cardiology, Addenbrooke's Hospital, Cambridge University Hospitals NHS Foundation Trust, University of Cambridge School of Clinical Medicine, Cambridge, UK

Thomas Slater Department of Paediatric Inherited Metabolic Diseases, Evelina London Children's Hospital, London, UK

Francesca Sperotto Department of Cardiology, Boston Children's Hospital, Harvard Medical School, Boston, MA, USA

Kentigern Thorburn PICU, Alder Hey Children's Hospital, Liverpool, UK

Department of Clinical Infection, Microbiology and Immunology, University of Liverpool, Liverpool, UK

Dick Tibboel Department of Intensive Care, Erasmus MC, Rotterdam, The Netherlands

First Faculty of Medicine, Department of Paediatrics and Inherited Metabolic Disorders, Charles University and General University Hospital, Prague, Czech Republic

Intensive Care and Department of Paediatric Surgery, Erasmus MC-Sophia Children's Hospital, Rotterdam, the Netherlands

Lyvonne Tume Faculty of Health, Social care & Medicine, Edge Hill University, Ormskirk, UK

Alder Hey Children's Hospital, Liverpool, UK

Lyvonne N. Tume Liverpool, UK

Faculty of Health, Social Care & Medicine, Edge Hill University, Ormskirk, UK

Gaurang Upadhyay Paediatric Intensive Care Unit, King's College Hospital NHS Foundation Trust, London, UK

Frédéric V. Valla Paediatric Intensive Care, Hôpital Femme Mère enfant, Hospices Civils de Lyon, Lyon, France

Roshni Vara Department of Paediatric Inherited Metabolic Diseases, Evelina London Children's Hospital, London, UK

Estelle Vergnaud, MD University Paris Cité, Paris, France

Anita Verma, Dr., MD Department of Infection Science and Institute of Liver Studies, King's College Hospital, NHS Trust, London, UK

Timothy Wait Intensive Care Medicine, Thames Valley Deanery, Oxford, UK

Jef Willems Paediatric Intensive Care Unit, University Hospital Ghent, Ghent, Belgium

Traci A. Wolbrink Department of Anesthesiology, Critical Care and Pain Medicine, Boston Children's Hospital, Boston, MA, USA

Leonie Wong Department of Paediatric Cardiology, Royal Brompton & Harefield NHS Foundation Trust, London, UK

Dora Wood Bristol Royal Hospital for Children, Bristol, UK

Gavin Wooldridge Paediatric Intensive Care Unit, Cambridge University Hospitals NHS Foundation Trust, Cambridge, UK

North West and North Wales Paediatric Transport team (NWTS), Manchester University Hospitals Foundation Trust, Mancheter, UK

Anna Zanin Pediatric Intensive Care Unit, San Bortolo Hospital, Vicenza, Italy

Department of Women and Children's health, Azienda Ospedaliera Università di Padova, Padova, Italy

Bogdana Zoica King's College Hospital, London, UK

Abbreviations

ADME	Absorption, distribution, metabolism, excretion
ALPS	Astrid Lindgren Children's Hospital Pain Scale
ARDS	Acute respiratory distress syndrome
AUC	Area under the curve
BIS	Bispectral index
BiVAD	Bi-ventricular assist device
CAAS	Cardiac Analgesic Assessment Scale
CHD	Congenital heart disease
CHEOPS	Eastern Ontario Children's Hospital Pain Scale
CL	Clearance
C_{max}	Maximum concentration
C_{min}	Minimum concentration
COMFORT-B	COMFORT Behavior Scale
COMFORT-neo	COMFORT score for neonates
CPAP	Continuous positive airway pressure
CPB	Cardiopulmonary bypass
Cpl	Plasma concentration
CRIES scale	Cry Requires oxygen, Increased vital signs, Expression, Sleeplessness Scale
CRRT	Continuous renal replacement therapy
CYP450	Cytochrome P450
DMS-5	Diagnostic and statistical manual of mental disorders, fifth edition
DT	Destination therapy
ECMO	Extracorporeal membrane oxygenation
E-CPR	Extra-corporeal cardiopulmonary resuscitation
ED	Emergency department
EEG	Electroencephalogram
ePAP	Expiratory positive airway pressure
EUROMACS	European Registry for Patients with Mechanical Circulatory Support
F	Bioavailability
FLACC	Face, Legs, Activity, Cry, Consolability scale
GA	Gestational age
GFR	Glomerular filtration rate
GTS	Glutathione S-transferase
HFNC	High-flow nasal cannula

HT	Hypothermia
i.m.	Intramuscular
i.v.	Intravenous
ICU	Intensive care unit
INTERMACS	Interagency Registry for Mechanically Assisted Circulatory Support
iPAP	Inspiratory positive airway pressure
k	Elimination rate constant
K_a	Absorption rate constant
LD	Loading dose
LV	Left ventricle
LVAD	Left ventricular assist device
MAPS	Multidimensional Assessment of Pain Scale
MCS	Mechanical circulatory support
MD	Maintenance dose
MIC	Minimum inhibitory concentration
NAS	Neonatal Abstinence Syndrome
NFCS	Neonatal Facial Coding System
NICU	Neonatal intensive care unit
NIPS	Neonatal Infant Pain Scale
NIV	Noninvasive ventilation
NONMEM	Non-linear mixed-effects modelling
NPASS	Neonatal Pain, Agitation, and Sedation scale
NRS	Numeric Rating Scale
OATPs	Organic anion transporting polypeptides
OATs	Organic anion transporters
OCTs	Organic cation transporters
OHTx	Orthotopic heart transplantation
p.o.	Oral administration
p.r.	Rectal administration
PaPaSS	Pediatric Palliative Screening Scale
PBPK	Physiology-based pharmacokinetics
PD	Pharmacodynamics
Pedimacs	Paediatric Interagency Registry for Mechanical Circulatory Support
PedsQL	Pediatric Quality of Life Inventory Scale
PG	Pharmacogenetics
PICU	Pediatric intensive care unit
PIPP-r	Premature Infant Pain Profile-Revised score

PK	Pharmacokinetics
PMA	Postmenstrual age
PNA	Postnatal age
POD	Post-operative day
RA	Right atrium
RR	Respiratory rate
RV	Right ventricle
RVD	Right ventricular dysfunction
s.c.	Subcutaneous administration
SIRS	Systemic inflammatory response syndrome
SOS	Sophia Observation Withdrawal Symptoms-Scale
SULTs	Sulfotransferases
$T_{1/2}$	Elimination half life
Ti	Inspiratory time
UDP	Uridine 5′-diphospho
UGTs	Uridine 5′-diphospho glucuronosyltransferases
VA	Veno-arterial
VAD	Ventricular assist device
VAS	Visual Analogue Scale
Vd	Volume of distribution
VNS	Verbal Numeric Scale
VT	Tidal volume
WAT-1	Withdrawal Assessment Tool version 1
WOB	Work of breathing

Introduction

Content

Paediatric and Neonatal Intensive Care: Quo Vadis

Dick Tibboel

Contents

Partly based on the opening lecture of the 21st ESPNIC meeting in Salzburg, Austria, 2019, and the Denis DeVictor award for lifelong achievement.

J. Brierley et al. (eds.), *ESPNIC Children's Intensive Care Textbook*,
https://doi.org/10.1007/978-3-031-64762-8_1

Learning Objectives

- To understand recent changes in patient case mix, and the consequences for the future.
- Be aware of the differences in knowledge needed and education for contemporary and future. Paediatric and Neonatal intensive care specialists.

1.1 Introduction

Over the last decades, paediatric intensive care medicine has developed into a mature speciality from different angles, such as anaesthesiology and paediatrics, depending on the history of individual countries. There are major differences in case mix between units worldwide, in particular with regard to the admission of newborns with or without a surgical problem to the PICU. Although the main initial focus was to reach a low mortality rate, this is now only around 3–5%, so more contemporary attention is paid to long-term complications or induced morbidity in different organ systems. Although many therapeutic modalities are still not investigated in detail (inter)national collaboration has resulted in guidelines such as for sepsis, nutrition, hemodynamic monitoring, perioperative case, transfusions and analgosedation, though with variable levels of evidence [1–8]. Moreover, new horizons emerge when dealing with patients considered unsalvageable in the past, or new cohorts admitted to PICU, such as COVID-19 patients recently [9, 10]. For obvious reasons, this results in new ethical dilemmas for treatment teams and the need for the integration of different specialities involved in decision-making and varying cultural, religious and societal points of view [11–17].

As research is the base of every (sub)speciality, it becomes increasingly crucial that achievements in basic and translational science are integrated and implemented in daily clinical practice, as illustrated by the following short medical history of six patients to help understand the potential changes in the PICU case mix.[1]

1 Reading counterclockwise.

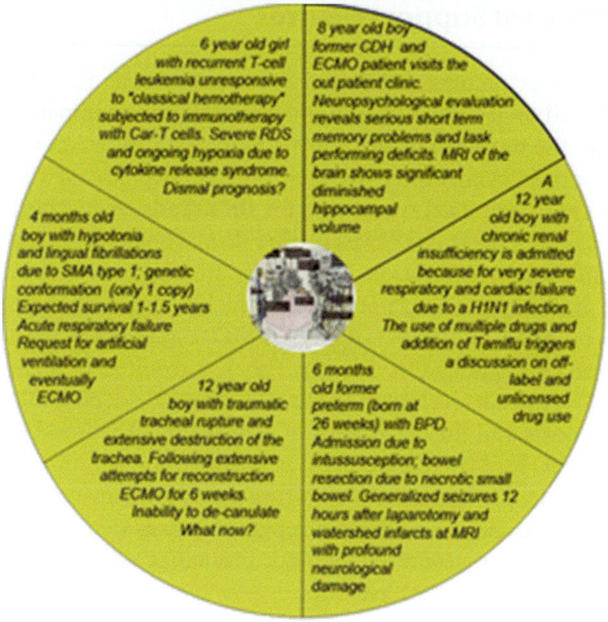

1.2 Cell-Based and Genetic Therapy

1. In cancer therapy, an intriguing development is the use of CAR-T (chimeric antigen receptor T) as cell therapy for malignancies of different origins [18, 19]. Although many patients who receive CAR-T cell therapy will never need admission to the PICU, a subset will develop the so-called cytokine release syndrome. This can result in multi-organ failure with the need for admission to the PICU and occasionally the need for organ support by ECMO therapy, although the results are debatable [20–22].
2. Another direct reflection of progress in research is represented by increased insight into the molecular-genetic base of neuro-muscular diseases such as spinal muscular atrophy. Although initially, the therapy of SMA type 1 used an antisense oligonucleotide (AS) with the promise of improved motor function, this therapy is burdensome, administrated indefinitely on a quarterly basis via intrathecal injection, and both requires a lengthy induction period prior to clinical effect and has safety considerations which need clinical monitoring. The newer viral vector-mediated gene therapy [23] based on genetically manipulated mouse strains is now the prime clinical application with a single treatment, though, of course, with limited outcome or safety data [24]. Gene therapy for metabolic conditions, such as Pompe's disease, is also becoming standard [25]. For sure, the application of gene therapy will evolve over the years for children with rare diseases and a previously limited life expectancy. Consequently, difficult decisions regarding admission and interventions for children with such conditions for whom ICU therapy was once considered futile can be anticipated [26–35].

1.3 Extracorporeal Support Devices

3. The use of extracorporeal support systems such as ECMO and VADs [36, 37] is based on technical developments of systems compatible with body tissues and the response of the body usually resulting in a systemic inflammatory response syndrome (SIRS) in the initial phase of therapy. Although ECMO has been used worldwide for thousands of newborns over the past two decades, indications for its use are decreasing, particularly for newborns with meconium aspiration syndrome. In children beyond the newborn period, solid inclusion criteria remain lacking, as well as international consensus on how and when to apply ECMO, especially in the case of different forms of malignancy [36, 38–44]. This has resulted in many complications and an overall survival ranging from 20% to 60% depending on the underlying diagnosis and the experience of the treatment teams. Under specific circumstances, ECMO can be used as a bridge for definitive therapy, such as with a child with myocarditis awaiting a cardiac transplant. The same holds true for tissue-engineered organ replacement, as demonstrated for tracheal reconstruction in severe congenital anomalies of the trachea, such as in selected pulmonary sling patients.

1.4 Brain and Critical Illness

4. As mortality is relatively low in PICUs worldwide, morbidity, both in the acute phase as well as in the long term, is increasingly important, with a particular focus on the brain. Although imaging (ultrasounds, CT and MRI) was initially performed in the case of overt clinical symptoms, such as convulsions, nowadays, more focus is being aimed at understanding the pathophysiological changes that occur in the brain under specific conditions. So far, not many neuro-monitoring modalities have been evaluated systematically [6, 45, 46], though NIRS is now being implemented, mainly in paediatric cardiac procedures as a trend monitor in the absence of predetermined treatment algorithms. In addition, multimodal neuro-monitoring taking into account the pharmacokinetic aspect of different drugs is a new direction in clinical research aiming to prevent even subtle neurological abnormalities. Only a few research groups have implemented these targets to understand the long-term neurological consequences of intensive care treatment and the resulting abnormalities in executive functions known as growing into deficit [47–57]. Within this context, it is essential that ICU-trained physicians and nurses form an integral part of the ICU outpatient clinic [58].

1.5 Evidence Base Pharmacotherapy

5. The majority of drugs used in the PICU are either prescribed off-label or unlicensed due to the shortage of well-conducted studies, even in the most frequently used groups of drugs such as analgosedative drugs and, to a lesser

extent, antibiotics. Due to restrictions in the volume of blood that is allowed to be taken for clinical research, new methodologies have emerged, such as dry blood spot technology (DBS); microdialysis and mathematical methods such as population pharmacokinetics-pharmacodynamics modelling (POP-PK) using samples from individual patients and more recently physiology-based PK modelling (PB-PK) [59]. In this way, new dosing regimens can be developed for groups of drugs using the same metabolic pathways and implemented in daily clinical practice by dosing adjustments [60]. This is especially relevant for analgosedative drugs given their high prescription rate in PICUs worldwide and relatively new drugs such as dexmedetomidine [61]. Both over- and under-dosing can have serious consequences for the outcome of the individual patient and also in the long run (pharmacovigilance) [2, 62]. The brain is severely prone to the potential adverse effects of drugs which have resulted in a mission statement of NIH to prevent general anaesthesia in children <3 years of age, although the level of evidence is really low [63]. At this moment, the use of microdialysis is promising, as shown in patients with traumatic brain injury [64]. For the development of new drugs, POP-PK data are nowadays an essential part of the evaluation process both by the FDA as well as by EMA. For the paediatric age group, we require clinical practice guidelines for the prevention and management of pain, agitation and delirium as published by the adult intensive care specialist [65, 66] and recently for the paediatric age group [2, 67]. Close collaboration with industry, paediatric ICU consultants and hospital pharmacists is essential [65, 66, 68–70].

1.6 Long-Term Outcome

6. Given the heterogeneity of the case mix of patients in the PICU, there is a need for international collaboration and the standardization of long-term follow-up. Apart from organ-specific points of interest (cardiac, pulmonary, etc.), general aspects of growth and development are essential for the developing child and surveillance of any deviations. Apart from the somatic aspects, psychosocial evaluation is equally vital, particularly related to brain development and executive functions into adolescence. For many mainly congenital anomalies operated on at birth or at a young age, adult congenital anomaly outpatient clinics have been instituted, given the long-term adverse effects and the need for repeated operative procedures (cardiac), surveillance of an increased risk for cancer (CPAM, oesophageal atresia) or ongoing severe morbidity (sexual dysfunction after anorectal malformations). The same holds true for the most critically ill children admitted to PICUs, such as survivors of ECMO or other assist devices. They can be confronted with both subtle and/or major brain abnormalities and resulting consequences for their quality of life, and with important decisions, such as about suitable careers in adulthood [45, 63, 71–77].

1.7 Reflection

As paediatric intensive care medicine has evolved into a mature speciality, reflections on the future with regard to case mix and the potential futility of therapies, together with the consequences for future staff, are needed. New technologies enable us to use machine learning for decision-making [78] and to develop core outcome sets [79], but do incur costs both direct and indirect [80] while we must consider environmental protective measures [81]. In this way, paediatric intensive care medicine as an entity can develop from a monodisciplinary and subspecialty structure towards real integration with the achievements in science, which usually takes place beyond the scope of the intensivist. Although in many units, consultants with special interest or training in, for instance, neurology, pharmacology, and pulmonology are in place, new fields of knowledge, as represented in the six index patients, warrant novel PICU-specialisation.

The actual situation:the future is near

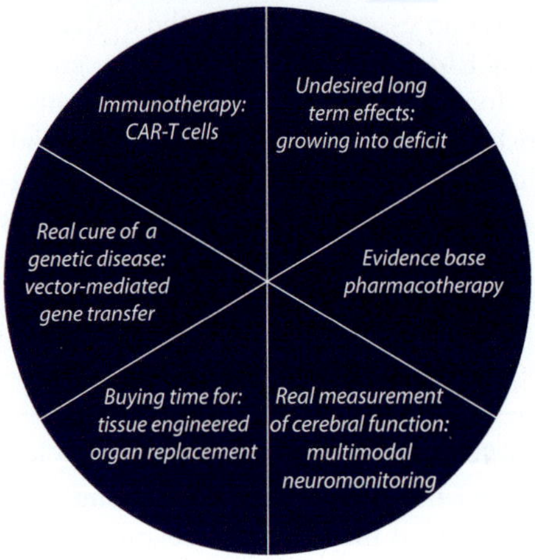

Differentation of staff in the future

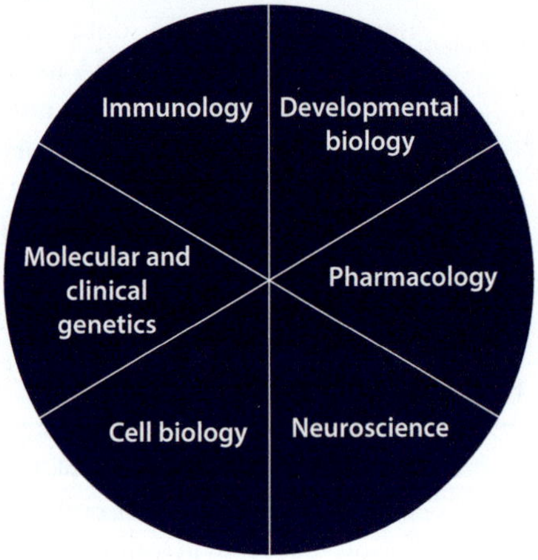

Taking the achievements of (translational) science in other fields of medicine into consideration, the following implications for the PICU in the future can be identified:

- Developments outside the PICU will change the case mix
- PICU teams have a significant responsibility beyond the actual stay of the individual patient
- Big data, machine learning and artificial intelligence will provide instruments for EU-broad treatment algorithms and benchmarking
- PICU specialists should also be knowledgeable in different areas of science
- Care providers are pivotal partners not only in daily care but also in the evolution of evidence-based therapy and care

Take-Home Message

Developments in translational science and its implementation for individual patients will determine the future case mix of children admitted to paediatric intensive care units worldwide.

References

1. Tume LN, et al. Nutritional support for children during critical illness: European Society of Pediatric and Neonatal Intensive Care (ESPNIC) metabolism, endocrine and nutrition section position statement and clinical recommendations. Intensive Care Med. 2020;46(3):411–25.
2. Smith HAB, et al. 2022 Society of Critical Care Medicine clinical practice guidelines on prevention and management of pain, agitation, neuromuscular blockade, and delirium in critically ill pediatric patients with consideration of the ICU environment and early mobility. Pediatr Crit Care Med. 2022;23(2):e74–e110.
3. Weiss SL, et al. Surviving sepsis campaign international guidelines for the management of septic shock and sepsis-associated organ dysfunction in children. Pediatr Crit Care Med. 2020;21(2):e52–e106.
4. Singh Y, et al. Recommendations for hemodynamic monitoring for critically ill children-expert consensus statement issued by the cardiovascular dynamics section of the European Society of Paediatric and Neonatal Intensive Care (ESPNIC). Crit Care. 2020;24(1):620.
5. Brindle ME, et al. Consensus guidelines for perioperative care in neonatal intestinal surgery: Enhanced Recovery After Surgery (ERAS®) Society recommendations. World J Surg. 2020;44(8):2482–92.
6. Yang MT. Multimodal neurocritical monitoring. Biom J. 2020;43(3):226–30.
7. Nellis ME, et al. Executive summary of recommendations and expert consensus for plasma and platelet transfusion practice in critically ill children: from the Transfusion and Anemia EXpertise Initiative-Control/Avoidance of Bleeding (TAXI-CAB). Pediatr Crit Care Med. 2022;23(1):34–51.
8. Iping R, Hulst JM, Joosten KFM. Research developments in pediatric intensive care nutrition: a research intelligence review. Clin Nutr ESPEN. 2022;50:1–7.
9. Piroth L, et al. Comparison of the characteristics, morbidity, and mortality of COVID-19 and seasonal influenza: a nationwide, population-based retrospective cohort study. Lancet Respir Med. 2021;9(3):251–9.
10. Rimensberger PC, et al. Caring for critically ill children with suspected or proven coronavirus disease 2019 infection: recommendations by the scientific sections' collaborative of the European Society of Pediatric and Neonatal Intensive Care. Pediatr Crit Care Med. 2021;22(1):56–67.
11. Duffett M, et al. Research collaboration in pediatric critical care randomized controlled trials: a social network analysis of coauthorship. Pediatr Crit Care Med. 2020;21(1):12–20.
12. Gelijns AC, Gabriel SE. Looking beyond translation--integrating clinical research with medical practice. N Engl J Med. 2012;366(18):1659–61.
13. Marini JJ, et al. Our favorite unproven ideas for future critical care. Crit Care. 2013;17(Suppl 1):S9.
14. Pearson GA. Intensive care: because we can or because we should? Arch Dis Child. 2018;103(6):527–8.
15. Peters MJ, et al. The intensive care medicine clinical research agenda in paediatrics. Intensive Care Med. 2017;43(9):1210–24.
16. Schwartz DA. Physician-scientists: the bridge between medicine and science. Am J Respir Crit Care Med. 2012;185(6):595–6.
17. Vincent JL, Hall JB, Slutsky AS. Ten big mistakes in intensive care medicine. Intensive Care Med. 2015;41(3):505–7.
18. Hucks G, Rheingold SR. The journey to CAR T cell therapy: the pediatric and young adult experience with relapsed or refractory B-ALL. Blood Cancer J. 2019;9(2):10.
19. Pettitt D, et al. CAR-T cells: a systematic review and mixed methods analysis of the clinical trial landscape. Mol Ther. 2018;26(2):342–53.

20. Sanford E, et al. Severe tumor lysis syndrome and acute pulmonary edema requiring extracorporeal membrane oxygenation following initiation of chemotherapy for metastatic alveolar rhabdomyosarcoma. Pediatr Blood Cancer. 2016;63(5):928–30.
21. Di Nardo M, et al. Extracorporeal membrane oxygenation in children receiving haematopoietic cell transplantation and immune effector cell therapy: an international and multidisciplinary consensus statement. Lancet Child Adolesc Health. 2022;6(2):116–28.
22. Gutierrez C, et al. The chimeric antigen receptor-intensive care unit (CAR-ICU) initiative: surveying intensive care unit practices in the management of CAR T-cell associated toxicities. J Crit Care. 2020;58:58–64.
23. Devaney J, Contreras M, Laffey JG. Clinical review: gene-based therapies for ALI/ARDS: where are we now? Crit Care. 2011;15(3):224.
24. Roper H, Quinlivan R, Workshop P. Implementation of "the consensus statement for the standard of care in spinal muscular atrophy" when applied to infants with severe type 1 SMA in the UK. Arch Dis Child. 2010;95(10):845–9.
25. Roger AL, et al. What's new and what's next for gene therapy in Pompe disease? Expert Opin Biol Ther. 2022;22(9):1117–35.
26. Geyer MB, Brentjens RJ. Review: current clinical applications of chimeric antigen receptor (CAR) modified T cells. Cytotherapy. 2016;18(11):1393–409.
27. Godel P, Shimabukuro-Vornhagen A, von Bergwelt-Baildon M. Understanding cytokine release syndrome. Intensive Care Med. 2018;44(3):371–3.
28. Merkle FT, Eggan K. Modeling human disease with pluripotent stem cells: from genome association to function. Cell Stem Cell. 2013;12(6):656–68.
29. Newick K, et al. CAR T cell therapy for solid tumors. Annu Rev Med. 2017;68:139–52.
30. Sasai Y. Next-generation regenerative medicine: organogenesis from stem cells in 3D culture. Cell Stem Cell. 2013;12(5):520–30.
31. Tian Y, et al. Nanomedicine as an innovative therapeutic strategy for pediatric lung diseases. Pediatr Pulmonol. 2013;48(11):1098–111.
32. Barnes FA, Bingle L, Bingle CD. Pulmonary genomics, proteomics, and PLUNCs. Am J Respir Cell Mol Biol. 2008;38(4):377–9.
33. Calvo SE, et al. Molecular diagnosis of infantile mitochondrial disease with targeted next-generation sequencing. Sci Transl Med. 2012;4(118):118ra10.
34. Thébaud B. Stem cell-based therapies in neonatology: a new hope. Arch Dis Child Fetal Neonatal Ed. 2018;103(6):F583–8.
35. Wilkinson DJ, et al. Genomic intensive care: should we perform genome testing in critically ill newborns? Arch Dis Child Fetal Neonatal Ed. 2016;101(2):F94–8.
36. MacLaren G, Brown KL, Thiagarajan RR. What's new in paediatric extracorporeal life support? Intensive Care Med. 2020;46(3):492–4.
37. Hoskote A, Stiller B, Thiagarajan RR. What's new in mechanical support strategies for the intensivist in children with severe cardiac failure. Intensive Care Med. 2021;47(10):1152–5.
38. Cashen K, et al. Extracorporeal membrane oxygenation outcomes in children with hemophagocytic lymphohistiocytosis. Perfusion. 2017;32(2):151–6.
39. Potratz J, et al. Successful extracorporeal life support in a pediatric hematopoietic stem cell transplant recipient with periengraftment respiratory failure. J Pediatr Hematol Oncol. 2018;40(4):e256–9.
40. Sacco O, et al. Long-term extracorporeal membrane oxygenation as bridging strategies to lung transplantation in rapidly devastating isolated Langerhans cell histiocytosis. Pediatr Blood Cancer. 2016;63(5):941–3.
41. Shankar V, et al. Ethical dilemma: offering short-term extracorporeal membrane oxygenation support for terminally ill children who are not candidates for long-term mechanical circulatory support or heart transplantation. World J Pediatr Congenit Heart Surg. 2014;5(2):311–4.
42. Vanderlaan RD, et al. Risk factors for specific causes of death following pediatric heart transplant: an analysis of the registry of the International Society of Heart and Lung Transplantation. Pediatr Transplant. 2015;19(8):896–905.
43. von Bahr V, et al. Long-term survival and causes of late death in children treated with extracorporeal membrane oxygenation. Pediatr Crit Care Med. 2017;18(3):272–80.
44. Williams FZ, et al. Successful use of extracorporeal life support in a hematopoietic stem cell transplant patient with neuroblastoma. J Extra Corpor Technol. 2018;50(1):61–4.

45. Brown KL, et al. The brain in pediatric critical care: unique aspects of assessment, monitoring, investigations, and follow-up. Intensive Care Med. 2022;48(5):535–47.
46. Costerus SA, et al. Towards integrative neuromonitoring of the surgical newborn: a systematic review. Eur J Anaesthesiol. 2020;37(8):701–12.
47. Brilli RJ, et al. A comprehensive patient safety program can significantly reduce preventable harm, associated costs, and hospital mortality. J Pediatr. 2013;163(6):1638–45.
48. Geoghegan S, et al. The experience of long-stay parents in the ICU: a qualitative study of parent and staff perspectives. Pediatr Crit Care Med. 2016;17(11):e496–501.
49. O'Brien S, et al. The impact of chronic health conditions on length of stay and mortality in a general PICU. Pediatr Crit Care Med. 2017;18(1):1–7.
50. Pollack MM, et al. Pediatric intensive care outcomes: development of new morbidities during pediatric critical care. Pediatr Crit Care Med. 2014;15(9):821–7.
51. Pollack MM, et al. Functional status scale: new pediatric outcome measure. Pediatrics. 2009;124(1):e18–28.
52. Russell JA. “She's out of the ICU now.” “That's a relief, isn't it?”: the growing problem of ICU recidivism. Am J Respir Crit Care Med. 2012;185(9):906–8.
53. Semenova O, et al. Coupling between mean blood pressure and EEG in preterm neonates is associated with reduced illness severity scores. PLoS One. 2018;13(6):e0199587.
54. Verstraete S, Van den Berghe G, Vanhorebeek I. What's new in the long-term neurodevelopmental outcome of critically ill children. Intensive Care Med. 2018;44(5):649–51.
55. Vijayaraghavan BKT, Willaert X, Cuthbertson BH. Should ICU clinicians follow patients after ICU discharge? No. Intensive Care Med. 2018;44(9):1542–4.
56. Westra AE. Ambiguous articles in new EU Regulation may lead to exploitation of vulnerable research subjects. J Med Ethics. 2016;42(3):189–91.
57. Schiller R, et al. Memory deficits following neonatal critical illness: a common neurodevelopmental pathway. Lancet Child Adolesc Health. 2018;2(4):281–9.
58. Maddux AB, et al. Postdischarge outcome domains in pediatric critical care and the instruments used to evaluate them: a scoping review. Crit Care Med. 2020;48(12):e1313–21.
59. Verscheijden LFM, et al. Physiologically-based pharmacokinetic models for children: starting to reach maturation? Pharmacol Ther. 2020;211:107541.
60. Ceelie I, et al. Effect of intravenous paracetamol on postoperative morphine requirements in neonates and infants undergoing major noncardiac surgery: a randomised controlled trial. JAMA. 2013;309(2):149–54.
61. Mahmoud M, Barbi E, Mason KP. Dexmedetomidine: What's new for pediatrics? A narrative review. J Clin Med. 2020;9(9):2724.
62. Stenkjaer RL, et al. Development of a non-pharmacologic delirium management bundle in paediatric intensive care units. Nurs Crit Care. 2022;27(6):867–76.
63. Andropoulos DB, Greene MF. Anesthesia and developing brains - implications of the FDA warning. N Engl J Med. 2017;376(10):905–7.
64. Ketharanathan N, et al. Combining brain microdialysis and translational pharmacokinetic modeling to predict drug concentrations in pediatric severe traumatic brain injury: the next step toward evidence-based pharmacotherapy? J Neurotrauma. 2019;36(1):111–7.
65. Devlin JW, et al. Clinical practice guidelines for the prevention and management of pain, agitation/sedation, delirium, immobility, and sleep disruption in adult patients in the ICU. Crit Care Med. 2018;46(9):e825–73.
66. Devlin JW, et al. Methodologic innovation in creating clinical practice guidelines: insights from the 2018 Society of Critical Care Medicine pain, agitation/sedation, delirium, immobility, and sleep disruption guideline effort. Crit Care Med. 2018;46(9):1457–63.
67. Daverio M, et al. Pain and sedation management and monitoring in pediatric intensive care units across Europe: an ESPNIC survey. Crit Care. 2022;26(1):88.
68. Dickinson R, Franks NP. Bench-to-bedside review: molecular pharmacology and clinical use of inert gases in anesthesia and neuroprotection. Crit Care. 2010;14(4):229.
69. Meyburg J, et al. Risk factors for the development of postoperative delirium in pediatric intensive care patients. Pediatr Crit Care Med. 2018;19(10):e514–21.
70. Ista E, et al. Validation of the SOS-PD scale for assessment of pediatric delirium: a multicenter study. Crit Care. 2018;22(1):309.

71. Cuthbertson BH, Wunsch H. Long-term outcomes after critical illness. The best predictor of the future is the past. Am J Respir Crit Care Med. 2016;194(2):132–4.
72. Edwards JD. Anticipatory guidance on the risks for unfavorable outcomes among children with medical complexity. J Pediatr. 2017;180:247–50.
73. Rennick JE, Childerhose JE. Redefining success in the PICU: new patient populations shift targets of care. Pediatrics. 2015;135(2):e289–91.
74. Seymour CW, et al. Precision medicine for all? Challenges and opportunities for a precision medicine approach to critical illness. Crit Care. 2017;21(1):257.
75. Gluckman PD, et al. Towards a new developmental synthesis: adaptive developmental plasticity and human disease. Lancet. 2009;373(9675):1654–7.
76. McCann ME, et al. Neurodevelopmental outcome at 5 years of age after general anaesthesia or awake-regional anaesthesia in infancy (GAS): an international, multicentre, randomised, controlled equivalence trial. Lancet. 2019;393(10172):664–77.
77. O'Leary JD, Orser BA. Neurodevelopment after general anaesthesia in infants. Lancet. 2019;393(10172):614–5.
78. Dong J, et al. Machine learning model for early prediction of acute kidney injury (AKI) in pediatric critical care. Crit Care. 2021;25(1):288.
79. Fink EL, et al. A core outcome set for pediatric critical care. Crit Care Med. 2020;48(12):1819–28.
80. Slater BJ, Vogel AM. The economics of a pediatric surgical ICU. Curr Opin Pediatr. 2020;32(3):424–7.
81. Zimmerman JJ, et al. Choosing wisely for critical care: the next five. Crit Care Med. 2021;49(3):472–81.

Why Do Children Need Critical Care

Content

Elective Admission to Critical Care

Lyvonne Tume and Kentigern Thorburn

Contents

J. Brierley et al. (eds.), *ESPNIC Children's Intensive Care Textbook*,
https://doi.org/10.1007/978-3-031-64762-8_2

Learning Objectives

At the end of this chapter the reader will be able to:

- Discuss both the organisational and clinical considerations when admitting a child electively to a critical care unit
- Discuss the physiological and monitoring criteria that require a critical care unit admission
- Critically discuss the issues around optimisation of the child's physical and psychological state prior to elective critical care unit admission
- Describe the parental education and involvement in planning for a critical care unit admission

2.1 Introduction

The admission of a child to a critical care unit is expensive both in terms of parental/child stress and anxiety as well as financially costly. With the cost of healthcare increasing, a paediatric critical care bed costing around €2500 per 24 h is a scarce resource in many countries, which must be utilised appropriately. Conversely, ensuring a safe environment where medical therapies can be delivered with an appropriate level of observation and monitoring, by appropriately trained staff, is essential to achieve the best outcomes for a critically ill child. This benefit needs to be balanced with recent questions over whether patients admitted to critical care are overtreated [1]. This chapter will consider the organisational and clinical considerations that the healthcare professional needs to consider for the admission of a child to a critical care unit. We invite the reader to consider this question for the two case study scenarios presented below.

Case Study 1

Sarah is a 10-year-old girl after an elective craniotomy and removal of a benign brain tumour. The surgery went as planned, and she was in the operating room for 4 h and received 2 units of packed red cells for some blood loss. Sarah is still drowsy in the operating theatre recovery area with a Glasgow Coma Score (GCS) of 14. It is now 6 pm at night. She has a surgical drain in situ, which is draining a little, a central venous line and a urinary catheter.

Consider the infrastructure and staffing set-up in your hospital regarding whether Sarah is admitted to the neurosurgical ward post-operatively or to the critical care unit.

Questions to Consider

Organisational Factors

- What is the registered nurse staffing ratio on the ward?
- What level of monitoring and observation does this child require?
- What skills do the nursing staff on the ward have to manage potential acute deterioration?

- What is the time of day of the admission and are medical staff readily available overnight on the ward?
- Is there a 'high dependency' area on the ward?
- How frequently do Sarah's observations need to be undertaken and can this be delivered in the ward?

Clinical Factors

- What is the risk of deterioration in this case?
- What are potential post-op complications and how likely are they to occur in Sarah's case?
- Is her Glasgow coma score (GCS) improving or deteriorating?
- Is her pain controlled? Could pain control become a clinical problem?

Family Factors

- Are Sarah's parents around? Can they stay overnight by the bed (in the ward)?

On the neurosurgery ward, the registered nurse (RN) to patient ratio is 1:5, there is no high dependency area and the only medical staff available on the ward overnight are the general hospital doctors (the neurosurgeons are on call from home). Sarah requires hourly observations (especially neuro-observations and GCS) for the first 4 h or until GCS is 15. She still has some bleeding from her neurosurgical drain and is complaining of some pain. It is 1800 h. Her parents are present and extremely anxious, Sarah previously had a respiratory arrest after anaesthesia, and they are concerned it might happen again.

- **Should Sarah be admitted to critical care unit overnight?**

It is helpful to consider the physiological and monitoring criteria in a post-operative child that require a critical care unit admission at this point compared to a ward admission. There is increasingly a merger between critical care and higher-level ward care (often called high dependency care) and the care a child receives is viewed as a continuum of critical care, regardless of where this is delivered [2]. A critical care unit provides both a higher level of registered nurse to patient ratio and continual specialist medical presence than a ward area [2]. The educational level and critical care skills of the staff in critical care are usually higher than that of ward staff. Although ward staff will be highly knowledgeable about their speciality, they may not be as skilled in managing an acutely deteriorating child. In addition to the staffing differences, the geographical set-up in a critical care unit ensures continuous visualisation and constant monitoring of patients, unlike many ward environments. So, although critical care therapies, such as high flow nasal cannula oxygen and sometimes non-invasive ventilation, can be delivered in a ward setting, the level of monitoring is not the same, nor are the staffing ratios or acute clinical skills and experience.

- **Sarah would best be cared for in a critical care unit, at least overnight.**

Case Study 2

Francois is a 4-month-old infant with a moderate-sized ventricular septal defect (VSD) being electively admitted to the PICU after his VSD closure. Despite being 4 months old, Francois only weighs 4.2 kg and has failed to gain weight. The parents, Jean-Paul and Delphine, have three other children aged 18 months to 7 years and have no immediate family able to look after their other children while Francois is in hospital. The cardiac ward in this hospital has all single enclosed rooms with a central monitoring station and the nurse:patient staffing ratio is around 1 RN to 6 children.

- **In this situation, let us consider how best we can optimally prepare Francois and his family for his impending critical care unit admission and surgery?**

Optimising Francois' physiological (and if he was older, psychological) state prior to critical illness and ICU admission is important to reduce complications and improve outcomes [3, 4]. Many paediatric critical care units now provide advice on how best to prepare a child for this admission. Undernutrition and 'failure to thrive' are common problems in infants like Francois, with heart failure [5]. Furthermore, increasing evidence supports worse outcomes in underweight infants after heart surgery, in terms of length of ventilation, length of stay and wound breakdown [6, 7]. The involvement of the broader multidisciplinary team, including specialist cardiac nurses and dieticians, is crucial pre-operatively. For older children and their families, the involvement of clinical psychology can be beneficial. This may be particularly valuable if the child has had previous hospitalisations and previous surgery.

- **Now consider the post-operative care of this child, Francois—Why the critical care environment is crucial and the most appropriate immediate post-operative location?**

Francois heart surgery (VSD repair) involves cardiopulmonary bypass (CPB), and after this large fluid shifts and third spacing occur as a result of both hemodilution and the systematic inflammatory response from CPB itself, thus requiring predictable intravascular volume replacement [8]. Central venous access is required for rapid volume replacement, medication administration and cardiovascular monitoring. Francois will require a continuous opiate infusion (to prevent pain), possibly some sedatives (to maintain calmness and to ensure lines and chest drains remain in situ) and may return on some inotropic support. Adequate assessment of pain and sedation levels, along with continuous monitoring of physiological parameters in the 'target' range for the child's age is essential for a safe recovery [8].

Improvements in paediatric cardiac anaesthesia have led to a more proactive 'fast-tracking' approach with early extubation, often on the operating table [9]. Despite being extubated early, these children (and especially infants like Francois) still require close observation of the airway, breathing and circulation, that is rarely available in a ward environment. The staff need to be skilled and experienced in managing post-operative cardiac children. Proactively identifying complications early, such as arrythmias or ongoing chest drain losses (common problems after VSD surgery), is essential [8].

- **These multiple time-critical factors make the critical care environment, with skilled staff, equipment and the high level of monitoring and observation, the safest place for Francois in the early post-operative period.**

2.2 Preparing the Child and Family Psychologically for an Elective Critical Care Unit (CCU) Admission

For some large and complex elective surgical procedures, such as cardiac or thoracic surgery and neurosurgery, critical care unit admissions are always planned. In these circumstances, there is an opportunity to prepare both the child physically and psychologically along with their parents for this admission [3, 10]. The critical care unit is a frightening place for the child and family. Many are open plan, allowing visualisation of other critically ill children and limited privacy for the child and family. There is increasing evidence to show that psychological preparation (through education and tours of the unit) of the child and parents reduces their anxiety [10]. Older children should have the option of 'seeing the critical care unit' themselves with the tubes, wires and monitors being explained to them, as well as the reasons for their use. They should be reassured that their pain and discomfort will be negated, and their parents allowed in PICU to be with them [3, 10]. For cardiac surgery, many countries have specialist cardiac nurses (called cardiac liaisons or specialist cardiac nurses) who lead the preparation of the child and family for surgery and critical care unit admission, with relatively few cases requiring the expert input of a clinical psychologist. However, if the child, has any specific phobias (as can often occur during previous hospitalisations) these will require a clinical psychologist. Likewise, if the family are extremely anxious, have mental health problems or learning disabilities themselves, this specialist input is essential. The child's developmental state also requires consideration, and any learning difficulties or specific needs they might have. Much of the child's fears can be anticipated by their developmental level and it should be considered [3, 10].

2.3 Optimising the Physical Condition of the Child Prior to Surgery and Critical Care Unit Admission

Especially after cardiac surgery, increasing evidence shows improved outcomes in children who are well nourished, with an optimal physical state (for their condition) prior to surgery and critical care unit admission. Knowing that children in intensive care receive, on average, less than half of their predicted energy needs [11], we can anticipate nutritional deficits during their CCU stay, thus optimising their nutrition and weight before admission is vital. Although in children, this is usually about increasing their weight, for some older children it may be reducing weight if they are obese. Both underweight and overweight children have worse outcomes [12], so the involvement of a dietician and working with the family in the pre-operative assessment process is important. Improving cardiorespiratory function may also be possible in some children pre-operatively, with the involvement of a physiotherapist or physician therapist.

Take-Home Messages

- Both clinical (patient-related) and organisational (hospital, ward, staff) factors must be considered when determining appropriate elective admissions to a paediatric critical care or intensive care unit.
- In elective admissions there is always a chance to prepare the child and their family both psychologically and physically. This should be undertaken to improve the family experience and satisfaction, to reduce anxiety and to enhance clinical outcomes for the child.

References

1. Zampieri F. Elective ICU admission after major surgery: can too much support be futile? J Thoracic Dis. 2018;10(Suppl):17. https://doi.org/10.21037/jtd.2018.05.154.
2. UK Paediatric Intensive Care Society standards. 2020 [cited 2020 Mar 4]. Available from: https://picsociety.uk/wp-content/uploads/2016/05/PICS_standards_2015.pdf
3. Gulec E, Ozcengiz D. Preoperative psychological preparation of children. Turk J Anaesth Reanim. 2015;43:344–6. https://doi.org/10.5152/tjar.2015.16768.
4. UK National Clinical Guideline Centre. Sedation for diagnostic and therapeutic procedures in young in children and young people. London: Royal College of Physicians; 2010 [cited 2020 Feb 19]. Available from: https://www.nice.org.uk/guidance/cg112/evidence/full-guideline-136287325.
5. Hoover J, Wong W, Adachil I, Brandt P, Jewa A. Energy intake and expenditure in children with heart failure. Ped Crit Care Med. 2018;9(11):e627–30. https://doi.org/10.1097/PCC.0000000000001697.
6. Curzon C, Milford-Beland S, Li J, et al. Cardiac surgery in infants with low birth weight is associated with increased mortality: analysis of the society of thoracic surgeons congenital heart database. J Thorac Cardiovasc Surg. 2008;135:546. Available from: https://core.ac.uk/download/pdf/82033109.pdf
7. Lim C, Lim J, Moorakonda R, et al. The impact of pre-operative nutritional status on outcomes following congenital heart surgery. Front Pediatr. 2019;7:429. https://doi.org/10.3389/fped.2019.00429.
8. Beke D, Braudis N, Lincoln P. Management of the pediatric postoperative cardiac surgery patient. Crit Care Nurs Clin North Am. 2005;17(4):405–16, xi.
9. Alghamadi A, Singh S, Hamilton B, et al. Early extubation after pediatric cardiac surgery: systematic review, meta-analysis, and evidence-based recommendations. J Card Surg. 2010;25(5):586–95. https://doi.org/10.1111/j.1540-8191.2010.01088.x.
10. Stremler R, Haddad S, Pullenayegum E, Parshuram C. Psychological outcomes in parents of critically ill hospitalized children. J Pediatr Nurs. 2017;34:36–43.
11. Moreno Y, Hauschild D, Barbosa E, Bresolin L, Mehta N. Problems with optimal energy and protein delivery in the pediatric intensive care unit. Nutr Clin Pract. 2016;31:5.
12. Tume LN, Valla FV, Joosten K, et al. Nutritional support for children during critical illness: European Society of Pediatric and Neonatal Intensive Care (ESPNIC) metabolism, endocrine and nutrition section position statement and clinical recommendations. Intensive Care Med. 2020;46:411. https://doi.org/10.1007/s00134-019-05922-5.

Mortality Predictions and Severity of Illness Scores

Contents

III

Mortality Predictions and Severity of Illness

Severity of Illness and Organ Dysfunction Scoring in Pediatric Intensive Care Units: Developments in 2020

Stéphane Leteurtre, Morgan Recher, and Stéphanie Delangue

Contents

J. Brierley et al. (eds.), *ESPNIC Children's Intensive Care Textbook*,
https://doi.org/10.1007/978-3-031-64762-8_3

Learning Objectives

The objectives of this chapter are to:

- provide an updated inventory of general severity scores and organ dysfunction in pediatric intensive care unit (PICU) settings
- clarify performance measures using discrimination and calibration
- analyze the usefulness, limits, and perspectives of severity scores in PICUs

3.1 Introduction

Mortality rates in adult and pediatric intensive care units (PICUs) have been reported to be approximately 20% and between 2.7% and 5%, respectively [1–6]. Mortality, as an objective endpoint, is determined in intensive care [7, 8] or at hospital discharge [6]. To quantify the severity of illness at PICU admission, severity scores have been developed and validated, considering physiological parameters collected during the first hours of intensive care. In pediatric intensive care, prognostic scores have been established that are almost independent of the diagnosis to account for the heterogeneity of patients [2, 3]. These scoring systems are called severity scores. In the 1990s, describing and quantifying organ dysfunction (OD) during an intensive care unit (ICU) or PICU stay became important information for inclusion [9, 10]. OD can be present at the time of admission or can occur during an ICU stay. Thus, OD scores have been validated to describe OD during an ICU stay and not as tools to predict mortality [11, 12]. The sequential organ failure assessment (SOFA) score to assess organ dysfunction during the first few days of ICU admission has been shown to be a good prognostic indicator. Independent of the initial score, an increase in the SOFA score during the first 48 h in the ICU predicts a mortality rate of at least 50% [13]. In children, an increase in the daily collection of Pediatric Logistic Organ Dysfunction (PELOD) scores between days 1 and 2 and between days 2 and 5 predicts a mortality rate of at least 50% [8]. However, a daily collection of OD scores is time consuming in terms of medical resources. Therefore, targeted days were determined as days with the best link to mortality during a PICU stay, namely, days 1, 2, 5, 8, 12, 16, and 18 [8]. OD scores have also been used to develop a new endpoint in clinical trials, namely, new or progressive multiple organ dysfunction syndrome [14, 15].

3.1.1 Which Severity Scores Are Available for Use in Pediatric Intensive Care?

In pediatric intensive care, interest in evaluating severity has increased due to the heterogeneity of pediatric populations, ranging from newborns to adolescents. Two scoring systems have been proposed for the pediatric population, excluding premature babies, as follows:

1. The Pediatric Risk of Mortality (PRISM) scoring system, which can be used for newborns through to adolescents. In 1984, the first version, namely, the Physiologic Stability Index, included 24 variables [16]. In 1988, Pollack et al. published a new version of the PRISM score (PRISM II) that included 14 variables [17]. In 1996, an updated version (PRISM III) included 17 variables with specific educational

features [18]. PRISM III score data were collected within the first 12–24 h after admission to the ICU. The most pathological value concerning each variable was considered over two periods (12 h or 24 h). Strengths of the PRISM III score are validation involving a large sample of 11,165 patients from 32 PICUs in the United States and regular adaptation using the myVPS network (▶ https://www.myvps.org/vps-picu) from United States PICUs [19]. PRISM III score values are calculated independent of the probability of death.

Limitations to the PRISM III score are as follows. First, the long data collection period (12–24 h) reflects initial severity and the effect of treatment provided during that period. Therefore, a patient receiving optimal care in one department may show improved parameters, whereas a similar patient in another department and receiving nonoptimal treatments may show deteriorating parameters. The latter patient will likely have a higher risk of death than a similar patient receiving optimal care. Therefore, predicted mortality in the department with sub-optimal care will appear to provide evidence of greater severity of illness in the patients, although such evidence is reflective of management rather than severity at PICU admission. Moreover, the coefficients of each variable required to calculate the probability of death are not in the public domain. In 2016, PRISM IV was published, which involved a prospective cohort of 10,078 patients (age range, newborn to 18 years) using data derived from seven North American PICUs between 2011 and 2013 [6]. The outcome was a measure of mortality at hospital discharge. Collection time ranged from 2 h before ICU admission (medical transport) to the first 4 h post-ICU admission. The collected variables and cutoffs were identical to the PRISM III score [20]. This freely available calculation of the probability of death takes into account age, medical characteristics, and educational features [6].

2. Second, the Pediatric Index of Mortality (PIM) scoring system can be used for newborns through to patients aged 16 years. In 1997, the PIM score included eight variables collected during the first hour after admission to the PICU [21]. In 2003, a new version was developed (PIM2) that included ten variables. This version was validated in a study of 20,787 patients in Australia and in the United Kingdom [22]. In 2013, a third version, namely, the PIM3 was developed from a sample of 53,112 patients and included ten variables [7]. PIM2 and PIM3 have identical variables, although items of the variables have been reorganized (low-risk and high-risk diagnoses in PIM2 have been reclassified as low-risk, high-risk, and very high-risk diagnoses in PIM3). The strengths of the PIM3 score include the large size of the validation population, early assessment from the first hour after admission to the PICU, and the equation to calculate the probability of death available at no cost. The main limitation of the PIM3 score is that no new variables were evaluated [23, 24].

3.1.2 What Organ Dysfunction Scores Are Currently Available?

In 1999, the PELOD score was developed for a population of 594 patients [25] and was validated on a population of 1806 patients in seven ICUs in Canada, France, and Switzerland [11, 12]. The PELOD score contains six organ dysfunctions and 12 variables. The main limitation of the PELOD score is the use of unobservable values on a discrete scale ranging from 0 to 71 (possible score values: 0, 1, 2, 3, 4, 10, 11, 12, 13,

14, and 20, for example) [26]. The PELOD-2 score, developed and validated in 2013 from 3761 patients from 15 PICUs in France and Belgium, included five ODs and ten variables [27]. In terms of the variables, the main differences between these two versions were the removal of hepatic OD, replacement of systolic blood pressure with mean blood pressure, and replacement of heart rate with lactatemia. Furthermore, in the PELOD-2 score, all discrete values between 0 and 33 points are possible. The PELOD score is based on a daily collection over a 24 h period, beginning from the admission schedule. The most relevant collection days, otherwise known as targeted days (days 1, 2, 5, 8, 12, 16, and 18), for predicting mortality have been determined for the PELOD and PELOD-2 scores [8, 28]. Equations to calculate the probability of death using the PELOD system are available for use at no cost.

The Pediatric Multiple Organ Dysfunction (P-MODS) score was developed and validated in 2005 in a single American service involving 6456 patients [29]. The P-MODS score includes five ODs, namely, cardiovascular, respiratory, renal, hematologic, and hepatic ODs, and excludes neurologic dysfunction. These five ODs are characterized according to biological variables. An equation for calculating the probability of death has not been published, and the P-MODS score is yet to be externally validated [29].

The pediatric Sequential Organ Failure Assessment (pSOFA) scores have been developed. A first version of the pSOFA score was proposed [30]. Later, in a large cohort study of 8711 pediatric intensive care unit encounters, a second version of the pSOFA score demonstrated excellent discrimination for in-hospital mortality. This second version of the pSOFA score was developed by adapting the original SOFA score through two approaches: first, the age-dependent cardiovascular and renal variables of the original SOFA score were modified using validated cutoffs from the PELOD-2 scoring system; second, the respiratory subscore was expanded to include the Spo_2:Fio_2 ratio as an alternative surrogate of lung injury [31]. Equations to calculate the probability of death using the pSOFAs are not available [30, 31].

Assessing pediatric patients with a pragmatic rapidly available score (one criterion for each neurological, cardiovascular, and respiratory dysfunction) is equally important to ensure the timely identification of sepsis with organ dysfunction [32]. These scoring systems named Quick Pediatric Sequential (Sepsis-Related) Organ Failure Assessment vary with the vital sign threshold used [33]. The quick PELOD-2 was composed of three binary variables (tachycardia, hypotension, and altered mentation) and the quick SOFA scores were composed of three binary variables (tachypnoea, altered mentation, and hypotension) [34, 35]. Their performance was moderate in the studies with external validation [36–38].

3.1.3 Probabilities of Death

There are two different methods in which to calculate the probability of death using ICU scores:

1. The PRISM and PELOD systems provide a score value for each patient. This score value is transformed into a probability of death using an equation that is readily available in the PELOD system, PRISM score, and PRISM IV at no cost.
2. In the PIM system, while it is not possible to calculate the value of the score, the probability of death can be directly calculated.

3.1.4 ICU Score Quality

Certain quality criteria are required for severity scores before their use. Variables must be relevant to the medical recommendations, as well as standard, objective, easy to collect, rapidly available, and obtained early after admission. The prognostic score must have good intra- and inter-observer reproducibility, be able to detect fine variations in severity between patients (indicating a sensitivity to change), be acceptable, easy to use, and low in cost for the patient, and be feasible for any service likely to apply it [24]. These quality criteria justify regular updating of severity and organ dysfunction scores [2, 14].

3.2 Performance and Adaptation of the Scores

3.2.1 Score Performance: What Is Evaluated and How to Measure Performance?

Scores used in ICUs should help clinicians answer the following questions:
1. Are the most ill patients the ones who die in my department?
2. Is this score able to predict the number of deaths in my department? and;
3. Does the predicted number of deaths adequately align with the level of severity evaluated using the score?

The statistical tools used to evaluate score performance and to provide successive answers to these three questions are described below:
1. Score discrimination evaluation enables the first question to be answered.

   For survivors, score values should be lower than those observed for nonsurvivors. Score discrimination measures the capacity of a score to assign the lowest score values (or probabilities of death for general severity scores) to survivors and to assign the highest score values (or probabilities of death) to nonsurvivors. Discrimination can be assessed either from the value of the score or the probability of death calculated from the score. Converting the score to a probability of death is a monotonic function (logarithmic function) that does not modify the order. In addition, score discrimination considers only the classification of patients and is independent of the values. Theoretically, therefore, it would be possible for all patients in a department to be perfectly classified between survivors and nonsurvivors on a probability range of death between 1% and 13%. In this example, if all the surviving patients were classified between 1% and 4% and all the deceased patients were classified between 5% and 13%, the score would have perfect discrimination, while no patient would have a probability of death >13%. Thus, this discrimination criterion is limited in that the classification of the score alone is considered.

   Discrimination can be assessed by calculating the area under the receiver operating curve (ROC and AUC). A ROC curve was obtained using successively varying thresholds and calculating sensitivities and specificities. The results from the AUC can be interpreted as follows: an AUC equal to 0.50 implies that the score is no more discriminating than chance, an AUC between 0.70 and 0.79 is considered to be correct, an AUC between 0.80 and 0.89 is considered to be good, and an AUC >0.90 is considered to be excellent [39, 40]. When a confidence interval is calculated, the upper limit cannot be >1 [41].

2. The standardized mortality ratio enables the second question to be answered.

   The standardized mortality ratio (SMR) is the ratio between observed and predicted deaths in the entire population. The observed death is the number of deaths in the sample during this period. Predicted death is the sum of the probabilities of death for each patient during the same period. If the SMR is <1, observed deaths are lower than the predicted deaths. If the SMR is >1, observed deaths are greater than the predicted deaths. A confidence interval is determined for each SMR: if the confidence interval includes 1, the difference between observed and predicted deaths is not significant.

3. Calibration enables the third question to be answered.

   Calibration evaluates the equation between observed and predicted deaths, taking into account the severity level in the whole population. Severity levels can be defined in several ways. In general, 10 deciles (or classes) of severity levels are considered, for example, 0–10%, 11–20%, etc., and patients are classified into subgroups according to their probability of death [42]. This classification can lead to an imbalance in the number of patients per subgroup. Sometimes, patients are sorted in ascending order of probability of death to allow consideration of between five and ten groups, including the same number of patients in each group [43]. In each group, the number of predicted deaths (sum of the predicted probabilities of death of patients), and the number of predicted survivors (1 minus the sum predicted of the probability of death) are determined. If we consider the deaths, two elements can usually be expected: (1) the number of observed and predicted deaths is lower in subgroups with a low probability of death, and; (2) in each of the groups, the number of deaths observed is close to the number of deaths predicted. The Hosmer–Lemeshow statistical goodness of fit test enables an overall comparison of observed and predicted deaths using the chi-square test [42, 43]. A *p*-value is calculated [44], and no difference between observed and predicted deaths is expected: calibration is good (or adequate) if the *p*-value is >0.05 [40, 45, 46].

3.2.2 Adaptation of the Scores

Severity scores are predictive (or prognostic) scores used to calculate the probability of death on admission to intensive care (during the first hour or within the first 24 h). Thus, discrimination and calibration are typically used for validation. OD scores aim to assess the OD during the ICU stay and are not predictive scores for mortality [1, 14]. Therefore, for OD scores, discrimination is a criterion for evaluating performance. However, calibration for both types of scores has been performed in some studies [47]. A general severity score or an OD score has been developed and validated in a general population. However, external validations have frequently shown poor calibration [48]. The most plausible explanation for such poor calibration is a different case mix between different services, due to regional or national specificities in care organizations [49, 50]. Thus, an adaptation (or customization in relation to studies to date) of the score to new populations is necessary [5], even if comparability with the original population is compromised [51]. There are three levels of score customization, as follows: first level, overall correction coefficient assigned to the calculated score without modifying variables or coefficients of each variable [5]; second level: new coefficients assigned to each variable; and third level or updated score, updated variables and coefficients assigned to the score, and the score version is then changed (PIM2, PIM3, PRISM III, PRISM IV, or PELOD-2).

3.2.3 Why Use a Severity or Organ Dysfunction Score in Pediatric Intensive Care?

3.2.3.1 Objective Assessment of the Severity and Organ Dysfunctions for Each Patient

Quantifying the severity of illness and OD is the primary goal in ICUs. The calculated probability of death cannot be used for therapeutic or ethical decisions concerning the management of a child.

3.2.3.2 Use in Studies

Description of Tools Used

Severity and OD scores are tools used to describe and characterize a study population [52].

Study Inclusion Criteria

Using the severity score as an inclusion criterion in trials remains controversial. Severity and OD scores should not be used for this purpose [53]. Stratification of severity assessed using scores should be undertaken in the analysis plan [54].

Comparing Illness Severity in Randomized Trials

PRISM, PIM, and PELOD systems have been used to compare severity in randomized trials [52]. Severity and OD scores have also been used as adjustment criteria in clinical trials [55–57].

3.3 Evaluation of the Recruitment and Performance of a Service

The SMR can be calculated each year in a single service to follow the evolution of this criterion. Similarly, a comparison between several services can be undertaken. Severity scores are primarily constructed to overcome patient diagnoses and can be applied to all ICU populations. However, case mix or organization of services (for example, cardiac surgery in a center, neonatal referral to another center, admissibility or discharge policy, and intermediate care) can modify the SMR and an adaptation of the scores in each center could be necessary to allow comparability [55–57].

3.4 Future Considerations

3.4.1 Health Quality of Life Scores

In the PICU, the mortality rate has decreased, while the morbidity rate remains consistent (4.6%) [58, 59]. Pollack et al. developed and validated a predictive tool that considers three criteria: living without new morbidity, living with morbidity, or death [60]. Morbidity status was quantified using the Functional Status Scale, based on six areas (consciousness, sensoriality, communication, motor skills, eating, and breathing) with a quantification ranging between 1 (normal) and 5 (very severe dysfunction) for each area [61]. Aspesberro et al. identified the following four available health quality of life scales for pediatric intensive care trials: (1) the Pediatric Quality of Life Inventory version 4.0 scale (Peds QL 4.0 Generix Core Scale), for children aged 2–18 years [62–64]; (2) the KIDSCREEN-27 scale, for children aged 8–18 years [65]; (3) the KINDL, for children aged 6–18 years; and (4) the Child Health Questionnaire-Parent Form 28 Questions, for children aged 5–18 years [62].

3.4.2 Evaluation of Practices in Pediatric Intensive Care Units

The need for annual national monitoring of medical and medico-economic activities has led to the development of national pediatric resuscitation service networks in many industrialized countries, including those in North America (Virtual PICU Performance System, ▶ https://portal.myvps.org/) [19], as well as in Great Britain (Pediatric Intensive Care Audit Network, ▶ http://www.picanet.org.uk/) [66], and in Australia and New Zealand (Australian and New Zealand Pediatric Intensive Care Society, ▶ http://www.anzics.com.au/pages/CORE/ANZPICR-registry.aspx) [67].

The aim of these collective networks is to constitute a database, with the following objectives: (1) identification of best practices; (2) benchmarking at local, regional, and national levels; (3) monitoring of disease epidemiology, case mix, and outcome indicators such as mortality, morbidity, and nosocomial infections; and (4) develop multicenter clinical studies.

3.5 Conclusion

Scores used in pediatric intensive care are constantly evolving. General severity and OD scores in pediatric intensive care are necessary to quantify the severity and OD at admission and during a PICU stay. Informatics, technological tools, and growing pediatric databases provide valuable assistance in constructing complex models linked to outcomes.

Learning Outcomes

- Improved understanding of pediatric severity (Pediatric Index of Mortality and Pediatric Risk of Mortality) and organ dysfunction scores.
- Understanding of which statistical tools are most useful to evaluate scoring systems.
- Enhanced awareness of the main uses of severity scores.

Educational Features

PIM3: ▶ https://espnic-online.org/Education/Professional-Resources/Paediatric-Index-of-Mortality-3
PELOD-2: ▶ https://espnic-online.org/Education/Professional-Resources/Paediatric-Logistic-Organ-Dysfunction-2-Score-Calculator
PRISM IV: ▶ https://www.cpccrn.org/calculators/prismiiicalculator/

References

1. Vincent J-L, Carvalho F. Severity of illness. Semin Respir Crit Care Med. 2010;31:31–8.
2. Lacroix J, Cotting J, Pediatric Acute Lung Injury and Sepsis Investigators (PALISI) Network. Severity of illness and organ dysfunction scoring in children. Pediatr Crit Care Med. 2005;6:S126–34.
3. Marcin JP, Pollack MM. Review of the acuity scoring systems for the pediatric intensive care unit and their use in quality improvement. J Intensive Care Med. 2007;22:131–40.
4. Martinot A, Leclerc F, Hue V. Les scores de gravité généraux en réanimation pédiatrique. Réanimation Urgences. 1995;4:335–63.
5. Bakhshi-Raiez F, Peek N, Bosman RJ. The impact of different prognostic models and their customization on institutional comparison of intensive care units. Crit Care Med. 2007;35:2553–60.
6. Pollack MM, Holubkov R, Funai T. The pediatric risk of mortality score: update 2015. Pediatr Crit Care Med. 2016;17:2–9.
7. Straney L, Clements A, Parslow RC. Paediatric index of mortality 3: an updated model for predicting mortality in pediatric intensive care. Pediatr Crit Care Med. 2013;14:673–81.
8. Leteurtre S, Duhamel A, Grandbastien B. Daily estimation of the severity of multiple organ dysfunction syndrome in critically ill children. CMAJ. 2010;182:1181–7.
9. Wilkinson JD, Pollack MM, Ruttimann UE. Outcome of pediatric patients with multiple organ system failure. Crit Care Med. 1986;14:271–4.
10. Proulx F, Fayon M, Farrell CA. Epidemiology of sepsis and multiple organ dysfunction syndrome in children. Chest. 1996;109:1033–7.
11. Leteurtre S, Martinot A, Duhamel A. Validation of the paediatric logistic organ dysfunction (PELOD) score: prospective, observational, multicentre study. Lancet. 2003;362:192–7.
12. Leteurtre S, Duhamel A, Grandbastien B. Paediatric logistic organ dysfunction (PELOD) score. Lancet. 2006;367:900–2.
13. Ferreira FL, Bota DP, Bross A. Serial evaluation of the SOFA score to predict outcome in critically ill patients. JAMA. 2001;286:1754–8.
14. Vincent J-L, Moreno R. Clinical review: scoring systems in the critically ill. Crit Care. 2010;14:207.
15. Villeneuve A, Joyal J-S, Proulx F. Multiple organ dysfunction syndrome in critically ill children: clinical value of two lists of diagnostic criteria. Ann Intensive Care. 2016;6:40.

16. Yeh TS, Pollack MM, Ruttimann UE. Validation of a physiologic stability index for use in critically ill infants and children. Pediatr Res. 1984;18:445–51.
17. Pollack MM, Ruttimann UE, Getson PR. Pediatric risk of mortality (PRISM) score. Crit Care Med. 1988;16:1110–6.
18. Pollack MM, Patel KM, Ruttimann UE. PRISM III: an updated pediatric risk of mortality score. Crit Care Med. 1996;24:743–52.
19. VPS PICU. In.
20. Pollack MM, Dean JM, Butler J. The ideal time interval for critical care severity-of-illness assessment. Pediatr Crit Care Med. 2013;14:448–53.
21. Shann F, Pearson G, Slater A, Wilkinson K. Paediatric index of mortality (PIM): a mortality prediction model for children in intensive care. Intensive Care Med. 1997;23:201–7.
22. Slater A, Shann F, Pearson G, Paediatric Index of Mortality (PIM) Study Group. PIM2: a revised version of the paediatric index of mortality. Intensive Care Med. 2003;29:278–85.
23. Wolfler A, Osello R, Gualino J. The importance of mortality risk assessment: validation of the pediatric index of mortality 3 score. Pediatr Crit Care Med. 2016;17:251–6.
24. Gulla KM, Sachdev A. Illness severity and organ dysfunction scoring in Pediatric intensive care unit. Indian J Crit Care Med. 2016;20:27–35.
25. Leteurtre S, Martinot A, Duhamel A. Development of a pediatric multiple organ dysfunction score: use of two strategies. Med Decis Mak. 1999;19:399–410.
26. Garcia PCR, Eulmesekian P, Branco RG. External validation of the paediatric logistic organ dysfunction score. Intensive Care Med. 2010;36:116–22.
27. Leteurtre S, Duhamel A, Salleron J. PELOD-2: an update of the PEdiatric logistic organ dysfunction score. Crit Care Med. 2013;41:1761–73.
28. Leteurtre S, Duhamel A, Deken V. Daily estimation of the severity of organ dysfunctions in critically ill children by using the PELOD-2 score. Crit Care. 2015;19:324.
29. Graciano AL, Balko JA, Rahn DS. The Pediatric multiple organ dysfunction score (P-MODS): development and validation of an objective scale to measure the severity of multiple organ dysfunction in critically ill children. Crit Care Med. 2005;33:1484–91.
30. Shime N, Kawasaki T, Nakagawa S. Proposal of a new pediatric sequential organ failure assessment score for possible validation. Pediatr Crit Care Med. 2017;18:98–9.
31. Matics TJ, Sanchez-Pinto LN. Adaptation and validation of a pediatric sequential organ failure assessment score and evaluation of the Sepsis-3 definitions in critically ill children. JAMA Pediatr. 2017;171:e172352.
32. Weiss SL, Balamuth F, Chilutti M, et al. Identification of pediatric sepsis for epidemiologic surveillance using electronic clinical data. Pediatr Crit Care Med. 2020;21:113–21.
33. Peters C, Murthy S, Brant R, Kissoon N, Görges M. Mortality risk using a pediatric quick sequential (sepsis-related) organ failure assessment varies with vital sign thresholds. Pediatr Crit Care Med. 2018;19:e394.
34. Leclerc F, Duhamel A, Deken V, Grandbastien B, Leteurtre S, Groupe Francophone de Réanimation et Urgences Pédiatriques (GFRUP). Can the pediatric logistic organ dysfunction-2 score on day 1 be used in clinical criteria for sepsis in children? Pediatr Crit Care Med. 2017;18:758–63.
35. Schlapbach LJ, Straney L, Bellomo R, MacLaren G, Pilcher D. Prognostic accuracy of age-adapted SOFA, SIRS, PELOD-2, and qSOFA for in-hospital mortality among children with suspected infection admitted to the intensive care unit. Intensive Care Med. 2018;44:179–88.
36. Chandna A, Tan R, Carter M, et al. Predictors of disease severity in children presenting from the community with febrile illnesses: a systematic review of prognostic studies. BMJ Glob Health. 2021;6(1):e003451.
37. van Nassau SC, van Beek RH, Driessen GJ, Hazelzet JA, van Wering HM, Boeddha NP. Translating Sepsis-3 criteria in children: prognostic accuracy of age-adjusted quick SOFA score in children visiting the emergency department with suspected bacterial infection. Front Pediatr. 2018;6:266. https://doi.org/10.3389/fped.2018.00266.
38. Görges M, Peters C, Murthy S, Pi S, Kissoon N. External validation of the "quick" pediatric logistic organ dysfunction-2 score using a large North American cohort of critically ill children with suspected infection. Pediatr Crit Care Med. 2018;19:1114–9.
39. Shann F. Are we doing a good job: PRISM, PIM and all that. Intensive Care Med. 2002;28:105–7.

40. Keegan MT, Gajic O, Afessa B. Severity of illness scoring systems in the intensive care unit. Crit Care Med. 2011;39:163–9.
41. Deeks JJ, Altman DG. Sensitivity and specificity and their confidence intervals cannot exceed 100%. BMJ. 1999;318:193–4.
42. Lemeshow S, Hosmer DW. A review of goodness of fit statistics for use in the development of logistic regression models. Am J Epidemiol. 1982;115:92–106.
43. Peek N, Arts DGT, Bosman RJ. External validation of prognostic models for critically ill patients required substantial sample sizes. J Clin Epidemiol. 2007;60:491–501.
44. Murphy-Filkins R, Teres D. Effect of changing patient mix on the performance of an intensive care unit severity-of-illness model: how to distinguish a general from a specialty intensive care unit. Crit Care Med. 1996;24:1968–73.
45. Pearson GA, Stickley J, Shann F. Calibration of the paediatric index of mortality in UK paediatric intensive care units. Arch Dis Child. 2001;84:125–8.
46. Tibby SM, Murdoch IA. Calibration of the paediatric index of mortality score for UK paediatric intensive care. Arch Dis Child. 2002;86:65–6.
47. Minne L, Abu-Hanna A, Jonge E. Evaluation of SOFA-based models for predicting mortality in the ICU: a systematic review. Crit Care. 2008;12:R161.
48. Metnitz PG, Lang T, Vesely H. Ratios of observed to expected mortality are affected by differences in case mix and quality of care. Intensive Care Med. 2000;26:1466–72.
49. Metnitz B, Schaden E, Moreno R. Austrian validation and customization of the SAPS 3 Admission Score. Intensive Care Med. 2009;35:616–22.
50. Kramer AA, Higgins TL, Zimmerman JE. Comparison of the mortality probability admission model III, national quality forum, and acute physiology and chronic health evaluation IV hospital mortality models: implications for national benchmarking. Crit Care Med. 2014;42:544–53.
51. Wolfler A, Silvani P, Musicco M. Pediatric index of mortality 2 score in Italy: a multicenter, prospective, observational study. Intensive Care Med. 2007;33:1407–13.
52. Lacroix J, Hébert PC, Hutchison JS. Transfusion strategies for patients in pediatric intensive care units. N Engl J Med. 2007;356:1609–19.
53. Vincent J-L, Opal SM, Marshall JC. Ten reasons why we should NOT use severity scores as entry criteria for clinical trials or in our treatment decisions. Crit Care Med. 2010;38:283–7.
54. Bernard GR, Vincent JL, Laterre PF. Efficacy and safety of recombinant human activated protein C for severe sepsis. N Engl J Med. 2001;344:699–709.
55. Glance LG, Osler T, Shinozaki T. Effect of varying the case mix on the standardized mortality ratio and W statistic: a simulation study. Chest. 2000;117:1112–7.
56. Leteurtre S, Grandbastien B, Leclerc F. International comparison of the performance of the paediatric index of mortality (PIM) 2 score in two national data sets. Intensive Care Med. 2012;38:1372–80.
57. Kramer AA, Higgins TL, Zimmerman JE. Comparing observed and predicted mortality among ICUs using different prognostic systems: why do performance assessments differ? Crit Care Med. 2015;43:261–9.
58. Namachivayam P, Shann F, Shekerdemian L. Three decades of pediatric intensive care: who was admitted, what happened in intensive care, and what happened afterward. Pediatr Crit Care Med. 2010;11:549–55.
59. Epstein D, Wong CF, Khemani RG. Race/ethnicity is not associated with mortality in the PICU. Pediatrics. 2011;127:e588–97.
60. Pollack MM, Holubkov R, Funai T. Simultaneous prediction of new morbidity, mortality, and survival without new morbidity from pediatric intensive care: a new paradigm for outcomes assessment. Crit Care Med. 2015;43:1699–709.
61. Pollack MM, Holubkov R, Glass P. Functional status scale: new pediatric outcome measure. Pediatrics. 2009;124:e18–28.
62. Aspesberro F, Mangione-Smith R, Zimmerman JJ. Health-related quality of life following pediatric critical illness. Intensive Care Med. 2015;41:1235–46.
63. Varni JW, Seid M, Kurtin PS. PedsQL 4.0: reliability and validity of the Pediatric Quality of Life Inventory version 4.0 generic core scales in healthy and patient populations. Med Care. 2001;39:800–12.

64. Tessier S, Vuillemin A, Lemelle J-L, Briançon S. Propriétés psychométriques du questionnaire générique français «Pediatric Quality of Life Inventory Version 4.0» (PedsQLTM 4.0) psychometric properties of the French Pediatric Quality of Life Inventory Version 4.0 (PedsQLTM 4.0) generic core scales. Eur Rev Appl Psychol. 2009;59:291–300.
65. Ravens-Sieberer U, Auquier P, Erhart M. The KIDSCREEN-27 quality of life measure for children and adolescents: psychometric results from a cross-cultural survey in 13 European countries. Qual Life Res. 2007;16:1347–56.
66. PICANet.
67. Straney LD, Clements A, Alexander J, Slater A. Measuring efficiency in Australian and New Zealand paediatric intensive care units. Intensive Care Med. 2010;36:1410–6.

Paediatric Early Warning Scores

Susan M. Chapman

Contents

J. Brierley et al. (eds.), *ESPNIC Children's Intensive Care Textbook*,
https://doi.org/10.1007/978-3-031-64762-8_4

Learning Objectives

In this chapter you will learn about:

- the function and key features of a PEWS
- the two main types of PEWS and their strengths and weaknesses
- how to assess the quality of a PEWS
- the evidence of the impact of PEWS in clinical practice
- the role of PEWS in the wider healthcare system
- practical tips to support you in using PEWS in the clinical environment

4.1 Introduction

Unrecognised deterioration in hospitalised children may lead to adverse events such as respiratory and cardiac arrest, emergency intubation, unplanned admission to the Paediatric Intensive Care Unit (PICU) and death. These events are considered to be largely preventable [1] as they are preceded by physiological and behavioural signs which indicate physiological derangement and developing critical illness.

From the mid-2000s clinicians began to develop tools to support clinical judgement in identifying the early signs of deterioration in children [2, 3]. They promoted standardisation in the recording of vital signs and other clinical observations and provided a structured framework to help clinicians recognise when these were considered to lie outside the 'normal threshold'. They were known as Paediatric Early Warning Scores or Systems, commonly referred to as the PEWS. These are now considered to be standard practice in paediatric wards with the majority of centres in Europe having a PEWS in place. Although PEWS are not generally used in the Paediatric Intensive Care Unit, it is important that critical care clinicians understand the types, indications, benefits, limitations and evidence base for PEWS as they are a key mechanism for identifying deteriorating children in hospital wards requiring critical care referral. As such clinicians in both the ward and critical care environment need to be familiar with their use.

4.2 What Is a Paediatric Early Warning Score?

As yet there is no universally agreed definition [4]. However, there is general agreement that PEWS support clinical judgement and help healthcare professionals identify children 'at risk' of clinical deterioration, prompting increased monitoring and escalation to staff with appropriate resuscitation and critical care expertise [4].

A number of different systems exist but they share some common features and characteristics. All use at least one (but often more) of the 'vital signs' and other clinical observations that are commonly used to monitor children for deterioration or other adverse events. The PEWS provides a standardised framework to assess, evaluate and 'track' the child's 'physiological health'. Clinicians are alerted to physiological abnormalities associated with clinical deterioration, which should 'trigger' the clinician to assess, intervene or escalate care. PEWS are generally integrated into observation charts and are utilised for the routine recording of vital signs and other 'core' clinical indicators [5, 6].

The most common clinical indicators in PEWS are heart rate, respiratory rate and oxygen saturation closely followed by assessment of consciousness, respiratory effort and systolic blood pressure [7]. Some PEWS include more subjective assessments such as nurse or staff concern [5]. In more recent years, some PEWS have formalised the contribution of parents and families to the PEWS. The inclusion of 'family concern' has demonstrated positive benefits and healthcare professionals' concerns that they would be overwhelmed by numerous calls for non-urgent situations do not appear to have been founded [8].

4.3 Why Might We Need a PEWS?

Studies have shown that the failure to detect or act upon deterioration can be a source of harm to hospitalised children [9]. A UK confidential enquiry found that of the 89 children who died in hospital, 19 (21%) had avoidable factors that contributed to their death and a further 44 (49%) had potentially avoidable factors [10]. The failure to appreciate the severity of the disease and inadequate observations were highlighted as particular areas requiring improvement. Recognition and response to children with sepsis have also been spotlighted as an area of particular concern. Sub-optimal care has been identified in up to 76% of children who died from severe bacterial infection [11].

Optimal care for deteriorating hospitalised children is complex due to a number of factors. These include child-related, physiological and system-related factors and are summarised in ◘ Table 4.1. The presence of a PEWS may mitigate some of these factors and support the healthcare team to recognise deterioration at an early stage [9].

◘ Table 4.1 Factors contributing to the challenge of recognising deterioration in children

Factor	Rationale
Physiological development	Children undergo vast changes in physiology, particularly during their early years which makes the identification of abnormal vital signs and clinical indicators more difficult [9]
Child's developmental age	Children, particularly infants and young children, may be unable to describe their symptoms or articulate when they feel unwell, making assessment more complex
Physiological compensation	Children tend to compensate physiologically in the early stages of critical illness [9]. This may mask the early stages of deterioration and make it more difficult for staff to recognise its presence
Chronic and complex illness	The presence of a chronic illness may result in long-term physiological changes. The child may have an altered response to deterioration or have baseline vital signs that always lie outside the normal range, even in health. This makes assessment more complex

(continued)

Table 4.1 (continued)

Factor	Rationale
Staff experience	More junior staff may find it more difficult to recognise the early signs of deterioration [10]. The lower rate of critical illness in children compared to adults may mean staff have not been exposed to a deteriorating child previously [9]
Staff skill mix	A weaker skill mix of staff, particularly nursing and medical professionals, may expose deteriorating children to staff with less expertise [12]. Staff may find it more difficult to access senior help from experienced staff
Increasing demand for high-dependency and critical care	Increasing demand for paediatric critical care, particularly in winter, makes it important to identify children at risk of deterioration at an early stage so that appropriate care can be sought. Timely admission may also reduce the length of stay which may release critical care capacity [13]
Lack of standardisation	Lack of a standardised PEWS may mean staff, particularly those in training, may not be familiar with the charts and tools that could support their decision-making [14]

4.4 Types of PEWS

Many different PEWS exist, and it can sometimes be difficult to differentiate between them as they often have similar names [5]. However, they broadly take two forms: score-based or trigger-based tools.

4.4.1 Score-Based System

Score-based tools such as the 'Brighton' PEW score [2] are commonly seen in paediatrics. Vital signs and other clinical parameters are recorded at periodic intervals. Each parameter is assessed against a scoring matrix and assigned a score. The scoring matrix is often embedded into the vital signs/PEWS chart using a colour-coded system. If the parameter value is considered to be in the normal range, it is assigned a 'zero' value. However, the more the parameter value lies out of the normal range, the greater the individual parameter score. These component scores are then combined to generate an overall score. This is commonly known as the PEWS score. Scores of zero generally indicate 'normal' or 'stable' status. Higher scores indicate greater physiological abnormality and greater risk of clinical deterioration. PEWS scores are usually linked to escalation algorithms that provide guidance on monitoring frequency and prompt interventions such as clinical review, critical care referral and clinical emergency calls.

4.4.2 Trigger-Based Systems

Trigger-based systems, such as MET activation criteria [3, 15], contain a number of pre-defined criteria. When the threshold for one or more of these are breached, this 'triggers' a pre-determined response. These thresholds can be measurable, objective criteria such as a 'respiratory rate of more than 50 in an infant from 4 to 12 months of age' [15]. They can also be more subjective such as 'severe respiratory distress, apnoea or cyanosis' [15]. Trigger-based PEWS may also include criteria that are more intuitive or judgement-based such as 'staff member or parent *worried* about clinical state' [15]. Unlike score-based PEWS, there is no associated algorithm and no score to calculate. Threshold-based systems result in a dichotomous 'all or nothing' response. For that reason, they are typically used to mobilise a team of expert clinicians with critical care skills to assess, treat and evaluate the child. These teams have varying compositions but can be described as a 'critical care outreach', 'rapid response' or 'medical emergency' team.

4.4.3 Which Type of PEWS Is Best?

The use of a score-based system facilitates a graded response as they are linked with an escalation algorithm to indicate the prescribed response to each score. Escalation algorithms represent a set of instructions to prompt monitoring and review by a doctor or specialist personnel, such as increasing the frequency of observations or activating a rapid response team. This may be more advantageous as escalation algorithms can be developed that are tailored to local needs and available resources. However, scoring systems are recognised as being more complex, requiring correct allocation of individual parameter scores and correct summation of the overall score [16, 17]. This may be particularly important for paediatric scoring systems, which may be more complicated due to the need to acknowledge age-appropriate vital sign thresholds which may result in clinicians needing to select the correct age-appropriate chart [16].

Not all settings that care for children have access to a rapid response team, and this may limit the utility of a trigger-based system. However, trigger systems are generally easier to use and eliminate the additional mathematical calculation required by score-based systems. A summary of the advantages and disadvantages of both types of systems can be seen in ◘ Table 4.2.

4

Table 4.2 Comparison of trigger and scoring systems

Type of system	Advantages	Disadvantages
Scoring system	The score can be tracked over time which gives an indicator of the child's clinical progress. Higher scores can facilitate an immediate 'senior' response without the need for a chain of escalation. This can preserve resources and support rapid access to critical care. May improve communication between professionals [18]. Widely used in paediatrics [5].	More complex than trigger systems to use. Each vital sign parameter needs to be assessed against the scoring matrix. If paper charts are used, this increases the time taken to record a set of observations [19]. Requires calculation of a total score, which introduces a risk of error. The need for age-appropriate thresholds to calculate the score requires the healthcare professional to select the correct chart for the child's age. This may introduce more errors [16]. May lack reproducibility and reliability due to human errors in calculating the PEWS score. A range of sensitivities and specificities depend on the cut-off score used, but it is possible to achieve high sensitivity and specificity at the defined cut-off point.
Trigger system	Simpler to use. Quicker to use as it does not require a score to be calculated. Less risk of errors as there is no score to calculate.	Does not allow a patient's progress to be tracked over time. As a trigger system can only provide an 'all or nothing' response, this may use critical care resources unnecessary. Evidence suggests that trigger systems have lower sensitivity and lower positive predictive value but higher specificity [20]. This could potentially cause increased triggers that are not related to an adverse event.

4.5 What Is the Evidence for PEWS?

Despite the widespread use of PEWS, there remains surprisingly little empirical evidence that supports their use. A number of systematic reviews of PEWS have examined the impact of PEWS in acute paediatric ward settings using a variety of clinical outcomes [5, 6, 18, 21, 22]. All have identified a weak evidence base to support PEWS. The majority of evidence has been derived from retrospective, uncontrolled observational studies with only two prospective randomised controlled trials [23, 24]. Most studies were conducted in tertiary specialist centres which may limit their applicability to secondary care hospitals. The differences in settings, outcome measures, patient populations and the diversity of PEWS studied have made it difficult to compare and synthesise the findings [6]. At present, all systematic reviews have concluded that there is insufficient evidence to support PEWS, particularly as a tool to prevent mortality. Secondary benefits such as improved communication, teamwork and empowerment of junior staff have been proposed, but the evidence to support this is still emerging [6].

4.5.1 A Landmark Study: The EPOCH Trial

Early 2011 saw the development of a study to examine the effect of the BedsidePEWS on all-cause mortality in hospitalised paediatric patients. Known as the EPOCH trial, it represented the first large-scale multi-centre randomised controlled study of a PEWS and was considered a milestone in the evidence base for PEWS.

The BedsidePEWS was developed in 2009 as a simple risk assessment tool to quantify the severity of illness at the bedside of hospitalised children. It is a score-based, age-dependent tool with seven parameters and the five age ranges. An overview of the component parameters and age ranges can be seen in ◘ Table 4.3.

The BedsidePEWS has been evaluated in a variety of settings using case-controlled and observational studies The EPOCH trial was a multicentre cluster randomized trial in 21 hospitals in seven countries to evaluate the effect of PEWS on all-cause mortality. The trial also evaluated the impact of the BedsidePEWS on 'significant clinical deterioration events' and frequency of observation recording. The BedsidePEWS was implemented in ten hospitals. An interprofessional team supported the ten intervention hospitals to implement the five age-specific BedsidePEWS charts, deliver a locally relevant training programme and adapt escalation protocols to match local care provision. The 11 control hospitals did not introduce a severity of illness tool but continued with 'usual care' which included pre-existing rapid response teams, ICU consultation mechanisms and resuscitation teams.

A total of 144,539 patient discharges and 559,443 patient days were seen during the intervention period. The frequency of documentation of five of the seven vital sign parameters increased at hospitals with the BedsidePEWS and 38% more observation sets were considered complete at BedsidePEWS hospitals compared to usual care centres. Hospitals with the BedsidePEWS had fewer significant clinical deterioration events compared to usual care hospitals; however, this difference was not statistically significant ($p = 0.3$). Despite these findings, implementing the BedsidePEWS did not significantly decrease all-cause mortality (1.93 per 1000 discharges vs 1.56 per 1000 discharges respectively, $p = 0.96$). The findings were considered surprising by many. The general decline in childhood deaths which has occurred over time may

◘ **Table 4.3** Parameters and age ranges in the BedsidePEWS

Parameters	**Age range**
Heart rate	<3 months
Respiratory rate	3–<12 months
Systolic blood pressure	1–4 years
Oxygen saturation	5–<12 years
Oxygen therapy	>12 years
Respiratory distress	
Capillary refill time	

have led to the study being underpowered and the choice of all-cause mortality as a primary outcome may have been 'unrealistic' [25]. However, this remains a landmark study in paediatric critical care.

Researchers in Denmark used the findings of the EPOCH trial to inform a subsequent randomised controlled trial. They highlighted the poor compliance in the EPOCH trial in obtaining complete sets of observations (5.1%) and the frequent absence of a blood pressure recording. They reasoned that both the difficulty in obtaining accurate blood pressure recordings in children and the limited value it had in the early identification of deterioration in children due to physiological compensatory responses made blood pressure a poor indicator [26]. They also highlighted the absence of an assessment of consciousness in the BedsidePEWS, which they proposed was an important indicator of evolving critical illness in childhood. They developed the Central Denmark Region (CDR) PEWS to address these issues and proposed that it may prove superior to the BedsidePEWS. The trial recruited patients from every paediatric department and one emergency department in Denmark. This resulted in recruitment of 16,213 patients from 31,337 admissions [24]. Similar to the EPOCH trial, this study also saw a lower number of unplanned transfers to intensive care than expected so was also considered to be under powered. The study also had poor compliance in the recording of PEWS, with around a third of children having no PEWS value recorded. This was despite training and protocols which mandated that PEWS should be recorded [24]. No difference was found in predicting unplanned transfer to intensive care although the CDR PEWS demonstrated a shorter median time to reassessment. This may represent the impact of staff preference and familiarity with the CDR PEWS.

4.6 How Might We Assess the Quality of a PEWS?

The idea PEWS would have high levels of predictive validity. In other words, it would accurately predict children who deteriorate at an early enough stage to allow healthcare professionals to intervene without falsely identifying children who are 'well'.

Sensitivity and specificity are important assessments of the predictive validity of 'diagnostic tests' such as PEWS [27]. Sensitivity represents the ability to correctly identify children who are deteriorating, while specificity is the ability to correctly identify children who are not deteriorating. For PEWS, this means a high PEWS score is found in children who are deteriorating (high sensitivity) and a low PEWS score is associated with children who are stable and do not deteriorate (high specificity).

Sensitivity and specificity are important characteristics for different reasons. High sensitivity protects patients by providing clinicians with an accurate indicator that a child is deteriorating (a true positive). No child who was deteriorating would be misclassified as 'stable' (a false negative) and clinicians can put their confidence in the PEWS to support their decision-making. High specificity protects resources. Children who are stable will not be identified as at risk of deterioration (a true negative) and the clinician will not be prompted to provide closer monitoring or inappropriately escalate a child who is 'stable' (a false positive). This allows critical care and experienced clinicians to use their skills appropriately and may prevent the 'stable' child from undergoing unnecessary examinations and tests.

No PEWS yet exist which has perfect sensitivity (100%) and perfect specificity (100%). However, the overall performance of a PEWS can be assessed using the area under the receiver operator characteristic curve (AUROC). An AUROC of 1.0 indicates the perfect PEWS. An AUROC of 0.5 indicates the PEWS is no better than the chance of differencing 'sick' from 'well' children. Several retrospective studies and systematic reviews have examined the sensitivity, specificity and AUROC of different PEWS [27, 28]. The AUROC for critical deterioration varies between 0.62 and 0.89 [27] although higher levels of 0.95–0.99 have been seen in predicting sepsis-related mortality [28].

Reliability is also an important characteristic of a high-performing PEWS. High levels of reliability mean that the PEWS will give consistent performance. This includes inter-rater reliability where different clinicians will agree on the PEWS score and intra-rater reliability, where the same clinician will document a consistent PEWS on repeated measures [29].

Finally, utility is an important consideration for assessing a PEWS. Utility can take into consideration the appropriateness, accessibility, practicability and acceptability of a PEWS [30]. In other words, a PEWS needs to be acceptable to patients, families and clinicians if it is going to be used in effective practice.

4.7 PEWS as Part of a Wider System Response

It has become increasingly recognised that PEWS are not a panacea to address missed deterioration. Nor can their use ensure that a child who is deteriorating will always receive optimal care. The Royal College of Paediatrics and Child Health in the UK have collaborated to develop a framework [31] which highlights the people and core elements that can create a safe system to recognise and respond to children at risk of deterioration (Fig. 4.1).

This framework recognises the complexities that exist when managing deterioration in hospitalised children. They note that a PEWS is just one part of this system of recognition and response to deterioration, and effective management requires more than the documentation of a PEWS score alone. They advocate that we should consider PEWS to be part of a wider system. They have identified six core elements and six individuals, groups and organisations that contribute and influence care. Table 4.4 provides a summary of the six core elements.

When considering the individuals, groups and organisations, at the centre is the patient (infant, child or young person). Their needs should be considered with the support and input of their family and/or carer. The child and family are surrounded by clinicians who provide direct care as well as the wider clinical team, such as laboratory staff, family doctors and social workers who indirectly provide support. These professionals are responsible for all aspects of assessment, care and support needed by the child and family. The outer circles represent the input from local services or organisations and regional and national services or networks such as professional bodies and royal colleges which guide and influence care delivery through local and national guidance and recommendations.

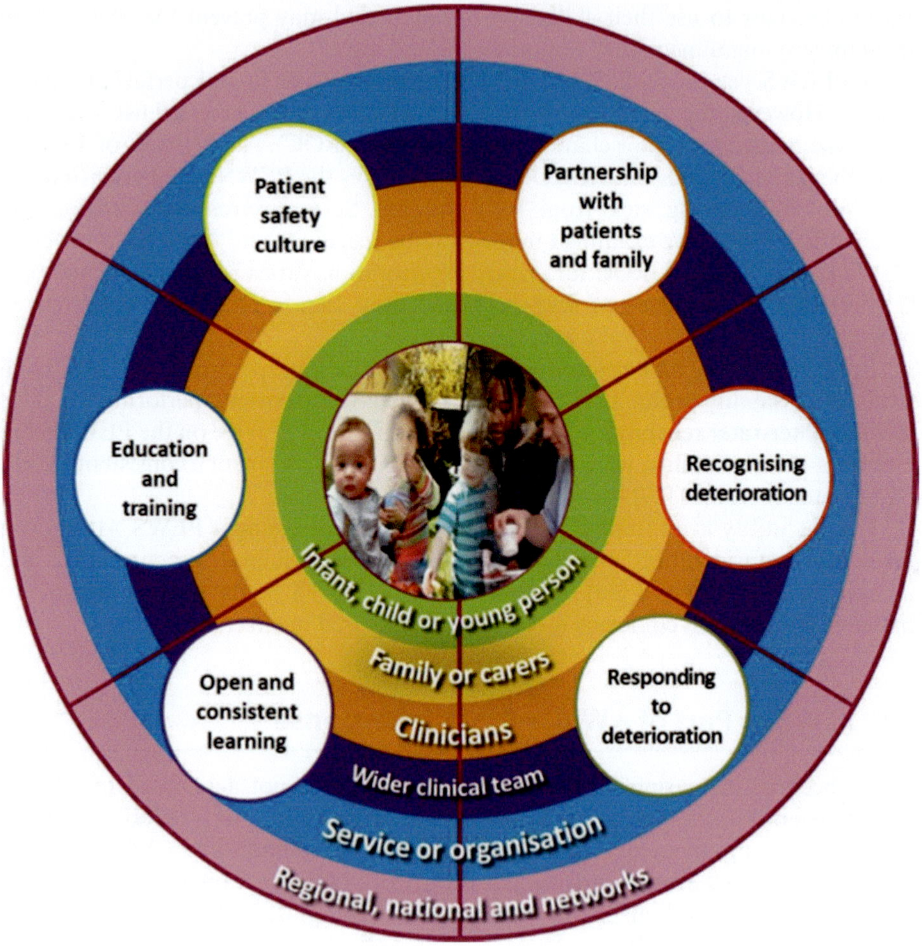

Fig. 4.1 Safe system for recognising and responding to children at risk of deterioration. Reproduced with permission from the Royal College of Paediatrics and Child Health [31]

Table 4.4 Core elements of the safe system framework

Core element	Safe system framework description
Recognising deterioration	Identifying the early signs of deterioration before significant changes in care are required or harm occurs. PEWS is an important part of this element but not to the exclusion of other aspects such as clinical judgement
Responding to deterioration	Ensuring a timely and accurate response encompassing all necessary support and treatment from all involved in the care of the patient
Patient safety culture	Monitoring and measuring patient safety and making a commitment to improving patient safety, prioritising safety, leadership and executive accountability
Partnership with patients and their family	Partnering with patients and families to maximise their contribution
Open and consistent learning	Creating an environment of continual improvement including assessing system errors and individual responsibility, recording, investigating and evaluating incidents, and promoting and sharing best practice
Education and training	Providing knowledge, skills and experience in core elements for staff, children and families

Adapted from the RCPCH and NHS Improvement Safe System Framework [31]

4.8 What's the Future for PEWS?

More hospitals are embracing the digital age and looking at ways that technology can support healthcare. Hospitals with an electronic patient record in place may see benefits particularly related to the accuracy and speed of PEWS scoring, the ability of clinicians to review PEWS wherever they are located, automated triggering of prompts and alerts to identify children at increased risk of deterioration and greater availability of data to support decision-making [19, 32]. Electronic patient records may also facilitate future research on PEWS by providing rich and timely data with greater ease than paper-based records.

SMART technology, self-monitoring and reporting technologies, such as electronic physiological surveillance systems may offer more effective methods to recognise and respond to deterioration in children [33]. Early studies in paediatrics indicate the potential benefits of electronic surveillance systems, but it is important that these tools are evaluated and are acceptable not only to clinicians but also to children and families.

Opportunities are also emerging for more novel approaches, including continuous monitoring of vital and clinical signs which may offer more effective oversight than intermittent measurements. These may be combined with machine learning-based analysis of physiological parameters to detect clinical deterioration [34]. Future developments may include the use of 'big data' to personalise track and trigger tools for individual patients.

4.9 Practical Tips for Maximising the Effectiveness of PEWS

Finally, here are some practical tips when working in the clinical environment to get the best out of yourself and the PEWS.

1. **Get familiar with your local PEWS**
   (a) Take a look at your PEWS as soon as possible. You never know when a child might deteriorate and it will be easier if you understand the PEWS you are working with.
   (b) Check if the same PEWS system is used across your hospital or if different areas use a different tool. Check the requirements in your paediatric ward, paediatric assessment unit, emergency department, neonatal unit and operating theatre. You may be surprised by what you find!
   (c) Is it recorded on paper, in the child's electronic health record or entered into a separate system? Do you have access to see the parts you need to do your role effectively?
   (d) Is your PEWS score or trigger-based? Is there an associated escalation protocol that helps interpret the findings?
   (e) Does the system vary with age? It is important to check the child's observations are being recorded on the correct chart during any assessment.
   (f) What vital sign parameters are included in your PEWS? What other indicators are part of the PEWS? Are they recorded consistently and at the correct frequency?
2. **Know your role in the system**
   (a) Understand your role in the system. What are you expected to do? This may vary depending on the staff on duty or the department you are working in.
   (b) Are there any policies or procedures you need to read or become familiar with before you are involved with a deteriorating child.
   (c) Seek out opportunities to become an expert in your role. Many centres use simulation as an opportunity to gain experience and skills.
3. **Understand the pathway for escalation of care**
   (a) Do you have an outreach or medical emergency team? If so, who do you contact if a child is deteriorating? See if you can work a shift with them to develop your understanding of their role.
   (b) If you don't have an outreach team, who do you call if a child needs an escalation of care? How do you get access to admit a child who needs PICU? Is your PICU on-site or located in another centre.
   (c) Know the escalation process during the day, at night and at weekends/public holidays. It may vary depending on the resources available and services provided.
4. **Participate in improving the system**
   (a) Participate in debriefs and reflective practice after significant events. Think critically about the performance of your PEWS. Look for the 'human factors' that might have impacted the system.

(b) Use incident reporting to highlight situations where PEWS didn't identify children who were deteriorating at an early stage. You may be able to adapt to the system or raise awareness of situations where PEWS performs less well.
(c) Encourage audit and evaluations of your PEWS. Participate if you can—you will learn a lot.

5. **Work in partnership**
   (a) Work in partnership with families and carers. Actively encourage their contribution when assessing and treating their child.
   (b) Take parents' and carers' concerns seriously. They know their child best.
   (c) Recognise everyone's contribution and be a team player.

Take-Home Message
- Detecting deterioration in hospitalised children is complex
- Despite the limited evidence to support their use, most paediatric centres in Europe have implemented a PEWS
- PEWS can provide a standardised framework support to clinicians in identifying hospitalised children at risk of deterioration
- Many PEWS exist and it is important to consider validity, reliability and utility when assessing or selecting a PEWS
- The PEWS score is part of a systemwide response to the deteriorating child

References

1. Parshuram CS, Hutchison J, Middaugh K. Development and initial validation of the Bedside Paediatric Early Warning System score. Crit Care. 2009;13:R135.
2. Monaghan A. Detecting and managing deterioration in children. Paediatr Care. 2005;17:32–5.
3. Tibballs J, Kinney S, Duke T, Oakley E, Hennessy M. Reduction of paediatric in-patient cardiac arrest and death with a medical emergency team: preliminary results. Arch Dis Child. 2005;90:1148.
4. Chapman SM, Maconochie IK. Early warning scores in paediatrics: an overview. Arch Dis Child. 2019;104:395.
5. Chapman SM, Wray J, Oulton K, Peters MJ. Systematic review of paediatric track and trigger systems for hospitalised children. Resuscitation. 2016;109:87–109.
6. Trubey R, Huang C, Lugg-Widger FV, et al. Validity and effectiveness of paediatric early warning systems and track and trigger tools for identifying and reducing clinical deterioration in hospitalised children: a systematic review. BMJ Open. 2019;9:e022105.
7. Roland D, Oliver A, Edwards ED, Mason BW, Powell CVE. Use of paediatric early warning systems in Great Britain: has there been a change of practice in the last 7 years? Arch Dis Child. 2014;99:26.
8. Gill FJ, Leslie GD, Marshall AP. Barriers and facilitators to implementing a process to enable parent escalation of care for the deteriorating child in hospital. Health Expect. 2018;21:1095–103.
9. Roland D, Stilwell PA, Fortune P-M, Alexander J, Clark SJ, Kenny S. Case for change: a standardised inpatient paediatric early warning system in England. Arch Dis Child. 2021;106:648–51.
10. Pearson GA, editor. Why children die: a pilot study 2006; England (North East, South West and West Midlands), Wales and Northern Ireland. London: CEMACH; 2008.
11. Launay E, Guen CG-L, Martinot A, et al. Suboptimal care in the initial management of children who died from severe bacterial infection: a population-based confidential inquiry. Pediatr Crit Care Med. 2010;11:469–74.

12. Tume LN, Sefton G, Arrowsmith P. Teaching paediatric ward teams to recognise and manage the deteriorating child. Nurs Crit Care. 2013;19:196–203.
13. Sefton G, McGrath C, Tume L, Lane S, Lisboa PJG, Carrol ED. What impact did a Paediatric Early Warning system have on emergency admissions to the paediatric intensive care unit? An observational cohort study. Intensive Crit Care Nurs. 2015;31:91–9.
14. Wheway J, Stilwell PA, Cook A, Roland D. A pre-implementation survey for a standardised approach to paediatric early warning systems. Arch Dis Child. 2020;106(6):620–2.
15. Tibballs J, Kinney S. Reduction of hospital mortality and of preventable cardiac arrest and death on introduction of a pediatric medical emergency team. Pediatr Crit Care Med. 2009;10:306–12.
16. Chapman SM, Oulton K, Peters MJ, Wray J. Missed opportunities: incomplete and inaccurate recording of paediatric early warning scores. Arch Dis Child. 2019;104:1208.
17. Prytherch DR, Smith GB, Schmidt P, et al. Calculating early warning scores—a classroom comparison of pen and paper and hand-held computer methods. Resuscitation. 2006;70:173–8.
18. Lambert V, OShea MT, Walshe C, et al. A systematic literature review to support the development of a national clinical guideline – Paediatric Early Warning System (PEWS). Technical report. Department of Health (Commissioned Research); 2014. p. 1–340.
19. Sefton G, Lane S, Killen R, et al. Accuracy and efficiency of recording pediatric early warning scores using an electronic physiological surveillance system compared with traditional paper-based documentation. Comput Inform Nurs. 2016;35:228–36.
20. NICE. Acutely ill patients in hospital: recognition of and response to acute illness in adults in hospital. NICE Clin Guidel. 2007;50:1–107.
21. Lambert V, Matthews A, MacDonell R, Fitzsimons J. Paediatric early warning systems for detecting and responding to clinical deterioration in children: a systematic review. BMJ Open. 2017;7:e014497.
22. Chapman SM, Grocott MPW, Franck LS. Systematic review of paediatric alert criteria for identifying hospitalised children at risk of critical deterioration. Intens Care Med. 2010;36:600–11.
23. Parshuram CS, Dryden-Palmer K, Farrell C, et al. Effect of a pediatric early warning system on all-cause mortality in hospitalized pediatric patients: the EPOCH randomized clinical trial. JAMA. 2018;319:1002.
24. Jensen CS, Olesen HV, Aagaard H, Svendsen MLO, Kirkegaard H. Comparison of two pediatric early warning systems: a randomized trial. J Pediatr Nurs. 2019;44:e58–65.
25. Chapman SM, Wray J, Oulton K, Peters MJ. 'Death is not the answer': the challenge of measuring the impact of early warning systems. Arch Dis Child. 2018;104:210.
26. Jensen CS, Aagaard H, Olesen HV, Kirkegaard H. A multicentre, randomised intervention study of the Paediatric Early Warning Score: study protocol for a randomised controlled trial. Trials. 2017;18:267.
27. Chapman SM, Wray J, Oulton K, Pagel C, Ray S, Peters MJ. 'The Score Matters': wide variations in predictive performance of 18 paediatric track and trigger systems. Arch Dis Child. 2017;102:487.
28. Romaine ST, Sefton G, Lim E, et al. Performance of seven different paediatric early warning scores to predict critical care admission in febrile children presenting to the emergency department: a retrospective cohort study. BMJ Open. 2021;11:e044091.
29. Jensen CS, Aagaard H, Olesen HV, Kirkegaard H. Inter-rater reliability of two paediatric early warning score tools. Eur J Emerg Med. 2017;26:34–40.
30. Smart A. A multi-dimensional model of clinical utility. Int J Qual Health Care. 2006;18:377–82.
31. Royal College of Paediatrics and Child Health and NHS Improvement. A safe system for recognising and responding to children at risk of deterioration. 2016. Available from: http://www.rcpch.ac.uk/safer-system-children-risk-deterioration.
32. Carter B, Saron H, Siner S, et al. Health professionals' initial experiences and perceptions of the acceptability of a whole-hospital, pro-active electronic paediatric early warning system (the DETECT study): a qualitative interview study. BMC Pediatr. 2022;22:365.
33. Sefton G, Carter B, Lane S, et al. Dynamic Electronic Tracking and Escalation to reduce Critical care Transfers (DETECT): the protocol for a stepped wedge mixed method study to explore the clinical effectiveness, clinical utility and cost-effectiveness of an electronic physiological surveillance system for use in children. BMC Pediatr. 2019;19:359.
34. Kim SY, Kim S, Cho J, et al. A deep learning model for real-time mortality prediction in critically ill children. Crit Care. 2019;23:279.

Further Reading

Parshuram CS, Dryden-Palmer K, Farrell C, et al. Effect of a pediatric early warning system on all-cause mortality in hospitalized pediatric patients: the EPOCH randomized clinical trial. JAMA. 2018;319:1002.

RCPCH. Safe System Framework for children at risk of deterioration. 2022 [cited 2022 Dec 16]. Available from: https://www.rcpch.ac.uk/resources/safe-system-framework-children-risk-deterioration.

RCPCH. Paediatric Early Warning System (PEWSystem) - developing a standardised tool for England. 2022 [cited 2022 Dec 16]. Available from: https://www.rcpch.ac.uk/resources/paediatric-early-warning-system-pewsystem-developing-standardised-tool-england#downloadBox.

Trubey R, Huang C, Lugg-Widger FV, et al. Validity and effectiveness of paediatric early warning systems and track and trigger tools for identifying and reducing clinical deterioration in hospitalised children: a systematic review. BMJ Open. 2019;9:e022105. https://doi.org/10.1136/bmjopen-2018-022105.

ICU Structure

Contents

ICU: Gas, Humidity, Power and Airflow

Daniele De Luca and Roberta Centorino

Contents

J. Brierley et al. (eds.), *ESPNIC Children's Intensive Care Textbook*,
https://doi.org/10.1007/978-3-031-64762-8_5

Learning Objectives

- Know the main characteristics of modern PICU/NICU design
- Understand the needs behind these characteristics
- Know critical threshold values of light, noise, power, and humidity for a PICU/NICU
- Understand how to choose between the different designs

5.1 Introduction

The design of a neonatal (NICU) or paediatric (PICU) intensive care unit might theoretically influence both short- and long-term outcomes and surely has a great impact on the teamwork and fitness of healthcare providers [1]. Evidence has shown that hospital design can significantly improve patient safety and make patient, staff and family environments healthier [2]. Achieving an optimal design for PICUs and NICUs is not easy, as several features and needs must be balanced. The majority of the literature available in this field is dedicated to NICU design, and it is understandable since NICUs are more than PICUs on average. However, for the majority of the issues discussed below, there is no clear reason to think that data would not be applicable to PICUs as well. We will discuss this and also the peculiarity of mixed PICU/NICU units when needed. The main characteristics are explained as follows.

Family-centred care is generally seen as a safe and optimal working condition for healthcare professionals and might be considered when designing new NICUs and PICUs [1]. The health benefits of continuous parents' participation and interaction are significantly improved if the environmental design allows privacy and reduces environmental sources of stress [3]. Further important elements of NICU design are the spatial division of facilities and appropriate lighting levels to optimise the ability of healthcare professionals to perform care while meeting the health needs of patients and their families [4]. These needs might be seen as contradictory but must be balanced and an ideal system must be flexible: space and possibilities should be provided to families, but they must also be easy to change quickly and dedicated to medical and surgical emergencies. Careful consideration should also be given to infection prevention and control, including sink availability and automatic washing frequency, water safety controls, airborne isolation facilities and logistic pathways [5]. In large NICU/PICU, an area dedicated to full isolation with negative-pressure rooms should also be available. Ideally, if a unit admits extremely preterm or immunocompromised patients, positive-pressure areas should also be available.

5.2 Single Family Rooms Versus Open-Bay Units

The choice between single rooms or open bay design is difficult and the debate is almost endless. It is not possible to give firm recommendations in favour of one or the other. However, we will list here the main characteristics of the two designs and their pros and cons.

Single family rooms (SFR) were noticed to improve sleep, increase privacy and parental involvement, and assist with infection control and noise reduction. Neonates were found to have fewer apnoeic events, reduced nosocomial sepsis and mortality as well as improved neonatal nutritional outcomes and earlier transition to enteral feeding [6]. When SFR and open-bay were compared for parental experiences, the SFR design resulted in greater parental satisfaction [7]. In contrast to the above studies, Pineda et al. expressed concerns that environmental sound and language exposure in single rooms may be reduced to levels that are detrimental to child development, with a diminution of normal hemispheric asymmetry, lower language scores and a trend towards lower motor scores later in infancy. However, more stress has been reported by mothers in single rooms [8].

Moreover, the open bay design has the advantage of developing communication and interaction with medical staff and nurses and the ability to monitor multiple infants simultaneously. This design may also facilitate the implementation of emergency procedures although SFR can also allow this, provided that adequate monitoring tools are installed. Multiple-bed rooms or an open bay area shall have a minimum of 8 ft (2.4 m) between patients' beds.

The US Consensus Committee on Recommended Design Standards for Advanced Neonatal Care recommends a minimum size of 165 ft^2 (15.3 m^2) of clear floor area for SFR. Each room shall be designed to allow visual and speech privacy for the infant and family. Family space should also include: (1) comfortable reclining chairs suitable for kangaroo/skin-to-skin care (for NICUs); (2) recumbent sleep surfaces for at least one parent; (3) desks or surfaces suitable for writing and/or use of a laptop computer for healthcare professionals; (4) at least four electrical outlets for use and charging of electronic devices and (5) no <6 ft^3 (0.2 m^3) of storage space. Within this space, there shall be sufficient furnishing to allow a parent to stay seated, reclining or fully recumbent at the bedside. There shall be an aisle adjacent to each infant space with a minimum width of 4 ft (1.2 m) in multiple-bed rooms.

Newer designs, with an intermediate nature between a single room and an open bay, have been recently realised. In these mixed designs, PICU/NICUs look like a sort of hive with 2–4 beds in a unique or partially divided room, which is connected by a corridor to the main bay area. Patient monitoring is ensured in the local area and re-transmitted in the open bay. This may represent the best solution although no studies evaluating this architecture are available yet.

5.3 NICU/PICU Location Within the Hospital

The NICU/PICU shall be a well-recognizable area within the healthcare facility, with controlled access and environment. This may be provided with video-surveillance systems or in-person safeguards, according to different needs and settings. The purpose is to provide safe and efficient transport of patients, as they are the more vulnerable ones and children with complex social problems or maltreatment can also be admitted.

PICU/NICU should also be adjacent to other related wards. For instance, paediatric emergency area or the delivery room should be closed. This may be a bit complicated if the intensive care unit is actually a mixed PICU/NICU. When delivery rooms and neonatal wards are on separate floors of the hospital, an elevator located adjacent to or within the PICU/NICU must be provided [9]. It is important to remember that the co-location of delivery rooms and the NICU has resulted in the reduction of moderate hypothermia and morbidity [10]. Anyhow pathways dedicated to the transportation of critically ill children and neonates to/from some related wards (such as operating rooms, general paediatric or radiology units) must be identified in order to reduce the transfer using public corridors [9]. Care should be taken to limit the number of exits and entrances to the unit. The control station should be located within close proximity and direct visibility of the entrance to the infant care area.

5.4 Support Areas

The units shall have a clearly identified entrance and reception area for families. Families shall have immediate and direct contact with staff when they arrive at this entrance and reception area. This area should have lockable storage facilities for personal belongings and a handwashing and gowning area. The units shall have dedicated areas for the storage and cleaning of medical devices and disposable materials. A clear pathway should be identified to separate clean and used materials. Adequate space shall be provided to realise meetings between physicians, nurses, other healthcare professionals and administrative staff. Obviously, rooms (and dedicated toilets) must be provided for attending physicians or fellows and residents on call. Space for preparation and storage of formula or additives to human milk and formula shall be available ideally within the unit [11]. In high-volume NICUs, a milk bank is also desirable, and this requires adequate space and sanitation protocols. Administrative space shall be provided within the unit and/or in the proximity of all physicians and some of these should be clearly reserved for research activities. Ideally (at least) some ancillary services such as respiratory therapy, laboratory, pharmacy, radiology and developmental therapy should also be included in the NICU/PICU facility, if possible.

5.5 Specialized Procedure Spaces

Special rooms designed for surgery or other particular procedures shall have a minimum clear floor area of 360 ft^2 (33.5 m^2) with a minimum dimension of 16 ft (4.9 m^2) exclusive of hand-washing stations and columns. These rooms shall be designed to comply with safety requirements for surgical or other procedures. The space requirements for these functions in multi-bed rooms shall have a minimum clear floor area of 225 ft^2 (21 m^2) exclusive of hand-washing stations, columns and aisles.

5.6 Noise, Light, Temperature and Humidity

In patients' rooms and adult sleep areas, the combination of continuous background sound and operational sound shall not exceed an hourly measurement of 45 dB. Transient sounds or peaks shall not exceed 65 dB. Different thresholds may be dictated by local regulations. In staff work, family and staff lounge areas, the combination of continuous background sound and operational sound shall not exceed an hourly measurement of 50 dB and a peak of 70 dB [9]. Median sound levels were significantly lower in the single room or enclosed space design compared to the open-bay models in four studies [12–15].

Ambient lighting levels in infant spaces shall be adjustable through a range of at least 10 to no more than 600 lux (B1 to 60 foot candles) as measured on a horizontal plane at each bedside. Both natural and electric light sources shall have controls that allow immediate darkening of any bed position sufficient for transillumination or ultrasound imaging when necessary. There are conflicting data regarding the light levels in single rooms versus open bay design, and it is not clear if one or the other provides a better illumination [13, 15].

The PICU/NICU shall be designed to provide an air temperature of 72.1F to 78.1F (22–26 °C) and relative humidity of 30–60% while avoiding condensation on walls and window surfaces. Temperature and humidity were assessed in only one study which found the single-room environment to be cooler and with greater temperature stability; however, mean humidity in the two environments was the same [13]. We believe that these characteristics might be influenced more by the implementation of adequate conditioning and humidification systems than by the facility design itself. The air delivered to the intensive care unit shall be filtered with at least the efficiency specified in the FGI (Facilities Guidelines Institute) guidelines [3]. Filters shall be located outside the infant care area so they can be changed easily and safely. High-efficiency particulate air filters should also be included in positive- or negative-pressure areas.

5.7 Electrical, Gas Supply and Mechanical Needs

Mechanical requirements at each bed, such as electrical and gas outlets, shall be organized to ensure safety, easy access and maintenance. There shall be a minimum of 20 simultaneously accessible electrical outlets. There should be a minimum of three outlets per air, oxygen and vacuum. There shall be a mixture of emergency and normal power for all electrical outlets according to the US National Fire Protection Association recommendations [16]. Periodical tests and maintenance should be performed and energy supply for vital outlets must be ensured at any time.

5.8 Handwashing Facilities

Two studies demonstrated significantly increased rates of nosocomial infection when infants were moved to smaller, temporary NICUs and subsequently decreased when infants were moved to a newly constructed facility with improved sink-to-bed ratios [17, 18]. We can presume the same effect for PICU patients. Every bed, whether in a single-bed or multiple-bed room, shall be within 20 ft (6 ms) of a hands-free handwashing station. Handwashing stations shall be no closer than 3 ft (0.9 m) from a bed, clean supply storage or counter/worksurface unless a splashguard is provided. Handwashing sinks shall be large enough to control splashing and designed to avoid standing or retained water [9].

5.9 Airborne Infection Isolation Room

A negative pressure airborne infection isolation room, with a clear floor space of 14 m^2, containing hand-washing facilities, space for storage, means of emergency communication and self-closing doors should be available [10]. At least one single-occupancy isolation room should be available for infants with airborne transmissible infections. A space should also be available to safely cohort a group of infants infected with or exposed to a common airborne pathogen. Airborne infection isolation rooms shall have a permanently installed visual mechanism to constantly monitor the pressure status of the room when occupied by a patient with an airborne infectious disease. The mechanism shall continuously monitor the direction of the airflow.

5.10 Access to Nature and Other Positive Distraction

Views of nature, toys and/or electronic entertainment shall be provided in the unit in at least one space that is accessible to all families and one space that is accessible to all staff. These may also be useful in rooms for children who are not sedated [9]. When possible, windows should have views of external environments or walls may be decorated with trees, plants, human and animal activity, gardens and landscapes. In urban settings, appropriate nature elements might include planters or water features. Family and staff lounge spaces are ideal locations for views of nature and other positive distractions [9].

5.11 Ceiling Finishes, Wall Surface and Floor Surface

Ceilings shall be easily cleanable and constructed in a manner to prohibit the passage of particles from the cavity above the ceiling plane into the clinical environment. Wall surfaces shall be easy to clean and provide protection at points where contact with movable equipment is likely to occur. Surfaces shall be free of substances known to be teratogenic, mutagenic, carcinogenic or otherwise harmful to human health. Floor surfaces shall be easily cleanable and shall minimize the growth of microorganisms. Flooring material with a reflectance of no >40% and a gloss value of no >30 gloss units shall be used to minimize the possibility that glare reflected from a bright procedure or work area light will impinge on the eyes of infants or caregivers.

Take-Home Messages

- There are different possible PICU/NICU designs, each with its own pros and cons
- The choice of a PICU/NICU design must be done according to local availability and needs but minimum characteristics in terms of power and gas supply, safety control, light, temperature and humidity stability must be respected. Critical thresholds for these parameters are provided

References

1. Örtenstrand A, Westrup B, Broström EB, et al. The Stockholm Neonatal Family Centered Care Study: effects on length of stay and infant morbidity. Pediatrics. 2010;125(2):e278–85.
2. Flacking R, Dykes F. Creating a positive place and space in NICUs. Pract Midwife. 2014;17(7):18–20.
3. Lester BM, Salisbury AL, Hawes K, et al. 18-Month follow-up of infants cared for in a single-family room neonatal intensive care unit. J Pediatr. 2016;177:84–9.
4. Raiskila S, Axelin A, Toome L, et al. Parents' presence and parent-infant closeness in 11 neonatal intensive care units in six European countries vary between and within the countries. Acta Paediatr. 2017;106(6):878–88.
5. O'Callaghan N, Dee A, Philip RK, et al. Evidence-based design for neonatal units: a systematic review. Maternal Health Neonat Perinatol. 2019;5:6.
6. Domanico R, Davis DK, Coleman F, Davis BO. Documenting the NICU design dilemma: comparative patient progress in open-ward and single family room units. J Perinatol. 2011;31(4):281–8.
7. Stevens DC, Helseth CC, Thompson PA, Pottala JV, Khan MA, Munson DP. A comprehensive comparison of Open-Bay and single-family-room neonatal intensive care units at Sanford Children's hospital. HERD. 2012;5(4):23–39.
8. Pineda RG, Stransky KE, Rogers C, et al. The single-patient room in the NICU: maternal and family effects. J Perinatol. 2012;32(7):545–51.
9. White RD, Consensus Committee on Recommended Design Standards for Advanced Neonatal Care. Recommended standards for newborn ICU design, 9th edition. J Perinatol. 2020;40(Suppl 1):2–4.
10. Terrin G, Conte F, Scipione A, et al. New architectural design of delivery room reduces morbidity in preterm neonates: a prospective cohort study. BMC Pregnancy Childbirth. 2016;16:63.
11. ADA Pediatric Nutrition Practice Group. Infant feedings: guidelines for preparation of human milk and formula in health care facilities. 2nd ed. Chicago: American Dietetic Association; 2011.
12. Liu WF. Comparing sound measurements in the single-family room with open-unit design neonatal intensive care unit: the impact of equipment noise. J Perinatol. 2012;32(5):368–73.
13. Van Enk RA, Steinberg F. Comparison of private room with multiple-bed ward neonatal intensive care unit. HERD. 2011;5(1):52–63.
14. Chen HL, Chen CH, Wu CC, Huang HJ, Wang TM, Hsu CC. The influence of neonatal intensive care unit design on sound level. Pediatr Neonatol. 2009;50(6):270–4.
15. Stevens DC, Akram Khan M, Munson DP, Reid EJ, Helseth CC, Buggy J. The impact of architectural design upon the environmental sound and light exposure of neonates who require intensive care: an evaluation of the Boekelheide neonatal intensive care nursery. J Perinatol. 2007;27(Suppl 2):S20–8.
16. NFPA. NFPA 99: health care facilities code, 2012 edition. Quincy, MA: National Fire Protection Association; 2012.
17. Lester BM, Hawes K, Abar B, et al. Single-family room care and neurobehavioral and medical outcomes in preterm infants. Pediatrics. 2014;134(4):754–60.
18. Von Dolinger de Brito D, de Almeida Silva H, Jose Oliveira E, et al. Effect of neonatal intensive care unit environment on the incidence of hospital-acquired infection in neonates. J Hosp Infect. 2007;65(4):314–8.

Basic Patient Safety and Quality in PICU

Mona Mahyub and Joe Brierley

Contents

J. Brierley et al. (eds.), *ESPNIC Children's Intensive Care Textbook*,
https://doi.org/10.1007/978-3-031-64762-8_6

Learning Objectives
- Appreciate how the human factors and ergonomic approaches developed from other industries such as aviation improve ICU care
- Understand how a flattened hierarchy and a blame-free approach to incident reporting and investigation can reduce healthcare-associated harm
- Explore how the ICU team can regularly review its performance by measuring important healthcare-associated episodes, and those of related services in measuring other related episodes of care

> Better is possible. It does not take genius. It takes diligence. It takes moral clarity. It takes ingenuity. And above all, it takes a willingness to try.
> —Atul Gawande, Better: A Surgeon's Notes on Performance

6

6.1 Introduction

At the turn of the century, a significant shift in healthcare was observed. As mortality rates from critical illness improved, it became evident that healthcare itself was contributing to morbidity and even mortality in our patients. In the ICU, hospital-acquired infections, bedsores and drug errors were no longer seen as unavoidable difficulties, but as avoidable harm. This marked a fundamental shift in our understanding of how to improve healthcare.

Research was no longer the only approach to improve patient outcomes, there was now a focus too on optimising clinical effectiveness and healthcare delivery.

Key steps in this paradigm shift included interest in obtaining and interpreting data about incidence and prevalence, but not of diseases as most are familiar with, but rather of healthcare episodes, for example central-venous catheters/line (CVC) infections.

Measurement was, of course, fundamental to this new approach of tackling avoidable healthcare-associated harm. As Sherlock Holmes said, 'Data, data, data, I can't make bricks without clay'. Yet one key epidemiological concept was required to give meaning: the idea of a denominator to assess not just incidence but also prevalence or rates of the issue. For example, two CVC infections in a unit with three central lines at a time may be more concerning than in a unit with 20—so the idea of 'line days' to quantify the number of CVC lines in a unit became part of the ICU terminology.

6.2 Culture

Once such measurements allowed an assessment of the magnitude of the problem, the efficacy of steps to reduce various issues became measurable. However, cultural change was and is required. The airline industry has been instrumental in other industries, learning how to adopt a safety culture. Of necessity following numerous high-profile air crashes with multiple fatalities, a safety culture approach was developed. A classic example is the 1989 UK Kegworth disaster when an almost new Boeing 737–400 on a routine flight from London Heathrow to Belfast had one of the two engines malfunction with fire visible. In response, the crew shut down what they thought was the malfunctioning engine, but was rather the functioning engine, with confusing feedback of improvement. Shortly afterwards, they realised their mistake, but the malfunctioning engine then completely failed, and they could not restart the shut-down engine, meaning the aircraft effectively had become a powerless glider without power, which crash-landed, killing 47 people and causing horrific injuries to the survivors, including the pilots. Sadly, a standard blame approach from the media attacked the pilots when it became public knowledge that they had shut down the wrong engine.

A fuller description of the investigation is available.[1] However, the key findings were that these human factors were part of a system-wide series of issues. One key observation was that the culture of the pilot being in charge and assumed to clearly know what they were doing prevented other crew members and passengers from speaking out when the pilots announced they were shutting down the unaffected engine, despite many outside the cockpit seeing it was the engine on the other side that had fire coming from it. From episodes such as this, the concept of a flattened hierarchy with anyone empowered to speak out about safety issues has become the norm.

Similarly, now in healthcare, a safety approach empowers anyone, including patients and their families, to speak out, superseding the traditional medical lead of the team being an unchallengeable authority. For anyone doubting the relevance of this to healthcare, the case of Elaine Bromiley is illustrative.[2] She was a fit and well lady undergoing an elective procedure under general anaesthesia. There was a failure to intubate and then oxygenate her, with various devices.

The consultant anaesthetist persisted in attempts to intubate with various devices, including via laryngeal mask ventilation despite worsening hypoxia ignoring the suggestions of the theatre nurses to desist and perform a surgical airway. Sadly, when the anaesthesia was reversed, it became clear that Elaine had suffered a severe hypoxic brain injury, from which she sadly died.

Her husband, Martin Bromiley an airline pilot, insisted on an independent, but crucially, no-blame review in which the human factors and ergonomics (HFE) which contributed were explored and openly analysed. From here, he set up the charity Clinical Human Factors Group and continues to advocate for an improved safety culture in healthcare.

In ICU such cultural change has specifically targeted those areas most affecting critically ill patients: healthcare-associated infections, drug errors and ventilation-induced lung injury.

In cardiac ICU, many units have worked with another safety-focussed industry, Formula one motor racing, to improve the transfer of complex information between the cardiac operating theatre and the ICU following congenital heart surgery. Learning from those who have striven to improve and indeed perfect the most vulnerable data transfer episode in their industry, to turn marginal gains into seconds that can win a race may seem very tangential to the ICU team, but can clearly be adapted to improve the team's performance.

---

1 ► https://humanfactors101.com/incidents/kegworth/
2 ► www.futurelearn.com/info/courses/airway-matters/0/steps/68647

6.3 Data, Data, Data!

As well as cultural change, the modern ICU has developed an entire system of measuring those parts of healthcare that might lead to harm to patients. As highlighted, it is crucial to measure both the incidence of adverse healthcare episodes and also the denominator underlying the episodes. So, the number of prescriptions errors should be divided by the number of prescriptions in the ICU per week, though this is still inadequate if the many prescriptions this week of high-risk complex biological agents, where errors may be fatal, rather than standard ICU drugs where the risk is arguably lower. Essentially, this is to allow measurements to be compared between each week on a single unit, between similar units in a city or country or between countries.

This is not to say that incidents themselves are not vital, but a standardised no-blame incident reporting system allows the recording of healthcare episodes that might have affected the patient or may do so in the future. The no-blame part of this is crucial in that it encourages reporting and accepts most episodes to have system issues rather than just human errors. In this way, effective change rather than a blame and cover-up approach can lead to improvements in patient safety. Crucially support rather than blame can be provided to healthcare professionals involved, thus preventing any second victim harm to healthcare professionals who will rarely commit any serious professional failure.

Taking such a human factors approach can help prevent future episodes in a system that can itself, therefore, learn.

Why did ICU doctors put central lines in without optimal insertion techniques and maintenance techniques? Largely because CVC infections were considered unavoidable complications of healthcare, and no one routinely measured their incidence.

Generic approaches such as the focus on hand hygiene have improved safety throughout medicine, and in our ICUs, as have specific reductions in wrong site surgery and surgical infections. The use of a simple approach has been crucial in all these improvements, the use of an independent checklist, enables a safety approach, adopted from the airline and other industries, to be used in crucial areas of healthcare. For example, WHO checklists before surgery. The key feature of this checklist approach is an independent live audit of practice, and a standard of getting things right not some of the time, or most of the time, but every time.

In the ICU, checklists now feature in more specific bundles of care regarding insertion and maintenance of CVC and endotracheal/tubes among other episodes of care. The bundle approach does not target a single intervention but rather a collection of agreed interventions that should ideally be met every time the treatment issue is faced. For example, an insertion bundle may feature skin preparation, draping, hand washing and gloves, insertion attempts before more senior help, X-ray, securing devices and documentation.

This type of approach has reduced hospital-acquired or nosocomial infections including CVC-related infections and ventilator-associated pneumonia in units that implement them. Such bundles of care are also now used to ensure surviving sepsis goals of care are delivered in a timely manner to children with severe infections, both in the ICU or during their presentation to the hospital.

Compliance with checklists can be readily audited, and any issues or non-compliant professionals addressed. In this, a flattened hierarchy is again crucial—nurses in the ICU and the families of children in the hospital are encouraged to challenge those who may not respect hand hygiene adequately. Suit jackets and white coats have no place in the modern ICU, shirt sleeves must be rolled up to facilitate hand hygiene.

Preventing interruptions during the prescribing and administration of drugs in the ICU is another vital behavioural approach shown to improve outcomes by reducing drug errors, one of the commonest causes of morbidity and mortality due to inadvertent harm in healthcare.

Controlling so-called professional freedom to protect patients is not always straightforward. It takes buy-in from the healthcare team, rather than imposition. Presenting weekly on the ICU measurable safety information from the previous week with a running total enables those involved to review the care they were involved in. Why was there an accidental extubation? Do our rates suggest a problem compared to our own data or national norms? Are delayed discharges getting better? Is the mortality rate within acceptable limits, compared to norms, or do we need to investigate cases more fully or call in an external review of our practice?

Areas that impact the ICU, but those that the ICU does not control can also be measured, presented and addressed. Examples include: re-admission to the ICU within a short period of discharge, ostensibly due to early discharge, but in reality, a feature of the quality of the ward care post ICU; elective unbooked admissions from theatre and delayed discharges when the child is fit.

After predominantly being used to reduce readily quantifiable issues such as infections or issues with the correct placement of equipment it became clear that the behavioural approach be applied to other areas. Many ICUs use a checklist acronym at the end of each ward round to ensure no important episode of care has been missed in the round. For example, this can enable an ICU team to help in the vital battle against antibiotic resistance by working within antibiotic stewardship processes to ensure antibiotics are stopped in a timely fashion. Also, this can be used to ensure the tidal volume on each child's ventilator is not excessive, given unnecessarily high levels are associated with ventilator-associated lung injury.

In recent years, referral by ICU teams to organ donation services according to basic screening processes can be automated, avoiding the need to remember to refer during what can be an intense clinical interaction, and removing concern about complaints following the referral of someone who survives.

So, this chapter has reviewed the vital healthcare improvement approach to securing better outcomes for the child in the ICU. Flattening hierarchies, and a no-blame approach as in other industries, allow a safe and effective analysis of serious incidents that may have caused harm to ensure learning and to address any contributing system issues. This includes allowing changes to systems to safeguard future patients.

Minimising harm by an approach that measures the incident and the ongoing prevalence of the number of measurables allows an assessment of the quality of healthcare delivery and provides an early warning marker for ICU teams.

Take-Home Messages

- Human factors and ergonomics are vital considerations in the delivery of a safe and effective ICU
- Behavioural changes supporting flattened hierarchy and a patient safety-based approach are important norms in modern healthcare
- Incident reporting and the measurement of healthcare-associated episodes, such as infections with a meaningful denominator, allow regular and ongoing assessment of the quality of ICU delivery
- Healthcare improvement has now broadened to include other areas such as antibiotic stewardship and organ donation

Further Reading

Anderson M. Introduction to human factors & work psychology. Human Factors 101. [cited 2024 Apr]. Available from: https://humanfactors101.com/incidents/kegworth/.

Bromiley M. The story of Elaine Bromiley. [cited 2024 Apr]. Available from: www.futurelearn.com/info/courses/airway-matters/0/steps/68647.

Scanlon MC, Densmore EM. Human factors and children: implications for patient safety. Healthcare systems ergonomics and patient safety: human factor, a bridge between care and cure - proceedings of the International Conference HEPS 2005. 2005; p. 123–6.

Handover from Operating Theatre

Aurélie Bardaji and Serge Grazioli

Contents

J. Brierley et al. (eds.), *ESPNIC Children's Intensive Care Textbook*,
https://doi.org/10.1007/978-3-031-64762-8_7

Learning Objectives

- Understand the importance of the handover process
- Review common errors and barriers to an effective handover process
- Learn different strategies to improve the handover process

7.1 Why Are Effective Handovers So Important for the Patient's Safety?

Handovers are defined as the transition of care, involving the transfer of responsibility, accountability, and authority [1–3]. This transition process involves the transmission of vital information to ensure continuity of care for each patient. It represents a real communication challenge, which can be a source of medical errors.

It is well established that these crucial moments represent high-risk processes that can lead to discontinuity of care, associated with misunderstanding, errors, and information omission. Literature reports that handover is linked to 80% of sentinel events, which are serious andpreventable. Furthermore, incomplete handovers were implicated in 28% of surgical errors, and 24% of malpractice cases in ambulatory and emergency departments [4]. Poor handover was the most prevalent cause leading to medical errors [5], and is associated with delayed or inappropriate treatment or testing, and overall prolonged hospital length of stay [1]. This task involves several skills across various domains including clinical medicine, communication, and team leadership, all of which must be executed simultaneously. Additionally, this process must be completed within a short period of time, often in a highly constrained environment.

Because of their small size and weight, pediatric patients are more susceptible to adverse events, which occur eight times more frequently in children than in adults [6]. The transition of a child from the operating room (OR) to the pediatric intensive care unit (PICU) represents a high-risk procedure prone to errors, where the quality of the handover process may have a significant impact on the patient safety and medical outcomes of this vulnerable patient population.

Ideally, the handover should deliver safe, effective, and up-to-date information without compromising continuity of care so that the incoming providers can function as if they had been present and engaged in all previous patient care activities (◘ Fig. 7.1).

Finally, handovers constitute also a great educational opportunity for medical students and student nurses who will learn the specificities of different surgical interventions and their postoperative care management [7].

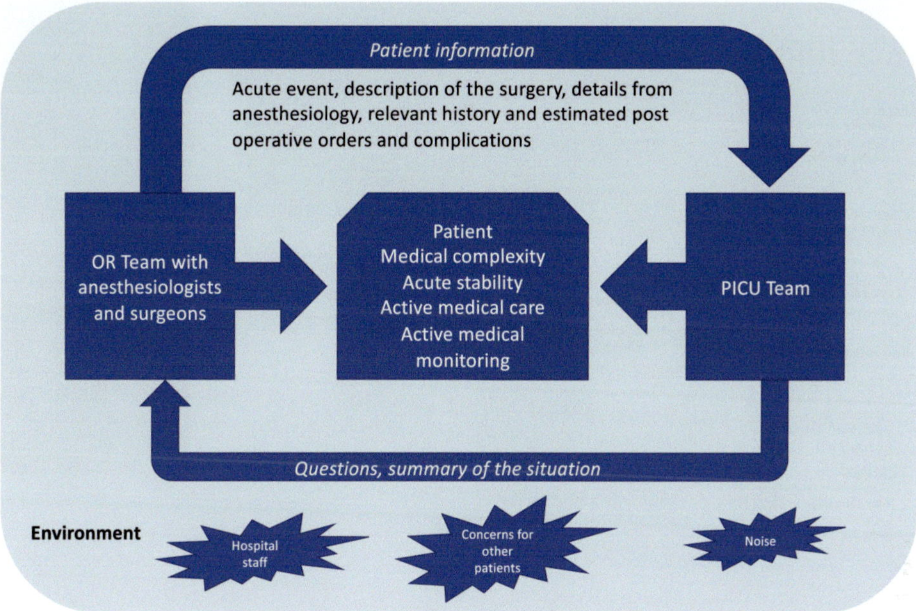

Fig. 7.1 Handover process between operating room team and PICU team

7.2 Team Performance and Commons Errors

Multidisciplinary teamwork is a fundamental component of the post-surgical handover process that involves surgical, anesthetic, and intensive care teams with different areas of expertise, hierarchical structure, and cultural differences.

Because the patient is often in a very unstable physiologic condition during the handover process, in particular children after surgery, there is a time pressure to transmit the maximum of information in a minimum of time with the conservation of maximum intelligibility. A better understanding of the barriers to effective handover will help improve handover quality and efficiency.

7.2.1 Communication Team Performance

Although good cooperation between medical teams is essential for an effective handover, it has been shown that other important factors are also essential for the success of this highly complex process.

Cognitive science has identified models of team functioning, sharing a three-part structure: **input**, **process**, and **outcome** framework (Fig. 7.2). The "input" represents the conditions prior to the discussion. The "process" describes how the inputs are transformed into outcomes. And the "outcome" is the result of the team's activity. Identifying parameters for each category in relation to the specific transition of care, in our case, from the OR to the PICU, helps to conduct an effective handover.

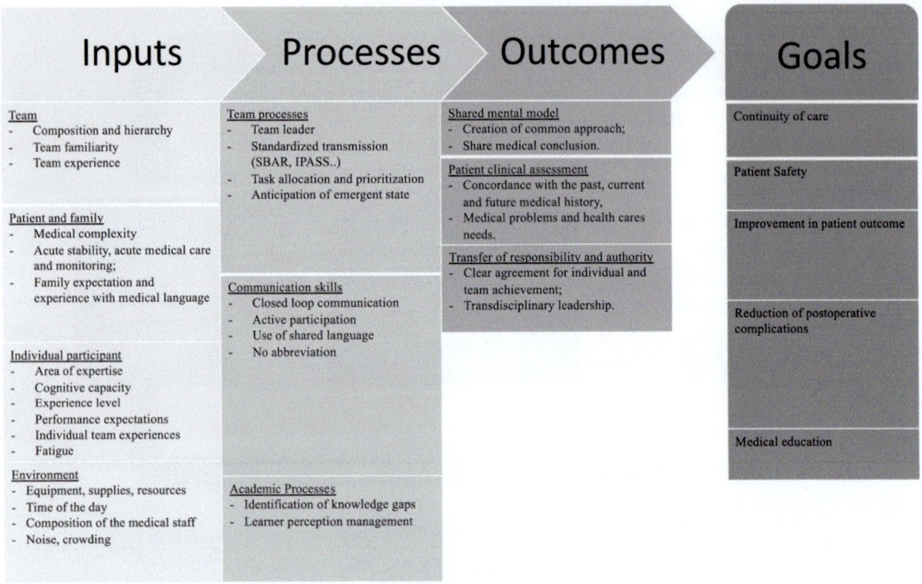

Fig. 7.2 Communication process and team functioning during handover

7.2.2 Inputs

The handover process consists of various important input factors with their own characteristics that can all be individually modified in order to improve the overall efficiency of the input-process-outcome framework of the handover. Input factors can be at the level of the group, the individual, or the environment. Group size, structure, and level of "cohesiveness" and composition have to be identified as important input factors on the group level with poor teamwork being directly linked to negative patient outcomes [8].

At the individual level, important factors related to characteristics of individual participants inside the different medical teams had been identified: for example, area of expertise, level of knowledge, performance expectations, experience level, cognitive capacity, as well as their attitudes (e.g., preference toward teamwork) and personality characteristics (e.g., extraversion, conscientiousness). If we look at the cognitive capacity that is required during this exchange, it appears that the working memory is very solicited, but this type of memory is limited by the number of information that it can hold and process at the same time which are between 4–7 and 2–5 elements, respectively [9]. Furthermore, working memory performance can be reduced by the distracting effect of external factors, highlighting the importance of a quiet environment during the handover process in order to maximize the working memory operation. Another individual input factor is related to the patient himself. The complexity of the medical history and the severity of the patient's condition associated with the caregiver's involvement may all contribute to the exchange of incomplete, inaccurate, or misunderstood handover information. Finally, input factors can also be found at the organization level, where unit location, resource availability in equipment, supplies, staffing, and safety culture may all contribute to improving the general process of handover by influencing all the other input factors.

7.2.3 Processes

To process the input, the team needs to learn to work together and rely on good communication skills. In particular, closed loop communication has been shown to be essential for an effective handover. A standardized handover requires the transmission of accurate medical information from the sender to the receiver and the ability of the receiver to ask the right question and to summarize the information at the end of the process. It has been shown that unidirectional communication is ineffective and may be the source of omissions and misunderstandings. Moreover, the information needs to be communicated in a clear, intelligible way without abbreviations.

7.2.4 Outcomes

From the input, thanks to a satisfactory process, can emerge the outcomes, from which can occur the continuity of care and the other goals for appropriate medical care. An important factor in this process is the concept of a shared mental model that has been used in the literature to explain team functioning. The idea is that team performance improves if team members have a shared understanding of the task that is to be performed. The notion of sharing the mental models is used when the condition of communication is difficult in the context of excessive workload and time pressure and allows people to draw inferences and make predictions [10].

The challenge of effective handover is to transmit his mental model to ensure the continuity of care. It is a moment of exchange, where two parts, the provider of care and the next provider construct a mutual understanding of the patient's condition and can decide together what will be the postoperative management plan.

Cognitive science has described how difficult it is to share one's own mental shape with others and this is further exacerbated when the involved participants (e.g., surgeons, anesthetists, and intensivists) have different mental models. Lack of a shared mental model during handover has been associated with ineffective handovers caused by misunderstanding and false consensus effect. It is important to build a communication strategy, based on a proper shared mental model between the surgical team and PICU team (◘ Fig. 7.3). The qualitative assessments of handover showed the importance of developing mental models to reduce communication errors [8].

7.2.5 Mains Parameters of Ineffective Handover

The ultimate goal of an effective handover is not to act as successive teams who relay information, but as a single wider team that provides care successively [4]. Missing or incomplete information during handover is associated with patient injury and is reported in 57% of surgical malpractice claims [11]. The main errors during handover and barriers to an effective handover are summarized in ◘ Table 7.1.

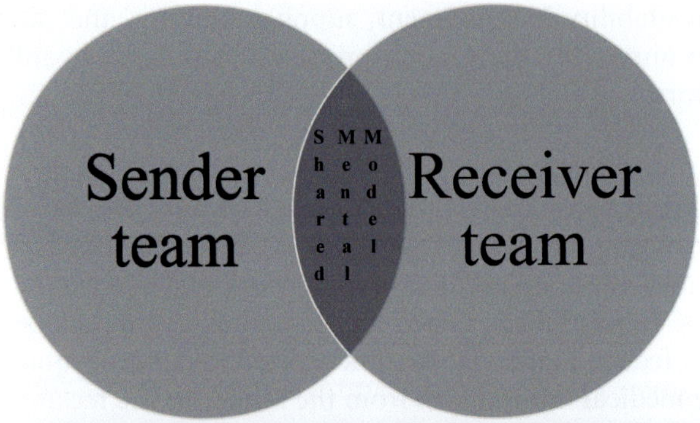

Mental Model
Awareness of the identity of the patient
Awareness of the clinical situation
Awareness of the monitoring
Awareness of existing healthcare needs
Same language, no abbreviation, written checklist, mnemotechnic tools
Anticipation of next healthcare needs

Fig. 7.3 Description of a shared mental model for OR to PICU handover

Table 7.1 Main barriers and errors to avoid during handovers

Main *errors* during Handover	Main *barriers* to effective Handover and solutions	
Omission	Distraction	Use a dedicated and quiet environment to do the handover.
Inaccurate information	Noise	Limit alarm levels, and do not allow other discussions during handover.
Irrelevant information	Interruptions	Prevent interruptions by consultants, avoid neighboring conversations, and delegate phone responsabilities.
Contradictory information	Crowding	Limit the number of people present.
Illegible, unclear sign-out	Multi-tasking	Focus attention on the handover, delegate other patient-related activities.
Faiurel to discuss the next problems	Hierarchical differences	Foster a culture of open communication.
Failure to discuss a decision	Passive listening	Encourage questions and postoperative care plan summaries by receiving team.
	Lack of standardized handover	Implement a structured communication framework.
	Lack of training	Proper training is essential for both the sender and the receiver to ensure an accurate handover.

7.3 How to Manage an Effective Handover?

Patient handovers have been recognized as a major healthcare challenge, and numerous efforts have been made to improve the quality of the handover process through standardization, structured framework, and written checklists [12]. The implementation of a structured handover process improves healthcare data exchange, reduces complications and errors, and enhance perceptions of handover quality [13]. Two examples of structured handovers are shown in ◘ Table 7.2 and ◘ Fig. 7.4 incorporating key elements of an effective handover: efficient teamwork, thorough preparation, and good communication. Teamwork can be learned and trained with multidisciplinary simulation and feedback. Preparing the handover in advance by synthesizing and ordering different diagnoses and treatments on paper can be very helpful, especially for the less-experienced clinicians.

In order to improve the efficiency of communication, different standardized handover tools have been developed (◘ Fig. 7.5) and shown to reduce medical errors and preventable adverse events [14] The application of one of these mnemotechnic tools is illustrated in ◘ Table 7.3 with the use of the SBAR (situation, background, assessment, and recommendation) tool for a postoperative handover. These mne-

◘ **Table 7.2** Example of the structure of a handover

Where	Dedicated place or at the bedside of the patient, quiet room.
How	Standardized procedure, incorporating mnemonics tools (SBAR, IPASS…).
Language	No abbreviation, common language, shared mental model.
Documents	Written files, checklists. Written documents help to reduce information omissions and improve handovers.
Communication skills	Active participation, closed-loop communication, and questions/summaries from the receiving team.

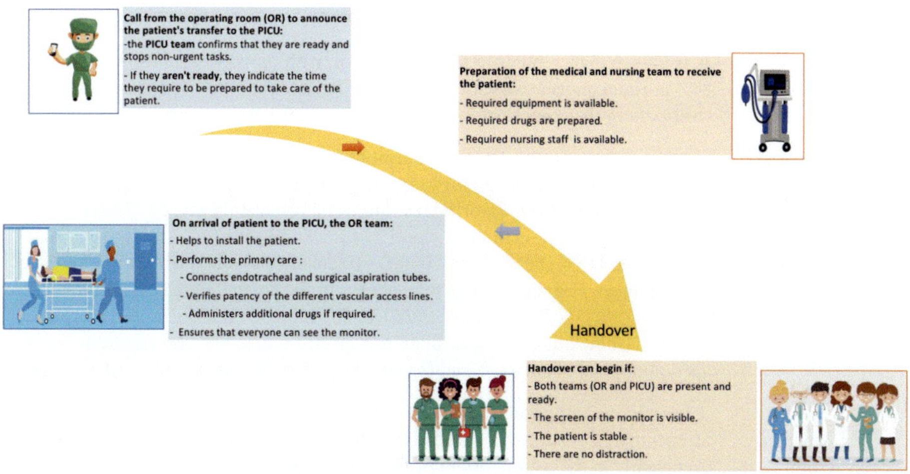

◘ **Fig. 7.4** Overview of the handover process

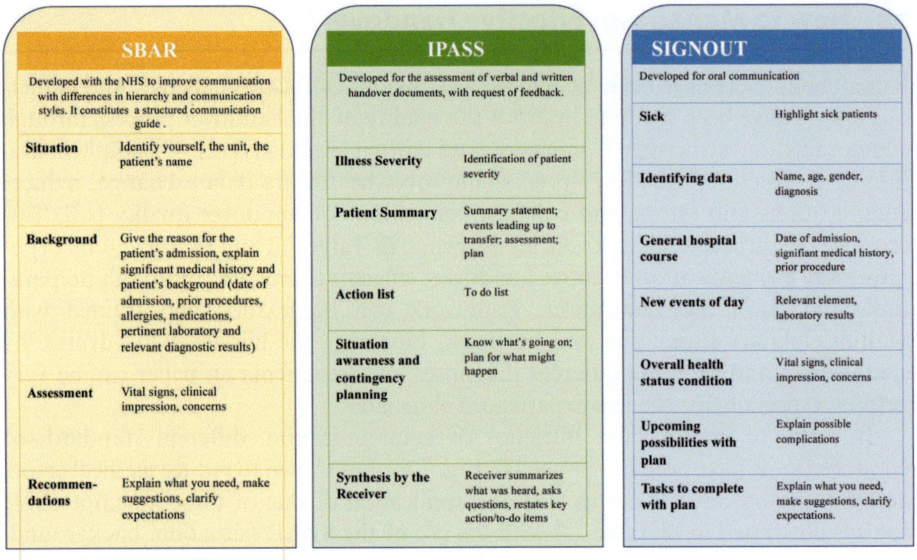

Fig. 7.5 Example of mnemotechnic tools for standardized handovers

Table 7.3 Example of a handover with the SBAR tool

Handover with the SBAR tool		
S	Situa-tion	B., is a 2-year-old girl, who underwent surgery for a regular tetralogy of Fallot under general anesthesia with an easy intubation (Cormack grade 1, tube 4,5 fixed at 13 cm blade 2). She is equipped with an arterial line in the left radial artery, a two-lumen 8Fr 8 cm central line in the right internal jugular vein, a urinary catheter, two chest tubes, and a naso-gastric tube. There were no significant complications during surgery. Cardiopulmonary bypass (CPB) and aortic cross-clamp time were, respectively, 75 and 45 min. The interventricular communication was closed, hypertrophic right ventricular muscle was resected, and the right infundibulum was enlarged, but the pulmonary valve was good and not touched. The last echocardiography showed diastolic right ventricular dys-function but no valvular dysfunction or residual interventricular communication
B	Back-ground	B. is known for a regular tetralogy of Fallot, with baseline saturation around 80% at room air. She was not known for allergies. She was on propranolol treatment in the context of cyanotic spells started 2 months ago
A	Assess-ment	Currently, she is supported with milrinone for diastolic right ventricular dys-function and noradrenaline for vasoplegia induced by anesthesia and CPB. She is ventilated with 8 mL/kg of tidal volume at a respiratory rate of 25/min without oxygen. The estimated blood loss is 200 mL, the first ACT was 120 and the last one 115 s, she received 180 mL of packed red blood cells and 70 mg/kg of fibrinogen. Her blood gases were always in the normal ranges. For sedation and analgesia, she is receiving continuous infusion of midazolam and morphine and the last injection of rocuronium was given 1 h ago. She also received acetaminophen 30 min ago and the last dose of antibiotic was given at 8:30 am
R	Recom-menda-tion	Chest drains and pacemaker can be removed in 24 h if there is not bleeding or arrhythmia. If a surgeon is needed call the resident at his number. The family is currently in the waiting room of the unit. Here are the checklist documents

motechnic tools help to structure the communication, enable preparation before the communication process, encourage interprofessional collaboration, and reduce hierarchical inhibition by encouraging the sender to provide a personal assessment and suggestion of the situation.

Take-Home Messages

- Handover is essential for the continuity of care.
- Uncorrected handover can be the origin of major medical errors and fatal events.
- It represents a real communication challenge between the operating room and the critical care team.
- Handover communication is a skill that must be learned.
- Effective and standardized communication during handover allows teams to develop mental models to create a shared understanding of the patient clinical condition and its needs for ongoing care.
- The implantation of tools to standardize the handover process is recommended to improve the safety of transitions from OR to ICU.

References

1. Sochet AA, Siems A, Ye G, Godiwala N, Hebert L, Corriveau C. Standardization of postoperative transitions of care to the pediatric intensive care unit enhances efficiency and handover comprehensiveness. Pediatr Qual Saf. 2016;1(2):e004. https://doi.org/10.1097/pq9.0000000000000004.
2. Pucher PH, Johnston MJ, Aggarwal R, Arora S, Darzi A. Effectiveness of interventions to improve patient handover in surgery: a systematic review. Surgery. 2015;158(1):85–95. https://doi.org/10.1016/j.surg.2015.02.017.
3. Agarwal HS, Saville BR, Slayton JM, et al. Standardized postoperative handover process improves outcomes in the intensive care unit: a model for operational sustainability and improved team performance. Crit Care Med. 2012;40(7):2109–15. https://doi.org/10.1097/CCM.0b013e3182514bab.
4. Cohen MD, Hilligoss B, Kajdacsy-Balla Amaral AC. A handoff is not a telegram: an understanding of the patient is co-constructed. Crit Care. 2012;16(1):303. https://doi.org/10.1186/cc10536.
5. Farhan M, Brown R, Woloshynowych M, Vincent C. The ABC of handover: a qualitative study to develop a new tool for handover in the emergency department. Emerg Med J. 2012;29(12):941–6. https://doi.org/10.1136/emermed-2011-200199.
6. Kaushal R, Bates DW, Landrigan C, et al. Medication errors and adverse drug events in pediatric inpatients. JAMA. 2001;285(16):2114–20. https://doi.org/10.1001/jama.285.16.2114.
7. Gumuchian ST, Pal NE, Young M, et al. Learner handover: perspectives and recommendations from the front-line. Perspect Med Educ. 2020;9(5):294–301. https://doi.org/10.1007/s40037-020--00601-4.
8. Lucrezia S, Noether J, Sochet AA. Standardized work rounds enhance teaming, comprehensiveness, shared mental model development, and achievement rate of end-of-shift goals. Pediatr Crit Care Med. 2021;22(4):354–64. https://doi.org/10.1097/PCC.0000000000002609.
9. Young JQ, Wachter RM, Ten Cate O, O'Sullivan PS, Irby DM. Advancing the next generation of handover research and practice with cognitive load theory. BMJ Qual Saf. 2016;25(2):66–70. https://doi.org/10.1136/bmjqs-2015-004181.
10. Mathieu JE, Heffner TS, Goodwin GF, Salas E, Cannon-Bowers JA. The influence of shared mental models on team process and performance. J Appl Psychol. 2000;85(2):273–83. https://doi.org/10.1037/0021-9010.85.2.273.
11. Methangkool E, Tollinche L, Sparling J, Agarwala AV. Communication: is there a standard handover technique to transfer patient care? Int Anesthesiol Clin. 2019;57(3):35–47. https://doi.org/10.1097/AIA.0000000000000241.

12. Sochet AA, Ryan KS, Miller W, Bartlett JL, Nakagawa TA, Bingham L. A longitudinal and sustainability assessment of pediatric interfacility transport handover standardization. Pediatr Qual Saf. 2018;3(6):e118. https://doi.org/10.1097/pq9.0000000000000118.
13. France DJ, Slagle J, Schremp E, et al. Impact of patient handover structure on neonatal perioperative safety. J Perinatol. 2019;39(3):453–67. https://doi.org/10.1038/s41372-018-0305-6.
14. Starmer AJ, Spector ND, Srivastava R, et al. I-pass, a mnemonic to standardize verbal handoffs. Pediatrics. 2012;129(2):201–4. https://doi.org/10.1542/peds.2011-2966.

Infection Prevention and Control in the Paediatric Intensive Care Unit

Anita Verma and Pam D'Silva

Contents

J. Brierley et al. (eds.), *ESPNIC Children's Intensive Care Textbook*,
https://doi.org/10.1007/978-3-031-64762-8_8

Learning Objectives

This book chapter highlights the essential components of infection prevention strategies to control healthcare-associated infections (HCAIs) in a paediatric intensive care unit (PICU):

- Understand HCAIs are highly prevalent in critically ill patients because of frequent contact with healthcare staff, multiple interventions and invasive devices
- Learn modes of transmission of HCAI
- Learn standard infection prevention and control (SIPC) measures and enhanced IPC measures
- Understand practice of hand hygiene and personal protective equipment (PPE)
- Learn about bundles for care to prevent ventilator-associated pneumonia (VAP) and central line-associated bloodstream infections (CLABSI)
- Learn aseptic non-touch technique (ANTT)
- Environment, materials and equipment for IPC at PICU
- Understand cleaning standards and waste disposal
- Importance of antimicrobial stewardship (AMS) and IPC education and training
- Case study—isolation and IPC measures for SARS CoV-2 in PICU

8.1 Introduction

Patients admitted to the paediatric intensive care unit (PICU) are critically ill and vulnerable. They continue to be at the greatest risk for health care-associated infections (HCAIs) by virtue of greater staff–patient contact with several healthcare workers (HCWs) and the presence of invasive medical devices [1–4]. Additionally, most patients undergo a variety of supportive treatments, including resuscitation, mechanical ventilation, fluid or blood transfusions, haemodialysis, and advanced surgical and diagnostic procedures. HCAIs represent a major problem in the PICU, and contribute to high morbidity, mortality and increased cost for hospitals [5–7]. The prevalence rate of HCAIs varies from centre to centre, and between resource-rich and resource-poor countries. The prevalence of HCAI in PICU from various countries has been reported to range from 1.3% to 40% [1–4]. The most common HCAIs are central line-associated bloodstream infections (CLABSI), ventilator-associated pneumonia (VAP), catheter-associated urinary tract infections (CAUTI) and surgical site infections (SSIs). A large proportion of these HCAIs can be prevented by early institution of effective infection prevention and control (IPC) measures. In this chapter, we describe the essential components of IPC measures in PICUs.

8.2 Prevention of Infection in PICU

IPC in healthcare settings is the responsibility of all healthcare providers. Although IPC teams and medical microbiologists provide essential expertise, it is important that the PICU teams collaborate in establishing infection control (IC) protocols in the unit. IPC training should be considered a mandatory component of healthcare worker competencies. The essential components of IPC are understanding how organisms spread, effective hand hygiene, appropriate use of personal protective equipment, use of care bundles to reduce CLABSI and VAP and building the right environment for a PICU. Training of staff, monitoring of IPC practice and feedback are other key components of IPC in any healthcare setting. However, although there are significant improvements and many IPC guidelines, most PICUs modify the protocols around the needs of their patient population, isolation facilities and staff [8–12].

8.3 Modes of Transmission of Infectious Agents

Knowledge of the modes of transmission of any infectious agent is critical for understanding IPC. IPC strategies are based on interruptions to the three main modes of transmission (Table 8.1).

Table 8.1 Routes of transmission of microorganisms

Mode of transmission	Examples	References
Direct contact	Direct physical contact between patient and person either colonised or infected with organisms, e.g. staff or visitors or parents infected with Herpes simplex virus; or contact with infected body fluid or by contaminated hands, e.g. SARS-CoV-2 virus. Physical transfer of organisms occurs through mucous membranes (e.g. eyes), open wounds or any abraded skin	[9, 11, 13, 14]
Indirect contact	Indirect transmission modes are contaminated via hands that are not cleaned between patients, via contaminated instruments or other inanimate objects contaminated in and around the patient environment, e.g. keyboards, bedrails, door handles, scales, stethoscope, etc. e.g. *Clostridium difficile*, Norovirus, respiratory tract pathogens, *Carbapenemase-producing Enterobactereacae* (CPE), vancomycin-resistant *Enterococcus faecium* (VRE) or methicillin-resistant *Staphylococcus aureus* (MRSA). This is the most common route of transmission to patients admitted in PICU	
Airborne	Dissemination of microorganisms by the airborne route. These organisms are carried and transmitted in droplets of different sizes Aerosol transmission: Airborne infections spread by droplet nuclei (≤5 um in diameter, referred to as aerosols). These can remain suspended indefinitely in air and can be transported over long distances, and be transmitted from the respiratory tract of an individual to the mucosa or conjunctiva of another host over distances >1 m. e.g. *Mycobacterium tuberculosis*, some viruses, e.g. measles, chicken pox and SARS-CoV-2 virus (ONGSW2020) Droplet transmission: When the droplet particles are >5 um in diameter they are referred to as respiratory droplets (WHO 2014, AA ICC). These large droplets are generated from the respiratory tract and spread in the air for a distance of at least 1 m during coughing and sneezing. These droplets can spread directly onto the mucosa or conjunctiva or be inhaled by a new host in close vicinity, e.g. SARS-CoV-2 virus. However, these droplets are large and do not remain suspended in the air for long. Therefore special ventilation systems are not required. E.g. influenza virus, adenovirus, bacteria like *Bordetella pertussis*	[9, 11, 13–15]

8.4 Prevention for Transmission of Infectious Agents

8.4.1 Standard Infection Control Precautions (SICPs)

The SICPs are basic infection control measures necessary to reduce the risk of the spread of recognised and unrecognised infection sources [8–10]. These sources include secretions and excretions, blood and body fluids, non-intact skin and mucous membranes, and equipment in the healthcare environment. SICPs should apply to all patient care, regardless of infection status and in every healthcare setting. SICPs include:

- Transmission based precautions: Hand hygiene, personal protective equipment (PPE)
- Patient screening and isolation
- Preventing device-related infections
- Appropriate waste disposal, cleaning and decontamination of the equipment, and linen
- Environment

8.4.1.1 Hand Hygiene

Although hand hygiene is more than a century-old concept, it is still one of the single most effective and simple methods for reducing the transmission of pathogenic micro-organisms to patients and personnel in healthcare settings [16].

- It should be performed at the right time by the right method with the right products. The ideal hand hygiene products are those that have high antimicrobial efficacy and moisturisation to maintain skin conditions. It has been shown that alcohol-based hand sanitisers are most effective in inactivating enveloped viruses like the new pandemic virus SARS-CoV-2 [16, 17].
- In practice, hands must be cleaned with soap and water or alcohol-based hand rub following five moments of care (◘ Fig. 8.1 below promoted by the World Health Organisation (WHO)'s Save Lives: Clean your Hands campaign [18].
- Alcohol-based hand rub is the most widely used sanitiser in acute healthcare settings, except when hands are visibly soiled or potentially contaminated with body fluids, or when caring for a patient with vomiting or diarrhoea. Hands must be washed with soap and water in these situations. Every staff should perform hand hygiene before and after the contact with patients, immediately after contact with objects in the patient environment and after glove removal (◘ Fig. 8.1). To achieve effective decontamination of hands, HCWs must not wear wrist or hand jewellery, should wear short-sleeved clothes 'bare below the elbows', have short, clean fingernails, free from nail polish or false nails, and cover cuts and abrasions with a waterproof dressing.

8.4.1.2 Personal Protective Equipment (PPE)

Personal protective equipment (PPE) is worn by a person to protect themselves from exposure to or contact with infectious or harmful agents that pose risks to their health and safety [10, 19, 20]. It is used based on the assessment of the risk of transmission of micro-organisms to the patient or healthcare worker (HCW), and

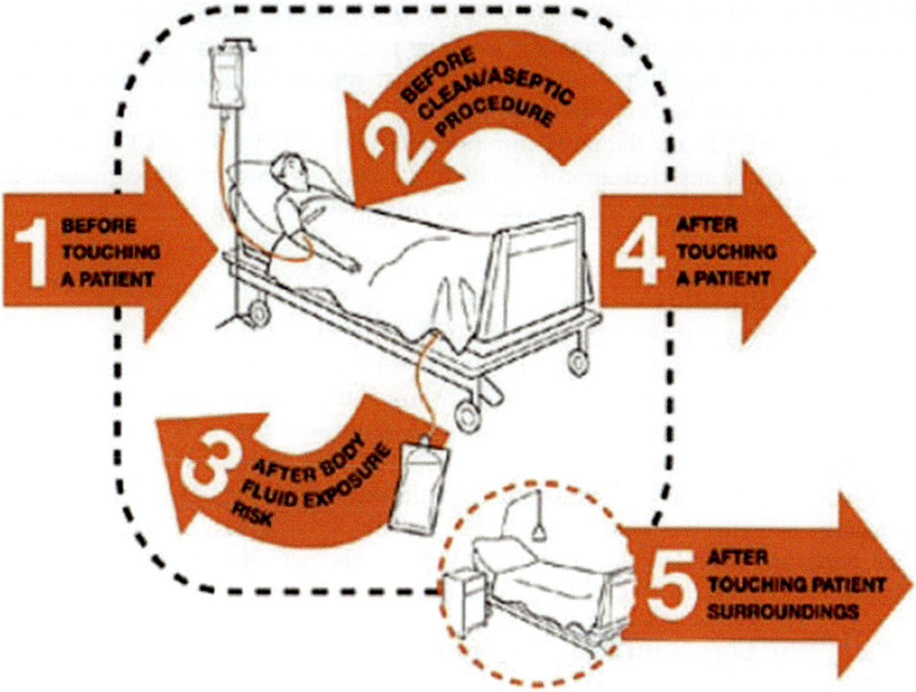

Fig 8.1 World Health Organisation's five moments for hand hygiene

the risk of contamination of the HCW's skin and clothes by patients' blood or body fluids, and the procedure being undertaken. HCWs should be educated and their competency assessed in the selection and the use of PPE. The PPE required to prevent HCAIs is listed below and must be worn as outlined.

- **Gloves** must be worn for contact with non-intact skin or mucous membranes, blood and other body fluids, sterile sites, invasive procedures, handling sharps or contaminated equipment.
- **Disposable plastic aprons** must be worn for close contact with a patient, equipment or surroundings, where there is a risk that clothes may become contaminated with microorganisms, blood or body fluids.
- **Full-body fluid-repellent gowns** must be worn when there is a risk of extensive splashing of blood or body fluids onto the skin or clothes of HCWs, including aerosol-generating procedures, e.g. SARS-CoV-2.
- **Eye or face protection (goggles or full-face visor)** must be worn when there is a risk of blood, body fluids, secretions or excretions splashing onto the face or eyes, including during aerosol-generating procedures.
- **Fluid-repellent surgical face masks (FRSMs)** must be worn when there is a risk of blood, body fluids, secretions or excretions splashing onto the nose and mouth. They protect against infectious droplets (spread via infectious particles >5 um or droplets).
- **FFP3 or N95 or respirator hoods** must be worn during aerosol-generating procedures in airborne infections (spread via infectious particles ≤5 um or droplet nuclei).

8.4.1.3 Prevention of Invasive Device-Associated Infections

Device-associated infections remain a major issue in paediatric patients' health, safety and outcomes [19]. Ventilator-associated pneumonia (VAP), central line-associated bloodstream infections (CLABSI) and catheter-associated urinary tract infections (CAUTI) are the most common HCAIs in PICU patients. All invasive devices should be inserted appropriately, monitored for need and discontinued as soon as possible to help in the prevention of infections.

8.4.2 Care Bundles

Increasing evidence suggests that care bundles are beneficial as part of a comprehensive improvement programme in the ICU. Adult and paediatric literature agree that care bundles are valuable tools in significantly reducing certain HCAIs [21, 22]. A care bundle is defined as a group of evidence-based interventions related to a specific condition, which when applied together significantly improves patient outcomes. In paediatric patients, the focus is usually on care bundles against VAP and CLABSIs. The paediatric care bundles have recently been updated and published by Safer Healthcare [21, 22].

8.4.2.1 VAP Care Bundle in Children

VAP is one of the most frequent HAIs in mechanically ventilated children.

- Systematic reviews have determined that ventilator bundles impact positively on the incidence of VAP in critically ill neonates and children in the PICU and neonatal intensive care unit [23–25]. The VAP bundle is aimed at avoiding the risk of aspiration in the lungs, colonisation of the respiratory tract with pathogenic microorganisms and contamination of respiratory equipment. Similarly, tracheostomised children are at increased risk of VA respiratory infections, but preventive measures have a greater impact on them.
- De Neef et al. conducted a meta-analysis study reviewing the literature on the effectiveness of ventilator care bundles in critically ill children. Eleven studies were included. Inclusion criteria were: (1) implementation of a ventilator care bundle in PICU settings; (2) quality improvement or multi-component approach with the (primary) objective of lowering the VAP rate; and (3) making a comparison, for example, with or without ventilator care bundle, using an experimental randomised or non-randomised study design or an interrupted-times series [24]. The median VAP incidence decreased from 9.8 (interquartile range, 5.8–18.5) per 1000 ventilator days to 4.6 (interquartile range, 1.2–8.6) per 1000 ventilator days after the implementation of a ventilator care bundle. The meta-analysis showed that the implementation of a ventilator care bundle resulted in significantly reduced VAP incidences (incidence risk ratio = 0.45; 95% CI, 0.33–0.60; $p < 0.0001$; $I = 55\%$).
- A VAP care bundle should include these elements:
  - Assess readiness to extubate daily using spontaneous breathing trials
  - Elevate the head of bed to 30–45° in infants and older, 15–30° for neonates, if no positioning limitations
  - Meticulous hand hygiene before and after any contact with ventilator circuits

  - Maintain tubing in a dependent position, drain water in vent circuits away from the patient at least every 2–4 h and prior to repositioning
  - Minimise circuit disruption. Only change circuits and in-line suctioning systems when visibly soiled or malfunctioning
  - Eliminate the routine use of saline instillation before suctioning of the endotracheal tube
  - Oral hygiene minimum every 12 h
  - Peptic ulcer prophylaxis is not recommended in children

8.4.2.2 Central Line Care Bundle (Insertion and Care and Maintenance)

CLABSIs result in approximately 28,000 deaths and approximately $2.3 billion in added costs to the U.S. healthcare system each year. Like the VAP bundle, the central line care bundle is used to reduce CLABSIs. The impact of central venous access device (CVAD) bundles has been studied extensively in children's hospitals and has demonstrated reductions in CLABSIs in PICU [26, 27].

- A Central Venous Line Insertion bundle should include the following elements:
  - Hand hygiene before and after palpating/assessing insertion sites, and before and after inserting an intravascular device
  - Skin antisepsis with >0.5% chlorhexidine preparation with alcohol for 30 s–2 min
  - Maximal sterile barrier precautions, i.e. cap, mask, sterile gown, sterile gloves and sterile full-body drape
  - Selection of the best site to minimise infections and mechanical complications, avoiding the femoral vein in adults
  - Chlorhexidene-impregnated sponge and suture-free securement device, if possible
  - Sterile semi-permeable dressing
- Central line care and maintenance bundle should incorporate the following elements:
  - Hand hygiene before and after any line manipulation or use
  - Clean the catheter hub, needle-free connector and injection port with chlorhexidine with alcohol for at least 15 s before accessing catheters
  - Review dressing daily to ensure clean, dry and intact; replace if damp, loose or soiled, or every 7 days
  - Change crystalloid tubing sets every 72 h, blood product and lipid infusion tubing sets every 24 h
  - Daily discussion of necessity and removal of unnecessary lines
  - Daily 2% chlorhexidine wipes for all children >2 months of age and daily bed linen change recommended
- Use of these bundles can reduce the infection rate to zero.
- Preventive measures for CLABSIs include the discontinuation of parenteral nutrition with early institution of enteral feeding, limitation of open catheter circuits, careful preparation of intravenous fluids and limiting blood products.
- Antiseptic such as chlorhexidine gluconate (CHG) baths have shown reduction in CLABSIs, multidrug-resistant organism colonisation and surgical site infections [28, 29]. Use of antiseptic-impregnated catheters, e.g. silver sulphadiazine-

impregnated catheters and cuffs, heparin-bonded catheters, antibiotic-coated (e.g. rifampin-minocycline) catheters and use of chlorhexidine sponges for cutaneous antisepsis haa also been shown to reduce CLABSIs [30].

8.5 Aseptic Technique

8

Good aseptic technique procedures help prevent and control HCAIs. The aseptic technique is a key component of the National Safety and Quality Health Service (NSQHS) Standards which are intended to prevent or minimise the risk of introducing harmful infectious agents into sterile areas of the body when undertaking clinical procedures. The principles of the aseptic technique remain the same for all procedures, the level of practice will change depending upon a standard risk assessment. Rowley et al. introduced the aseptic technique 'ANTT (aseptic non-touch technique)' which aims to prevent the contamination of wounds or other susceptible sites by removing variation in practice. It provides a comprehensive set of principles including ANTT, which can be applied for several invasive procedures, including insertion of urinary catheters and peripheral cannulas, phlebotomy and the administration of intravenous drugs [31].

8.6 Aseptic Non-Touch Technique (ANTT)

ANTT refers to the technique and infection prevention actions used during invasive clinical procedures to protect the patient from infection by preventing the transfer of microorganisms from the healthcare worker, equipment or the environment to the patient [31]. This is achieved by ensuring the asepsis of key parts and key sites at all times during all procedures, including during the handling of indwelling medical devices. It is one of the most important and commonly performed infection prevention procedures in healthcare.

- Key parts are the critical parts of procedure equipment or medical devices that come into direct or indirect contact with any key sites. This includes any part of the equipment that will be in direct or indirect contact with the infusion fluid in intravenous lines.
- Key sites are the areas of skin penetration and include open wounds, surgical sites and insertion/exit sites of indwelling catheters or drains.
- Key parts and key sites are portals of entry for bacteria. ANTT involves the basic precautions of hand hygiene, PPE use, effective skin disinfection, use of sterilised equipment, an aseptic field and a non-touch handling technique to protect these key parts and sites.
- The term 'aseptic' means an absence of pathogenic microorganisms in sufficient numbers to cause infection. This is achievable in the typical healthcare setting. The term 'sterile' means the absence of all microorganisms. This is not achievable in typical healthcare settings due to microorganisms in the air.
- An aseptic field is used to ensure that all equipment is maintained in an aseptic state during a procedure by protection from the environment. Depending on the procedure, this can be a sterile drape to hold and protect all sterile equipment, or

a decontaminated disinfected surface/procedure tray/dressing trolley with key parts inside a recently opened sterile packaging.

- Non-touch indicates that critical parts of equipment and vulnerable parts of the patient are not directly touched, where practically possible, in both standard and surgical ANTT.
- There are two types of ANTT:
  - Standard ANTT: is used for procedures that are technically less complicated, short in duration <20 min, and involve small key sites and key parts. Peripheral venous catheter insertion can be performed using this technique, wearing non-sterile gloves if the access site is not touched following skin antisepsis.
  - Surgical ANTT: is used when procedures are technically complex and last for >20 min, and involves large open key sites and large key parts. This is the technique to be used for central venous catheter insertion, which requires maximal sterile barrier precautions. All equipment is handled as key parts in surgical ANTT.
- The aseptic technique represents the last line of defence for patients from micro-organisms during invasive clinical procedures. A safe aseptic technique relies on effective staff training, safe environments and equipment that is fit-for-purpose.
- The Health and Social Care Act 2008 requires healthcare providers to have a standardised aseptic technique in which education and compliance audit can be demonstrated. The Aseptic Non-touch Technique (ANTT) is the standard aseptic technique in the UK, adopted by most NHS organisations. As a result, it has helped in the significant reduction of HCAIs [31].

8.7 Environment Build, Materials and Equipment for IPC in PICU

The environment can have several concerns for IPC. The most relevant are those that deal with some features of the building design and cleaning conditions. A well-designed ICU with adequate bed space, isolation rooms, hand hygiene stations, ventilation and filtration systems, waste disposal and equipment storage can help lower the spread of infections [32–36]. The guidance on the design of critical care units in terms of infection control should have the following requirements.

- The total ICU area of a unit should be 2.5–3 times the patient care area, which would allow for adequate service areas and circulation space. It should have appropriate air change rates, ventilation systems and air conditioning, with controls for temperature and humidity.
- The unit design should provide appropriate movement pathways for contaminated equipment and access to the utility room for waste disposal and cleaning appliances.
- Each patient bed space in an open-plan area should be at least 20 m^2, with at least one wash basin with elbow-operated taps for every 1–2 bed spaces. Unobstructed circulation at each bed space is mandatory to maintain separation for infection control reasons, to provide adequate space for equipment and furniture and space for up to five members of staff to attend to the patient in emergencies. The working area must be adequate for staff to work in comfort while maintaining visual

contact with the patient, and have space for monitoring, equipment and medical storage.

- An P ICU should have adequate single rooms for the isolation of infectious patients and protection of immunocompromised patients. The recommendation is that at least 20% of beds in an ICU should be single rooms, increasing up to 50% in units that routinely admit immunocompromised patients, e.g. neutropenic haematology patients.
- An isolation facility is aimed to control airflow in the room so that the number of airborne infectious particles is reduced to a level so that cross-infection is avoided [36]. This can be achieved by controlling the quality and quantity of intake or exhaust air, by maintaining different air pressure between adjacent areas, designing airflow patterns for specific clinical procedures and diluting infectious particles with large air volume and air filtration using HEPA filters.
- Isolation facilities can be of different types: (1) neutral or standard room air pressure, (2) positive room air pressure and (3) negative room air pressure with anteroom.
- All isolation rooms should have sealed ceilings and windows, self-closing doors with tight-fitting seals, its own wash basin and en-suite facilities.
- **Standard isolation rooms:** Ventilated single rooms with en-suite facilities can be used as standard isolation rooms for contact precautions.
- **Positive pressure rooms** allow positive airflow from the room to the adjacent area, and are used to isolate immunocompromised patients and transplant patients. The ideal pressure differential recommended is >+2.5 Pa (ideal >+8 Pa) for the outward flow of air from the room to the adjacent areas. The room should have high-efficiency particulate air (HEPA) filters capable of removing 99.97% of particles ≥0.3 um in diameter for incoming air, ≥12 air changes per hour with extract ventilation, with the en-suite at negative pressure to the room. The ante-room should have a positive pressure of 8–12 pascals with respect to the corridor.
- **Negative pressure isolation rooms** prevent the escape of contaminated air from the room to the surrounding areas, and are required for the isolation of patients with airborne infections, e.g. haemorrhagic fever. These isolation rooms should have ≥6–10 for existing ICU (≥12 for new construction as of 2001) air changes per hour, and an air extract, preferably to the outside. A pressure differential >−2.5 Pa is sufficient to indicate a definite inward flow of air from the adjacent areas into the room. Negative pressure rooms should be located at the entry to the ward so that patients requiring isolation do not need to pass other patient areas to access the room.
- **An anteroom** should be a minimum 25 m^2 with a 3–5 m^2. The anteroom functions as an airlock and should have a wash basin, PPE storage and waste disposal. It requires a high supply and extract air change rate (≥10 air changes per hour) to avoid the spread of airborne organisms from the isolation room and adjacent spaces. Isolation rooms without an ante-room should have a minimum pressure differential of 15 pascals with the adjoining area.

- **Isolation policy in PICU:** The risk of transmission can be minimised by using patient isolation and cohorting procedures, as has been demonstrated in many studies [36–38]. Although isolation and cohorting strategies are beneficial, they cannot be implemented in all cases, especially in open-plan PICUs. The universal use of contact precautions potentially prevents the horizontal transmission of pathogens in a high disease severity and high colonisation with multidrug-resistant organisms (MDROs) in ICUs [37, 38]. Continued increase in the incidence of HCAIs caused by MDROs and new respiratory pathogens, e.g. SARS-CoV has created a need for more specific recommendations for surveillance and transmission-based infection control precautions.

Case Study: IPC for SARS CoV-2 in PICU

SARS-CoV-2 is primarily transmitted between people through respiratory (droplet and aerosol) and contact routes. In addition to respiratory secretions, SARS-CoV-2 has been detected in blood, faeces and urine. Transmission risk is the highest when people are in close proximity (within 2 m). Airborne transmission can occur in healthcare settings where procedures or support treatments that generate aerosols are performed in poorly ventilated indoor spaces. Public Health England (PHE) Coronavirus (COVID-19) guidance [20]:

Patients **Known/Suspected COVID or contact**	**Patients** **Low risk or test results unavailable** **Used as transitional area pending viral testing results**	**Patients** **Low risk/test results available**
• +ve COVID-19 test result • Known close contact of positive COVID-19 patients • Unexpected fever >37.8 °C • Loss of senses of taste or smell • Respiratory symptoms	• COVID-19 test result unavailable • No close contact with known or suspected cases • No unexplained fever >37.8 °C • No changes in senses of taste or smell • No respiratory symptoms	• COVID-19 test result negative. • No close contact with known or suspected cases. • No unexplained fever >37.8 °C or respiratory symptoms • No changes in senses of taste or smell.

- All patients admitted to PICU should be screened for SARS CoV-2 via combined throat and nasal swab on admission and weekly. An endotracheal aspirate should be tested if the patient is intubated.
- Public Health England recommends risk-based patient cohorting in pandemic situations, which can be split into red (known/suspected COVID or contact), amber (low risk/test results unavailable) and green (low risk/test results available) areas depending on a formal clinical risk assessment. Patients can then be moved between red, amber or green areas as risk assessment and viral testing results develop
- The other sources of (potential) infection include any equipment or items in the care environment that could have become contaminated. Enhanced IPC precautions are therefore important for both suspected and confirmed cases. All SIPC

(continued)

measures are necessary to reduce the risk of transmitting infectious agents from both recognised and unrecognised sources of infection across all COVID-19 pathways. Enhanced IPC measures include patient placement and assessment for infection risk—screening for COVID 19, hand hygiene, respiratory and cough hygiene, routine wearing of airborne PPE, including surgical mask and visor, safe management of the care environment, equipment and healthcare linen, blood and body fluids, safe disposal of waste (including sharps), occupational safety: prevention and exposure management, and maintaining social/physical distancing. This negates the requirement for the routine wearing of airborne PPE including a respirator in the low risk COVID-19 pathway.

8.8 Cleaning Standards

ICUs should implement standard cleaning and disinfection protocols to control environmental contamination with multidrug resistant organisms (MDRO), e.g. methicillin-resistant *Staphylococcus aureus* (MRSA) or vancomycin-resistant *Enterococcus* (VRE), and respiratory or enteric viruses. Cleaning is a pre-requisite to effective disinfection, it means the removal of organic matter including dirt, debris, blood and bodily fluids with detergent. Disinfection is the process of eliminating or reducing harmful micro-organisms from inanimate objects and surfaces. Whereas sterilisation is the process of killing all micro-organisms through physical or chemical means. Cleaning, disinfection and sterilisation are all decontamination processes.

- More frequent cleaning of high-touch areas (e.g. bed rails, bedside carts/trolleys, doorknobs, light switches, faucet handles, patient call-bells, phones, computer equipment, communication devices, patient commodes and communal toilets), at least twice daily, is recommended during outbreaks.
- Disposable patient-care items (e.g. blood pressure cuffs) should be used where possible, to minimise the risk of cross-infection. Policies and procedures for cleaning and disinfection of reusable non-invasive devices as per the manufacturer's recommendations should be adhered to.
- Policies and procedures should also cover appropriate cleaning and decontamination of blood and body fluid spills and be readily available to staff.
- An infection-control risk assessment must be conducted before any construction, renovation or repairs in a healthcare area to identify and minimise the risks from dust or water aerosols generated by these activities. Environmental opportunistic (e.g. *Aspergillus* spp.) pathogens can lead to significant infections. Dust and moisture-control measures and physical barriers along with the presence of negative airflow within these areas during the works are required.
- Needles and sharps should be handled with care. Safer needle disposal units that are impermeable and puncture proof should be available next to areas used for injections and venipuncture.

Antimicrobial Stewardship

- Judicious use of antimicrobials is now seen as an essential component of preventing HCAIs and the emergence of multidrug-resistant organisms especially in PICUs [39].
- Clear guidelines for antimicrobial use should be available, which are also based on local resistance patterns.
- Antimicrobials should be prescribed and supported with clear evidence for infection, rationalised on organism identification and stopped on completion of a clearly defined treatment period.

Preventable Disease

- It is recommended that all staff working in ICUs and healthcare settings should be fully immunised against vaccine-preventable disease.
- Annual influenza immunisation should be strongly advised for staff working with vulnerable patient groups.
- Other vaccine-preventable infections including chickenpox, hepatitis B, measles, mumps, rubella, pertussis and COVID-19 vaccine should be given.

Education and Audits

- All IPC practices should be effectively translated to the bedside. For this, it requires a robust safety culture, the incorporation of high-reliability principles, and patient and family engagement [40].
- IPC training and education must be applied consistently by all healthcare workers (HCWs) taking care of patients, and must be embedded into routine daily clinical practice. Adherence to IPC must be monitored and regular feedback provided, along with surveillance of infections.

Take-Home Messages

- The IPC strategies may only be effective over prolonged periods if they can be integrated into the behaviour of all staff members who are involved in patient care.
- All IPC measures should be viewed as a priority and have to be integrated fully into the continuous process of improvement of the quality of care.
- The written policies and procedures concerning IPC should be developed in collaboration with IPC teams, infectious diseases or microbiology consultants. These should be available to all staff and reviewed at least every 2 years.
- An educational programme should be implemented to train all staff in IPC policies.
- Standard ICP should be performed in every interaction with a patient.
- Patients with potentially contagious diseases should be promptly isolated.
- Hand hygiene is the most important means of preventing HCAI. Compliance with hand hygiene should be audited on a regular basis.

(continued)

- PPE, blood-borne pathogens and sharp disposal protocols should be available in all units.
- Protocols and guides should be established for communicating with staff, patients and families in case of infectious disease outbreaks and seasonal increases of infections (influenza and respiratory syncytial viruses).
- In PICU, parents and visitors also should be educated in IPC protocols to help prevent infection in their children.
- Although there is a significant variation between organisations in the contents of various medical device care bundles, the focus should be on avoiding device utilisation unless absolutely necessary, device removal when no longer required and minimising access to the device.
- All IPC should be effectively translated to bedside practice. For that, it should require a robust safety culture, the incorporation of high-reliability principles, and patient and family engagement.

References

1. Northway T, Langley JM, Skippen P. Health care–associated infection in the pediatric intensive care unit. Pediatr Crit Care. 2011;2011:1349–63. https://doi.org/10.1016/B978-0-323-07307-3.10097-7.
2. Abulhasan YB, Rachel SP, Châtillon-Angle MO, et al. Healthcare-associated infections in the neurological intensive care unit: results of a 6-year surveillance study at a major tertiary care center. Am J Infect Control. 2018;46:656–62.
3. Gupta A, Kapil A, Lodha R, et al. Burden of healthcare-associated infections in a paediatric intensive care unit of a developing country: a single centre experience using active surveillance. J Hosp Infect. 2011;78:323–6.
4. Kepenekli E, Soysal A, Yalindag-Ozturk N, et al. Healthcare-associated infections in pediatric intensive care units in Turkey: a national point-prevalence survey. J Infect Dis. 2015;68(5):381–6.
5. Stockwell JA. Nosocomial infections in the pediatric intensive care unit: affecting the impact on safety and outcome. Pediatr Crit Care Med. 2007;8(2):S21–37.
6. Slonim AD, Kurtines HC, Sprague BM, Singh N. The costs associated with nosocomial bloodstream infections in the pediatric intensive care unit. Pediatr Crit Care Med. 2001;2:170–4.
7. Elward AM, Hollenbeak CS, Warren DK, Fraser VJ. Attributable cost of nosocomial primary bloodstream infection in pediatric intensive care unit patients. Pediatrics. 2005;115:868–72.
8. NICE. NICE Quality Standard 61. Infection prevention and control. 2021. Available from: https://www.nice.org.uk/guidance/qs61.
9. Rathore MH, Jackson MA, AAP Committee on Infectious Diseases. Infection prevention and control in pediatric ambulatory settings. Pediatrics. 2017;140(5):e20172857.
10. Loveday HP, Wilson JA, Pratt RJ, et al. UK Department of Health epic3: national evidence-based guidelines for preventing healthcare-associated infections in NHS hospitals in England. J Hosp Infect. 2014;86(Suppl 1):S1–70.
11. Wagh A, Sinha A. Prevention of healthcare-associated infections in paediatric intensive care unit. Childs Nerv Syst. 2018;34:1865–70.
12. Bion J, Richardson A, Hibbert P, et al. Matching Michigan Collaboration & Writing Committee. "Matching Michigan": a 2-year stepped interventional programme to minimise central venous catheter-blood stream infections in intensive care units in England. BMJ Qual Saf. 2013;22:110–23.
13. World Health Organization. Infection prevention and control of epidemic- and pandemic-prone acute respiratory infections in health care. Geneva: World Health Organization; 2014. Available from: https://apps.who.int/iris/bitstream/handle/10665/112656/9789241507134
14. Ocansey S, Abu EK, Abraham CH, et al. Ocular symptoms of SARS-CoV-2: indication of possible ocular transmission or viral shedding. Ocul Immunol Inflamm. 2020;28(8):1269–79.

15. Ong SW, Tan YK, Chia PY, et al. Air, surface environmental, and personal protective equipment contamination by severe acute respiratory syndrome coronavirus 2 (SARS-CoV-2) from a symptomatic patient. JAMA. 2020;323(16):1610–2.
16. Boyce JM, Pittet D. Guideline for hand hygiene in health-care settings: recommendations of the Healthcare Infection Control Practices Advisory Committee and the HICPAC/SHEA/APIC/IDSA Hand Hygiene Task Force. Infect Control Hosp Epidemiol. 2002;23:S3–40.
17. Golin AP, Choi D, Ghahary A. Hand sanitizers: A review of ingredients, mechanisms of action, modes of delivery, and efficacy against coronaviruses. Am J Infect Control. 2020;48(9):1062–7.
18. WHO guidelines on hand hygiene in health care 2009, ISBN: 9789241597906 WHO/IER/PSP/2009/01.
19. Coffin SE, Zaoutis TE. Infection control, hospital epidemiology, and patient safety. Infect Dis Clin N Am. 2005;19:647–65.
20. Public Health England Coronavirus (COVID-19) guidance. Available from: https://www.gov.uk/government/publications/wuhan-novel-coronavirus-infection-prevention-and-control/wuhan-novel-coronavirus-wn-cov-infection-prevention-and-control-guidance.
21. Lachman P, Yuen S. Using care bundles to prevent infection in neonatal and paediatric ICUs. Curr Opin Infect Dis. 2009;22:224–8.
22. Mack EH, Stem CT. Prevention of CAUTIs, CLABSIs, and VAPs in children. Curr Treat Options Peds. 2017;3(3):221–35.
23. Niedzwiecka T, Patton D, Walsh S, et al. What are the effects of care bundles on the incidence of ventilator-associated pneumonia in paediatric and neonatal intensive care units? A systematic review. J Spec Pediatr Nurs. 2019;24:e12264. https://doi.org/10.1111/jspn.12264.
24. de Neef M, Bakker L, Dijkstra S, Raymakers-Janssen P, Vileito A, Ista E. Effectiveness of a ventilator care bundle to prevent ventilator-associated pneumonia at the PICU: a systematic review and meta-analysis. Pediatr Crit Care Med. 2019;20(5):474–80.
25. Muszynski JA, Sartori J, Steele L, et al. Multidisciplinary quality improvement initiative to reduce ventilator-associated tracheobronchitis in the PICU. Pediatr Crit Care Med. 2013;14(5):533–8.
26. Nowak JE, Brilli RJ, Lake MR, et al. Reducing catheter-associated bloodstream infections in the pediatric intensive care unit: business case for quality improvement. Pediatr Crit Care Med. 2010;11(5):579–87.
27. Rosenthal VD, Ramachandran B, Villamil-Gómez W, et al. Impact of a multidimensional infection control strategy on central line-associated bloodstream infection rates in pediatric intensive care units of five developing countries: findings of the International Nosocomial Infection Control Consortium (INICC). Infection. 2012;40:415–23.
28. Musuuza JS, Guru PK, O'Horo JC, et al. The impact of chlorhexidine bathing on hospital-acquired bloodstream infections: a systematic review and meta-analysis. BMC Infect Dis. 2019;19(1):416. https://doi.org/10.1186/s12879-019-4002-7.
29. Donskey CJ, Deshpande A. Effect of chlorhexidine bathing in preventing infections and reducing skin burden and environmental contamination: a review of the literature. Am J Infect Control. 2016;44(Suppl 2):e17–21.
30. Lai NM, Chaiyakunapruk N, Lai NA, O'Riordan E, Pau WSC, Saint S. Catheter impregnation, coating or bonding for reducing central venous catheter-related infections in adults. Cochrane Database Syst Rev. 2013; Available from: http://onlinelibrary.wiley.com/doi/10.1002/14651858.CD007878.pub3/full
31. Rowley S, Clare S. ANTT: a standard approach to aseptic technique. Nurs Times. 2011;107(36):12–4.
32. Zingg W, Holmes A, Dettenkofer M, et al. Hospital organisation, management, and structure for prevention of health-care-associated infection: a systematic review and expert consensus. Lancet Infect Dis. 2015;15:212–24.
33. Eggimann P, Pittet D. Infection control in the ICU. Environment- the environment in PICU is high risk for transmission of organisms because of involvement of variety of healthcare staff and heavy traffic flow. Chest. 2001;120:2059–93.
34. Health Building Note 04-02 Critical Care Units. Guidance on designing critical care units, including bed space requirements and the location of a unit in a hospital. Available from: https://www.england.nhs.uk/publication/critical-care-units-planning-and-design-hbn-04-02/
35. Paediatric Intensive Care Society. Standards for the care of critically ill children. London: Paediatric Intensive Care Society; 2015.

36. Siegel JD, Rhinehart E, Jackson M, Chiarello L. Health Care Infection Control Practices Advisory Committee. Guideline for isolation precautions: preventing transmission of infectious agents in health care settings. Am J Infect Control. 2007;35(10 Suppl 2):S65–164.
37. CDC. MDRO prevention and control. Management of multidrug-resistant organisms in health-care settings. 2006 [cited 2018 Oct]. Available from: http://www.cdc.gov/infectioncontrol/guidelines/mdro/prevention-control.html.
38. Iordanou S, Palazis L, Timiliotou-Matsentidou C, Mendris M, Raftopoulos V. When multidrug-resistant organism (MDRO)-positive ICU patient isolation and cohorting is not feasible, what comes next? Cureus. 2021;13(3):e13636.
39. Department of Health, Advisory Committee on Antimicrobial Resistance and Healthcare Associated Infection. Antimicrobial prescribing and stewardship competencies. Start smart - then focus antimicrobial stewardship toolkit for English hospitals [updated 2015 Mar]. Available from: https://assets.publishing.service.gov.uk/government/uploads/system/uploads/attachment_data/file/417032/Start Smart Then Focus.
40. Ibrahim AM, Al-Rafay SS, Tantawi HR. Application of care bundle approach for preventing device associated infections: a training program for pediatric and neonatal nurses. Medico-legal Update. January–March 2021;21(1):744–1751.

Information Technology in PICU

Samiran Ray and Padmanabhan Ramnarayan

Contents

J. Brierley et al. (eds.), *ESPNIC Children's Intensive Care Textbook*,
https://doi.org/10.1007/978-3-031-64762-8_9

Learning Objectives

- Understand the various uses of information technology in paediatric intensive care
- Gain an appreciation of the potential benefits but also the pitfalls of electronic systems
- An introduction to the potential of machine learning techniques in paediatric intensive care
- Understanding of the human–computer interface in systems design

9.1 Introduction

Intensive care units (ICUs) are data-rich environments, and intensive care involves highly complex decision-making in the face of rapidly changing patient conditions. These challenges are particularly accentuated in paediatric intensive care units (PICUs), where vast amounts of data have to be interpreted by clinicians in children with a wide range of ages, weights, diagnoses, underlying co-morbidities and physiological characteristics. In the PICU, data are collected from a multitude of sources: clinical documentation (ward rounds, admission and discharge notes, and procedure notes), investigations (point-of-care tests, laboratory and electrophysiological investigations, and imaging), medical devices (monitors, ventilators and infusion pumps), medication details (sedation, antibiotics and vasoactive agents) as well as structured data at patient-level (age, weight and diagnosis) and unit-level (staffing levels, risk prediction scores and quality indicators). Data are generated at different frequencies—for example, vital signs are monitored continuously, with waveform data containing information at resolutions of <1 s. In contrast, ward rounds may take place 2–3 times a day, and imaging only once or twice during the patient stay.

The large amounts of data generated raise several potential questions relating to its use for clinical decision-making: how much of the generated data can be processed and how to filter out noise; what is the most user-friendly way to present the data for patient care; how data systems improve safety and may also increase risk; and whether electronic systems can provide us with novel and better understanding of our patients. The adoption of information technology (IT) solutions to acquire, store and analyse data, influence patient care, and to learn and disseminate knowledge is a key priority in intensive care, including in the PICU setting. In this chapter, we will discuss how IT systems are used in paediatric intensive care, focusing on electronic health records, incorporation of computerised prescriber order entry (CPOE) systems, clinical decision support systems (CDSS) and telemedicine, and the future potential of machine learning and artificial intelligence (AI) systems to augment clinical care by harnessing data that are traditionally 'lost' during decision-making.

9.2 Electronic Health Records

Although intensive care units have been at the forefront of the IT revolution in healthcare for many decades, more recently, the proliferation of electronic health systems was driven in the United States following the 2009 Health Information Technology for Economic and Clinical Health (HITECH) Act, which aimed to improve quality, safety and efficiency in healthcare through the use of electronic health records (EHRs) and associated tools [1]. Similar initiatives to promote AHR adoption have been announced in the European Union and the United Kingdom. Many PICUs have implemented EHRs—either as part of a hospital-wide solution or a stand-alone system used in the PICU only [2].

9.2.1 Clinical Documentation

One of the main functions of an EHR in the PICU is clinical documentation. Clinical documentation serves the purpose of recording healthcare encounters, procedures and significant events. During the PICU admission, the patient encounter is a continuous process within which data are generated, accessed and evaluated continuously. The bulk of medical documentation is usually based around fixed time points—admission and discharge, ward rounds, recognised deterioration, procedures such as intubation or extubation and conversations with families. Nursing documentation may be more sporadic and focused on shift handovers, while the multidisciplinary team (physiotherapists, dieticians and pharmacists) documentation is usually linked to regular visits. Clinical documentation serves the purpose of communicating information to the wider team and also to signal the rationale behind decision-making informed by a synthesis of the available data.

Clinical documentation benefits from being standardised to build an accurate representation of a patient's state. Standardisation allows data to be organised logically and improves the consistency of recorded information. Standardised documentation lends itself well to formatted note templates in EHRs. Aids to help with this include drop-down menus, smart text (shortcuts to auto-fill commonly typed words or phrases) and shared documentation (allowing data such as problem lists to be shared between several data templates). Drop-down menus validate documentation fields. For example, when documenting in a procedure note, a drop-down menu can limit the choice for central venous line insertion to 'femoral vein' rather than possible alternatives such as 'groin'. By limiting free text, it can reduce spelling and typing errors. All of this serves to allow the logical organisation of data items in separate cells or fields. Therefore, when searching for all femoral central venous lines inserted, EHRs can easily collate data using site fields populated by the same term. In contrast, free text documents would rely on search functions which could be hampered by spelling and typing errors or a variation of terms used. Non-electronic notes are unable to offer this benefit (even with the most sophisticated optical character recognition systems!) (◘ Fig. 9.1).

Shared documentation such as problem lists both improves efficiency and safety. Data can be lost with written or free text notes over time because of the effort of replicating the same list several times a day. This could lead to less-active problems being forgotten or missed, even though they may have implications for long-term treatments and follow-up arrangements. This can be important in children with long stays in PICU and with multiple co-morbidities. Shared problem lists across notes prevent this; at a more basic level, copy-and-paste functions on EHRs may also mitigate data loss. Hospital-wide systems can also help by making data easily accessible before PICU admission, such as procedure notes or medication records from the ward (◘ Table 9.1).

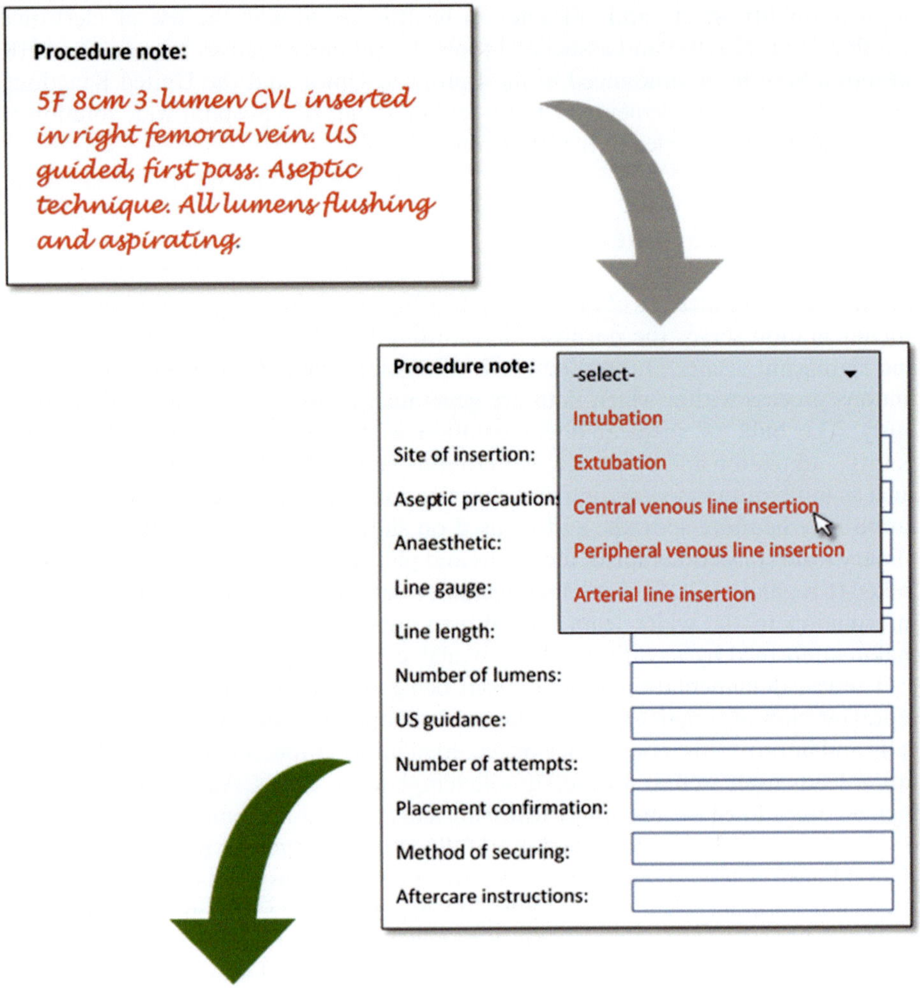

Right femoral vein	Left femoral vein	Right internal jugular vein	Left internal jugular vein	Right subclavian vein	Left subclavian vein	4 French gauge
1	0	0	0	0	0	1
0	0	0	1	0	0	0
0	1	0	0	0	0	0

Fig. 9.1 Organisation of data from documentation. The top panel shows an example of free-text documentation for a central venous line insertion. This could be handwritten or typed into an electronic health record. The text contains several bits of discrete information, e.g. the size of the line, the site of the line insertion, how many lumens present, etc. EHRs in particular enable entering these discrete bits of information separately in a form—the use of an electronic medium allows for tools such as drop-down menus to be used to save time. Forms allow for consistency of information to be entered—for example, the free-text note does not mention anything about the anaesthetic. Data from forms can then automatically populate a database. This allows for information to be collated and processed later—in the future, it will be easy to search for the number of central venous lines inserted in the internal jugular vein for example

Table 9.1 Benefits and risks of structured electronic documentation in the PICU

Benefits	Risks
– Promotes a 'paperless' information system	– May take much longer than free-text documentation
– Improves the logical flow and presentation of information	– Form fatigue among clinicians
– Improves consistency of documentation and validates data entered	– Burnout and stress increased with longer duration spent on electronic medical records
– Assists novice users with the completion of documentation through the structured process	– Risk of reinforcing prior errors (e.g. by copying old problem lists)
– Enables faster documentation through the use of drop-down menus, selection of pre-configured options	– Non-compliance with documentation or poor-quality documentation
– Avoids spelling errors, unwarranted abbreviations	– Inability to search/retrieve information outside structured data elements
– Allows sharing of fragments of information (e.g. problem lists) between users and patients	
– Allows information to be searched for easy retrieval	

Nevertheless, electronic documentation comes with trade-offs [3]. To facilitate the capture of a wide range of options, documentation forms can become cumbersome. This introduces the risk of 'form fatigue' with clinicians opting not to fill in all the fields. Some fields could be made mandatory to fill in but this can lead to clinician dissatisfaction and further non-compliance. Clinical burnout related to cumbersome data entry into EHRs is an important current area of debate in the United States [4]. The act of writing or typing also involves the processing of information in human working memory. Auto-population of fields or shared problem lists may not be verified regularly, and important problems may still be left unconsidered, resulting in errors. Medico-legally, the documentation of shared documentation assumes verification unless explicit processes are in place to indicate verification. This can be mitigated by including tools such as checkboxes to indicate verification or electronic sign-off. This can further add to documentation time and may paradoxically reduce efficiency. A comparison of clinician documentation times with and without EHRs suggests an increase in documentation time with electronic documentation (albeit most studies were outside the ICU setting). There is insufficient evidence to know whether the extra time spent improves communication and patient safety or reduces time spent on more essential patient care tasks [5].

9.2.2 Electronic Charting

One of the hallmarks of ICUs is the continuous multi-parameter monitoring of patients. At the most basic level, this includes vital sign monitoring at the bedside such as heart rate, oxygen saturations, blood pressure and respiratory rate, which are displayed as waveforms and summarised by numbers. Traditionally, these summary numerics have been transcribed at discrete time points to summarise vital signs' trends in the patient, reflecting their recovery. This is usually done manually by the bedside nurse on paper charts that allow trends to be easily visible.

ICU charting systems were developed in the early 2000s. These provide several benefits, most immediately the ability to visualise the entire patient's stay continuously. Paper charts do not allow this as there is a continuity problem at the end of each shift or each 24-h period. Changes that happen around the times the paper charts are changed may not be recognised. Some trends may develop slowly—for example, a heart rate gradually rising over 24–48 h may not be recognised using paper charts that change every 12 h. Electronic charts can also provide an option of representing the numerical data graphically or as figures. Graphs may also be optimised, for example, by changing the time resolution so that short- and long-term trends may be seen, without being distracted by short-term variation (◘ Fig. 9.2). Hospital-wide systems may extend the continuum of charting—a child's vital signs can be seen before they arrive on PICU.

Charting with paper systems requires a bedside nurse to transcribe a number from a screen onto paper. This is labour intensive—for each hour, the bedside nurse may have to chart 20–25 data items. With the cognitive load of having to also provide other aspects besides nursing care, the risk of charting errors is high. Electronic charting can allow for automated charting, either through wired (e.g. local area networks) or wireless connections between the bedside monitor and the charting computer terminals. This can save nursing time. However, charting is not only for posterity—it ensures a person has seen and hopefully processed observations. Automated charting can lead to trends and abnormal values being missed. A compromise solution may be automated charting which still needs human verification as a safety net.

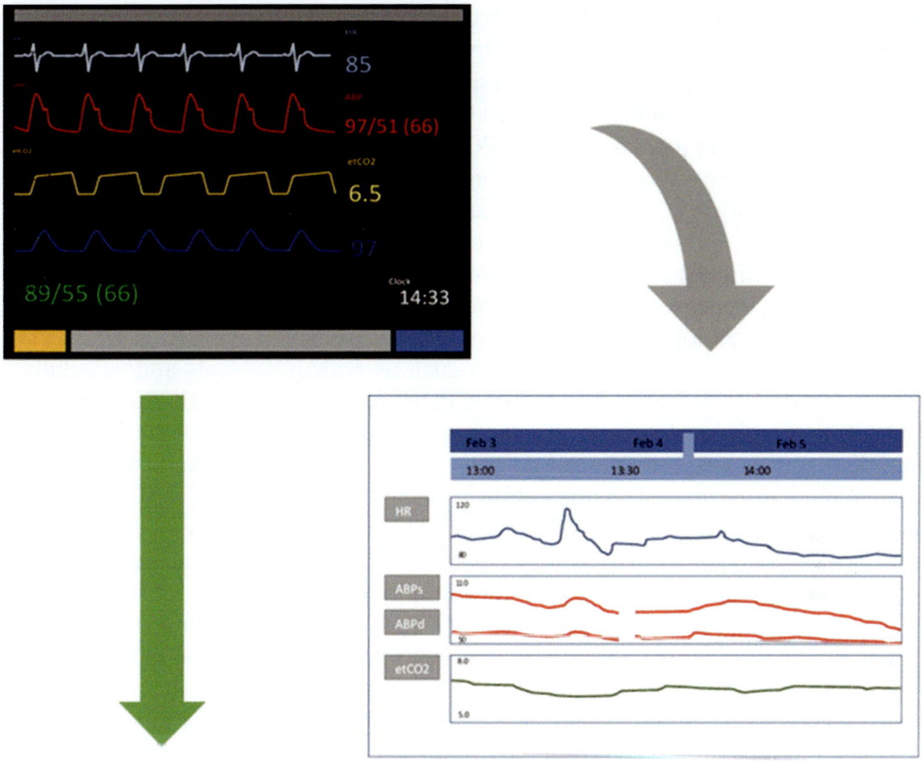

Flowsheet	04/04/2020 12:00	04/04/2020 13:00	04/04/2020 14:00	04/04/2020 15:00	04/04/2020 16:00	04/04/2020 17:00	04/04/2020 18:00
Weight (working)	18	18	18	18	18	18	18
Height (working)							
No of days on ITU	2	2	2	2	2	2	2
Heart rate	110	100	95	90	96	94	97
Heart Rhythm	SR	SR	SR	SR	SR	SR	SR
Art BP	101/53 (69)	100/53 (69)	105/50 (68)	97/47 (64)	97/52 (67)	100/52 (68)	101/52 (68)
NIBP	89/54 (66)		89/55 (66)		81/54 (63)		91/54 (66)
Temp	37.7				36.9		
Respiratory Rate	24	22	22	20	20	22	22
Capillary Refill	<2	<2	<2	<2	<2	<2	<2
Pupils	3: equal	3: equal	3: equal	3: equal	3: equal	3: equal	3: equal

Fig. 9.2 Data organisation in the ICU. Data continuously generated through continuous monitoring (top panel). These data may be observed by clinicians to help with decision-making. The data are typically recorded as hourly 'snapshots' on paper charts or electronic health records (EHR, bottom panel). This may demonstrate trends in data but some features may be missed, for example significant changes in heart rate or desaturation. Recording of higher resolution data (middle panel) may accurately capture this information but too much information may also drown out any signal in the noise of the 'normal' variability of data. An interactive display that allows variation of the time axis may be ideal

9.3 Computerised Physician Order Entry (CPOE) Systems

Medication errors are one of the greatest risks to healthcare delivery, particularly in the ICU environment. In PICU the need for age- or weight-adjusted dosing increases the risk even further [6]. The use of CPOE has been driven by health professionals and the technology industry as a response to this risk. CPOE allows an order (an electronic request) to be entered into a computer system which is immediately transferred to the relevant department or patient bedside and it can be seen by multiple users, thereby allowing the responder to update the status of the order (e.g. item being checked, dispensed and administered) in real-time. CPOE is not limited to prescribing—investigations and imaging requests can also be incorporated within CPOE systems, as well as more logistical tasks such as patient referrals and scheduling. There are several potential benefits of CPOE: handwriting errors are eliminated; delay from the physical transfer of a written order between the ICU and the relevant recipient can be reduced; clinical decision support systems can be used to reduce drug dosage, duplication and interaction errors; drug dosing and administration data can be integrated into the rest of the EHR allowing more accurate documentation; and vice versa information from the EHR can be shared, e.g. the problem list informing the order recipient of the order indications [7, 8].

The most frequently reported benefit of CPOE has been in reducing drug errors. Most studies evaluating CPOE have used before-after comparisons to demonstrate its effect. This limits the interpretation of results which are biased by indication: often CPOE is introduced as part of a larger EHR system meaning the effect of the CPOE cannot be dissociated from the overall introduction of the system. The effect of time and other advancements in treatment may not be considered. Before-after comparisons are also not agnostic to the type of system being used: locally developed systems have the advantage of being tailored to the local working infra-structure but are vulnerable to problems identified by larger commercial systems that have been used more widely. Some studies have also tried to assess the effect on length of stay. While a shorter length of stay is associated with CPOE introduction in some reports, when subject to meta-analysis in ICU studies, this finding has not been translated. There may be a small reduction in ICU mortality associated with CPOE use, although this was not found in PICU studies [9, 10].

The introduction of CPOE can also uncover new problems: for example, drug prescriptions being discontinued after a certain period as default even though not intended as such. Similarly, drug chart visualisation may also be difficult, with drug prescriptions not fitting on a single screen. One study found that over time following CPOE introduction medication errors increased. Subsequent changes to Clinical Decision Systems were able to bring the error rate back down to below baseline levels [11]. This highlights the complexity and evolving interaction between the user-technology interface.

9.4 Clinical Decision Support Systems (CDSS)

Clinical Decision Support Systems are computerised tools that integrate at least one piece of patient data with medical knowledge to provide patient-specific advice. Examples include electronic systems that provide a risk score for venous thromboembolism based on the patient's age and diagnosis, or an alert that warns clinicians not to prescribe amoxicillin to someone with documented penicillin allergy. CDSS are invaluable in an era where medical knowledge has exploded and guidelines have proliferated. Adherence to guidelines ensures standardisation of care based on best quality evidence. However, this has had unintended consequences: the sheer number of guidelines available, often from multiple bodies with conflicting information, poor accessibility and problems with version control can make adhering to guidelines difficult [12]. CDSS offer the potential to deliver guideline knowledge at the point of clinical care (◘ Table 9.2).

CDSS can be integrated within EHRs and CPOEs to provide prompts to clinicians when carrying out clinical tasks. This can reduce task load and reduce cognitive bias. For example, electronic prescribing systems can prompt a prescriber to monitor drug levels at the time of prescription. In some cases, this may be in the future: better clinical decision support may be to prompt a bedside nurse to check the drug level prior to administering the dose. CDSS can draw information from other parts of the EHR: for example, for a patient on digoxin a CDSS can cross check the potassium level before drug prescription or administration.

CDSS can also link EHR problem lists to available current guidelines, nudging the clinician towards providing standardised evidence-based care. More complex systems can aid diagnostic decisions: systems such as ISABEL have been demonstrated to consider a clinically important diagnosis in 1 in 8 cases and request an extra investigation in 1 in 10 cases in emergency care [13]. Computerised CDSS in theory improves access to information, makes decision making more standardised and pro-

◘ Table 9.2 Types of clinical decision support systems and their function in the PICU

Type	Role	Examples
Diagnostic CDSS	To provide differential diagnosis or diagnostic suggestions based on clinical features, either entered manually or drawn automatically from the EHR. See ◘ Fig. 9.3	Commercial systems such as Isabel [13], Visual Dx [14]
Prescribing alerts	To provide alerts to clinicians when prescribing medications, either based on drug–drug interaction, allergy alerts, dose-range checking or drug–disease interaction	Usually embedded as part of CPOE systems
Clinical management	To guide clinicians during patient management	Antibiotic stewardship [15] Ventilator weaning [16] Venous thromboembolism risk [17] Blood glucose control [18]

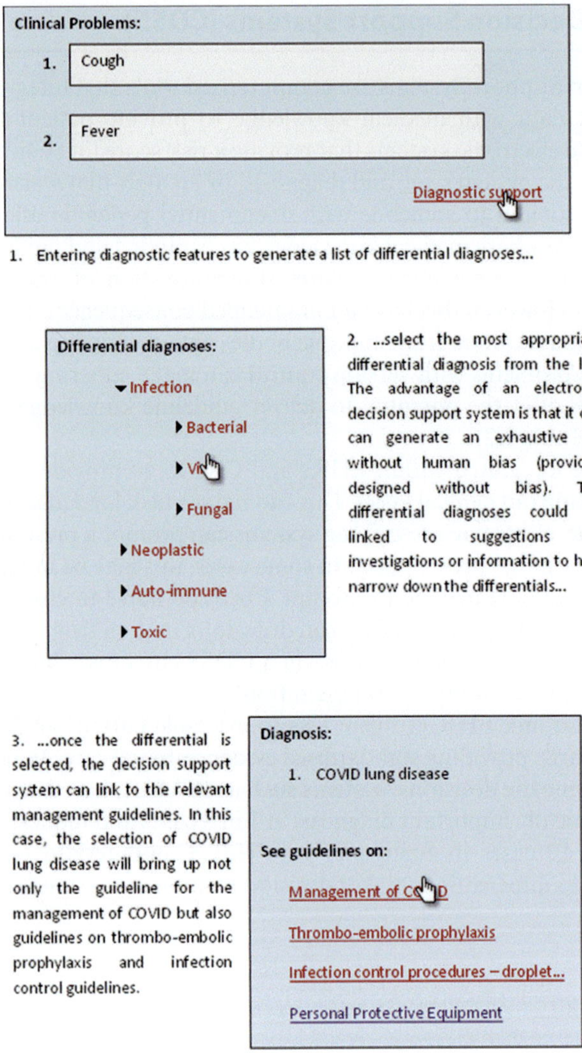

Fig. 9.3 An example of a Clinical Decision Support System. In this example, clinical symptoms can be entered to generate an exhaustive list of differential diagnoses, from which the likeliest differential can be selected. A more sophisticated system may be able to present an interactive decision tree, narrowing down the likelier differentials by asking for more specific information. Once a diagnosis is selected as the likeliest, the system can automatically link to relevant guidelines to help the user tailor management. Such systems safeguard against inconsistencies in diagnosis thereby providing a safety net against cognitive biases. However, the system will only perform as well as it is designed—success or failure of the system will still rely on human input—the computer provides a memory bank

vides an important safety net. All of these are relevant to environments such as the ICU where large volumes of data need to be assimilated to deliver patient care. Nevertheless, such systems have not gained popularity. An extensive evaluation of the literature about CDSS shows that an average absolute improvement was evident in only 5.8% (95% confidence intervals of 4.0–7.6%) of patients receiving the desired process of care. Paediatric studies report a slightly greater effect with CDSS, possibly reflecting the complexity around decision-making due to age and weight differences, rare diagnoses and lack of specialisation [19]. Overall, factors such as human–computer interface problems, 'medical alert' fatigue and the deployment of a CDSS inappropriately to a problem that may require a different solution may explain the smaller than desired effect of CDSS on clinical care.

9.5 Automated Alerting Systems and Early Warning Scores

All hospital inpatients have the potential to have unexpected deterioration during their hospital stay. In the vast majority, these can be detected retrospectively through monitored vital signs. This forms the basis of early warning scores (EWS)—to combine multiple physiological markers, detect abnormal values consistent with deterioration and alert a clinician to evaluate further or intervene [20].

There are several scoring systems developed for children, which have iteratively been adapted and improved to suit local demands. Most scoring systems in existence use thresholds for individual physiological markers such as heart rate or blood pressure, to categorise into an ordinal scale. A composite score from these ordinal values indicates the action required. Using paper-based systems these scores are calculated when each set of observations are documented. Electronic charting systems can allow EWS to be calculated from charted values. Alerts and alarms can be activated accordingly—for example, through notifications on mobile devices. While most EWS are used to prevent admission to the ICU through early intervention, EWS can still be valuable in the ICU. This may reduce potential cognitive bias by using an objective heuristic: a rising blood pressure in a patient with brain injury for example alerting to potential rising intra-cranial pressure. A possible problem with this may be in the interpretation and the number of false alarms. Electronic charting systems can monitor EWS continuously, providing a continuous representation of the patient state, which may still allow a clinician to detect trends in observations. Such composite scores are particularly useful in the cardiac ICU where multiple channels of data need to be analysed over time to identify deteriorating trends. Some centres have demonstrated these to be able to alert clinicians to impending cardiac arrest in neonates post cardiac bypass [21].

However, while the ability to continuously track the progress of a patient in the ICU and provide an early warning for an impending adverse event seems attractive, the added value does need to be contextualised. Many report a base assessment of a scoring system on retrospective data, a validation of the ability to detect a problem. Few studies, particularly in the ICU where patients are very closely monitored, compare the performance of an EWS against a clinician not equipped with an EWS. When tested, albeit retrospectively, continuous scoring systems of paediatric wards have not improved clinician performance in detecting deterioration [22]. This is consistent with the finding that even paper-based EWS systems do not reduce mortality when tested by a well-designed large-scale randomised controlled trial [23]. This may be due to inadequate sensitivity of the scoring systems—i.e. the score at which action is required may need to be lower, although this comes with a trade-off of too many false alarms.

9.6 Telemedicine

Regionalisation of paediatric intensive care services means that critically ill children presenting to non-specialist centres may not be able to access specialist care and advice early on—telemedicine has been implemented in many critical care settings to address this issue. While early versions of telemedicine solutions offered asynchronous 'store and forward' solutions (e.g. echocardiograms and other imaging), modern telemedicine solutions allow real-time advice to be sought, with full audiovisual capabilities. In addition, electronic documentation may be shared during the telemedicine encounter. The literature relating to the benefits of telemedicine in the PICU setting is still evolving and appears to show improved clinical satisfaction during remote assessment (versus standard telephone assessment), improved clinical assessment, and in some studies, improvements in process measures such as adherence to guidelines [24, 25].

9.7 Machine Learning, Big Data and Artificial Intelligence

ICUs are data-rich environments. It is beyond the human working memory to assimilate and process several channels of numerical data, analyse trends over different time intervals and detect signals among the noise introduced by artefacts, inter- and intra-individual variability. The volume of data involved are too large: data for each patient can require hundreds of megabytes of computer memory.

Machine learning involves the use of powerful computing and statistical techniques to learn from large data sets. While often presented as a 'black box', the essence of machine learning is an iterative sampling from data and the use of classification and regression sampling repetitively to converge upon a model to fit the data provided. Learning can be 'unsupervised' where the model identifies latent similarities in data features and arranges the data into clusters, or 'supervised' where the data are labelled into certain categories such as survival, and the data features are selected by the model to fit the label [26]. Medical imaging has so far leaned itself to machine learning techniques most frequently to date and the most promising breakthroughs have been in this field: for example, in the diagnosis of macular degeneration based on retinal images. This is a form of supervised learning. Similar methods are being used to improve early warning using monitor data in children in hospitals or within the ICU. In contrast, unsupervised learning has been applied to 'omic' data for example to identify phenotypes in sepsis, identifying those who may be steroid responsive [27].

Within the ICU, recent attempts have been made to understand optimal treatment strategies for sepsis—by training a model to emulate clinical decision-making. These examples use techniques known as reinforcement learning, where decision rules are trained to attain a desired outcome—in this case shock resolution or survival. Such tools may be able to reduce inconsistencies in treatment and promote personalised treatment strategies, such as when deciding when to use fluid and when to use vaso-active drugs in shock [28, 29]. While the technology is some way off to replace human decision-making and may never, there may be potential to use such tools in the future to augment clinical decision-making. Ultimately the clinician may decide to deviate from suggested treatment options based on dynamic feedback: in that respect machine learning are more sophisticated forms of guidelines that can take input from patient-level data and produce an output to match it. Whether this can improve clinical outcomes in the future remains to be seen.

While most of the methods described have focussed on numerical or categorical data, increasingly Natural Language Processing (NLP) tools are being used in medicine to detect or predict risk. NLP attempts to apply machine learning to identify meaning from unstructured language data. This can be applied to medical documentation that is not formatted, for example, free-text ward round notes or accounts of conversations with families. EHR makes such data more accessible to NLP processes as the data do not need to be converted to text and can be validated for example using spell-check functions to reduce errors. Although in its infancy, NLP techniques are being used to identify risks such as dementia and psychosis in some patient groups. Within the ICU there is potential to use NLP techniques to predict outcomes such as length of stay or mortality from the language used by clinicians at admission.

9.8 Human–Technology Interface

Although most of the applications discussed theoretically carry the possibility of revolutionising medicine, particularly within the data-rich environment of PICU, none have done so, despite the increase in the adoption of electronic health systems. While some of this is due to the technology, much of the success of technology adoption is reliant on the human–technology interface. This is not limited to the hardware available to healthcare workers, or the way a program looks, but how the human interacts with the machine and vice versa. Healthcare technology still forms a relatively small proportion of the technology industry and may not see a large return on investment. This may explain an evident lag between the creation of technology and translation to healthcare including the ability for healthcare professionals to adopt and embrace innovation. Many of today's doctors and nurses are trained before the era of the internet—while we have become dependent on technology in most aspects of our lives, the use of information technology in medicine almost demands a level of expertise in information technology as it does in medicine. This remains a barrier to a majority of healthcare workers. Equally, healthcare technology cannot be created in a vacuum. Developers need to understand the specific needs of an environment: for example, systems built for PICU need to account for weight and physiological variations. Locally developed systems can provide this advantage but this compromises consistency and connectivity between systems and will always have budget restrictions. A good illustration of this is demonstrated by contrasting reports of the effect of a CPOE system in two PICUs: one reported an increase in hospital mortality, and another a decrease, despite the use of the same system! [1] A better model may be the local configuration of standard commercial systems to fit local needs. However, healthcare systems are complex: the impact of a new electronic system will need continued evaluation, and optimisation to try and respond to evolving demands, and patterns of use.

9.9 Conclusion

Information technology is central to the delivery of intensive care in children in the present. The role and reliance on information technology will only increase. The evolution of machine learning holds promise in improving processes of care and potentially improving outcomes. Healthcare professionals have a vital role to play in information technology design, adoption and optimisation to fully leverage the advantages of electronic systems. This provides a challenge but also an opportunity to improve patient care.

Take-Home Messages

- Information technology systems often offer attractive solutions to data organisation, allowing automation, processing and analytical functions
- Information technology systems aim to reduce personal time through electronic charting, smart text entry and shared notes
- Systems such as Computerised Physician Order Entry, Clinical Decision Support System and early warning systems all potentially offer safety nets against inconsistency in care and clinician biases
- Machine learning techniques offer the opportunity to leverage data, many of which are not used in decision-making as human processing capacity is rapidly exceeded in the ICU environment
- However, few electronic systems have shown definite measurable tangible benefits across clinical contexts
- All information technology systems require a human–computer interface to function well to realise the full potential a system can offer
- Clinicians must be involved in the design of systems to optimise the human–computer interface that suits the use environment best

9

References

1. Frederick SA. Advanced technology in pediatric intensive care units: have they improved outcomes? Pediatr Clin N Am. 2016;63(2):293–301.
2. Thiru K, Rowe S, Shaw N, Durward A, Inwald DP, Ramnarayan P. Survey of clinical information system usage by paediatric intensive care units in the UK. Intensive Care Med. 2010;36(9):1616–7.
3. Schiff GD, Bates DW. Can electronic clinical documentation help prevent diagnostic errors? N Engl J Med. 2010;362(12):1066–9.
4. Kroth PJ, Morioka-Douglas N, Veres S, et al. Association of electronic health record design and use factors with clinician stress and burnout. JAMA Netw Open. 2019;2(8):e199609.
5. Baumann LA, Baker J, Elshaug AG. The impact of electronic health record systems on clinical documentation times: a systematic review. Health Policy. 2018;122(8):827–36.
6. Alghamdi AA, Keers RN, Sutherland A, Ashcroft DM. Prevalence and nature of medication errors and preventable adverse drug events in paediatric and neonatal intensive care settings: a systematic review. Drug Saf. 2019;42(12):1423–36.
7. Koppel R, Metlay JP, Cohen A, et al. Role of computerized physician order entry systems in facilitating medication errors. JAMA. 2005;293(10):1197–203.

8. Abraham J, Kitsiou S, Meng A, Burton S, Vatani H, Kannampallil T. Effects of CPOE-based medication ordering on outcomes: an overview of systematic reviews. BMJ Qual Saf. 2020;29(10):1–2.
9. Lyons AM, Sward KA, Deshmukh VG, Pett MA, Donaldson GW, Turnbull J. Impact of computerized provider order entry (CPOE) on length of stay and mortality. J Am Med Inform Assoc. 2017;24(2):303–9.
10. Prgomet M, Li L, Niazkhani Z, Georgiou A, Westbrook JI. Impact of commercial computerized provider order entry (CPOE) and clinical decision support systems (CDSSs) on medication errors, length of stay, and mortality in intensive care units: a systematic review and meta-analysis. J Am Med Inform Assoc. 2017;24(2):413–22.
11. Kadmon G, Pinchover M, Weissbach A, Kogan Hazan S, Nahum E. Case not closed: prescription errors 12 years after computerized physician order entry implementation. J Pediatr. 2017;190:236–240.e2.
12. Carthey J, Walker S, Deelchand V, Vincent C, Griffiths WH. Breaking the rules: understanding non-compliance with policies and guidelines. BMJ. 2011;343:d5283.
13. Ramnarayan P, Roberts GC, Coren M, et al. Assessment of the potential impact of a reminder system on the reduction of diagnostic errors: a quasi-experimental study. BMC Med Inform Decis Mak. 2006;6:22.
14. Tleyjeh IM, Nada H, Baddour LM. VisualDx: decision-support software for the diagnosis and management of dermatologic disorders. Clin Infect Dis. 2006;43(9):1177–84.
15. Catho G, De Kraker M, Waldispühl Suter B, et al. Study protocol for a multicentre, cluster randomised, superiority trial evaluating the impact of computerised decision support, audit and feedback on antibiotic use: the COMPuterized Antibiotic Stewardship Study (COMPASS). BMJ Open. 2018;8(6):e022666.
16. Jouvet PA, Payen V, Gauvin F, Emeriaud G, Lacroix J. Weaning children from mechanical ventilation with a computer-driven protocol: a pilot trial. Intensive Care Med. 2013;39(5):919–25.
17. Kucher N, Koo S, Quiroz R, et al. Electronic alerts to prevent venous thromboembolism among hospitalized patients. N Engl J Med. 2005;352(10):969–77.
18. Faraon-Pogaceanu C, Banasiak KJ, Hirshberg EL, Faustino EV. Comparison of the effectiveness and safety of two insulin infusion protocols in the management of hyperglycemia in critically ill children. Pediatr Crit Care Med. 2010;11(6):741–9.
19. Kwan JL, Lo L, Ferguson J, et al. Computerised clinical decision support systems and absolute improvements in care: meta-analysis of controlled clinical trials. BMJ. 2020;370:m3216.
20. Duncan H, Hudson AP. Implementation of a paediatric early warning system as a complex health technology intervention. Arch Dis Child. 2021;106(3):215–8.
21. Futterman C, Salvin JW, McManus M, et al. Inadequate oxygen delivery index dose is associated with cardiac arrest risk in neonates following cardiopulmonary bypass surgery. Resuscitation. 2019;142:74–80.
22. Winter MC, Kubis S, Bonafide CP. Beyond reporting early warning score sensitivity: the temporal relationship and clinical relevance of "true positive" alerts that precede critical deterioration. J Hosp Med. 2019;14(3):138–43.
23. Parshuram CS, Dryden-Palmer K, Farrell C, et al. Effect of a pediatric early warning system on all-cause mortality in hospitalized pediatric patients: the EPOCH randomized clinical trial. JAMA. 2018;319(10):1002–12.
24. Harvey JB, Yeager BE, Cramer C, Wheeler D, McSwain SD. The impact of telemedicine on pediatric critical care triage. Pediatr Crit Care Med. 2017;18(11):e555–60.
25. Ellenby MS, Marcin JP. The role of telemedicine in pediatric critical care. Crit Care Clin. 2015;31(2):275–90.
26. Sanchez-Pinto LN, Luo Y, Churpek MM. Big data and data science in critical care. Chest. 2018;154(5):1239–48.
27. Antcliffe DB, Burnham KL, Al-Beidh F, et al. Transcriptomic signatures in sepsis and a differential response to steroids. From the VANISH randomized trial. Am J Respir Crit Care Med. 2019;199(8):980–6.
28. Komorowski M. Artificial intelligence in intensive care: are we there yet? Intensive Care Med. 2019;45(9):1298–300.
29. Komorowski M, Celi LA, Badawi O, Gordon AC, Faisal AA. The artificial intelligence clinician learns optimal treatment strategies for sepsis in intensive care. Nat Med. 2018;24(11):1716–20.

The Lung and Mechanical Ventilation in ICU

Contents

Basic Respiratory Physiology

Theodore Dassios and Anne Greenough

Contents

J. Brierley et al. (eds.), *ESPNIC Children's Intensive Care Textbook*,
https://doi.org/10.1007/978-3-031-64762-8_10

Learning Objectives

To understand:

- The phases of intrauterine and postnatal lung development
- The roles of foetal lung fluid and pulmonary surfactant
- How gases are transferred and exchanged at the alveolar membrane
- How an abnormal ventilation-perfusion ratio leads to hypoxaemia
- That respiratory disorders are characterised by abnormal lung mechanics such as low compliance and increased airway resistance
- That ventilator waveforms can serve as a real-time window to monitor evolving respiratory disease

10.1 Foetal and Postnatal Development

The foetal development of the lungs is divided in five phases [1]. During the ***embryonic phase*** (until the eighth week of gestation) the two primary lung buds appear from the anterior foregut. The five lobar buds that will later correspond to the three right and two left lung lobes appear on day 32. Following repeated consecutive dichotomisation of the airways in the ***pseudoglandular phase*** (5th–17th week) the foetal lungs will have 16–25 generations of primitive airways. No new airways will develop after this stage, although the existing ones will elongate and widen. During the ***canalicular phase*** (16th–26th week) epithelialized airways grow rapidly and penetrate the mesenchymal tissue. The epithelial cells also differentiate into either type-I or type-II pneumocytes that are responsible for forming the blood–air interface and the production of surfactant, respectively. Limited gas exchange, and thus viability, can be achieved by the end of this stage. During the ***saccular phase*** (24th week of gestation birth), the airspaces increase in size and the airspace walls become thinner. The development of the alveoli starts in the ***alveolar phase*** (36th week of gestation birth) by a division of the primary to secondary septa which will form the alveolar membrane. This membrane consists of the thin epithelial wall of the type I pneumocytes, the basal membranes of the epithelial and endothelial cells and the thin-walled endothelial cells.

10.2 Surfactant and Foetal Lung Fluid

Pulmonary surfactant is a lipoprotein synthesised by type-II pneumocytes which reduces the surface tension in the lungs and prevents alveolar collapse. It consists mostly of phospholipid and cholesterol and four surfactant proteins [2]. The pulmonary surfactant system develops in the second half of the gestation and continues to mature until birth, making the lack of endogenous surfactant a major determinant of respiratory disease in prematurely born infants. In utero, the foetal lungs are filled with a fluid, which is not inhaled amniotic fluid but is formed by the active secretion of the lung cells [3]. The foetal lung fluid stimulates lung growth by distending the developing lung units: this is the rationale of the foetoscopic endoluminal tracheal occlusion procedure in infants with congenital diaphragmatic hernia [4]. In those infants, it is hypothesised that tracheal occlusion will increase the distending pressure and hence facilitate lung growth. Foetuses make breathing movements and the combination of these and adequate foetal lung liquid contribute to lung development and maturation [5].

10.3 Transition from Foetal to Postnatal Cardiorespiratory Function

The source of oxygenation transitions rapidly after birth from the placenta to the newborn lungs. In utero, the lungs are not performing a gas exchange, thus they receive a small fraction of the right ventricular output while the majority is shunted to the left circulation via the foramen ovale and the ductus arteriosus. The pulmonary vessels are also functionally dormant in utero as they have high vascular resistance and accommodate a smaller blood volume. At birth, following the first breath, the newborns achieve clearance of the foetal lung fluid via ejection from the upper airways and absorption via the pulmonary lymphatics. They expand their lungs with air and establish a functional residual capacity. The clamping of the cord causes an increase in the systemic pressure with the effect of closing the foramen ovale which acts as a one-way flap valve. Simultaneously, the flow of blood through the umbilical vein ceases which causes the ductus arteriosus to collapse. The pulmonary vasculature also responds to the increased oxygen tension by vasodilation and a decrease in the pulmonary artery pressure [1]. The combination of the increased systemic and decreased pulmonary pressures leads to a functional reversal of the flow through the foramen ovale from right-to-left to left-to-right. During foetal life, due to the mixing of blood via the foramen ovale and the ductus arteriosus, the foetal peripheral oxygen saturation is in the range of 60% but increases gradually to above 90% within the first 10 min after birth [6].

10.4 Postnatal Development

The development of new alveoli (alveolarisation) starts in utero and continues following birth. At birth, a term-born infant has approximately 150 million alveoli [7]: the final number of 400–600 million is reached later in childhood [8]. Lung volume also increases throughout childhood to approximately 25 years of age. Longitudinal trajectory studies have shown that lung function at age 4–6 years is determined by lung function soon after birth and thereafter follows a predefined trajectory (tracking) at least up to the age of 50 years. The postnatal development of lung function in childhood can be negatively affected by prenatal factors such as prematurity and intrauterine growth retardation and postnatal factors such as exposure to tobacco or air pollution, early viral infections, development of asthma or atopy and potentially over-nutrition or exposure to abnormal microbiomes [9].

10.5 How Structure Serves Function

The structure of the respiratory system is largely explained by the need to provide a large interface for gas exchange. The alveolar membrane has a surface of 50–100 m^2 in a healthy adult which is accommodated in a contained volume of approximately 6 L in an

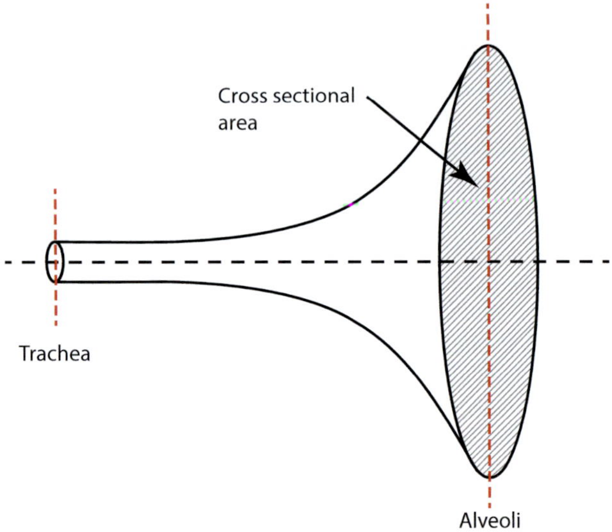

■ **Fig. 10.1** The total cross-sectional area of the airways increases from the trachea towards the terminal bronchioles

energy-efficient way that serves oxygen needs at rest and in increased demands such as during strenuous aerobic activity [10]. This is achieved by a sophisticated system of repeated subdivisions starting from the trachea down to the alveoli. Consecutive subdivisions lead to approximately 500 million alveoli in a fully developed human lung [11]. The diameter of the airways decreases with every division (i.e. the diameter of the trachea is larger than the diameter of the left or right main bronchus and so on), the total cross-sectional area of the airways, however, increases from the trachea to the terminal bronchioles in a way that schematically resembles the bell of a trumpet (■ Fig. 10.1). This structure facilitates the transfer of gases in the last divisions of the bronchial tree.

10.6 Ventilation and Lung Volumes

Ventilation is the process of transporting inspired and expired gas to and from the alveoli. The volume of air which enters the upper airways and consequently the lungs is called the tidal volume and is approximately 500 mL in adults. The product of the tidal volume and the breathing rate over a minute is called minute ventilation and is the major determinant of the clearance of carbon dioxide. A fraction of the tidal volume comes from the non-gas-exchanging parts of the lungs such as the upper airways and large bronchi and will not participate in gas exchange. This is called anatomical dead space (■ Fig. 10.2). Dead-space ventilation also includes parts of the lung that are ventilated but not perfused by pulmonary circulation and thus cannot accommodate gas exchange (alveolar dead space). The aggregate of the anatomical and alveolar dead space is the physiological dead space [12].

The anatomical dead space can be calculated by plotting the expired carbon dioxide against the expired volume in a graph which is called a volumetric capnogram (■ Fig. 10.3). This graph has three phases: one that corresponds to the initial expired

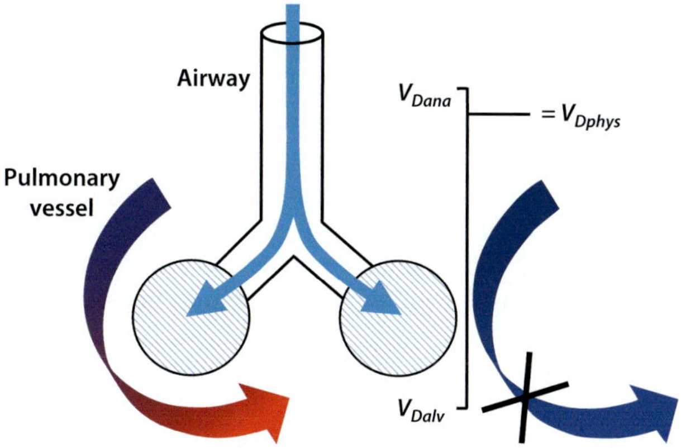

Fig. 10.2 The aggregate of the anatomical (V_{Dana}) and the alveolar (V_{Dalv}) dead space is the physiological dead space (V_{Dphys})

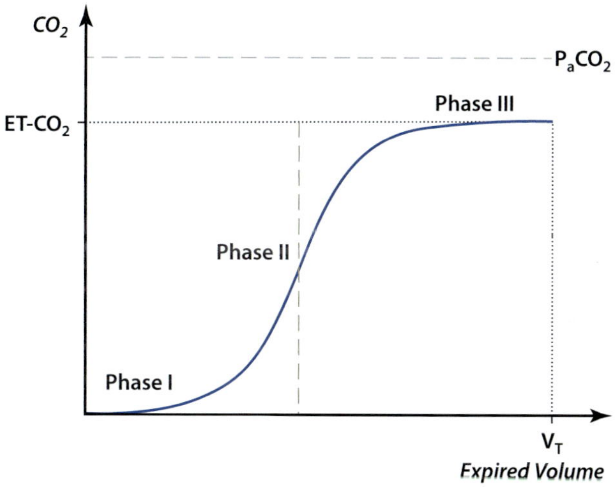

Fig. 10.3 The three phases of a volumetric capnogram and the two equal triangles used to estimate the anatomical dead space. The arterial pressure of CO_2 ($PaCO_2$) and the end tidal CO_2 (ET-CO_2) are depicted

air from the large airways that contains no carbon dioxide (phase I), the last phase which corresponds to the exhalation of pure alveolar gas (phase III) and a transitional phase between phases I and III which corresponds to the mixing of air from the large airways and the alveoli (phase II). By constructing such a diagram and using a method that separates phases I and III by creating two equal triangles, the anatomical dead space can be calculated [13, 14].

The physiological dead space can be estimated with the Bohr–Enghoff equation:

$$V_D = V_T \times \left(1 - P_ECO_2 / PaCO_2\right)$$

where V_D is the physiological dead space, V_T the expired tidal volume, P_ECO_2 the mean expired carbon dioxide and $PaCO_2$ the arterial partial pressure of carbon dioxide [15]. By deducting the anatomical dead space from the total physiological dead space, the alveolar dead space can be determined. While the anatomical dead space is primarily influenced by size and demographics, the alveolar dead space is an index of disease severity that is increased in subjects with severe lung injury [12]. The fraction of the dead space to tidal volume is also an index of respiratory disease with a higher fraction representing more damaged lungs and a less efficient breathing strategy as the work of breathing is 'wasted' in ventilating non-functional lung parenchyma [16].

The total volume of gas contained in the lungs after a deep inspiration is called total lung capacity and the volume of gas left in the lungs after a forced maximal expiration is the residual volume. The volume of gas that remains in the lungs after a non-forced expiration is the functional residual capacity (FRC). Lung volumes can be measured by spirometry, but forced manoeuvres that are required to measure lung volumes can usually not be performed by children younger than 5–6 years of age. FRC is a useful lung function test that can give information about air trapping (high FRC) or atelectasis (low FRC) but cannot be measured with simple spirometry and requires a dilution technique of a gas such as helium or body plethysmography [10].

10.7 Diffusion

The process of transfer of gas across the alveolar membrane is called diffusion and is a passive phenomenon where a gas moves from a compartment with a higher concentration to one with a lower concentration; for example, carbon dioxide diffuses from the pulmonary capillaries where it has a partial pressure of 40 mmHg to the atmosphere where the concentration is practically negligible. The diffusion of a gas through tissue is described by Fick's law:

$$V_A = \frac{S_A}{d} D(P_1 - P_2)$$

where V_A is the alveolar ventilation, S_A is the alveolar surface area, D the diffusion coefficient of the gas and $P_1 - P_2$ the pressure difference of the gas across the two sides of the alveolar membrane.

The rate of transfer of a gas through a tissue is proportional to the surface area of the tissue and the difference in the partial pressures of the gas across the tissue and inversely proportional to the thickness of the tissue. Adult human, fully developed lungs have a surface area of 50–100 m^2 and a thickness of only 0.3 μm making the alveolar membrane ideal for gas exchange [17]. Diffusion will be impaired in any disease that is characterised by decreased alveolar surface area, thickened alveolar membrane and decreased gradient of gases across the membrane. For example, a prematurely born infant assessed at term has a five-fold smaller surface area than a term-born infant owing to arrested alveolarisation following prematurity and chronic respiratory morbidity [18]. This might not be clinically apparent in an otherwise well developing child who is not using the entirety of its functional reserves for everyday activities, but might cause significant functional limitations later in life such as exercise intolerance and decreased reserves [19]. The diffusing capacity of the lungs is measured using Fick's law assessing the diffusing capacity for carbon monoxide (DLCO) where a single inspiration of a dilute mixture of carbon monoxide is followed by the measurement of the rate of disappearance of carbon monoxide from the expired alveolar gas.

10.8 Pulmonary Perfusion

The pulmonary artery carries deoxygenated blood from the right ventricle and branches repeatedly to form the pulmonary capillaries. The oxygenated blood is then collected by the small pulmonary veins that transfer oxygenated blood to the left atrium. The pressures in the pulmonary circulation are significantly lower than in the systemic circulation: while the mean pressure in the aorta is 100 mmHg, the mean pressure in the pulmonary artery is only about 15 mmHg. The pulmonary capillaries are also thin walled with little smooth muscle compared to the systemic circulation. The main pathology that can affect pulmonary circulation following birth is the failure to transition to a low-pressure system (persistent pulmonary hypertension of the newborn or persistent foetal circulation) or the de novo development of increased pressures. The pulmonary vascular bed is very sensitive to a number of postnatal irritant factors that can cause vasoconstriction and pulmonary hypertension. Such factors typically include meconium aspiration, pneumonia, respiratory distress syndrome, hypoxia–ischemia and polycythaemia. In the presence of an open ductus arteriosus and a patent foramen ovale, the increased pulmonary pressures cause the shunting of deoxygenated blood from the right to the left circulation and the development of cyanosis. This condition is called persistent pulmonary hypertension in the newborn. Pulmonary hypertension in the postnatal period can also develop as a consequence of chronic respiratory disease in prematurely born infants or as a result of inadequate intrauterine lung development such as in cases of severe congenital diaphragmatic hernia [20]. In these disorders, pulmonary hypertension has a fixed/structural component as the otherwise normal blood volume of the systemic circulation will have to be accommodated in series by a smaller 'container' which is the smaller-volume pulmonary circulation that accompanies pulmonary hypoplasia [21]. In the paediatric setting, conditions such as congenital heart disease, interstitial lung disease, altitude hypoxia and haemolytic anaemias can also cause pulmonary hypertension [20].

When the balance of osmotic pressure that keeps the fluid in the capillaries against the hydrostatic pressure that draws fluid out of the capillaries is disrupted, fluid can extravasate from the capillaries to the pulmonary interstitium and the alveolar spaces (pulmonary oedema). For example, a neonate with a large patent ductus arteriosus can develop left heart failure and pulmonary congestion followed by interruption of gas exchange secondary to filling of the alveolar spaces with fluid. This will manifest clinically with increased oxygen and ventilatory needs.

10.9 Ventilation–Perfusion Relationships

When ventilation to perfusion (V_A/Q) matching ($V_A/Q = 1$) is disrupted, this results in V_A/Q mismatch and hypoxaemia. Decreased ventilation can be caused by a decreased alveolar surface area either permanently (chronic lung disease) or temporarily (acute pulmonary infection), by hypoventilation secondary to sedative drugs such as morphine, by a thickened alveolar membrane (lung fibrosis) or by a decreased gradient of the gas across the two sides of the membrane (environmental hypoxia). Emphysematous lungs will be normally ventilated but poorly perfused due to the destruction of the lung architecture that results in an abnormally high V_A/Q. Areas of the lungs that are not ventilated but perfused (for example in atelectasis) will cause deoxygenated blood to bypass the lungs (intrapulmonary shunting). Completely atelectatic but perfused lung units have a V_A/Q of zero. Contrarily, areas of the lungs that are not perfused but retain their ventilation (for example in pulmonary embolism) have a V_A/Q ratio of infinite (alveolar dead space). The end result of any abnormality of V_A/Q, either high or low, will be a decreased delivery of oxygen to the peripheral tissues. In health, children have a V_A/Q ratio of approximately one, similar to healthy adults, but severely abnormal values ranging as low as 0.1–0.2 have been reported in children with bronchopulmonary dysplasia [22, 23].

10.10 Mechanics of Breathing

The diaphragm is the most important muscle of inspiration. It is a dome-shaped skeletal muscle that contracts caudally and generates negative intrathoracic pressure which draws air in the chest. In neonates, the function of the diaphragm is negatively affected by prematurity, poor nutrition, congenital abnormalities of the chest or abdomen and systemic or respiratory infection [24]. Diaphragmatic function later in childhood can be affected by chronic diseases that cause airway obstruction or hyperinflation such as asthma, cystic fibrosis or neuromuscular diseases [25]. Prolonged mechanical ventilation also affects the strength and function of the diaphragm [26]. The strength of the diaphragm increases throughout childhood and adolescence [27]. Expiration in health is passive, where the chest wall and the lungs return to their resting state after having been actively expanded by the respiratory muscles during inspiration. Expiration can become active in strenuous exercise and in diseases that are characterised by a prolonged expiration such as asthma.

The relation of the pressure required to generate a specific change in lung volume either in quietly breathing or mechanically ventilated subjects is described by the pressure–volume (PV) curve (◘ Fig. 10.4). The curve follows a different route during inhalation/inflation compared to exhalation/deflation. The difference between the two limbs of the curve is called hysteresis and is increased in diseases with increased airway resistance such as asthma, bronchiolitis, respiratory distress syndrome due to surfactant insufficiency and bronchopulmonary dysplasia. The compliance can be calculated by the slope of the PV curve. Compliance is also decreased in diseases that involve the pulmonary parenchyma such as pneumonia, pulmonary oedema, pulmonary haemorrhage and acute respiratory distress syn-

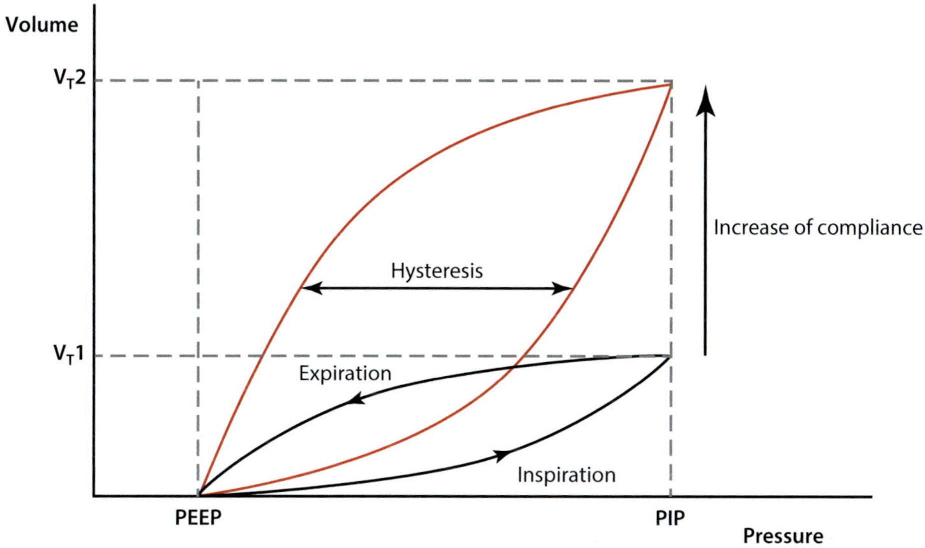

Fig. 10.4 The pressure–volume curve of a ventilated patient: the positive end expiratory pressure (PEEP), peak inflation pressure (PIP) and tidal volumes (V_T) are depicted. If a very large pressure is required to generate a small change in volume, the curve appears depressed towards the pressure (x) axis. This is a condition of low compliance. The change between the inspiratory and expiratory limb represents the hysteresis. Typically, a PV curve of a newborn infant with respiratory distress syndrome will be initially depressed and will move upwards after the administration of exogenous surfactant and an increase in compliance

drome. Compliance can be abnormally high, typically in emphysematous changes due to loss of elastic tissue [10].

The resistance of a fluid moving through a tube with laminar flow is proportional to the length of the tube and inversely proportional to the fourth power of the radius [10]. In mechanically ventilated infants and children, the resistance can be read on the ventilator screen and increased resistance can be attributed either to the airways as in asthma, bronchiolitis or bronchopulmonary dysplasia, or to the endotracheal tube that often is the narrowest part of the ventilator circuit. Decreasing, thus, the length of the endotracheal tube and using a wider-diameter endotracheal tube will decrease the resistance and facilitate gas exchange. Increased resistance is initially apparent in expiration but in severe obstruction, it extends to inspiration. Airway resistance owing to lung pathology can be overcome by agents that relax the airway smooth muscles (beta-2 agonists or anticholinergic agents). During mechanical ventilation in a setting of increased airway resistance, slow rates are usually used to allow for long inflation and provide adequate expiratory time for the lungs to fully deflate.

The product of compliance and resistance is the time constant which is the time required for inflation up to 63% of the final volume. The clinical utility of the index lies in that it can help estimate the required duration of inspiration. Three to five time constants are required for sufficient inflation; for example, lungs with a time constant of 0.15 s will require an inflation time of at least 0.45 s [28].

10.11 Control of Respiration

The respiratory system is controlled by the respiratory centres in the pons and the medulla. These centres gather information from a rich network of receptors that are located centrally, peripherally (carotid and aortic bodies) or in the lung (stretch, irritant and other receptors). The peripheral chemoreceptors located in the carotid and aortic bodies respond rapidly to an increased partial pressure of carbon dioxide or pH and to a decreased partial tension of oxygen. The ventilatory response to the stimulation of the pulmonary stretch receptors is a decrease in the respiratory frequency due to an increase in the expiratory time and is called the Hering–Breuer inflation reflex. The control of respiration is not fully developed in newborn infants and this phenomenon is more pronounced in prematurely born infants who suffer from periodic breathing and long pauses of breathing known as apnoea of prematurity [29]. Prematurely born infants have altered control of breathing and a blunted hypoxic ventilatory response in early postnatal life [30]. Infants of smoking and/or substance misusing mothers also have dampened ventilatory responses to hypoxia and the dampening of the ventilatory responses to hypoxia is more pronounced in the prone compared to the supine position [31].

10.12 Ventilator Waveform Monitoring

One area of intensive care medicine where respiratory physiology finds a direct clinical application is the monitoring of the respiratory waveforms on the ventilator screen. The commonly used waveforms are flow, volume, pressure or carbon dioxide over time, the pressure–volume curve and the flow–volume curve. Real-time ventilator waveform monitoring has become possible with the introduction of flow, pressure and carbon dioxide sensors and the incorporation in ventilators of central processing capabilities that can construct and display the graphics [32].

Using the waveform of flow versus time (◘ Fig. 10.5), the adequacy of the expiratory time can be evaluated: if the expiratory flow has not returned to zero before the next inflation, this is an indication that the ventilator rate is too high and will need to decrease to allow for full deflation of the lungs. If this adjustment is not made, consecutive episodes of air trapping might lead to air leaks. A very prolonged expiratory flow is an indicator of increased airway resistance. The same waveform can inform the clinician that the spontaneous patient effort to trigger inflation is not reaching the set flow threshold. This can be overcome by a decrease in the trigger sensitivity.

In the volume versus time waveform (◘ Fig. 10.6), a sudden decrease of the tidal volume to approximately half of that previously delivered might signify intubation of the right lung by an endotracheal tube that has slipped into the right main bronchus. The position of the endotracheal tube might thus need checking and adjusting. Different modes of ventilation will manifest with different volume waveforms: in volume-targeted ventilation, the delivered volume will be fairly constant and the pressure requirement will fluctuate to accommodate the changing pressure needed to achieve the set volume. In pressure-controlled ventilation, the pressure waveform will appear fairly unchanged and the volume will fluctuate from breath to breath. An

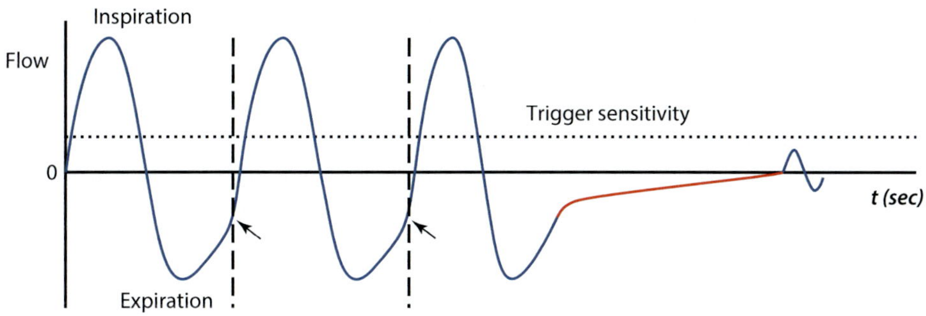

Fig. 10.5 Flow versus time: insufficient time for deflation, a prolonged expiratory phase and failure to trigger are presented

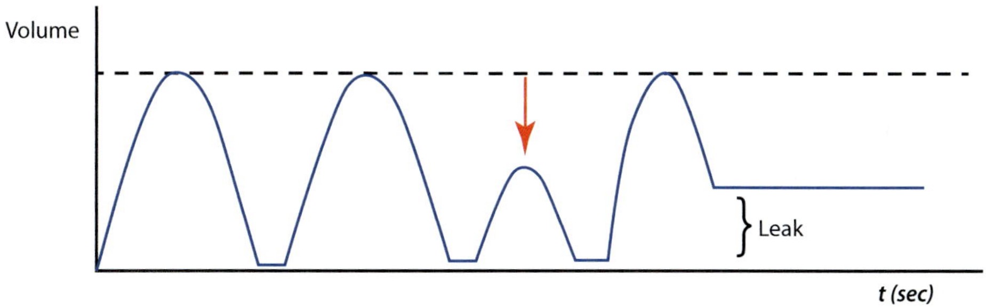

Fig. 10.6 Volume versus time: intubation of the right main bronchus (arrow) and endotracheal leak

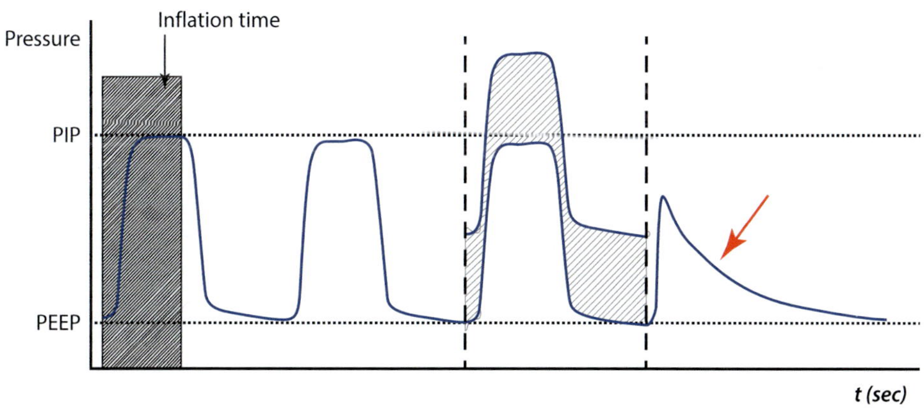

Fig. 10.7 Pressure versus time: The effect of increasing the peak inflation pressure (PIP) or the positive end expiratory pressure (PEEP) on the mean airway pressure is highlighted. A delay of the pressure signal to return to baseline (arrow) represents respiratory muscle fatigue

expiratory volume waveform that does not return to zero indicates endotracheal tube leak.

In the pressure versus time waveform (Fig. 10.7), the area under the pressure waveform represents the mean airway pressure and an increase in the peak or positive end expiratory pressures or inflation time will cause an increase in the mean airway pressure. The rate of decline of the pressure waveform following a spontaneous breath is an indicator of respiratory muscle function as fatigued respiratory muscles will exhibit a more gradual return to baseline owing to impaired relaxation [26, 33].

The difference between the arterial and the end-tidal carbon dioxide is an index of respiratory disease severity with a larger difference signifying more severe respiratory disease [34]. A sharply rising waveform of carbon dioxide against time ('shark-fin' capnogram, ◘ Fig. 10.8) signals uneven and delayed alveolar emptying [35] that can be caused by bronchoconstriction as happens in asthma or bronchiolitis.

The flow-volume waveform (◘ Fig. 10.9) is very useful in assessing airway obstruction. Due to the enlargement of the airways during inspiration, the inwards flow of air to the lungs is usually unobstructed, but during expiration when the air-

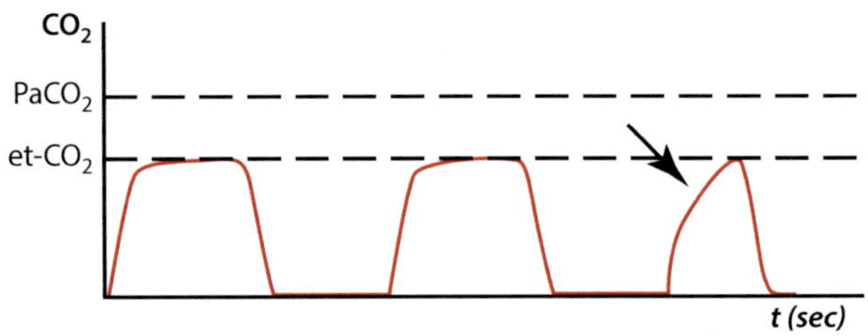

◘ **Fig. 10.8** Carbon dioxide versus time: The shark fin appearance of the capnogram (arrow) represents bronchoconstriction and uneven alveolar emptying

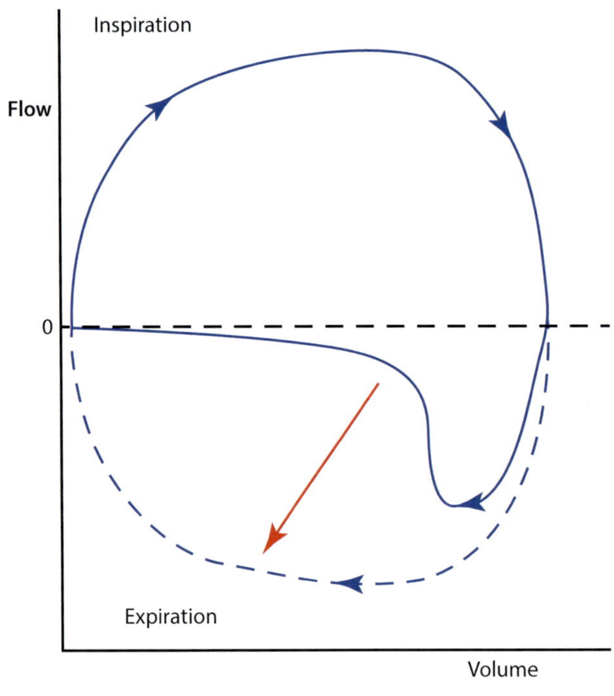

◘ **Fig. 10.9** Flow versus volume: increasing the positive end expiratory pressure (arrow) prevents airways collapse during expiration

ways narrow due to dynamic compression, expiratory flow can be obstructed. This will manifest in a flow-volume waveform by a fairly round inspiratory limb and a steep expiratory limb. In diseases characterised by expiratory flow limitation such as tracheomalacia or inhalation of a foreign body, this waveform can guide the clinician in titrating the amount of positive end-expiratory pressure required to stent open the airway at the end of expiration [36].

Summary

Ventilation is the process of transferring oxygen and carbon dioxide to the alveolar membrane. Oxygen and carbon dioxide passively diffuse across the side of the alveolar membrane depending on the differences in the levels on either side of the membrane. The pulmonary circulation then carries oxygenated blood to the heart and the systemic circulation. Hypoxaemia occurs when the process of ventilation and perfusion are not well matched. The part of the tidal volume that does not participate in gas exchange is called the dead space and it can either be the anatomical dead space corresponding to the upper airways and the main bronchi or the alveolar dead space when it describes areas of the lung that receive ventilation but are not perfused by the pulmonary circulation. A low compliance describes stiff lungs that require high pressures to achieve a volume change. High airway resistance describes narrow airways that make the movement of gas problematic in expiration when the airways become narrower. The respiratory waveforms as displayed on a ventilator screen can offer information on the changing lung mechanics and underlying lung disease.

Take-Home Messages

- The airways develop during the pseudoglandular intrauterine phase, after which no new airways will develop but the existing ones will elongate and widen.
- The alveoli start developing during intrauterine life but continue to increase in number during childhood.
- Assessment of ventilation needs to take into account that some areas of the lungs are ventilated but not perfused (dead space).
- Diffusion of oxygen can be impaired by a decreased alveolar surface area, thickened alveolar membrane and a decreased gradient of oxygen across the membrane.
- Ventilation waveform monitoring can serve as an open window to observe changing lung mechanics and the evolution of respiratory disease.

References

1. Schoenwolf GC, Larsen WJ. Larsen's human embryology. 4th ed. Philadelphia: Churchill Livingstone/Elsevier; 2009. xix, 687 p.
2. Soll RF, Blanco F. Natural surfactant extract versus synthetic surfactant for neonatal respiratory distress syndrome. Cochrane Database Syst Rev. 2001;(2):CD000144.
3. Olver RE, Walters DV, Wilson SM. Developmental regulation of lung liquid transport. Annu Rev Physiol. 2004;66:77–101.
4. Jani JC, Nicolaides KH, Gratacos E, Vandecruys H, Deprest JA, FETO Task Group. Fetal lung-to-head ratio in the prediction of survival in severe left-sided diaphragmatic hernia treated by fetal endoscopic tracheal occlusion (FETO). Am J Obstet Gynecol. 2006;195(6):1646–50.
5. Adzick NS, Harrison MR, Glick PL, Villa RL, Finkbeiner W. Experimental pulmonary hypoplasia and oligohydramnios: relative contributions of lung fluid and fetal breathing movements. J Pediatr Surg. 1984;19(6):658–65.

6. Dildy GA, van den Berg PP, Katz M, et al. Intrapartum fetal pulse oximetry: fetal oxygen saturation trends during labor and relation to delivery outcome. Am J Obstet Gynecol. 1994;171(3):679–84.
7. Hislop AA, Wigglesworth JS, Desai R. Alveolar development in the human fetus and infant. Early Hum Dev. 1986;13(1):1–11.
8. Narayanan M, Owers-Bradley J, Beardsmore CS, et al. Alveolarization continues during childhood and adolescence: new evidence from helium-3 magnetic resonance. Am J Respir Crit Care Med. 2012;185(2):186–91.
9. Bush A. Lung development and aging. Ann Am Thorac Soc. 2016;13(Suppl 5):S438–46.
10. West JB. Respiratory physiology: the essentials. 9th ed. Philadelphia: Wolters Kluwer Health/Lippincott Williams & Wilkins; 2012. viii, 200 p.
11. Weibel ER. Morphometry of the human lung. Berlin: Springer; 1963. xi, 151 p.
12. Dassios T, Kaltsogianni O, Greenough A. Determinants of pulmonary dead space in ventilated newborn infants. Early Hum Dev. 2017;108:29–32.
13. Fletcher R. Airway deadspace, end-tidal CO2, and Christian Bohr. Acta Anaesthesiol Scand. 1984;28(4):408–11.
14. Fowler WS, Comroe JH. Lung function studies. I. The rate of increase of arterial oxygen saturation during the inhalation of 100 per cent O_2. J Clin Invest. 1948;27(3 Pt 1):327–34.
15. Dassios T, Dixon P, Hickey A, Fouzas S, Greenough A. Physiological and anatomical dead space in mechanically ventilated newborn infants. Pediatr Pulmonol. 2018;53(1):57–63.
16. Nuckton TJ, Alonso JA, Kallet RH, et al. Pulmonary dead-space fraction as a risk factor for death in the acute respiratory distress syndrome. N Engl J Med. 2002;346(17):1281–6.
17. Zeltner TB, Caduff JH, Gehr P, Pfenninger J, Burri PH. The postnatal development and growth of the human lung. I. Morphometry. Respir Physiol. 1987;67(3):247–67.
18. Dassios T, Dassios KG, Dassios G. Functional morphometry for the estimation of the alveolar surface area in prematurely-born infants. Respir Physiol Neurobiol. 2018;254:49–54.
19. Lovering AT, Elliott JE, Laurie SS, et al. Ventilatory and sensory responses in adult survivors of preterm birth and bronchopulmonary dysplasia with reduced exercise capacity. Ann Am Thorac Soc. 2014;11(10):1528–37.
20. Abman SH, Hansmann G, Archer SL, et al. Pediatric pulmonary hypertension: guidelines from the American Heart Association and American Thoracic Society. Circulation. 2015;132(21):2037–99.
21. Nair J, Lakshminrusimha S. Update on PPHN: mechanisms and treatment. Semin Perinatol. 2014;38(2):78–91.
22. Dassios T, Kaltsogianni O, Hickey A, Bhat R, Greenough A. Chronology and determinants of respiratory function changes following administration of systemic postnatal corticosteroids in extremely preterm infants. J Pediatr. 2019;215:17–23.
23. Dassios T, Curley A, Morley C, Ross-Russell R. Using measurements of shunt and ventilation-to-perfusion ratio to quantify the severity of bronchopulmonary dysplasia. Neonatology. 2015;107(4):283–8.
24. Dassios T, Kaltsogianni O, Dixon P, Greenough A. Effect of maturity and infection on the rate of relaxation of the respiratory muscles in ventilated, newborn infants. Acta Paediatr. 2018;107(4):587–92.
25. Dassios T. Determinants of respiratory pump function in patients with cystic fibrosis. Paediatr Respir Rev. 2015;16(1):75–9.
26. Dassios T, Kaltsogianni O, Greenough A. Relaxation rate of the respiratory muscles and prediction of extubation outcome in prematurely born infants. Neonatology. 2017;112(3):251–7.
27. Dassios T, Dimitriou G. Determinants of inspiratory muscle function in healthy children. J Sport Health Sci. 2019;8(2):183–8.
28. Henderson WR, Dominelli PB, Molgat-Seon Y, et al. Effect of tidal volume and positive end-expiratory pressure on expiratory time constants in experimental lung injury. Physiol Rep. 2016;4(5):e12737.
29. Poets CF, Samuels MP, Southall DP. Epidemiology and pathophysiology of apnoea of prematurity. Biol Neonate. 1994;65(3–4):211–9.
30. Debevec T, Pialoux V, Millet GP, Martin A, Mramor M, Osredkar D. Exercise overrides blunted hypoxic ventilatory response in prematurely born men. Front Physiol. 2019;10:437.

31. Rossor T, Ali K, Bhat R, Trenear R, Rafferty G, Greenough A. The effects of sleeping position, maternal smoking and substance misuse on the ventilatory response to hypoxia in the newborn period. Pediatr Res. 2018;84(3):411–8.
32. Donn SM, Mammel MC. Neonatal pulmonary graphics: a clinical pocket atlas. New York, NY: Springer; 2015. xv, 175 p.
33. Dassios T, Kaditis A, Katelari A, Chrousos G, Doudounakis S, Dimitriou G. Time constant of inspiratory muscle relaxation in cystic fibrosis. Pediatr Res. 2015;77(4):541–5.
34. Williams E, Dassios T, Greenough A. Assessment of sidestream end-tidal capnography in ventilated infants on the neonatal unit. Pediatr Pulmonol. 2020;55:1468.
35. Gravenstein JS. Capnography. 2nd ed. Cambridge, NY: Cambridge University Press; 2011. xiv, 474 p.
36. Mok Q. Airway problems in neonates-a review of the current investigation and management strategies. Front Pediatr. 2017;5:60.

Basics of Mechanical Ventilation

Peter Rimensberger

Contents

J. Brierley et al. (eds.), *ESPNIC Children's Intensive Care Textbook*,
https://doi.org/10.1007/978-3-031-64762-8_11

Learning Objectives

- Review the physiologic effects of positive airway pressure application on the respiratory system
- Review basic respiratory mechanics relevant during mechanical ventilation
- Review basic monitoring of ventilator waveforms and loops

In simple means, the respiratory system can be reduced to a straw (endotracheal tube and airways exhibiting resistance) and a balloon on the end of this straw (network of alveoli exhibiting compliance). This balloon is placed somewhat in a semi-rigid cage (the thorax exhibiting elastic recoil forces) opposing the distending forces by the negative intrathoracic pressure effect during spontaneous breathing, or the positive pressure effect on the balloon volume during positive pressure application to the system (i.e. positive pressure ventilation). The movement of gas is determined by the force (i.e. pressure, or more precisely in physiologic terms pressure/surface area) applied, gas displacement kinetics, resistive forces exhibited against flow by the airways (resistance determined by the size and length of the straw, and the viscosity of the gas), and the rate of change of displacement of the components that are distensible (balloon). Alterations in the composition of the lung parenchyma and the airways due to alveolar and/or interstitial oedema, cellular infiltrates, or fibrosis will not only reduce **distensibility** of the lung but also increase elastic recoil forces exhibited by the lung parenchyma.

The behaviour of the total respiratory system is best described mathematically by the equation of motion of the respiratory system. It states that the force utilized to drive ventilation (by the respiratory muscles and/or the ventilator) is equal to the force applied by the respiratory system in the opposite direction.

11

Opposing forces of the respiratory system are as follows:

1. The resistive load (i.e. the product of resistance (R_{rs}) and flow: R_{rs} × flow).
2. The elastic load (i.e. the product of elastance (E_{rs}) and volume (V): $E_{rs} \times V$ or $1/C_{rs} \times V$, as elastance is the inverse of compliance (C_{rs})).
3. The pressure of the system before initiation of inspiration, which corresponds to the PEEP level in ventilated patients.
4. The inertial components to move gas (inertance).

Equation of motion:

$$\boldsymbol{P_{musc} + P_{vent} = (R_{rs} \times \text{flow}) + (1 / C_{rs} \times V) + \text{PEEP} + \text{inertance}}$$

where P_{musc} is the pressure generated by the respiratory muscles and P_{vent} is the total pressure delivered by the ventilator, R_{rs} = resistance, C_{rs} = compliance, V = volume, PEEP = end-expiratory pressure. Inertance can be ignored with gas flow rates during conventional mechanical ventilation but becomes important during high frequency oscillation.

Although this equation indicates that at each point in time, the pressure in the respiratory system has an elastic component needed for distension of the lung parenchyma, a resistive component needed for the air flow to advance against the resistances of the airway, and an inertial component due to the changes in the lung parenchyma caused by volume acceleration.

11.1 The Mechanical Behaviour of the Respiratory System (in the Ventilated Patient)

To assess respiratory mechanics in a quantitative way in spontaneous breathing neonates and children is complex and requires special knowledge and equipment; therefore, it remains in the domain of the paediatric pulmonologist. Bedside assessment of mechanics remains qualitative by observing clinical signs focusing on classical signs of respiratory distress (e.g. respiratory rate and pattern, signs of indrawing, thoracoabdominal balancing, and presence of a stridor or wheezing). However, in patients on mechanical ventilation, airway graphics (mainly the flow-time curve, the pressure-volume loop, and the flow-volume loop) will give essential information on respiratory mechanics and help guiding ventilator settings. For all measurements to be most accurate, the primary signals (i.e. airway pressure and gas flow) have to be measured proximal to airway opening. Integration of gas flow over time provides the volume change (i.e. tidal volume).

The flow-time curve gives essentially the information whether respiratory cycle time settings (inspiratory and expiratory time) are chosen adequately. According to the respiratory system's time constant, the product of compliance and resistance is $T = C_{rs} \times R_{rs}$. Calculating the time constant, giving the information on the time needed to reach full filling or emptying with the delta pressure set (i.e. about 5–6 time constants) is cumbersome at bedside. Searching for a no-flow condition at end-inspiration and expiration indicating that no further volume will be delivered to or exhaled by the patient (i.e. pressure equilibrium reached) is simple and practical for adjusting respiratory cycle times (◘ Fig. 11.1).

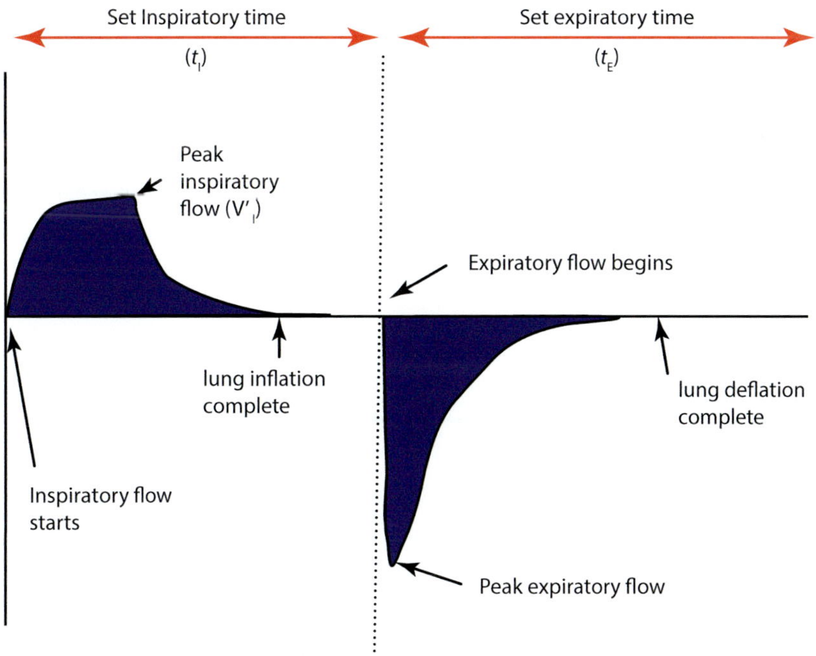

◘ **Fig. 11.1** Illustration of correct cycle time settings according the patients respiratory system behavior on inflation and during passive exhalation as can be observed on the flow-time curve. Note that at end-inspiration and end-expiration a short period of Zero-flow can be identified

During mechanical ventilation, dynamic (often mislabelled as static) respiratory system compliance can be calculated as $C_{rs_{dyn}} = V_t / (P_{plat} - \text{PEEP})$, where P_{plat} = Plateau pressure, PEEP = positive end-expiratory pressure. To have readings of effective airway pressure, an inspiratory pause or hold manoeuver is required. During volume-controlled ventilation, presence of a plateau phase on the pressure-time curve confirms a no-flow condition (i.e. short inspiratory hold), and in pressure control mode, a no-flow condition at end-inspiration confirms a short inspiratory pause as well, rendering the PIP value measured at end-inspiration equal to P_{plat} during volume control. Under such a no-flow condition, the calculation can be made according to $C_{rs_{dyn}} = V_t / (\text{PIP} - \text{PEEP})$. Yet in the absence of a no-flow condition during pressure control ventilation, Plat needs to be measured during an inspiratory hold manoeuver in absence of any spontaneous respiratory activity (◘ Figs. 11.2 and 11.3).

Furthermore, absence of a no-flow condition at end-inspiration and/or expiration indicates that respiratory system time constants have not been respected, which will lead during pressure control ventilation to incomplete filling (outside pressures as

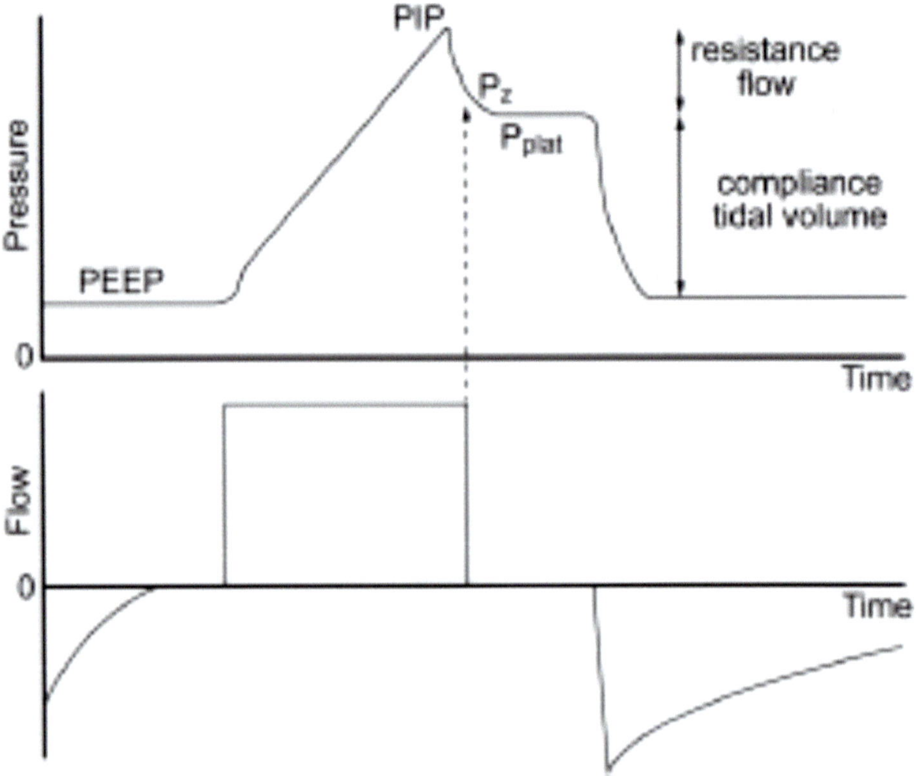

◘ **Fig. 11.2** Illustration on how to estimate/measure respiratory system compliance during mechanical ventilation: With a period of no flow (i.e. plateau pressure period), the difference between P_{plat} and PEEP is determined by tidal volume and respiratory system compliance, i.e. $C_{rs} = V_t/(P_{plat} - \text{PEEP})$, P_z = pressure at zero flow. With permission from Hess (2014) [1]

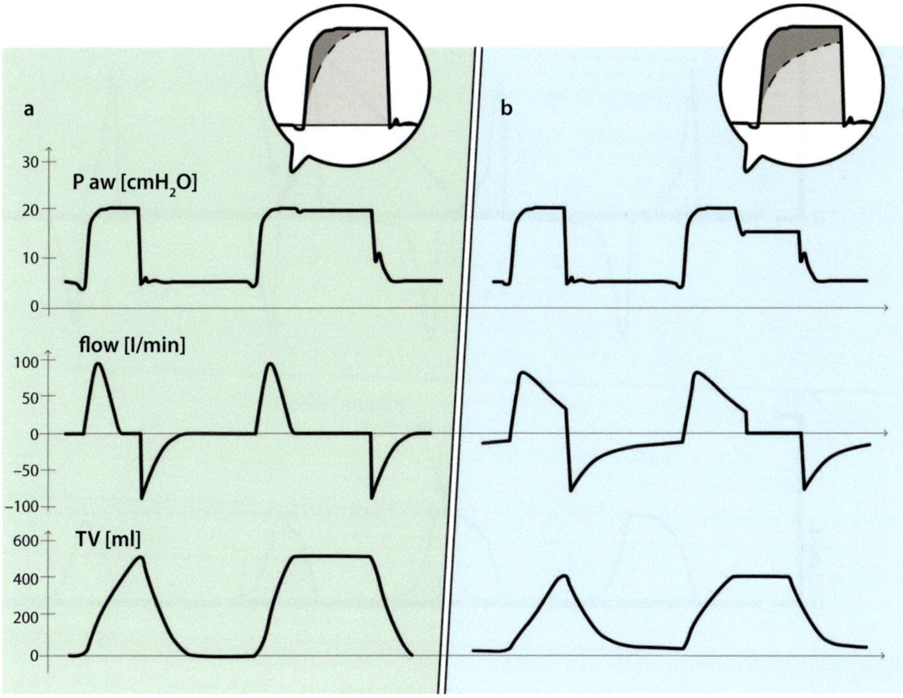

Fig. 11.3 P_{plat} during pressure control ventilation: The airway pressure normally seen on the ventilator screen is the total pressure applied on the respiratory system. It is the sum of the elastic and the resistive pressures. In the balloons this is shown in detail, the pressure that inflates the alveoli is shown in light grey, and the pressure that is spent to generate the flow is shown in dark grey. The pressure applied to the alveoli, net of the resistive pressure, can be revealed by an inspiratory pause; once the flow reduces to zero, only the elastic pressure distending the lung is seen. This is the correct Plateau pressure (P_{plat}). In subject A, due to low resistance, flow reaches zero during normal respiratory cycles also, so that P_{peak} coincides with P_{plat}. In subject B, due to resistive load, flow does not reach zero value at the end of inspiration and P_{plat} (revealed by inspiratory hold) is lower than P_{peak}. With permission from Sosio and Bellani (2019) [2]

displayed by the ventilator will not correspond to the inside pressure on the alveolar level) leading to a smaller resulting V_t that could be achieved at this pressure settings while respecting the time behaviour or lung filling (as testimonied by a no-flow condition at end-inspiration) (Fig. 11.4), or which will lead to an incomplete emptying during expiration (inside PEEP being higher than extrinsic PEEP set by the operator) with the consequence of air-trapping and again smaller V_t that could be achieved while respecting the time behaviour of passive lung emptying (as testimonied by a no-flow condition at end-inspiration). In short, not respecting the in- and expiratory time constant will render ventilation less efficient that could be achieved with set pressures.

During volume control ventilation, non-respecting the expiratory time required for full emptying, i.e. allowing for intrinsic PEEP, may become rapidly dangerous, because the ventilator will deliver the set V_t at each breath, which will finally increase at each breath the trapped expiratory lung volume, as long as upper pressure safety limits are not set very strictly.

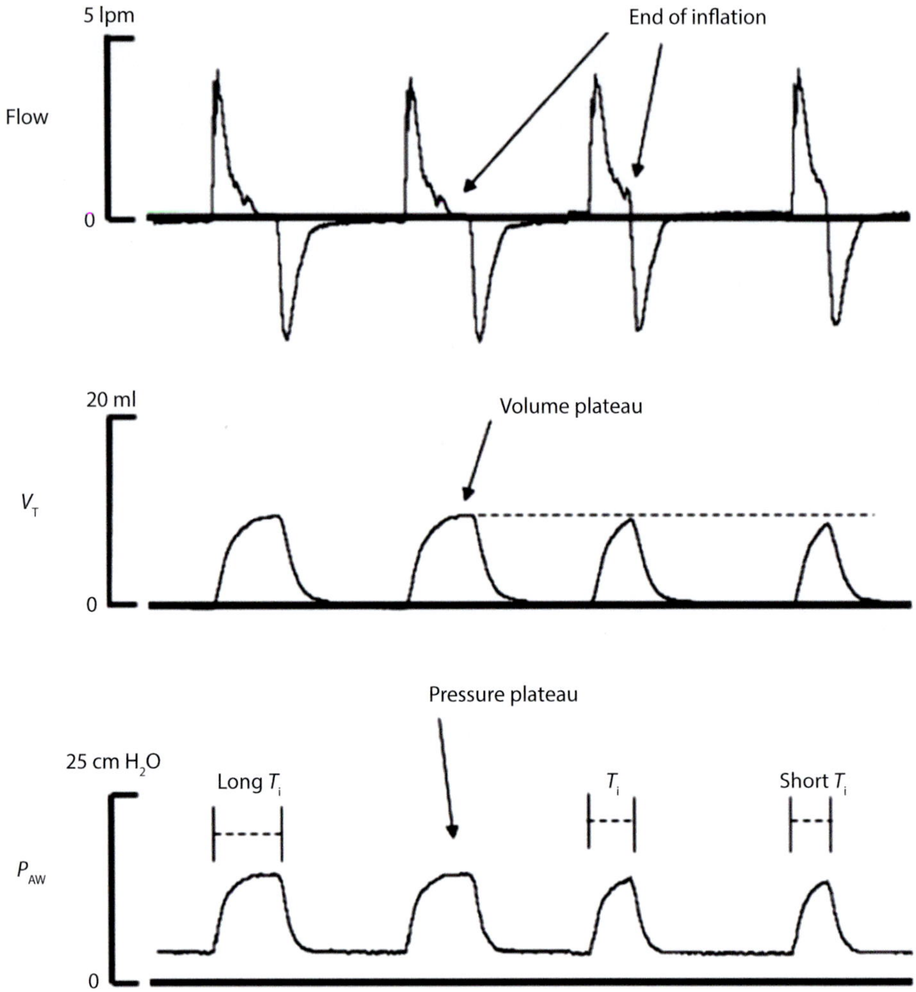

Fig. 11.4 Flow-, volume-, and pressure-time curves illustrating the effect of volume delivery when shortening inappropriately inspiratory times, i.e. no more allowing for a zero flow condition on end-inspiration. Note also that the volume curve displayed on the ventilator screen shows no plateau (i.e. is peaking) with a too short i-time. Note also that in this example even the set pressure rise time does not allow the ventilator to build up the requested inspiratory pressure (i.e. absence of a pressure plateau) within the given time frame. With permission from Heulitt et al. (2015) [3]

The pressure-time and volume-time curves are of much less interest and certainly give no major information on the respiratory system's behaviour. However, the volume-time curve allows to detect easily the presence of leak, which will lead to erroneous $C_{rs_{dyn}}$ measures too.

Analysis and careful monitoring of the shape of the inspiratory and expiratory limb of the dynamic pressure-volume (PV) loop is only of some limited interest when trying to minimize ventilator-induced lung injury by avoiding (1) overdistention and (2) alveolar recruitment/derecruitment. However, dynamic PV-loop interpretations must be done with caution and awareness for the limitations of this method (see below).

1. Pulmonary overdistention occurs when the volume limit of some component of the lungs is approached. It can be manifested as a reduction in compliance at the terminal end of the breath. This is commonly referred to as "beaking" and can be quantified by the C20/Cdyn ratio (i.e. the compliance of the last 20% of the dynamic pressure-volume curve divided by the total dynamic compliance) (◘ Fig. 11.5). However, this method allows only to detect major overdistention, which should be avoided as it have several deleterious effects on the cardiovascular and pulmonary system. First, overdistention puts the patient at risk for baro/volutrauma. Second, overdistention can increase dead space and therefore render ventilation less efficient. Third, overdistention will result in an increase in pulmonary vascular resistance from compression and in a reduction of cardiac output.
2. Commonly the presence of a so-called lower inflection point (point of maximal change in curvature) on the lower part of the inflation limb of the dynamic PV-loop is interpreted as the point where lung opening (i.e. recruitment) starts, and it has been repeatedly recommended to overcome this point by increasing PEEP, slightly above this point (◘ Fig. 11.6). However, this concept of optimizing PEEP by graphic analysis is of very limited value. In fact one needs to look carefully at some details of this inflation limb before applying it to all patients without caution. A flat horizontal dynamic pressure-volume (PV) curve (0 volume reading between the set PEEP and a higher pressure level at which airway opening will start to happen) (in ◘ Fig. 11.6 from 0 cmH_2O to the crossing of the a and b lines) might eventually indicate that below that PEEP airway collapse does occur. Whereas when the first part of the PV-curve from set PEEP shows a slow and a second part a fast increase in volume, this will not indicate that PEEP settings are too low allowing for cyclic collapse. Such a phenomenon is a result of initial fast flows in a high resistive system (endotracheal tube) during rapid increase of airway pressures, because pressures are measured in the respiratory circuit at the ETT connection and not on the tracheal level (◘ Fig. 11.7).

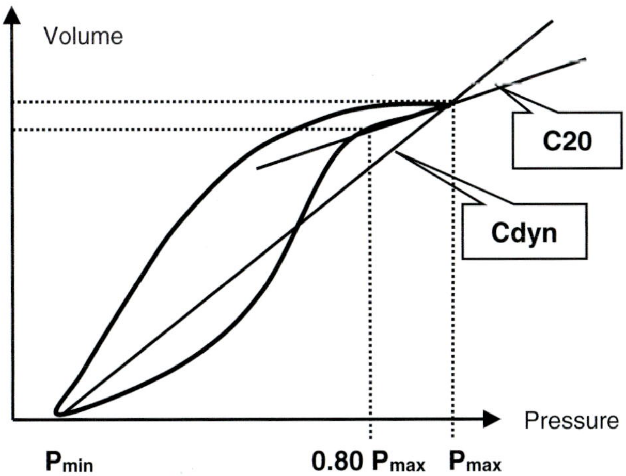

◘ **Fig. 11.5** Overdistention index C20/Cdyn according to Nève et al. (2000) [4], where $C_{20} = \left(V_T - V_{0.80\,P_{\max}}\right) / \left(P_{\max} - 0.80\,P_{\max}\right)$ and Cdyn = $V_T/P_{\max} - P_{\min}$

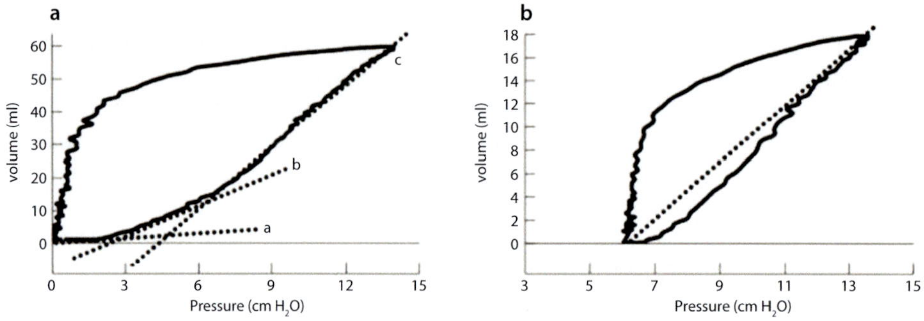

Fig. 11.6 The pressure-volume curve for a ventilated infant. When the lung is ventilated at 0 positive end-expiratory pressure (PEEP) (**a**), a lower inflection point can be seen (crossing of line *a* and *b*). With increasing inspiratory pressure, the lungs are inflated and the pressure-volume relation becomes linear (line *c*). If PEEP is set to 6 (**b**), most of the inspiratory limb of the pressure-volume curve is linear from Schibler and Frey (2002) [5]. Comment: However, setting PEEP slightly above the point where the flat part of the curve ends (crossing of line *a* and *b* in Figure **a**), in this case at 4 cmH2O, would have been sufficient to observe the same effect. The second inflection at the point where line b and c cross is a result of airway resistance (see Fig. 11.7)

11

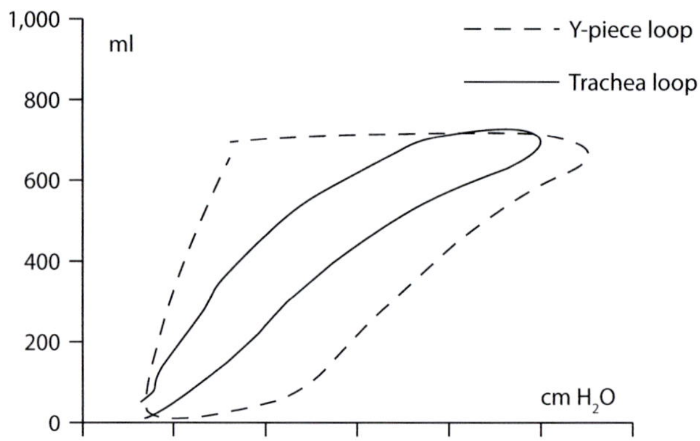

Fig. 11.7 PV-loop during mechanical ventilation with an extrinsic PEEP of 8 cmH2O. The dashed line shows the dynamic PV-loop with pressure measurement at the airway opening (i.e. at endotracheal tube connector, the solid line shows the dynamic PV-loop derived from a pressure measurement at the endotracheal tube tip, i.e. carinal level. Note the difference in the amount of PV-hysteresis and the appearance of a lower inflection point (LIP) on the inflation limb of the PV-loop derived from pressure measurements at airway opening. This LIP cannot be identified on the PV-loop derived from pressure measurements at the carina level. Similarly, there is appearance of a deflection point on the deflation limb of the PV-loop, derived from pressure measurements at airway opening. Again, this deflection point cannot be identified on the PV-loop derived from pressure measurements at the carina level. However, on the inflation limb, there is appearance of an upper inflection point with a flattening of the PV-curve at the upper end (lower compliance at the higher pressure end, which may indicate overinflation of the lungs). However, this is not a very marked point but rather a successive phenomenon. With permission from Kárason et al. (2000) [6]

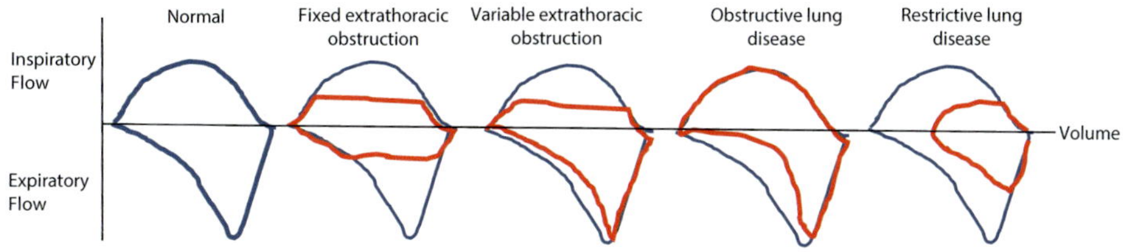

Fig. 11.8 Classical flow-volume patterns as displayed on the ventilator screen for identifying the type and level of airway obstruction, or restrictive lung disease

The recognition and treatment of increased airway resistance (inspiratory and/or expiratory airway obstruction) are essential, and the flow-volume loop can be diagnostic. In contrary to the classical presentation of lung function measurements in the pneumology department, flow-volume loops are presented on a ventilator with inspiration above the 0 flow line (positive flow value) and expiration below the 0 flow line (negative flow value). Limitation of the inspiratory flow (flattening of the inspiratory limb) can be seen with an extrathoracic obstruction. Airway obstruction can be categorized as either fixed (e.g. tracheal stenosis, extratracheal compression, tracheal mass, and an occluded or kinked endotracheal tube) or variable (e.g. tracheobronchomalacia, asthma, and bronchiolitis). Fixed airway obstructions show absence of an initial peak phase, and the flow-volume curve is much flatter (during in- and expiration) in general than the one of normal airway's conditions. Variable (i.e. dynamic) expiratory obstruction is characterized by a classical shape of the expiratory flow-volume curve that presents in a first part with a reduced peak flow when compared to a normal condition with normal airway resistance, and in the second part a flattening of the expiratory flow-volume curve (Fig. 11.8).

For flow measures and tidal volume calculations (by integration of the flow over time) to be accurate, it is mandatory to measure flow (and volume) at the endotracheal tube connector. Furthermore, any air leak situation (usually around the endotracheal tube), which can be easily recognized without inbuilt leak compensating algorithms activated on the flow-volume loop or the volume-time curve, will not allow to know the exact V_t delivered to the patients lung and will lead to incorrect derived parameters from V_t measures.

References

1. Hess DR. Respiratory mechanics in mechanically ventilated patients. Respir Care. 2014;59(11):1773–94.
2. Sosio S, Bellani G. Plateau pressure during pressure control ventilation. AboutOpen. 2019;6(1):76–7.
3. Heulitt MJ, Bancalari E, Keszler M, Sanders RC, Claure N. Respirator cycle control modes. In: Rimensberger P, editor. Pediatric and neonatal mechanical ventilation. Berlin, Heidelberg: Springer; 2015.
4. Nève V, de la Roque ED, Leclerc F, et al. Ventilator-induced overdistension in children: dynamic versus low-flow inflation volume-pressure curves. Am J Respir Crit Care Med. 2000;162(1):139–47. https://doi.org/10.1164/ajrccm.162.1.9906091.
5. Schibler A, Frey U. Role of lung function testing in the management of mechanically ventilated infants. Arch Dis Child Fetal Neonatal Ed. 2002;87(1):F7–10.
6. Kárason S, Søndergaard S, Lundin S, Wiklund J, Stenqvist O. Evaluation of pressure/volume loops based on intratracheal pressure measurements during dynamic conditions. Acta Anaesthesiol Scand. 2000;44:571–7.

Oxygen Therapy and Acute Noninvasive Ventilation in Children

Marti Pons Odena, Christophe Milési, Sundaram Manu, Julien Baleine, and Gilles Cambonie

Contents

J. Brierley et al. (eds.), *ESPNIC Children's Intensive Care Textbook*,
https://doi.org/10.1007/978-3-031-64762-8_12

Learning Objectives

- To initiate NIV following a structured approach (I.C.E.M.A.N acronym)
- To identify the indications and contraindications of NIV
- To select the appropriate equipment
- Interfaces
- Ventilator
- To select the mode of ventilation and the initial settings
- To analyze efficiency and tolerance
- To identify failure criteria
- To identify the indications and limitations of HFNC

12.1 Noninvasive Ventilation

12.1.1 Introduction

The number of children treated with NIV has increased in the last decades.

This chapter provides a structured approach in order to facilitate the initiation of acute noninvasive ventilation in children.

NIV is defined as the application of ventilatory support that does not include an invasive airway device, such as an endotracheal or a tracheostomy tube. Various studies in pediatric and adult populations have supported the benefits of NIV in selected patients [1]. This support is able to relieve respiratory distress symptoms, to reduce the work of breathing (WOB), to improve gas exchange, and to reduce risks of ventilator-associated pneumonia [2–4]. NIV acts through different mechanisms: reduction of airway resistances, ventilation/perfusion (V/Q) mismatch and respiratory muscle fatigue, and increase in functional residual capacity and lung compliance. This results in improvement of the respiratory function, i.e., gas exchange.

We propose to follow a structured approach for NIV initiation. This approach can be summarized through the **I.C.E.M.A.N** acronym:

- **I** Indications
- **C** Contraindications
- **E** Equipment
- **M** Ventilation modes
- **A** Analyze
- **N** Next step

12.1.2 Indications

12.1.2.1 Long-Term Ventilatory Support

NIV is used for long-term ventilatory support in chronic or progressive respiratory failure such as Duchenne muscular dystrophy, spinal muscular dystrophy, and other type II respiratory failures. Its use is associated with improved quality of life, lower risk of hospitalization, and prolonged survival [5].

12.1.2.2 Short-Term Ventilatory Support

NIV is initiated for conditions that are reversible within a few days. Usually, in this context, NIV is used continuously until the patient improves or requires escalation of therapy.

Hypoxemic Respiratory Failure (Type I)

Type 1 respiratory failure is caused by diseases that affect the *V*/*Q* at the alveolar level and results in low PaO_2 with usually normal $PaCO_2$.

Common examples of type I respiratory failures are neonatal respiratory distress syndrome, bronchiolitis, pneumonia, cardiogenic or noncardiogenic pulmonary edema, and pulmonary hemorrhage.

The NIV success rate in acute respiratory distress syndrome (ARDS) is lower (50%) than its average success rate in other situations (75–80%). In children with severe ARDS, early intubation should be considered if no improvement is observed after a 2–6 h NIV trial.

Hypercapnic Respiratory Failure (Type II)

Type II respiratory failure is caused by hypoventilation. It is characterized by early increased $PaCO_2$ and low PaO_2 at a later stage.

The common diseases associated with type II respiratory failure are neuromuscular disease, chest wall abnormalities, drug overdose, and some severe airway disorders such as asthma and chronic obstructive pulmonary disease.

NIV success rate in type II respiratory failure is high (80%–85%).

Asthma exacerbation leads to air trapping and auto-positive end-expiratory pressure (auto-PEEP). The use of NIV helps to overcome dynamic airway obstruction, to decrease respiratory muscle overload, and to improve gas exchange. Hence, NIV is increasingly accepted as a bridge to support these patients while waiting for pharmacotherapy to be effective. The success rate for NIV in severe asthma has been quoted as about 80% [6].

NIV is also used for the weaning of mechanical ventilation. In that instance, NIV is especially interesting for patients with neuromuscular or chronic lung diseases, who are at higher risk of reintubation. In these patients, prophylactic NIV has been associated with higher successful weaning rates than rescue NIV [7].

12.1.3 Contraindications

The **N.A.B.C** acronym provides a structured approach to check the different contraindications (◘ Table 12.1).

Table 12.1 NIV contraindications

	Absolute	Relative
Neuro	– Unconscious: Patient unable to protect airways	– Noncompliant patients
Airways	– Compromised airways – Severe upper gastro-intestinal bleeding	– Oro-facial anomalies
Breathing	– High risk of inhalation	– Moderate ARDS – Nondrained pneumothorax
Circulation	– Imminent cardiac or respiratory arrest – Hemodynamic instability	

Table 12.2 NIV ventilators

	Characteristics
Home NIV ventilators	– Portable devices – Turbine-driven ventilators – Single limb circuit, good leak compensation – Need for vented mask or exhalation port – Maximum FiO_2 limited – Internal batteries for greater mobility
NIV specific PICU ventilator	– Turbine-driven ventilators – Single-limb tubing, performant leak compensation – Need for vented mask or exhalation port – Maximum FiO_2 = 100%
PICU ventilator with NIV option	– Double limb circuit – Need for nonvented interface – Maximum FiO_2 = 100%

12.1.4 Equipment

12.1.4.1 Types of NIV Ventilators

NIV devices can be divided into three groups (Table 12.2).

12.1.4.2 Circuits (Fig. 12.1)

The circuit choice depends on the ventilator.

- **Single limb circuit**: home ventilator and NIV-specific PICU ventilator + vented mask.
- **Dual limb circuit**: PICU ventilator + nonvented mask.

12.1.4.3 Humidification

The air from the machine is dry. This can be uncomfortable and may reduce secretion clearance. Heated humidification is necessary to improve secretion clearance and prevent associated side effects [8].

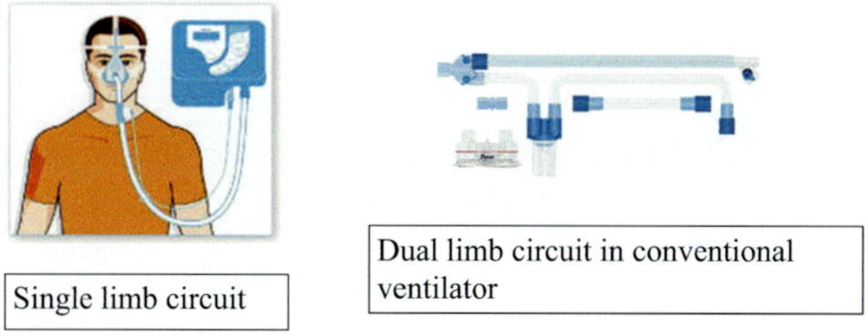

Fig. 12.1 Circuits

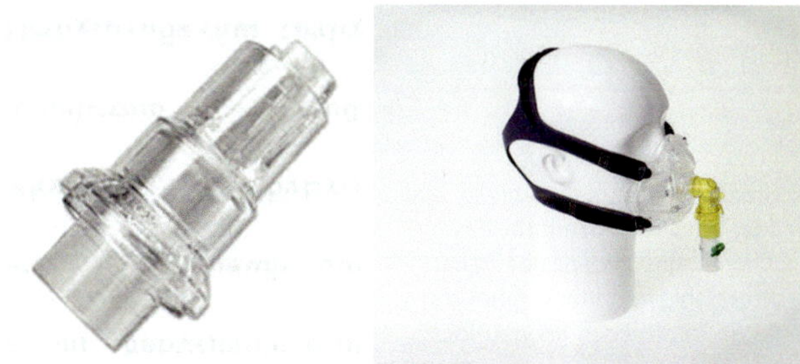

Fig. 12.2 Exhalation ports

12.1.4.4 Exhalation Port (Fig. 12.2)

When NIV is delivered through a single ventilator tubing system with a nonvented mask, an exhalation port must be used for CO_2 removal and to prevent rebreathing. In this situation, a vented mask should be preferred.

12.1.4.5 Anti-Asphyxia Valve (Fig. 12.3)

An anti-asphyxia valve is a bias flow flap valve. It is different from an expiratory port. It prevents the patient from asphyxia if there is a mechanical failure or power cut. At the loss of pressure, the pressure valve opens to ambient air so that the patient can breathe in and out of environmental air. Those valves are designed as security for outpatients where power cuts may be frequent.

12.1.4.6 Interfaces (Table 12.3)

A good mask fit is essential to ensure patient comfort, compliance, synchrony, and effective ventilation [9, 10]. The ideal interface must be lightweight, have minimal dead space, minimal resistance to airflow, and must be easy to remove in case of vomiting. These interfaces must be available in various sizes and should be affordable. Attention should be paid to reduce pressure sores and eye irritation. There are two types of interfaces.

- **Vented masks**: The expiration occurs through the holes present on the mask itself. A single-limb circuit should have a vented interface for CO_2 removal and the intentional leak needs to be compensated by the ventilator. This mask is used mainly with home ventilators and NIV-specific ventilators.
- **Nonvented masks**: The expiration occurs through the exhalation limb in double-limb circuits. This mask is used mainly with PICU ventilators.

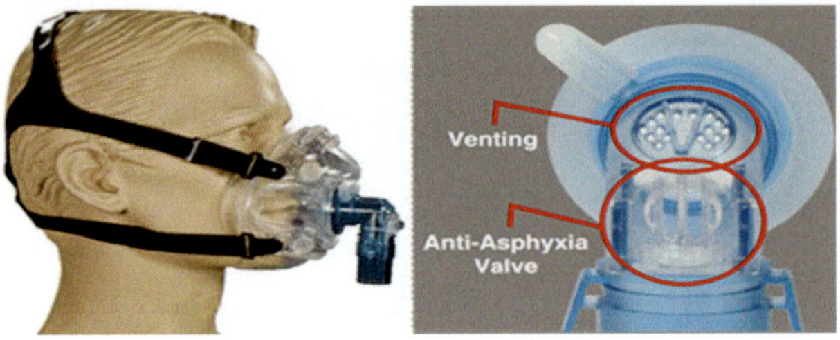

Fig. 12.3 Anti-asphyxia valve

Table 12.3 Interfaces

Interface	Pro	Con
Nasal pillows	– Small and unobtrusive – Ideal to wear during the day – The patient can speak and eat – Preferable for claustrophobics – Main interface in neonatology	– Can be uncomfortable as all air is directed into the nostrils – Can cause irritation/dryness inside the nose – Not effective for mouth breathers
Nasal mask	– Relatively small and unobtrusive – Preferable for claustrophobics – Long-term ventilation, as the risk of aspiration is lower and the mouth is not covered – The patient can speak	– Can cause dryness inside the nose – Not effective for mouth breathers – Long-term mid-face hypoplasia – Inadequate pressurization if the mouth is open, this can be managed with chin straps and pacifiers
Oro-nasal masks	– Ideal for acute NIV – Ideal for mouth breathers	– Risk of aspiration if the patient vomits – Increased incidence of pressure sores on the nasal bridge – Patients are unable to eat and drink – Long-term mid-face hypoplasia
Total face mask	– Ideal for acute NIV – Ideal for mouth breathers	– Can be difficult to accept if claustrophobic – Condensation and rainout in mask
Helmet	– Ideal for patients with dysmorphic face, craniofacial anomalies – Ideal for mouth breathers	– Less effective than standard interfaces in situations of resistive load – Claustrophobia – Absence of synchronization: CPAP is the only available mode – Risk of rebreathing if flow <30 L/min

12

12.1.5 Ventilation Modes

12.1.5.1 Volume-Controlled Modes

In the volume ventilation mode, a fixed tidal volume (VT) is delivered to the patient with a fixed inspiratory time. The pressure required to deliver the tidal volume is independent of the patient's effort, but depends on respiratory compliance and resistance as long as there are no leaks. This mode does not compensate correctly leaks.

12.1.5.2 Pressure-Controlled Modes (Table 12.4)

Currently, this mode is favored whatever the disease. The tidal volume is adjusted by increasing or decreasing the pressure limit (iPAP), the pressure gradient, and the ramp slope. The pressure is controlled, but the volume depends on lung compliance and airway resistance.

Table 12.4 Pressure modes

Continuous positive airway pressure	
CPAP Continuous positive airway pressure	– No inspiratory support – The pre-set pressure keeps the airway open – It reduces the work of breathing – This mode has the lowest asynchrony rate – The recruitment achieved with this mode helps to correct hypoxemia in patients with type I acute respiratory failure – This mode is not appropriate for patients with type II respiratory failure, except for obstructive apnea Best indications: bronchiolitis, obstructive apnea, transport
Bi-level ventilation modes [11, 12]	
S Spontaneous mode:	– The patient activates (trigger) the inspiration support – The patient controls inspiratory time (Ti) – The patient controls the respiratory rate – The physician controls the expiratory pressure (ePAP) and inspiratory pressure (iPAP) – In case of leaks, Ti increases inadequately creating asynchrony **This mode is not adapted for patients unable to trigger all their breaths**
S/T Spontaneous/timed mode	– In addition to spontaneous mode, this mode delivers additional controlled (timed) breaths if the patient's breath rate falls below the clinician's set "backup" breath rate – Ti is set accordingly to these backup breaths **If the machine does not detect the patient's breath, a mandatory (timed) breath will be delivered**
Assisted/controlled pressure control	In addition to the S/T mode, Ti is set for both assisted (triggered by the patient) and mandatory breaths
AVAPS (average volume-assured pressure support)	– Hybrid mode – Volume-targeted pressure control ventilation – The pressure support is adapted from measures of exhaled VT in order to deliver a programmed average TV
IVAPS (intelligent volume assured pressure support)	– Hybrid mode – Targeted alveolar minute volume by adjusting inspiratory pressures and backup respiratory rate on the size of the patient
NIV NAVA (neurally adjusted ventilatory assist)	This mode uses the electrical activity of the diaphragm (Edi) in order to synchronize and support proportionally to the patient's respiratory drive. Several studies confirm that neural trigger assures better synchrony, although the impact on other important clinical outcomes has not been demonstrated

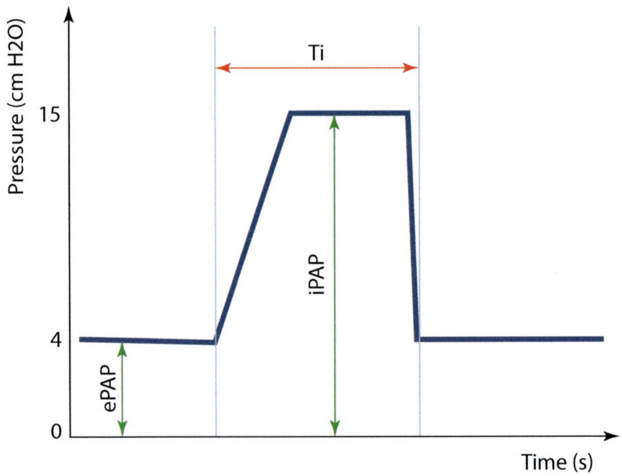

Fig. 12.4 Bilevel ventilation. *ePAP* expiratory Positive Airway Pressure, *iPAP* inspiratory Positive Airway Pressure, T_i inspiratory time

12.1.5.3 Initial Settings

- **CPAP**
  - ePAP: 5–10 cm H_2O (bronchiolitis: 7 cm H_2O)
- **Bi-level ventilation modes** (Fig. 12.4)
  - iPAP: 7–8 cm H_2O
  - ePAP: 5–6 cm H_2O
  - Ti max: close to the patient's needs (one-third of the cycle)
  - Inspiratory trigger: sensitivity +++ (but without auto-triggering)
  - Cycling (expiratory trigger): 40–80% of the maximum flow

12

The first objective is the comfort of the patient, then ePAP and iPAP will be titrated to optimize oxygenation and CO_2 removal.

- Δ iPAP: +2 cm H_2O every 5 min according to thorax extension (VT: 8–10 mL/kg, target iPAP setting: 10–20 cm H_2O)
- Δ ePAP: +1 cm H_2O (according to the FiO_2, target ePAP setting: 5–8 cm H_2O).

12.1.6 Installation

Two caregivers are needed for the first installation. The first keeps the interface centered on the child's face. The second one starts the ventilation and adapts the straps.

- Select the appropriate ventilator and interface (size; vented/nonvented; nasal/oro-nasal/total face):
  - If CPAP is required, we propose to select a nasal or oro-nasal mask
  - If bi-level support is required, we propose as first choice oro-nasal or total facemask
- Provide a good fitting of the interface, maintaining an appropriate oxygenation

- Connect to the circuit and turn on the ventilator
- Check for leaks and adjust the straps. A finger should pass between the strap and the skin

12.1.7 Analysis

During the first hour, comfort is the main objective. We propose to start with low parameters, and to increase them later according to the ventilation goals.

12.1.7.1 Efficiency

Efficacy criteria will be checked according to the acronym **R.T.W.O** (◘ Table 12.5).

12.1.7.2 Tolerance

- We encourage the presence of the parents, the use of a "cuddly toy," and/or a pacifier
- Fight against the leaks, especially those toward the eyes
- Check and improve the synchrony patient ventilator (◘ Table 12.6)
- A sedative may be used, such as hydroxyzine (1 mg/kg oral) or dexmedetomidine (4 µg/kg intranasal)

12.1.8 Next Steps

- When to escalate

  In situations with no improvement regarding **R.T.W.O** after a couple of NIV hours, escalation should be discussed [13]. In addition, factors such as decreased level of consciousness, inability to clear secretion, and interface intolerance increase the risk of NIV failure.
- When to wean

  As soon as **R.T.W.O** improves and remains stable after a few hours, a weaning protocol should be initiated.

◘ Table 12.5 Efficacy criteria

	Success	Action in case of failure
RR	Decrease	Increase iPAP by 2 cm H_2O steps
Thoracic extension	Significant thoracic extension (target VT: 8 mL/kg)	Increase iPAP by 2 cm H_2O steps
WOB	Decrease	Increase iPAP by 2 cm H_2O steps
Oxygenation	Decrease	Increase ePAP by 1 cm H_2O steps

Table 12.6 Asynchrony

Asynchrony	Curves	Management
Ineffective effort	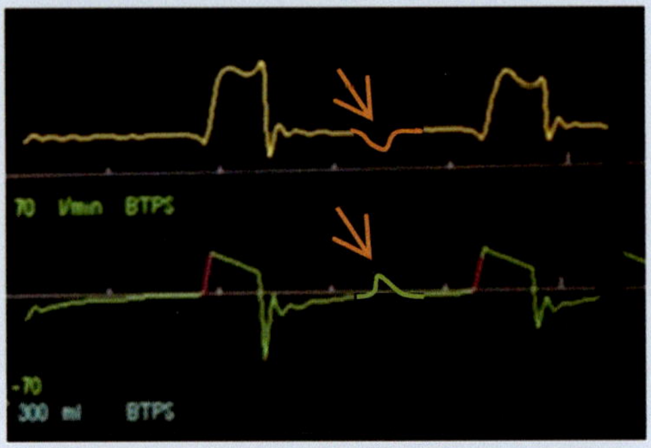	Absence of triggering: – Reduce leaks, sensitize the trigger, change interface, change ventilator
Autotriggering		A cycle is delivered, although the patient did not trigger it: – Reduce leaks, reduce trigger sensitivity
Pressurization asynchrony		The patient is "thirsty for air": – Increase the flow speed (decrease the ramp time)
Double triggering	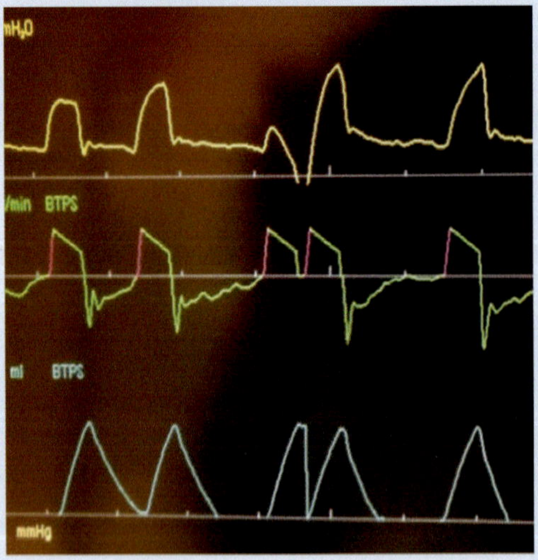	The patient "asks for more": a second cycle is triggered before the end of the previous one – Increase either the flow speed, Ti, or iPAP

(continued)

12

Table 12.6 (continued)

Asynchrony	Curves	Management
Inspiration time too long	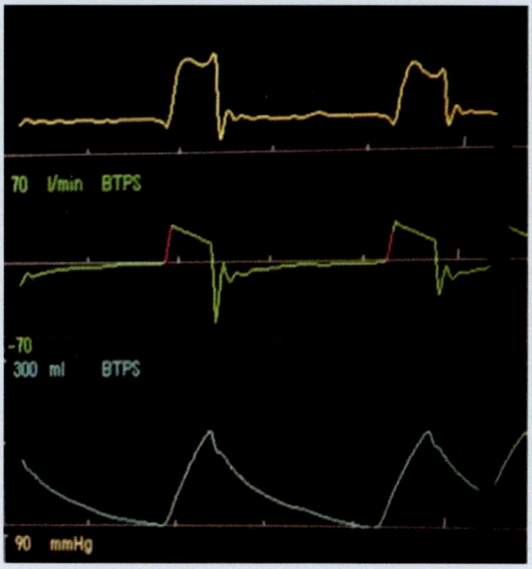	The patient wants to exhale against the machine (increase at the end-part of the inspiratory pressure curve): – Decrease Ti or cycling – Check for leaks

12.2 HFNC

12.2.1 Introduction

Over the last decade, HFNC has increasingly been used for oxygen delivery in neonatology departments, gradually replacing nasal CPAP. Its use in pediatrics departments is more recent. The HFNC was first employed in intensive care units, then in emergency departments, and today is finding use during pre- or inter-hospital transport.

Clinicians are quite rightly raising questions about where it should be positioned among the systems of oxygenation and noninvasive respiratory support, such as high concentration face masks and nasal CPAP. Its mode of action is original and complex. Initiating HFNC is relatively simple, but close monitoring is essential.

12.2.2 Mechanism of Action

HFNC is designed to administer a heated and humidified mixture of air and oxygen at a flow higher than the patient's inspiratory flow [14]. There is currently no single, simple definition of high flow.

The flow should therefore be at least equal to the peak tidal inspiratory flow (PTIF). This PTIF is of the order of 30 L/min in adults, and 1.7–2 L/min/kg in infants with bronchiolitis [15]. Several studies suggest the presence of an upper threshold. Indeed, beyond this threshold, no improvement was observed [16, 17].

12.2.2.1 Gas Mixture Conditioning

HFNC provides a relative humidity of nearly 100% with the gas warmed between 34 °C and 37 °C. Compared with "low-flow oxygenation" or the high-concentration oxygen mask, HFNC improves patient tolerance by reducing the sensation of respiratory distress and mouth dryness. Furthermore, it improved muco-ciliary clearance. Heated and humidified gas diminishes the resistance in the nasal mucosa induced by dry and cold gas, a point that should not be neglected given that these resistances make up nearly 50% of the total resistance of the respiratory system.

12.2.2.2 High Flow

A flow higher than the patient's inspiratory flow provides better oxygen delivery than "low flow" oxygen therapy or the high-concentration oxygenation mask. This observation has been explained as the effect of a high flow on the oropharyngeal dead space. Dead space washout also reduces CO_2 rebreathing. The extra-thoracic dead space is proportionally two to three times greater in children than in adults. It may measure up to 3 mL/kg in newborns and becomes similar to the adult volume only after 6 years of age (0.8 mL/kg) [18]. Consequently, the younger a child, the greater the effect of a high flow on oxygenation and CO_2 clearance [19].

12.2.2.3 Generated Pressures

A high-flow mixture is likely to create a modest positive pharyngeal pressure of about 4 cm H_2O during expiration [20]. The pressure is determined not only by the flow but also by the ratio of the prong/nostril fit and whether or not the mouth is closed. The inter- and intra-individual variations are nevertheless quite wide [18]. Recent work suggests that this effect should not be the primary mechanism of action in bronchiolitis, and that HFNC should not be used for lung recruitment, but rather to reduce obstructive apnea [21]. The effects of the continuous positive pressure generated by HFNC differ with the ventilation phase. Positive pressure at the beginning of inspiration may compensate for the inspiratory burden related to auto-PEEP and facilitate inspiratory flow (▶ Sect. 2.5.1). Positive pressure during expiration prevents small airway collapse (stenting effect), increases the expiratory time, and reduces the auto-PEEP. The favorable effect of this technique on the ventilation/perfusion ratio has not been clearly established. This suggests the need for caution when HFNC is used in the management of respiratory failure type 1.

12.2.3 Side Effects and Monitoring

Compared with other systems delivering CPAP, cutaneous tolerance is better with fewer skin lesions reported. However, like any respiratory support system, this device has drawbacks. For example, the noise level reaches about 80 dB. The decibel level is correlated with the flow and may be higher than that generated by other CPAP systems [22].

Some pneumothorax and pneumo-mediastinum were reported during HFNC use [23]. The risk of air leak syndrome could be associated with an inappropriate prong size that occludes the nostril lumen.

Finally, the greatest risk in using HFNC, as for the NIV strategy, is that recourse to more invasive management may be delayed in cases of respiratory decompensation. In children, the risk of HFNC failure, defined as intubation requirement, ranges from 8% to 19% and reaches nearly 30% when escalation in respiratory support is also taken into consideration. In children younger than 2 years, HFNC failure may occur within 7–14 h [24]. HFNC should therefore be initiated in an emergency department or a pediatric intensive care unit that has sufficient staff to closely monitor the patient's clinical course and who are well trained to recognize the early signs of failure. After several hours of stability, the infant may be transferred to a conventional ward, depending on hospital policy.

12.2.4 HFNC Initiation in Practice (◘ Fig. 12.5)

The HFNC system has a few parts: the cannula, a flow generator, an air/oxygen blender, and a respiratory gas humidifier.

12.2.4.1 Where to Initiate HFNC

Most HFNC studies took place in ICUs, emergency departments, and a few during pre- or inter-hospital transport [25]. The ward admitting the child will nevertheless need to provide close surveillance and be equipped with a centralized alarm system for early detection of respiratory failure or signs of decompensation.

12.2.4.2 Cannula

The prong caliber is adapted to the nostril size in order to allow for leakage and avoid overpressure phenomena. The prong diameter should be about half that of the nostril [24]. It may be useful for infants to reduce mouth leaks with a pacifier.

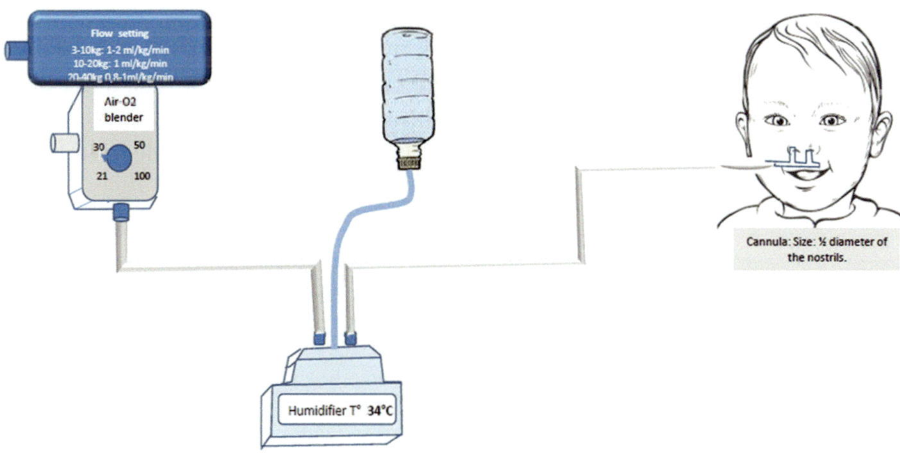

◘ **Fig. 12.5** Equipment to administer high-flow nasal cannulae

12.2.4.3 Generator

Three types of gas generators are currently available:

- The first type uses an air/oxygen blender and is connected to a system to humidify and heat the gas. Several devices are available: Optiflow System® (Fisher and Paekel, Auckland, New Zealand), Precision Flow® (Vapotherm, Exeter, UK), and Comfort-Flo® (Teleflex Medical, Durham, NC, USA).
- The second type uses a turbine + humidifier (Airvo2®, Fisher and Paekel, Auckland, New Zealand). This system has the advantage of not requiring an external source of gas, except oxygen. This device cannot be used with neonates and its start-up is sometimes a bit long compared with other types.
- The third type is based on a CPAP or conventional ventilator with an HFNC breathing circuit connected to the humidifier.

12.2.4.4 Settings (▫ Table 12.7)

12.2.5 Indications for HFNC

Despite the advantages of this technique, the quality of the literature dealing with a pediatric population remains poor.

The most prudent course would be to restrict HFNC therapy to mild forms of respiratory distress and situations of discomfort or interface intolerance. Whatever the etiology of the respiratory distress, observational studies suggest significant success rates [15, 26–29].

12.2.5.1 Acute Viral Bronchiolitis

12

HFNC has most often been evaluated in populations with acute viral bronchiolitis, with several studies comparing the efficacy and tolerance of HFNC with different CPAP systems [26], including a decreased rate of intubation as compared with historical controls prior to HFNC [26]. Four RCTs compared HFNC vs CPAP. In the largest one, Milési et al. found a higher failure rate of HFNC [30]. The other three studies, with variable outcomes, did not confirm these results [31–33].

A recent meta-analysis (15 studies, 1127 patients) showed that prophylactic use of HFNC did not reduce PICU admission [34–36].

▫ Table 12.7 Proposition of flow setting according to the weight of the patient

Weight (kg)	Flow setting (L/kg/min)
3–10	1–2
10–20	1
20–40	0.8–1
>40	0.5–1

Therefore, it seems reasonable to reserve NIV/CPAP for severe bronchiolitis and to limit HFNC use to moderate forms of the disease.

Overall, the studies showed that HFNC is safe in pediatric wards and not associated with higher rates of significant adverse events.

12.2.5.2 Withdrawal of Invasive Ventilation

In the neonatal population, weaning from invasive ventilation is one of the main indications for HFNC, [37]. This result has not been confirmed in the pediatric population [27].

12.2.5.3 Asthma

From a physiological point of view, HFNC for asthmatic patients seems attractive. The use of heated and humidified high-flow gas rates may reduce the burden on the inspiratory muscles related to auto-PEEP, and limit bronchoconstriction induced by cold dry gas. Few studies demonstrated the interest of this device [28]. An observational study suggested that the failure rate was higher with HFNC than with NIV (8/20 patients vs 0/22 patients) [29]. The multicenter randomized controlled open-label study CANULASTHME has the objective to evaluate the efficacy of HFNC in reducing first-line treatment failure in children with status asthmaticus, in comparison to standard oxygen therapy. This trial is currently in the recruiting phase.

If HFNC is used in this indication, special attention should be paid to inhalation therapy. The dose of bronchodilator received varies from 0.5% to 25% of the administered dose. Distal bronchodilator delivery might be improved by decreasing the flow, positioning the aerosol upstream of the humidifier, and choosing an ultrasonic nebulizer over a pneumatic nebulizer [38].

12.2.5.4 ARDS

This is a controversial point. Indeed, HFNC has little effect on lung recruitment, thus NIV or even invasive ventilation should be preferably used. Nevertheless, the quality of oxygenation, higher comfort, and the results of the FLORALI study which found lower intubation rates in the most severe forms of ARDS have fueled the discussion [39].

In the adult population, a meta-analysis suggests that the efficacy of high flow is comparable to that of NIV in terms of intubation rates, escalation of respiratory support, and mortality [40]. In patients with low work of breathing or low risk of PSILI (Patient Self-Inflicted Lung Injury), a trial of HFNC support may be considered. However, if SpO_2 to FiO_2 ratio does not improve in the following hours, the situation should be reevaluated, in order to avoid delayed intubation and worse clinical outcomes [41].

12.2.5.5 Preoxygenation and Intubation

This is an important part of an intubation procedure. It is intended to reduce the incidence of desaturation, bradycardia, procedural failure, and cardiorespiratory arrest. This step is even more important in young infants; as their oxygen stores are lower [42].

In the adult population, a meta-analysis showed the superiority of HFNC compared to conventional oxygen therapy, and a nearly comparable efficacy to NIV

[43]. In neonatology, a recent study showed the superiority of high flow compared to standard care for successful intubation on the first attempt without physiological instability [44].

Finally, the high flow has an interesting place in this indication, which argues for the presence of a high-flow module on ICU ventilators.

12.2.6 Conclusion

HFNC use is increasing in pediatric wards, despite the lack of clearly established benefits in the medical literature. The most cited indication in the literature is moderate to severe bronchiolitis in infants, but recent reports suggest HFNC may also be effectively and safely applied to a broader spectrum of patient ages and diseases [28, 29, 31]. The device is very attractive because of its simplicity and excellent tolerance. On a practical level, this treatment should be initiated in the emergency department or the pediatric ICU in order to evaluate its effectiveness and identify as early as possible the signs of failure requiring more appropriate respiratory support.

References

1. Morris JV, Ramnarayan P, Parslow RC, Fleming SJ. Outcomes for children receiving noninvasive ventilation as the first-line mode of mechanical ventilation at intensive care admission: a propensity score-matched cohort study. Crit Care Med. 2017;45(6):1045–53.
2. Lazner MR, Basu AP, Klonin H. Non-invasive ventilation for severe bronchiolitis: analysis and evidence. Pediatr Pulmonol. 2012;47(9):909–16.
3. Borckink I, Essouri S, Laurent M, et al. Infants with severe respiratory syncytial virus needed less ventilator time with nasal continuous airways pressure then invasive mechanical ventilation. Acta Paediatr. 2014;103(1):81–5.
4. Javouhey E, Barats A, Richard N, Stamm D, Floret D. Non-invasive ventilation as primary ventilatory support for infants with severe bronchiolitis. Intensive Care Med. 2008;34(9):1608–14.
5. Gomez-Merino E, Bach JR. Duchenne muscular dystrophy: prolongation of life by noninvasive ventilation and mechanically assisted coughing. Am J Phys Med Rehabil. 2002;81(6):411–5.
6. Thill PJ, McGuire JK, Baden HP, Green TP, Checchia PA. Noninvasive positive-pressure ventilation in children with lower airway obstruction. Pediatr Crit Care Med. 2004;5:337–42.
7. Mayordomo-Colunga J, Medina A, Rey C, et al. Non invasive ventilation after extubation in paediatric patients: a preliminary study. BMC Pediatr. 2010;10:29.
8. Schettino GP, Chatmongkolchart S, Hess DR, Kacmarek RM. Position of exhalation port and mask design affect CO_2 rebreathing during noninvasive positive pressure ventilation. Crit Care Med. 2003;31(8):2178–82.
9. Mortamet G, Amaddeo A, Essouri S, Renolleau S, Emeriaud G, Fauroux B. Interfaces for noninvasive ventilation in the acute setting in children. Paediatr Respir Rev. 2017;23:84–8.
10. Conti G, Spinazzola G, Gregoretti C, et al. Comparative bench study evaluation of different infant interfaces for non-invasive ventilation. BMC Pulm Med. 2018;18(1):57.
11. Rabec C, Emeriaud G, Amadeo A, Fauroux B, Georges M. New modes in non-invasive ventilation. Paediatr Respir Rev. 2016;18:73–84.
12. Pavone M, Verrillo E, Caldarelli V, Ullmann N, Cutrera R. Non-invasive positive pressure ventilation in children. Early Hum Dev. 2013;89(Suppl 3):S25–31.
13. Mayordomo-Colunga J, Medina A, Rey C, et al. Predictive factors of non invasive ventilation failure in critically ill children: a prospective epidemiological study. Intensive Care Med. 2009;35(3):527–36.

14. Lee JH, Rehder KJ, Williford L, Cheifetz IM, Turner DA. Use of high flow nasal cannula in critically ill infants, children, and adults: a critical review of the literature. Intensive Care Med. 2013;39:247–57.
15. Milési C, Requirand A, Douillard A, et al. Assessment of peak inspiratory flow in young infants with acute viral bronchiolitis: physiological basis for initial flow setting in patients supported with high-flow nasal cannula. J Pediatr. 2021;231:239–45.
16. Milési C, Pierre AF, Deho A, et al. A multicenter randomized controlled trial of a 3-L/kg/min versus 2-L/kg/min high-flow nasal cannula flow rate in young infants with severe viral bronchiolitis (TRAMONTANE 2). Intensive Care Med. 2018;44(11):1870–8.
17. Weiler T, Kamerkar A, Hotz J, Ross PA, Newth CJL, Khemani RG. The relationship between high flow nasal cannula flow rate and effort of breathing in children. J Pediatr. 2017;189:66–71.
18. Numa AH, Newth CJ. Anatomic dead space in infants and children. J Appl Physiol. 1996;80:1485–9.
19. Dysart K, Miller T, Wolfson M, Marla R, Shaffer TH. Research in high flow therapy: mechanisms of action. Respir Med. 2009;103:1400–5.
20. Milési C, Baleine J, Matecki S, et al. Is treatment with a high flow nasal cannula effective in acute viral bronchiolitis? A physiologic study. Intensive Care Med. 2013;39:1088–94.
21. Guglielmo RD, Hotz JC, Ross PA, et al. High-flow nasal cannula reduces effort of breathing but not consistently via positive end-expiratory pressure. Chest. 2022;162(4):861–71.
22. König K, Stock EL, Jarvis M. Noise levels of neonatal high-flow nasal cannula devices--an in-vitro study. Neonatology. 2013;103:264–7.
23. Hegde S, Prodhan P. Serious air leak syndrome complicating high-flow nasal cannula therapy: a report of 3 cases. Pediatrics. 2013;131:e939–44.
24. Abboud PA, Roth PJ, Skiles CL, Stolfi A, Rowin ME. Predictors of failure in infants with viral bronchiolitis treated with high-flow, high-humidity nasal cannula therapy. Pediatr Crit Care Med. 2012;13:e343–9.
25. Schlapbach LJ, Schaefer J, Brady AM, Mayfield S, Schibler A. High-flow nasal cannula (HFNC) support in interhospital transport of critically ill children. Intensive Care Med. 2014;40:592–9.
26. Schibler A, Pham TM, Dunster KR, et al. Reduced intubation rates for infants after introduction of high-flow nasal prong oxygen delivery. Intensive Care Med. 2011;37:847–52.
27. Ramnarayan P, Richards-Belle A, Drikite L, et al. Effect of high-flow nasal cannula therapy vs continuous positive airway pressure following extubation on liberation from respiratory support in critically ill children: a randomized clinical trial. JAMA. 2022;327:1555–65.
28. Baudin F, Buisson A, Vanel B, Massenavette B, Pouyau R, Javouhey E. Nasal high flow in management of children with status asthmaticus: a retrospective observational study. Ann Intensive Care. 2017;7(1):55.
29. Pilar J, Modesto I Alapont V, Lopez-Fernandez YM, Lopez-Macias O, Garcia-Urabayen D, Amores-Hernandez I. High-flow nasal cannula therapy versus non-invasive ventilation in children with severe acute asthma exacerbation: an observational cohort study. Med Intensiva. 2017;41(7):418–24.
30. Milési C, Essouri S, Pouyau R, et al. High flow nasal cannula (HFNC) versus nasal continuous positive airway pressure (nCPAP) for the initial respiratory management of acute viral bronchiolitis in young infants: a multicenter randomized controlled trial (TRAMONTANE study). Intensive Care Med. 2017;43(2):209–16.
31. Cesar RG, Bispo BRP, Felix P, et al. High-flow nasal cannula versus continuous positive airway pressure in critical bronchiolitis: a randomized controlled pilot. J Pediatr Intensive Care. 2020;9(4):248–55.
32. Sarkar M, Sinha R, Roychowdhoury S, et al. Comparative study between noninvasive continuous positive airway pressure and hot humidified high-flow nasal cannulae as a mode of respiratory support in infants with acute bronchiolitis in pediatric intensive care unit of a tertiary care hospital. Indian J Crit Care Med. 2018;22(2):85–90.
33. Vahlkvist S, Jürgensen L, la Cour A, Markoew S, Petersen TH, Kofoed PE. High flow nasal cannula and continuous positive airway pressure therapy in treatment of viral bronchiolitis: a randomized clinical trial. Eur J Pediatr. 2020;179(3):513–8.
34. Dafydd C, Saunders BJ, Kotecha SJ, Edwards MO. Efficacy and safety of high flow nasal oxygen for children with bronchiolitis: systematic review and meta-analysis. BMJ Open Respir Res. 2021;8(1):e000844.

35. Durand P, Guiddir T, Kyheng C, et al. A randomised trial of high-flow nasal cannula in infants with moderate bronchiolitis. Eur Respir J. 2020;56(1):1901926.
36. Franklin D, Babl FE, Schlapbach LJ, et al. A randomized trial of high-flow oxygen therapy in infants with bronchiolitis. N Engl J Med. 2018;378(12):1121–31.
37. Manley BJ, Owen LS, Doyle LW, et al. High-flow nasal cannulae in very preterm infants after extubation. N Engl J Med. 2013;369:1425–33.
38. Perry SA, Kesser KC, Geller DE, Selhorst DM, Rendle JK, Hertzog JH. Influences of cannula size and flow rate on aerosol drug delivery through the Vapotherm humidified high-flow nasal cannula system. Pediatr Crit Care Med. 2013;14:e250–6.
39. Frat J-P, Thille AW, Mercat A, et al. High-flow oxygen through nasal cannula in acute hypoxemic respiratory failure. N Engl J Med. 2015;372(23):2185–96.
40. Zhao H, Wang H, Sun F, Lyu S, An Y. High-flow nasal cannula oxygen therapy is superior to conventional oxygen therapy but not to noninvasive mechanical ventilation on intubation rate: a systematic review and meta-analysis. Crit Care. 2017;21(1):184.
41. Kang BJ, Koh Y, Lim C-M, et al. Failure of high-flow nasal cannula therapy may delay intubation and increase mortality. Intensive Care Med. 2015;41(4):623–32.
42. Hardman JG, Wills JS. The development of hypoxaemia during apnoea in children: a computational modelling investigation. Br J Anaesth. 2006;97(4):564–70.
43. Fong KM, Au SY, Ng GWY. Preoxygenation before intubation in adult patients with acute hypoxemic respiratory failure: a network meta-analysis of randomized trials. Crit Care. 2019;23(1):319.
44. Hodgson KA, Owen LS, Kamlin COF, et al. Nasal high-flow therapy during neonatal endotracheal intubation. N Engl J Med. 2022;386:1627–37.

Paediatric Acute Respiratory Distress Syndrome (pARDS)

Yolanda M. López-Fernández

Contents

J. Brierley et al. (eds.), *ESPNIC Children's Intensive Care Textbook*,
https://doi.org/10.1007/978-3-031-64762-8_13

Learning Objectives

- To identify pARDS using paediatric-specific criteria that allow the syndrome to be recognised and diagnosed in children.
- To understand the pathophysiology of pARDS in the context of the heterogeneity of this syndrome.
- To review the clinical practice recommendations of the second Paediatric Acute Lung Injury Consensus-Conference (PALICC-2) for the management and treatment of pARDS.

13.1 Introduction

Acute respiratory distress syndrome (ARDS) is a heterogeneous clinical syndrome associated with high morbidity and mortality. It is recognised as a non-cardiogenic lung oedema causing hypoxaemic respiratory failure following a systemic inflammatory response that damages the pulmonary alveolar-capillary membrane. Risk factors contributing to the development of ARDS may be of pulmonary (e.g., pneumonia) or extrapulmonary (e.g., sepsis) origin.

ARDS was first described by Ashbaugh et al. in 1967 in a case series of 12 patients (five of whom were less than 20 years old) with severe hypoxaemic acute respiratory failure, poor lung compliance and diffuse alveolar infiltrates on chest radiograph [1]. Because of the clinical and histological similarities (hyaline membrane formation) with the infant respiratory distress syndrome described in premature infants, they named this entity adult respiratory distress syndrome.

The original definition of ARDS was revised and renamed at the American-European Consensus Conference (1994), and almost 20 years later, the Berlin definition (2012) replaced the previous one [2, 3]. The Berlin definition classifies the severity of ARDS according to the degree of hypoxaemia, requires the use of the PaO_2/FiO_2 ratio as oxygenation metrics with a minimum PEEP of 5 cmH_2O, and advocates the use of cardiac ultrasonography to rule out a cardiac origin of the oedema. An update of the Berlin definition has recently been published (2023) to reflect changes in evidence and has been renamed the global definition of ARDS as it makes more flexible the diagnostic criteria depending on the availability of resources [4].

ARDS is often under-recognised by clinicians. This problem is aggravated in paediatrics because for years paediatric intensivists have used definitions of ARDS designed by adult intensivists for adult subjects. However, there are important differences between ARDS in children and adults owing to variations in the stage of lung development, risk factors, epidemiology, co-morbidities, and response to supportive therapies and outcomes. Therefore, limitations in the applicability of the adult criteria to children prompted the Paediatric Acute Lung Injury Consensus Conference (PALICC) group to publish a specific definition and guidelines for the management of ARDS in children in 2015. Since the publication of the pARDS definition, there has been a large increase in the number of studies using the PALICC criteria. The PALICC guidelines were updated in 2023 (PALICC-2) to reflect changes in clinical practice [5].

13.2 Definition of Paediatric ARDS (pARDS) (Table 13.1)

The PALICC pARDS definition is certainly based on the Berlin definition, but it also has unique differences. First, the radiographic criteria have been simplified by removing the requirement for bilateral infiltrates to reflect the high interobserver variability in reading radiographs and their limited prognostic relevance in pARDS [6]. Second, for intubated patients, severity is quantified by the oxygenation index (OI), which includes mean airway pressure (MAP) in addition to arterial partial pressure of oxygen (PaO_2) and fraction of inspired oxygen (FiO_2). Finally, fewer arterial

Table 13.1 The new PALICC definition of paediatric acute respiratory distress syndrome (pARDS)

Paediatric acute respiratory distress syndrome		
Age	<18 years, excluding patients with perinatal lung disease	
Timing	Within 7 days of a clinical insult	
Chest imaging	New opacities (unilateral or bilateral), not due primarily to atelectasis or pleural effusions on chest radiograph or thorax CT	
Origin of oedema	Not fully explained by cardiac failure or fluid overload	
Oxygenation	[a]Invasive MV: OI ≥4 or OSI ≥5	[b]NIV: PaO_2/FiO_2 ≤300 or SpO_2/FiO_2 ≤250
Stratification of PARDS severity: ≥4 h after initial diagnosis		
	Mild/moderate	**Severe**
IMV PARDS	OI <16 or OSI <12	OI ≥16 or OSI ≥12
NIV PARDS (full face mask)	PaO_2/FiO_2 >100 or SpO_2/FiO_2 >150	PaO_2/FiO_2 ≤100 or SpO_2/FiO_2 ≤150
Possible PARDS	HFNC (1.5 L/kg/min or >30 L/min) or <u>nasal</u> NIV (PaO_2/FiO_2 ≤300 or SpO_2/FiO_2 ≤250) Missing lung imaging/resource limited settings	
At-risk for PARDS	O_2 required to maintain SpO_2 ≥88% with any interface.	

CXR chest radiograph, *CPAP* continuous positive airway pressure, *CT* computed tomography scan, *FiO_2* fraction of inspired oxygen, *HFNC* high flow nasal cannula, *MAP* mean airway pressure, *NIV* non-invasive ventilation, *MV* mechanical ventilation, *O_2* oxygen, *OI* oxygenation index, *OSI* oxygenation saturation index, *PaO_2* partial pressure of arterial oxygen, *PEEP* positive end-expiratory pressure, *SpO_2* pulse-oximetric oxygen saturation

$OI = FiO_2/PaO_2 \times MAP \times 100$. $OSI = FiO_2/SpO_2 \times MAP \times 100$

Special populations: Cyanotic cardiac disease/chronic lung disease: above criteria, with acute deterioration in oxygenation from baseline. Stratification of pARDS severity does not apply to these populations

Additional note: pARDS should not be diagnosed in children with respiratory failure solely from airways obstruction (e.g., critical asthma, virus-induced bronchospasm)

[a]IMV-PARDS requires continuous positive airway pressure (CPAP) (or end-expiratory positive airway pressure [PEEP]) ≥ 5 cm H_2O.

[b]NIV-PARDS requires full facemask interface with CPAP or PEEP ≥ 5 cm H_2O.

blood gas tests are used in children to diagnose and assess the severity of hypoxaemia, which led the PALICC group to allow a metric of oxygenation severity using pulse oximetry oxygen saturation (SpO_2), such as the oxygenation saturation index (OSI) for children on invasive mechanical ventilation or the SpO_2/FiO_2 ratio for those on non-invasive ventilation.

The PALICC definition excludes perinatal lung disease, which is addressed by the neonatal definition of ARDS (Montreux definition) [7]. The paediatric definition also includes the diagnosis of pARDS in children with cyanotic congenital heart disease or chronic lung disease and has established specific criteria to identify children treated with non-invasive respiratory support (NRS) who are at risk of pARDS. A category of possible pPARDS has been created for those patients receiving high flow nasal cannula (HFNC) or nasal modes of NIV, since these modes of NRS are increasingly being used in the paediatric intensive care units (PICUs), even in children who are likely to have an ARDS pathophysiology. The possible pARDS category also includes patients who meet the pARDS criteria but are in resource-limited settings where chest X-ray is not readily available.

13.3 Epidemiology

A systematic review of the incidence and mortality of paediatric ARDS revealed a low incidence but high mortality. Incidence of pARDS was 3.5 cases/100,000/year and PICU incidence was 2.3% whereas mortality rate was 33.7%. These results also indicate that both the incidence and mortality of pARDS have not changed over the last two decades and that mortality depends on the geographical location of the studies [8]. In an international, prospective and cross-sectional study (PARDIE study) [9] involving 145 PICUs from 27 countries, 744 of 23,280 (3.2%) PICU patients were identified as having pARDS in approximately 6% of mechanically ventilated children according to PALICC definition. In contrast, the incidence of ARDS in the adult population is higher, ranging from 17.9 to 81 cases/100,000/year.

The most common causes of pARDS in children are pneumonia or lower respiratory tract infection followed by non-pulmonary sepsis. However, other relevant clinical conditions involve aspiration, trauma, pulmonary contusion and pulmonary haemorrhage, among others. Pre-existing comorbidities are also common, including chronic lung disease, prematurity, congenital heart disease or immunosuppression.

13.4 Pathophysiology

The pathophysiology of ARDS is characterised by inflammatory damage to the pulmonary endothelium and epithelium which leads to an increased vascular permeability, accumulation of protein-rich fluid inside the alveoli and interstitium, dysregulated inflammation and coagulation, and fibrosis [10]. Mechanical ventilation may aggravate this process especially if high volumes and pressures are applied (ventilator-induced lung injury, VILI).

Multiple risk factors can trigger lung injury marked by diffuse alveolar damage and subsequent release of proinflammatory cytokines. Cytokines recruit neutrophils into the lungs where they are activated and release toxic inflammatory mediators which damage the lung endothelium and epithelium leading to disruption of cell tight-junctions, cell apoptosis and necrosis of alveolar type-1 and -2 cells. Oncotic gradients disappear and prevent fluid reabsorption which leaks into the interstitial space and subsequently blood, protein-rich fluid and cell detritus occupy the alveolar space. Therefore, the barrier function of the endothelium and surfactant production is impaired.

All these microscopic changes result in:

- Impaired gas exchange due to ventilation/perfusion mismatch with hypoxaemic respiratory failure. Increased dead space impairs carbon dioxide (CO_2) exchange.
- Reduced lung distensibility due to lung stiffness and poor lung aeration. Extensive consolidation and atelectasis contribute to the "baby lung" concept.
- Pulmonary hypertension occurs in over 25% of patients with pARDS on mechanical ventilation due to hypoxic vasoconstriction, parenchymal destruction, airway collapse and hypercapnia.

The heterogeneity inherent to pARDS may reflect the existence of distinct subgroups of patients with respect to treatment response and prognosis, often referred to as subphenotypes or endotypes [10]. Patients belonging to a particular subphenotype share a risk factor, diagnostic characteristic, mortality risk or treatment response that distinguishes them from other subgroups. Endotypes are defined as subgroups with a common underlying pathophysiology. In adults, two subphenotypes have been identified with distinct clinical patterns: hyperinflammatory and hypoinflammatory. A recent paediatric study also confirms the presence of these two subphenotypes in pARDS, although with some differences between children and adults [11]. Plasma biomarkers (proteomics, metabolomics, transcriptomics) would be the markers of the underlying pathophysiology that would allow differentiation of one subphenotype from the other.

Understanding the pathophysiological mechanisms will allow to enrich studies of those patients at greatest risk of an outcome such as mortality (prognostic enrichment) and the identification of those who are likely to respond to a treatment based on their underlying pathobiology (predictive enrichment). Therefore, part of the future direction in pARDS research could be the characterisation of subgroups most likely to benefit from therapies that target common underlying biological mechanisms, to provide more personalized treatments.

13.5 Monitoring

13.5.1 General

- *Physical examination*: including clinical assessment of effort of breathing and patient–ventilator synchrony.
- *Respiratory rate (RR), heart rate (HR), blood pressure (BP) and* SpO_2: pulse oximetry alarms should be programmed to alert for oxygen saturations below the lower and upper limits and minimize the detrimental effects of hypoxia/hyperoxia. To calculate the OSI and SpO_2/FiO_2 ratio, it is necessary to reduce FiO_2 for SpO_2 <98%.

- *Exhaled tidal volume (V_T)*: to monitor protective MV strategies. Obese children have lung volumes that reflect their ideal body weight (IBW), whereas children with a low or normal body mass index have lung volumes that reflect actual body weight (ABW). The lower of ABW and IBW should be used to assess V_T [12].

13.5.2 Respiratory System Mechanics

- *Plateau pressure (P_{Plat}) and driving pressure (DP)*: P_{Plat} measurement requires a stable static or quasi-static manoeuvre with no flow and an end-inspiratory pause to allow pressure equilibration in the lung. In patients managed with pressure-controlled ventilation, P_{Plat} and peak pressure may be similar if inspiratory flow reaches zero prior to exhalation [12].
- *Intrinsic positive end-expiratory pressure (PEEPi)*: PEEPi can be quantified during quasi-static conditions using an end-expiratory *occlusion*.
- *Flow–time (and pressure–time) waveforms*: PEEPi can be identified by examination of the expiratory flow–time curve.

13.5.3 Oxygenation and CO_2 Monitoring

- *Severity of pARDS*: OI/OSI for intubated patients; PaO_2/FiO_2 and SpO_2/FiO_2 ratios for patients on non-invasive respiratory support (NRS).
- *Blood gas monitoring* (ideally arterial sample): not only for oxygenation assessment, but also for evaluation of pH and $PaCO_2$, especially in the context of permissive hypercapnia.
- *Capnography*: *end-tidal CO_2* ($PetCO_2$) reflects significant changes to $PaCO_2$, although may add anatomic dead space contributing to hypoventilation in young infants. In children on NRS or High Frequency Oscillatory Ventilation (HFOV), *transcutaneous CO_2 monitoring* can be used instead of the end-tidal CO_2.

13

Elevation of alveolar dead space can be related to low pulmonary perfusion (i.e., cardiac output) or alveolar overdistension and is associated with worse outcomes. Alveolar dead space fraction ($AVDSf = [PaCO_2 - PetCO_2]/PaCO_2$) allows an estimate of dead space to be calculated in the absence of volumetric capnography [10, 12].

13.5.4 Chest Imaging

- *Chest X-ray*: mandatory criterion for the diagnosis of pARDS.
- *Lung ultrasonography (LUS) and Electrical Impedance Tomography (EIT)*: radiation-free modalities that enable bedside assessment of the pathophysiology and complications of pARDS in real time.
- *Chest CT* allows quantification of functional residual capacity, lung strain and lung recruitment potential, but it has risks associated with transport to the radiology room and radiation.

13.5.5 Hemodynamic Monitoring

- *Arterial catheter* for haemodynamic monitoring and blood gas analysis in severe pARDS.
- *Echocardiogram* to assess left and right ventricular function, preload and pulmonary arterial pressure.
- *Central venous saturation* when the target SpO_2 is low (88–92%).
- *Cumulative fluid balance*, including insensible fluid losses, fluid administration prior to ICU admission and diuresis monitoring using a urinary catheter.

13.6 Treatment

13.6.1 Non-Invasive Respiratory Support (NRS)

13.6.1.1 High Flow Nasal Cannula (HFNC)

The new PALICC-2 definition adds a Possible pARDS category, which includes patients who meet pARDS criteria but receive HFNC at >1.5 L/kg/min or >30 L/min.

HFNC is increasingly used in children with possible pARDS and at risk for pARDS due to the ease of application and perceived improvement in tolerance compared to NIV. However, there is little data to support the physiologic mechanism behind HFNC in pARDS. PEEP generation does not seem to be the main mechanism of action, but rather the effect of dead space washout in the upper airway or improved airway flow dynamics [13].

13.6.1.2 Non-Invasive Ventilation (NIV): Continuous Positive Airway Pressure (CPAP) and Bilevel Positive Airway Pressure (BiPAP)

NIV is increasingly used in children with acute hypoxaemic respiratory failure to avoid intubation. However, severe hypoxaemia is an important risk factor for NIV failure and determining who may require intubation is challenging. In the largest observational study of children with pARDS (PARDIE study) that included 744 children, 160 were treated initially with NIV with a failure rate of 50% [9].

Children with pARDS may benefit from a time-limited trial of NIV. Potential harms of NIV in pARDS include intubation delay and patient self-inflicted lung injury (P-SILI) when the ventilatory drive is high. Intubation is recommended in children who do not show clinical improvement or have signs of worsening disease as reflected by increased RR, HR and work of breathing and worsening gas exchange as measured by SpO_2/FiO_2 ratio within <6 h of initiation of NIV. In addition, there are two subpopulations of patients who are more likely to NIV failure; therefore, intubation should be initiated earlier [13]:

- Immunosuppressed patients, in whom prolonged exposure (more than 6 h) to NIV and HFNC has been associated with worse outcomes, including increased mortality.
- Children with severe NIV-PARDS or with other severe organ dysfunction.

CPAP can be an effective mode of initial ventilatory support, but if inspiratory muscle effort and work of breathing are increased, the addition of inspiratory pressure (BiPAP) is recommended to maximise the potential benefit of NIV. NIV should be used by trained staff and closely monitored in a safe environment (ideally the PICU). Furthermore, an adequate interface provides efficient patient–ventilator synchronisation. Heated humidification should be routinely used to avoid nasal mucosal injury, increased work of breathing and decreased interface tolerance. In certain circumstances, sedation (e.g., dexmetomidine) may improve both synchrony and interface tolerance in a monitored environment and with experienced practitioners.

13.6.1.3 NRS in Resource-Limited Settings (RLS)

CPAP (bubble-CPAP), HFNC or low-flow oxygen are the primary methods of respiratory support in these settings. Five RCTs comparing the use of these modes of NRS favour CPAP over HFNC and low-flow oxygen. All trials were conducted in heterogeneous populations of children, likely including patients with pARDS although the definition criteria were not specifically assessed. Of note, CPAP also implies a risk of adverse events if it is used without oversight or without staff adequately trained in the use of CPAP devices [13].

13.6.2 Invasive Mechanical Ventilation (IMV)

The strategy of lung-protective ventilation is built on physiologic V_T delivery to avoid ventilator-induced lung injury (VILI), and PEEP titration to prevent cyclic alveolar collapse (de-recruitment).

13.6.2.1 V_T

13

A physiologic V_T between 6 and 8 mL/kg should be used in patients with pARDS, but further reduction of V_T <6 mL/kg may be required to maintain lung-protective limits on plateau pressure (P_{Plat}) and driving pressure (DP). V_T <4 mL/kg should be used with caution because of a U-shape curve in the relationship between V_T and mortality, with higher mortality at both low (<4 mL/kg) and high (>8 mL/kg) V_T [14].

13.6.2.2 Pressures

Plateau pressure (P_{Plat}) should be limited to 28 cmH_2O (up to 32 cmH_2O for patients with reduced chest wall compliance) and Driving Pressure (DP) to 15 cmH_2O. It should be kept in mind that the relationship between P_{Plat} and peak inspiratory pressure (PIP) are influenced by mode of ventilation, flow characteristics, airway resistance and patient effort. P_{Plat} and DP (P_{Plat}–PEEP) should be measured under static conditions that includes an inspiratory pause to measure P_{Plat} and an expiratory pause to ensure there is no intrinsic PEEP [12].

13.6.2.3 PEEP

PEEP should be titrated at or above the lower PEEP/higher FiO_2 table according to the ARDS Network protocol. Subsequently, PEEP can be adjusted to balance oxygen delivery, haemodynamics and lung compliance to prevent P_{Plat} and/or DP limits being exceeded [13].

FiO_2	0.3	0.4	0.5	0.6	0.7	0.8	0.9	1
PEEP cmH_2O	5	6–8	8–10	10	10–14	14	14–18	18–24

13.6.2.4 Lung-Protective Ventilation (LPV) Bundles

Adherence to LPV protocols prioritizes maintaining multiple ventilator settings (V_T, FiO_2, P_{Plat}, DP, PEEP) within the suggested limits as well as using electronic tools (detection algorithms) and educational programmes.

13.6.2.5 Oxygenation Target

SpO_2 should be maintained between 92% and 97% for mild/moderate pARDS, whereas for severe pARDS SpO_2 between 88% and 92% can be accepted to reduce FiO_2 exposure (permissive hypoxaemia).

13.6.2.6 Ventilation Target

Permissive hypercapnia (pH ≥7.20) allows ventilator settings to be maintained within recommended pressure and tidal volume limits to prevent VILI. Exceptions to this ventilatory strategy might be intracranial hypertension, severe pulmonary hypertension, selected congenital heart disease, haemodynamic instability and significant ventricular dysfunction. Bicarbonate supplementation should also not be used routinely except in patients with severe metabolic acidosis or pulmonary hypertension that adversely affects cardiac function or haemodynamic stability.

13.6.2.7 Mode of Ventilation

There are no outcome data on the influence of a determined mode during conventional MV. Other less conventional modes, such as airway pressure release ventilation (APRV), have been tested in pARDS showing no superiority or even equivalence compared to conventional low V_T ventilation [15].

High frequency oscillatory ventilation (HFOV): Paediatric studies show no clear improvement in outcomes with the use of HFOV compared with conventional MV in pARDS. Therefore, the PALICC-2 recommendation was neutral, neither for nor against. However, HFOV may be considered in circumstances where adequate gas exchange cannot be maintained with conventional lung-protective ventilation. When using HFOV in patients with pARDS, lung volume should be optimised with a stepwise increase and decrease in MAP while monitoring oxygenation, CO_2 and haemodynamic parameters [14].

13.6.2.8 Recruitment Manoeuvres (RMs)

RMs can prevent lung collapse and improve oxygenation. Paediatric observational studies have shown that children tolerate RMs without haemodynamic compromise, significant barotrauma, hypoxaemia or arrhythmia. However, data from adult RCTs highlight the potential for harm when aggressive RMs are performed. PALICC-2 recommendation was neutral, neither for nor against the use of RMs in pARDS. However, in selected patients with severe pARDS, cautious stepwise RMs (i.e., incremental PEEP increases of 2 cmH_2O followed by decremental PEEP titration) may be performed while continuously monitoring oxygenation, lung compliance and haemodynamics. Sustained manoeuvres are not recommended in pARDS [14].

13.6.3 Ancillary Treatments [16, 17]

13.6.3.1 Prone Positioning

There is strong evidence to support the use of prone positioning in adults with ARDS. The paediatric literature supports this inexpensive treatment, which does not require any special equipment other than the presence of experienced staff. Furthermore, prone positioning is readily implemented across different geo-economic healthcare settings. The procedure has been reported to be safe in children, despite the inherent risks associated with loss of vascular access or endotracheal tube displacement. However, there is a lack of data demonstrating improved clinical outcomes in pARDS, so PALICC-2 does not have sufficient data to support or refute the use of prone positioning in patients with pARDS and should only be considered in patients with hypoxaemia refractory to other interventions.

13.6.3.2 Inhaled Nitric Oxide (iNO)

iNO provides a vasodilatory effect in the lungs, which improves ventilation/perfusion matching. However, the effect of improved oxygenation appears to be only temporary. Moreover, this treatment is costly, may cause renal failure and prolonged exposure is associated with methemoglobinemia. Therefore, PALICC-2 recommends against the routine use of iNO in patients with pARDS, although it may be considered in patients with known pulmonary hypertension, severe right ventricular dysfunction or as a rescue or bridge to ECMO. To minimise toxicity and costs associated with unnecessary exposure, the effect of iNO should be assessed serially, especially during the first hours of administration.

13.6.3.3 Surfactant

PALICC-2 recommends against the routine use of surfactant therapy in patients with pARDS, and there is still insufficient evidence to know which subpopulations may benefit. Several well-conducted multicentre paediatric trials show no significant benefit on clinical outcomes, combined with the potential adverse events associated with surfactant administration (hypotension, hypoxia and bradycardia).

13.6.3.4 Corticosteroids

PALICC-2 recommends against the routine use of corticosteroids in patients with pARDS. Although some studies show that glucocorticoid administration leads to a reduction in inflammatory markers, there are insufficient data to support improved outcomes in children with pARDS. However, recent studies in adults and emerging data from patients with COVID-19 suggest that may be beneficial in ARDS. Therefore, corticosteroids may be considered in patients with pARDS caused by SARS-CoV-2.

13.6.3.5 Neuromuscular Blockade (NMB)

NMBs help to optimise protective ventilation, improve patient–ventilator synchrony, prevent self-induced lung injury (pSILI), reduce barotrauma and decrease metabolic rate and oxygen consumption in severe pARDS. However, prolonged exposure to NMBs masks assessment of pain, sedation, level of consciousness and delirium, may cause ventilator-induced diaphragm dysfunction and is associated with long-term neuromuscular weakness. PALICC-2 recommends the combined use of NMB and sedation when the goals of protective MV cannot be achieved with sedation alone.

13.6.4 Other Ancillary Treatments [17]

13.6.4.1 Fluid Management

Fluid resuscitation in pARDS allows for the maintenance of adequate intravascular volume to achieve adequate oxygen delivery and optimal end-organ perfusion. However, data in paediatric patients have shown that fluid overload (>20%) and cumulative positive fluid balance on day 3 are associated with increased morbidity, particularly in the setting of acute kidney injury (AKI). The fluid strategy should aim to prevent and treat fluid overload to reduce pulmonary oedema and improve oxygenation.

13.6.4.2 Nutrition

Enteral nutrition reduces bacterial translocation through the gastrointestinal tract and prevents mucosal atrophy. Therefore, early initiation of enteral nutrition (<72 h) is recommended in pARDS when feasible. In addition, patients with pARDS may have altered metabolism and often increased protein catabolism, so protein intakes ≥1.5 g/kg/day are the goal to achieve a positive protein balance.

13.6.4.3 Transfusion

Critically ill patients often require transfusion of red blood cells (RBCs), but transfusion is associated with risks including infections, transfusion-related acute lung injury (TRALI) and fluid overload. Although the optimal transfusion threshold for patients with pARDS is unknown, PALICC-2 recommends against RBC transfusion in patients with haemoglobin ≥7 g/dL, haemodynamically stable, without severe hypoxaemia, cyanotic heart disease or haemolytic anaemia.

13.7 ECMO

13.7.1 Indications/Initiation

ECMO support should be considered in severe pARDS when the underlying condition is thought to be reversible or as a bridge to lung transplantation. ECMO in severe pARDS enables the reduction of toxic ventilator settings associated with VILI and provides better control of hypercapnia. Despite this, ECMO is associated with inherent risks, notably haemorrhage, thrombosis and neurological damage.

There is no evidence to support strict criteria for the selection of patients who will benefit from ECMO in severe pARDS, but serial assessments of OI/OSI, gas exchange, MV settings and organ severity scores may be helpful to minimise delays in ECMO initiation or prevent unnecessary ECMO support.

Veno-venous ECMO should be used over veno-arterial ECMO in patients with pARDS who have adequate cardiac function. Although it is challenging to define inadequate cardiac function at the time of cannulation, left ventricular failure (high lactate, hypotension, poor perfusion) and the need for high doses of vasoactive support may be warning signs of cardiac dysfunction [18].

13.7.2 Ventilation Management

In ECMO-supported pARDS patients, ventilator pressures must be within lung-protective limits to allow resolution of lung injury and reduce complications. However, the precise modes and settings remain imprecise. It seems reasonable to avoid plateau pressure >25 cmH_2O as clinical trials in perinatal lung disease and adult ARDS have used this approach.

The target for gas exchange should be to maintain a normal PaO_2 and a slow decline in $PaCO_2$, especially in the context of hypercapnia. Observational studies in ECMO-supported children suggest that hyperoxia (PaO_2 >100 mmHg) or rapid reduction of hypercapnia are risk factors for adverse outcomes [18].

13.8 Outcomes

Mortality in pARDS ranges from 18% to 27%, whereas in the adult population mortality ranges from 27% to 45%. The PARDIE study found a mortality rate of 17%, with mortality exceeding 30% in those with severe hypoxaemia [9]. Patients with extrapulmonary pARDS have an increased risk of death. Immunocompromised state, multisystem organ failure and neurological failure are likewise associated with a high percentage of deaths, while a smaller percentage die from persistent hypoxaemia. Therefore, children die with pARDS rather than from pARDS.

Long Outcomes: according to PALICC-2, patients who survive pARDS should be assessed by their primary care provider within 3 months of discharge from hospital to screen for lung function abnormalities and neurocognitive function. If pulmonary or neurodevelopmental deficits are detected, patients should be referred to the appropriate specialist for further evaluation and follow-up [5].

Take-Home Messages

- PARDS is a heterogeneous clinical syndrome associated with high mortality and long-term morbidity.
- Triggering factors, comorbidities and changes in lung development and maturation distinguish pARDS from adult ARDS.
- The paediatric-specific PALICC definition of ARDS facilitates improved identification and prognosis of patients with PARDS.
- There is no specific treatment for PARDS and management is supportive, focusing on mechanical ventilation and ancillary treatments.

References

1. Ashbaugh DG, Bigelow DB, Petty TL, Levine BE. Acute respiratory distress in adults. Lancet. 1967;2(7511):319–23.
2. Bernard GR, Artigas A, Brigham KL, et al. Report of the American-European consensus conference on ARDS: definitions, mechanisms, relevant outcomes and clinical trial coordination. The Consensus Committee. Intensive Care Med. 1994;20(3):225–32.
3. ARDS Definition Task Force, Ranieri VM, Rubenfeld GD, et al. Acute respiratory distress syndrome: the Berlin definition. JAMA. 2012;307(23):2526–33.
4. Matthay MA, Arabi Y, Arroliga AC, et al. A new global definition of acute respiratory distress syndrome. Am J Respir Crit Care Med. 2023; https://doi.org/10.1164/rccm.202303-0558WS. Epub ahead of print.
5. Emeriaud G, López-Fernández YM, Iyer NP, et al. Executive summary of the second international guidelines for the diagnosis and management of pediatric acute respiratory distress syndrome (PALICC-2). Pediatr Crit Care Med. 2023;24(2):143–68.
6. López-Fernández YM, Smith LS, Kohne JG, et al. Prognostic relevance and inter-observer reliability of chest-imaging in pediatric ARDS: a pediatric acute respiratory distress incidence and epidemiology (PARDIE) study. Intensive Care Med. 2020;46(7):1382–93.
7. De Luca D, van Kaam AH, Tingay DG, et al. The Montreux definition of neonatal ARDS: biological and clinical background behind the description of a new entity. Lancet Respir Med. 2017;5(8):657–66.
8. Schouten LR, Veltkamp F, Bos AP, et al. Incidence and mortality of acute respiratory distress syndrome in children: a systematic review and meta-analysis. Crit Care Med. 2016;44(4):819–29.
9. Khemani RG, Smith L, Lopez-Fernandez YM, Kwok J, et al. Paediatric acute respiratory distress syndrome incidence and epidemiology (PARDIE): an international, observational study. Lancet Respir Med. 2019;7(2):115–28.
10. Grunwell JR, Dahmer MK, Sapru A, et al. Pathobiology, severity, and risk stratification of pediatric acute respiratory distress syndrome: from the second Pediatric Acute Lung Injury Consensus Conference. Pediatr Crit Care Med. 2023;24(12 Suppl 2):S12–27.
11. Dahmer MK, Yang G, Zhang M, et al. Identification of phenotypes in paediatric patients with acute respiratory distress syndrome: a latent class analysis. Lancet Respir Med. 2022;10(3):289–97.
12. Bhalla A, Baudin F, Takeuchi M, et al. Monitoring in pediatric acute respiratory distress syndrome: from the second Pediatric Acute Lung Injury Consensus Conference. Pediatr Crit Care Med. 2023;24(12 Suppl 2):S112–23.
13. Carroll CL, Napolitano N, Pons-Òdena M, et al. Noninvasive respiratory support for pediatric acute respiratory distress syndrome: from the second Pediatric Acute Lung Injury Consensus Conference. Pediatr Crit Care Med. 2023;24(12 Suppl 2):S135–47.
14. Fernández A, Modesto V, Rimensberger PC, et al. Invasive ventilatory support in patients with pediatric acute respiratory distress syndrome: from the Second Pediatric Acute Lung Injury Consensus Conference. Pediatr Crit Care Med. 2023;24(12 Suppl 2):S61–75.
15. Lalgudi Ganesan S, Jayashree M, Chandra Singhi S, et al. Airway pressure release ventilation in pediatric acute respiratory distress syndrome. A randomized controlled trial. Am J Respir Crit Care Med. 2018;198:1199–207.
16. Rowan CM, Randolph AG, Iyer NP, et al. Pulmonary specific ancillary treatment for pediatric acute respiratory distress syndrome: from the Second Pediatric Acute Lung Injury Consensus Conference. Pediatr Crit Care Med. 2023;24(12 Suppl 2):S99–S111.
17. Valentine SL, Kudchadkar SR, Ward S, et al. Nonpulmonary treatments for pediatric acute respiratory distress syndrome: from the Second Pediatric Acute Lung Injury Consensus Conference. Pediatr Crit Care Med. 2023;24(12 Suppl 2):S45–60.
18. Rambaud J, Barbaro RP, Macrae DJ, et al. Extracorporeal membrane oxygenation in pediatric acute respiratory distress syndrome: from the Second Pediatric Acute Lung Injury Consensus Conference. Pediatr Crit Care Med. 2023;24(12 Suppl 2):S124–34.

Physiology of Modes of Ventilation in Severe Acute Lung Injury (ALI)

Pauline de Jager, Alette Koopman, Robert G. T. Blokpoel, and Martin C. J. Kneyber

Contents

J. Brierley et al. (eds.), *ESPNIC Children's Intensive Care Textbook*,
https://doi.org/10.1007/978-3-031-64762-8_14

Learning Objectives

- To understand the taxonomy of mechanical ventilation.
- To understand how to use conventional mechanical ventilation in the presence of acute lung injury.
- To understand the working principles of high-frequency oscillatory ventilation (HFOV), airway pressure release ventilation (APRV) and liquid ventilation.
- To understand how to apply these non-alternative modes of ventilation.

14.1 Introduction

Mechanical ventilation (MV) is intimately linked with the daily care of critically ill children and has added significantly to survival. It is used to ensure oxygenation and ventilation and to decrease patient respiratory effort during the period in which the underlying (non-) pulmonary disorders can (partially) resolve. However, MV is also linked to the initiation or even aggravation of lung injury, termed ventilator-induced lung injury (VILI) The inflammation is not limited to the lung; inflammatory mediators can enter the systemic circulation and lead to organ failure and multiple system organ failure (MSOF) linked to VILI [1–3]. Several mechanisms have been attributed to play a role in VILI, including ventilating at high lung volumes following the delivery of inappropriately sized tidal volumes (V_t) in relation to the amount of inflatable lung volume (i.e. the "baby lung"), and ventilating at low lung volumes leading to repetitive alveolar opening and closure (also known as atelectrauma) [4, 5]. A better understanding of these mechanisms led to the concept of lung and diaphragm protective ventilation (LPV), a strategy that focuses on the delivery of small V_t to avoid excessive lung strain (the changes in volume in relation to its resting volume) and a certain level of positive end-expiratory pressure (PEEP) to maintain alveolar patency [6, 7]. When conventional mechanical ventilation (CMV) fails, high-frequency oscillatory ventilation (HFOV) and airway pressure release ventilation (APRV) can be considered alternative modes of ventilation as they are, at least theoretically, justifiable modes to be used in the context of LPV because they target the two major determinants of VILI.

14.2 Taxonomy of Mechanical Ventilation

Technological advancements and ongoing research in the field of mechanical ventilation made mechanical ventilators evolve quickly from very simple machines offering limited modes to sophisticated devices with complex microprocessors offering a wide variety of modes. However, the terminology used nowadays is very confusing and sometimes outdated, meaning that each ventilator brand has its "unique" ventilation modes.

Chatburn and colleagues developed a taxonomy for mechanical ventilation based on 10 maxims [8]. Simplified, a breath is assisted if the ventilator provides some or all the work of breathing. This is done using pressure control (PC) or volume control (VC) based on the equation of motion. Importantly, breaths are classified according to the criteria that trigger (start) and cycle (stop) inspiration. These can be either patient-initiated or ventilator-initiated. Breaths are spontaneous or mandatory based on the trigger and cycle events. Thus, ventilators deliver three types of breath sequences: continuous mandatory ventilation (CMV), intermittent mandatory ventilation (IMV) and continuous spontaneous ventilation (CSV). These breaths can either be in PC or VC, so there are five basic ventilatory patterns: PC-CMV, PC-IMV, PC-CSV, VC-CMV and VC-IMV (spontaneous breaths can only be controlled by pressure). In PC ventilation, the control variable is pressure, whereas in VC ventilation this is volume. PC-CMV and VC-CMV are often referred to as assist/control (A/C), as the patient can trigger the ventilator breaths. IMV modes allow for the possibility of having mandatory and spontaneous breaths. Most ventilators are designed to have a triggering window, that is the ventilator aims to detect patient inspiratory effort to allow synchronization before the mandatory breath is delivered. This is known as synchronized IMV (SIMV). It is important to note that SIMV differs across ventilator brands. Pressure support (PS) ventilation is an example of PC-CSV.

So far, in paediatrics no ventilator mode has been shown to be superior over the other [9]. Hence, the choice of a particular ventilator mode is mainly driven by personal experiences and institutional preferences.

14.3 Conventional Mechanical Ventilation Approaches During Acute Lung Injury

Tidal alveolar deformation and cyclic opening and collapse of recruitable lung units are important contributors to VILI. Therefore, measures to mitigate VILI are aimed at preventing excessive alveolar deformation due to the delivery of high V_t and the delivery of positive-end expiratory pressure to prevent alveolar derecruitment. Many of the mechanisms underlying VILI come together in lung strain and stress. Deformation in the lung is measured as strain, which is defined by the change in volume in relation to its resting volume (i.e. V_t in relation to EELV). The force per unit area to produce is called stress, which is the transpulmonary pressure (i.e. difference between the airway and pleural pressure). Lung stress and strain are intimately linked through the specific lung elastance which is similar for children and adults [10, 11]. Driving pressure (i.e. the difference between airway pressure and positive end-expiratory pressure) is strongly correlated with lung stress [12].

Inspiratory pressures must be limited to prevent excessive lung stress. In general, it is recommended to limit plateau pressure (i.e. the airway pressure at zero flow) to 28 cmH_2O (or 32 cmH_2O in patients with increased chest wall elastance such as obese patients or patients with stiff chest walls due to oedema). Excessive lung strain can be prevented by either decreasing V_t and/or increasing end-expiratory lung volume (EELV). Physiologic V_t is 5–8 mL/kg, but the actual V_t set should be scaled by respiratory system compliance (C_{rs}). Gattinoni proposed the "baby lung" concept which states that C_{rs} has a linear relationship with the amount of inflatable lung volume. Thus, the lower the C_{rs}, the stiffer the lung and the lower the allowable V_t would be. The importance of scaling V_t to C_{rs} can be appreciated from the landmark Acute Respiratory Distress Syndrome (ARDS) Network trial published in 2000 [13]. In this trial, a low V_t strategy (6 mL/kg predicted body weight [PBW]) resulted in significantly lower mortality compared to a "traditional" V_t strategy (i.e. 12 mL/kg PBW).

The mortality benefit was the strongest in subjects with reduced compliance as 6 mL/kg PBW may lead to injurious end-inspiratory regional tidal hyperinflation [13, 14]. Pooling adult V_t trials underscored the assumption that baseline C_{rs} is an important variable in V_t selection [15]. How can at the bedside "best" V_t be selected? Amato et al. reported that increased driving pressure >15 cmH_2O was associated with increased mortality risk in adults with ARDS [16]. Decreasing driving pressure by limiting P_{plat} and increasing PEEP was associated with decreased risk of mortality and limiting driving pressure was a stronger predictor for outcome than V_t. Therefore, scaling V_t with concurrent targeting driving pressure <15 cm_2O and limiting P_{plat} <28 cmH_2O is the most justified approach. This can most easily be achieved while ventilating the patient in PC mode. In PC ventilation, inspiratory pressures are set so it is easier to reach the target DP; the V_t that will be delivered depends on the C_{rs} and resistance of the respiratory system. The drawback of PC is that there is no inspiratory pause, hence P_{plat} is not measured. This requires a manual hold by the operator. Peak inspiratory pressure overestimates P_{plat} (especially in disease conditions with increased airway resistance) and can therefore not be used to calculate DP [17]. Pressure Regulated Volume Control (PRVC) is a much-cherished mode among paediatric critical practitioners as this combines the benefits of PC ventilation with volume targeting. However, the operator remains challenged by V_t selection with this mode.

Positive end-expiratory pressure (PEEP) is used to promote more homogenous ventilation by preventing alveolar collapse at end expiration [18]. The drawback of PEEP is that it may also cause circulatory depression and contribute to VILI through alveolar overdistention. The overall effect of PEEP is primarily related to the balance between the number of alveoli that are recruited to participate in ventilation and the amount of lung that is overdistended [19]. The ratio of benefit to harm from PEEP cannot be seen independent from the amount of lung that can be recruited, which varies widely among patients especially those with ARDS [20]. In the above-mentioned ARDSNetwork trial, PEEP was titrated according to a table of PEEP and FiO_2 combinations. In a comparative study, this table proved to be the best approach to PEEP setting in ARDS. In children with more severe lung injury, it was also observed that non-adherence to this table was associated with increased mortality [21–23]. It is therefore recommended, especially in patients with more severe lung disease, to initially set PEEP according to the grid and then individualize PEEP setting balancing oxygenation and haemodynamics. Lung recruitment manoeuvres (RM) may help to identify which patients might benefit from a higher level of PEEP. The concept of RMs includes an intentional transient increase in transpulmonary pressure aimed at reopening non-aerated or poorly aerated alveoli [24]. There are various types of RM, including sighs, sustained inflation (SI) and a stepwise incremental (± decremental) PEEP titration [25]. There are various approaches to SI, including the amount of pressure applied and the duration of the SI. With a staircase incremental (± decremental) PEEP titration, with a fixed V_t or DP depending on which ventilation mode is used, PEEP is gradually increased. Evidence for recruitability includes a decrease in P_{plat} (if in VC mode) or an increase in V_t (in PC mode). From a practical perspective, "optimal" PEEP is where dead space is the lowest, C_{rs}

is the highest and DP is <15 cmH_2O [26]. Improvements in oxygenation may also be an indicator of lung recruitability with higher PEEP [27]. Pressure–volume curves to titrate PEEP are of limited value. Others have proposed to titrate PEEP using oesophageal pressure manometry, targeting an end-expiratory PEEP minus oesophageal pressure (P_{oes}) >0 [28]. Such an approach may improve oxygenation and lung mechanics without increasing lung stress but warrants exploration in children. PEEP setting based on lung ultrasound or electrical impedance tomography is increasingly being studied.

14.4 High-Frequency Oscillatory Ventilation

14.4.1 What Is HFOV?

HFOV is a mode of ventilation that makes use of an oscillatory pump that generates a continuous distending pressure (CDP), often referred to as mean airway pressure (mP_{aw}). This CDP generates and maintains end-expiratory lung volume (EELV). Pressure oscillations are superimposed on the CDP at a frequency (F) of 3–15 Hz; the oscillatory pressure amplitude (ΔP) is highly attenuated over the endotracheal tube and the proximal and distal airways and results in the delivery of a very small stroke volume, usually lower than anatomical dead space (1–2 mL/kg) [29].

HFOV allows the decoupling of oxygenation and ventilation. For this purpose, the operator has to set the CDP, F, power, inspiratory to expiratory (I:E) ratio, FiO_2 and circuit bias flow. Simplified, oxygenation is dependent on EELV which is controlled by the CDP and the FiO_2. The power of the piston membrane is set to generate pressure oscillations (displayed on the device as ΔP) that determine the delivered V_t; CO_2 clearance ($\dot{V}_{CO2}$) is relatively independent of lung volume but influenced by F and the square of V_t ($\dot{V}_{CO2} = F \times V_t^2$) [18–21]. The I:E ratio is usually set at 1:2.

HFOV systems generate a simple harmonic oscillatory motion (SHM) that transforms the laminar or bias flow into a turbulent flow. The SHMs generated induce a series of secondary waves (e.g. harmonics) in all the structures with which they come in contact. Some of these resonance waves vibrate at a much lower frequency and why patients on HFOV wiggle. Ventilators that are capable of high-frequency ventilation have different characteristics. Some have an active in- and expiration, whereas others are so-called flow interrupters (i.e. the flow stops after inspiration). In this chapter, we mainly focus on oscillators with active in- and expiration.

The mechanisms of gas exchange during HFOV are complex and include pendelluft (i.e. movement of gas between lung regions with different time constants), convective gas transport (i.e. transport of gas into alveoli secondary to the vacuum left after absorption of oxygen into capillaries), Taylor dispersion (i.e. passage of oxygenated gas from rapid central jet into the deeper bronchial tree), enhanced molecular diffusion near the alveolo-capillary membrane and enhanced mixing in the large airways due to turbulence (■ Fig. 14.1) [30]. Pendelluft is of importance for lung units with long-time constants and for those alveoli that are not reached by V_t, whereas convective gas transport plays an important role in larger airways.

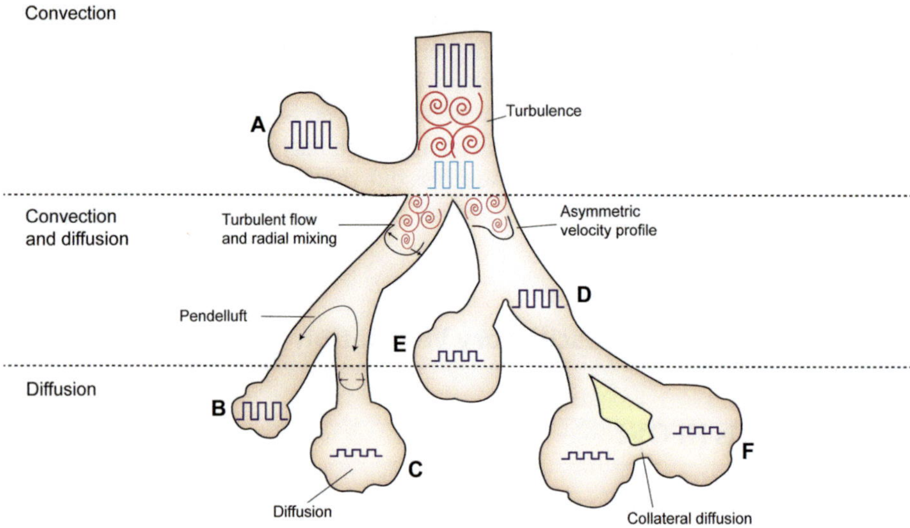

Fig. 14.1 Mechanisms of gas exchange and pressure transmission during high-frequency oscillatory ventilation. Mechanisms include pendelluft (i.e. movement of gas between lung regions with different time constants), convective gas transport (i.e. transport of gas into alveoli secondary to the vacuum left after absorption of oxygen into capillaries), Taylor dispersion (i.e. passage of oxygenated gas from the rapid central jet into the deeper bronchial tree), enhanced molecular diffusion near the alveolo-capillary membrane and enhanced mixing in the large airways due to turbulence. The oscillatory pressure applied at the airway opening is dampened by the resistance and inertance of the endotracheal tube and central airways. Proximal alveoli (A) are subjected to the same oscillatory pressure as the central airways, but the more distal from the airway opening, the more the oscillatory pressure is dampened, especially in compliant alveoli (C) but to a lesser extent in poorly compliant or not fully recruited alveoli (B). Increased peripheral airway resistance causes a higher pressure transmission to more proximal alveoli (E) but a lower pressure amplitude in alveoli distal of the airway resistance (F). (Modified with permission from [30, 85])

14.4.2 Clinical Evidence in Children

From a recent systematic review, including among other four small paediatric RCTs, it was concluded that HFOV in children does not improve relevant patient outcomes when compared with CMV [31]. The largest RCT was performed 25 years ago and designed as a cross-over study including 58 patients of whom 55% had PARDS according to the American European Consensus Conference (AECC definition) and an oxygenation index (OI) >13 [32]. The intention-to-treat analysis showed that HFOV did not improve survival (HFOV 66% vs 59%) or total ventilator-free days (VFD) (HFOV 20 ± 27 vs 22 ± 17) compared with CMV, but the percentage of survivors requiring supplemental oxygen at 30 days was significantly lower in the HFOV group (21% vs 59%). Samransamruajkit *et al.* conducted two small single-centre trials in children with AECC and Berlin-defined ARDS although both trials were not designed to study clinical outcomes. Additionally, the CMV strategy was not clear in the first trial from this group [33, 34]. Only in their second RCT, the authors reported their CMV approach could be appreciated as lung-protective [34]. The most recent (and largest) paediatric RCT was published in 2017 and included 200 children with moderate-to-severe Berlin-defined PARDS [35]. Mortality rates were comparable between HFOV and CMV (45% vs 43%) and the length of MV was not different. Importantly, the oscillator used in this trial was different than the three other RCTs. Instead of the SensorMedics (which is the most used oscillator [Vyaire, Mettawa, IL, USA]), in this trial, a neonatal hybrid ventilator/oscillator (Fabian [Vyaire, Mettawa, IL, USA]) was used. The Fabian device has different respiratory wave characteristics and is thought not to be sufficiently powerful to adequately oscillate children >6 kg.

Adding to these RCTS are two reports of propensity score analyses. The first is an observational study reporting increased mortality and morbidity in patients managed with HFOV compared with CMV through propensity score matching analyses of data from 9177 patients registered in the virtual PICU (vPICU) database [36]. Comparisons between matched patients showed higher mortality (overall HFOV vs CMV 17% vs 8%; early HFOV [i.e. within 24 h] vs conventional MV 18% vs 8%) and a significantly longer time on the ventilator among HFOV patients. However, this particular study is difficult to interpret since important clinical variables that influence the decision to initiate HFOV, such as metrics of oxygenation and ventilator settings were not available for propensity matching, thus challenging the relevance and clinical impact of this study [37–39]. Similarly, in a post-hoc propensity score matching analysis of data from the Randomized Evaluation of Sedation Titration for Respiratory Failure (RESTORE) study, where the mode of mechanical ventilation and ventilator weaning strategy was left to the discretion of the treating physician, it was found that while 90-day mortality rates were not different between HFOV and CMV (25% vs 17%), patients managed with the oscillator spend significantly more time on the ventilator [40]. Additionally, Wong and colleagues reported that the use of HFOV was associated with increased 28-day mortality after analyses of data from patients with PARDS from 10 paediatric intensive care units across Asia from 2009 to 2015 [41]. However, information on HFOV and CMV approaches are lacking in their report.

14.4.3 Clinical Evidence in Adults

Animal studies reported the superiority of HFOV over CMV in terms of better oxygenation, lung compliance and alveolar stability with less pulmonary inflammation and histological injury [42, 43]. However, these beneficial effects became less clear when control groups were modelled to a more LPV approach as currently used in daily clinical practice [44].

The use of HFOV in adults became highly controversial following the outcome of two large RCTs. No benefit on patient outcome was observed in the Oscillate for Acute Respiratory Distress Syndrome (OSCAR) trial that compared HFOV using a novel device with non-protocolized CMV in 795 patients admitted to centres with little HFOV experience [45]. More worrisome however were the outcomes of the Oscillation for Acute Respiratory Distress Syndrome Treated Early (OSCILLATE). This study was stopped prematurely after the inclusion of 548 out of 1200 planned patients for increased mortality (47% vs 35%, $p = 0.005$) and worse secondary outcomes in the HFOV group [46]. Unlike OSCAR, OSCILLATE was conducted in centres with previous HFOV and made use of a strictly protocolized CMV control arm. Including the results of these two later trials, an updated meta-analysis confirmed no outcome benefit of HFOV over CMV, challenging the routine use of HFOV in adults with moderate-to-severe ARDS [47, 48].

14.4.4 Indications for and Timing of HFOV

The indications for HFOV are ill defined and are usually dictated by personal preferences of the attending physician and institutional beliefs. In general, HFOV is only considered as a rescue approach when CMV fails but it could be argued that it should be considered early in the PARDS trajectory to minimize VILI and to prevent ventilator settings from becoming toxic. There is virtually no paediatric data supporting this concept, except for one small observational study of 26 patients reporting significantly higher 30-day survival rates (58.8% vs 12.5%) when HFOV was employed within 24 h rather than as rescue [49].

Some authors have proposed to use a specific oxygenation index (OI) or the PaO_2/FiO_2 ratio as a threshold in the decision-making when to move the patient to HFOV. Two paediatric trials used respectively an OI >13 and 15 as cut-off values [32, 33]. A recent re-evaluation of the OSCILLATE trial showed that a mortality benefit of HFOV could only be expected in adults with severe ARDS (i.e. PaO_2/FiO_2 <100) [50], suggesting that HFOV as (rescue) intervention should only be considered in the sickest of patients.

Some investigators have adopted a liberal threshold for HFOV when PIP (in case of PC ventilation) or P_{plat} >28–32 cmH_2O and PEEP >8 cmH_2O and FiO_2 >0.6 and a rise in the oxygenation index (OI) on three consecutive measurements that are 1 h apart [51].

The Pediatric Mechanical Ventilation Consensus Conference (PEMVECC) recommends that HFOV may be considered if conventional ventilation fails, using an open lung strategy to maintain optimal EELV [9]. These recommendations reflect the second iteration of the Pediatric Acute Lung Injury Consensus Conference (PALICC) recommendations for paediatric acute respiratory distress syndrome [52]. Their best practice statement stated that HFOV may be considered in patients with PARDS in whom the ventilatory goals are not achieved with a lung protective strategy on conventional mechanical ventilation.

14.4.5 Lung Volume Optimization Manoeuvres

Lung volume is the main determinant of oxygenation in DAD during HFOV. Simplified, PaO_2 increases linearly with lung volume up to a certain point when alveoli become overdistended [53]. This suggests that an open lung strategy (i.e. opening the lung and keeping it open) by (repeated) recruitment manoeuvres (RM) should be considered when switching to HFOV. Remarkable, RMs seem not to be the standard of care when switching to HFOV [54]. A stepwise pressure incremental–decremental CDP titration produced the greatest increase in lung volume and resolution of atelectasis in an animal model [55]. In children, an individualized, staircase incremental–decremental CDP titration as part of an open-lung approach to HFOV is feasible and safe in terms of hemodynamic consequences while allowing for sufficient gas exchange [51].

Additional benefits of optimization of the end-expiratory lung volume include a better distal dampening of the pressure oscillations. This is because pressure oscillations are less dampened in lungs with ongoing atelectasis, thus exposing the conducting airways and alveoli to higher injurious pressure swings (◘ Fig. 14.1) [30]. With reduced compliance in unresolved atelectasis, there is a marked increase in transmission of the peak-to-trough ΔP to the alveoli and bronchi. Another, at least theoretical, benefit of RMs is that they allow oscillating the patient on the deflation limb of the *P–V* curve thereby (partially) avoiding injurious hyperinflation and atelectasis [56–59]. By doing so, a lower CDP is needed to maintain the same amount of EELV than on the inflation limb because of the hysteresis of the respiratory system (◘ Fig. 14.2).

PALICC recommendations for PARDS include that when using HFOV, the optimal lung volume should be achieved by exploration of the potential for lung recruitment with a stepwise increase and decrease of the mean airway pressure under continuous monitoring of the oxygen and CO_2 response and hemodynamic parameters [52].

14.4.6 Achieving the Lowest Stroke Volume

The delivered stroke volume during HFOV is determined by numerous factors, including resistance of the respiratory system (R_{rs}) and oscillator settings such as oscillatory power (magnitude of membrane displacement), *F* in Hertz (Hz), I:E ratio, position of the membrane, endotracheal tube (ETT) length and diameter, and the presence of ETT leakage [60–64]. The ETT constitutes the major workload to the oscillator and is an important determinant of V_t [65]. V_t is proportional to the ETT's

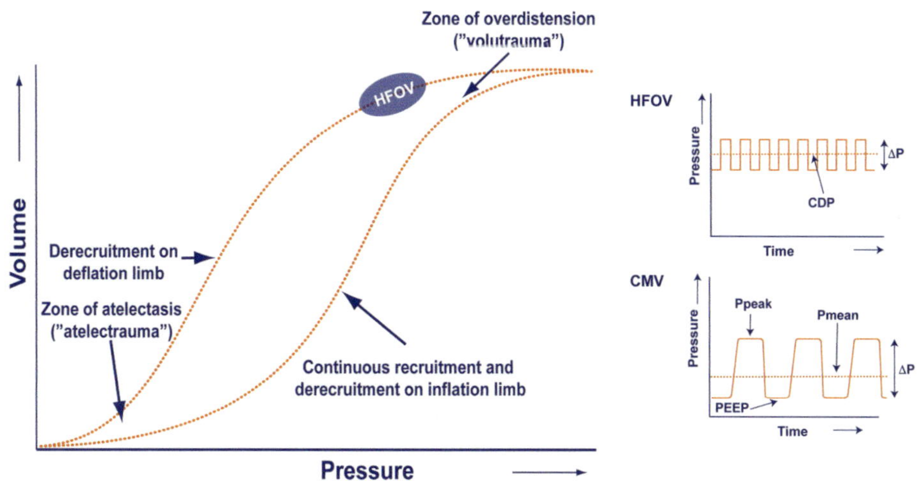

◘ **Fig. 14.2** Position of high-frequency oscillatory ventilation (HFOV) on the pressure–volume loop. Optimal use of HFOV means that it is positioned on the deflation limb after a lung volume optimization manoeuvre

inner cross-sectional area because the impedance of the ETT exceeds the impedance of the lung [66, 67].

In clinical practice, it is common to set *F* and power according to the patient's age, ventilator settings and observation of chest wiggle. However, from a physiological perspective, it seems more appropriate to use the highest possible *F* in PARDS. First, the higher the *F*, the smaller the V_t because changes in *F* are inversely proportional to the distal oscillatory pressure amplitude [68]. It will subsequently be easier to stay within the limits of the safe zone (i.e. the zone with the smallest risk of injurious hyperinflation or atelectasis) of the *P*–*V* loop. Second, collapsed lung regions are more easily opened at higher *F* [69]. Third, the delivered V_t is more equally distributed as it becomes less dependent on regional compliance at higher *F* [70]. However, finding the best *F* is challenging. Venegas et al. have proposed that setting the oscillatory *F* is dictated by the corner frequency (F_c) of the lung, $F_c = 1/(2\pi RC)$, where *R* is resistance and *C* compliance [71]. F_c defines the optimal frequency at which there is adequate gas transport during HFOV in combination with the least injurious pressures and is influenced by the underlying disease (◘ Fig. 14.3). It is increased in lung diseases characterized by short time constants and low compliance such as in PARDS. Importantly, *F* is intimately linked with ΔP. Basically, the higher the ΔP,

14

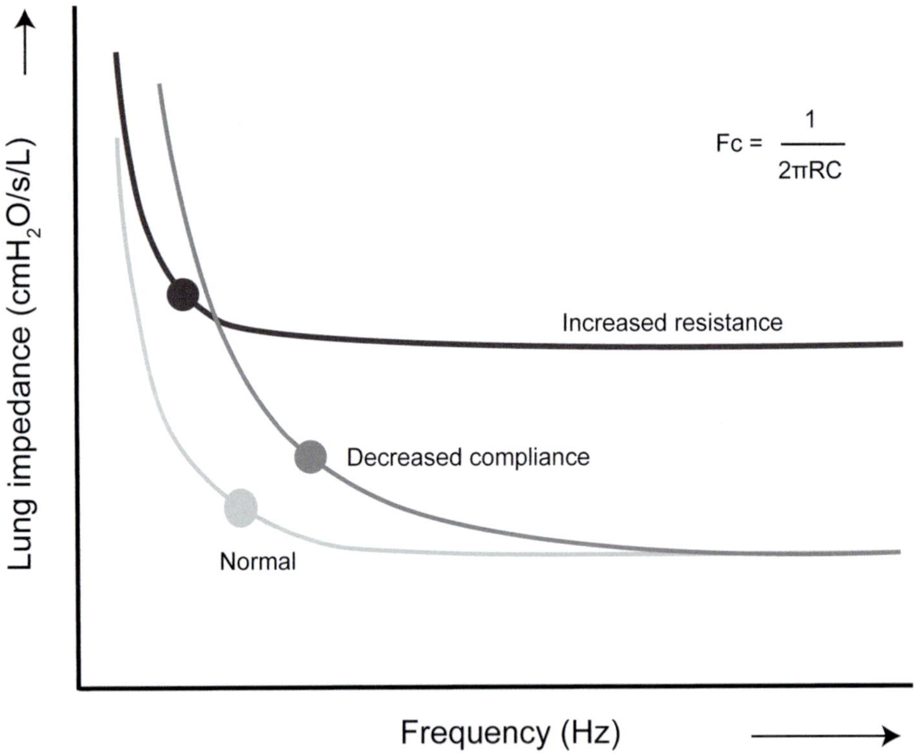

◘ **Fig. 14.3** Concept of corner frequency (F_c) of the lung in patients with decreased compliance, such as PARDS and increased resistance, such as obstructive airway disease. F_c (graphically depicted by the dot) defines the optimal frequency at which there is adequate gas transport during HFOV in combination with the least injurious pressures. F_c is calculated by $1/2\pi RC$, where *R* is resistance and *C* compliance. (Modified with permission from [71])

the larger the V_t. Yet, we (unpublished data) and others have observed in bench test studies that V_t was smaller when combining high F (15 Hz) and high power (set to achieve a ΔP of 90) compared with low F (5 Hz) and low power settings as the distal pressure amplitude was much lower but still associated with a sufficient CO_2 elimination [72].

14.4.7 HFOV Titration Weaning

When stabilized, twice daily CDP challenges should be performed for aggressive HFOV weaning in addition to commonly used approaches including small decreases in CDP if the FiO_2 is above a pre-defined threshold and the SpO_2 is in an acceptable range. With this CDP challenge, the CDP is decreased until the SpO_2 also decreases, indicating the onset of lung derecruitment. Ventilation is managed by titrating F to adhere to pre-defined ventilation goals. In general, a patient can be transferred back to CMV at CDP 15–20 cmH_2O and FiO_2 0.40.

14.5 Airway Pressure Release Ventilation

14.5.1 Description of APRV

Airway Pressure Release Ventilation (APRV) was first described in 1987 as a mode to deliver two levels of continuous positive airway pressure (CPAP) while allowing for spontaneous breathing throughout the respiratory cycle (◘ Fig. 14.4) [73]. Unlike traditional CPAP, both oxygenation and ventilation are supported during APRV. A continuous high flow is delivered to the patient, only interrupted by intermittent opening of the expiratory valve resulting in a decrease in circuit pressure allowing gas outflow and thereby CO_2 removal from the lungs as well as emptying of the anatomic

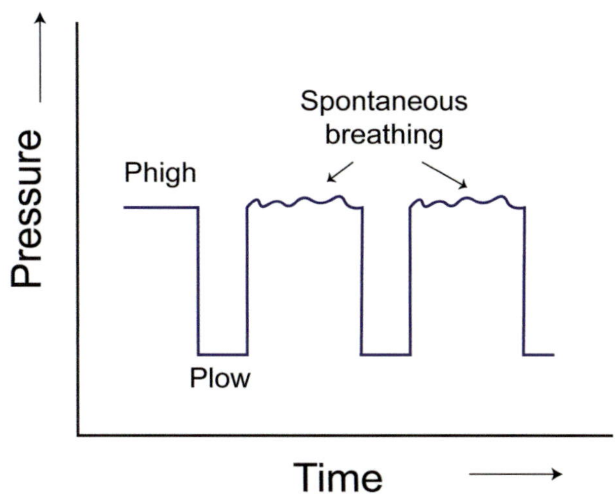

◘ **Fig. 14.4** Pressure–time scalar of airway pressure release ventilation (APRV)

dead space. Unlike CMV, the breath begins at an elevated baseline and ends with the deflation from high pressure to low pressure. This driving pressure gradient establishes the delivered V_t allowing for ventilation, which is (as with PCV) affected by C_{rs} and R_{rs}. Hence, APRV is considered a time-triggered, pressure-limited and time-cycled intermittent mode of ventilation with an inversed inspiratory to expiratory ratio [74]. Of note, APRV is in fact an inversed ratio mode of PCV if spontaneous breathing is absent.

The operator must set the high (P_{high}) and low pressure (P_{low}) as well as the time (T) intervals of these pressures (T_{high} and T_{low}). Oxygenation is determined by the FiO_2 and T_{high}. Usually, P_{high} is set to match the plateau pressure (P_{plat}) during CMV (targeting P_{plat} <30 cmH_2O), but the approach to setting P_{low} and T_{high} and T_{low} is highly variable [75]. T_{high} can be set somewhere between 4 and 10 s and is dictated by oxygenation. For P_{low} and T_{low}, there are roughly two concepts, being (a) using a constant T_{low} and non-zero P_{low} to prevent complete end-expiratory lung deflation and a T_{high} that is approximately 90% of the total cycle time, or (b) setting T_{low} dictated by lung mechanics (to achieve an end-expiratory flow: peak expiratory flow (PEF) ratio of ±50–75%), P_{low} at zero and T_{high} >90% of the total cycle time—the inherent short T_{low} thus prevents complete end-expiratory lung emptying [76, 77]. How both are ultimately set is dictated by the desired level of CO_2 elimination. The combination of these settings results in a mP_{aw} calculated by $((P_{high} * T_{high}) + (P_{low} * T_{low}))/(T_{high} + T_{low})$. The prolonged inspiratory time may lead to the development of intrinsic PEEP (PEEPi), which should be avoided because of the inherent cardiovascular compromise although published reported adult data seemed to suggest that the use of APRV was safe.

14.5.2 Physiologic Benefits

The potential benefits of APRV are linked to a presumed reduced risk of volutrauma inherent to the pressure limitation with this mode, and therefore the delivered V_t being affected by C_{rs} and R_{rs} (as with PCV). In line with the open-lung concept, the risk for atelectrauma may be reduced because APRV delivers a higher mP_{aw} than on PCV. Numerous animal studies have shown improved oxygenation and some reduced lung injury with APRV [75]. In addition, the true potential benefit of APRV is probably linked to spontaneous breathing resulting in a reduced shunt fraction, improved distribution of V_t towards the lung-dependent zones, less lung inflammation [78–80] and a better patient–ventilator synchrony.

14.5.3 Clinical Evidence in Children

The paediatric literature on APRV is mainly limited to case reports, case series and retrospective and prospective observational cohort studies with small sample sizes except for one RCT comparing APRV with CMV in Berlin-defined PARDS [76]. Children aged 1 month–12 years were randomized within 24 h of the PARDS diagnosis and 72 h of ventilation to APRV or CMV. The study was stopped prematurely at 50% enrolment because of increased mortality in the APRV group (53.8%) compared to CMV (26.9%), yielding a relative risk for death of 2.0 (95% CI

0.97–4.41). The cause of death in these patients was refractory hypoxemia in almost half of the patients, whereas the remaining patients died from multiple system organ failure (MSOF).

14.6 Liquid Ventilation

Liquid ventilation (LV) is a technique of MV in which the lungs are not insufflated with an oxygen-containing gas mixture but a perfluorochemical liquid is used instead. Compared to nitrogen gas mixtures, perfluorochemicals are inert carriers of oxygen and carbon dioxide having theoretical advantages of reducing surface tension, alveolar recruitment through hydraulic pressure with a lower risk of barotrauma, and functioning as a high-efficiency heat exchanger. Perflubron (LiquiVent), the only medical-grade PFC available for use in human LV trials, consists of a long, linear-fluorinated hydrocarbon chain. Perflubron contains one bromide atom, making it radiopaque. The complete range of toxicity due to perfluorochemicals (PFCs) is not known.

LV can be either total (TLV) or partial (TLV). In TLV, the entire lung is filled with an oxygenated PFC liquid and a liquid tidal volume of PFC is actively pumped into and out of the lungs with extra-corporeal oxygenation and removal of CO_2 [81, 82]. It is initiated by insufflating the desired volume of pre-oxygenated PFC liquid (functional residual capacity plus tidal volume) into the lungs. Ventilation and oxygenation depend upon minute ventilation coupled with sufficient time for the diffusion of respiratory gases to and from the PFC liquid. A low respiratory rate is set with an inspiratory-to-expiratory (I:E) ratio of 1:2 to 1:3 [83]. This gives sufficient time for the PFC fluid to dwell in the lung long enough for the diffusion of respiratory gases. Tidal volumes and peak inspiratory and positive end-expiratory pressures (PEEP) are adjusted based on pulmonary mechanics and blood gases in the same manner as when gas ventilation is employed. The return to gas ventilation is accomplished by a transition through a period of partial LV.

In partial liquid ventilation PLV, the lungs are slowly filled with a volume of PFC equivalent or close to the FRC during gas ventilation. The PFC within the lungs is oxygenated and carbon dioxide is removed by means of gas breaths cycling in the lungs by a conventional gas ventilator. It is initiated by insufflating 20–30 mL/kg PFC liquid into the lungs using an intravenous syringe pump or by slowly pushing the fluid in over a 15-min to 1-h period. End-expiratory lung volume capacity is reached when at end expiration a meniscus of PFC is present within the endotracheal tube [84]. As the fluid evaporates out of the lungs, it is intermittently and gradually replaced with additional PFC at approximately 2–8 mL/kg/h to maintain a total liquid volume of functional residual capacity [81, 82]. Pressure-controlled ventilation with the addition of PEEP is used to deliver gas ventilation, and fraction of inspired oxygen (FiO_2) and PEEP are adjusted based on pulmonary mechanics and blood gases [18]. Airway suctioning is still required with PLV.

The benefit of TLV is that it allows the lavage and removal of lung secretions, meconium or alveolar oedema from the lower airways better than PLV. Distribution of PFC may be more uniform. The drawback of TLV is that it requires a specific apparatus. PLV shares some of the same benefits as TLV and does not require specialized equipment.

Indications for LV include acute respiratory distress syndrome, meconium aspiration syndrome, persistent pulmonary hypertension of the newborn and to provide lung protection during cardiopulmonary bypass. To date, the limited clinical human data available do not support routine use of TLV or PLV. Adverse effects include an increase in pulmonary vascular resistance, mucus plug formation, pneumothorax and bleeding complications. Hence, LV is currently not recommended for use in children [9].

14.7 Conclusions

Non-conventional modes of ventilation such as HFOV and APRV are just another mode of ventilation. The use of these modes makes sense from a physiologic perspective, but these theoretical benefits have so far not been translated into improved outcomes in children. Liquid ventilation is not recommended outside research settings.

Take-Home Messages

- Conventional mechanical ventilation settings during acute lung injury are targeted at preventing excessive lung stress and strain by limiting inspiratory pressures and scaling tidal volume of respiratory system compliance.
- Lung recruitment manoeuvres may help identify patients who benefit from higher positive end-expiratory pressure to maintain alveolar patency.
- HFOV can be considered a second-tier intervention when on conventional mechanical ventilation oxygenation and/or ventilation goals cannot be met. If instituted, an open lung approach targeting the highest possible oscillatory frequency offers the best physiological advantages of HFOV.
- APRV is a complicated alternative mode of ventilation that allows the patient to breathe spontaneously on two different pressure levels.
- Use of liquid ventilation is limited to research settings.

References

1. Tremblay LN, Slutsky AS. Ventilator-induced lung injury: from the bench to the bedside. Intensive Care Med. 2006;32:24–33. https://doi.org/10.1007/s00134-005-2817-8.
2. Pinhu L, Whitehead T, Evans T, Griffiths M. Ventilator-associated lung injury. Lancet. 2003;361:332–40. pii: S0140-6736(03)12329-X. https://doi.org/10.1016/S0140-6736(03)12329-X.
3. Ranieri VM, Giunta F, Suter PM, Slutsky AS. Mechanical ventilation as a mediator of multisystem organ failure in acute respiratory distress syndrome. JAMA. 2000;284:43–4. https://doi.org/10.1001/jama.284.1.43.
4. Slutsky AS, Ranieri VM. Ventilator-induced lung injury. N Engl J Med. 2013;369:2126–36. https://doi.org/10.1056/NEJMra1208707.
5. Gattinoni L, Pesenti A. The concept of "baby lung". Intensive Care Med. 2005;31:776–84. https://doi.org/10.1007/s00134-005-2627-z.
6. Fan E, et al. An official American Thoracic Society/European Society of Intensive Care Medicine/Society of Critical Care Medicine Clinical Practice Guideline: mechanical ventilation in adult

patients with acute respiratory distress syndrome. Am J Respir Crit Care Med. 2017;195:1253–63. https://doi.org/10.1164/rccm.201703-0548ST.
7. Goligher EC, et al. Clinical strategies for implementing lung and diaphragm-protective ventilation: avoiding insufficient and excessive effort. Intensive Care Med. 2020;46:2314–26. https://doi.org/10.1007/s00134-020-06288-9.
8. Chatburn RL, El-Khatib M, Mireles-Cabodevila E. A taxonomy for mechanical ventilation: 10 fundamental maxims. Respir Care. 2014;59:1747–63. https://doi.org/10.4187/respcare.03057.
9. Kneyber MCJ, et al. Recommendations for mechanical ventilation of critically ill children from the Paediatric Mechanical Ventilation Consensus Conference (PEMVECC). Intensive Care Med. 2017;43:1764–80. https://doi.org/10.1007/s00134-017-4920-z.
10. Chiumello D, et al. Lung stress and strain during mechanical ventilation for acute respiratory distress syndrome. Am J Respir Crit Care Med. 2008;178:346–55. https://doi.org/10.1164/rccm.200710-1589OC.
11. Chiumello D, Chidini G, Calderini E, Colombo A, Crimella F, Brioni M. Respiratory mechanics and lung stress/strain in children with acute respiratory distress syndrome. Ann Intensive Care. 2016;6:11. https://doi.org/10.1186/s13613-016-0113-0.
12. Chiumello D, Carlesso E, Brioni M, Cressoni M. Airway driving pressure and lung stress in ARDS patients. Crit Care. 2016;20:276. https://doi.org/10.1186/s13054-016-1446-7.
13. Network A. Ventilation with lower tidal volumes as compared with traditional tidal volumes for acute lung injury and the acute respiratory distress syndrome. The Acute Respiratory Distress Syndrome Network. N Engl J Med. 2000;342:1301–8.
14. Chiumello D, et al. Lung recruitment assessed by respiratory mechanics and computed tomography in patients with acute respiratory distress syndrome. What is the relationship? Am J Respir Crit Care Med. 2016;193:1254–63. https://doi.org/10.1164/rccm.201507-1413OC.
15. Goligher EC, et al. Effect of lowering Vt on mortality in acute respiratory distress syndrome varies with respiratory system elastance. Am J Respir Crit Care Med. 2021;203:1378–85. https://doi.org/10.1164/rccm.202009-3536OC.
16. Amato MB, et al. Driving pressure and survival in the acute respiratory distress syndrome. N Engl J Med. 2015;372:747–55. https://doi.org/10.1056/NEJMsa1410639.
17. Ilia S, et al. Effect of endotracheal tube size, respiratory system mechanics, and ventilator settings on driving pressure. Pediatr Crit Care Med. 2020;21:e47–51. https://doi.org/10.1097/PCC.0000000000002186.
18. van der Zee P, Gommers D. Recruitment maneuvers and higher PEEP, the so-called open lung concept, in patients with ARDS. Crit Care. 2019;23:73. https://doi.org/10.1186/s13054-019-2365-1.
19. Sahetya SK, Goligher EC, Brower RG. Fifty years of research in ards. setting positive end-expiratory pressure in acute respiratory distress syndrome. Am J Respir Crit Care Med. 2017;195:1429–38. https://doi.org/10.1164/rccm.201610-2035CI.
20. Gattinoni L, et al. Lung recruitment in patients with the acute respiratory distress syndrome. N Engl J Med. 2006;354:1775–86. https://doi.org/10.1056/NEJMoa052052.
21. Khemani RG, Markovitz BP, Curley MA. Characteristics of children intubated and mechanically ventilated in 16 PICUs. Chest. 2009;136:765–71. https://doi.org/10.1378/chest.09-0207.
22. Santschi M, et al. Acute lung injury in children: therapeutic practice and feasibility of international clinical trials. Pediatr Crit Care Med. 2010;11:681–9. https://doi.org/10.1097/PCC.0b013e3181d904c0.
23. Khemani RG, Parvathaneni K, Yehya N, Bhalla AK, Thomas NJ, Newth CJL. PEEP lower than the ARDS network protocol is associated with higher pediatric ARDS mortality. Am J Respir Crit Care Med. 2018; https://doi.org/10.1164/rccm.201707-1404OC.
24. Suzumura EA, Amato MBP, Cavalcanti AB. Understanding recruitment maneuvers. Intensive Care Med. 2016;42:908–11. https://doi.org/10.1007/s00134-015-4025-5.
25. Hess DR. Recruitment maneuvers and PEEP titration. Respir Care. 2015;60:1688–704. https://doi.org/10.4187/respcare.04409.
26. Kneyber MCJ. Positive end-expiratory pressure in the pediatric intensive care unit. Paediatr Respir Rev. 2024;49:5–8. https://doi.org/10.1016/j.prrv.2023.11.003.
27. Gattinoni L, Carlesso E, Cressoni M. Selecting the 'right' positive end-expiratory pressure level. Curr Opin Crit Care. 2015;21:50–7. https://doi.org/10.1097/MCC.0000000000000166.

28. Talmor D, et al. Mechanical ventilation guided by esophageal pressure in acute lung injury. N Engl J Med. 2008;359:2095–104. https://doi.org/10.1056/NEJMoa0708638.
29. Gerstmann DR, Fouke JM, Winter DC, Taylor AF, deLemos RA. Proximal, tracheal, and alveolar pressures during high-frequency oscillatory ventilation in a normal rabbit model. Pediatr Res. 1990;28:367–73.
30. Pillow JJ. High-frequency oscillatory ventilation: mechanisms of gas exchange and lung mechanics. Crit Care Med. 2005;33:S135–41.
31. Junqueira FMD, Nadal JAH, Brandao MB, Nogueira RJN, de Souza TH. High-frequency oscillatory ventilation in children: a systematic review and meta-analysis. Pediatr Pulmonol. 2021;56:1872–88. https://doi.org/10.1002/ppul.25428.
32. Arnold JH, Hanson JH, Toro-Figuero LO, Gutierrez J, Berens RJ, Anglin DL. Prospective, randomized comparison of high-frequency oscillatory ventilation and conventional mechanical ventilation in pediatric respiratory failure. Crit Care Med. 1994;22:1530–9.
33. Samransamruajkit R, Prapphal N, Deelodegenavong J, Poovorawan Y. Plasma soluble intercellular adhesion molecule-1 (sICAM-1) in pediatric ARDS during high frequency oscillatory ventilation: a predictor of mortality. Asian Pac J Allergy Immunol. 2005;23:181–8.
34. Samransamruajkit R, Rassameehirun C, Pongsanon K, Huntrakul S, Deerojanawong J, Sritippayawan S, Prapphal N. A comparison of clinical efficacy between high frequency oscillatory ventilation and conventional ventilation with lung volume recruitment in pediatric acute respiratory distress syndrome: a randomized controlled trial. Indian J Crit Care Med. 2016;20:72–7. https://doi.org/10.4103/0972-5229.175940.
35. El-Nawawy A, Moustafa A, Heshmat H, Abouahmed A. High frequency oscillatory ventilation versus conventional mechanical ventilation in pediatric acute respiratory distress syndrome: a randomized controlled study. Turk J Pediatr. 2017;59:130–43. https://doi.org/10.24953/turkjped.2017.02.004.
36. Gupta P, et al. Comparison of high-frequency oscillatory ventilation and conventional mechanical ventilation in pediatric respiratory failure. JAMA Pediatr. 2014; https://doi.org/10.1001/jamapediatrics.2013.4463.
37. Kneyber MC, van Heerde M, Markhorst DG. It is too early to declare early or late rescue high-frequency oscillatory ventilation dead. JAMA Pediatr. 2014;168:861. https://doi.org/10.1001/jamapediatrics.2014.961.
38. Rimensberger PC, Bachman TE. It is too early to declare early or late rescue high-frequency oscillatory ventilation dead. JAMA Pediatr. 2014;168:862–3. https://doi.org/10.1001/jamapediatrics.2014.940.
39. Essouri S, Emeriaud G, Jouvet P. It is too early to declare early or late rescue high-frequency oscillatory ventilation dead. JAMA Pediatr. 2014;168:861–2. https://doi.org/10.1001/jamapediatrics.2014.937.
40. Bateman ST, et al. Early high-frequency oscillatory ventilation in pediatric acute respiratory failure. A propensity score analysis. Am J Respir Crit Care Med. 2016;193:495–503. https://doi.org/10.1164/rccm.201507-1381OC.
41. Wong JJ, et al. The impact of high frequency oscillatory ventilation on mortality in paediatric acute respiratory distress syndrome. Crit Care. 2020;24:31. https://doi.org/10.1186/s13054-020-2741-x.
42. Imai Y, Nakagawa S, Ito Y, Kawano T, Slutsky AS, Miyasaka K. Comparison of lung protection strategies using conventional and high-frequency oscillatory ventilation. J Appl Physiol. 1985;2001(91):1836–44.
43. Carney D, DiRocco J, Nieman G. Dynamic alveolar mechanics and ventilator-induced lung injury. Crit Care Med. 2005;33:S122–8. https://doi.org/10.1097/01.ccm.0000155928.95341.bc.
44. Rotta AT, Gunnarsson B, Fuhrman BP, Hernan LJ, Steinhorn DM. Comparison of lung protective ventilation strategies in a rabbit model of acute lung injury. Crit Care Med. 2001;29:2176–84. https://doi.org/10.1097/00003246-200111000-00021.
45. Young D, et al. High-frequency oscillation for acute respiratory distress syndrome. N Engl J Med. 2013;368:806–13. https://doi.org/10.1056/NEJMoa1215716.
46. Ferguson ND, et al. High-frequency oscillation in early acute respiratory distress syndrome. N Engl J Med. 2013;368:795–805. https://doi.org/10.1056/NEJMoa1215554.
47. Gu XL, Wu GN, Yao YW, Shi DH, Song Y. Is high-frequency oscillatory ventilation more effective and safer than conventional protective ventilation in adult acute respiratory distress syndrome

patients? A meta-analysis of randomized controlled trials. Crit Care. 2014;18:R111. https://doi.org/10.1186/cc13900.
48. Malhotra A, Drazen JM. High-frequency oscillatory ventilation on shaky ground. N Engl J Med. 2013;368:863–5. https://doi.org/10.1056/NEJMe1300103.
49. Fedora M, Klimovic M, Seda M, Dominik P, Nekvasil R. Effect of early intervention of high-frequency oscillatory ventilation on the outcome in pediatric acute respiratory distress syndrome. Bratisl Lek Listy. 2000;101:8–13.
50. Meade MO, et al. Severity of hypoxemia and effect of high-frequency oscillatory ventilation in acute respiratory distress syndrome. Am J Respir Crit Care Med. 2017;196:727–33. https://doi.org/10.1164/rccm.201609-1938OC.
51. de Jager P, et al. Feasibility of an alternative, physiologic, individualized open-lung approach to high-frequency oscillatory ventilation in children. Ann Intensive Care. 2019;9:9. https://doi.org/10.1186/s13613-019-0492-0.
52. Fernandez A, et al. Invasive ventilatory support in patients with pediatric acute respiratory distress syndrome: from the second Pediatric Acute Lung Injury Consensus Conference. Pediatr Crit Care Med. 2023;24:S61–75. https://doi.org/10.1097/PCC.0000000000003159.
53. Suzuki H, Papazoglou K, Bryan AC. Relationship between PaO2 and lung volume during high frequency oscillatory ventilation. Acta Paediatr Jpn. 1992;34:494–500.
54. Kneyber MC, van Heerde M, Markhorst DG. Reflections on pediatric high-frequency oscillatory ventilation from a physiologic perspective. Respir Care. 2012;57:1496–504. https://doi.org/10.4187/respcare.01571.
55. Pellicano A, Tingay DG, Mills JF, Fasulakis S, Morley CJ, Dargaville PA. Comparison of four methods of lung volume recruitment during high frequency oscillatory ventilation. Intensive Care Med. 2009;35:1990–8.
56. Froese AB. High-frequency oscillatory ventilation for adult respiratory distress syndrome: let's get it right this time! Crit Care Med. 1997;25:906–8.
57. Markhorst DG, van Genderingen HR, van Vught AJ. Static pressure-volume curve characteristics are moderate estimators of optimal airway pressures in a mathematical model of (primary/pulmonary) acute respiratory distress syndrome. Intensive Care Med. 2004;30:2086–93. https://doi.org/10.1007/s00134-004-2446-7.
58. Tingay DG, Mills JF, Morley CJ, Pellicano A, Dargaville PA. The deflation limb of the pressure-volume relationship in infants during high-frequency ventilation. Am J Respir Crit Care Med. 2006;173:414–20.
59. Goddon S, Fujino Y, Hromi JM, Kacmarek RM. Optimal mean airway pressure during high-frequency oscillation: predicted by the pressure-volume curve. Anesthesiology. 2001;94:862–9.
60. Pillow JJ, Sly PD, Hantos Z, Bates JH. Dependence of intrapulmonary pressure amplitudes on respiratory mechanics during high-frequency oscillatory ventilation in preterm lambs. Pediatr Res. 2002;52:538–44.
61. van Genderingen HR, Versprille A, Leenhoven T, Markhorst DG, van Vught AJ, Heethaar RM. Reduction of oscillatory pressure along the endotracheal tube is indicative for maximal respiratory compliance during high-frequency oscillatory ventilation: a mathematical model study. Pediatr Pulmonol. 2001;31:458–63.
62. Slutsky AS, et al. Effects of frequency, tidal volume, and lung volume on CO2 elimination in dogs by high frequency (2-30 Hz), low tidal volume ventilation. J Clin Invest. 1981;68:1475–84.
63. Scalfaro P, Pillow JJ, Sly PD, Cotting J. Reliable tidal volume estimates at the airway opening with an infant monitor during high-frequency oscillatory ventilation. Crit Care Med. 2001;29:1925–30.
64. Hamel DS, Katz AL, Craig DM, Davies JD, Cheifetz IM. Carbon dioxide elimination and gas displacement vary with piston position during high-frequency oscillatory ventilation. Respir Care. 2005;50:361–6.
65. Gavriely N, Solway J, Loring SH, Butler JP, Slutsky AS, Drazen JM. Pressure-flow relationships of endotracheal tubes during high-frequency ventilation. J Appl Physiol. 1985;59:3–11.
66. Niederer PF, Leuthold R, Bush EH, Spahn DR, Schmid ER. High-frequency ventilation: oscillatory dynamics. Crit Care Med. 1994;22:S58–65.
67. Hirao O, Iguchi N, Uchiyama A, Mashimo T, Nishimura M, Fujino Y. Influence of endotracheal tube bore on tidal volume during high frequency oscillatory ventilation: a model lung study. Med Sci Monit. 2009;15:MT1–4.

68. Wong R, Deakers T, Hotz J, Khemani RG, Ross PA, Newth CJ. Volume and pressure delivery during pediatric high-frequency oscillatory ventilation. Pediatr Crit Care Med. 2017;18:e189–94. https://doi.org/10.1097/PCC.0000000000001089.
69. Bauer K, Brucker C. The role of ventilation frequency in airway reopening. J Biomech. 2009;42:1108–13.
70. Tsuzaki K, Hales CA, Strieder DJ, Venegas JG. Regional lung mechanics and gas transport in lungs with inhomogeneous compliance. J Appl Physiol. 1993;75:206–16.
71. Venegas JG, Fredberg JJ. Understanding the pressure cost of ventilation: why does high-frequency ventilation work? Crit Care Med. 1994;22:S49–57.
72. Van de Kieft M, Dorsey D, Morison D, Bravo L, Venticinque S, Derdak S. High-frequency oscillatory ventilation: lessons learned from mechanical test lung models. Crit Care Med. 2005;33:S142–7.
73. Downs JB, Stock MC. Airway pressure release ventilation: a new concept in ventilatory support. Crit Care Med. 1987;15:459–61.
74. Chatburn RL, Primiano FP Jr. A new system for understanding modes of mechanical ventilation. Respir Care. 2001;46:604–21.
75. Jain SV, et al. The 30-year evolution of airway pressure release ventilation (APRV). Intensive Care Med Exp. 2016;4:11. https://doi.org/10.1186/s40635-016-0085-2.
76. Lalgudi Ganesan S, Jayashree M, Chandra Singhi S, Bansal A. Airway pressure release ventilation in pediatric acute respiratory distress syndrome. A randomized controlled trial. Am J Respir Crit Care Med. 2018;198:1199–207. https://doi.org/10.1164/rccm.201705-0989OC.
77. Habashi NM. Other approaches to open-lung ventilation: airway pressure release ventilation. Crit Care Med. 2005;33:S228–40.
78. Xia J, Sun B, He H, Zhang H, Wang C, Zhan Q. Effect of spontaneous breathing on ventilator-induced lung injury in mechanically ventilated healthy rabbits: a randomized, controlled, experimental study. Crit Care. 2011;15:R244. https://doi.org/10.1186/cc10502.
79. Putensen C, Hering R, Muders T, Wrigge H. Assisted breathing is better in acute respiratory failure. Curr Opin Crit Care. 2005;11:63–8.
80. Putensen C, Muders T, Varelmann D, Wrigge H. The impact of spontaneous breathing during mechanical ventilation. Curr Opin Crit Care. 2006;12:13–8.
81. Cox CA, Wolfson MR, Shaffer TH. Liquid ventilation: a comprehensive overview. Neonatal Netw. 1996;15:31–43.
82. Sarkar S, Paswan A, Prakas S. Liquid ventilation. Anesth Essays Res. 2014;8:277–82. https://doi.org/10.4103/0259-1162.143109.
83. Koen PA, Wolfson MR, Shaffer TH. Fluorocarbon ventilation: maximal expiratory flows and CO2 elimination. Pediatr Res. 1988;24:291–6. https://doi.org/10.1203/00006450-198809000-00003.
84. Hirschl RB. Advances in the management of respiratory failure. Liquid ventilation in the setting of respiratory failure. ASAIO J. 1996;42:209–10.
85. Slutsky AS, Drazen JM. Ventilation with small tidal volumes. N Engl J Med. 2002;347:630–1.

Paediatric Ventilator Liberation

Yolanda M. López-Fernández and Analía Fernández

Contents

J. Brierley et al. (eds.), *ESPNIC Children's Intensive Care Textbook*,
https://doi.org/10.1007/978-3-031-64762-8_15

Learning Objectives

- To review the current evidence and rationale for the development of the first guidelines for mechanical ventilation liberation in paediatrics.
- To identify the operational definitions associated with the MV liberation process in order to use a common and homogeneous language.
- To understand how the MV liberation process should be developed in clinical practice according to international clinical guidelines.

15.1 Introduction

Invasive mechanical ventilation (IMV) is commonly used as a supportive therapy in children admitted to paediatric intensive care units (PICUs) [1]. The longer the patient remains on IMV, the more likely they are to experience ventilator-associated events (VAEs), and paediatric patients with VAEs have an almost threefold increased risk of mortality [2]. Therefore, as the patient's clinical condition begins to improve, the focus should be on weaning the patient from IMV as soon as possible. However, this liberation process requires rigorous assessment, as too early liberation may expose patients to a high risk of extubation failure (EF), which in turn is associated with increased mortality and PICU length of stay [3].

EF rate in PICUs ranges from 1.5% to 19%, depending on patient-related factors such as underlying disease, duration of IMV and associated complications [1, 3, 4]. Furthermore, this wide range in EF is also related to the significant variation in practice between institutions and practitioners involved in the MV liberation process [5, 6], largely attributable to the lack of specific weaning protocols and guidelines.

The first international clinical practice guidelines for paediatric ventilation liberation were published in 2022 [7]. An international multi-professional panel was convened to provide 15 clinical practice recommendations for patients requiring >24 h of IMV. The expert panel also generated operational definitions (ODs) related to the weaning process [8]. In this chapter, we will discuss both the guidelines and the ODs and their application in daily practice.

15.2 Operational Definitions: A Common Language

ODs help to reduce variability between studies to ensure that the results are generalizable. It also allows the identification of patients who may benefit from the implementation of proven strategies and technologies [8].

15.2.1 Respiratory Support

Respiratory support includes IMV and non-invasive respiratory support (NRS) (Non-invasive ventilation [NIV], continuous positive airway pressure[CPAP], negative pressure ventilation [NPV], and high flow nasal cannula [HFNC]). These terms are often used as interchangeable, and because they have different mechanisms and levels of support and associated risks, clinical guidelines recommend differentiating the type of respiratory support in the literature [8] (■ Table 15.1).

Table 15.1 Paediatric ventilator liberation operational definitions. Respiratory support [8]

IMV	Positive pressure ventilation delivered via an artificial airway (endotracheal tube or tracheostomy)
NRS	Non-invasive respiratory support
NIV	Positive pressure with variable levels of pressure delivered without an artificial airway via any interface which aims to provide an occlusive fit (nasal mask, nasal pillows/prongs, full face mask or helmet)
CPAP	Positive pressure with a single continuous distending pressure delivered without an artificial airway via any interface which aims to provide an occlusive fit (nasal pillows/prongs, full face mask or helmet, etc.)
NPV	Respiratory support in which the surface of the thorax and/or abdomen is exposed to sub-atmospheric pressure (negative pressure)
HFNC	Flow that is delivered through a heated humidified nasal cannula circuit and interface at a flow rate which is: (a) ≥1 L/kg/min for patients up to 10 kg; (b) ≥10 L/min for patients >10 kg. When the HFNC flow falls below the above rates, the patient is considered to be receiving conventional oxygen therapy
COT	Provision of >0.21 oxygen by any of the following devices applied to a spontaneously breathing patient regardless of presence of humidification via: non-occlusive facial mask, nasal cannula at flow rates less than HFNC or tracheostomy collar

COT conventional oxygen therapy, *CPAP* continuous airway positive pressure, *HFNC* high flow nasal cannula, *IMV* invasive mechanical ventilation, *NRS* non-invasive respiratory support, *NIV* non-invasive ventilation, *NPV* negative pressure ventilation

15.2.2 Liberation from Invasive MV

A patient is liberated from invasive MV when:

(a) The endotracheal tube (ETT) is removed and is not reinserted within 48 h (excluding use for temporary procedures)
(b) Positive pressure ventilation is no longer being delivered through a tracheostomy tube and is not reinitiated within 48 h

15.2.3 Assessment for Liberation from Invasive MV

Spontaneous breathing trial (SBT) and Extubation readiness test (ERT) have been used interchangeably in the literature, although they are different concepts. An SBT is often part of an ERT [8].

(a) SBT: reduction of invasive MV support to predetermined settings to assess the likelihood that a patient will be able to independently maintain adequate minute ventilation and gas exchange without excessive respiratory effort if liberated from invasive MV. This reduction to predetermined values should be differentiated from the gradual reduction of ventilatory support.
(b) ERT: is defined as a bundle of elements used to assess the patient's eligibility to be liberated from invasive MV. In addition to the SBT, this may include assessment of

sedation level, adequacy of neurologic control of the airway (cough and gag), likelihood of post-extubation upper airway obstruction, assessment of respiratory muscle strength, magnitude of airway secretions, haemodynamic status and a plan for post-extubation respiratory support.

15.2.4 Post-extubation NRS

(a) Planned: to be initiated immediately after extubation.
(b) Rescue: within 48 h after extubation and not planned prior to the IMV liberation attempt.

15.3 The Liberation Process

The weaning process can be divided into two phases [9]:
- The gradual adjustment of ventilatory support, with periodic assessment of whether is feasible to separate the patient from the ventilator.
- The weaning phase itself.

The use of standardized MV liberation protocols may reduce the length of PICU stay and/or improve the rate of extubation success, whereas the liberation process guided by clinical judgement of the physician in charge may lead to unnecessary and prolonged mechanical ventilation. Protocols should be determined in each PICU according to institutional factors, human resources and patient characteristics. These protocols should involve the whole team (nurses, respiratory therapists and physicians) and be integrated with sedation protocols [10–12].

15.3.1 Gradual Adjustment of Respiratory Support

Once the patient's clinical condition has stabilized or improved, weaning from the ventilator should be actively promoted. Daily goals should include adjusting ventilatory support by facilitating assisted over controlled modes, avoiding asynchronies and assessing work of breathing. Sedoanalgesia, nutrition, metabolic and infection control will also influence the duration of MV and outcomes and should therefore be managed appropriately [9]. Ventilatory modes commonly used during this period are as follows:
- Synchronized intermittent mandatory ventilation (SIMV) combined with pressure support (PS): Mandatory respiratory rate (RR) is reduced. This mode has been associated with prolonged duration of ventilatory support and high rates of asynchronies [13].
- Self-regulating or automatic modes (mandatory minute ventilation [MMV] and adaptive support ventilation [ASV]): The mandatory breath rate is automatically adjusted according to the patient.

- Continuous spontaneous sequence: Pressure support (PS) and volume support (VS).
- Continuous spontaneous sequence with proportional support: Neural trigger adjusted assist ventilation (NAVA) and proportional assist ventilation (PAV). NAVA improves synchrony and allows monitoring of diaphragm electrical activity (Edi), while PAV adapts to the patient's respiratory effort.

During this phase, periodic assessment should be performed at regular intervals (at least daily but may be more frequent) to identify patients with potential for IMV liberation, in which case they will be further assessed with the extubation readiness testing (ERT) [7].

15.3.2 Protocol-Based Screening

The first clinical guidelines for paediatric MV liberation recommend a protocolized screening to assess eligibility for an ERT. Such screening should be performed at regular intervals and should meet pre-specified targets in relation to the patient's clinical status and ventilator settings [7]. The aim of such assessment should not be to achieve complete normalization of gas exchange, but sufficient improvement. More stringent oxygenation and ventilation indices do not improve the predictive value of failure.

15.3.2.1 Clinical Criteria

- Improvement of the process that led to IMV.
- Haemodynamic stability with minimal support. Some patients (e.g. with heart disease) may require inotropic support.
- Neurological status: The patient must have a level of consciousness sufficient to maintain respiratory effort and protective airway reflexes (cough and gag). Factors associated with the discontinuation of sedoanalgesia (delirium, withdrawal syndrome) should be assessed. In patients with traumatic brain injury (TBI) or severe neurological injuries, the presence of airway protective reflexes should be assessed even if the level of consciousness is decreased.
- Haematological status: absence of active bleeding; assess haemoglobin level individually.
- Afebrile or without signs of uncontrolled infection or sepsis.

15.3.2.2 Respiratory Support

- $FiO_2 \leq 0.5$ for a $SpO_2 \geq 92\%$ (except in cyanotic heart disease where baseline SpO_2 should be considered), PEEP <8 cmH_2O and PIP <25 cmH_2O.
- In patients with neuromuscular disease, SpO_2 >94% with FiO_2 0.21 combined with non-invasive ventilation (NIV) and respiratory physiotherapy is recommended.

15.3.3 Extubation Readiness

Once the pre-specified screening criteria have been met, the patient's ability to resume and maintain spontaneous ventilation without invasive ventilatory support should be assessed by performing an ERT. Among the assessments to be performed, the clinical guidelines recommend a test of spontaneous ventilation [7]. It is important to identify at this stage whether the patient being assessed falls into two categories that may require specific interventions: (a) patients at high risk of upper airway obstruction (UAO) (Table 15.2) and (b) patients at risk of extubation failure (Table 15.3). The following interventions are suggested in the clinical guidelines for paediatric ventilation liberation as part of an ERT:

Table 15.2 Population at high-risk factors of upper respiratory obstruction

High-risk factors of upper airway obstruction
ETT size larger than recommended for age
Leak test >25 cmH_2O (cuffed ETT)
Several intubation attempts
Intubation-related trauma or injury
Upper airway anatomical abnormalities
Others: aspiration, paralysis of vocal cords, etc.

ETT endotracheal tube

Table 15.3 Population at high risk of extubation failure

Population to be considered at high risk of EF
Borderline SBT
Chronic disease: Chronic pulmonary disease, neuromuscular disease, previous CPAP/NIV
Failure previous extubation
Genetic disorders: Trisomy 21 and others
Myocardial dysfunction
Neurological impairment.
Prolonged mechanical ventilation (>14 days)
Upper airway abnormalities or surgery
Younger patients

CPAP continuous positive airway pressure, *EF* extubation failure, *NIV* non-invasive ventilation, *SBT* spontaneous breathing test

15.3.3.1 Anticipate and Prevent Post-extubation UAO

- Administration of dexamethasone at 0.5 mg/kg dose (maximun dose 10 mg) at least 6 h prior to extubation decreases the risk of post-extubation UAO, with a decreased risk of extubation failure in patients at high risk of developing UAO. One network meta-analysis supports this recommendation [14].
- As the risk of UAO does not outweigh the risk of delaying extubation, extubation should not be delayed for this reason in standard-risk patients who have not been started on corticosteroids.
- Screening and indication for steroid therapy should be based on the criteria detailed in ◘ Table 15.2. In patients intubated with cuffed ETT, particularly if they are at high risk of post-extubation UAO, a leak test is suggested. We emphasize the importance of not performing this test at the time of extubation, but at least 6 h prior to extubation to allow timely prescription of dexamethasone. In patients with uncuffed ETT, this test has not been shown to be predictive of UAO.
- To perform the leak test, the patient is placed in the supine position with the head in the midline. The cuff is deflated completely, allowing time for suctioning if required. The patient is manually ventilated to a maximal pressure of 30 cmH_2O. If no air leak is heard at maximum pressures of 25–30 cmH_2O, it is considered a failed test and an increased risk for post-extubation UAO [7].

15.3.3.2 Airway Protection

- The level of sedation, presence of cough and gag reflexes and the magnitude of oropharyngeal secretions should be assessed. An adequate level of consciousness is required to initiate an SBT, as impaired consciousness is associated with absence of airway protection mechanisms. In patients with neurological sequelae in whom full assessment is not always possible, the presence of protective reflexes should be prioritized.
- Validated scores/scales allow for appropriate evaluation of the level of sedation. In addition to assess adequate respiratory drive, other factors that also affect the liberation process can be analysed, such as comfort, response to stimuli, presence of pain and delirium.
- Clinical guidelines are neutral on the use of sedation protocols (neither for nor against). Two randomized clinical trials on sedoanalgesia protocols in patients with more than 24 h of IMV found no significant differences in the dose of sedoanalgesia between intervention/control groups and no significant differences in the rate of extubation failure [15, 16].

15.3.3.3 Anticipate Post-extubation Non-invasive Respiratory Support

- Muscle strength: The clinical guidelines suggest measurement of maximal inspiratory pressure (PiMax). No clear cut-off point can be established to define the risk of extubation failure, but a PiMax <20 cmH_2O is associated with higher EF, whereas a PiMax >50 cmH_2O suggests lower risk of EF.

  A standardized PiMax measurement consists of using a manometer inserted between the ETT and the ventilator circuit. The manoeuvre comprises a sustained (5–8 breaths) end-expiratory occlusion performed by using a valve or gloved hand. The maximum negative inspiratory pressure achieved should be repeated three times, each time documenting the maximum pressure. If an inspiratory effort >50 cmH_2O is observed, it is not required to repeat the occlusion.

There are other tools that assess muscle strength, such as ultrasound (diaphragm thickening fraction) and electromyography, but further evidence is still needed to be included as a recommendation.

- In patients at high risk of extubation failure (Table 15.3), pre-planned use of non-invasive respiratory support is suggested. NRS may be delivered via HFNC, CPAP or BiPAP immediately after extubation. A meta-analysis that included two randomized control trials comparing HFNC vs CPAP and five RCTs comparing NRS vs conventional oxygen therapy (COT) reported that NRS decreases the risk of EF [7].
- In patients <1 year of age, CPAP is preferred to HFNC, whereas in patients >1 year of age, both CPAP and HFNC can be used depending on the clinical scenario, except in patients with previous NIV requirement due to chronic disease, in which case BiPAP is preferred. In patients in whom CPAP/HFNC does not reduce work of breathing, escalation to BiPAP is recommended [17].
- If a patient at standard risk of EF presents respiratory distress on COT, it is suggested escalation to NRS.

15.3.4 Spontaneous Breathing Test (SBT)

An SBT should be performed after assessing the ability to protect the airway, level of analgesia, magnitude of secretions, likelihood of UAO (corticosteroid therapy if indicated), assessed muscle strength and risk factors for extubation (with a NRS plan if needed). An SBT objectively assesses the patient's ability to independently maintain minute ventilation and adequate gas exchange without excessive respiratory effort. Approximately 75% of patients successfully pass the first SBT and are extubated.

- T-piece: The patient is disconnected from the ventilator. The T-piece is connected to the ETT and to a circuit that circulates a gas supply. The T-piece allows early detection of diaphragm dysfunction (e.g. paresis or paralysis due to phrenic nerve injury following cardiac surgery). Moreover, it also allows the patient to be assessed without ventilatory support and without the increased work of breathing associated with valve opening and circuit resistance. It is more costly due to additional equipment and increased work loading. Of note, flows below inspiratory demand should not be used as this may cause rebreathing of expired air.
- Minimal pressure support: PS does not require any additional equipment as it involves switching from one ventilation mode to the other. The programmed level of support is intended to compensate for the resistance presented by the circuit and the opening and closing of valves required for breathing. The most used setting is a PEEP of 5 cmH_2O and PS of 5 cmH_2O above PEEP, although PS settings have been suggested according to the size of the ETT (PS of 10 cmH_2O for ETT 3.5; PS of 8 cmH_2O for ETT 4–4.5, or PS of 6 cmH_2O for ETT ≥5). An alternative is the automatic tube compensation (ATC) mode, not available on all ventilators, which consists of a variable PS that compensates for the pressure drop caused by the resistance of the ETT.

- CPAP: A positive pressure of 5 cmH_2O is maintained throughout the respiratory cycle with the aim of avoiding alveolar collapse due to loss of physiological PEEP, thus preserving functional residual capacity.

Clinical guidelines for MV liberation in paediatrics [7] suggest that SBT should be performed with PS with CPAP or CPAP alone in children at standard risk of extubation failure. In high-risk patients (◘ Table 15.3), the guidelines recommend avoiding PS as a method of SBT, as it may overestimate the patient's ventilatory function [18].

With respect to the duration of SBT, the guidelines do not specifically recommend a short (30 min) or long (1–2 h) test, as there is insufficient evidence. A short test is likely to allow standard-risk patients to be properly assessed and avoid unnecessary prolongation of ventilatory support. However, patients at high risk of EF may develop signs of failure within 60–120 min and a long test is recommended for these patients (◘ Table 15.3). Pre-defined criteria for SBT failure are helpful to avoid subjective assessments. Once SBT has been passed, extubation should not be delayed and should be performed immediately.

Take-Home Messages

- The first clinical guidelines for paediatric ventilation liberation propose an objective and standardized assessment of patients who have received IMV for at least 24 h, based on currently available evidence.
- PICU protocols using clinical practice guidelines for liberation from MV improve the quality of practice.
- Implementation of paediatric MV guidelines has the potential to reduce morbidity and mortality, as well as delayed weaning and extubation failure.

References

1. Farias JA, Fernández A, Monteverde E, et al. Mechanical ventilation in pediatric intensive care units during the season for acute lower respiratory infection: a multicenter study. Pediatr Crit Care Med. 2012;13:158–64.
2. Klompas M, Anderson D, Trick W. The preventability of ventilator-associated events. The CDC Prevention Epicenters Wake Up and Breathe Collaborative. Am J Respir Crit Care Med. 2015;191(3):292–301.
3. Gaies M, Tabbutt S, Schwartz SM. Clinical epidemiology of extubation failure in the pediatric cardiac ICU: a report from the Pediatric Cardiac Critical Care Consortium. Pediatr Crit Care Med. 2015;16(9):837–45.
4. Newth CJ, Venkataraman S, Willson DF, et al. Weaning and extubation readiness in pediatric patients. Pediatr Crit Care Med. 2009;10(1):1–11.
5. Newth CJ, Hotz JC, Khemani RG. Ventilator liberation in the pediatric ICU. Respir Care. 2020;65:1601–10.
6. Loberger JM, Campbell CM, Colleti J Jr, et al. Ventilation liberation practices among 380 international PICUs. Crit Care Explor. 2022;4(6):e0710.
7. Abu-Sultaneh S, Iyer NP, Fernández A, et al. Executive summary: international clinical practice guidelines for pediatric ventilator liberation, a Pediatric Acute Lung Injury and Sepsis Investigators (PALISI) network document. Am J Respir Crit Care Med. 2023;207(1):17–28.

8. Abu-Sultaneh S, Iyer NP, Fernández A, et al. Operational definitions related to pediatric ventilator liberation. Chest. 2023;163(5):1130–43.
9. Sklar MC, Burns K, Rittayamai N, et al. Effort to breathe with various spontaneous breathing trial techniques. A physiologic meta-analysis. Am J Respir Crit Care Med. 2017;195(11):1477–85.
10. Abu-Sultaneh S, Hole AJ, Tori AJ, et al. An interprofessional quality improvement initiative to standardize pediatric extubation readiness assessment. Pediatr Crit Care Med. 2017;18:e463–71.
11. Krawiec C, Carl D, Stetter C, et al. With implementation of a respiratory therapist-driven protocol of spontaneous breathing trials in the pediatric ICU. Respir Care. 2017;62:1233–40.
12. Loberger JM, Jones RM, Prabhakaran P. A respiratory therapist-driven pathway improves timeliness of extubation readiness assessment in a single PICU. Pediatr Crit Care Med. 2020;21:e513–21.
13. Kacmarek RM, Branson RD. Should intermittent mandatory ventilation be abolished? Respir Care. 2016;61(6):854–66.
14. Iyer NP, López-Fernández YM, González-Dambrauskas S, et al. A network meta-analysis of dexamethasone for preventing postextubation upper airway obstruction in children. Ann Am Thorac Soc. 2023;20(1):118–30.
15. Blackwood B, Tume LN, Morris KP, et al., SANDWICH Collaborators. Effect of a sedation and ventilator liberation protocol vs usual care on duration of invasive mechanical ventilation in pediatric intensive care units: a randomized clinical trial. JAMA. 2021;326:401–10.
16. Curley MA, Wypij D, Watson RS, et al. Protocolized sedation vs usual care in pediatric patients mechanically ventilated for acute respiratory failure: a randomized clinical trial. JAMA. 2015;313:379–89.
17. Ramnarayan P, Richards-Belle A, Drikite L, et al., Step-Down RCT Investigators and the Paediatric Critical Care Society Study Group. Effect of high-flow nasal cannula therapy vs continuous positive airway pressure following extubation on liberation from respiratory support in critically ill children: a randomized clinical trial. JAMA. 2022;327(16):1555–65.
18. Khemani RG, Hotz J, Morzov R, et al. Pediatric extubation readiness tests should not use pressure support. Intensive Care Med. 2016;42:1214–22.

Ventilation of the Infant

Daniele De Luca, Lucilla Pezza, and Barbara Loi

Contents

J. Brierley et al. (eds.), *ESPNIC Children's Intensive Care Textbook*,
https://doi.org/10.1007/978-3-031-64762-8_16

Learning Objectives

- Know the most common causes of respiratory failure in infants.
- Understand primary indications for mechanical ventilation in infants.
- Understand the mechanical characteristics of infants with the most common types of respiratory failure.
- Understand possible ancillary therapies in mechanically ventilated infants.
- Understand the need for clinical monitoring of mechanically ventilated infants.

16.1 Introduction

Infants may be usually ventilated for a few primarily respiratory disorders and this makes their ventilatory management relatively easy to learn, at least, as long as they do not have rare disorders or malformations. However, patients' size entails some peculiarities and opens questions that we will try to discuss in this chapter.

16.2 Indications

The main indication for mechanical ventilation in infants is acute respiratory distress syndrome (ARDS), which may be diagnosed by using the pediatric (PARDS) [1] or neonatal (NARDS) [2] definitions. NARDS and PARDS definitions should be used, respectively, during and beyond the first month of life, although for former preterm infants, it is unclear if one or the other is more suitable [3].

Suggested risk factors for PARDS in infants are sepsis, near-drowning, congenital immunodeficiencies, thoracic trauma, pneumonia, bronchiolitis, pertussis, bronchopulmonary dysplasia (BPD), cancer, milk aspiration, major surgery, and gastroesophageal reflux [4].

ARDS is a typical restrictive disorder: accordingly, the ventilation goal in this category of patients is to open up the diseased alveoli with the best technique of alveolar recruitment, as described by PEMVECC guidelines in another chapter [5].

It is unclear what is the best strategy for ventilation and recruitment in PARDS; however, the same considerations apply to infants and older children [5].

A mixed mechanical disorder is uncommon in infants, as an obstructive pattern is relatively rare in these patients: it is described only in ARDS following severe bronchiolitis or in former preterm infants with severe BPD and dynamic airway obstruction or with airway malformations. These cases are more complex to be ventilated, ideally more prone to ventilator-induced lung injury (VILI) and may sometimes require nonconventional approaches. There is not a single unanimously acknowledged ventilatory strategy for this complicated category: a tailored approach may be needed and, anyway, there are no peculiarities for the infant population compared to older children.

Bronchiolitis is the second most common reason for infant ventilation. It is supposed to arise from an infection with a particularly intense inflammatory response primarily localized in the lower airways. Almost everyone on the planet is exposed to respiratory syncytial virus (RSV), which is the commonest cause of bronchiolitis, by the age of 2 years [6]. The main predictors of severe outcome in previously healthy infants appear to be the young age (i.e., <4 months, because of poor respiratory mechanical reserve), prematurity, congenital heart defects, and pulmonary consolidations suggesting an extension of inflammation to the alveolar tissue [7, 8].

A small proportion of cases of RSV bronchiolitis develop severe respiratory failure that needs to be managed in neonatal or pediatric intensive care units (respectively, NICUs or PICUs). About 4–15% of infants with bronchiolitis needing NICU/PICU care were previously healthy and 10–40% of cases are former preterm infants [9].

These patients are characterized by mainly obstructive lung mechanics; the work of breathing in bronchiolitis is two-to-six times that of normal infants because elastic and nonelastic resistances need to be overcome [10]. However, abnormality in compliance may coexist when the inflammatory process is diffused to the alveolar tissue and not only to the airways [10, 11]. This may happen when bronchiolitis is complicated by superinfections or anyway RSV is not the only etiologic agent. Moreover, when the inflammatory process is enough extended, it may trigger ARDS, so that the restrictive pattern adds to the airway obstruction [11].

In bronchiolitis, inspiratory muscles are unable to produce the necessary reduction in intrapleural pressure because of hyperinflation [10]. "Exhaustion" in infants with bronchiolitis usually results from the inability to perform the necessary workload for breathing with hyperinflated lungs. Another physiopathologic problem of severe bronchiolitis is transpulmonary fluid shift and the development of pulmonary edema, which follows obstructive breathing with large negative intrathoracic pressure swings [12].

The majority of PICU-admitted infants with bronchiolitis may be easily and successfully managed with continuous positive airway pressure (CPAP) and/or noninvasive ventilation (NIV) although solid trials are still lacking in this field [13, 14]. The best level of CPAP is around 7 cmH_2O in order to optimally discharge the work of breathing in these patients [15]. Javouhey et al. interestingly used a progressive approach from CPAP to NIV by using CPAP at 5–10 cmH_2O and, if this failed, switching to biphasic CPAP with a higher pressure level set at 12 cmH_2O and gradually increased to 18 cmH_2O [16]. This ensured a significantly lower intubation rate; unsurprisingly, the percentage of ventilator-associated pneumonia was also much reduced [16]. This approach should be submitted to short "trials" on a case-by-case scenario, knowing that oxygenation improvement after 1 h of CPAP/NIV usually predicts its success and that the co-existence of other organ failure beyond the respiratory insufficiency indicates the need for invasive ventilation [17, 18].

16.3 Ancillary Therapies During Infant Ventilation

Some ancillary measures, which are typical of this age and more uncommon in older children, have been proposed in addition to mechanical ventilation in infants and that are typical of this age and more uncommon in older children. We will cover them here and give some guidance.

Surfactant has been used in infants more easily than in older children since the volume of distribution in the lung is lower and it is easier to give a higher dose. A Cochrane meta-analysis of randomized controlled trials showed improved clinical outcomes in mechanically ventilated infants with bronchiolitis treated with surfactant [19]. There is enough physiopathological and pathobiological background to translate the use of surfactant in bronchiolitis to direct (i.e., "primary") PARDS in infants, particularly if younger than 6 months, to whom a correct surfactant dose can be easily administered [20–22]. In fact, infants with bronchiolitis treated so far with surfactant were likely having bronchiolitis-induced PARDS and not only a pure airway disease [21, 22]. We still wait for large multicenter, high-quality, randomized controlled trials to better define the population that may benefit from this intervention. The Bronchiolitis Endotracheal Surfactant Study (BESS) trial is ongoing in the United Kingdom and will be helpful to give more insight into this issue during 2021.

Helium, a naturally inert gas with a low molecular weight, when mixed with 21% oxygen produces a mixed gas (Heliox) with one-third the density of air and thus more capable to trespass airway obstructions. In bronchiolitis, Heliox when used with CPAP reduces clinical severity significantly more than CPAP alone [23]. The response to Heliox is rapidly seen within the first hour and is maintained during treatment. Despite interesting experiences, no well-established indications exist for the use of Heliox, its advantages are unclear and its high cost must also be factored in. The main indication may be the necessity to delay invasive ventilation as much as possible (i.e., in patients with immunodeficiencies, malignancies, or major malformation) while not achieving adequate levels of oxygenation or gas exchange during CPAP and/or NIV alone.

Chest physiotherapy has been commonly proposed for mechanically ventilated infants, at least in some countries, but evidence-based data have demonstrated its lack of usefulness [24, 25].

16.4 Monitoring During Infant Ventilation

Monitoring during mechanical ventilation has some peculiarities in infants due to the small patients' size.

The majority of infants requiring respiratory support are not in a such critical state; sometimes, instead, severe ARDS may occur and hemodynamic impairment may be observed. Thus, it is crucial to adapt not only to the aggressiveness of respiratory support but also physiological monitoring. A difficulty may come from the relative lack of suitable techniques for small infants. However, targeted point-of-care ultrasound is now the reference for hemodynamics and lung aeration monitoring, and ESPNIC guidelines are now available to guide its use [26]. Alternative techniques to be considered, where available, although they should be mainly used for research purposes, are electrical cardiometry [27] and electrical impedance tomography [28].

In general, monitoring during mechanical ventilation should follow a pyramidal approach and be as noninvasive as possible for most infants who only need noninvasive respiratory support (bottom of the pyramid) [29]. Conversely, infants with severe disease may need more complex and invasive monitoring including indwelling arterial lines, but they represent a minority of patients and this is well described by PEMVECC guidelines [5].

Take-Home Messages

- Mechanical ventilation in infants presents few peculiarities compared to pediatric general population.
- Infants are more often ventilated for PARDS and bronchiolitis, although this latter may often require CPAP or NIV only.
- Some ancillary therapies are commonly considered for infants with PARDS or bronchiolitis such as surfactants and Heliox.
- It is crucial to monitor mechanically ventilated infants using a pyramidal approach: monitoring should be as noninvasive as possible for most infants who only need noninvasive respiratory support and more accurate and aggressive for the few severest patients.

References

1. Khemani RG, Smith LS, Zimmerman JJ, Erickson S. Pediatric acute respiratory distress syndrome: definition, incidence, and epidemiology. Pediatr Crit Care Med. 2015;16:S23–40.
2. De Luca D, van Kaam AH, Tingay DG, et al. The Montreux definition of neonatal ARDS: biological and clinical background behind the description of a new entity. Lancet Respir Med. 2017;5:657–66.
3. De Luca D. Personalising care of acute respiratory distress syndrome according to patients' age. Lancet Respir Med. 2019;7:100–1.
4. On behalf of Respiratory Section of the European Society for Pediatric Neonatal Intensive Care (ESPNIC), De Luca D, Piastra M, et al. The use of the Berlin definition for acute respiratory distress syndrome during infancy and early childhood: multicenter evaluation and expert consensus. Intensive Care Med. 2013;39:2083–91.
5. On behalf of the section Respiratory Failure of the European Society for Paediatric and Neonatal Intensive Care, Kneyber MCJ, de Luca D, et al. Recommendations for mechanical ventilation of critically ill children from the Paediatric Mechanical Ventilation Consensus Conference (PEMVECC). Intensive Care Med. 2017;43:1764–80.
6. Hasegawa K, Goto T, Hirayama A, et al. Respiratory virus epidemiology among US infants with severe bronchiolitis: analysis of 2 multicenter, multiyear cohort studies. Pediatr Infect Dis J. 2019;38:e180–3.
7. Fauroux B, Hascoët J-M, Jarreau P-H, et al. Risk factors for bronchiolitis hospitalization in infants: a French nationwide retrospective cohort study over four consecutive seasons (2009-2013). PLoS One. 2020;15:e0229766.
8. López Guinea A, Casado Flores J, Martín Sobrino MA, et al. Bronquiolitis grave. Epidemiología y evolución de 284 pacientes. An Pediatr. 2007;67:116–22.
9. Carbonell-Estrany X, Figueras-Aloy J, Law BJ. Identifying risk factors for severe respiratory syncytial virus among infants born after 33 through 35 completed weeks of gestation: different methodologies yield consistent findings. Pediatr Infect Dis J. 2004;23:S193–201.
10. Newth CJ, Hammer J. Pulmonary function in ventilated infants with bronchiolitis. Pediatr Pulmonol. 1998;26:438–41.
11. Hammer J, Numa A, Newth CJ. Acute respiratory distress syndrome caused by respiratory syncytial virus. Pediatr Pulmonol. 1997;23:176–83.
12. Rimensberger PC. Mechanical ventilation in paediatric intensive care. Ann Fr Anesth Réanim. 2009;28:682–4.
13. Jat KR, Mathew JL. Continuous positive airway pressure (CPAP) for acute bronchiolitis in children. Cochrane Database Syst Rev. 2019. Published online Jan 31; https://doi.org/10.1002/14651858.CD010473.pub3.
14. Combret Y, Prieur G, Roux LE, P, Médrinal C. Non-invasive ventilation improves respiratory distress in children with acute viral bronchiolitis: a systematic review. Minerva Anestesiol. 2017;83:624–37.

15. Essouri S, Durand P, Chevret L, et al. Optimal level of nasal continuous positive airway pressure in severe viral bronchiolitis. Intensive Care Med. 2011;37:2002–7.
16. Javouhey E, Barats A, Richard N, Stamm D, Floret D. Non-invasive ventilation as primary ventilatory support for infants with severe bronchiolitis. Intensive Care Med. 2008;34:1608–14.
17. Piastra M, De Luca D, Marzano L, et al. The number of failing organs predicts non-invasive ventilation failure in children with ALI/ARDS. Intensive Care Med. 2011;37:1510–6.
18. Piastra M, De Luca D, Pietrini D, et al. Noninvasive pressure-support ventilation in immunocompromised children with ARDS: a feasibility study. Intensive Care Med. 2009;35:1420–7.
19. Jat KR, Chawla D. Surfactant therapy for bronchiolitis in critically ill infants. Cochrane Database Syst Rev. 2015. Published online Aug 24; https://doi.org/10.1002/14651858.CD009194.pub3.
20. Taut FJH, Rippin G, Schenk P, et al. A search for subgroups of patients with ARDS who may benefit from surfactant replacement therapy. Chest. 2008;134:724–32.
21. De Luca D, Piastra M, Tosi F, et al. Pharmacological therapies for pediatric and neonatal ALI/ARDS: an evidence-based review. Curr Drug Targets. 2012;13:906–16.
22. Boet A, Brat R, Aguilera SS, Tissieres P, De Luca D. Surfactant from neonatal to pediatric ICU: bench and bedside evidence. Minerva Anestesiol. 2014;80:1345–56.
23. Liet J-M, Ducruet T, Gupta V, Cambonie G. Heliox inhalation therapy for bronchiolitis in infants. Cochrane Database Syst Rev. 2015. Published online Sept 18; https://doi.org/10.1002/14651858.CD006915.pub3.
24. Perrotta C, Ortiz Z, Roque M. Chest physiotherapy for acute bronchiolitis in paediatric patients between 0 and 24 months old. In: The Cochrane Collaboration, editor. Cochrane database of systematic reviews. John Wiley & Sons, Ltd.: Chichester; 2005. https://doi.org/10.1002/14651858.CD004873.pub2.
25. Anand R, McAuley DF, Blackwood B, et al. Mucoactive agents for acute respiratory failure in the critically ill: a systematic review and meta-analysis. Thorax. 2020;75:623–31.
26. Singh Y, Tissot C, Fraga MV, et al. International evidence-based guidelines on Point of Care Ultrasound (POCUS) for critically ill neonates and children issued by the POCUS Working Group of the European Society of Paediatric and Neonatal Intensive Care (ESPNIC). Crit Care. 2020;24 https://doi.org/10.1186/s13054-020-2787-9.
27. Boet A, Jourdain G, Demontoux S, et al. Basic hemodynamic monitoring using ultrasound or electrical cardiometry during transportation of neonates and infants. Pediatr Crit Care Med. 2017;18:e488–93.
28. Frerichs I, Amato MBP, van Kaam AH, et al. Chest electrical impedance tomography examination, data analysis, terminology, clinical use and recommendations: consensus statement of the TRanslational EIT developmeNt stuDy group. Thorax. 2017;72:83–93.
29. De Luca D, Romain O, Yousef N, et al. Monitorages physiopathologiques en réanimation néonatale. J Pédiatr Puéricult. 2015;28:276–300.

Fluids and Hemodynamics

Contents

Hemodynamic Physiology

Joris Lemson

Contents

J. Brierley et al. (eds.), *ESPNIC Children's Intensive Care Textbook*,
https://doi.org/10.1007/978-3-031-64762-8_17

Learning Objectives

- Gain insight into basic physiological cardiovascular principles.
- Appreciate the dynamics of the hemodynamic physiology.

17.1 Introduction

The function of blood circulation is diverse but is mainly focused on transporting various substances to and from the tissues, for instance, oxygen from the lung alveoli to the cells of the liver, carbon dioxide from the quadriceps muscle to the lungs, and also hormones from endocrine organs to multiple sites of the body. Some of these transport functions require more than a minimum amount of blood flow over time. Specifically, oxygen delivery to the tissues requires a considerable amount of oxygen molecules per minute to be transported, while hormones, antibodies, or white blood cells would themselves require a lesser blood flow.

Many centuries ago parts of the blood circulatory system of the human body have already been described by the ancient Ayurveda masters, the native Indian system of healthcare, between 400 BCE and 500 CE [1]. However, William Harvey, for the first time, compiled all known available information in a logical system and published in 1628 a book called *On the Motion of the Heart and Blood in Animals*, describing the complete process of blood circulation [2].

It is essential to understand (hemodynamic) physiology to appreciate its dynamic character. The circulatory system is a complex and ever-changing continuous flowing system with constant adaptations in order to meet the tissue's demands.

Case Study 1

Tommy (5 years) is admitted to the PICU with bacterial pneumonia. He has moderate respiratory insufficiency, is in need of oxygen, and has a high fever. His heart rate is 180 bpm, blood pressure is 65/40. What could be the origin of his hypotension? In the next part, we will see what determines blood pressure and why it is important to understand basic physiology in order to be able to institute the correct resuscitative measures.

17.2 The Heart

17

The heart is the pump that pushes the blood through the lungs (right heart) and the systemic circulation (left heart). As such the heart is only capable of doing so when enough venous blood is present in the atrial part of the heart itself that can be pumped out. The pumping capacity of the heart is determined by heart rate and stroke volume (◘ Fig. 17.1). While heart rate is dependent on many factors (◘ Table 17.1), stroke volume is determined by three factors: preload, afterload, and contractility (◘ Fig. 17.1) [3, 4]. If we want to understand and treat the hemodynamic condition of Tommy (Case 1), we now know that his low blood pressure is caused by either a low cardiac output, a low vascular resistance, or both. This is essential information since each cause requires a different therapeutic approach.

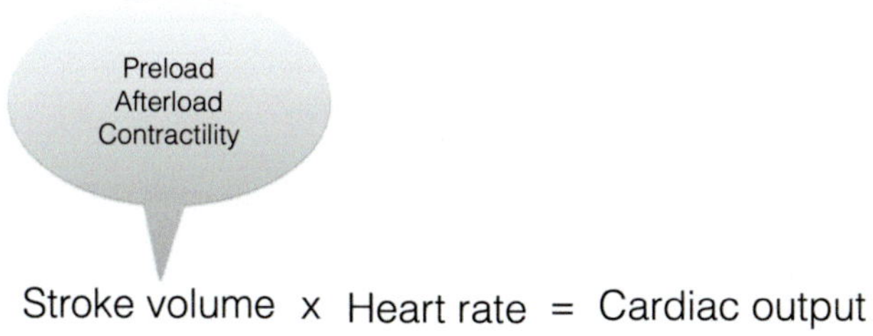

Fig. 17.1 Basic hemodynamic relations

Table 17.1 Some factors that influence heart rate
• Body temperature • Pain • Anxiousness • Emotions • Physical activity • Hypotension • Hypertension • Hormonal influence • Left ventricular function • Altitude • Respiratory dysfunction • Intracranial pressure • Cerebral dysfunction • Intrinsic cardiac factors

17.2.1 Preload

Preload is defined as the wall tension in the ventricular wall at the end of the diastole. This is determined by the amount of blood filling the ventricle in relation to the stiffness of the ventricular wall. It can be calculated by

$$\text{Preload} = (\text{end} - \text{diastolic pressure} \times \text{radius}) / 2 \times \text{wall thickness}$$

The relation between radius (R) and volume (V) of a sphere is reflected by

$$\text{Radius} = \sqrt[3]{\ } (3V / 4\pi)$$

Therefore, it becomes visible that volume plays a more important role than pressure, meaning that right atrial or central venous pressure does not reliably reflect the preload of the right ventricle. Neither does left atrial pressure (or pulmonary capillary wedge pressure) reflect the preload of the left ventricle. The most important component of preload is therefore the volume of blood in the ventricle at the end of the diastole together with the diastolic (relaxing) function of the ventricular wall [3, 4]. The relation between preload and stroke volume is reflected by the so-called starling curve as this was demonstrated more than 100 years ago by Patterson and Starling [5] (Fig. 17.2).

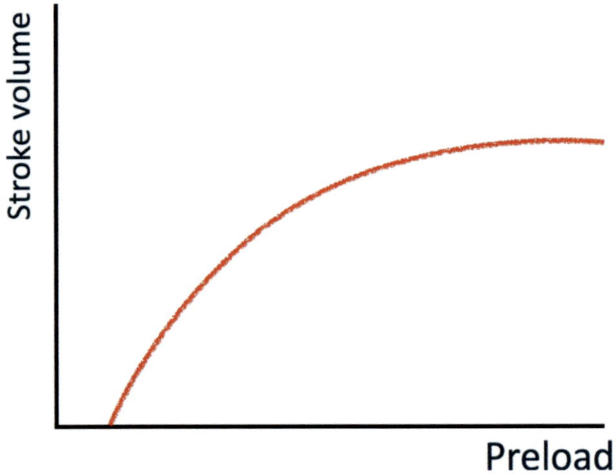

Fig. 17.2 The starling curve

17.2.2 Afterload

Like preload, the afterload can be calculated as

$$\text{Afterload} = (\text{ejection pressure} \times \text{radius}) / 2 \times \text{wall thickness}$$

Since, opposite to preload, the end-systolic volume is very small, the major determinant of afterload is the blood pressure during the ejection phase. In general, systolic arterial pressure is used as a reasonable measure of afterload.

17.2.3 Contractility

The contraction force of the ventricles is the last factor that contributes to the stroke volume. Contractility is measured using various methods. Routinely, the measurement of ejection fraction or shortening fraction using echocardiography is performed at the bedside.

17.2.4 Other Aspects

The diastolic function of the ventricle is primarily aimed at relaxing the myocardial muscle in order to prepare for a large blood volume. Therefore, diastolic dysfunction is considered to have a negative effect on myocardial performance and can be the cause of a lower stroke volume.

All of the above might lead to the impression that heart rate, stroke volume, and its determinants preload, afterload, and contractility are separate entities. However, all the factors involved have an influence on each other, for example, a stretch of the atria may cause an increase in heart rate, an increase in heart rate itself can cause an increase in contractility, and an increase in afterload may also increase contractility. Therefore, heart rate, blood pressure, preload, contractility, etc. are far more dynamic than we often think [6]. It is important to appreciate the dynamics in treating patients with hemodynamic derangements.

17.3 Venous Return

The blood that flows back to the heart is driven by an upstream pressure. This pressure is called mean systemic filling pressure [4, 5, 7–9]. When the blood flow seizes completely, the pressure in all vessels would reach the same value, which is higher than the central venous pressure. This pressure is determined by the blood volume and the compliance of the venous (and arterial) system. Venous return is therefore determined by

$$\text{Venous return} = \left(P_{\text{msf}} - P_{\text{ra}}\right) / R_{\text{v}}$$

P_{msf} = mean systemic filling pressure; P_{ra} = right atrial pressure; R_{v} = resistance to venous flow.

Figure 17.3 shows the relationship between P_{ra} and venous return as described by Guyton many years ago [9]. When P_{ra} is lower than P_{msf}, blood flow starts until a certain low pressure when negative venous pressures cause the collapse of the vessels and flow cannot increase anymore.

The above illustrates the importance of venous return in providing preload to the heart. Venous return can be increased by increasing the blood volume (most importantly fluid loading) but also by decreasing the compliance as a result of endogenous catecholamines or the administration of vasopressors. At the same time, a low right atrial pressure will contribute to an optimal venous return.

Combining the starling curve and the venous return curve shows how the present or actual cardiac output is determined as shown in Fig. 17.4 [3].

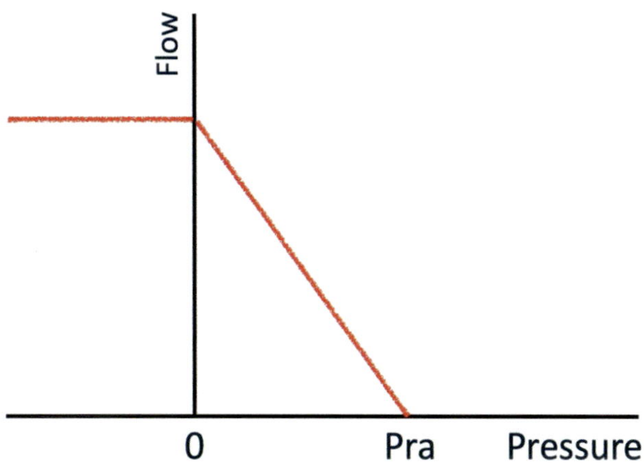

Fig. 17.3 The venous return curve

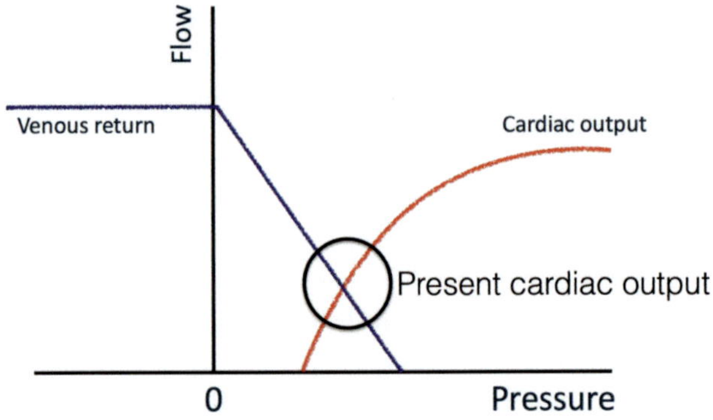

Fig. 17.4 The venous return curve and starling curve combined

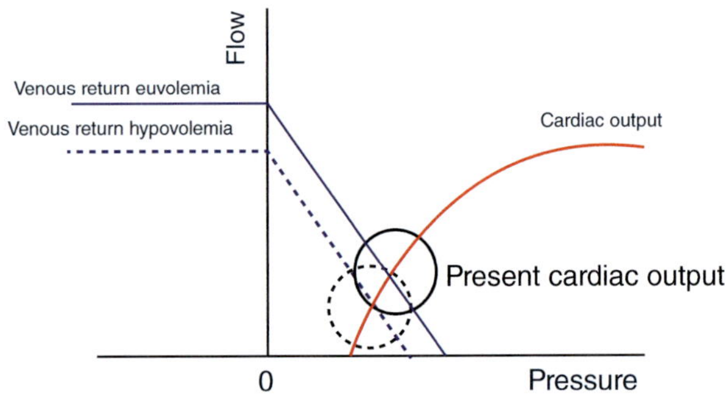

Fig. 17.5 The venous return curve and starling curve combined with hypovolemia

In the case of Tommy (Case 1), let us presume he suffers from hypovolemia due to sepsis with capillary leakage of intravascular volume. In that case, the P_{msf} will be reduced leading to a reduced venous return and thereby a reduced stroke volume as depicted in Fig. 17.5. The lower stroke volume cannot entirely be compensated by a higher heart rate leading to a low cardiac output resulting in hypotension.

17.4 Arterial Pressure

The arterial pressure waveform reflects multiple phenomena (Fig. 17.6) [10].

- the systolic wave caused by the amount of blood being pumped into the aorta with every heartbeat,
- the reflection of this wave that "bounces" against the arteriolar system and travels backward to the heart,
- the stiffness of the arterial system as a result of multiple factors like age, vascular disease, inflammation, and medication,
- the location in the body where the wave is registered.

The above implies that in general, systolic and diastolic blood pressures are determined by cardiac output and vascular resistance (Fig. 17.1). However, the location of measurement (and method) and many factors influencing "resistance" play an

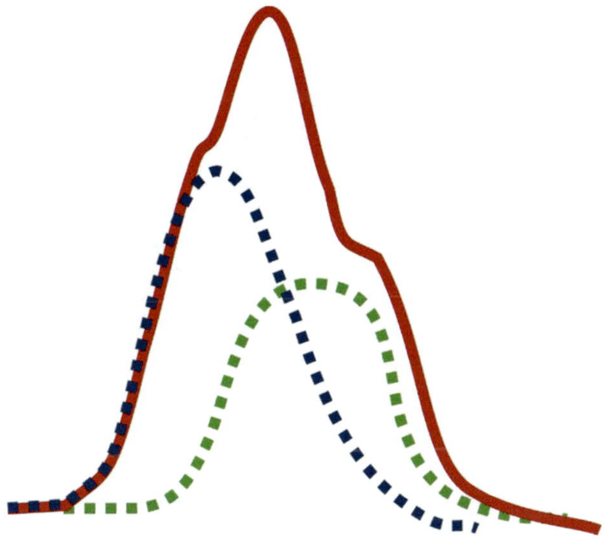

Fig. 17.6 The arterial pressure wave. Blue dotted line: forward traveling wave caused by left ventricular stroke volume, green dotted line: backward traveling reflection wave, and red solid line: combined (= observed) arterial pressure wave

important role. Therefore, blood pressure is a difficult variable to interpret. Since methods of measuring blood pressure are notoriously unreliable in children at the PICU, we often use mean arterial pressure (MAP) since measured MAP seems less influenced by technical factors. Also, MAP can be calculated from systolic (SAP) and diastolic arterial pressures (DAP) as

$$MAP = \left[SAP + 2 \times DAP\right] / 3$$

Normal values are age dependent and many algorithms have been published, but there are no strict cutoff values [11]. The threshold value of blood pressure below which hypoperfusion develops is dependent on many dynamic patient-related factors. Therefore, blood pressure must always be interpreted together with other measurements and clinical signs.

One could ask why blood pressure is relatively high. The "normal" blood pressure values are not necessary to drive blood through the capillary system since this is also accomplished through the pulmonary system with much lower pressures. Probably, these levels of pressure are a prerequisite to guarantee tissue perfusion when in many (large) tissues vasodilation occurs. Therefore, a lower-than-normal pressure is often well tolerated as long as the flow is sufficient and oxygen demand does not increase.

The body inhibits strong mechanisms to regulate blood pressure. Movements of the body, specifically in relation to gravity like standing up, require a fast regulatory system. In critically ill children, these mechanisms are still active.

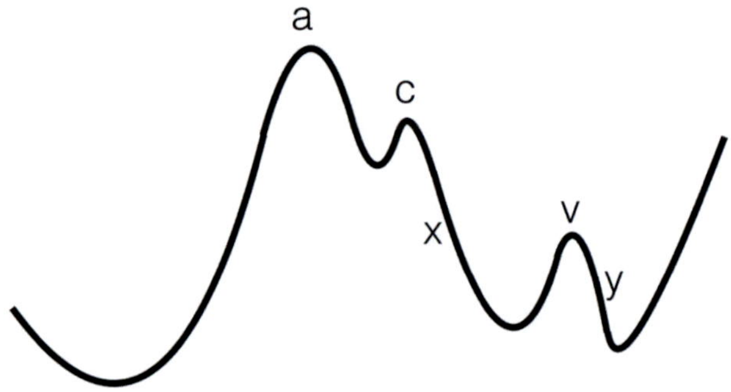

Fig. 17.7 The central venous pressure curve. a: atrial contraction, c: bulging T valve with ventricular contraction, x: atrial relaxation, v: before closing the T valve, and y: atrial emptying

17.5 Venous Pressure

Central venous pressure (CVP) can be measured using a catheter inserted in the upper central veins with the tip located close to the right atrium. It closely reflects right atrial pressure, and a typical central venous curve is depicted in Fig. 17.7 [4]. As we have seen earlier, P_{ra} is not the only determinant of venous return. Therefore, CVP cannot be used as a measure of preload although there is a relation. Neither does CVP reflect the need for fluid therapy. Closely studying the central venous pressure wave can provide useful information regarding right ventricular function (specifically in relation to fluid therapy) and also right heart valvular function.

Case Study 2

Sheena is 2 years old and suffers from viral myocarditis. She has an arterial and central venous catheter in place. After initial treatment with inotropic drugs, the arterial saturation is 98%, CVP is 10 mmHg, and blood pressure is 80/40 with a heart rate of 160 bpm. Is her hemodynamic condition sufficient?

Additional parameters show that central venous saturation ($ScvO_2$) is 53%. In the following parts, we will discover the usefulness of the last parameter.

17.6 Oxygen Transport

17

Oxygen transport (DO_2) can be estimated with

$$DO_2 \approx \text{cardiac output} \times \text{Hb} \times SaO_2$$

Hb = hemoglobin level and SaO_2 = arterial oxygen saturation.

In practice, DO_2 can be calculated although the absolute number is difficult to interpret. The same applies to oxygen consumption (VO_2). This parameter reflects the amount of oxygen that is being utilized by the body.

The relation between DO_2 and VO_2 is depicted in Fig. 17.8 [12]. There is a flat part of the curve when there is more than sufficient DO_2. However, when DO_2

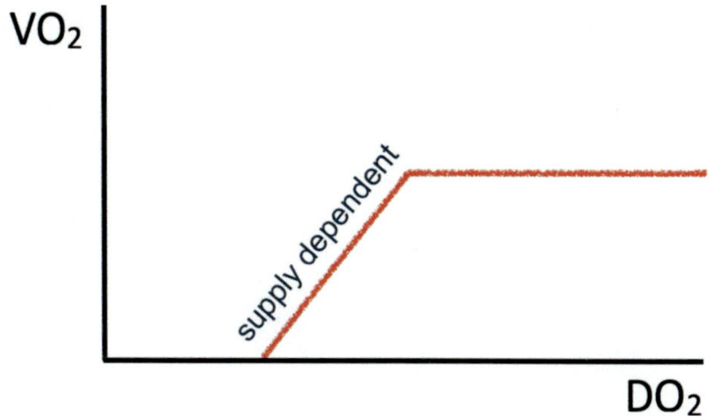

Fig. 17.8 The DO_2–VO_2 relation. DO_2: oxygen delivery to tissues and VO_2: oxygen utilization by tissues

declines below a critical level, VO_2 will start to decrease and anaerobic metabolism will develop in this so-called supply-dependent stage.

In daily practice, calculated values of DO_2 and VO_2 are hardly helpful in hemodynamic management. However, the relationship is helpful as a hemodynamic concept. Instead, as a measure of the relation between oxygen utilization and oxygen delivery, venous oxygen saturation (SvO_2) can be helpful. Drawing a blood sample from a central venous catheter can provide useful information. Normally, approximately 25% of the arterial oxygen content is offloaded and utilized (extracted) at the tissues resulting in a mean venous saturation of around 70%. Strongly reduced values indicate an increased extraction ratio often caused by a too low cardiac output. However, SvO_2 is not an indirect measurement of cardiac output itself. In the case of Sheena (Case 2), the low $ScvO_2$ might point to an insufficient systemic blood flow.

17.7 Microcirculation

All the above parameters concern the macrocirculation and the transfer of oxygen, carbon dioxide, and nutrition takes place at the level of the microcirculation. The capillaries are extremely small in order to minimize the distance between plasma, erythrocytes, etc. and the tissue surrounding the vessel. Capillaries have a diameter of 5–10 µm, red blood cells 6–8 µm, and white blood cells 7–30 µm [13, 14].

Since oxygen transport from the erythrocyte to the mitochondrion is a passive process, driven by a difference in partial oxygen pressure, the distance must be as short as possible. In the microcirculatory system, the delivery of oxygen to the cells is dependent on two principles:

- **Convection**. How many molecules are being transported through the capillaries? Blood flow is one of the essential factors.
- **Diffusion**. This is a passive process driven by the difference in partial pressure.

Microcirculation can be visualized using a special camera (Fig. 17.9). The quantification of microcirculatory blood flow at the bedside is still difficult and not

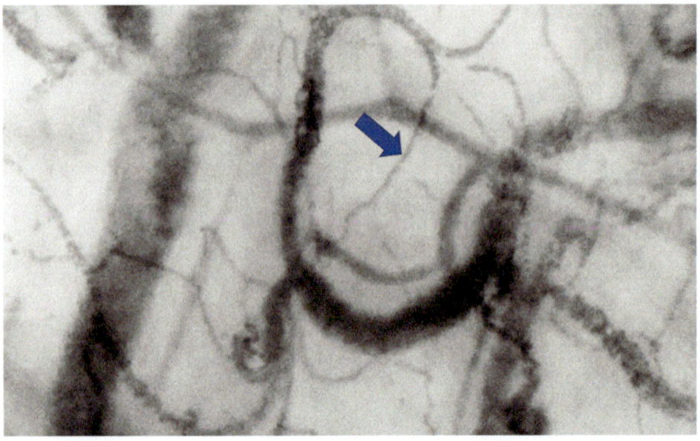

Fig. 17.9 Microcirculation. Image obtained from a healthy human subject using a video microscope. The dark spots are erythrocytes, they depict the capillaries and slightly larger vessels. The white spots within the vessels are white blood cells. The capillaries (example arrow) are only slightly larger than the erythrocytes. It must be remembered that at the capillary level, all un- and uploading of oxygen and carbon dioxide has to take place as well as the transport of nutrients

readily available. An approximation of the latter can be made using the difference between the arterial and central venous CO_2 levels (CO_2 gap or Pv-aCO_2) that should, under normal conditions, be lower than 7 mmHg [15].

17.8 Specific Aspects of Young Children

Basic hemodynamic physiology after birth is equal to the one in older children or adults. However, at birth, specifically, the myocardial and vascular systems are not fully developed. The myocardial cells are not as organized as in adult life and are not yet positioned to deliver maximum contractional performance. As a result, newborns have a lesser preload reserve, exhibit a smaller margin with respect to a potential increase in contractility, and have a greater dependence on afterload. During human growth and development, this slowly changes which is reflected in Fig. 17.10. The clinical relevance is that in situations with a reduced right or left ventricular function, specifically in newborns, an increase in preload (with fluids) or the delivery of inotropic drugs might not be very efficient. Instead, afterload reduction might be a better strategy [16, 17].

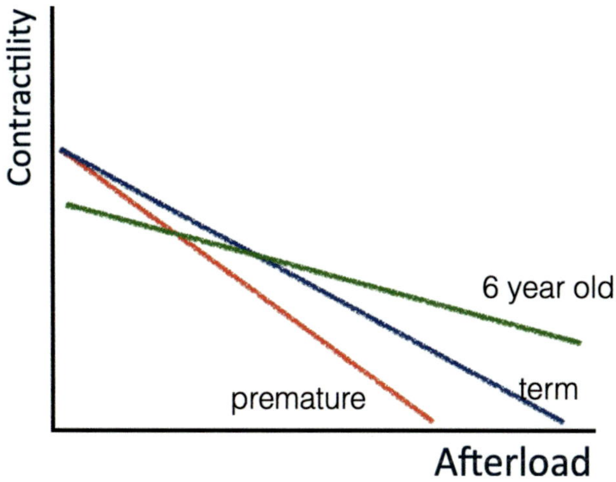

Fig. 17.10 Relation between afterload and contraction force

Take-Home Message

- Knowledge of basic hemodynamic physiology is essential in treating children with circulatory instability.

Summary

This chapter has depicted how commonly used hemodynamic parameters like heart rate and blood pressure relate and interact. These relations are dynamic and subject to regulatory mechanisms that strive for a status quo. Knowledge of physiology makes it possible to understand hemodynamic clinical conditions and disorders, interpret monitoring results, and ultimately endorse the selection of the right therapy.

References

1. Patwardhan K. The history of the discovery of blood circulation: unrecognized contributions of Ayurveda masters. Adv Physiol Educ. 2012;36:77–82.
2. Ribatti D. William Harvey and the discovery of the circulation of the blood. J Angiogenesis Res. 2009;1:3.
3. Magder S. Volume and its relationship to cardiac output and venous return. Crit Care. 2016;20:271.
4. Magder S. Understanding central venous pressure: not a preload index? Curr Opin Crit Care. 2015;21:369–75.
5. Patterson SW, Starling EH. On the mechanical factors which determine the output of the ventricles. J Physiol. 1914;48:357–79.
6. Magder SA. The ups and downs of heart rate. Crit Care Med. 2012;40:239–45.
7. Beard DA, Feigl EO. Understanding Guyton's venous return curves. Am J Physiol Heart C. 2011;301:H629–33.
8. Guyton AC. Determination of cardiac output by equating venous return curves with cardiac response curves. Physiol Rev. 1955;35:123–9.

9. Guyton AC, Polizo D, Armstrong GG. Mean circulatory filling pressure measured immediately after cessation of heart pumping. Am J Phys. 1954;179:261–7.
10. Magder S. The meaning of blood pressure. Crit Care. 2018;22:1–10.
11. Marlais M, Lyttle MD, Inwald D. Ten concerns about blood pressure measurement and targets in paediatric sepsis. Intensive Care Med. 2016;43:433–5.
12. Baker J, Vincent JL. The oxygen supply dependency phenomenon is associated with increased blood lactate levels. J Crit Care. 1991;6:152–9.
13. Top AP, Tasker RC, Ince C. The microcirculation of the critically ill pediatric patient. Crit Care. 2011;15:213.
14. Bateman RM, Sharpe MD, Ellis CG. Bench-to-bedside review: microvascular dysfunction in sepsis—hemodynamics, oxygen transport, and nitric oxide. Crit Care. 2003;7:359–73.
15. Mekontso-Dessap A, Castelain V, Anguel N, et al. Combination of venoarterial PCO2 difference with arteriovenous O2 content difference to detect anaerobic metabolism in patients. Intensive Care Med. 2002;28:272–7.
16. Rowland DG, Gutgesell HP. Myocardial contractility, preload, and afterload in healthy newborn infants. Am J Cardiol. 1995;75:1–4.
17. Teitel DF, Brett C, Chin T, et al. Developmental changes in myocardial contractile reserve in the lamb. Pediatr Res. 1985;19:948–55.

Hemodynamic Monitoring in the PICU

Yogen Singh and Joe Brierley

Contents

J. Brierley et al. (eds.), *ESPNIC Children's Intensive Care Textbook*,
https://doi.org/10.1007/978-3-031-64762-8_18

Learning Objectives

- Understand how basis clinical assessment of the circulatory system combines with advanced hemodynamic tools to assess critically ill children and the response to the treatment of shock such as intravenous fluids and vaso-active therapies.

18.1 Introduction

Hemodynamic monitoring is the monitoring of the changes in cardiovascular physiology as they occur. It includes both basic cardiovascular system observations and the so-called advanced parameters (such as NIRS, non-invasive continuous cardiac output monitoring, and functional echocardiography), some of which are measured invasively. Cardiovascular dysfunction is one of the commonest organ system failures that occur in critically ill children, whether as the primary derangement such with severe sepsis, or as a secondary feature of other organ system dysfunction. Specific relevant chapters on other organ systems feature throughout this book, e.g. congenital heart disease and surgical chapters. In this chapter, we focus on generic basic and advanced hemodynamic assessment and management during resuscitation, stabilization, and ongoing critical care.

A crucial concept to highlight at the outset is that the most basic parameters of hemodynamic assessment are not replaced by more advanced quantification once PIC expertise is available, but rather they are adjunct to basic parameters; they are added with repeat assessments of all hemodynamic parameters used to assess progress and the child's response to treatment.

18.2 Cardiovascular Instability Is Common in Critically Ill Children

Circulatory shock has been defined as a life-threatening generalized maldistribution of blood flow resulting in failure to deliver and/or utilize the adequate amount of oxygen to/by the end organs, leading to tissue dysoxia. Cardiovascular instability, with or without shock, is common in children admitted to paediatric intensive care, with over half of those with hemodynamic instability having multiple-organ dysfunction, commonly due to sepsis. A recent multi-centre international study (Sepsis Prevalence, Outcomes, and Therapies; SPROUT) reported that over two-thirds of children with sepsis had multiorgan dysfunction, associated with high mortality.

Although several studies suggest that early recognition and treatment of paediatric circulatory insufficiency or shock are crucial to improved survival, the optimal way to resuscitate children with circulatory failure remains controversial. The optimal order and quantity of fluids and vasoactive drug administration in critically ill children with shock are supported by little high-grade evidence. More didactic consensus statements have been superseded by a less prescriptive evidence-based approach in the recent paediatric surviving sepsis publications, which arguably serve more to direct research than assist the clinician at the bedside.

Hypotension and hypovolemia are associated with poor outcomes; however, too much fluid is detrimental to some children in shock and increases their mortality. The same is certainly true for inotropes and probably for any other treatment intervention in shock. This Goldilocks' principle is useful for anyone in critical care—not too little, not too much—but how can we determine 'just right'? A precise 'hemodynamic evaluation' and continuous monitoring to understand underlying pathophysiology, and targeted specific intervention based upon deranged physiology would appear to be the answer for shock, allowing quantifications of the physiological derangements and bedside individualized precise titration of therapies.

Significantly, more children in contemporary paediatric medicine receive complex immune-modulatory treatment, and cellular therapies which involve periods of immunosuppression and therefore carry a risk of infection and septic shock. Similarly, the increasing numbers of children living with advanced technological organ support whether ventilation, ventricular-assist devices, parenteral or artificial enteral nutrition, or indwelling vascular access catheters are all at greater risk of severe infection.

The approach we suggest in this chapter is safe and effective, and in line with the current understanding of hemodynamic resuscitation, but of course, is subject to change as research improves our understanding.

18.3 Basic Bedside Assessment

All paediatric resuscitation courses (such as EPALS, APLS, and ETAT) have emphasized early recognition of shock and provide an excellent framework for the initial assessment of the shocked child. The key step is the early recognition of shock, then delineating its type and underlying pathophysiology while resuscitation occurs. However, this can be challenging due to the dynamic status in shock, and even more difficult given the described changes in the background population with increased complexity and chronic community organ support, as well as the increased prevalence of children with life-limiting conditions which now account for a significant proportion of PIC admissions in some countries.

To optimally commence treatment, it is crucial to determine whether the child is in compensated or decompensated shock. Most care providers will be familiar with the clinical signs in the initial hemodynamic assessment of children, including heart rate (HR), blood pressure, respiratory rate (RR), state of consciousness, diuresis, core and peripheral temperature, capillary refill time (CRT), and peripheral perfusion. Deterioration in these parameters heralds a worsening state of shock unless treatment is provided, in the form of intravenous fluids, intravenous antibiotics, and cardio-respiratory support. Many parameters have age-related normal ranges in children, and some are also altered by other factors such as ambient temperature, pain, and anxiety which means familiarity with holistic child assessment is vital. The mission of the primary resuscitation team is to identify the shocked child in need of urgent intervention and to provide initial treatment with optimal fluid therapy (not too little and not too much), if there is an inadequate response to initiate vasoactive drugs progressively in a combination based on the morphology of shock, and response to treatment. In some children with established cardiogenic shock associated with severely impaired cardiac contractility, excessive fluid therapy can be detrimental but differentiating between hypolemia and poor contractility can be challenging on clinical examination or with traditional hemodynamic assessment. However, advanced hemodynamic monitoring tools such as point-of-care echocardiography, if available at the bedside, can be very helpful in choosing initial therapy and guiding treatment.

Children with congenital or acquired cardiac disease or metabolic causes of collapse require specific treatments covered in other chapters.

18.4 Blood Pressure

Both low and high blood pressure (BP) on admission are associated with increased mortality. BP measurement is one of the most used hemodynamic parameters for diagnostic and therapeutic decisions in critically ill children. BP can be measured invasively but also using several less reliable non-invasive methods. Invasive continuous BP monitoring is more reliable and it provides additional benefits of arterial blood sampling and continuous data sampling. Accurate measurement of BP is essential for the diagnosis and treatment of both hypotension and hypertension and in the management of shock given the frequent lability seen in children with shock.

We recommend the use of continuous invasive intra-arterial blood pressure (IBP) monitoring when there is a need for reliable measurement in children with shock who have not responded to initial fluid therapy, requiring inotropes or vasoactive medication. It is also preferable in children with intracranial hypertension undergoing intracranial pressure monitoring to measure cerebral perfusion pressure; during major surgery and in those with malignant hypertension/hypertensive emergencies to monitor the effects of continuous intravenous inotropes or vasoactive medications.

Hypotension presents late in paediatric shock, so BP should never be used as the only therapeutic target. Hemodynamic status should be evaluated by integrating BP with other clinical and hemodynamic parameters.

18.4.1 Central Venous Pressure (CVP)

CVP should be continuously measured as accurately as possible as part of multimodal hemodynamic monitoring aiming to assess intravascular volume and cardiac function. Isolated measurements are of limited value but CVP trends, including response to therapeutic manoeuvres with fluids or vasoactive agents, and wave morphology are more useful. CVP is not a reliable indicator of intravascular hypovolemia and in isolation often unhelpful, but in conjunction with other hemodynamic parameters can provide useful information. CVP should, therefore, be considered as part of the overall hemodynamic assessment of a child, for example, to quantify dynamic systemic vascular resistance (SVR).

18.4.2 Central Venous Oxygen Saturation Measurement

Central venous oxygen saturation ($ScvO_2$) sampled from the superior vena cava approximates mixed oxygen saturation ($SmvO_2$) derived from the invasive pulmonary artery sampling, which is not feasible at the bedside. The normal ranges for $ScvO_2$ and $SmvO_2$ are 70–80% and 60–70%, respectively, in the setting of normal aortic saturation. Trends between $ScvO_2$ and $SmvO_2$ are often interchangeable, although $SmvO_2$ values are generally around 7–10% lower. Low $ScvO_2$ typically indicates a mismatch between oxygen supply and demand. On the other hand, a normal or high $ScvO_2$ does not necessarily mean adequate supply–demand balance as tissue dysoxia (which may occur in sepsis) can cause high $ScvO_2$. We do not think $ScvO_2$ in isolation is a surrogate of other hemodynamic parameters such as cardiac index/cardiac output, though resuscitation targeted by $ScvO_2$ normalization has been shown to be beneficial in some studies of children with septic shock.

18.4.3 Cardiac Output Monitoring and Transpulmonary Indicator Dilution

Cardiac output (CO) is the product of heart rate and stroke volume. Stroke volume depends on preload, contractility, and afterload. The physical examination and simple commonly used hemodynamic parameters are surrogate markers of cardiovascular well-being, but they do not provide a direct assessment of the cardiovascular hemodynamic status of the patient, and clinical estimation of cardiac output is inaccurate. Hence, advanced hemodynamic monitoring seems sensible to titrate therapies, specifically when volume expansion or vasoactive drugs are used to improve cardiac output or systemic vascular resistance. In patients with refractory shock, when an effective and accurate measurement of CO is needed, the following methods have been advocated depending upon available resources and expertise: (1) measurement of CO using transthoracic ultrasound (echocardiography) and (2) transpulmonary dilution (TPD).

Ultrasonography is non-invasive, easily available, and can provide a fairly accurate and serial estimation of cardiac output at the bedside to monitor the initial response to therapy, but does require specific skills and is operator dependent. Despite arguably the most reliable clinical method to measure cardiac output, TPD is challenging in clinical practice because of resources, technical difficulties, and lack of expertise, and it is invasive and not suited to emergency resuscitation. Moreover, because of their intermittent measurement technique, TPD methods are not suitable for the detection of rapid, frequent changes in hemodynamic status as required in some critically ill children.

In clinical practice, cardiac output ultrasound/Doppler methods can be easily applied to estimate CO and serial assessments to guide the treatment. Cardiac output can also be estimated at the bedside using other non-invasive methods like bioimpedance, bioreactance, and pulse contour.

The validation of any of these methods in critically ill children is sparse, and no method has achieved broad consensus to be considered accurate enough to estimate absolute values of CO in the intensive care setting in children.

18.4.4 Pulmonary Artery Pressure

The pulmonary artery catheter (PAC) can provide continuous measurement of right atrial, PAP, measurement of CO, and pulmonary arterial occlusion pressure (wedge pressure). Left atrial pressure can be measured using surgically inserted left atrial catheters (LAC). However, because of invasiveness these are not used or recommended in children and are rarely used in the ICU. Transthoracic ultrasound echocardiography can be easily used to estimate pulmonary artery systolic pressure (PASP) at the bedside non-invasively, and it can provide serial assessment to monitor the response to therapy or disease process (as below).

18.4.5 Serum Lactate Measurement

In critically ill patients or children with shock, serum lactate provides an indirect assessment of tissue hypoxia or poor perfusion. A serum lactate of >2.0 mmol/L is generally considered abnormal and should be further investigated. Serial lactate blood sampling from a reliable site such as a central venous or arterial indwelling catheter is feasible and an easy bedside parameter that has demonstrated utility to predict the outcome or to change the targeted intervention in shock states. Studies report an association between failure to normalize lactate levels to a certain threshold (3.0 ± 1.0 mmol/L) during the first 12–24 h of ICU admission, and adverse outcomes regardless of the reason for ICU admission. However, as a hemodynamic monitoring tool, serum lactate lacks sensitivity and specificity. Like other hemodynamic monitoring parameters, serum lactate levels should be used in conjunction with other clinical indicators of poor systemic perfusion and hemodynamic monitoring. Persistently elevated lactate levels may reflect other mechanisms rather than those derived from poor tissue perfusion in shock and instead reflect aerobic glycolytic mechanisms including catecholamine administration or endogenous release.

18.4.6 Near-Infrared Spectroscopy

Near-infrared spectroscopy (NIRS) is a non-invasive, bedside technique to estimate regional capillary-venous haemoglobin saturation (rSO_2). The mean baseline cerebral rSO_2 is >70% in healthy children. Infants and children with cyanotic heart disease may have a cerebral rSO_2 between 46% and 57%. NIRS is mainly used to measure rSO_2 in the brain, but it is now commonly being applied to kidneys or abdomen. Like other hemodynamic parameters, a single absolute value provides little information but the trend in NIRS might be a useful haemodynamic monitoring tool in treating children with shock, post-cardiac arrest, post-traumatic brain injury, and infants with hypoxic–ischemic encephalopathy. A decline of cerebral rSO_2 under 40–50% or a change in baseline of more than 20% may be considered significant.

18.4.7 Microcirculation

Microcirculatory assessment by video-microscopy using side-stream or incident dark field is expensive and not widely available. It does not allow for the assessment of rapid circulatory changes during resuscitation. This is a good research tool and in the future may provide more insight into end-organ tissue perfusion but currently, it is not a valuable bedside hemodynamic monitoring tool.

18.4.8 Echocardiography/Ultrasonography

Cardiac ultrasound or functional echocardiography is non-invasive and easily available at the bedside in the intensive care setting and allows rapid real-time evaluation of hemodynamic status. It can assess cardiac contractility (function) and preload (cardiac filling) and as above can measure cardiac output and assess fluid responsiveness. It also can measure pulmonary artery systolic pressure. Hence, it can be a valuable adjunct to other parameters in children with hemodynamic instability to gain additional information to help clinical decisions such as in shock, hypovolemia, myocardial failure, pulmonary hypertension, or cardiac tamponade.

Bedside echocardiography can help in understanding the specific pathophysiology of shock in children, and to help choose the optimal timely, targeted specific, intervention. However, it does not provide continuous measurements, so serial intermittent assessments are required to assess disease progression or response to therapy. When available, it should be used in children with hemodynamic instability and may be considered as a modern hemodynamic tool for the intensive care setting.

18.4.9 Prediction of Volume Resuscitation and Fluid Responsiveness

Volume resuscitation remains one of the most used therapeutic interventions in sepsis; however, there is clear evidence that excessive fluid administration may impair tissue perfusion by promoting oedema and third-space fluid accumulation and increases mortality in ICU. Fluid therapy is effectively an attempt to improve cardiac output, which works well in children with normal cardiac function. However, as per the Frank–Starling rule in the presence of poor cardiac function, fluid therapy may fail to increase cardiac output and can actually decrease cardiac output.

A rise in cardiac output (or stroke volume) as a result of volume resuscitation is called fluid responsiveness. To prevent unnecessary fluid administration and target-specific interventions, fluid responsiveness should be assessed. Unfortunately, there is no proven reliable method to predict fluid responsiveness in children, static measures, mostly CVP and IVC size, are not appropriate to test fluid responsiveness in children, especially those on mechanical ventilators. In self-breathing adults, the IVC collapsibility index is a good parameter of fluid predictiveness but it is less sensitive and specific in younger children, especially those receiving mechanical ventilation. The published evidence suggests that respiratory variation in aortic blood flow peak velocity {(ΔVPeak/velocity time integral (VTI)} is the most reliable indicator of fluid responsiveness. Other dynamic methods, like the passive leg raising test, liver pressure, and IVC collapsibility index, have not been adequately assessed in children of all ages.

By first principles, if stroke volume is being measured, the effect of fluid administration is directly measured, so any decrease means fluid must be stopped.

In the absence of measuring stroke volume, recurrent smaller fluid boluses (maximal 5–10 mL/kg) in a short time interval in patients with hemodynamic instability while tracking changes in cardiac output, blood pressure, and CVP to confirm or assess fluid responsiveness are recommended. Fluid therapy in patients with an increasing CVP and no significant increase in blood pressure or cardiac output as a result of previous fluid therapy should be withheld.

Take-Home Messages

- Comprehensive hemodynamic monitoring can accurately determine the severity of circulatory derangement and help identify the underlying pathophysiology so enabling the clinician to choose the most appropriate treatment and guide individualized precise therapy. Furthermore, hemodynamic monitoring can provide useful information about the circulation in all types of life-threatening shock such as secondary to trauma, blood loss, major surgery, cardiac failure, sepsis, or others.
- The current management guidelines focus on early recognition and treatment but do not specify the type of hemodynamic monitoring to use under various circumstances which is the key to detecting the underlying deranged pathophysiology. There is a wide range of devices and techniques available to evaluate hemodynamic status, and an increasing number of these methods are now available for use in children. Recently published recommendations for hemodynamic monitoring for critically ill children, such as the expert consensus statement issued by the cardiovascular dynamics section of the European Society of Paediatric and Neonatal Intensive Care (ESPNIC), provide further guidance on hemodynamic monitoring in neonates and children.

Further Reading

Davis AL, Carcillo JA, Aneja RK, Deymann AJ, Lin JC, Nguyen TC, et al. American College of Critical Care Medicine Clinical Practice parameters for hemodynamic support of pediatric and neonatal septic shock. Crit Care Med. 2017;45:1061–93. https://doi.org/10.1097/CCM.0000000000002425.

de Oliveira CF, de Oliveira DS, Gottschald AF, Moura JD, Costa GA, Ventura AC, et al. ACCM/PALS haemodynamic support guidelines for pediatric septic shock: an outcomes comparison with and without monitoring central venous oxygen saturation. Intensive Care Med. 2008;34:1065–75.

Gan H, Cannesson M, Chandler JR, Ansermino JM. Predicting fluid responsiveness in children: a systematic review. Anesth Analg. 2013;117:1380–92.

Singh Y, et al. Recommendations for hemodynamic monitoring for critically ill children—expert consensus statement by the Cardiovascular Dynamics of the European Society of Pediatric and Neonatal Intensive Care (ESPNIC). Crit Care. 2020;24:620.

Singh Y, Tissot C, Fraga M, Yousef N, Cortes RM, Lopez J, et al. International evidence-based guidelines on Point of Care Ultrasound (POCUS) for critically ill neonates and children issued by the

POCUS Working Group of the European Society of Paediatric and Neonatal Intensive Care (ESPNIC). Crit Care. 2020;24:65.

Weiss SL, Fitzgerald JC, Pappachan J, Wheeler D, Jaramillo-Bustamante JC, Salloo A, Singhi SC, Erickson S, Roy JA, Bush JL, Nadkarni VM, Thomas NJ, Sepsis Prevalence, Outcomes, and Therapies (SPROUT) Study Investigators and Pediatric Acute Lung Injury and Sepsis Investigators (PALISI) Network. Global epidemiology of pediatric severe sepsis: the sepsis prevalence, outcomes, and therapies study. Am J Respir Crit Care Med. 2015;191(10):1147–57.

Weiss SL, Peters MJ, Alhzanni W, Agus MSD, Flori HR, Inwald DP, et al. Surviving sepsis campaign international guidelines for the management of septic shock and sepsis-associated organ dysfunction in children. Pediatr Crit Care Med. 2020;21:e52–106. https://doi.org/10.1097/PCC.0000000000002198.

Fluids on PICU (Paediatric Intensive Care Unit)

Gavin Wooldridge and David Philip Inwald

Contents

J. Brierley et al. (eds.), *ESPNIC Children's Intensive Care Textbook*,
https://doi.org/10.1007/978-3-031-64762-8_19

Learning Objectives

- Appraise the history of therapy with intravenous fluids.
- Consider the body fluid compartments.
- Regulation of extracellular fluid osmolarity and sodium.
- Compare and contrast intravenous fluids commonly used on PICU.
- Evaluate the evidence for and against fluid resuscitation in shock.
- Describe the use of intravenous fluid maintenance in PICU.
- Consider phases of fluid therapy—the "ROSE" concept.

19.1 Introduction

Therapy with intravenous fluids is an integral part of paediatric critical care. However, no ideal intravenous fluid exists, and it is only very recently that randomised controlled trials have been conducted to evaluate their role in the critically ill child. As our understanding of cell physiology and disease pathophysiology developed, so too has our approach to fluid therapy and a recognition that fluids should be considered like any other drug, maximising efficacy, and minimising disbenefits [1]. This chapter will explore the history of intravenous fluids and fluid physiology and consider the selection, timing, and doses of intravenous fluids in the critically ill child.

19.2 History of Intravenous Fluids

The first documented use of intravenous fluids was during the British cholera epidemic of 1830s [2]. O'Shaughnessy had found that the blood of cholera patients was dehydrated, acidotic and deplete of electrolytes and surmised that "treatment must depend on intravenous replacement of the deficient salt and water" [3]. Only two months later, the first cases of cholera were treated with an intravenous saline solution by Latta, who was in practice in Leith, near Edinburgh. The solution used consisted of "two to three drachms of muriate of soda and two scruples of the subcarbonate of soda in six pints of water"—a hypotonic solution [4]. It was not sterile; it had been strained through a chamois leather. Despite this, three of the initial five patients treated survived [5]. As a precursor to modern-day practice, Latta described how repeated injections of solution were guided by the patient's pulse and symptoms. Latta died of tuberculosis in 1833 and the cholera epidemic ended shortly thereafter; the use of intravenous fluids also ended for several decades.

In 1883, Ringer, at University College London, was studying the isolated frog heart and found that a 0.75% saline solution "makes an excellent circulating fluid in experiments with the detached heart" [6]. He later discovered that the saline solution used was made using piped water supplied by the New River Water Company and not distilled water as intended. On repeating the experiments, he found that bathing the heart muscle in saline solution made with distilled water made the ventricle grow "weaker and weaker" leading to cessation of contractility in about 20 minutes. He concluded that the effects he had previously obtained were "due to some of the inorganic constituents of the pipe water," later shown to be calcium. Ringer's solution was developed based on these observations, later modified by Hartmann, who added sodium lactate as a buffer [7]. These were the first "balanced crystalloids;" which have a sodium, potassium, and chloride content close to that of extracellular fluid and, when given intravenously, have few adverse effects on acid–base balance.

It was not until 1888, that the term "normal saline" was first used by Churton, in a case report about a "prostrate and pulseless" patient with pyloric stenosis due to gastric cancer, in whom he actually used a fluid with striking similarities to PlasmaLyte 148 but very different to 0.9% saline [8]. In the same decade, Hamburger discovered, by looking at the freezing point of human serum and haemolysis with solutions of different tonicities, that "the blood of the majority of warm-blooded animals, including man, was isotonic with a NaCl solution of 0.9%..." [9]. Over the next 10–20 years, the term "normal saline" came to apply to 0.9% saline (NaCl 154 mmol/L), even though it is neither "normal" (which would imply a concentration of 1000 mmol/L = 58.5 g NaCl/L), nor does its composition reflect that of extracellular fluid.

Fluid therapy with solutions based on 0.9% saline became routine in the early twentieth century. However, intravenous access was initially used rarely; the oral, rectal, or subcutaneous route were preferred. The intravenous route became commonly used only later. With rapid development in the understanding of cell, fluid, and blood group physiology and the progression of conflict medicine during both world wars, resuscitation fluids also evolved. During the First World War, blood transfusion was pioneered by Lawrence Bruce Robertson and Oswald Hope Robertson, who were not related. At the same time Bayliss developed the first colloid, "Bayliss gummy solution," which was used on the front from 1917. Using a cat model of shock Bayliss had demonstrated that if the saline used for volume resuscitation contained 5% gelatin or gum arabic, the rise in blood pressure observed was more sustained than if saline alone was used, due to the oncotic pressure exerted by the protein in solution [10]. Liquid and dried plasma were used for volume expansion in the Second World War and the first use of human albumin solution was during the attack on Pearl Harbour.

The first use of a "continuous drip" was by Matas in 1924 [11]. The use of 0.9% saline for maintenance fluid became widespread in the 1920s and 1930s despite increasing concern about fluid retention [12], particularly after surgery when the ability to excrete excess sodium and water load is reduced [13].

By the 1990s a wide variety of intravenous fluids were on the market, including crystalloids such as 0.9% saline, Ringer's solution, and Hartmann's solution; fluids based on 0.18% and 0.45% saline; dextrose alone and in combination with varying concentrations of saline; and colloids based on gelatin (gelofusin), starch (hetastarch), dextran (dextran 40 and dextran 70); and human albumin. PlasmaLyte 148, another balanced crystalloid (using acetate, which is converted to bicarbonate rather than lactate as a buffer), was also developed in the 1980s.

Some of these fluids are no longer recommended due to clinical trials which have indicated disbenefit; these will be discussed below. Intravenous hypotonic saline (0.18% saline/4% glucose solution) has been withdrawn from widespread use in children in the United Kingdom, after being shown to be associated with dangerous levels of hyponatraemia, which in some cases led to cerebral oedema and death [14].

In this review, the evidence for and against different fluid types and fluid management strategies will be explored in detail. Firstly, however, the review will turn to fluid physiology.

19.3 The Body Fluid Compartments

Water is essential for human life and maintaining fluid homeostasis is fundamental for cellular and organ function. An understanding of fluid physiology is critical in paediatric intensive care.

19.3.1 What Is the Total Body Water Content of a Child?

The total body water (TBW) is divided across two compartments, separated by a cell membrane: intra- and extracellular fluid (◘ Fig. 19.1).

- Intracellular fluid (ICF)
  - ICF volume remains relatively constant.
  - Cell membranes retaining ICF allow the free passive diffusion of water.
  - Active transport mechanisms maintain an internal solute milieu different from that found outside the cells. The major cations in ICF are potassium (K^+) and magnesium (Mg^{2+}); major anions are proteins and organic phosphates.
  - Changes in the ICF volume result from alterations in the osmolarity of the ECF but do not respond to isosmotic changes in extracellular volume, i.e., it is "regulated" by the movement of free water.

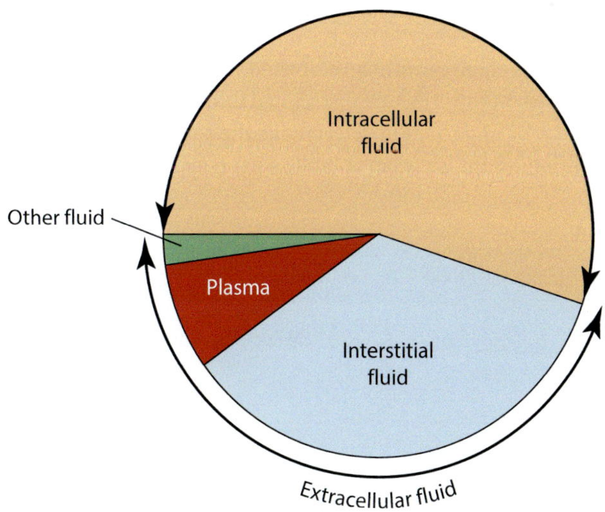

◘ **Fig. 19.1** Total body water composition

- Extracellular fluid (ECF)
  - ECF volume is regulated by the movement of sodium chloride. Water follows salt.
  - ECF volume as a proportion of TBW decreases in the first few years of life. Some of this is accounted for by an increase in body fat.
  - The major cation in ECF is sodium (Na^+); major anions are chloride (Cl^-) and bicarbonate (HCO_3^-).
  - ***The total solute concentration (osmolarity) is the same in ICF and ECF.***
  - ECF is composed of four compartments:
    - Plasma volume (25% ECF)
    - Interstitial fluid and lymphatics (75% ECF)
    - Transcellular fluid (1–2% TBW)—fluid formed by the secretory activity of cells existing within epithelium-lined spaces, e.g., CSF, bile, bowel contents, pleural fluid

Plasma makes up 25% of TBW and is also called the functional ECF. It is this "functional" ECF that receives isotonic fluid boluses, which should not cause any change in ICF volume. In contrast, infusion of hypotonic fluids will result in fluid shift from ECF to ICF, resulting in increased ICF volume. This may be dangerous in some circumstances, for example, cerebral oedema.

Body water content and blood volume as a proportion of body weight decreases with age in children (◘ Table 19.1). The high total body water (TBW) content is proportionally higher in the premature infant (80%) due to the relatively larger extracellular fluid compartment, and reduces to 75% during the neonatal period, 65% at 6 months, and approaches adult proportions at 5 years of age (60%).

Significance in PICU

- As water content changes with development, the volume of distribution of drugs may also change. Many drugs are distributed throughout the extracellular fluid and its volume may be important in determining the concentration of drugs at receptor sites. This is important for water soluble drugs (such as aminoglycosides).

◘ Table 19.1 Circulating blood volume of children

Age of child	Blood volume (mL/kg)
Neonate	85–90
Infant	75–80
Child	70–75
Adult	65–70

19.3.2 Fluid Input and Output

Stability of body fluid volume and composition is essential for homeostasis. This stability is achieved by matching the input and output of both fluid and electrolytes. In health, water is gained by ingestion or synthesis due to oxidation of carbohydrates by the respiratory pathways. Water is lost *insensibly* (evaporation from the respiratory tract and skin) or *sensibly* through sweat, faeces, and urine. The kidneys adjust the excretion of water and electrolytes to match the intake. Daily fluid requirement at rest varies over childhood (fluid requirements are discussed in detail in ► Sect. 19.7 below).

- *Insensible losses*: Insensible losses are those of which there is no conscious awareness, i.e., evaporation of electrolyte-free water from the skin and respiratory tract comprise the insensible losses.
- *Sensible losses*: In most hospitalised children, urinary water loss accounts for most sensible losses, with water loss from sweat and from the gastrointestinal tract minimal.
- *Electrolyte losses*: In the absence of vomiting and diarrhoea, or large gastric aspirates, there is minimal electrolyte loss from the gastrointestinal tract. In children in PICU, urinary losses account for most of the electrolyte loss, with limited losses in sweat.

19.3.2.1 Definitions

- **Osmole**: The number of osmotically active particles in a solution rather than the molar concentration. As sodium chloride dissociates into sodium and chloride ions in solutions, 1 mol/L NaCl is a 2 Osm/L solution.
- **Osmolality and osmolarity**: Osmolality is expressed as osmoles per kilogram of water; osmolarity is expressed as osmoles per litre. In clinical practice, osmolarity is most frequently measured and used. Plasma osmolarity is usually maintained at 280–305 mOsm/L. It may be estimated as [glucose] + [urea] + (2 × [Na]) in mmol/L.
- **Osmotic pressure**: Osmosis of water molecules across a semi-permeable membrane can be prevented by applying pressure in the direction opposite that of the osmosis. The pressure required to prevent the osmosis is called the osmotic pressure. From van't Hoff's Law, it can be calculated that for each milliosmole concentration gradient across the cell membrane, 19.3 mmHg osmotic pressure is exerted.
- **Oncotic pressure**: The osmotic pressure generated by large molecules (especially proteins) in solution, which do not freely cross the capillary basement membrane.

The distribution of extracellular fluid distributed between the plasma and interstitial spaces is determined mainly by the balance of hydrostatic and colloid osmotic forces across the capillary membranes.

This relationship is described by the Starling equation [15], which describes the net flow of fluid across a semi-permeable membrane:

$$Q_f = K_f\left[\left(P_c - P_i\right) - \sigma\left(\pi_c - \pi_i\right)\right]$$

where Q_f is the net filtration of fluid from the lung microvasculature to the interstitium, K_f is the capillary filtration coefficient or leakiness of the endothelium to water, P_c is the capillary hydrostatic pressure, P_i is the interstitial hydrostatic pressure, σ is the protein reflection coefficient, π_c is the plasma oncotic pressure, and π_i is the interstitial fluid oncotic pressure.

Increases in (1) capillary hydrostatic pressure, (2) reduction in capillary oncotic pressure, or (3) a decrease in the reflection coefficient, will result in net flow from the plasma into the interstitium resulting in extracellular fluid oedema. In clinical practice in PICU, the most common causes of these scenarios are (1) elevated atrial pressure due to pump failure or fluid overload, (2) hypoalbuminaemia, and (3) inflammation.

The distribution of fluid between intracellular and extracellular compartments is determined by the osmotic effect of small solutes—sodium, chloride, and other electrolytes—acting across the cell membrane. The reason for this is that cell membranes are highly permeable to water but relatively impermeable to small ions such as sodium and chloride. Therefore, water moves across the cell membrane, so that the intracellular fluid remains isotonic with the extracellular fluid. Minor changes in the concentration of solutes in the extracellular fluid can cause substantial changes in cell volume.

19.3.3 Isotonic, Hypotonic, and Hypertonic Fluids

If a cell is placed in a solution of solutes having an osmolarity of 282 mOsm/L, the cells will not shrink or swell because the water concentration in the intracellular and extracellular fluids is equal. Such a solution is ***isotonic***. Examples of isotonic solutions include 0.9% sodium chloride or 5% dextrose. If a cell is placed into a ***hypotonic*** solution that has a lower concentration of solute (less than 282 mOsm/L), water will diffuse into the cell, causing it to swell. If a cell is placed in a ***hypertonic*** solution with a higher concentration of solute, water will flow out of the cell into the extracellular fluid. This is the basis upon which cerebral oedema is treated with hypertonic saline (3% saline) or mannitol (◘ Fig. 19.2).

In some pathological conditions, the intracellular osmolarity changes, or the cell membrane no longer acts as an effective semi-permeable membrane. The former may result from tissue ischaemia, when the function of the main ATP-dependent membrane ion pump, the Na/K ATPase, is impaired and as a result, intracellular [Na] increases and causes osmosis of water into the cells, cell swelling and oedema. The latter may also result from inflammation, which may directly affect the permeability of cell membranes to ions, resulting in a similar picture.

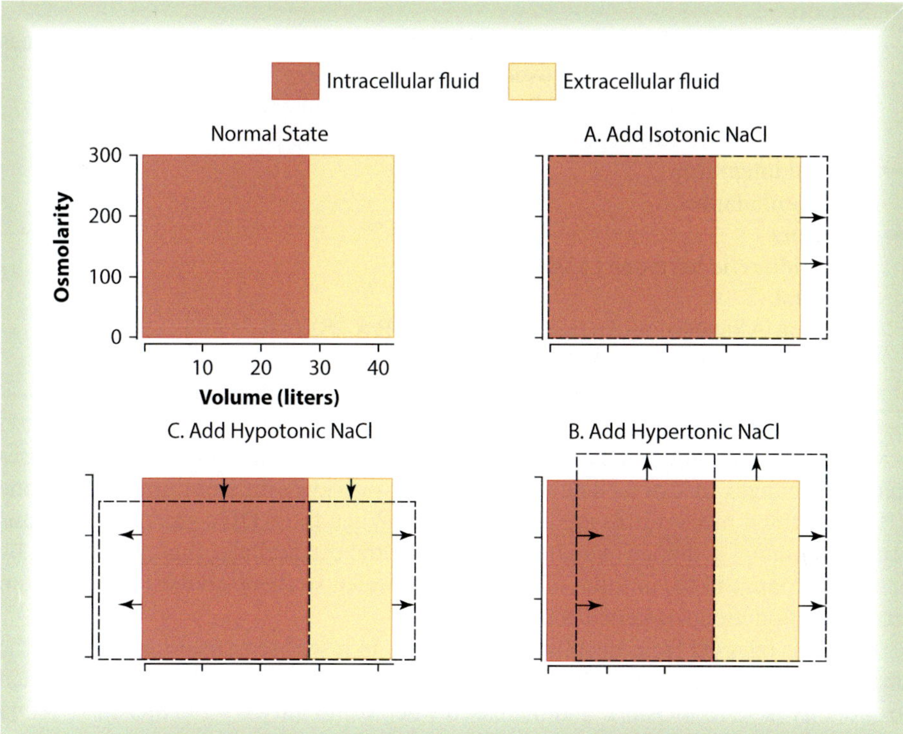

Fig. 19.2 Effect of adding isotonic, hypertonic, and hypotonic solutions to the extracellular fluid after osmotic equilibrium. The normal state is indicated by the solid lines, and the shifts from normal are shown by the hyphenated areas. (From: Guyton, Arthur C. Textbook of medical physiology/Arthur C. Guyton, John E. Hall., 11th ed., Elsevier, Philadelphia, PA, USA, 2006)

19.4 Regulation of Extracellular Fluid Osmolarity and Sodium

ECF volume is determined by the balance between intake and output of water and salt. In the kidney and in the body fluid compartments, water follows salt. ECF volume is usually regulated by the kidneys, which adapt their excretion of salt and water to match intake. However, salt and water intake may be highly variable in an intensive care setting. In many disease states, when renal function is impaired, effective renal regulation may not be possible; hence, the importance of meticulous attention to plasma [Na], which reflects [NaCl], and fluid balance in the critically ill child.

The overall regulatory mechanism is a closed-loop system involving sensors, integrators, and effectors. It is outside the remit of this chapter to examine renal physiology in detail, but the main elements of the system in relation to the regulation of osmolarity and volume status are shown below. The system tends to prioritise the maintenance of constant osmolarity over volume, for the reasons outlined above.

- Sensors
  - **Osmoreceptors in the hypothalamus that respond to changes in cellular volumes caused by changes in ECF osmolarity**
  - **Volume receptors (atrial walls, SVC, IVC, and pulmonary circulation)**
  - High-pressure baroceptors (aortic arch and carotid sinus)
- Central integrator
  - Hypothalamus
- Effectors
  - **Antidiuretic hormone (ADH)**
  - **Thirst**
  - Renin-Aldosterone-Angiotensin System (RAAS)
  - Natriuretic peptides (ANP/BNP)
  - The sympathetic nervous system

In health, regulation of extracellular fluid sodium chloride content usually causes parallel changes in extracellular fluid volume, provided the antidiuretic hormone (ADH)—thirst mechanisms are also operative. When the ADH—thirst mechanisms are functioning, a change in sodium chloride in the extracellular fluid is matched by a similar change in the amount of extracellular water, so that osmolarity and sodium concentration are maintained constant.

ADH is released from the posterior pituitary in response to osmoreceptors in the hypothalamus, detecting a change in osmolality. ADH release is decreased when osmolality is <275 mOsm/L and increased when osmolality is >290 mOsm/L. ADH release is also controlled by cardiovascular reflexes that respond to decreases in blood pressure and/or blood volume, including (1) the high-pressure baroreceptors and (2) the volume receptors. ADH acts upon V2 receptors in the collecting ducts to increase water reabsorption. Osmoreceptors also activate the urge of thirst above an osmolality of 290 mOsm/kg, when the maximal ADH effect is achieved.

ADH production is impaired in central diabetes insipidus, resulting in the production of copious quantities of dilute urine. Syndrome of inappropriate ADH (SIADH) describes the opposite situation, in which ADH secretion is increased, with consequent retention of water, increased ECF and hyponatraemia. In PICU, the most common causes are surgical trauma, acute pulmonary infection, or meningoencephalitis. Both scenarios require meticulous attention to diagnosis and management.

The renin-aldosterone-angiotensin system is a signalling pathway involving several hormones responsible for the regulation of blood pressure and ECF volume. Renin is produced by the kidneys in response to β1 adrenoceptor stimulation or hypotension and cleaves angiotensinogen to angiotensin I. Angiotensin Converting Enzyme (ACE) cleaves angiotensin I to angiotensin II, which has multiple functions related to water homeostasis. Angiotensin II increases sodium reabsorption in the proximal convoluted tubule and stimulates aldosterone secretion from the adrenal cortex, increasing thirst and ADH release. Aldosterone acts on the distal convoluted tubule to increase reabsorption of Na^+ and water and secretion of potassium.

Stimulation of atrial and ventricular stretch receptors activates atrial and brain natriuretic peptide release. These act to reduce blood pressure by decreasing aldosterone release, causing vasodilatation of peripheral smooth muscle. ECF volume is decreased by increasing glomerular filtration rate and decreasing tubular reabsorption of sodium and chloride.

Changes in sympathetic activity can also alter renal sodium and water excretion and hence ECF volume. For example, when blood volume falls in haemorrhage, volume receptors (and eventually, baroreceptors) cause reflex activation of the sympathetic nervous system. This in turn increases renal sympathetic nerve activity, which has several effects to decrease sodium and water excretion: (1) constriction of the renal arterioles, with resultant decreased GFR; (2) increased tubular reabsorption of salt and water; and (3) stimulation of renin release and increased angiotensin II and aldosterone formation, both of which further increase tubular reabsorption.

Significance in PICU

- Critically ill children have altered physiology in relation to fluid homeostasis. This is due to changes in the patient's sensible or insensible losses or alteration to the normal homeostatic mechanisms including ADH release:
  - Changes to sensible losses
    - Patients with vomiting, diarrhoea or polyuria have excess water losses.
    - Infants and young children have a higher metabolic rate and therefore greater fluid requirements.
    - Losses will be greater if higher solute load, inadequate ADH release or renal response to ADH.
  - Changes to insensible losses
    - Patients with burns, fever, or excessive sweating will have excess water loss from the insensible route.
    - Infants, especially those born preterm, have poorly developed dermal layers, a high surface area to body weight ratio and therefore higher insensible losses.
    - Humidification reduces insensible respiratory losses by 80%.
  - Changes to ADH release
    - ADH release is triggered by many common situations on PICU including positive pressure ventilation.

19.5 Intravenous Fluids Commonly Used on PICU

Intravenous fluids used in paediatric intensive care include blood products, crystalloids, and colloids (◘ Table 19.2). The use of blood products other than albumin is outside the scope of this review.

19.5.1 Crystalloid

A crystalloid fluid is an aqueous solution of mineral salts and other small, water-soluble molecules. [16]. Crystalloids include a variety of concentrations of solutes and can be saline, balanced or dextrose based. Most commercially available crystalloid solutions are isotonic.

Table 19.2 Composition of intravenous fluids

	Fluid	Osmo-lality	Tonicity	NA+	K+	Cl−	Other
	Plasma	**290**	**N/A**	**140**	**4**	**100**	**24 HCO_3^-**
Saline based crystalloids	0.9% Saline	308	Isotonic	154	0	154	0
	0.45% Saline*	155	Hypo-tonic	77	0	77	0
	0.18% Saline*	86	Hypo-tonic	39	0	39	0
	3% Saline	1027	Hyper-tonic	1027	0	0	0
Balanced crystalloids	Hartmann's	273	Isotonic	130	4	109	Ca 3 mmol/L Lactate 28 mmol/L
	Plasmalyte	294	Isotonic	140	5	98	Acetate 27 mmol/L Gluconate 23 mmol/L Magnesium 3 mmol/L
Dextrose based crystalloid	5% Dextrose*	253	Hypo-tonic	0	0	0	50 g/L dextrose
	10% Dextrose	506	Hyper-tonic	0	0	0	100 g/L dextrose
Colloid	5% Human albumin solution	290	Isotonic	145	0	150	50 g/L albumin
	Gelofusine*	274	Hypo-tonic	154	0	120	40 g/L gelatin

Note: * denotes fluids which are no longer routinely used, composition shown for reference purposes

Hypertonic solutions such as 3% saline solutions contain higher concentrations of solutes than those found in human serum. These fluids are osmotically active and will cause fluid shifts. Their primary indication is for treatment of cerebral oedema.

The terms balanced and buffered solution are often used interchangeably, but in this chapter, "balanced solution" will be used to refer to a crystalloid which has a "sodium, potassium and chloride content closer to that of ECF, and when given intravenously, has fewer adverse effects on acid base balance" [17]. Balanced solutions contain molecules that metabolise in vivo to bicarbonate. These solutions have physiological pH. The three commonly used molecules are lactate, acetate, and gluconate. Lactate and gluconate are metabolised by the liver to bicarbonate, while acetate is metabolised by skeletal muscle.

19.5.2 Colloid

A colloid is a homogeneous, non-crystalline substance consisting of large molecules or ultramicroscopic particles of one substance (e.g., albumin) dispersed through a second substance (e.g., 0.9% saline). In the case of plasma, proteins cannot pass through intact semi-permeable membranes and therefore maintain a higher intravascular osmotic pressure. The portion of that pressure due to protein is known as the "colloid oncotic pressure." The theoretical advantage of these solutions is that they should stay in circulation for longer than isotonic crystalloids. Colloids can be derived from human blood, i.e., albumin, based on naturally occurring substances such as gelatin (gelofusine, volplex or haemaccel) or starch (hetastarch) or synthetic glucose polymers (dextran 40 and dextran 70). These latter solutions are cheaper than albumin but more expensive than crystalloids.

19.5.2.1 5% Human Albumin Solution

"HAS" is a heat-sterilised blood product containing human albumin dissolved in normal saline. The theoretical advantage of albumin is that it has a much longer half-life than crystalloid in circulation—around 6 h—due to the oncotic pressure exerted by albumin, which tends to keep the fluid in circulation. Despite these theoretical advantages, there are no randomised controlled trials supporting the use of albumin in critically ill children. The largest study in adults, the SAFE study, demonstrated no benefit overall but benefit for patients with sepsis in the subgroup analysis and dis-benefit for those with traumatic brain injury [18]. In children, the FEAST trial investigated 3141 African children with infection and impaired perfusion, randomly assigned to resuscitation with albumin or saline boluses or no boluses on admission to hospital. Resuscitation with either albumin bolus or saline fluid bolus resulted in increased mortality compared to a no-bolus strategy, but there was no difference in mortality when comparing albumin to saline [19]. As a result of this trial, albumin is no longer recommended in the current paediatric surviving sepsis guidelines [20]. However, albumin remains in use for other indications and is still widely used in many paediatric intensive care units.

19.5.2.2 Gelatin-Based Solutions

These contain either succinylated or modified (e.g., volplex and gelofusine) or urea-cross-linked (e.g., haemaccel) gelatin. The gelatin is presented as a 4% solution in electrolytes—volplex and gelofusine in Na 154 mmol/L and Cl 125 mmol/L, haemaccel in Na 145 mmol/L, K 5 mmol/L, Ca 6 mmol/L, and Cl 145 mmol/L. Advantages include a longer time in circulation than crystalloid due to the colloid oncotic pressure of gelatin—3–4 h. However, gelatin may remain in the body up to 7 days and is excreted by the kidneys. Hyperchloraemic acidosis is a complication due to the composition of the solution in which it is suspended. A recent meta-analysis including 30 randomised controlled trials of gelatin-based fluids showed an increased risk of anaphylaxis and a non-significant signal to increased mortality, renal failure, and bleeding due to extravascular uptake and coagulation impairment [21, 22]. Gelatin-based fluids are not recommended in the current paediatric surviving sepsis guidelines [20] and are no longer used in paediatric critical care.

19.5.2.3 Starch-Based Solutions

These solutions remain in the circulation for longer than albumin and have a lower cost. However, several large-scale clinical trials demonstrated disbenefit in a variety of scenarios [23–25], and they have therefore been withdrawn in the United Kingdom in 2013 and in the European Union in 2022. They will not be considered further here.

19.5.3 What Happens During Rapid Infusion 10–20 mL/kg 0.9% Saline into a Patient?

19.5.3.1 Distribution

0.9% saline distributes rapidly from the intravascular (plasma) to the interstitial compartment; this phase takes about 25–30 min [26]. Because 0.9% saline is isoosmotic with the extracellular fluid, water distributes itself according to the proportional distribution of sodium (i.e., about 25% of it stays intravascular and 75% enters the interstitial fluid).

19.5.3.2 Changes to Plasma Oncotic Pressure

Neither baroreceptors nor low-pressure volume receptors are likely to react to the change in plasma volume caused by this amount of fluid. Osmoreceptors do not reduce ADH secretion as the fluid is isotonic. The homeostatic mechanism which results in renal elimination of the fluid bolus is via the change in oncotic pressure. As intravascular protein concentration decreases, plasma oncotic pressure decreases.

19.5.3.3 Excretion

Glomerulotubular balance ensures a return to homeostasis by increasing water and salt excretion (the decrease in peritubular capillary oncotic pressure decreases the rate of water and salt reabsorption from the proximal tubule) (◘ Fig. 19.3).

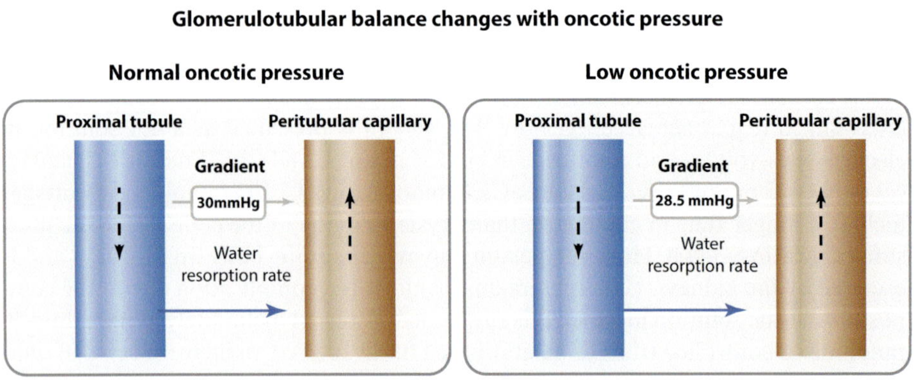

◘ **Fig. 19.3** Glomerulotubular balance changes with oncotic pressure. (From ► https://derangedphysiology.com/main/cicm-primary-exam/required-reading/body-fluids-and-electrolytes/Chapter%20233/response-1l-normal-saline)

After a saline bolus, the rate of water reabsorption declines, and more water is excreted in the urine. As more water is excreted, oncotic pressure gradually returns to normal.

The half-life of a bolus of normal saline in health is around 20–40 min [27], 2–4 h for critically ill patients, and up to 8 h in mechanically ventilated or shocked patients.

19.5.3.4 Acid–Base Effects

Infusion of fluids can influence the acid–base balance of plasma. Administration of chloride-rich solutions, such as normal saline, is a well-recognised cause of a normal anion gap hyperchloraemic metabolic acidosis. The mechanism for this chloride-driven metabolic acidosis is explained by the strong ion theory of acid–base proposed by Stewart. A detailed discussion of the Stewart hypothesis is beyond this text; the reader is referred to his original work for a detailed explanation [28].

If 0.9% saline is used for fluid resuscitation, inexperienced staff may continue to administer further fluid boluses based on the finding of the acidosis which develops, assuming that it is driven by tissue hypoperfusion rather than hyperchloraemia. The key to avoiding this unfortunate situation is to check the anion gap:

$$\text{Anion gap} = [\text{Na}] + [\text{K}] - [\text{HCO}_3] - [\text{Cl}]$$

A normal anion gap is around 8–12 mmol/L. A normal anion gap and hyperchloraemia, in the context of administration of 0.9% saline, is iatrogenic. If the lactate is in the normal range and peripheral perfusion is adequate, no further fluid boluses should be given.

19.5.3.5 Possible Deleterious Effects

It has been postulated that hyperchloraemia may be detrimental by causing a reduction in renal cortical blood flow [29], acute kidney injury [30, 31] and even a pro-inflammatory state [32]. There is emerging data that balanced or buffered crystalloids are associated with better clinical outcomes and these are now generally preferred over normal saline both for acute resuscitation and for maintenance (see below).

19.5.3.6 Rationale for Intravenous Fluids

The oral route is the preferred and safest route for rehydration and maintenance therapy. If the patient is unable to tolerate oral fluids or feeding is contraindicated, intravenous fluids are warranted. Intravenous fluid should be treated like any other medication, and only prescribed after consideration of the potential benefits and harms from its use.

Intravenous fluids are given to patients for three main reasons:

- **Resuscitation in shock**
  - To correct intravascular volume or acute hypovolaemia, augment circulatory volume and improve preload, with the aim to improve cardiac output.
- **Maintenance therapy**
  - Provision of daily requirements of water, electrolytes, and dextrose if patient unable to take anything orally.

- **Rehydration therapy**
  - To correct existing or developing deficits of water and electrolytes that lost through vomiting, diarrhoea, or insensible losses that cannot be replaced by oral intake alone [4]. Rehydration therapy, e.g., gastroenteritis and diabetic ketoacidosis are not considered here.

19.6 Fluid Resuscitation in Shock

Early, rapid fluid resuscitation is the integral to the supportive management of shock [1]. Early and aggressive initial fluid resuscitation was promoted in the 1990s for children with sepsis [33] based on observational studies in children with meningococcal sepsis. However, the FEAST trial [19] demonstrated increased mortality in febrile African children with impaired perfusion treated with a fluid bolus compared with no fluid bolus, which has resulted in a reappraisal of this strategy. To date, the FEAST trial is the only large-scale trial of fluid bolus therapy in children and although the context of the trial and patients may differ from those in the global North, the benefit of fluid bolus therapy in paediatric critical care is now unclear. Despite the findings of the FEAST trial, there is still a consensus that fluid bolus therapy is of benefit to critically ill children in resource-rich environments [20]. However, more restrictive fluid strategies and early use of inotropes are currently being explored [34].

19.6.1 What Is a Fluid Bolus? How Much to Give?

Fluid bolus therapy, rapid infusion of boluses of intravenous fluid of 10–20 mL/kg, is often administered to patients with hypotension or those with markers of poor systemic perfusion, whatever the cause. The assumption being made by the treating clinician is that these patients have relative hypovolaemia, resulting in cardiovascular physiology on the ascending portion of the Frank-Starling curve (A1 below); hence it makes physiological sense to continue to deliver fluid bolus therapy to get them to point A or A2 [35]. The aim is to increase preload and hence cardiac output, improving organ and tissue perfusion (◘ Fig. 19.4).

The problem is that there is poor correlation of bedside clinical assessment to cardiovascular parameters measured using advanced monitoring [36, 37], and advanced monitoring is often unavailable in an emergency setting. Hence it is not possible to know clinically where an individual patient is on the Frank-Starling curve. At the point of assessment, the patient may be at any of the points on the graph; fluid bolus therapy may be of no benefit. In the context of a failing myocardium (e.g., in a patient with severe sepsis or myocarditis) the patient may be at point D or D2 at the point of presentation and fluid bolus therapy may be harmful. Inotropic drugs may be of more benefit.

In sepsis, the current ACCM-ESPNIC guidelines recommend up 40–60 mL/kg fluid bolus therapy in the first hour of resuscitation, in aliquots of 10–20 mL/kg, for children with septic shock diagnosed by abnormal perfusion or hypotension in healthcare systems with availability of advanced supportive and intensive care. Fluid

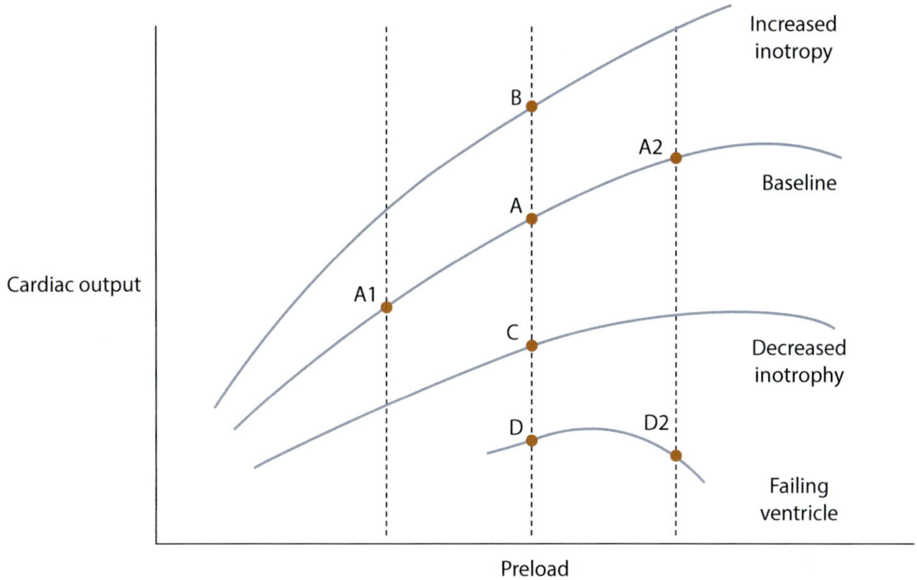

Fig. 19.4 The Frank-Starling curve demonstrating the relationship between cardiac output and preload. The vertical (dashed) lines demonstrate similar levels of preload at different levels of ventricular inotropy. A1, A, and A2 demonstrate how increasing preload may lead to increased cardiac output along a baseline Frank-Starling curve. D and D2 demonstrate how increasing preload can lead to reduced cardiac output in the failing ventricle. A, B, C, D compare how changing the inotropy of the heart with a fixed preload can result in different cardiac outputs. (Reproduced from Mann D. (2017) "Frank-Starling Curve." In: Raj TD (Ed.) Data Interpretation in Anaesthesia—A Clinical Guide. Springer, Cham, with permission from Springer Nature)

resuscitation should be titrated to clinical markers of cardiac output (even though they are unreliable) and discontinued if signs of fluid overload develop [20].

Based on the FEAST trial in healthcare systems with no availability of intensive care, up to only 20 mL/kg fluid bolus fluid (10 20 mL/kg per bolus) over the first hour is suggested, titrated to the same endpoints.

Following the initial fluid bolus, the need for further bolus fluid should be guided by frequent reassessment of clinical markers of cardiac output, serial lactate measurement and advanced monitoring when available. Signs of fluid overload may include clinical signs of pulmonary oedema or new or worsening hepatomegaly.

19.6.2 Haemodynamic Targets of Fluid Bolus Therapy

Clinical markers of cardiac output may include level of consciousness, heart rate, blood pressure, capillary refill time and urine output [20]. Heart rate and blood pressure are the most used markers [38]. There SCCM-ESPNIC sepsis guidelines recommend targeting a mean arterial pressure between the 5th and 50th centile [20]. Permissive hypotension in paediatric trauma patients is not advocated once bleeding has been addressed, and supraphysiologic blood pressure may be targeted in conditions requiring neurointensive care and in pulmonary hypertension.

Measurement of blood lactate as a guide to fluid resuscitation is recommended in the SCCM-ESPNIC sepsis guideline and is indirectly supported by adult evidence [39]. A systematic review in adults suggested a decreased blood lactate was associated with an improved outcome [40].

If advanced haemodynamic monitoring is available, e.g., invasive arterial blood pressure monitoring with pulse contour analysis; ultrasound Doppler of the ascending or descending thoracic aorta (suprasternal or oesophageal Doppler); echocardiography; or measurement of central venous oxygen saturations ($ScvO_2$); then it may also be helpful to target parameters such as CI, SVRI and $ScvO_2$. Such techniques may also reveal which patients are "fluid responsive," i.e., exhibit an increase in stroke volume (or cardiac output/index) of 10–15% after fluid bolus administration.

19.6.3 What Fluid to Use for Acute Resuscitation?

Because of the FEAST study, albumin has fallen out of favour in PICU. Outside trauma, when blood products are preferred, crystalloids are now in general used for fluid bolus therapy. There is some evidence from observational studies and RCTs in adults that crystalloids containing high chloride concentrations are associated with hyperchloraemic acidosis, increased mortality and/or with acute kidney injury when compared to resuscitation with balanced crystalloids [41]. There are two observational studies in children with sepsis [42, 43], demonstrating balanced fluids were associated with a reduced risk of death and AKI. Therefore, the 2020 ACCM-ESPNIC guidance conditionally recommends balanced crystalloids over normal saline for resuscitation of children with sepsis-associated organ dysfunction or septic shock [20]. However, a more recent meta-analysis found three randomised controlled trials comparing balanced and unbalanced crystalloid. There was no difference in chloride serum level, acute kidney injury, renal replacement therapy, or mortality [44]. Further studies are required to develop a robust evidence base upon which to recommend a particular isotonic fluid for bolus therapy in critically ill children.

19.6.4 What Are the Potential Harms of Fluid Bolus Therapy?

Fluid bolus therapy may lead to a variety of complications in a critically ill child, from positive fluid balance, which is associated with detrimental outcomes (see below), to acute excess of pulmonary and systemic fluid leading to (1) pulmonary oedema leading to impaired gas exchange due to fluid in the alveolar space (2) interstitial oedema causing impaired oxygen diffusion between capillaries and cells. The FEAST trial showed that an early resuscitation protocol involving intravenous bolus therapy was associated with increased mortality in a resource-poor setting. In a post hoc analysis of the data from FEAST, it was demonstrated that both albumin and saline boluses caused respiratory and neurological dysfunction, hyperchloraemic acidosis, and reduction in haemoglobin concentration, supporting the possibility that both fluid resuscitation and the use of unbuffered electrolyte solutions may have caused harm [45]. Further evaluation of the effects of buffered and unbuffered solutions is required.

19.7 Intravenous Fluid Maintenance in PICU

19.7.1 Paediatric Fluid Requirements

In 1957, Holliday and Segar [46] calculated the amount of parenteral fluid required by hospitalised children and adults based on their body weight and energy expenditure. A total of 100 mL/100 cal/day was deemed the requirement to meet the water losses of patients on parenteral fluid therapy. Holliday and Segar's '4,2,1' is the most widely used formula to calculate maintenance requirements in children (Table 19.3).

In general, the maximum 24-h fluid requirement for males is 2500 mL and females is 2000 mL. Maintenance fluid requirements vary between children and will depend upon several factors (Fig. 19.5).

▶ Example

A 24 kg child is ventilated on PICU with Paediatric Acute Respiratory Distress and is currently on intravenous fluids due to an ileus and is fully sedated and paralysed.

- 0–10 kg 10 × 100 = 1000 mL
- 10–20 kg 10 × 50 = 1500 mL
- 20–24 kg 4 × 20 = 80 mL
  - Therefore 100% maintenance = 1580 mL
- The child is ventilated, sedated, and paralysed and will therefore have minimal insensible losses via the respiratory route and minimal energy expenditure so should receive less than 100% maintenance, for example, 70%
  - 1580/100 × 70 = 1106 mL in 24 h
  - 1106/24 h = 46 mL/h ◀

Holliday and Segar based their paper on the work of Darrow and Pratt [47], who recognised the important relationship between energy expenditure and water requirement. This is because energy expenditure causes carbon dioxide production, resulting in increased insensible losses due to increased minute ventilation (and hence respiratory evaporative losses) and skin evaporative losses due to heat. Energy (caloric) expenditure was originally calculated according to body surface area. Holliday and Segar simplified this approach, relating energy expenditure to one of three weight-based categories (<10, 10–20, and >20 kg). Electrolyte requirements were calculated based on those seen in human and cow's milk, resulting in a recom-

Table 19.3 Maintenance fluid rates

Body weight	Hourly infusion rate	Total fluid amount in 24 h
0–10 kg	4 mL/kg/h	100 mL/kg/day
10–20 kg	2 mL/kg/h	50 mL/kg/day
>20 kg	1 mL/kg/h	20 mL/kg/day

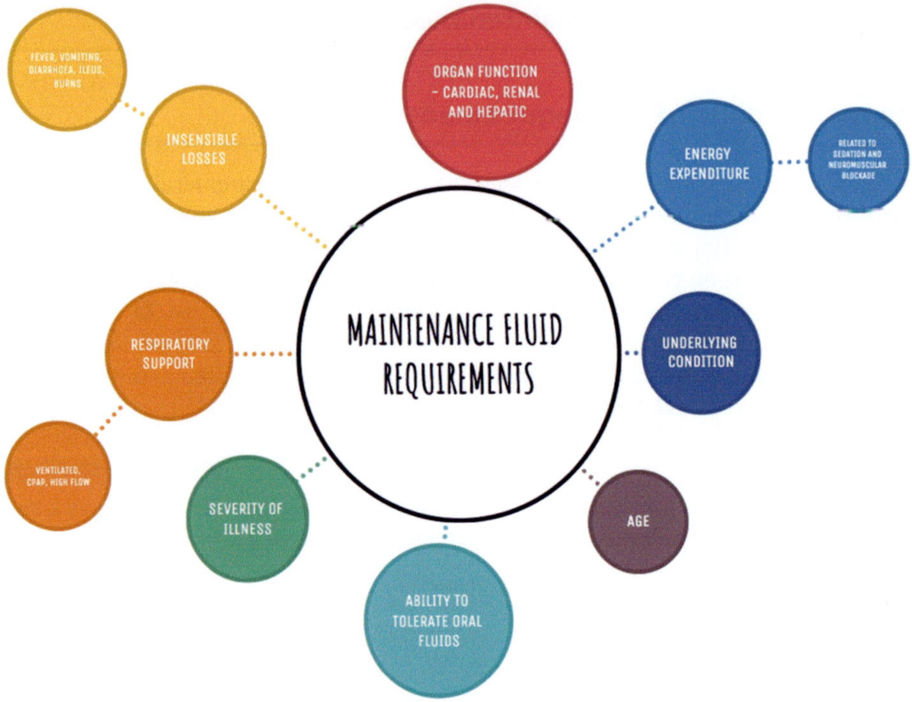

Fig. 19.5 Determinants of maintenance fluid requirements

mendation for maintenance sodium, chloride and potassium of 3.0, 2.0 and 2.0 mEq/100 cal/day, resulting in hypotonic maintenance fluid. Unfortunately, many of the assumptions of Holliday and Segar were incorrect, particularly in an intensive care environment. Energy expenditure is often much lower than expected; insensible losses are lower as a consequence of humidification of gas in the ventilator circuit; renal losses are lower due to increased ADH in response to stress (pain, fever, surgery) or drugs [48]; electrolyte needs were calculated based on observed intake rather than the need to maintain isotonic plasma.

For these reasons, full maintenance fluid, according to the Holliday-Segar formula, is rarely prescribed to critically ill children in PICU. Fluid requirements are often prescribed as a percentage of "full" maintenance, i.e., 70%. In conditions associated with inappropriate ADH secretion, maintenance fluids are often restricted to 50–80% of "full" maintenance needs; in oligo-anuric renal failure, they may be calculated based on insensible losses (e.g. 300–400 mL/m^2/24 h) plus urine output [49]. No single rate of administration or composition of maintenance fluid is appropriate in all circumstances [50]; these should be continually tailored to the patient's observed fluid balance and plasma electrolytes.

19.7.2 Neonatal Fluid Requirements

It is outside the scope of this chapter to consider neonatal fluid requirements in detail. However, a brief overview of the maintenance fluid requirements in the term infant is given as these infants sometimes come to the PICU. Intravenous fluids and electrolytes should be prescribed with care in the newborn term infant. Sodium and water requirements in the first few days of life are low. Urine output is low due to the elevated levels of circulating ADH at birth. In the first days after birth, pulmonary vascular resistance falls and pulmonary venous return increases, causing release of atrial natriuretic peptide, which in turn results in diuresis [51]. Hence, fluid requirements slowly increase (◘ Table 19.4).

Newborn infants are prone to hypoglycaemia and require intravenous glucose if enteral feeds are withheld. Blood glucose falls after birth but rises in the first few hours due to endogenous glucose production or feeding. Neonates metabolise ketones as well as glucose as a brain energy substrate, so they are protected from hypoglycaemia. However, prolonged hypoglycaemia <2.6 mmol/L is associated with abnormal neurological outcomes [52]. Intravenous glucose should be provided to babies at risk of hypoglycaemia at a starting rate of 5–7 mg/kg/min (10% dextrose 70–100 mL/kg/day), and blood glucose should be monitored.

Sodium (or potassium) is rarely required in the first 24 h of life. After the first 24 h, a newborn baby requires 2–3 mmol/kg/day of sodium and 1–2 mmol/kg/day of potassium [53].

Intravenous crystalloids are effective in treating hypotension, and albumin and other colloids are not recommended. Balanced solutions should be used to replace losses during surgery (and blood or coagulation factors as indicated).

19.7.3 Dealing with Fluid Losses

Critically ill children with, for example, high nasogastric losses or diarrhoea may become rapidly dehydrated if losses are not accounted for. The electrolyte composition of different body fluids varies (◘ Table 19.5) and needs to be taken into consideration when prescribing replacement fluids.

◘ Table 19.4 Neonatal daily fluid requirements

Age	Fluid requirements
Birth	50–60 mL/kg/day
D2	70–80 mL/kg/day
D3	80–100 mL/kg/day
D4	100–120 mL/kg/day
D5	120–150 mL/kg/day

Table 19.5 Contents of body fluids

	Na (mmol/L)	K (mmol/L)	Cl^- (mmol/L)	HCO_3^- (mmol/L)
Sweat	50	5	55	0
Saliva	30	20	35	15
Bile	145	5	110	40
Gastric fluid	20–80	5–20	100–150	0
Ileal fluid	100–140	5	110	30
Colonic fluid	30–140	30–70	40	20
Pancreatic fluid	120–140	5–15	40–80	Up to 140

In the recovery phase of acute tubular necrosis, when tubular function is still impaired, water and electrolyte losses can be extreme—careful replacement with fluid tailored to match the content of the urine may be required. These replacement fluids should be given in addition to estimated insensible losses if necessary, replacing urine losses on an hourly basis (e.g. 300–400 mL/m^2/day + previous hour's urine losses every hour). Urinary electrolyte measurement can be helpful in this situation.

19.7.4 What Maintenance Fluid to Use?

The choice of maintenance fluid will depend on many of the factors previously alluded to, including age of patient, underlying condition, availability, and biochemistry. However, the general quantity and quality of evidence to guide choice remains low and is compounded by the significant heterologous nature of conditions and patients in intensive care. In general, isotonic crystalloid is best used, to limit the risk of iatrogenic hyponatraemia [54]. Close electrolyte monitoring is required for all patients on intravenous fluids. In the United Kingdom, the National Institute for Clinical Excellence (NICE) guidance recommends measuring blood glucose and plasma electrolyte concentrations prior to starting intravenous maintenance therapy and at least every 24 h thereafter [49]. A recent survey involving members of the European Society of Pediatric and Neonatal Intensive Care (ESPNIC) showed considerable variation in the type of maintenance fluid prescribed [55]. Subsequently, consensus guidelines have been issued by ESPNIC with recommendations on intravenous maintenance fluid therapy in acute and critically ill children. These guidelines, which were based on a systematic review and meta-analysis, supported the use of balanced isotonic fluid for maintenance [56].

19.7.5 Glucose Requirements

A healthy child maintains their plasma glucose levels using glycogen stores if insufficient energy intake for at least the first 24 h, before switching to gluconeogenesis. Glucose can be provided in parenteral fluids, in the form of dextrose, to provide 4–8 mg/kg/min of glucose, which is sufficient to meet most children's caloric requirements and limit tissue catabolism, but it does not provide complete nutritional support [50].

The addition of 5% or 10% dextrose to the isotonic solution may be required depending on the patient's age and underlying condition and is supported by ESPNIC recommendations [56]. Certain patients require glucose supplementation to prevent hypoglycaemia, e.g., prolonged fasting, neonates, and children with liver dysfunction. A neonate will usually require 10% dextrose; 5% may be sufficient for older infants and children.

Dextrose is rapidly taken up by cells and metabolised and is therefore not a significant contributor to plasma osmolarity [57]. Solutions in which dextrose is the only osmotically active substance are equivalent to administering water ("free water"). The water in 5% dextrose is distributed evenly throughout the intracellular and extracellular spaces. Outside the newborn period, solutions only containing dextrose should not be given to children due to the risk of hyponatraemia [49].

19.7.6 What Maintenance Fluid to Use Postoperatively?

Patients requiring maintenance fluids should receive isotonic fluids with appropriate potassium and dextrose, as recommended by NICE, ESPNIC and American Association of Paediatrics (AAP), due to the significant risk of hyponatraemia [57].

19.7.7 How Is Fluid Balance Assessed?

The assessment of fluid balance in the critically ill child is challenging but important, especially with emerging evidence of detrimental outcomes in those patients with cumulative positive fluid balance.

- Daily fluid balance = Daily fluid intake – daily fluid output.
- Cumulative fluid balance = Sum of fluid balance over a defined time, usually from admission.

Current methods of assessing fluid volume status include weight, daily intake and output recordings, and clinical assessment of body oedema. These methods are often unreliable [58]. Accurate documentation of daily output can be particularly challenging. Additionally, there is a reluctance to weigh critically ill children due to perceived safety concerns [59] (◘ Table 19.6).

New methodology is being developed for assessment of total body water including bio-impedance spectroscopy [60] and bioelectrical impedance vector analysis [61], but these are still experimental.

Table 19.6 Fluid balance measurement methods

Method	Description	Advantages	Disadvantages
Clinical—oedema, pulmonary oedema, haemodynamic parameters	Clinical assessment of oedema, enlarged liver, pulmonary oedema, heart rate, blood pressure, capillary refill	Can be done at bedside	Inaccurate Low specificity
Balance chart	Hourly inputting of fluid input and output	Widespread Easy to do	Inaccurate—does not account for insensible losses
Body weight	Daily weight of child can be compared to admission weight	Useful in uncomplicated patient	Time consuming Labour intensive Safety concerns in ventilated children

19.8 Phases of Fluid Therapy: The "ROSE" Concept

Four dynamic phases of fluid therapy have been proposed. Malbrain et al.'s ROSE acronym (Resuscitation, Optimisation, Stabilisation, Evacuation) was the preferred term adopted for the phases of critically illness and fluid therapy during the international fluid academy day (IFAD). [62].

The varying phases of fluid therapy reflect the dynamic changes in the critically ill patient and will vary in length depending upon individual patient's needs. The phases range from a few hours' duration in the acute resuscitation and optimisation stage during restoration and maintenance of tissue perfusion through to several days in the stabilisation and evacuation phase, when normal fluid maintenance therapy is delivered, and excessive fluid removed (Fig. 19.6).

- Resuscitation phase (R)
  - Rescue treatment with fluids administered quickly as a bolus
  - Aim is correction of shock and restoration of adequate perfusion pressure with early goal directed fluid management
  - Fluid balance should be positive
- Optimisation (O)
  - Occurs within hours
  - Patient is no longer in obvious hypovolaemia but remains haemodynamically unstable
  - Aim is to optimise and maintain adequate tissue perfusion
  - Fluid challenges will be required and administered based on individual needs and their markers of cardiac output
- Stabilisation phase (S)
  - Occurs over days
  - Fluid therapy required for normal maintenance, replacement of losses and provide organ support
  - No shock is present
  - Daily weight and fluid balance important

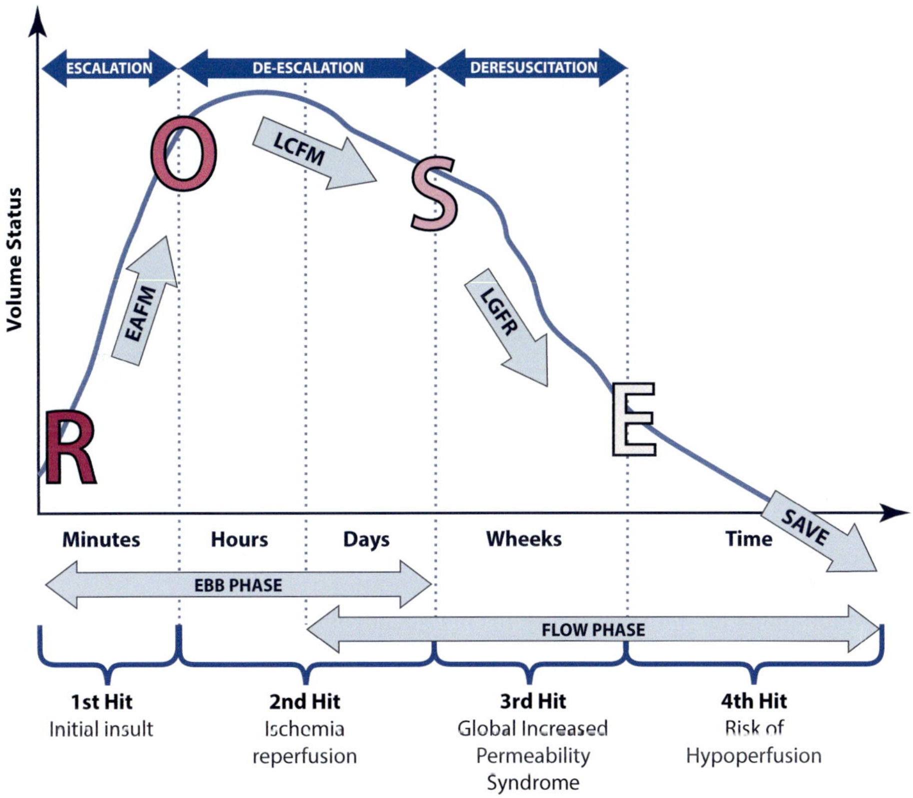

Fig. 19.6 The four-hit model of shock with evolution of patients' cumulative fluid volume status over time during the five phases of resuscitation: Resuscitation (R), Optimisation (O), Stabilisation (S), and Evacuation (E) (ROSE), followed by a risk of Hypoperfusion in case of too aggressive deresuscitation. On admission patients are often hypovolemic, followed by euvolaemia after fluid resuscitation (escalation or EAFM, early adequate fluid management), and fluid overload, again followed by a phase returning to euvolaemia with de-escalation via achieving zero fluid balance or late conservative fluid management (LCFM) and followed by late goal directed fluid removal (LGFR) or deresuscitation. (Malbrain MLNG et al. 2022. [63]

- Evacuation phase (E) or de-escalation phase (D)
  - Removal of excessive fluid
  - Can be achieved through spontaneous diuresis
  - Patient may require ultrafiltration or diuretics

19.8.1 What Is Fluid Overload and Is It Important?

Multiple definitions of fluid overload exist. Malbrain et al. defined it in adults as "a cut off value of 10% of fluid accumulation as this is associated with worse outcomes", with the percentage of fluid accumulation defined "by dividing the cumulative fluid balance in litre by the patient's baseline body weight and multiplying by 100%" [42].

Recently, in adult practice, the term "fluid accumulation" has been suggested—denoting a pathological state of overhydration associated with clinical impact and worse outcomes, which may vary depending on age, comorbidity, and phase of illness [63].

The most common way to calculate the degree of fluid overload is based on the method described by Goldstein [64]:

- % Fluid overload = Sum of daily (fluid in – fluid out)/ICU admission weight × 100
  - Formula depends on the accuracy of the fluid chart

A threshold of 10% over the baseline weight appears to be the most widely used paediatric definition.

Increasing evidence shows that fluid overload in critically ill children is associated with adverse outcomes. A recent systematic review and meta-analysis showed that fluid overload in critically ill children admitted to the paediatric intensive care unit (PICU) was associated with fewer ventilator-free days, a higher risk of acute kidney injury and even an increased risk of mortality [65]. There are no published clinical trials comparing liberal to restrictive fluid therapy strategies in critically ill children.

Maintaining an optimal fluid status in critically ill children is challenging. Fluid bolus therapy can be lifesaving and is recommended in septic shock [20]. Fluid overload can develop because of excess fluid administration and/or a continuous high fluid intake in combination with syndrome of inappropriate production of ADH (SIADH) or renal failure. This often leads to the accumulation of extravascular fluid, further aggravated by degradation of the endothelial glycocalyx (EGL). EGL, a web of membrane-bound glycoproteins and proteoglycans on the luminal surface of endothelium, excludes proteins from the sub-endothelial cleft, thereby resulting in a local oncotic gradient between plasma and cleft, which opposes trans-capillary efflux [66]. Once the EGL is damaged, fluid efflux becomes primarily dependent on capillary hydrostatic pressure culminating in the formation of oedema in several tissues including the lung. This is the main cause of adverse effects of fluid overload (◘ Fig. 19.7).

19.8.2 How Do I Deresuscitate My Patient?

Measures to remove excess fluid can be pharmacological and non-pharmacological, along with fluid restriction. Diuretics are usually tried first. In case of low serum albumin levels or low serum total protein level, hyper-oncotic albumin 20–25% may be added for synergistic effect, but this will not be effective if the EGL has not recovered. Mechanical fluid removal should be considered when fluid overload has not responded to diuretics or in anuric renal failure. Slow continuous ultrafiltration (SCUF) or Renal Replacement Therapy may be required. Occasionally it may be necessary to increase vasoactives to support the blood pressure to facilitate fluid removal.

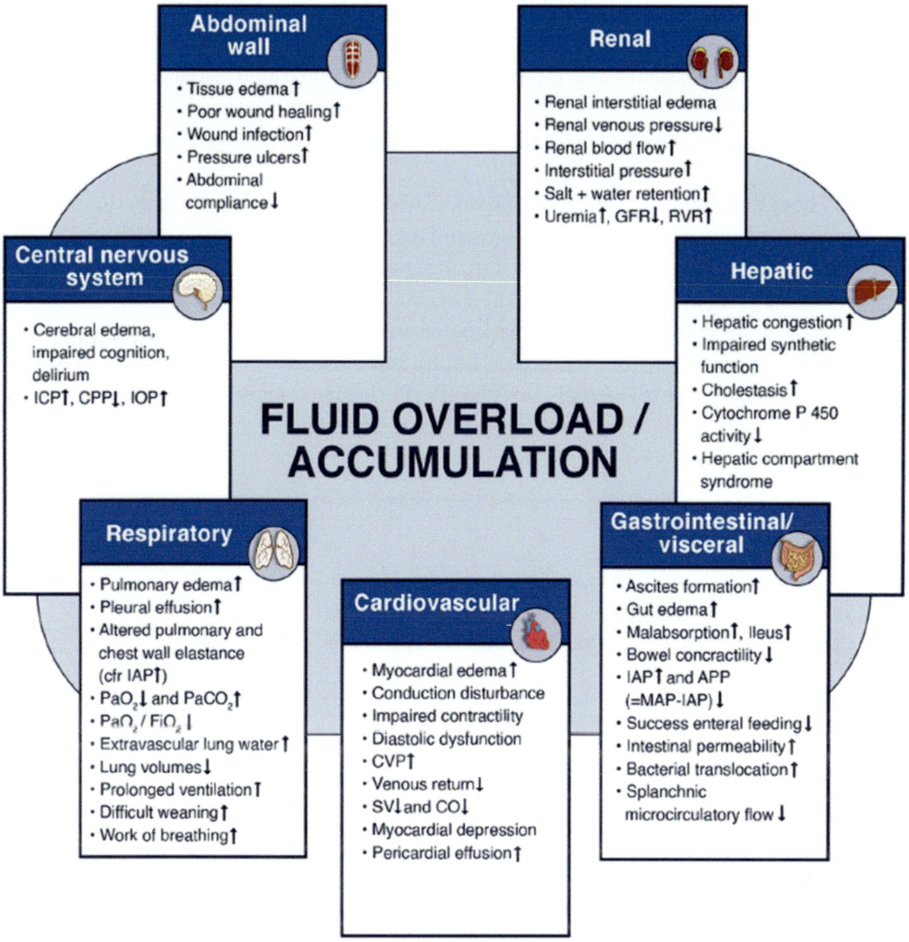

Fig. 19.7 Possible adverse effects of fluid accumulation. (After Malbrain MLNG et al. 2022 [63])

Deresuscitation should be stopped when the patient is clinically euvolaemic, or earlier if complications arise. It is difficult to assess euvolaemia, however, and often fluid balance or weight are targeted; or other markers of improving fluid status (e.g. resolving peripheral oedema, improving oxygenation, extubation). There is no specific marker to indicate euvolaemia.

A recent meta-analysis showed that a fluid restrictive/deresuscitation strategy in adults and children with acute respiratory distress syndrome, sepsis, or systemic inflammatory response syndrome, resulted in an increased number of ventilator-free days and a decreased length of ICU stay compared with a liberal strategy or standard care. The effect on mortality was uncertain [67].

Take-Home Messages
- Isotonic fluid should be used for bolus and maintenance fluid. Balanced (buffered) solutions are favoured over non-balanced solutions.
- Blood glucose and electrolytes should be checked at least daily if on intravenous fluids.
- Though maintenance fluids can be calculated using the "4,2,1" formula, in intensive care, fluid requirements are substantially reduced.
- The rate of maintenance fluids for intensive care patients should be regularly assessed and adjusted according to individual need.
- Assessment of fluid balance is challenging and rarely accurate.
- Fluid overload is associated with mortality and morbidity.
- Randomised controlled trials are needed to determine optimal fluid type and resuscitation and deresuscitation strategies in paediatric critical illness.

References

1. Myburgh JA, Mythen MG. Resuscitation fluids. N Engl J Med. 2013;369:1243–51.
2. Cosnett JE. The origins of intravenous fluid therapy. Lancet. 1989;333:768–71.
3. O'Shaughnessy WB. Report on the chemical pathology of the malignant cholera. London: S. Highley; 1832. p. 1–72.
4. Latta TA. Lancet. 1832;2:275.
5. Latta TA. Injections into the veins in cholera. London Med Gaz. 1832;379–82.
6. Ringer SA. A further contribution regarding the influence of the different Constituents of the Blood on the Contraction of the Heart. J Physiol. 1883;4:29–42.3.
7. Hartmann AF, Senn MJ. Studies in the metabolism of sodium r-lactate. III. Response of human subjects with liver damage, disturbed water and mineral balance, and renal insufficiency to the intravenous injection of sodium r-lactate. J Clin Invest. 1932;11:345–55.
8. Awad S, Allison SP, Lobo DN. The history of 0.9% saline. Clin Nutr. 2008;27:179–88.
9. Hamburger HJ. A discourse on permeability in physiology and pathology. Lancet. 1921;198:1039–45.
10. Van der Kloott W. William Maddock Bayliss's therapy for wound shock. Notes Rec R Soc Lond. 2010;64:271–86.
11. Matas R. A the continued intravenous "drip": with remarks on the value of continued gastric drainage and irrigation by nasal intubation with a gastroduodenal tube (jutte) in surgical practice. Ann Surg. 1924;79:643–61.
12. Coller FA, Dick VS, Maddock WG. Maintenance of normal water exchange with intravenous fluids. JAMA. 1936;107:1522–7.
13. Wilkinson AW, Billing BH, Nagy G, Stewart CP. Excretion of chloride and sodium after surgical operations. Lancet. 1949;1:640–4.
14. MHRA UK Public Assessment Report. Intravenous 0.18% saline/4% glucose solution ('hypotonic saline'): do not use in children except in specialist settings under expert supervision, Oct 2012, London, UK.
15. Starling EH. On the absorption of fluids from the connective tissue spaces. J Physiol. 1896;19:312–26.
16. Finfer S, Liu B, Taylor C, Bellomo R, Billot L, Cook D, et al., SAFE TRIPS Investigators. Resuscitation fluid use in critically ill adults: an international cross-sectional study in 391 intensive care units. Crit Care. 2010;14:R185.
17. Semler MW, Kellum JA. Balanced crystalloid solutions. Am J Respir Crit Care Med. 2019;199:952–60.

18. Finfer S, Bellomo R, Boyce N, French J, Myburgh J, Norton R, SAFE Study Investigators. A comparison of albumin and saline for fluid resuscitation in the intensive care unit. N Engl J Med. 2004;350(22):2247–56.
19. Maitland K, Kiguli S, Opoka RO, Engoru C, Olupot-Olupot P, Akech SO, et al., FEAST Trial Group. Mortality after fluid bolus in African children with severe infection. N Engl J Med. 2011;364:2483–95.
20. Weiss SL, Peters MJ, Alhazzani W, Agus MSD, Flori HR, Inwald DP, et al. Surviving sepsis campaign international guidelines for the management of septic shock and sepsis-associated organ dysfunction in children. Pediatr Crit Care Med. 2020;21:e52–106.
21. Moeller C, Fleischmann C, Thomas-Rueddel D, Vlasakov V, Rochwerg B, Theurer P, et al. How safe is gelatin? A systematic review and meta-analysis of gelatin-containing plasma expanders vs crystalloids and albumin. J Crit Care. 2016;35:75–83.
22. Lewis SR, Pritchard MW, Evans DJ, Butler AR, Alderson P, Smith AF, et al. Colloids versus crystalloids for fluid resuscitation in critically ill people. Cochrane Database Syst Rev. 2018;8:CD000567.
23. Brunkhorst FM, Engel C, Bloos F, Meier-Hellmann A, Ragaller M, Weiler N, et al., German Competence Network Sepsis (SepNet). Intensive insulin therapy and pentastarch resuscitation in severe sepsis. N Engl J Med. 2008;358:125–39.
24. Perner A, Haase N, Guttormsen AB, Tenhunen J, Klemenzson G, Åneman A, et al., 6S Trial Group, Scandinavian Critical Care Trials Group. Hydroxyethyl starch 130/0.42 versus Ringer's acetate in severe sepsis. N Engl J Med. 2012;367:124–34.
25. Wilkes MM, Navickis R. Postoperative renal replacement therapy after hydroxyethyl starch infusion: a meta-analysis of randomised trials. Netherlands J Crit Care. 2014;18:4–9.
26. Hahn RG, Warner DS. Volume kinetics for infusion fluids. J Am Soc Anesthesiol. 2010;113:470–81.
27. Hahn RG, Lyons G. The half-life of infusion fluids: an educational review. Eur J Anaesthesiol. 2016;33:475.
28. Stewart PA. Modern quantitative acid base chemistry. Can J Physiol Pharmacol. 1983;61:1444–61.
29. Wilcox CS. Regulation of renal blood flow by plasma chloride. J Clin Invest. 1983;71:726–35.
30. Chowdhury AH, Cox EF, Francis ST, Lobo DN. A randomized, controlled, double-blind crossover study on the effects of 2-L infusions of 0.9% saline and plasma-lyte® 148 on renal blood flow velocity and renal cortical tissue perfusion in healthy volunteers. Ann Surg. 2012;256:18–24.
31. Mitting RB, Ramnarayan P, Inwald D. Hyperchloremia on admission to pediatric intensive care in mechanically ventilated children is associated with impaired renal function. J Paediatr Intensive Care. 2021; https://doi.org/10.1055/s-0041-1728788.
32. Kellum JA, Song M, Almasri E. Hyperchloremic acidosis increases circulating inflammatory molecules in experimental sepsis. Chest. 2006;130:962–7.
33. Carcillo JA, Davis AL, Zaritsky A. Role of early fluid resuscitation in pediatric septic shock. JAMA. 1991;266:1242–5.
34. Parker MJ, Thabane L, Fox-Robichaud A, Liaw P, Choong K, Canadian Critical Care Trials Group and the Canadian Critical Care Translational Biology Group. A trial to determine whether septic shock-reversal is quicker in pediatric patients randomized to an early goal-directed fluid-sparing strategy versus usual care (SQUEEZE): study protocol for a pilot randomized controlled trial. Trials. 2021;17:556.
35. Long E, Duke T. Fluid resuscitation therapy for paediatric sepsis. J Paediatr Child Health. 2016;52:141–6.
36. Tibby SM, Hatherill M, Marsh MJ, Murdoch IA. Clinicians' abilities to estimate cardiac index in ventilated children and infants. Arch Dis Child. 1997;77:516–8.
37. Razavi A, Newth CJL, Khemani RG, Beltramo F, Ross PA. Cardiac output, and systemic vascular resistance: clinical assessment compared with a noninvasive objective measurement in children with shock. J Crit Care. 2017;39:6–10.
38. Gelbart B, Schlapbach L, Ganeshalingham A, Ganu S, Erickson S, Oberender F, et al. Fluid bolus therapy in critically ill children: a survey of practice among paediatric intensive care doctors in Australia and New Zealand. Crit Care Resusc. 2018;20:131–8.
39. Gu WJ, Zhang Z, Bakker J. Early lactate clearance-guided therapy in patients with sepsis: a meta-analysis with trial sequential analysis of randomized controlled trials. Intensive Care Med. 2015;41:1862–3.

40. Vincent JL, Quintairos E, Silva A, Couto L Jr, Taccone FS. The value of blood lactate kinetics in critically ill patients: a systematic review. Crit Care. 2016;20:257.
41. Semler MW, Self WH, Wanderer JP, Ehrenfeld JM, Wang L, Byrne DW, et al., SMART Investigators and the Pragmatic Critical Care Research Group. Balanced crystalloids versus saline in critically ill adults. N Engl J Med. 2018;378:829–39.
42. Weiss SL, Keele L, Balamuth F, Vendetti N, Ross R, Fitzgerald JC, et al. Crystalloid fluid choice and clinical outcomes in pediatric sepsis: a matched retrospective cohort study. J Pediatr. 2017;182:304–10.
43. Emrath ET, Fortenberry JD, Travers C, McCracken CE, Hebbar KB. Resuscitation with balanced fluids is associated with improved survival in pediatric severe sepsis. Crit Care Med. 2017;45:1177–83.
44. Lehr AR, Rached-d'Astous S, Barrowman N, Tsampalieros A, Parker M, McIntyre L, Sampson M, Menon K. Balanced versus unbalanced fluid in critically ill children: systematic review and meta-analysis. Pediatr Crit Care Med. 2022;23:181–91.
45. Levin M, Cunnington AJ, Wilson C, Nadel S, Lang HJ, Ninis N, et al. Effects of saline or albumin fluid bolus in resuscitation: evidence from re-analysis of the FEAST trial. Lancet Respir Med. 2019;7:581–93.
46. Holliday MA, Segar WE. The maintenance need for water in parenteral fluid therapy. Pediatrics. 1957;19:823.e32.
47. Darrow DC, Pratt EL. Fluid therapy; relation to tissue composition and the expenditure of water and electrolyte. JAMA. 1950;143:432–9.
48. Sharples PM, Seckl JR, Human D, et al. Plasma and cerebrospinal fluid arginine vasopressin inpatients with and without fever. Arch Dis Child. 1992;67:998–1002.
49. National Institute for Health and Care Excellence. Intravenous fluid therapy in children and young people in hospital. NICE guideline [NG29]. 2015. https://www.nice.org.uk/guidance/ng29/chapter/recommendations. Accessed 5 Apr 2020.
50. Moritz ML, Ayus JC. Maintenance intravenous fluids in acutely ill patients. N Engl J Med. 2015;373:1350–60.
51. Modi N, Bétrémieux P, Midgley J, Hartnoll G. Postnatal weight loss and contraction of the extracellular compartment is triggered by atrial natriuretic peptide. Early Hum Dev. 2000;59:201–8.
52. Adamkin DH. Neonatal hypoglycemia. Semin Fetal Neonatal Med. 2017;22:36–41.
53. O'Brien F, Walker IA. Fluid homeostasis in the neonate. Paediatr Anaesth. 2014;24:49–59.
54. Almeida HI, Mascarenhas MI, Loureiro HC, Abadesso CS, Nunes PS, Moniz MS, Machado MC. The effect of NaCl 0.9% and NaCl 0.45% on sodium, chloride, and acid-base balance in a PICU population. J Pediatr (Rio J). 2015;91:499–505.
55. Morice C, Alsohime F, Mayberry H, Tume LN, Brossier D, Valla FV, ESPNIC IVMFT Group. Intravenous maintenance fluid therapy practice in the pediatric acute and critical care settings: a European and Middle Eastern survey. Eur J Pediatr. 2022;181:3163–72.
56. Brossier DW, Tume LN, Briant AR, Chaparro CJ, Moullet C, Rooze S, et al. ESPNIC clinical practice guidelines: intravenous maintenance fluid therapy in acute and critically ill children—a systematic review and meta-analysis. Intensive Care Med. 2022; https://doi.org/10.1007/s00134-022-06882-z.
57. Feld LG, Neuspiel DR, Foster BA, Leu MG, Garber MD, Austin K, Basu RK, Conway EE Jr, Fehr JJ, Hawkins C, Kaplan RL, Rowe EV, Waseem M, Moritz ML. Clinical practice guideline: maintenance intravenous fluids in children. Pediatrics. 2018;142:e20183083.
58. Bontant T, Matrot B, Abdoul H, Aizenfisz S, Naudin J, Jones P, Dauger S. Assessing fluid balance in critically ill pediatric patients. Eur J Pediatr. 2015;174:133–7.
59. Mehta NM. Bringing back the (weighing) balance in the PICU—for good measure. Pediatr Crit Care Med. 2015;16:301–2.
60. Farr BJ, Bechard LJ, Rice-Townsend SE, Mehta NM. Bio-impedance spectroscopy for total body water assessment in pediatric surgical patients: a single center pilot cohort study. J Pediatr Surg. 2022. pii: S0022-3468(22)00462-6. https://doi.org/10.1016/j.jpedsurg.2022.07.014.
61. Stagi S, Silva AM, Jesus F, Campa F, Cabras S, Earthman CP, Marini E. Usability of classic and specific bioelectrical impedance vector analysis in measuring body composition of children. Clin Nutr. 2022;41:673–9.
62. Malbrain MLNG, Langer T, Annane D, Gattinoni L, Elbers P, Hahn RG, et al. Intravenous fluid therapy in the perioperative and critical care setting: executive summary of the International Fluid Academy (IFA). Ann Intensive Care. 2020;10:64.

63. Malbrain MLNG, Martin G, Ostermann M. Everything you need to know about deresuscitation. Intensive Care Med. 2022;48:1781–1786. https://doi.org/10.1007/s00134-022-06761-7.
64. Goldstein SL, Currier H, Graf JM, Cosio CC, Brewer ED, Sachdeva R. Outcome in children receiving continuous venovenous hemofiltration. Pediatrics. 2001;107:1309–12.
65. Alobaidi R, Morgan C, Basu RK, Stenson E, Featherstone R, Majumdar SR, et al. Association between fluid balance and outcomes in critically ill children: a systematic review and meta-analysis. JAMA Pediatr. 2018;172:257–68.
66. Woodcock TE, Woodcock TM. Revised Starling equation and the glycocalyx model of transvascular fluid exchange: an improved paradigm for prescribing intravenous fluid therapy. Br J Anaesth. 2012;108:384–94.
67. Silversides JA, Major E, Ferguson AJ, Mann EE, McAuley DF, Marshall JC, Blackwood B, Fan E. Conservative fluid management or deresuscitation for patients with sepsis or acute respiratory distress syndrome following the resuscitation phase of critical illness: a systematic review and meta-analysis. Intensive Care Med. 2017;43:155–70.

Vasoactive Agents

Aarti Pandit and Joe Brierley

Contents

J. Brierley et al. (eds.), *ESPNIC Children's Intensive Care Textbook*,
https://doi.org/10.1007/978-3-031-64762-8_20

Learning Objectives

- To understand the physiology and mechanism of action of Inotropes.
- To understand the cardiovascular physiology of shock in the paediatric population, including recognition of shock.
- To identify the need for inotropes and the choice of inotrope in various clinical situations.

20.1 Introduction

'Which inotrope?' for the sick child is a question that suggests the existence of a ready answer. But, with critically ill children, the 'answer' is context-specific. What is the clinical situation? Is the predominant problem impaired myocardial function post cardiopulmonary bypass, decreased systemic vascular resistance in sepsis or diastolic dysfunction in restrictive cardiomyopathy? What about age and ethnicity? In fact, the optimal inotrope relies on factors that medical science has not yet entirely elucidated—such as genomic/genetic and developmental variations in inotrope receptor distribution and function and underlying variability in host responses to varying clinical situations.

Overall, the evidence-base to guide the choice of inotrope in children is sparse, so extrapolations from adult medicine and direct physiological assessment predominate. In daily practice, a combination of experience, 'usual regimes' and local clinical practice guidelines—often derived from resuscitation courses or international guidelines provide identifiable standards for inotrope use. A few clinicians actively measure the direct effect of inotropes on the cardiovascular system using hemodynamic monitoring, though there is little consensus about the optimal technique.

This means that the use of inotropes is based on expert opinion, animal data and the use of surrogate endpoints, such as reversal of the shock state and oxygen delivery as a proxy for decreased morbidity and mortality.

This chapter provides a background to using inotropes in critically ill children and offers suggestions to help decision-making regarding their use.

20.2 What Are Inotropes?

Inotropy is the condition of contractility of the myocardium, and inotropes are substances that *increase* the force or energy of ventricular muscle contraction. Inotropes are often used in critically ill children to improve cardiac output (CO) and increase oxygen delivery (DO_2) to tissues.

No inotrope exerts its action solely by altering myocardial contraction; all have other effects—whether on systemic or pulmonary vascular resistance (SVR or PVR), heart rate or ventricular relaxation. Furthermore, the relative effects depend on blood concentration and often unresolved host variability issues, such as receptor distribution.

20.3 Some Terms

Inotropes: *increase* force or energy of ventricular muscle contraction (**Inotropy**—the condition of contractility of the myocardium).

Vasopressors: increase vascular tone and therefore increase *systemic vascular resistance* (SVR).

Vasodilators: reduce vascular tone and therefore reduce the (SVR).

Inodilators: have both inotropic and vasodilator effects.

Chronotropes: influence heart rate.

Lusitropes: improve ventricular diastolic relaxation.

The choice of 'which inotrope' ought to be determined by specific therapeutic goals, which should seldom be just the elevation of systemic blood pressure. Manipulating *haemodynamics* in acutely unwell children should be directed at optimising DO_2 to vital tissues to treat or prevent shock.

20.4 Cardiovascular System

Cardiovascular system failure is one of the most frequent organ system failures encountered in critically ill children.

It is associated with shock, the state in which DO_2 is insufficient to meet metabolic demand. This mismatch between tissue metabolic requirements and DO_2 stems from three main, often co-existing, mechanisms: increased metabolic demand, primary circulatory failure of DO_2 and other nutrients delivery to the tissues and an inability to utilise delivered oxygen at the cellular level. Although decreasing metabolic demand can be useful, medical treatments overwhelmingly address circulatory failure's second mechanism, optimising CO and global/regional perfusion.

There are a few basic hemodynamic terms that are useful to consider when addressing circulatory failure:

Cardiac output (CO) is the blood flow ejected by the heart in 1 min and divided by body surface area, gives **cardiac index (CI)**. It is the product of **stroke volume** (SV) and heart rate (HR), so: **CO = SV × HR**.

SV is directly related to pre-load (volume status, atrioventricular synchrony) and myocardial function, which depends on both ventricular systolic and diastolic function. It is inversely related to afterload (increased by outflow tract obstruction or increased SVR).

In children, decreased pre-load due to volume loss is a commonly encountered cause of shock, for example, due to diarrhoea and vomiting, sepsis or inadequate fluid intake. Because blood pressure is affected by SVR and CO (a version of Ohm's law), knowing BP in isolation cannot tell us CO without knowing SVR: **BP = CO × SVR**. Multiple neural, humoral and chemical factors regulate SV, HR and SVR. However, it is not uncommon for this regulation to fail, e.g. vasodilated septic shock and inotrope choice may be aided by understanding their likely action on the physiological derangement: drugs influencing heart rate are known as chronotropes, whilst lusitropy pertains to ventricular diastolic relaxation. Vasopressors raise the vascular tone, thereby increasing systemic vascular resistance, whereas vasodilators reduce it, and inodilators possess both inotropic and vasodilator effects.

▪ **Table 20.1** Types of shock

Type of shock	Examples	Physiology
Hypovolemic	Vomiting/diarrhoea Bleeding/trauma	Decreased CO Increased SVR
Cardiogenic	Myocarditis Cardiomyopathies Pulmonary oedema	Decreased CO Increased SVR Pump failure
Distributive	Anaphylaxis Sepsis	Decreased CO Decreased SVR
Obstructive	Tamponade Tension pneumothorax	Decreased CO Increased SVR
Neurogenic	Spinal trauma/surgeries	Decreased CO Decreased SVR

As all drugs have more than one effect, perhaps vasoactive drug is a better term than *inotrope* per se.

Although shock states are categorised according to the primary aetiological process (▪ Table 20.1), there is an overlap between the various mechanisms and frequent changes in children's predominant pathophysiological manifestation as shock evolves [1].

20.4.1 Recognition and Assessment of Shock

Recognition of shock is well covered in resuscitation courses (ALSG) [2]; however, it is essential to understand how cardiovascular system failure is quantified and assessed before discussing vasoactive drugs.

In children presenting with circulatory compromise, heart rate, blood pressure, capillary refill and core-peripheral temperature gradient can be readily assessed and repeated. As children with shock deteriorate, the effects of hemodynamic compromise on *end organs* can be assessed—such as decreased urine output and conscious level.

Adequate volume expansion is an essential primary step in the shocked child. However, the FEAST randomised trial of fluid without inotrope in children in a low resource (non-PICU) environment showed volume expansion to be harmful [3].

Whilst pre-load optimisation with volume resuscitation is still generally recommended in settings with intensive care provision, early concurrent inotrope therapy, as suggested in the last iteration of the international ACCM hemodynamic guidelines [4], and the less didactic more evidence based paediatric surviving sepsis guidelines [5], is also recommended. Further studies are urgently needed to clarify optimum fluid therapy in shock.

20.4.2 Targets

In paediatric shock, compromised DO_2 is often the primary problem rather than oxygen extraction, as in adults. Therefore, tissue perfusion seems a critical parameter to quantify in children in shock. However, to date, there is no 'tissue perfusion monitor' in widespread use. Near-infrared spectroscopy and microcirculation assessment devices are interesting, but it remains unclear how they can contribute to circulatory optimisation in children with severe shock.

BP is the most commonly measured hemodynamic parameter in PICU despite being an inaccurate measure of DO_2. In children, hypotension is a late event in the cascade of shock, unsurprising to those taught it is a pre-terminal sign in resuscitation courses. Whilst not strictly accurate—children in vasodilated shock can maintain relative hypotension for a time—this 'truism' underpins an essential biological fact: children have pristine systemic vasculature compared to adults and can readily compensate for changes in myocardial performance with either vasodilation or pronounced vasoconstriction. However, in reality, it is far from established whether vascular or myocardial derangements are the primary pathophysiological alteration in paediatric shock. In children, the concept of measuring hemodynamic parameters—such as CO—has not received widespread acceptance compared to adults, possibly due to the early risks of the initial measurement devices and expense and paucity of evidence. However, they remain recommended on consensus statements [6].

Whilst the International Paediatric Consensus definition for sepsis and organ dysfunction have defined cardiovascular system dysfunction as hypotension despite fluid resuscitation, the ALSG and the American Academy of Critical care Medicine focus on other parameters on targeting early resuscitation against decreased mental status, decreased urine output, capillary refill time (CRT) >2 s, cool mottled extremities and diminished pulses in 'cold' shock and brisk CRT and bounding pulses for 'warm' shock.

However, for post 60-min/PICU on-going care, optimisation of perfusion pressure in 'catecholamine-resistant shock' is advised. This is mean arterial pressure—central venous pressure, or the pressure drop across the circuit. Later, a CI between 3.3 and 6.0 L/min/m^2 is advised if the shock is not reversed.

Lactate, which accumulates during anaerobic metabolism, is one of the biomarkers used to assess global tissue metabolism, and lactate clearance is a widespread resuscitation target in shock. However, certain drugs such as adrenaline or specific inborn metabolic derangements and deranged local *waste removal* from tissues also influence lactate levels.

Central venous oxygen saturation ($CVC\text{-}O_2$) is another global measure of circulatory performance, with low levels suggesting increased tissue oxygen extraction due to poor circulation. The normalisation of $CVC\text{-}O_2$ has been used adult and paediatric shock as a target for shock therapy, with improved survival when this target was included in therapy goals; however, central venous saturation may be falsely high when the O_2ER is severely impaired, such as in mitochondrial disease.

Table 20.2 Distribution of adrenergic receptors and their action

Type of receptor	Typical location	Action
α1	Vascular smooth muscle, visceral smooth muscle, radial smooth muscle of iris and CNS neurons	Contraction of vessels, pupillary dilatation
α2	Some presynaptic terminals, pancreatic islets, ciliary smooth muscles, CNS neurons	Inhibits release of neurotransmitter
β1	Myocardium, JG cells, some presynaptic terminals and CNS neurons	Increased rate and force of contraction
β2	Visceral smooth muscle, liver, pancreas, uterus	Smooth muscle relaxation
β3	Adipose tissue and urinary bladder	Activation of lipolysis

20.4.3 How Do Inotropes Work

Inotropes primarily mediate their actions via stimulation of α1, β1, β2 adrenoceptors and dopaminergic receptors varyingly distributed throughout the tissues (Table 20.2).

The paediatric evidence base for the use of vasoactive agents is sparse, so there is a lack of data regarding developmental pharmacodynamics and the various adverse effects. Some adverse effects are secondary to an agent's hemodynamic profile, such as regional vasoconstriction leading to tissue ischaemia; others result from interactions with cellular energy metabolism and the inflammatory response mechanism.

20.4.3.1 Polymorphisms

With rapid advances in molecular biology, knowledge of polymorphisms within the genetic code has increased dramatically. Adrenergic receptors are expressed on virtually every cell type in the body and are the receptors for adrenaline and noradrenaline within the sympathetic nervous system. They serve critical roles in maintaining homeostasis in normal physiologic settings as well as pathologic states. These receptors are also targets for therapeutically administered agonists and antagonists. Recent studies have shown that at least seven adrenergic receptor subtypes display variation in amino acid sequence in the human population due to common genetic polymorphisms. Variations in potential regulatory domains in the noncoding sequence are also present. The consequences of these polymorphisms are linked in terms of signalling, human physiology and disease and response to therapy, e.g. enhanced ionotropic potency in response to noradrenaline and higher resting heart rate and diastolic blood pressure in patients with Arg 389 allele®.

20.4.3.2 Receptor Downregulation

Various mechanisms affecting the sensitivity of target cells to both endogenous and exogenous catecholamines can modify the overall system's activity in numerous sites. Some of these receptor modifications are clinically important to the critical care physician; the best documented involves agonist-mediated receptor desensitisation.

Exposure of receptors to agonists markedly reduces the sensitivity of the target cell to the agonist. These changes are mediated by changes in intracellular phosphorylation of various receptor kinases, i.e. protein kinase A/C (PKA/PKC) and G receptor kinases (GRKS). The role of GRKS has been established for β1, β2 and α2 receptors®. In addition to agonist-mediated desensitisation, other stimuli also have been implicated in downregulation, including endotoxin, tumour necrosis factor and congestive heart failure (CHF)®. Lymphocyte β adrenergic receptor density in children with CHF was reduced in proportion to the degree of elevation in plasma norepinephrine concentration®. Several pharmacological agents such as corticosteroids and ketotifen are thought to upregulate β adrenergic receptors, and evidence exists that both immaturity and senescence are associated with β adrenergic receptor desensitization®.

20.4.4 Physiologic Mechanisms of Vasoconstriction

α1—adrenoceptors stimulation on arterial vascular smooth muscle cells leads to smooth muscle contraction, and an increased SVR.

β1—adrenoceptor stimulation increases myocardial contractility via Ca^{2+}-mediated actin-myosin complex binding with troponin C and increases heart rate through Ca^{2+} channel activation.

β2—adrenoceptor stimulation causes vasodilation due to relaxation of vascular smooth muscle cells following increased Ca^{2+} uptake by the sarcoplasmic reticulum.

D1 and D2 dopaminergic receptor stimulation in the renal and splanchnic vascular beds results in respective vasodilation via activation of second-messenger systems.

V1—V1a stimulation in vascular smooth muscle causes vasoconstriction.

Calcium sensitisers—some agents increase the myocardial contractile apparatus's sensitivity to calcium, causing increased myofilament tension development and myocardial contractility (e.g., pimobendan and levosimendan). These agents have additional pharmacologic properties, such as phosphodiesterase inhibition, which may increase inotropy and vasodilation and contribute significantly to their clinical profile, the details of which are discussed separately.

Angiotensin—angiotensin receptors (AT_1 and AT_2) are G-coupled protein receptors with angiotensin II as their ligand. Angiotensin II is a vasoconstrictor that is part of the renin-aldosterone-angiotensin (RAAS) system. When receptors are stimulated, cytosolic calcium concentration increases to mediate vasoconstrictive effects as well as aldosterone and vasopressin secretion.

However, whilst genetic variations in adrenoceptor distribution are being explored in both hypertension and asthma, little is known about how this influences inotrope efficacy.

20.5 Endogenous Inotropes and Vasoactive Agents: Sympathomimetic Amines

Virtually all sympathomimetics currently used to treat hemodynamic problems are catecholamines. This class includes endogenous compounds such as adrenaline, noradrenaline and dopamine. Catecholamines include a β-phenylethylamine core with hydroxyl (OH) substitutes at the 3 and 4 aromatic ring positions. Tyrosine serves as the base compound for the synthesis of catecholamines. Tyrosine hydroxylase catalyses the conversion of tyrosine to Dopa, which undergoes decarboxylation, producing dopamine. Dopamine β hydroxylase converts dopamine to norepinephrine. In the adrenal medulla, norepinephrine is converted to epinephrine by *n*-methyl transferase.

Catecholamines are subject to several different elimination processes®. Infused dopamine is an example of elimination through a variety of processes. A small proportion is excreted unchanged in the urine, and a small proportion undergoes neuronal reuptake. The principal means of elimination appears to be *O*-methylation by catechol-*o*-methyl transferase (COMT) to form metanephrines, followed by either sulfoconjugation (by phenyl sulfotransferase) or by deamination by monoamine oxidase (MAO) to homovanillic acid®. The contribution of these pathways to total body clearance of catecholamines varies with age and the particular circulatory bed.

20.5.1 Adrenaline

Adrenaline is an endogenous catecholamine secreted by the adrenal gland, which is an agonist to all adrenoceptors. It causes a wide array of cardiovascular, metabolic, endocrine and immunological effects. In the cardiovascular system, low-dose adrenaline infusion (0.05–0.1 mcg/kg/min) mainly affects cardiac β1 receptors, resulting in increased contractility, heart rate and coronary blood flow and a theoretically detrimental increase in myocardial oxygen requirement. At these doses, there is also β2 receptor-activated vasodilatation that decreases both SVR and PVR, contributing to improved CO. Between 0.1 and 1 mcg/kg/min, α receptor-mediated constriction is counterbalanced by β2-receptor-mediated vasodilatation, but at greater doses, vasoconstriction predominates potentially compromising organ perfusion, for example in severe septic shock adrenaline decreases splanchnic blood flow in comparison with NA.

Adrenaline has considerable non-hemodynamic effects: hyperglycaemia is induced by inhibition of insulin release, stimulation of glucagon release and hepatic glycogenolysis and gluconeogenesis; lipolysis raises plasma free fatty acid levels, and β2 receptor activation mediates increased lactate secondary to increased oxygen consumption. In the immune system, β2 receptor stimulation induces leucocytosis from the marginal pool, though adrenaline is also associated with late-phase immunosuppression. Adrenaline has also been shown to be pro-thrombotic, inducing the release of factor 8 and von Willebrand factor and promoting platelet aggregation.

- Whereas low-dose adrenaline can be safely administered through a peripheral intravenous line, central or even intraosseous access is recommended for high-dose adrenaline because of the risk of extravasation and tissue necrosis due to local vasoconstriction. The overall recommended dose ranges between 0.05 and 2 mcg/kg/min.

20.5.2 Noradrenaline

Noradrenaline is a potent α1 and β1 agonist with minimal effects on β2 receptors, so the main cardiovascular effect is vasoconstriction, leading to increased SVR and blood pressure. The expected cardiac β1 adrenoceptors mediated chronotropic effect is blunted by increased blood pressure-induced vagal responses so that although SV increases, CO is relatively unchanged. Although coronary blood flow is increased owing to β1-mediated vasodilatation and increased BP, splanchnic, cutaneous, pulmonary and renal blood flow decreases with increasing concentration of NA. Cerebral blood flow is preserved as the distribution of adrenoceptors in the CNS vasculature is minimal.

Whilst noradrenaline has fewer non-hemodynamic effects than adrenaline, causing only a modest rise in serum glucose and no lactate increase, it does increase bacterial iron uptake and, hence, growth rate. A recent prospective study of adults with septic shock demonstrated noradrenaline to be inversely associated with IL-8 and TNF-α levels, and hence less pro-inflammatory than adrenaline.

Noradrenaline should usually be administered through central venous access due to possible extreme vasoconstriction. The infusion rate is 0.05–2 mcg/kg/min.

20.5.3 Vasopressin

Vasopressin is a hormone released from the posterior pituitary gland in response to stimuli from chemical, osmotic and baroreceptors and exerts its effect on V1 and the higher affinity V2 receptors. In the normovolaemic state, circulating vasopressin has little effect on vascular tone but maintains BP during hypovolaemia. The hemodynamic effects of vasopressin are mediated through V1 receptors, causing significant vasoconstriction and an increase in SVR. The resulting decrease in splanchnic blood flow is so substantial that vasopressin is used to treat GI bleeding. Through the stimulation of V2 receptors, vasopressin triggers water absorption in the kidneys, and procoagulant factors release from the endothelium. Increased vasopressin levels have been found in haemorrhagic shock, but this compensatory response is blunted in septic shock.

Vasopressin should be administered through central venous access in a dose ranging from 0.01 to 0.12 units/kg/h.

20.5.4 Dopamine

Dopamine is rarely used and features here for completeness. A precursor of noradrenaline and adrenaline, it acts as a neurotransmitter in the nervous system and as a humeral factor when secreted from the adrenal gland. It agonises both dopaminergic and adrenergic receptors, although the latter requires higher plasma concentration due to lower affinity.

Dopaminergic receptors in the kidneys, mesenteric vasculature and coronary arteries are activated by infusion rates up to 5 mcg/kg/min, leading to vasodilatation with improved coronary, renal and splanchnic blood flow and increased CO. A direct effect on renal tubules leading to diuresis and natriuresis has been argued but is now largely dismissed.

At infusion rates 5–10 mcg/kg/min β-adrenoceptor-mediated inotropy and chronotropy lead to improved CO and higher systolic BP.

With infusions exceeding 10 mcg/kg/min (maximum 20 mcg/kg/min), α adrenoceptor-induced vasoconstriction prevails, which can increase SVR to the extent that CO and regional blood are compromised. Furthermore, increased arrhythmia has been reported during dopamine use in septic shock.

Extra-hemodynamic effects are problematic and include suppression of growth hormone, thyroid-stimulating hormone and prolactin release in addition to lymphocytic apoptosis, immunosuppression and an overall pro-inflammatory cytokine profile. Due to this dopamine use has decreased though is occasionally still, used in neonates. A diluted solution can be safely given peripherally before central access is secured.

Table 20.3 Inotropes—mechanisms and dosed in shock

Inotrope	Mechanism	Effects	Clinical usage	Dosing range
Dopamine	DA at lower dosing range β1 and 2 at increasing doses α at the higher end of dosing	Increased cardiac output; vasoconstriction at higher doses	**Septic shock** (low cardiac output shock)	**5–20 μg/kg/min**
Epinephrine	β1 and 2 at increasing doses α at the higher end of dosing	Increased cardiac output; vasoconstriction at higher doses	**Moderate to severe septic shock** (low cardiac output shock)	**0.05–5 μg/kg/min** (doses greater than 1 μg/kg/min indicate extremely severe dysfunction)
Norepinephrine	Predominance of α, even at lower doses β1 and 2 at increasing doses	Increased vasoconstriction and some increased cardiac output	**Moderate to severe "warm" septic shock** (high cardiac output with vasodilation)	**0.05–5 μg/kg/min** (doses greater than 1 μg/kg/min indicate extremely severe dysfunction)
Dobutamine	β1 and 2 at increasing doses	Increased cardiac output	**Septic shock** (low cardiac output shock) ***or* myocarditis/cardiomyopathy** (often with dopamine)	**2.5–20 μg/kg/min**
Milrinone	Increases cAMP via inhibition of phosphodiesterase, modulating intracellular Ca^{2+}	Increased diastolic relaxation, increased cardiac output and vasodilation	**Myocarditis/ cardiomyopathy** (often with dopamine)	**2.5–1.0 μg/kg/min**
Vasopressin	Increases levels of IP_3 and DAG, which in turn increase intracellular Ca^{2+}	Increased peripheral vasoconstriction	**Moderate to severe "warm" septic shock** (high cardiac output with vasodilation)	**0.04–0.1 U/min** (adult) or **0.0005–0.001 U/kg/min**

20.6 Exogenous Inotropes and Vasoactive Agents

20.6.1 Dobutamine

Dobutamine is a synthetic catecholamine binding β1 and β2 receptors in a 3:1 ratio, with some α receptor agonism. It is available as a compound of two isomers: the (+) isomer is a potent β1 agonist and α1 antagonist, and the (−) isomer is a weak β1 antagonist and a potent α1 agonist. Due to the opposing α effects, inotropy predominates, but with increased myocardial oxygen demand and marked chronotropy, which can limit ventricular filling time and therefore use in septic shock. The main indication is short-term cardiac support in cardiogenic and septic shock with infusion rates of 5–20 mcg/kg/min, which may be given dilute via a peripheral vein.

20.6.2 Phenylephrine

Phenylephrine is an extremely potent selective α1 agonist, leading to vasoconstriction with increased SVR and BP but occasional reflex bradycardia and significantly reduced splanchnic blood flow. It is used to restore vascular tone in spinal/neurogenic shock and can be given as an intravenous bolus, most frequently to mitigate short term pharmacologically-induced vasodilation, or by continuous infusion titrated to response.

20.6.3 Phosphodiesterase Inhibitors

Milrinone, a potent, selective inhibitor of phosphodiesterase III, causes an increase in cAMP and PKA levels in a non-receptor-dependent fashion. It is an inodilator causing inotropy, lusitropy and, to a lesser extent, chronotropy, along with vasodilatation of the pulmonary and systemic vasculature. As a result of the decrease in the afterload to both ventricles, there is no significant increase in cardiac oxygen demand despite increased contractility and heart rate. The use of milrinone is widespread in cardiac intensive care to treat heart failure and post-cardiac surgery. It is also used to treat pulmonary hypertension and as an adjunctive medication in cardiogenic shock to support the failing heart e.g., 'cold' shock with reasonable blood pressure. Adverse effects include hypotension, arrhythmia, thrombocytopenia (rare) and impaired liver enzymes.

Milrinone is administered in a continuous infusion ranging from 0.25 to 1 mcg/kg/min. Due to the long half-life, a loading dose (20–50 mcg/kg) may be given, depending on blood pressure. Milrinone may be administered through peripheral venous access but due to renal excretion must be used with caution in renal impairment.

Enoximone is a PDE III inhibitor with greater affinity to β1 cAMP hydrolysis inhibition, consequently exerting its inotropic effect mainly in the myocardium with minimal vasodilatation.

20.6.4 Levosimendan

Levosimendan binds to troponin c and acts as a myofilament calcium sensitiser and opens ATP-dependent potassium channels. It is inotropic and also vasodilates both coronary and peripheral vessels. Levosimendan has minimal effects on myocardial oxygen consumption and does not interfere with diastolic relaxation. There is a hemodynamic benefit in adults in cardiogenic shock after myocardial infarction, but no survival benefit in either cardiogenic shock or acute heart failure. In adult septic shock, Levosimendan improves ejection fraction, SV, CI, urine output and gastric mucosal perfusion compared with dobutamine improving both right ventricular performance and mixed venous oxygen saturation.

In children, levosimendan is as effective as milrinone after congenital cardiac surgery.

A loading dose of 6–12 μg/kg over 10 min is followed by an infusion of 0.05–0.2 μg/kg/min, with a hemodynamic effect within 5 min.

20.7 Selection of Inotropic and Vasoactive Agents in Shock

Three fundamental concepts guide the rational use of vasopressors and inotropes:

- One drug, many receptors—A given drug often has multiple effects due to actions upon more than one receptor. For example, dobutamine increases cardiac output by beta-1 adrenergic receptor activation, but also acts upon beta-2 adrenergic receptors inducing vasodilation and possibly hypotension.
- Dose-response curve—Many agents have dose-response curves, such that the primary adrenergic receptor subtype activated by the drug is dose-dependent. For example, dopamine stimulates beta-1 adrenergic receptors at doses of 2–10 mcg/kg/min and alpha-adrenergic receptors when in excess of 10 mcg/kg/min.
- Direct versus reflex actions—A given agent can affect mean arterial pressure (MAP) both by immediate actions on adrenergic receptors and by reflex actions triggered by the pharmacologic response. Norepinephrine-induced beta-1 adrenergic stimulation alone would usually cause tachycardia, however the elevated MAP from norepinephrine's alpha-adrenergic receptor-induced vasoconstriction causes a reflex decrease in heart rate. The net result may be a stable or slightly reduced heart rate.

Traditionally, in paediatric septic shock, the first and most crucial step is timely adequate volume resuscitation, with repeated boluses of 20 mL/kg of isotonic fluids given until clinical parameters such as peripheral perfusion and heart rate improve. The FEAST study demonstrated increased mortality in a developing world population with lone administration of fluids in septic shock, arguably confirming the ACCM suggestion of early inotropes during fluid resuscitation.

In definite cardiogenic shock, judicious fluid management is needed due to the risk of causing pulmonary oedema with severe left ventricular dysfunction. This approach, mindful of the Starling curve of the LV, may offer optimal shock, though the skill to quantify SV at the bedside is not widespread.

Acidosis, frequently encountered in shock states, decreases adrenoceptor responsiveness, hence correction of acidosis should be considered.

Given the therapeutic properties and adverse events of the various vasoactive and inotropic agents, the dynamic nature of shock and the differences between adult and paediatric shock states, it is sensible to tailor the hemodynamic support to the individual child, until a better evidence base emerges.

20.7.1 Septic Shock

Previous shock definition have evolved but arguably the state is characterised by circulatory organ system failure in the presence of systemic inflammatory response syndrome, immune dysregulation, microcirculatory derangements and end-organ dysfunction. The major pathophysiological abnormalities are vasoconstriction or dilation, inflammation, and increased microvascular permeability, leading to leukocyte accumulation in tissues remote to the infective source. All these derangements affect the pharmacokinetics and pharmacodynamics of vasoactive drugs. The metabolism and clearance of drugs may be altered due to redistribution of flow, resulting in splanchnic hypoperfusion in addition to the altered cellular metabolism secondary to the 'cytokine storm'. The volume of distribution of any infused drug is also affected by increased capillary permeability. Sustained activation of adrenoceptors in sepsis can result in downregulation and desensitisation of both α and β receptors reduced generation of new adrenoceptors, all worsened by any endotoxins that downregulate adenylate cyclase. As a result, any recommended vasoactive dose should be regarded as a starting point, with titration to individual response necessary.

Furthermore, the manifestation of shock in children evolves over time, with the hemodynamic pattern changing over time, necessitating frequent re-assessment and change of vasoactive agents [1]. Children often present in "cold" shock with decreased CO and often increased SVR, rather than in the adult pattern of high-output vasodilatation.

Low-dose adrenaline and nor-adrenaline can be safely administered via peripheral cannula and therefore are the first-line vasoactive agents recommended to reverse shock. If shock persists, the addition of another agent is recommended.

If the shock then continues (catecholamine-resistant shock), steroids should be administered if steroid deficiency is suspected. Adding a third agent should be considered according to the evolution of the shock. In normotensive "cold" shock with low CO, the circulation may improve by administering an inodilator such as milrinone or a direct vasodilator to decrease SVR. Hypotensive "cold" shock may benefit from titrating adrenaline, dobutamine and noradrenaline. Noradrenaline may be used early in hypotensive "warm" shock to increase SVR or as a countermeasure to milrinone-induced hypotension. In most adults with septic shock and some children, the hemodynamic presentation is "warm shock" with low SVR, hypotension and increased CO. Noradrenaline is the recommended first-line agent in adults in fluid refractory vasodilated shock, and use is increasing in paediatrics.

In refractory vasodilatory paediatric shock, vasopressin administration improves the hemodynamic state, although urine output and creatinine can be reversibly compromised, and thrombocytopenia can occur.

In shock states, refractory to catecholamines and vasopressors, enoximone and levosimendan may be added.

20.7.2 Cardiogenic Shock

Excluding cardiac surgery patients, cardiogenic shock in the PICU is most frequently due to severe sepsis, myocarditis, dilated cardiomyopathy (DCMP) or arrhythmia. Arrhythmia should be treated with rate and rhythm control measures, not least because inotropes can be detrimental. In myocarditis/DCMP, inotropes and vasodilators are the primary agents used, though increased myocardial oxygen consumption can be a problem. For cardiac tamponade, whilst aggressive fluid therapy to restore right ventricular filling pressure is useful, evacuation of pericardial fluid is the mainstay of treatment.

In a low CO state with reasonable low dose AD has a positive inotropic effect while causing vasodilation, though low diastolic pressure can impair coronary perfusion. Milrinone can improve diastolic function and provide positive inotropy whilst reducing SVR and PVR without increased myocardial oxygen demand.

In hypotensive cardiac shock, titration AD, or even judicious NA can achieve positive inotropy and vasoconstrictor support whilst adequate pre-load is restored.

20.7.3 Neurogenic Shock

Neurogenic/spinal shock results in profound hypotension secondary to sympathetic denervation of the vasculature and heart. There is extreme vasodilatation, with some decreased inotropy and chronotropy. Initial fluid resuscitation to ensure adequate circulatory volume is recommended before inotrope use, with NA recommended due to strong α mediated vasoconstriction and some inotropy and chronotropy. In contrast, AD or Dopamine, even at high doses, do not adequately reverse peripheral vascular failure. Alternatively, a combination of an inotrope with a potent vasoconstrictor such as Phenylephrine can be used.

20.8 Failure of Shock Reversal

If shock cannot be reversed, mechanical support/ECMO may be indicated, depending on the likelihood of eventual reversal of the pathophysiology.

20.9 Conclusion

Selecting the appropriate vasoactive agent in any shock state is influenced by many variables. The dynamic evolution of shock and its effects on the pharmacodynamics and pharmacokinetics of the different agents, the vast array of non-hemodynamic effects exerted by various agents, and the lack of evidence from paediatric randomised control trials all contribute to the complexity of shock treatment. The key message is to start with a reasonable agent, given the manifestation of shock at presentation and then frequently reassess and alter the hemodynamic support.

There is little direct high grade evidence to guide the management of shock in children, and this I arguably weaker regarding inotrope use.

Take-Home Messages

- Inotropes and vasoactive agents are potent drugs that increase myocardial contractility and have pronounced vasoactive effects, impacting cardiovascular physiology in health and sickness.
- These drugs work at different doses on different receptors, variably distributed in the body, to cause variable hemodynamic responses. In general, stimulation of alpha-1 adrenergic receptors induces vasoconstriction beta-1 receptors inotropy and chronotropy and beta-2 receptors vasodilation.
- Alternative mechanisms include increasing the myocardial contractile apparatus's sensitivity to calcium and direct vasoconstriction via angiotensin II receptor stimulation.
- Genetic polymorphism receptor types exist together with variable downregulation mechanisms and tachyphylaxis, which plays an unclear role in the dose-response relationship in different age groups and ethnic populations.
- Choice of an initial agent should ideally be based upon the suspected underlying aetiology and the underlying pathophysiologic mechanism of shock, though generic guidance exists.
- Clinical acumen should guide the desired inotropic and vasoactive effects required, with frequent re-assessment as the shock morphology in children can change.

References

1. Deep A, Goonasekera CD, Wang Y, Brierley J. Evolution of haemodynamics and outcome of fluid-refractory septic shock in children. Intensive Care Med. 2013;39(9):1602–9. https://doi.org/10.1007/s00134-013-3003-z.
2. APLS. https://www.alsg.org/en/files/PFactsheet.pdf.
3. Maitland K, Kiguli S, Opoka RO, Engoru C, Olupot-Olupot P, Akech SO, Nyeko R, Mtove G, Reyburn H, Lang T, Brent B, Evans JA, Tibenderana JK, Crawley J, Russell EC, Levin M, Babiker AG, Gibb DM, FEAST Trial Group. Mortality after fluid bolus in African children with severe infection. N Engl J Med. 2011;364(26):2483–95.
4. Davis AL, Carcillo JA, Aneja RK, Deymann AJ, Lin JC, Nguyen TC, Okhuysen-Cawley RS, Relvas MS, Rozenfeld RA, Skippen PW, Stojadinovic BJ, Williams EA, Yeh TS, Balamuth F, Brierley J, de Caen AR, Cheifetz IM, Choong K, Conway E Jr, Cornell T, Doctor A, Dugas MA, Feldman JD, Fitzgerald JC, Flori HR, Fortenberry JD, Graciano AL, Greenwald BM, Hall MW, Han YY, Hernan LJ, Irazuzta JE, Iselin E, van der Jagt EW, Jeffries HE, Kache S, Katyal C, Kissoon N, Kon AA, Kutko MC, MacLaren G, Maul T, Mehta R, Odetola F, Parbuoni K, Paul R, Peters MJ, Ranjit S, Reuter-Rice KE, Schnitzler EJ, Scott HF, Torres A Jr, Weingarten-Abrams J, Weiss SL, Zimmerman JJ, Zuckerberg AL. The American College of Critical Care Medicine clinical practice parameters for hemodynamic support of pediatric and neonatal septic shock: executive summary. Pediatr Crit Care Med. 2017;18(9):884–90.
5. Weiss SL, Peters MJ, Alhazzani W, Agus MSD, Flori HR, Inwald DP, Nadel S, Schlapbach LJ, Tasker RC, Argent AC, Brierley J, Carcillo J, Carrol ED, Carroll CL, Cheifetz IM, Choong K, Cies

JJ, Cruz AT, De Luca D, Deep A, Faust SN, De Oliveira CF, Hall MW, Ishimine P, Javouhey E, Joosten KFM, Joshi P, Karam O, Kneyber MCJ, Lemson J, MacLaren G, Mehta NM, Møller MH, Newth CJL, Nguyen TC, Nishisaki A, Nunnally ME, Parker MM, Paul RM, Randolph AG, Ranjit S, Romer LH, Scott HF, Tume LN, Verger JT, Williams EA, Wolf J, Wong HR, Zimmerman JJ, Kissoon N, Tissieres P. Surviving sepsis campaign international guidelines for the management of septic shock and sepsis-associated organ dysfunction in children. Pediatr Crit Care Med. 2020;21(2):e52–106.

6. Singh Y, Villaescusa JU, da Cruz EM, Tibby SM, Bottari G, Saxena R, Guillén M, Herce JL, Di Nardo M, Cecchetti C, Brierley J, de Boode W, Lemson J. Recommendations for hemodynamic monitoring for critically ill children-expert consensus statement issued by the cardiovascular dynamics section of the European Society of Paediatric and Neonatal Intensive Care (ESPNIC). Crit Care. 2020;24(1):620.

Specific Organ System Failure

Contents

The Lung

Peter Rimensberger

Contents

J. Brierley et al. (eds.), *ESPNIC Children's Intensive Care Textbook*,
https://doi.org/10.1007/978-3-031-64762-8_21

Learning Objectives

- Understand the PICU-physician/nurse-relevant characteristics in respiratory physiology and mechanics in the neonate and the growing child.
- Understand principals of pulmonary gas exchange in healthy and sick children.
- Understand basic concepts of cardiopulmonary interactions.
- Some specific lung pathologies.

21.1 Introduction

Most frequent pathology seen in a general paediatric ICU is respiratory failure of various aetiology and severity. Respiratory support is often needed, requiring a good knowledge of relevant specificities of respiratory physiology and mechanics in the neonate and growing child. To optimise respiratory support to the patient's individual condition, respiratory monitoring can be helpful and should be thoughtfully used at bedside to anticipate changes in patient's condition. This chapter reviews and discusses the lung as a functional unit with focus on physiology, pathophysiology and respiratory system mechanics, knowledge that should allow the PICU physician/nurse to optimise respiratory care and support, independent of an individual's specific diagnosis/disease that was leading to respiratory insufficiency.

21.2 Basics of Respiratory Physiology and Mechanics in the Neonate and the Growing Child

During lung development, the lung reaches a functional stage, allowing for a vital gas exchange from the saccular stage (at around 24 weeks of gestation) when the air-blood interphase is sufficiently developed with terminal airways as primitive saccules, differentiation of the epithelium into pneumocytes and capillary layers developed sufficiently to share the basement membrane as air-blood interface, resulting in functional lung units [1]. At about the same time (i.e. around 22–24 weeks of gestation), intracellular surfactant synthesis begins and surfactant can be secreted. Yet normal lung function requires further alveolarisation (i.e. alveologensis) to maximise the surface area of the air-blood barrier at minimal thinness for development of an air-blood barrier of maximal surface area, which is achieved around 36 weeks; however, growth and maturation of alveoli and the intra- and extrapulmonary vessels continues postnatally and cease only years after birth [2, 3]. Another major step towards a functional lung occurs during transitional circulation [4].

Any disturbances during intrauterine (e.g. infections, exposure to toxic substances including maternal medications, delayed alveorisation and/or angiogensis) or early postnatal lung development (e.g. infection, extreme prematurity, surfactant deficiency, injurious mechanical ventilation, delayed alveorisation and/or angiogensis), or in the transition of circulation after birth (e.g. asphyxia, sepsis, intrauterine closure or persistent patency postnatally of the ductus arteriosus) can lead to various pathologies in the newborn and infant (e.g. persistent pulmonary hypertension, bronchopulmonary dysplasia (BPD), lung hypoplasia syndromes, alveolar-capillary dysplasia and others).

For pulmonary ventilation, a functional neuromechanical unit for the operation of the respiratory system requires a generator (brain steam), an output (neural conductance and neuro-muscular innervation), and a feedback control (via carbon dioxide and oxygen chemoreceptors, response to changes in pH, and mechanoreceptors, i.e. chest wall proprio-receptors and pulmonary stretch receptors) [5]. Although normal respiration is driven mostly by the levels of carbon dioxide, the respiratory drive will begin to rely more on the oxygen receptors (hypoxic drive) in the presence of important chronic hypercarbia [6] (e.g. in patients with chronic hypercarbic lung disease, like in some severe BPD cases). In such chronic condition (excessive), oxygen administration can reduce the respiratory drive.

Activation of the respiratory muscles (diaphragm and intercostal muscles) will lead to a muscle contraction (muscle force), which is proportional to the neuronal input; however, this force depends mainly on the efficiency of neuromuscular coupling, the muscle mass and the functionality of the muscle fibres. With normal muscle fibres the muscle mass (i.e. cross-sectional area) is proportionally related to the muscle force that can be generated. Although the muscle mass is small in neonates and infants, the pleural pressure generated is not less than in older children and adults, given the smaller surface on which the force has to be applied [7, 8]. Furthermore, the neonate can compensate for the weaker diaphragmatic muscle when compared to the adult, by the smaller diameter of the diaphragm, since the resulting force (i.e. the trans-diaphragmatic pressure (P_{di})) depends on the radius of curvature of the diaphragm, which is according to the law of Young-Laplace inversely related to the force generated ($P_{di} - T/r$). With that, it is not really true that neonate and infants have less efficient respiratory muscles than adults.

The major difference between infants and adults is, however, given by the chest wall distortion, i.e. newborns, infants and young children have a softer chest wall (i.e. higher compliance/lower elastance) in view of incomplete ribcage ossification than in older children or adults. As a consequence, the outward recoil of the chest wall is low, while the inward lung recoil is similar to that of an adult. The resting volume (V_r), i.e. the lung volume at the end of passive expiration (respiratory system under zero pressure condition), point at which the outward recoil of the chest wall balances that of the inward recoil of the lungs, corresponds in older children and in adults to functional residual capacity (FRC). Yet in neonates, infants and young children (up to the age of 6–8 years) the V_r is, because of the relatively high chest wall compliance, much lower, i.e. below FRC. This will prone them to airway collapse (with a closing volume above residual volume), which is overcome by keeping end-expiratory volume dynamically elevated by

1. "Laryngeal control" with dynamic partial glottis closure (laryngeal breaking) during expiration.
2. Fast breathing rates (keeping the volume at end-expiration high).
3. Active diaphragmatic and intercostal expiratory tone.

Allowing to keep FRC above closing volume to avoid collapse and consequently hypoxemia. In the presence of surfactant deficiency, this becomes more difficult to achieve because of the decreased surface tension of alveoli and small airways, lead-

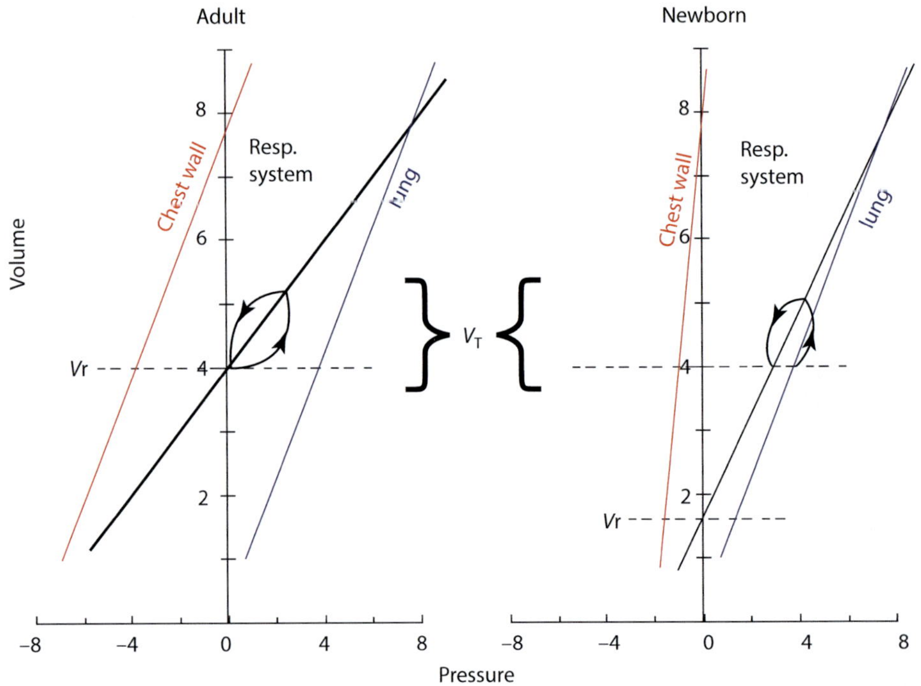

Fig. 21.1 Schematic pressure-volume (*P*–*V*) relations of the lungs, chest wall, and respiratory system (*heavy line*) in adult (*left*) and newborn (*right*). For simplicity, the *P*–*V* relations are indicated by *straight lines*, the slope of which represents the compliance. On left, the compliance of the chest wall (C_w) is similar to that of the lungs (C_L). At right, the C_w–C_L ratio is about five times higher. The result is that in the newborn the resting volume of the respiratory system (V_r, *dashed line*) is lower than in adults. Tidal volume (V_T, with inspiratory-expiratory loops indicated by *arrows*) is approximately at the same absolute lung volume in both newborns and adults because newborns keep their end-expiratory level dynamically elevated. (With permission from Mortola [5])

ing to low lung compliance and increased tendency to small airway and alveolar collapse. Similarly, with sedation, during anaesthesia, and especially with an endotracheal tube in place, it will be more difficult for the newborn to maintain his FRC sufficiently elevated by the above-mentioned mechanisms (Fig. 21.1).

Given the smaller size of airways of newborns, infants and small children airway resistance to overcome is higher when compared to adults. This may become rapidly a problem with a reduction in airway radius ($R = \eta L/r^4$; according to transformation and simplification of the law of Hagen-Poiseuille, where airway resistance (R) becomes directly proportional to the length (L) and the viscosity (η) of the air–gas mixture, and inversely proportional to the radius to the fourth power (r^4)) in any inflammatory airway disease leading to mucosal swelling at various levels of the upper and/or lower airways, obstructive airway disease of various aetiology including malformations, or extrinsic airway compression (e.g. double arc aortic).

Higher minute ventilation (MV = V_t × RR) demands (normal MV for term infants is around 200–300 mL/kg/min, two to three times that of adults) because of

Table 21.1 Lung mechanics and respiratory variables of the neonate compared with the adult

Variable	Neonate	Adult
Compliance ($mL/cmH_2O/kg$)	1.2–1.5 (premature infants: up to 2.0)	0.6–0.8 (typical practical number used in adult ICUs: 50 mL/cmH_2O)
Resistance ($cm/H_2O/L/s$)	Up to 30	2
Tidal volume	6–8 mL/kg	6–8 mL/kg
Respiratory rate (breaths/min)	30–40	12–15
Minute ventilation[a] ($V_t \times RR$)	200–300 mL/kg/min	80–120 mL/kg/min
Alveolar minute ventilation $(V_t - V_D) \times RR$	140–200 mL/kg/min	50–80 mL/kg/min
Physiologic dead space	2.0–2.5 mL/kg (approx. 30% of V_t)[b]	2.0–2.5 mL/kg (approx. 30% of V_t)
FRC	30 mL/kg (while keeping end-expiratory volume dynamically elevated)	1800–2200 mL (approx. 30 mL/kg)
Closing volume	Above V_r	Below V_r

V_r residual volume

[a] Minute volume comprises the sum of alveolar ventilation and dead space ventilation. $V = V_A + V_D$, where V_A is alveolar ventilation, and V_D represents dead-space ventilation

[b] Any increase caused by apparatus dead space has a proportionally greater effect on small children than on adults

a higher metabolic rate in newborns, infants and children explain their higher breathing rates compared to adolescents and adults, given that physiologic tidal volumes (V_t) are in the range of about 6–8 mL/kg for all ages (Table 21.1).

21.3 Gas Exchange and Its Measures

Arterial blood gas measurements (PO_2, SaO_2 and PCO_2) and/or transcutaneous measures (mainly for SO_2 and $P_{tc}CO_2$), are the main measures to assess the degree of pulmonary gas exchange abnormality. The O_2 carrier in the blood, i.e. the red blood cell, exhibits various affinities to O_2-molecules, depending on the type of haemoglobin (e.g. HbF, HbA or other pathologic Hb), pH, temperature and 2,3-diphosphoglycerate (2,3-DPG) levels in the blood, shifting the position of the sigmoid shaped oxyhaemoglobin dissociation curve (Fig. 21.2).

The fact, that dissolved oxygen comprises a very small (insignificant) portion of the total arterial oxygen content, renders the utility of measuring PaO_2 as an isolated value in the clinical setting questionable. However, measuring SaO_2 and PaO_2 simultaneously allows to know on which part of the curve the patient is and will be helpful

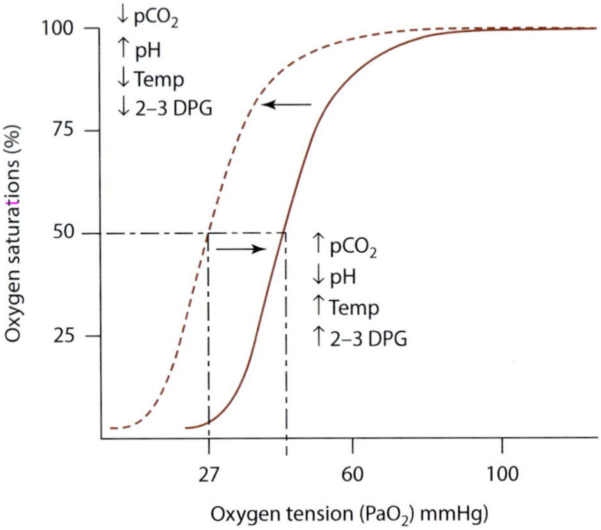

Fig. 21.2 Oxygen dissociation curve. (With permission from Turner and Cheifetz [9])

to predict the response on small changes in PaO_2 on SO_2. However, with high values of SaO_2 above 92% (on the flat portion of the dissociation curve), a small change in SaO_2 might be associated with a large change in PaO_2, which might underestimate the risk of toxic O_2 levels. To keep in mind that transcutaneous SO_2 measures or measures with blood gas analysers that calculate SO_2 according an assumed dissociation curve may overestimate real oxygen saturations, as measured by a direct method (i.e. co-oxymetry), for example, in the presence of methaemoglobin or carboxyhaemoglobin (CO-intoxication), are relatively unreliable.

For CO_2 measures, various methods exist ($PaCO_2$ by blood gas analysers, transcutaneous $P_{tc}CO_2$, capnometry measuring end-tidal CO_2 ($P_{et}CO_2$) giving the peak value of expired CO_2 at end-expiration, and volumetric capnography giving an information on effective CO_2 elimination per minute ($V_{min}CO_2$)). Despite some limited information that can be drawn from $P_{et}CO_2$, without repeated calculations of dead space requiring regular arterial blood gas samples, it is recommended and almost universally monitored in critically ill children on mechanical ventilatory support in the PICU [10]. It allows primarily to continuously monitor respiratory rate and rhythm, confirm proper tracheal tube placement and position, and monitor patient-ventilator asynchrony [11, 12]. Yet, changes of $P_{et}CO_2$, either slow or rapid, should prompt a search for potential causes (Table 21.2).

$$\text{Physiological dead space}: V_D / V_T = \left(PaCO_2 - P_{et}CO_2\right) / PaCO_2$$
$$= 1 - \left(PaCO_2 - P_{et}CO_2\right)$$

Pulmonary gas exchange involves (1) alveolar ventilation, (2) diffusion and (3) perfusion. In order to simplify at bedside, we can reason mainly in terms of intrapulmonary shunt fraction and dead-space ventilation. Intrapulmonary shunt is primarily reflected by hypoxaemia and can be rapidly estimated (Fig. 21.3). The percent of shunt can be calculated with the following equation:

$$Q_s / Q_t = \frac{C_{CO2} - C_{aO2}}{C_{CO2} - C_{VO2}}$$

or estimated from the ISO shunt diagram that is based on the relationship between FiO_2 and PaO_2 (◘ Fig. 21.3).

◘ **Table 21.2** Conditions associated with changes in $P_{et}CO_2$

	Increase in $P_{et}CO_2$	Decrease in $P_{et}CO_2$	Absent $P_{et}CO_2$
Rapid change	• Increase in cardiac output (e.g. seizure)	• Decreased cardiac output (e.g. cardiac arrest) • Pulmonary embolus • Air embolus • Tracheal tube obstruction • Large tracheal tube leak	• Oesophageal intubation • Inadvertent extubation • Ventilator disconnection
Slow change	• Inadequate minute ventilation • Increased CO_2 production (e.g. fever) • Equipment malfunction • CO_2-rebreathing (e.g. in presence of Auto-PEEP)	• Increased minute ventilation • Decreased CO_2 production (e.g. sedation, paralysis, hypothermia) • Increased dead-space ventilation • Auto-triggering	

Adapted with permission from: Wheeler DS, Rimensberger P. Respiratory Monitoring. In: Derek S. Wheeler, Hector R. Wong, Thomas P. Shanley (eds), Pediatric Critical Care Medicine: Basic Science and Clinical Evidence, 2nd edition/Volume 1: Care of the Critically Ill or Injured Child. Springer-Verlag, London. pp. 521–542. ▸ https://doi.org/10.1007/978-1-4471-6362-6_39

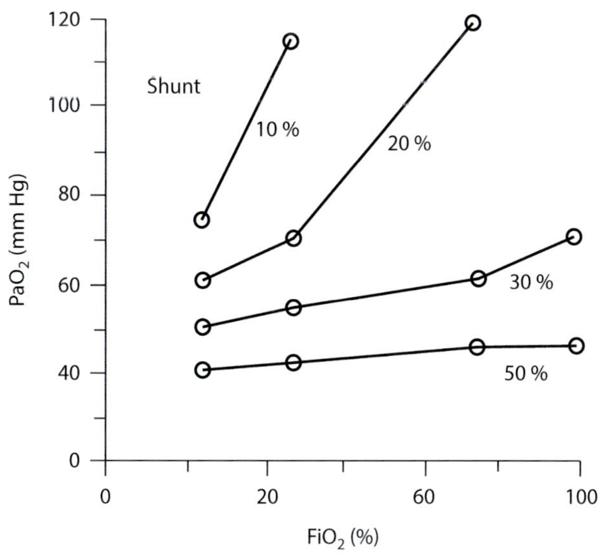

◘ **Fig. 21.3** Response to increasing FiO_2 with variation in intrapulmonary shunt fraction. (With permission from Turner and Cheifetz [9])

However, reasons for hypoxaemia are manifold including inspiratory hypoxia, hypoventilation, ventilation/perfusion inequality, diffusion limitation, shunting and reduced mixed venous oxygenation. The latter reflects the body's ability to compensate for insufficient O_2 transport of various origins by greater O_2 extraction. Other mechanisms to compensate for gas exchange disturbances are increasing ventilation or cardiac output [13]. However, the first step for gas exchange is alveolar ventilation. Yet the gas volume that finally participates in gas exchange is the inspired tidal volume minus the total (physiological, anatomical and apparatus) dead-space volume. The alveolar concentrations of O_2 and CO_2, expressed as P_AO_2 and P_ACO_2, correspond because of the high diffusion capacity disease of CO_2 to the $PaCO_2$ in the absence of significant lung disease, depending on this dead-space effect. Therefore, the $PaCO_2$ has to be taken into account for P_AO_2 calculations, according to the alveolar gas equation, and ultimately, the a/A ratio—the ratio of PaO_2 to P_AO_2, as the most reliable measure of the degree of impairment of oxygen transfer across the lung. A normal a/A ratio is normally greater than 0.9. The classical PaO_2/FiO_2 ratio or the oxygenation index ($OI = (FiO_2 \times MAP)/PaO_2$) as used for the severity definition of ARDS and PARDS, respectively, do both not take into account the dead-space effect on oxygen kinetics. However, the dead-space fraction can be important in severe ARDS [14]:

$$\text{Alveolar gas equation:}\quad P_AO_2 = P_iO_2 - P_aCO_2 / R \quad PiO_2 = FiO_2 \times \left(P_B - P_{H2O}\right)$$

where P_iO_2 is the partial pressure of oxygen in the inspired gas mixture (P_iO_2 incorporates both barometric (P_B) and vapour pressure (P_{H2O}), at 37 °C P_{H2O} is 47 mmHg) and R is the respiratory quotient (i.e. the ratio of CO_2 elimination to O_2 consumption, estimated in most circumstances to be 0.8).

21.4 Respiratory Physiology, Mechanics and Gas Exchange Disturbances in Disease

Most paediatric lung disease or pathologies leading to an involvement of the lung requiring PICU admission are of a restrictive pattern (e.g. atelectasis, pneumonia, bronchopneumonia, bronchiolitis (often with a mixed restrictive and obstructive pattern), PARDS and NARDS, respectively, lung oedema of cardiac origin, inflammatory or toxic lung oedema) characterised by a reduced FRC with the hallmark sign of hypoxaemia because of increased intrapulmonary shunt, whereas obstructive lung disease of various aetiology (e.g. asthma, bronchiectasis, cystic fibrosis, bronchiolitis, bronchopulmonary dysplasia, the latter three classically with a mixed restrictive and obstructive pattern) requires relatively seldom PICU care when acute hypoxaemia is not present.

FRC can be reduced not only in restrictive lung disease but also when there is an alteration in the elastic recoil relationship between the lungs and the chest wall. In this latter condition, there is either an increased elastic inward recoil of the lung (e.g. with interstitial (chronic) lung disease) or a reduced elastic recoil of the chest wall (e.g. kyphoscoliosis, obesity, chest wall oedema) or major abdominal distention (e.g. important ascites), or a combination of those. Reduced FRC leads to reduced respiratory system compliance, which leads to a reduced tidal volume for the same amount of distending pressure. In the spontaneous breathing patient trying to maintain the "same" tidal volume, a greater inspiratory muscle effort (i.e. work of breathing) is required, which may lead, when becoming too important, to fatigue and hypercapnic respiratory insufficiency.

With obstructive airway disease, FRC may be normal or elevated (air trapping). Classical gas-exchange abnormalities that can be observed in obstructive lung disease are ventilation/perfusion (V/Q) mismatch, intrapulmonary shunt and hypoventilation. Airway obstruction may induce regional hypoventilation, leading to a V/Q mismatch and subsequent hypoxaemia. Dynamic hyperinflation, as observed with major airway narrowing, places the respiratory muscles at a mechanical disadvantage, requiring an increased inspiratory effort to maintain adequate ventilation, likely to become insufficient in severe disease or acute deterioration of chronic obstructive lung disease leading to hypoventilation and hypercapnia [15].

With upper airway obstruction of various aetiology, the main mechanical issue is an increase in airway resistance, mainly inspiratory or mixed (in- and expiratory), when the process extends below the larynx, i.e. in the trachea or the main bronchi. With a fixed stenosis or compression of the airways, airflow might become limited. Stenting the airways by PEEP titration may sometimes help to alleviate, to some extent, the obstruction and allow for better ventilation, i.e. allowing mainly for more complete exhalation. Continuous analysis of the flow-volume curve does sometimes help to optimise ventilator settings accordingly. As to the various aetiologies of intrinsic- or extrinsic upper airway obstruction it must be referred to in the paediatric literature/textbooks.

21.5 Cardiopulmonary Interactions

Since the lung and the heart are through the circulation two connected systems that also share the same body cavity, it is obvious that any alterations in intrathoracic pressures will have an influence on pre- (systemic and pulmonary venous return) and afterload (systemic and pulmonary vascular resistance) of the heart, yet having mainly an effect on right heart filling and subsequent systemic output. Furthermore, the circulation is placed in a two-compartment system, i.e. the intrathoracic and the extrathoracic compartment (◘ Fig. 21.4).

This two-compartment model helps to understand the various effects of a negative (during spontaneous breathing) or positive (during positive pressure ventilation) intrathoracic, i.e. pleural pressure, on venous return (preload). Inspiration during spontaneous ventilation will decrease pleural pressure and, by this, increase the pressure gradient for venous return, leading to an increased right atrial filling and an increase in right ventricular stroke volume. Concomitantly, the left ventricular stroke volume drops slightly because of blood pooling in the pulmonary vasculature given the negative pressure environment, ventricular interdependence (the right heart filling causes a change in left ventricular diastolic compliance leading to less LV filling), and an increase in left ventricular afterload because of negative intrathoracic pressure. This effect is usually minor, and clinical signs (respiratory cycle-dependent fluctuation of the systolic pressure, i.e. pulse-pressure variation (deltaPP)) can normally

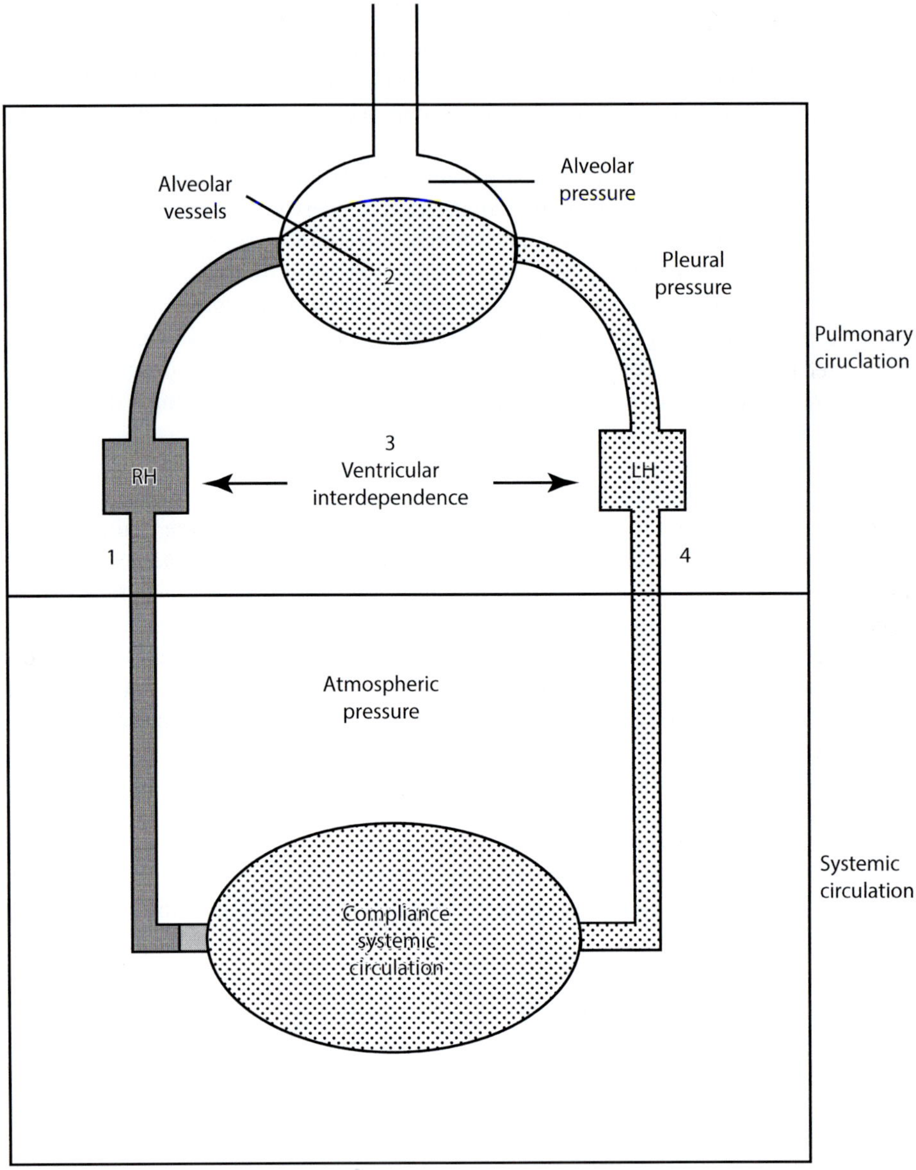

Fig. 21.4 Model of the circulation in a two-compartment with the right and left heart as well the pulmonary vasculature located in the intrathoracic compartment, subjected to intrathoracic (i.e. pleural pressure) and the systemic vasculature in the extrathoracic compartment, subjected to atmospheric/intra-abdominal pressure. (With permission already reused as Fig. 53.1 in Bohn [16])

only be seen when negative pressures become important (i.e. with severe respiratory distress) or with major intravascular hypovolemia.

With the application of positive pressures either during the (end-)inspiratory phase of a mechanical positive pressure breath [17] or during a Valsalva manoeuvre, hemodynamic effects might become important with a decrease in cardiac output, i.e. by reducing venous return and therefore RA filling pressure (RV-inflow) and an increased pulmonary vascular resistance leading to a reduced RV-outflow, both at end-inspiration. Yet, this is primarily influenced by the tidal volume size [17].

However, positive pressure application can in some conditions improve cardiac output. An increased intrathoracic pressure will reduce the transmural pressure of the left heart (LV afterload) required during contraction to reach a certain systolic pressure. This latter becomes clinically relevant and even a therapeutic tool (use of CPAP) in the failing left heart.

Not only intrathoracic pressures but also lung expansion (i.e. the lung volume) may alter pulmonary blood flow (by changes of the capacitance of the pulmonary venous system). This effect may become clinically relevant in severe obstructive lung disease, e.g. status asthmaticus with important overinflation of the lungs. This might be worsened further by application of positive pressure ventilation, especially with rapid respiratory rates and inadequate expiratory times. Ventilation-induced overexpansion of lung volumes (by application of high PEEP values and/or generously large tidal volumes) is in general hemodynamically not well tolerated. Also, the effects of positive pressure ventilation may unmask intravascular hypovolemia. Additional assessment, for example by ultrasonography looking at the collapsibility of the vena cava depending on the respiratory cycle phase or by transthoracic flow Doppler looking at ventilator setting dependent variations of the anterograde aortic flow might help to recognise hypovolemia or signs of important cardiopulmonary interactions in an individual patient.

On the other side, predominant lung collapse will lead to an increased pulmonary vascular resistance and therefore an increase in the RV afterload, yet the interest to restore functional residual capacity (by PEEP application and/or ev a recruitment approach) in the sick lung with predominant atelectasis [18, 19].

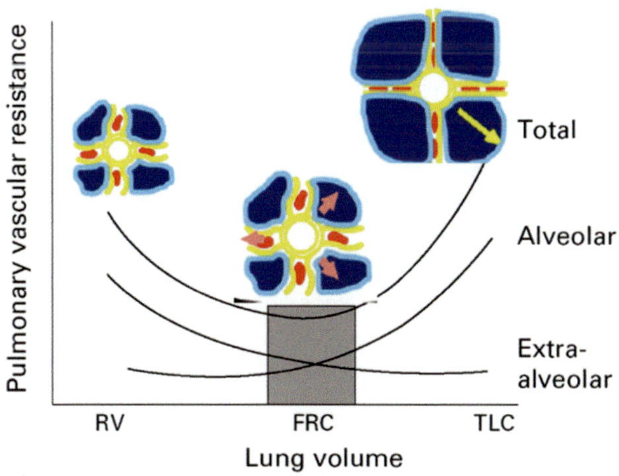

In summary, the application of positive pressure ventilation can become harmful for the right heart (reduced RV preload, i.e. venous return, and increased RV afterload, i.e. increased pulmonary vascular resistance), and as ventricles pump in series, reduce

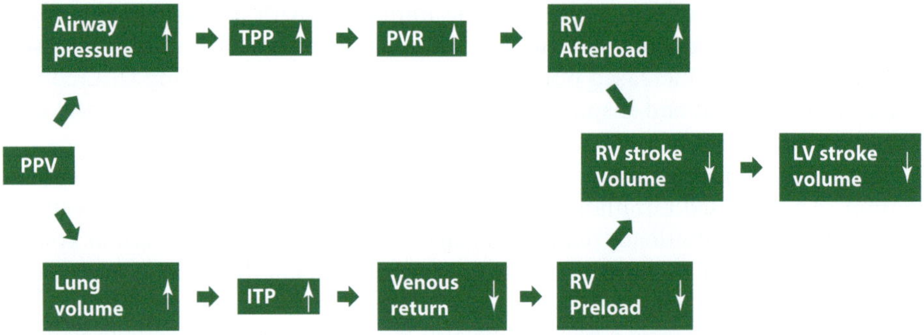

Fig. 21.5 Positive pressure ventilation primarily affects the right ventricular output and secondary the left ventricular output as the ventricles pump in series. *PPV* positive pressure ventilation, *TPP* transpulmonary pressure, *PVR* pulmonary vascular resistance, *RV* right ventricle, *LV* left ventricle, *ITP* intrathoracic pressure

systemic cardiac output (Fig. 21.5). However positive pressure application might be a therapeutic cornerstone for left ventricular failure, by reducing required transmural pressures of the left ventricle during contraction [20].

In summary, the keys for understanding on how to optimise ventilator management in the setting of a right heart failure are transpulmonary pressure and lung volume/intrathoracic pressure effects on venous return and pulmonary vascular resistance and their effects on pre- and afterload of the RV. In the setting of a left heart failure, the key to understanding is the transmural pressure of the LV.

References

1. Adamson IY. Development of lung structure. In: Crystal RG, editor. The lung: scientific foundations. 2nd ed. Philadelphia: Lippincott-Raven; 1997. p. 993–1001.
2. Burri PH. Structural aspects of prenatal and postnatal development and growth of the lung. In: McDonald J, editor. Lung growth and development. New York: Marcel Dekker; 1997. p. 1–35.
3. Joza S, Post M. Development of the respiratory system (including the preterm infant). In: Rimensberger PC, editor. Pediatric and neonatal mechanical ventilation. Berlin: Springer-Verlag; 2016. p. 3–26. https://doi.org/10.1007/978-3-642-01219-8_1.
4. Cuneo B. Transition from fetal to neonatal circulation. In: Da Cruz E, Ivy D, Jaggers J, editors. Pediatric and congenital cardiology, cardiac surgery and intensive care. London: Springer; 2014. https://doi.org/10.1007/978-1-4471-4619-3_155.
5. Mortola JP. The neonatal neuromechanical unit: generalities of operation. In: Rimensberger PC, editor. Pediatric and neonatal mechanical ventilation. Berlin: Springer-Verlag; 2015. p. 27–42. https://doi.org/10.1007/978-3-642-01219-8_1.
6. Brinkman JE, Toro F, Sharma S. Physiology, respiratory drive. StatPearls Publishing; 2020. Last update: 24 May 2020. https://www.statpearls.com/as/pulmonary/28414/.
7. Sieck GC, Vandenboom R, Mantilla CB, et al. Chapter 10. Structural and functional development of the respiratory muscles. In: Haddad GG, Abman SH, Chernick V, editors. Basic mechanisms of pediatric respiratory disease. 2nd ed. Hamilton: BC Decker Inc.; 2002. p. 139–53.
8. Mortola JP. Respiratory physiology of newborn mammals. A comparative perspective. Baltimore: The Johns Hopkins University Press; 2001.

9. Turner DA, Cheifetz IM. Basics of gas exchange. In: Rimensberger PC, editor. Pediatric and neonatal mechanical ventilation. Berlin: Springer-Verlag; 2015. p. 43–54. https://doi.org/10.1007/978-3-642-01219-8_1.
10. Hamel DS, Cheifetz IM. Do all mechanically ventilated pediatric patients require continuous capnography? Respir Care Clin N Am. 2006;12:501–13.
11. Carlton GC, Ray CJ, Miodownik S, Kopec I, Groeger JS. Capnography in mechanically ventilated patients. Crit Care Med. 1988;16:550–6.
12. Walsh BK, Crotwell DN, Restrepo RD. Capnograph/capnometry during mechanical ventilation: 2011. Respir Care. 2011;56:503–9.
13. Wagner PD. The physiological basis of pulmonary gas exchange: implications for clinical interpretation of arterial blood gases. Eur Respir J. 2015;45:227–43. https://doi.org/10.1183/09031936.00039214.
14. Yehya N, Bhalla AK, Thomas NJ, Khemani RG. Alveolar dead space fraction discriminates mortality in pediatric acute respiratory distress syndrome. Pediatr Crit Care Med. 2016;17(2):101–9. https://doi.org/10.1097/PCC.0000000000000613.
15. Dahnd R. Ventilator graphics and respiratory mechanics in the patient with obstructive lung disease. Respir Care. 2005;50(2):246–59.
16. Bohn D. Cardiopulmonary interactions in the ventilated patient. In: Rimensberger PC, editor. Pediatric and neonatal mechanical ventilation. Berlin: Springer-Verlag; 2014. p. 1332–66. https://doi.org/10.1007/978-3-642-01219-8_1.
17. Vieillard-Baron A, et al. Cyclic changes in right ventricular output impedance during mechanical ventilation. J Appl Physiol. 1999;87:1644–50.
18. Duggan M, et al. Atelectasis causes vascular leak and lethal right ventricular failure in uninjured rat lungs. Am J Respir Crit Care Med. 2003;167:1633–40.
19. Schmitt JM, et al. Positive end-expiratory pressure titration in acute respiratory distress syndrome patients: impact on right ventricular outflow impedance evaluated by pulmonary artery Doppler flow velocity measurements. Crit Care Med. 2001;29:1154–8.
20. Bradley TD, et al. Cardiac output response to continuous positive airway pressure in congestive heart failure. Am Rev Respir Dis. 1992;145:377.

Acute Kidney Injury in the PICU

Zaccaria Ricci, Francesco Guzzi, and Akash Deep

Contents

J. Brierley et al. (eds.), *ESPNIC Children's Intensive Care Textbook*,
https://doi.org/10.1007/978-3-031-64762-8_22

Learning Objectives

- This text will present the basic concepts to be appraised regarding acute kidney injury in critically ill patients with a specific focus on the pediatric setting. The reader will be informed about current diagnostic and classification methods, the importance of predicting the occurrence of renal dysfunction, and the application of some biomarkers. Preventive and pharmacological approaches to the management of pediatric acute kidney injury will also be covered.

22.1 Introduction

AKI is a common event in all hospitalized patients, with varying incidence rates according to age. From the emergency department to internal medicine and elective surgery wards, any patient can be exposed to the risk of developing AKI proportionally to the severity of their admission disease or eventual complications. The cascade of events that characterize overt AKI ultimately leads to a SCr increase and/or UO reduction, accumulation of waste products, and potentially fatal dysregulation of electrolytes, acid-base balance, and extracellular volume homeostasis. In-hospital AKI is independently correlated with mild to severe short-term complications (e.g., the need for diuretic therapy, prolongation of hospital stay, distal organ dysfunction, and renal replacement therapy), long-term complications (e.g., chronic kidney disease (CKD) and cardiovascular disease), and mortality [1]. Establishing a consensus for a common definition and staging of AKI helped ameliorate the general understanding of this clinical entity in the nephrology and critical care fields. With respect to the previous confusing terminology, the new AKI definition [2] helped to standardize epidemiologic research and to highlight the spectrum of progressive damage of this heterogeneous syndrome. However, community-acquired AKI, especially in middle- and low-income countries, is severely under-reported and has a huge burden of mortality for previously healthy young individuals [3]. To gather a comprehensive pediatric perspective on AKI and to establish the future research agenda, in November 2021, the first Pediatric Acute Disease Quality Initiative (pADQI), the 26th ADQI Consensus conference, with a panel of 46 pAKI global experts, was convened in Napa, California, US [4, 5]. The present chapter will discuss several aspects of pediatric AKI (pAKI), including recent advances in the correct diagnosis, epidemiology, prevention and medical strategies to take care of critically ill children with AKI.

22.2 pAKI Definition

Currently accepted criteria for AKI definition according to Kidney Disease Improving Global Outcomes (KDIGO) [6] and its relative classification are summarized in ◘ Table 22.1. AKI staging is built on two parameters: the reduction of the estimated glomerular filtration rate (eGFR) (or rise in SCr levels), and UO reduc-

Table 22.1 KDIGO and neonatal KDIGO criteria for acute kidney injury

	Serum creatinine (SCr) criteria	Urine output criteria
KDIGO criteria (ref SCr is premorbid or estimated value)		
Stage 1	≥0.3 mg/dL (≥26.5 μmol/L) increase within 48 h OR 1.5–1.9 times baseline within 7 days	<0.5 mL/kg/h for 6–12 h
Stage 2	2.0–2.9 times baseline	<0.5 mL/kg/h for ≥12 h
Stage 3	3.0 times baseline OR Increase in SCr to ≥4.0 mg/dL (≥354 μmol/L) OR KRT initiation OR In patients >18 years, decrease in eGFR to <35 mL/min/1.73 m^2	<0.3 mL/kg/h for ≥24 h OR Anuria for ≥12 h
Neonatal KDIGO criteria (ref SCr is the lowest prior measurement)		
Stage 1	≥0.3 mg/dL (≥26.5 μmol/L) increase within 48 h OR 1.5–1.9 times baseline (previous lowest value) within 7 days	≤1 mL/kg/h for 24 h
Stage 2	2.0–2.9 times baseline	≤0.5 mL/kg/h for 24 h
Stage 3	3.0 times baseline OR Increase in SCr ≥2.5 mg/dL (≥221 μmol/L) OR KRT initiation	≤0.3 mL/kg/h for 24 h

tion, measured as volume per body weight over time. Past and present definitions focused on SCr levels and highlighted the importance of time from baseline to peak SCr, daily creatinine monitoring, and accurate UO measuring [7]. Three stages of increasing severity (AKI stage 1–3) were introduced and different definition systems were reconciled [8]. The KDIGO criteria are currently accepted in the pediatric population, with the exception of neonates [9]. Neonates have peculiar characteristics in terms of renal physiology, kidney function maturity (according to gestational age), variable "normal" SCr levels due to lack of standardized references, and the influence of maternal creatinine. Moreover, it is often difficult to obtain daily SCr measurements and accurate hourly UO monitoring unless a bladder catheter is used. For all these reasons, in 2017, the National Institute of Diabetes and Digestive and Kidney Diseases (NIDDK) proposed an alternative classification for neonatal AKI (nAKI), which follows modified KDIGO criteria (Table 22.1) [10]. The KDIGO and neonatal KDIGO criteria in the PICU population have been recently applied in two multinational observational cohort studies, respectively, the Assessment of Worldwide Acute Kidney Injury, Renal Angina and Epidemiology in Critically Ill Children (AWARE) and Assessment of Worldwide Acute Kidney injury Epidemiology in Neonates (AWAKEN) [11, 12].

22.3 Epidemiology

The 2014 International Society of Nephrology (ISN) Global Snapshot revealed the hidden burden of AKI with lack of diagnosis, poor awareness of its impact and shortness of therapeutic options in developing countries, linked to increased mortality rate compared to industrialized countries [3]. The AKI-EPI study was the first epidemiologic research collecting AKI episodes per KDIGO criteria in the first week after ICU admission. 57% of 1800 patients developed AKI (18% stage 1, 9% stage 2, 30% stage 3) [13]. AKI occurrence, especially severe AKI, was independently associated with mortality, increased length of stay, renal non-recovery and higher SCr at discharge [13]. The AWARE and AWAKEN studies, revealed a high prevalence of AKI in the PICU setting, respectively in children (26.9%) and neonates (29.9%), often linked to complex diseases and multi-organ failure. In particular, in AWARE, shock, heart failure, and trauma were identified as main risk factors for AKI at admission, and a history of transplantation (both solid and bone marrow) together with the utilization of nephrotoxins (Box ▶ 22.1) were the most frequent variables associated with AKI throughout PICU discharge. AKI was an independent risk factor for length of hospital stay and mortality, with the association being progressively more significant with the increase of AKI severity (both in children and in neonates). The incidence of severe AKI (stage 2–3) was 11.6% in children and 16.0% in neonates while mortality rate in AKI patients was respectively 6.5% and 9.8% versus 2.4% and 1.4% in non-AKI children and neonates [11, 12] (◘ Fig. 22.1). AWARE study excluded by protocol patients with congenital heart diseases undergoing cardiac surgery being a specific cohort at highest risk of AKI, especially in the post-cardiac

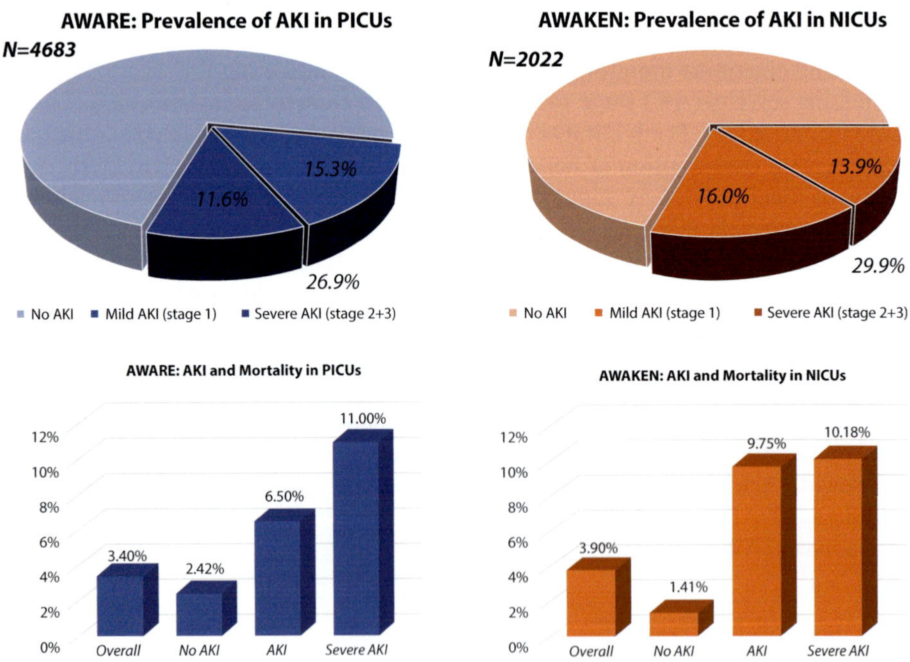

◘ **Fig. 22.1** AKI prevalence and related mortality in the PICU and NICU

surgery phase. As a matter of fact, a recent observation, conducted in three centers of the United States, concluded that cardiac surgery-associated AKI (CS-AKI) occurred in 36%, most of whom had stage II or III disease (72%). Cardiac patients at higher risk of CS-AKI were younger, underwent more complex surgery and had longer cardiopulmonary bypass (CPB) times. Interestingly, within centers incidence varies significantly (from 16% to 65%), possibly depending on case mix and the presence of different risk factors among patients [14]. The need to expand the knowledge about pAKI epidemiology also to the non-ICU and ambulatory settings as well as to middle- and low-income countries, to better investigate pAKI pathobiology and the causal link between AKI and its outcomes, and the importance of epidemiology to improve pAKI prevention and to mitigate its complications have been recently addressed by the first pADQI [15, 16].

Box 22.1: Most Common AKI-Inducing Nephrotoxins

Drug category	Nephrotoxins
Antibiotics	Aminoglycosides, Vancomycin, Ciprofloxacin, Sulfamethoxazole-trimethoprim, Piperacillin-tazobactam, Amphotericin B, Ceftriaxone
Antivirals	Acyclovir, Valacyclovir, Tenofovir
NSAIDs	Rofecoxib, Ibuprofen, Diclofenac, Celecoxib, Naproxen, Aspirin
Immunosuppressive	Cyclosporine, Tacrolimus, Sirolimus, Micofenolate mofetil, Rituximab
Antineoplastic	Ifosfamide, Cisplatin, Carboplatin, Check-point inhibitors, Methotrexate
Antihypertensive	Ramipril, Lisinopril, Enalapril, Valsartan, Olmesartan
Diuretics	Furosemide, Thiazides, Spironolactone
Other	Contrast medium, Metformin, Lithium, Sodium phosphate-containing purgatives, Bisphosphonates, Proton-pump inhibitors, Intravenous immunoglobulin

22.4 Specific Aspects of pAKI Diagnosis

AWARE and AWAKEN studies highlighted the importance of accurately collecting data on both creatinine levels/eGFR and UO to correctly diagnose AKI. In fact, as many as 67% and 80% of AKI patients per UO criteria would not have been identified by SCr alone, as in infants (AWARE) and in neonates (AWAKEN) [11, 12]. Unfortunately, both SCr and UO have important limitations as AKI markers. Creatinine levels are highly influenced by extra-renal conditions such as gender, age, muscle mass, metabolic state (e.g., sepsis), drugs, fluid or protein load [7]. Moreover, a baseline SCr is often difficult to obtain, and creatinine levels remain often unchanged until half of the nephrons are lost, due to renal functional reserve (RFR) [17]. Finally, the importance of development as a biologic variable, since kidney development and nephrogenesis (with a variable number of functioning nephrons at birth) are largely influenced by gestational age and other biopsychosocial factors, while glomerular and tubular function undergo constant maturation throughout the first 2 years of life [16]. Interpretation of the UO criteria is also characterized by practical difficulties being often confounded by diuretic administration, lack of consensus over the use of ideal/actual body weight indexing, benign and transient oliguria, especially in the ICU setting. Indeed, both SCr and UO lack specificity and sensitivity for AKI diagnosis. Such limitations could be overcome by the use of alternative renal biomarkers. New biomarkers could ameliorate AKI risk stratification, prediction, and early detection, add details about pathophysiology (glomerular, tubular, inflammatory, or hemodynamic injury), possibly inform about etiology, indicate specific treatments, and improve prognostic data. Among others, cystatin C (CysC), Neutrophil Gelatinase-Associated Lipocalin (NGAL), kidney injury molecule-1 (KIM-1), interleukins, liver-type fatty acid binding protein (L-FABP), and combinations of these biomarkers have been proposed for prediction and early diagnosis of AKI (also called subclinical AKI) prior to established AKI occurrence (◘ Table 22.2). While researchers are intensively working on such renal biomarkers, the clinical significance of subclinical AKI is still unclear [18], especially in the pediatric setting. In children undergoing CPB and cardiac surgery, preoperative plasma IL-6 concentration was associated with stage 2–3 AKI development [19] while plasma preoperative IL-8 and postoperative TNFα were associated with the risk of AKI, longer hospital stay, and mechanical ventilation in children ≥2 years [20]. Some authors have proposed the integration of biomarkers analysis and AKI diagnostic systems. In a recent report, Stanski and coworkers performed the measurements of urine neutrophil gelatinase-associated lipocalin (uNGAL) and SCr samples from PICU admission and created four groups for comparison: uNGAL−/SCr−, uNGAL+/SCr, uNGAL−/SCr+, and uNGAL+/SCr+. They found that uNGAL+/SCr− patients, with respect to those

◘ **Table 22.2** Biomarkers of AKI

Type of injury	**Biomarkers**
Functional injury	Serum creatinine, eGFR, urinary output, cystatin C, FeNa
Structural injury	Neutrophil gelatinase-associate lipocalin (NGAL), Kidney injury molecule-1 (KIM-1), Liver type fatty acid binding protein (L-FABP), *N*-acetyl-beta-glucosamide (NAG), Alpha glutathione-s-transferase (α-GST)
Inflammatory injury	IL-18, IL-6, IL-8, TNFα, INFγ
Cell-cycle arrest	Insulin-like growth factor binding protein-7 (IGFBP-7), Tissue inhibitor of metalloproteinase-2 (TIMP-2)
Combinations	uNGAL/SCr, Nephrocheck (TIMP-2 + IGFBP-7), RAI score

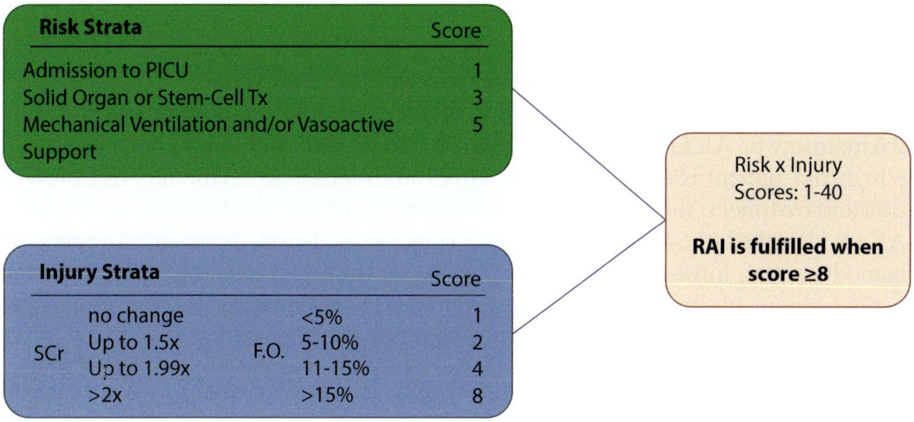

Fig. 22.2 Renal angina index

with the negativity of both diagnostic tests, had increased risk for all-stage Day 3 AKI (≥KDIGO stage 1). Furthermore, uNGAL+/SCr+ patients had an increased risk for severe Day 3 AKI (≥KDIGO stage 2) with respect to those with SCr positivity and negative uNGAL. These classifications may enable a more personalized approach to the early management of AKI [21, 22].

However, in the everyday PICU clinical practice it might be useful to stratify the population according to AKI risk, with the aim of reducing false-positive results and to properly select those who could benefit by having a biomarker dosed. With this purpose, the Renal Angina Index (RAI) was proposed [23] (Fig. 22.2). The RAI, a bedside scoring system which combines baseline and clinical characteristics, ranges from 1 to 40. An RAI score ≥8 identifies a subset population at increased risk for AKI in the following 72 h, while an RAI <8 yields a negative predictive value >92%. With such a clinical scoring, a RAI positive patient might deserve further testing with AKI biomarkers were a RAI negative score would discourage the use of biomarkers [23, 24]. A sub-study of the AWARE prospective observational multicenter study, tested the RAI performance in a cohort of almost 1600 children admitted to the ICU. A RAI score ≥8 (RA+) was compared to SCr increase relative to baseline (SCr > Base) in the first 12 h of ICU stay. Severe AKI (stage 2–3 KDIGO) on the third day of ICU stay occurred in 42.3% of RA+ patients versus 26.4% of SCr > Base. While the SCr criteria appeared more sensitive, with the identification of a greater number of patients, the RAI predictive accuracy was superior (specificity 87% vs. 70%, PPV 31% vs. 25%) [25]. Recently, a modified "acute" RAI was proposed and successfully tested in children admitted to the emergency department [26].

Moreover, severe pAKI detection rate is improved when RAI is associated with urinary NGAL measurement [27] and when a multi-dimensional approach is utilized such as in the recently proposed Fluid Overload Kidney Injury Score (FOKIS) [28].

The possibility to anticipate the occurrence and severity of an AKI episode through novel diagnostic and risk stratification tools which could bring improvements in the timeliness and precision of pAKI diagnosis appear of crucial importance for its management that is currently based on primary and secondary prevention [22, 29].

22.5 Prevention

Prevention of AKI occurrence (primary prevention) or prevention of AKI worsening (i.e., stage modification from mild to severe—secondary prevention) is currently the mainstay of AKI management. Since time to the first appropriate intervention in a high-risk patient is one of the most important modifiable factors in AKI prevention and treatment, the focus on early identification of this condition is crucial. After AKI is identified or a high risk of its occurrence is predicted, timely improvement of hemodynamics, intravascular volume, cardiac output, and renal blood flow are the main weapons on hand to reduce both the risk of developing AKI and its severity together with avoidance of nephrotoxic drugs and contrast media.

To contrast AKI unawareness in the hospitalized population, the use of e-alert systems based on early detection of SCr variations has been increasingly proposed. Big data and electronic health records made it possible to develop computer programs for AKI early detection, alert, and risk stratification, but reports of their applicability and cost-effectiveness in the clinical practice are conflicting [30–32]. Early AKI detection, compliance with dedicated care bundle and nephrologist referral proved to significantly reduce AKI severity and related complications [33]. A single-center randomized trial assigned 2393 hospitalized (ICU and not-ICU) adult patients to either an "AKI alert" group or a "usual care" group and found that maximum change in SCr levels, need for kidney replacement therapy (KRT), and death at 7 days did not differ [34]. A new multicenter RCT from the same research group found that e-alerts did not reduce the risk of progression of acute kidney injury, receipt of dialysis, or death within 14 days of randomization [35]. The ICE-AKI study demonstrated improved in-hospital outcomes by combining an electronic clinical prediction score with an AKI e-alert in patients admitted to the emergency department for medical conditions [36], while a multicenter randomized trial evaluating AKI e-alerts and care bundles demonstrated a reduction in hospital length of stay but not mortality rate [37]. In the pediatric setting, a cross-sectional multicenter study evaluated an AKI e-alert algorithm to study AKI incidence and to retrospectively evaluate its recognition and management [38]. Interestingly only approximately one out of four e-alert AKI episodes were correctly recognized by the clinicians.

E-alert systems also have the ability to flag those patients who are at increased AKI risk because of nephrotoxic drug exposure. Indeed, exposure to nephrotoxic medications is ubiquitous, representing one of the most frequent causes of in-hospital preventable AKI (Box ▶ 22.1). Withdrawal of the nephrotoxic medication, reduction of the duration of the exposure or reduction of the cumulative dose could reduce AKI incidence and related complications. According to a recent analysis of the Food and Drug Administration Adverse Event Reporting System (FAERS) database, the most commonly reported nephrotoxic drugs were aprotinin, sodium phosphate, furosemide, vancomycin, and metformin, but also interestingly, more than half of the reported drug-related AKI episodes were from medications not currently recognized as nephrotoxic highlighting the need for further research [39]. A 2013 study implemented a systematic electronic record screening with clinical decision-support process in hospitalized, non-critically ill children [40]. Among more than 20,000, 726 patients had high exposure to nephrotoxic medication during 945 hospital admissions. Highly nephrotoxic exposure was defined as the administration of three or more nephrotoxic medications or a prolonged (more than 3 consecutive days) therapy with aminoglycoside antibiotics. AKI occurred in 25% of exposed patients and 31% of hospital admissions with an initial average rate of 30 AKI episodes per 100 days of exposure. The implementation of the surveillance program was able to reduce AKI intensity below 20 episodes per 100 days of exposure [40]. This study led to the development of a prospective AKI monitoring program called Nephrotoxic Injury Negated by Just-in-time-Action (NINJA) that has been tested in non-critically and critically ill hospitalized children and neonates. In 3 years of prospective implementation of the NINJA program, the exposure to nephrotoxic medications decreased by 38% and nearly 400 AKI episodes were avoided (a decrease of more than 60% of expected AKI episodes) in a cohort of non-critically ill children in almost 2400 separate hospital admissions [41]. In a retrospective cohort of 154 critically ill children undergoing congenital heart surgery, 21% received more than three nephrotoxic medications but no significant association was found between high nephrotoxic exposure and AKI. Of notice, in this study AKI was defined as per KDIGO stage ≥2 [42]. In the neonatal intensive care unit, the NINJA program was able to identify high-risk infants and prevent nephrotoxic-induced AKI with a significant reduction of nephrotoxic medications exposure, a 20% reduction in AKI episodes, and a reduction of the intensity of AKI episodes [43]. Recently, the NINJA program was successfully applied to a multicenter prospective cohort of more than 4500 non-critically ill hospitalized children and demonstrated an improvement of AKI prevalence rates per 1000 patient-day (23.8% reduction) and per exposure (36.7% reduction) [44]. According to the first pADQI Consensus conference, given the immediate and lifelong adverse outcomes, more should be done by the community for the prevention of pAKI episodes. Coordinated efforts from governmental and non-governmental organizations, industry, and professional societies should raise awareness, education and advocacy for the identification of those at-risk for AKI, enhance early diagnosis and develop damage mitigation strategies [45].

22.6 Pharmacological Treatment

No specific pharmacological interventions are available for established AKI treatment. Nevertheless, much effort and research have been dedicated to this issue with controversial results. In addition to timely identification of patients at risk and reduction of nephrotoxic exposure, numerous interventions can halt AKI progression, ease recovery, and reduce complications' rate. Fluid management has a significant role in both prevention and treatment of AKI episodes, especially in post-surgical patients. Postoperative fluid overload (Box ▶ 22.2) was significantly linked to AKI development, prolonged hospital stay, and mortality in a meta-analysis of studies among pediatric patients undergoing cardiac surgery [46]. In the PICU, fluid overload proved to be detrimental in critically ill children in terms of in-hospital mortality, time to wean from mechanical ventilation, PICU length of stay, and AKI development [47]. The first pADQI Consensus conference convened an expert multidisciplinary working group dedicated to the standardization of terminology and reporting of fluid assessment in the PICU [48]. Importantly, the pADQI working group proposed utilizing the terms *daily fluid balance*, *cumulative fluid balance*, and *percent cumulative fluid balance* to describe the fluid status both in clinical care and research setting despite inherent assumptions commonly utilized. Also, the group collected evidence regarding fluid balance disorders epidemiology, established the best targets for intervention, and identified areas for future research and endpoints for clinical trials [48].

Diuretics may at times, be useful for managing fluid overload in oliguric patients before starting KRT. Although not recommended for the treatment oligo-anuric AKI, furosemide per se does not cause AKI when appropriately administered and is not contraindicated in AKI patients when, on the contrary, higher doses may be needed [49]. In a prospective double-blinded RCT, etacrynic acid, also a loop diuretic inhibiting the NKCC2 channel, proved superior to furosemide in terms of early postoperative UO, fluid overload reduction, cardiac index, length of mechanical ventilation, and PICU stay [50]. In 2013 a Furosemide Stress Test (FST) was developed to help predict the occurrence of severe AKI (AKIN stage 3). In the setting of early AKI, a one-time dose of 1–1.5 mg/kg predicted the development of progressive AKI in critically ill patients with a sensitivity and specificity of around 85% for a cutoff of 100 mL/h UO in the first 2 h [51]. FST-induced UO proved to be more significant than biochemical biomarkers for AKI progression risk stratification, but assessing FST UO in patients with increased biomarker levels further improved risk stratification [52]. Recently, in a multicenter, prospective, observational study, FST ability to predict AKI worsening was validated in a cohort of 92 critically ill patients and then confirmed in a systematic review and meta-analysis [53, 54]. The same test has proved useful in the pediatric setting [55].

Sepsis is also frequently associated with AKI, ranging from 16% to 50% in pediatric patients [56, 57]. A key goal to managing septic AKI is to maintain hemodynamic stability, avoiding whenever possible fluid overload, anticipating fluid de-resuscitation as soon as possible and administering vasoconstrictors if required. Recent preclinical and clinical studies demonstrated septic AKI to also be a disease of the microcirculation, resulting in kidney medulla hypoxia and tubular stress. Kidney medulla tissue oxygenation, and the surrogate marker of urinary oxygenation, were improved by resuscitation with angiotensin II with respect to norepinephrine [58, 59]. The administration of angiotensin II before starting KRT improved 28-day survival, KRT discontinuation, and mean arterial pressure with respect to placebo in septic shock patients with severe AKI [60]. Consistent data on the effects of vasoactive drugs in the general PICU population and specifically in pAKI are currently lacking. Researchers investigated the role of perioperative anesthetic drugs in AKI prevention. Dexmedetomidine halved AKI incidence and reduced AKI severity with positive effect on morbidity and length of ICU stay compared to placebo [61]. Decreased AKI incidence was also demonstrated in pediatric patients after congenital heart surgery in the PICU [62]. A recent systematic review and meta-analysis of 14 studies including 2625 pediatric patients confirmed significantly lower AKI incidence after congenital heart surgery in those treated with dexmedetomidine and acetaminophen [63]. Recently, a single-center, placebo-controlled, RCT showed reduced AKI incidence and shorter length of hospital stay in the dexmedetomidine group with no side effects in a cohort of 108 patients undergoing aortic surgery and CPB [64]. Levosimendan, an inotropic drug administered to cardiac surgery patients with low cardiac output syndrome, showed a decrease in AKI incidence and the need for KRT [65, 66]. Fenoldopam, an antihypertensive D1 receptor partial agonist, has been used for AKI prevention in pediatric settings, and it has been shown to reduce AKI incidence, but the evidence is not strong enough to support its systematic use [67, 68]. Its application at high doses during CPB in pediatric cardiac patients confirmed a potential role in reducing sub-

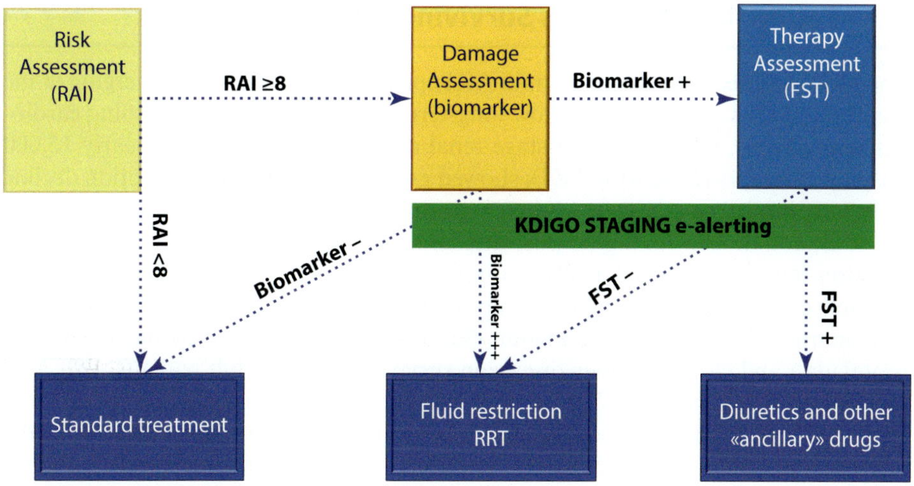

Fig. 22.3 Tentative pragmatic approach in AKI diagnosis and management. Biomarker and FST could be alternatively tested after RAI. KDIGO classification for AKI detection should be constantly checked on all RAI positive patients

clinical AKI and a positive effect on postoperative AKI [69]. Recent work has been finally conducted by the AWAKEN investigators who found some protective effects of caffeine on kidney function of critically ill neonates [70], while other authors found acetaminophen being beneficial in the early post-cardiac surgery phase in a large cohort of infants [71], even if the role of these commonly administered drugs has to be further evaluated. A tentative approach to diagnosis and management of pAKI is described in Fig. 22.3. Future research in the field of pharmacological treatment will focus on the characterization of the pharmacology modifications of high-value medications eliminated by the kidney during pAKI episodes, on the prioritization of nephrotoxin stewardship and of targeted nutritional interventions in the short- and long-term period to improve patient-centered outcomes [72].

Box 22.2: Fluid Overload

Fluid overload is usually calculated between two time points (*A*–*B*). Frequently used time points in the literature are for example PICU admission to CKRT initiation or Pre-operative to Post-operative. Once the two time points are established, fluid overload can be calculated with a fluid-based or weight-based formulas:

- Fluid-based formula: (fluid intake *A*–*B* [L] – fluid output *A*–*B* [L])/(weight *A* [kg]) × 100%
- Weight-based formula: (weight *B* [kg] – weight *A* [kg])/(weight *A* [kg]) × 100%

The RAI score considered a time frame of the first 8 h after PICU admission: *A* = PICU admission, *B* = 8 h after PICU admission. Based on previous results, mainly from pCKRT studies, four injury strata of fluid accumulation were considered of increasing severity (<5%, 5–10%, 10–15%, >15%).

22.7 Follow-Up of Patients Surviving AKI

Long-term consequences of even mild AKI episodes are increasingly emerging in the literature. AKI survivors often show long-term adverse outcomes including cardiovascular disease, CKD, and end-stage renal disease [73]. A study of nearly 15,000 hospital survivors (1966 with AKI), showed greater long-term renal function decline from post-discharge eGFR in AKI patients and, interestingly, that renal decline was worse among those with higher post-discharge eGFR. Therefore, even when kidney function returns to normal at PICU discharge, increased risk for renal disease progression persists in AKI patients for up to 10 years, irrespective of AKI severity or proteinuria [74]. Long-term follow-up demonstrated a high rate of mortality with proteinuria and chronic kidney disease in survivors among adult patients with AKI requiring KRT in the ICU [75]. For pediatric patients surviving AKI episodes, long-term follow-up and nephrologist referral could be even more important. Both the AWARE and the AWAKEN study described, together with increased mortality, increasing length of stay, and need for mechanical ventilation in hospitalized and PICU AKI patients [11, 12]. While short-term complications have very likely some impact over long-term outcomes, data from pediatric cohorts are not extensive. A recent comprehensive review summarized the available data about mid- and long-term outcomes after AKI in neonates and children [76]. Six months after one in-hospital nephrotoxic associated AKI episode, 70% of children had residual kidney damage in terms of reduced eGFR, hyperfiltration, proteinuria, or hypertension, but few had been referred to a nephrologist for CKD evaluation [77]. A retrospective study from two PICUs at tertiary centers found that renal recovery after AKI was 92.5% when defined as serum creatinine level less than 1.5 times baseline, and 75.9% when defined as less than 1.15 times baseline. Stage 3 AKI (KDIGO) was associated with no renal recovery by both definitions. The overall awareness of the importance of AKI monitoring was low since less than half of the PICU population had serum creatinine measured before hospital discharge [78].

The peculiar situation of very low birth weight neonates was addressed in a small cohort of children aged 3–7 years. The risk for renal dysfunction, defined as eGFR <90 mL/min/1.73 m^2, proteinuria, or blood pressure ≥95th percentile, was higher in those patients who experienced AKI in the PICU [79].

In high-risk settings such as pediatric cardiac surgery patients, long-term CKD, proteinuria, and hypertension are even commoner. In a prospective multicenter cohort study, children between 1 month and 18 years of age who underwent CPB were followed for 5 years. Despite perioperative AKI was not significantly associated with long-term CKD development and hypertension, follow-up was relatively short, and their occurrence was common (8% and 17%), but only 5/131 (4%) children were referred to a nephrologist [80].

Despite the increasing knowledge of AKI-related long-term effects, and the chances to improving outcomes, only a minority of patients receive nephrology referral and follow-up [81]. An important nationwide, population-based, historical cohort study of 1,521,501 adolescents examined before military service showed that a history of any kidney disease during childhood had a fourfold hazard ratio for end-stage renal disease. Interestingly, a sensitivity analysis including only patients with "mild or resolved renal disease" did not significantly change the association with adulthood kidney disease [82]. Children who survive an AKI episode requiring KRT are at high risk of long-term outcomes [83], but yet only a minority receive pediatric nephrologist follow-up [84], it is unclear how to identify the ones a greater risk, and with which tests and frequency they should be monitored [85]. Future research will be focused to identify tools for clinical risk stratification in these patients to guide appropriate referral and guidance at the time of PICU discharge [85].

Take-Home Messages

- AKI is a silent enemy of all hospitalized patients. Other than adults, children are also affected by this syndrome. There is a high risk in the medical community to overlook the problem.
- AKI should be timely diagnosed and classified because the management of this disease is based essentially on primary and secondary prevention (being avoidance of nephrotoxins a priority).
- Fluid overload is a cause and a consequence of pediatric AKI and a major clinical aspect to be prevented and aggressively treated in this context.
- The occurrence of an AKI episode is an independent risk factor of mortality, prolonged mechanical ventilation, and duration of PICU stay in critically ill children.
- AKI is the first scar on children's kidneys. An AKI episode may be the starting point for chronic kidney disease development at any age. Any AKI episode should be followed up exactly as it is done for recovered heart failure and respiratory failure.
- Management of AKI requires a multidisciplinary team. "Acute" nephrologist referral and his/her consult in the PICU is very important to increase the awareness level. Clinicians should avoid being reassured by a normal serum creatinine at PICU discharge, and nephrologists should keep following up these children.

References

1. Coca SG, Yusuf B, Shlipak MG, Garg AX, Parikh CR. Long-term risk of mortality and other adverse outcomes after acute kidney injury: a systematic review and meta-analysis. Am J Kidney Dis. 2009;53(6):961–73.
2. Bellomo R, Ronco C, Kellum JA, Mehta RL, Palevsky P. Acute Dialysis Quality Initiative workgroup. Acute renal failure—definition, outcome measures, animal models, fluid therapy and information technology needs: the Second International Consensus Conference of the Acute Dialysis Quality Initiative (ADQI) Group. Crit Care. 2004;8(4):R204–12.
3. Mehta RL, Burdmann EA, Cerdá J, Feehally J, Finkelstein F, García-García G, et al. Recognition and management of acute kidney injury in the International Society of Nephrology 0by25 Global Snapshot: a multinational cross-sectional study. Lancet. 2016;387(10032):2017–25.
4. Goldstein SL. The twenty-sixth Acute Disease Quality Initiative: the Pediatric ADQI (pADQI)—a dream realized. Pediatr Nephrol. 2024;39(3):917–8.
5. Goldstein SL, Akcan-Arikan A, Alobaidi R, Askenazi DJ, Bagshaw SM, Barhight M, et al. Consensus-based recommendations on priority activities to address acute kidney injury in children: a modified Delphi consensus statement. JAMA Netw Open. 2022;5(9):e2229442.
6. Kidney Disease: Improving Global Outcomes (KDIGO) Acute Kidney Injury Work Group. KDIGO clinical practice guideline for acute kidney injury. Kidney Int Suppl. 2012;2:1–138.
7. Ricci Z, Romagnoli S. Acute kidney injury: diagnosis and classification in adults and children. Contrib Nephrol. 2018;193:1–12.
8. Akcan-Arikan A, Zappitelli M, Loftis LL, Washburn KK, Jefferson LS, Goldstein SL. Modified RIFLE criteria in critically ill children with acute kidney injury. Kidney Int. 2007;71(10):1028–35.

9. Sutherland SM, Byrnes JJ, Kothari M, Longhurst CA, Dutta S, Garcia P, et al. AKI in hospitalized children: comparing the pRIFLE, AKIN, and KDIGO definitions. Clin J Am Soc Nephrol. 2015;10(4):554–61.
10. Zappitelli M, Ambalavanan N, Askenazi DJ, Moxey-Mims MM, Kimmel PL, Star RA, et al. Developing a neonatal acute kidney injury research definition: a report from the NIDDK neonatal AKI workshop. Pediatr Res. 2017;82(4):569–73.
11. Kaddourah A, Basu RK, Bagshaw SM, Goldstein SL. Epidemiology of acute kidney injury in critically ill children and young adults. N Engl J Med. 2017;376(1):11–20.
12. Jetton JG, Boohaker LJ, Sethi SK, Wazir S, Rohatgi S, Soranno DE, et al. Incidence and outcomes of neonatal acute kidney injury (AWAKEN): a multicentre, multinational, observational cohort study. Lancet Child Adolesc Health. 2017;1(3):184–94.
13. Hoste EAJ, Bagshaw SM, Bellomo R, Cely CM, Colman R, Cruz DN, et al. Epidemiology of acute kidney injury in critically ill patients: the multinational AKI-EPI study. Intensive Care Med. 2015;41(8):1411–23.
14. Blinder JJ, Asaro LA, Wypij D, Selewski DT, Agus MSD, Gaies M, et al. Acute kidney injury after pediatric cardiac surgery: a secondary analysis of the safe pediatric euglycemia after cardiac surgery trial. Pediatr Crit Care Med. 2017;18(7):638–46.
15. Sutherland SM, Alobaidi R, Gorga SM, Iyengar A, Morgan C, Heydari E, et al. Epidemiology of acute kidney injury in children: a report from the 26th Acute Disease Quality Initiative (ADQI) consensus conference. Pediatr Nephrol. 2024;39(3):919–28.
16. Starr MC, Barreto E, Charlton J, Vega M, Brophy PD, Ray Bignall ON, et al. Advances in pediatric acute kidney injury pathobiology: a report from the 26th Acute Disease Quality Initiative (ADQI) conference. Pediatr Nephrol. 2024;39(3):941–53.
17. Ronco C, Bellomo R, Kellum J. Understanding renal functional reserve. Intensive Care Med. 2017;43(6):917–20.
18. Koyner JL, Zarbock A, Basu RK, Ronco C. The impact of biomarkers of acute kidney injury on individual patient care. Nephrol Dial Transplant. 2019;35:1295.
19. Greenberg JH, Whitlock R, Zhang WR, Thiessen-Philbrook HR, Zappitelli M, Devarajan P, et al. Interleukin-6 and interleukin-10 as acute kidney injury biomarkers in pediatric cardiac surgery. Pediatr Nephrol. 2015;30(9):1519–27.
20. de Fontnouvelle CA, Greenberg JH, Thiessen-Philbrook HR, Zappitelli M, Roth J, Kerr KF, et al. Interleukin-8 and tumor necrosis factor predict acute kidney injury after pediatric cardiac surgery. Ann Thorac Surg. 2017;104(6):2072–9.
21. Stanski N, Menon S, Goldstein SL, Basu RK. Integration of urinary neutrophil gelatinase-associated lipocalin with serum creatinine delineates acute kidney injury phenotypes in critically ill children. J Crit Care. 2019;53:1–7.
22. Fuhrman DY, Stanski NL, Krawczeski CD, Greenberg JH, Arikan AAA, Basu RK, et al. A proposed framework for advancing acute kidney injury risk stratification and diagnosis in children: a report from the 26th Acute Disease Quality Initiative (ADQI) conference. Pediatr Nephrol. 2024;39(3):929–39.
23. Basu RK, Zappitelli M, Brunner L, Wang Y, Wong HR, Chawla LS, et al. Derivation and validation of the renal angina index to improve the prediction of acute kidney injury in critically ill children. Kidney Int. 2014;85(3):659–67.
24. Menon S, Goldstein SL, Mottes T, Fei L, Kaddourah A, Terrell T, et al. Urinary biomarker incorporation into the renal angina index early in intensive care unit admission optimizes acute kidney injury prediction in critically ill children: a prospective cohort study. Nephrol Dial Transplant. 2016;31(4):586–94.
25. Basu RK, Kaddourah A, Goldstein SL. Assessment of a renal angina index for prediction of severe acute kidney injury in critically ill children: a multicentre, multinational, prospective observational study. Lancet Child Adolesc Health. 2018;2(2):112–20.
26. Hanson HR, Carlisle MA, Bensman RS, Byczkowski T, Depinet H, Terrell TC, et al. Early prediction of pediatric acute kidney injury from the emergency department: a pilot study. Am J Emerg Med. 2020;40:138.
27. Goldstein SL, Krallman KA, Kirby C, Roy JP, Collins M, Fox K, et al. Integration of the renal angina index and urine neutrophil gelatinase-associated lipocalin improves severe acute kidney injury prediction in critically ill children and young adults. Kidney Int Rep. 2022;7(8):1842–9.

28. Akcan-Arikan A, Gebhard DJ, Arnold MA, Loftis LL, Kennedy CE. Fluid overload and kidney injury score: a multidimensional real-time assessment of renal disease burden in the critically ill patient. Pediatr Crit Care Med. 2017;18(6):524–30.
29. Fuhrman D. The use of diagnostic tools for pediatric AKI: applying the current evidence to the bedside. Pediatr Nephrol. 2021;36(11):3529–37.
30. James MT, Garg AX. Acute kidney injury: do electronic alerts for AKI improve outcomes? Nat Rev Nephrol. 2015;11(6):322–3.
31. Lachance P, Villeneuve PM, Rewa OG, Wilson FP, Selby NM, Featherstone RM, et al. Association between e-alert implementation for detection of acute kidney injury and outcomes: a systematic review. Nephrol Dial Transplant. 2017;32(2):265–72.
32. Kashani KB. Automated acute kidney injury alerts. Kidney Int. 2018;94(3):484–90.
33. Kolhe NV, Staples D, Reilly T, Merrison D, Mcintyre CW, Fluck RJ, et al. Impact of compliance with a care bundle on acute kidney injury outcomes: a prospective observational study. PLoS One. 2015;10(7):e0132279.
34. Wilson FP, Shashaty M, Testani J, Aqeel I, Borovskiy Y, Ellenberg SS, et al. Automated, electronic alerts for acute kidney injury: a single-blind, parallel-group, randomised controlled trial. Lancet. 2015;385(9981):1966–74.
35. Wilson FP, Martin M, Yamamoto Y, Partridge C, Moreira E, Arora T, et al. Electronic health record alerts for acute kidney injury: multicenter, randomized clinical trial. BMJ. 2021;372:m4786.
36. Hodgson LE, Roderick PJ, Venn RM, Yao GL, Dimitrov BD, Forni LG. The ICE-AKI study: impact analysis of a clinical prediction rule and electronic AKI alert in general medical patients. PLoS One. 2018;13(8):e0200584.
37. Selby NM, Casula A, Lamming L, Stoves J, Samarasinghe Y, Lewington AJ, et al. An organizational-level program of intervention for AKI: a pragmatic stepped wedge cluster randomized trial. J Am Soc Nephrol. 2019;30(3):505–15.
38. Bhojani S, Stojanovic J, Melhem N, Maxwell H, Houtman P, Hall A, et al. The incidence of paediatric acute kidney injury identified using an AKI E-alert algorithm in six English hospitals. Front Pediatr. 2020;8:29.
39. Welch HK, Kellum JA, Kane-Gill SL. Drug-associated acute kidney injury identified in the United States food and drug administration adverse event reporting system database. Pharmacotherapy. 2018;38(8):785–93.
40. Goldstein SL, Kirkendall E, Nguyen H, Schaffzin JK, Bucuvalas J, Bracke T, et al. Electronic health record identification of nephrotoxin exposure and associated acute kidney injury. Pediatrics. 2013;132(3):e756–67.
41. Goldstein SL, Mottes T, Simpson K, Barclay C, Muething S, Haslam DB, et al. A sustained quality improvement program reduces nephrotoxic medication-associated acute kidney injury. Kidney Int. 2016;90(1):212–21.
42. Uber AM, Montez-Rath ME, Kwiatkowski DM, Krawczeski CD, Sutherland SM. Nephrotoxin exposure and acute kidney injury in critically ill children undergoing congenital cardiac surgery. Pediatr Nephrol. 2018;33(11):2193–9.
43. Stoops C, Stone S, Evans E, Dill L, Henderson T, Griffin R, et al. Baby NINJA (Nephrotoxic Injury Negated by Just-in-Time Action): reduction of nephrotoxic medication-associated acute kidney injury in the neonatal intensive care unit. J Pediatr. 2019;215:223–8.e6.
44. Goldstein SL, Dahale D, Kirkendall ES, Mottes T, Kaplan H, Muething S, et al. A prospective multi-center quality improvement initiative (NINJA) indicates a reduction in nephrotoxic acute kidney injury in hospitalized children. Kidney Int. 2020;97(3):580–8.
45. Mottes T, Menon S, Conroy A, Jetton J, Dolan K, Arikan AA, et al. Pediatric AKI in the real world: changing outcomes through education and advocacy—a report from the 26th Acute Disease Quality Initiative (ADQI) consensus conference. Pediatr Nephrol. 2024;39(3):1005–14.
46. Bellos I, Iliopoulos DC, Perrea DN. Association of postoperative fluid overload with adverse outcomes after congenital heart surgery: a systematic review and dose-response meta-analysis. Pediatr Nephrol. 2020;35(6):1109–19.
47. Alobaidi R, Morgan C, Basu RK, Stenson E, Featherstone R, Majumdar SR, et al. Association between fluid balance and outcomes in critically ill children: a systematic review and meta-analysis. JAMA Pediatr. 2018;172(3):257–68.

48. Selewski DT, Barhight MF, Bjornstad EC, Ricci Z, de Sousa TM, Akcan-Arikan A, et al. Fluid assessment, fluid balance, and fluid overload in sick children: a report from the Pediatric Acute Disease Quality Initiative (ADQI) conference. Pediatr Nephrol. 2024;39(3):955–79.
49. Joannidis M, Klein SJ, Ostermann M. 10 myths about frusemide. Intensive Care Med. 2019;45(4):545–8.
50. Ricci Z, Haiberger R, Pezzella C, Garisto C, Favia I, Cogo P. Furosemide versus ethacrynic acid in pediatric patients undergoing cardiac surgery: a randomized controlled trial. Crit Care. 2015;19:2.
51. Chawla LS, Davison DL, Brasha-Mitchell E, Koyner JL, Arthur JM, Shaw AD, et al. Development and standardization of a furosemide stress test to predict the severity of acute kidney injury. Crit Care. 2013;17(5):R207.
52. Koyner JL, Davison DL, Brasha-Mitchell E, Chalikonda DM, Arthur JM, Shaw AD, et al. Furosemide stress test and biomarkers for the prediction of AKI severity. J Am Soc Nephrol. 2015;26(8):2023–31.
53. Rewa OG, Bagshaw SM, Wang X, Wald R, Smith O, Shapiro J, et al. The furosemide stress test for prediction of worsening acute kidney injury in critically ill patients: a multicenter, prospective, observational study. J Crit Care. 2019;52:109–14.
54. Chen JJ, Chang CH, Huang YT, Kuo G. Furosemide stress test as a predictive marker of acute kidney injury progression or renal replacement therapy: a systemic review and meta-analysis. Crit Care. 2020;24(1):202.
55. Penk J, Gist KM, Wald EL, Kitzmiller L, Webb TN, Li Y, et al. Furosemide response predicts acute kidney injury in children after cardiac surgery. J Thorac Cardiovasc Surg. 2019;157(6):2444–51.
56. Starr MC, Banks R, Reeder RW, Fitzgerald JC, Pollack MM, Meert KL, et al. Severe acute kidney injury is associated with increased risk of death and new morbidity after pediatric septic shock. Pediatr Crit Care Med. 2020;21:e686.
57. Fitzgerald JC, Basu RK, Akcan-Arikan A, Izquierdo LM, Piñeres Olave BE, Hassinger AB, et al. Acute kidney injury in pediatric severe sepsis: an independent risk factor for death and new disability. Crit Care Med. 2016;44(12):2241–50.
58. Lankadeva YR, Kosaka J, Evans RG, Bailey SR, Bellomo R, May CN. Intrarenal and urinary oxygenation during norepinephrine resuscitation in ovine septic acute kidney injury. Kidney Int. 2016;90(1):100–8.
59. Lankadeva YR, Kosaka J, Evans RG, Bellomo R, May CN. Urinary oxygenation as a surrogate measure of medullary oxygenation during angiotensin II therapy in septic acute kidney injury. Crit Care Med. 2018;46(1):e41–8.
60. Tumlin JA, Murugan R, Deane AM, Ostermann M, Busse LW, Ham KR, et al. Outcomes in patients with vasodilatory shock and renal replacement therapy treated with intravenous angiotensin II. Crit Care Med. 2018;46(6):949–57.
61. Cho JS, Shim JK, Soh S, Kim MK, Kwak YL. Perioperative dexmedetomidine reduces the incidence and severity of acute kidney injury following valvular heart surgery. Kidney Int. 2016;89(3):693–700.
62. Kwiatkowski DM, Axelrod DM, Sutherland SM, Tesoro TM, Krawczeski CD. Dexmedetomidine is associated with lower incidence of acute kidney injury after congenital heart surgery. Pediatr Crit Care Med. 2016;17(2):128–34.
63. Bellos I, Iliopoulos DC, Perrea DN. Pharmacological interventions for the prevention of acute kidney injury after pediatric cardiac surgery: a network meta-analysis. Clin Exp Nephrol. 2019;23(6):782–91.
64. Soh S, Shim JK, Song JW, Bae JC, Kwak YL. Effect of dexmedetomidine on acute kidney injury after aortic surgery: a single-centre, placebo-controlled, randomised controlled trial. Br J Anaesth. 2020;124:386.
65. Sanfilippo F, Knight JB, Scolletta S, Santonocito C, Pastore F, Lorini FL, et al. Levosimendan for patients with severely reduced left ventricular systolic function and/or low cardiac output syndrome undergoing cardiac surgery: a systematic review and meta-analysis. Crit Care. 2017;21(1):252.
66. Guerrero Orriach JL, Navarro Arce I, Hernandez Rodriguez P, Raigón Ponferrada A, Malo Manso A, Ramirez Aliaga M, et al. Preservation of renal function in cardiac surgery patients with low cardiac output syndrome: levosimendan vs beta agonists. BMC Anesthesiol. 2019;19(1):212.

67. Ricci Z, Stazi GV, Di Chiara L, Morelli S, Vitale V, Giorni C, et al. Fenoldopam in newborn patients undergoing cardiopulmonary bypass: controlled clinical trial. Interact Cardiovasc Thorac Surg. 2008;7(6):1049–53.
68. Costello JM, Thiagarajan RR, Dionne RE, Allan CK, Booth KL, Burmester M, et al. Initial experience with fenoldopam after cardiac surgery in neonates with an insufficient response to conventional diuretics. Pediatr Crit Care Med. 2006;7(1):28–33.
69. Ricci Z, Luciano R, Favia I, Garisto C, Muraca M, Morelli S, et al. High-dose fenoldopam reduces postoperative neutrophil gelatinase-associated lipocaline and cystatin C levels in pediatric cardiac surgery. Crit Care. 2011;15(3):R160.
70. Harer MW, Askenazi DJ, Boohaker LJ, Carmody JB, Griffin RL, Guillet R, et al. Association between early caffeine citrate administration and risk of acute kidney injury in preterm neonates: results from the AWAKEN study. JAMA Pediatr. 2018;172(6):e180322.
71. Van Driest SL, Jooste EH, Shi Y, Choi L, Darghosian L, Hill KD, et al. Association between early postoperative acetaminophen exposure and acute kidney injury in pediatric patients undergoing cardiac surgery. JAMA Pediatr. 2018;172(7):655–63.
72. Wong Vega M, Starr MC, Brophy PD, Devarajan P, Soranno DE, Akcan-Arikan A, et al. Advances in pediatric acute kidney injury pharmacology and nutrition: a report from the 26th Acute Disease Quality Initiative (ADQI) consensus conference. Pediatr Nephrol. 2024;39(3):981–92.
73. Hoste EAJ, Kellum JA, Selby NM, Zarbock A, Palevsky PM, Bagshaw SM, et al. Global epidemiology and outcomes of acute kidney injury. Nat Rev Nephrol. 2018;14(10):607–25.
74. Sawhney S, Marks A, Fluck N, Levin A, McLernon D, Prescott G, et al. Post-discharge kidney function is associated with subsequent ten-year renal progression risk among survivors of acute kidney injury. Kidney Int. 2017;92(2):440–52.
75. Gallagher M, Cass A, Bellomo R, Finfer S, Gattas D, Lee J, et al. Long-term survival and dialysis dependency following acute kidney injury in intensive care: extended follow-up of a randomized controlled trial. PLoS Med. 2014;11(2):e1001601.
76. Uber AM, Sutherland SM. Acute kidney injury in hospitalized children: consequences and outcomes. Pediatr Nephrol. 2020;35(2):213–20.
77. Menon S, Kirkendall ES, Nguyen H, Goldstein SL. Acute kidney injury associated with high nephrotoxic medication exposure leads to chronic kidney disease after 6 months. J Pediatr. 2014;165(3):522–7.e2.
78. Hessey E, Ali R, Dorais M, Morissette G, Pizzi M, Rink N, et al. Renal function follow-up and renal recovery after acute kidney injury in critically ill children. Pediatr Crit Care Med. 2017;18(8):733–40.
79. Harer MW, Pope CF, Conaway MR, Charlton JR. Follow-up of Acute kidney injury in Neonates during Childhood Years (FANCY): a prospective cohort study. Pediatr Nephrol. 2017;32(6):1067–76.
80. Greenberg JH, Zappitelli M, Devarajan P, Thiessen-Philbrook HR, Krawczeski C, Li S, et al. Kidney outcomes 5 years after pediatric cardiac surgery: the TRIBE-AKI study. JAMA Pediatr. 2016;170(11):1071–8.
81. Mehta R, Bihorac A, Selby NM, Quan H, Goldstein SL, Kellum JA, et al. Establishing a continuum of acute kidney injury—tracing AKI using data source linkage and long-term follow-up: workgroup statements from the 15th ADQI Consensus Conference. Can J Kidney Health Dis. 2016;3:102.
82. Calderon-Margalit R, Golan E, Twig G, Leiba A, Tzur D, Afek A, et al. History of childhood kidney disease and risk of adult end-stage renal disease. N Engl J Med. 2018;378(5):428–38.
83. Robinson CH, Jeyakumar N, Luo B, Wald R, Garg AX, Nash DM, et al. Long-term kidney outcomes following dialysis-treated childhood acute kidney injury: a population-based cohort study. J Am Soc Nephrol. 2021;32(8):2005–19.
84. Hessey E, Morissette G, Lacroix J, Perreault S, Samuel S, Dorais M, et al. Healthcare utilization after acute kidney injury in the pediatric intensive care unit. Clin J Am Soc Nephrol. 2018;13(5):685–92.
85. Neumayr TM, Bayrakci B, Chanchlani R, Deep A, Morgan J, Arikan AA, et al. Programs and processes for advancing pediatric acute kidney support therapy in hospitalized and critically ill children: a report from the 26th Acute Disease Quality Initiative (ADQI) consensus conference. Pediatr Nephrol. 2024;39(3):993–1004.

Further Reading

Deep A, Goldstein S, editors. Critical care nephrology and renal replacement therapy in children. Springer; 2018.
Ronco C, Kellum JA, Bellomo R, Ricci Z. The critical care nephrology book. 3rd ed. Elsevier; 2012.

Additional Resources

NephTwitterArchive.com.

The Gut

Frédéric V. Valla and Corinne Jotterand Chaparro

Contents

J. Brierley et al. (eds.), *ESPNIC Children's Intensive Care Textbook*,
https://doi.org/10.1007/978-3-031-64762-8_23

Learning Objectives

Readers will learn how gut function adapts during critical illness and how it may be impaired as a consequence of critical illness; we will mainly focus on gut motility issues which impact on feed tolerance, and on the role of the microbiota in this particular setting.

23.1 Introduction

The main function of the gut is to digest and assimilate feeds, to maintain corporeal homeostasis. Besides, the gut is also one of the major barriers that protects the body from its environment and from various pathogens. Finally, the gut hosts the intestinal microbiota which is now recognised as a major player in homeostasis and immunological defence. In the acutely ill child, gut function may be altered, directly after gut injury (trauma, ischaemia, infection, drug toxicity, etc.) or indirectly in case of gut cell hypoxia (haemodynamic failure, acute respiratory distress syndrome, multiple organ failure, severe oedema, etc.), which will impact on all the functions cited above. Other factors (e.g. sedative drugs, antibiotics and immobility) which are frequently encountered in paediatric intensive care units (PICUs) also affect gut structure and gut motility, which may lead to GI symptoms.

This chapter begins with a brief overview of gut functions and addresses gut dysfunctions in critically ill children including gut dysmotility. We will discuss the main gastrointestinal symptoms, their causes, prevention and treatment, and review the available data on gut microbiota including the role of probiotics supplementation.

23.2 The Gut: A Key Organ of Nutrition Physiology

The gut is responsible for feed digestion and nutrient absorption. Oral feeds or enteral feeding provide complex macronutrients (carbohydrates, proteins, and lipids) which are transformed into small nutrients by digestive enzymes, and micronutrients (vitamins and trace elements), electrolytes, minerals and water. All absorbed nutrients will enter the global body pool to be metabolised, being incorporated in complex molecules (amino acids, lipids, carbohydrates, trace elements, etc.), serving as co-enzymes (e.g. vitamins), or serving as energy sources (carbohydrates, lipids, and amino acids).

The digestion begins with salivary enzyme action on nutrients and continues along the GI tract until simple nutrients are absorbed. Each organ of the GI tract has specific and complex roles. The stomach acts as a reservoir for food and has a motor and a secretory function (alkaline mucus, hydrochloric acid, pepsin, intrinsic factor, gastric lipase, etc.) [1]. The contractions of the stomach and the pylorus mix the food content and regulate the flow so that it will be released into the duodenum at a slow rate that is optimal for digestion and absorption. This regulatory function must be taken into account in patients who are post-pyloric fed: nutrition solution osmolarity should be controlled and bolus feeding avoided to prevent dumping syndrome occurrence.

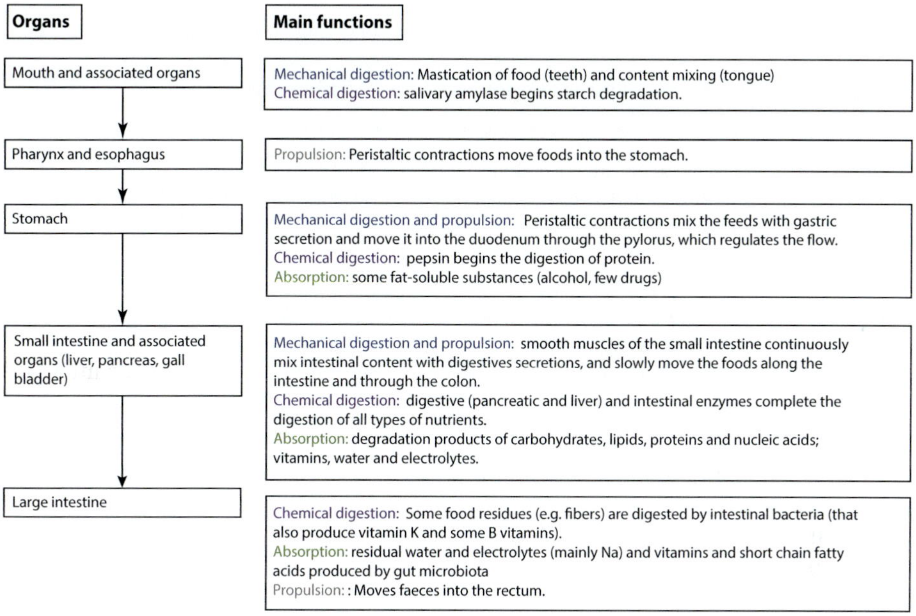

Fig. 23.1 Main functions of the organs of the GI tract, adapted from Marieb & Hoehn [3]

Most of digestion and absorption processes occur in the small intestine with the actions of the pancreatic, biliary and intestinal secretions [2]. The small intestine receives 6–10 L of chyme (nutrition and gut secretions) per day, but only 0.5–1 L will enter the colon: almost all nutrients, 80% of electrolytes and most of the water are absorbed by the small intestine (Fig. 23.1).

Large flows of water are secreted in the proximal digestive tract to dilute oral/enteral feeds. Na^+, K^+, Cl^-, and HCO^{3-} are also excreted in large amounts in various digestive fluids (Tables 23.1 and 23.2). The composition of gut secretion should be taken into consideration in children with gut resection, stomia, gut drainage, biliary drainage, continuous gastric suctioning, etc., as nutrient losses may lead to nutrient deficiencies. Monitoring of electrolyte plasma levels is recommended, and supplementation should be adapted based on the type of intestinal losses.

In case of intestinal failure, digestion and absorption functions may be altered [4]. If this phenomenon lasts, it may lead to malnutrition and severe nutritional deficiencies. Parenteral nutrition, which is usually indicated in case of intestinal failure, bypasses the gut, providing nutrients intravenously, but its indications and optimal timing in PICU are still debated. Early parenteral nutrition may be associated with an increase in adverse outcomes in critically ill children [5, 6]. Enteral nutrition (EN) should remain the first-line nutritional therapy in PICU when oral nutrition is not possible. Providing adequate amounts of nutrition has been shown to improve outcomes; both underfeeding and overfeeding are harmful in this setting [7, 8].

Table 23.1 H_2O, Na and K secretion and absorption throughout the intestine

	Intakes and significant endogenous secretions	Gut absorption
H_2O	Oral/enteral nutrition/hydration Saliva (0.7–1 L/d in adults) Gastric secretions (1.5–3.5 L/d in adults) Pancreatic and biliary secretions (2.2–3.7 L/d in adults)	Continuous absorption throughout the intestine: 90% reabsorption at the end of the colon
Na^+	Oral/enteral nutrition/hydration Saliva (15 mmol/d in adults) Gastric secretions (125 mmol/d in adults) Pancreatic Secretions (350 mmol/d in adults) Biliary secretions (105 mmol/d in adults)	Continuous absorption throughout the intestine: 99% reabsorption at the end of the colon
K^+	Oral/enteral nutrition/hydration Saliva (15 mmol/d in adults) Gastric secretions (35 mmol/d in adults)	Continuous absorption throughout the intestine, mainly in duodenum and jejunum: 85% reabsorption at the end of the colon

Table 23.2 Main electrolytes contained in various digestive tract fluids

Saliva	H_2O, Na^+, K^+, Cl^-, HCO_3^-
Gastric secretions	H_2O, HCl, K^+
Biliary secretions	H_2O, HCO_3^-

23.3 Gut Dysfunction in Critically Ill Children

The digestion of macronutrients requires gut enzyme secretion and gut motility to transfer feeds from the upper digestive tract to the small intestine where absorption occurs. Both secretion and motility function can be altered during critical illness.

- **Enzyme production and secretion may be reduced**. However, enzyme supplementation is not recommended for the critically ill child. Semi-elemental enteral formulas (or elemental formulas) which correspond to "pre-digested feeds" are not recommended as first-line nutritional support but in case of patient history such as chronic enteropathy or feed allergy [7].

  Severe pancreatitis is not a contraindication to enteral feeding nor to the use of polymeric enteral formula. In this particular setting, pancreatic enzymes are still produced in sufficient amounts to allow the digesting of macronutrients. Fasting or use of semi-elemental nutrition should only be proposed in case of polymeric feed intolerance or in case of increased abdominal pain in relation to enteral feeding.

- **Gut motility is severely altered in critically ill children**. Multiple factors have been identified in adult, neonatal or paediatric studies:
  - ***Gut hormone secretion shift***: Increased secretion of ghrelin, motilin, cholecystokinin, peptide-YY, and glucagon-like peptide 1 will lead to altered migrating motor complex, proximal to distal stomach motor discoordination, decreased phasic contractions, and antroduodenal discoordination [9, 10].
  - ***Use of drugs*** impacting on gut motility: opioids and benzodiazepines.
  - ***Fasting and delayed administration of EN.***
  - ***Total parenteral nutrition:*** in volunteers, total parenteral nutrition is associated with altered gut motility and morphology.
  - ***Immobility, decubitus.***
  - ***Electrolyte disturbances*** (dyskaliaemia, dysphosphoraemia, dysmagnesaemia). Fluid overload as well as potassium and magnesium disturbances have been associated with slowing of gastric emptying in adult after surgery [9].
  - ***Mechanical ventilation:*** The mechanism by which positive pressure ventilation affects gut motility in critically ill patients is poorly understood and likely multifactorial. Reduced gastric blood flow has been observed in neonates on continuous positive pressure [11].
  - ***Effect of inflammation and disease.*** Conditions of critical illness such as hemodynamic instability, multiple organ failure, multi-trauma, or shock have been identified as high-risk factors for gut dysmotility [9]. A recent prospective pilot study has examined the associations between post-operative changes in inflammatory cytokines, markers of gut barrier integrity, gastric emptying and zonulin (reversible regulator of gut barrier tight junctions) in 20 critically ill children (median age 14 years) [12].

> Gut dysfunction, mostly gut dysmotility, is common in critically ill children. This is mainly due to PICU conditions and to various drugs commonly used in PICU.

23.4 Main Symptoms of GI Dysfunction in Critically Ill Children: Prevalence, Causes, Prevention and Treatments

Symptoms of GI dysfunction are common in critically ill patients [13, 14]. Altered GI motility is the principal mechanism underlying delayed gastric emptying, ileus and constipation [14].

The published occurrence rate of GI symptoms and complications in critically ill children varies due to the absence of a consensus in their definitions. Lopez et al. have found that constipation occurred in 47% of 150 children (mean age, 34 months) [13]. The major factors associated with constipation were higher body weight and severity score, post-surgery admission, and vasoconstrictor therapy. In a recent study, Martinez et al. observed that the majority of children had delayed gastric emptying and that delayed gastric emptying predicted slow EN advancement [15].

Diarrhoea is also common in PICU: the first bowel opening, that usually happens 2–3 days after admission, often consists of loose/watery stools. Lasting diarrhoea is rarely a sign of feeding intolerance but rather the consequence of non-feed related issues such as infection (e.g. clostridium difficile) or withdrawal syndrome.

Gut dysmotility will impact on PICU complications (aspiration and ventilator-associated pneumonia occurrence rates are increased in case of gastric delayed emptying), on nutritional intake and on malnutrition occurrence during PICU stay. GI symptoms and complications should be prevented proactively, detected early and actively treated (◘ Table 23.3). Consensus must be reached on the definition of the criteria of excessive gastric residues, constipation and diarrhoea.

GI symptoms and complications, more specifically delayed gastric emptying and constipation, are frequent in critically ill children and mostly due to gut dysmotility. These should be diagnosed early, treated proactively and prevented. Early enteral feeding is recommended following local written guidance.

◘ **Table 23.3** Main GI symptoms occurring during critical illness in children

	Cause	Prevention	Treatment
Delayed gastric emptying	Gut hormone secretion shift Electrolyte disturbances Opioids, benzodiazepines	Correct K, P and Mg plasma levels Limit sedative drugs Limit enteral feeding osmolarity (prefer non-enriched and polymeric feeds)	Use prokinetics (erythromycin) Use post-pyloric tube feeding
Ileus	Gut hormone secretion shift Electrolyte disturbances Opioids, benzodiazepines	Correct K, P and Mg plasma levels Limit sedative drugs	Use prokinetics (erythromycin)
Constipation	Opioids, benzodiazepines Fasting Microbiota disturbance	Limit sedative drugs Use enteral nutrition with fibres Laxatives	Laxatives, enemas
Diarrhoea	Infection (clostridium difficile colitis) Withdrawal syndrome Post constipation diarrhoea Microbiota disturbance	Limit antibiotic use Prevent withdrawal syndrome Use EN with both hydro and non-hydro soluble fibres	Confirm and treat clostridium difficile infection Treat withdrawal syndrome

23.5 Enteral Feeding Intolerance as a Result of GI Dysfunction

EN intolerance may be the result of an underlying disease or of a side effect of some treatments used in critical care. Eveleens et al. have recently proposed a definition of feeding intolerance that still requires validation in future studies [16]. (◘ Table 23.4).

However, it is important, as highlighted by Tume et al. to distinguish feed related intestinal symptoms which may require feeding interruption, to non-feed related symptoms whose treatment should rather be based on the identification and treatment of its cause (withdrawal syndrome, gut infection, tracheal tube related coughing, etc.) [17].

The utility of gastric residual volume (GRV) assessment is currently being reconsidered. In adult critically ill patients, GRV measurement did not protect from aspiration and ventilator-associated pneumonia but reduced nutritional intakes [18]. In both adult [19] and children [15], no correlation was observed between high GRV and EN intolerance or delayed gastric emptying.

In paediatrics, no randomised control trial has been published so far, but an observational study found no difference on vomiting, ventilation-associated pneumonia and nutrition goal achievement between two centres: one using GRV as standard practice and the other centre not using it [20]. Besides, laboratory studies question the accuracy of suctioning stomach content, in relation to the technique used (suction level, syringe size, stomach content thickness, tube material, etc.) [21]. The latest nutrition guidelines for critically ill children and adults do not recommend the routine measurement of GRV to drive EN advancement decisions [7, 22].

◘ Table 23.4 Proposed definition by Eveleens et al. for enteral feeding intolerance in critically ill children in whom EN is indicated and attempted [16]

1. Insufficient enteral intake	Two-third of prescribed daily target or EN is withheld for >48 h or EN is not increased for >48 h Excluding interruptions due to procedures
AND 2. At least one of the following GI symptoms:	
(a) GI symptoms	
Large Gastric residual volume (GRV)	>50% of the EN delivered in the last 4 h
Vomiting	>2 times with gastric content in 24 h period
Diarrhoea	>4 times loose stool with negative fluid balance in 24 h period
(b) Severe GI symptoms with concern for intestinal ischaemia	Abdominal distention, abdominal pain, melena, haematochezia

Enteral feeding intolerance may occur in critically ill children. It is, however, important to distinguish GI symptoms related to feeds which may require feeding interruption, from non-feed-related symptoms, whose treatment should rather be based on the identification and treatment of their cause.

23.6 Gut Damages in Case of Critical Illness

The gut may be damaged, like any other organ, while facing hemodynamic failure or respiratory failure (i.e. gut cell hypoxia). Regional hypoxia may alter and/or destroy gut cells, but we are still lacking accurate, specific biomarkers of gut failure [4]. In a study assessing abdominal NIRS monitoring (near-infrared spectroscopy), Kaufman et al. found a correlation of NIRS with SvO2 and plasma lactates in critically ill children [23]. However, the impact of critical illness on gut perfusion remains unclear. Sim et al. reported in critically ill adults that fasting small intestinal blood flow was 50% greater in hemodynamically stable patients (which is the opposite of what is currently found in fasting healthy subjects) [24]. However, the expected increment in blood flow in response to the small intestinal infusion of nutrients was decreased, and the increment was related to small intestinal glucose absorption; this suggests this may contribute to, or be a result of, reduced absorption. Oedema and overhydration may also impact on gut absorption function, and strict fluid balance monitoring may also help maintain gut function.

Sertaridou et al. have recently published a review paper on gut failure in critically ill patients [25]. They proposed a concept that first involves visceral hypoperfusion, which releases gut-derived proinflammatory factors. Then, haemodynamic resuscitation leads to ischaemia-reperfusion gut injury, loss of gut barrier function (increase in gut inflammatory response) and bacterial and endotoxin crossing of mucosal barrier. Finally, the release of chemokines and cytokines leads to systemic inflammatory response syndrome and multiple organ dysfunction syndrome. Events occurring as the normal intestinal barrier becomes impaired in sepsis, ischaemia and other harmful conditions: enterocytes go on to apoptosis, tight junctions are breached and microbes penetrate the intestinal wall. The latter are further taken up by phagocytes, innate immune receptors are activated, chemokines and proinflammatory cytokines are released, innate and adaptive immune cells are attracted to the site, and the immune response is further propagated.

Health care professionals fear gut complications in case of haemodynamic instability and especially the occurrence of gut ischaemia or necrotising enterocolitis (NEC). Real gut ischaemia is however rarely reported in children. NEC is a well describe condition in preterm infants, but remains rare in PICUs. New-borns and children with a history of congenital heart disease (CHD) are at higher risk of NEC, but its severity and occurrence rate reported in various studies remain low [26, 27].

The implication of enteral feeding in NEC occurrence is still unclear but recent international guidelines on critically ill children nutrition do not contra-indicate EN in stabilised children on vaso-active medications or extracorporeal hemodynamic support, or in children receiving prostaglandin to maintain the ductus arteriosus open [7, 8]. Close monitoring of feeding tolerance is, however recommended, as detailed above.

The Pediatric Organ Dysfunction Information Update Mandate (PODIUM) Collaborative recently developed consensus criteria to define GI dysfunction in critically ill children [28]. The experts found that a definition for paediatric GI dysfunction necessitates use of signs and symptoms of GI dysfunction rather than biomarkers or specific scoring systems to directly interrogate loss of primary GI functions. They proposed the following criteria for severe GI dysfunction (which was a weak recommendation): 1a) bowel perforation, 1b) pneumatosis intestinalis, or 1c) bowel ischaemia, present on plain abdominal radiograph, computed tomography scan, magnetic resonance imaging, or gross surgical inspection, or 2) rectal sloughing of gut mucosa. There was insufficient evidence to define consensus criteria to diagnose mild or moderate GI dysfunction [28].

Like any other organ, the gut may be damaged in case of circulatory or respiratory failure. However, severe complications remain rare in critically ill children.

23.7 Children with History of Intestinal Condition

Some children presenting with a history of altered gut conditions deserve some particular attention.

Children presenting with CHD are often malnourished because of swallowing issues, eating fatigability due to heart and respiratory chronic failure, fluid restriction, and slight malabsorption in relation to gut mucosa oedema. CHD is not a contraindication to EN in PICU, but as the occurrence rate of NEC is higher in this population, strict monitoring of feeding tolerance is required [26, 27].

In case of a history of malabsorption or feed intolerance or allergy, the common recommendation of providing polymeric feeds as first-line feeding regimen should of course be adapted to the specific needs of each child [7].

Special attention should be paid on children with congenital heart diseases, as they are a high risk group for feeding intolerance and gut complications.

23.8 The Gut Microbiota

23.8.1 The Role of Gut Microbiota

The gut hosts between 10^{12} and 10^{14} bacteria and yeasts which constitute the gut microbiota. The gut microbiota is strongly involved in overall homeostasis, as it protects the host from infections, interacts in various physiological pathways, impacts on metabolic status, modulates immune responses at systemic sites, and contributes to energy supply and carbohydrate, lipid and protein homeostasis and metabolism [29–31]. The gut microbiota is composed of various bacterial species in balanced proportions (symbiosis). The gut is also one of the major immune-competent organs: it contains more immunological tissues and lymphocytes than any other organ. Its interaction with gut microbiota allows for immune signalisation, defence, and tolerance processes. The optimal balance, composition and function of gut microflora depend on food intake (fermentable fibres and complex proteins) and may fluctuate in case of antibiotic use, diarrhoeas, and during critical illness.

23.8.2 Impact of Critical Illness on Gut Microbiota

Critical illness has been shown to alter gut integrity by increasing epithelial apoptosis and permeability and by decreasing epithelial proliferation and mucus integrity [32]. This is related to an imbalance of the gut microbiota composition due to the use of antibiotics and other drugs that alter the microbiota environment. This is also probably due to other factors like local hemodynamic failure and cell hypoxia in case of global circulatory or respiratory failure. This impairs the gut-microbiota symbiosis (gut dysbiosis) and the microbiota-host beneficial interaction, while virulence factors enhanced in the microbiome can perpetuate or worsen critical illness, impacting on distant organs. Local inflammation can also be worsened by an altered microbiota [33]. Observational studies have shown highly heterogeneous patterns of intestinal microbiota in both septic and non-septic critically ill patients. Nevertheless, some general patterns were observed, including disappearance of bacterial genera with important functions in host metabolism [34]. Limited data is currently available in critically ill children. Wijeyesekera et al. have published a large observational study confirming the occurrence of a functional activity disruption of the intestinal microbiome in critically ill children [35], which may result in worsening organ failure. The same group explored the time course of the relationship between the microbiome and bile acid profile in faecal samples. The findings suggested that gut microbiota recovery can be readily assessed via measurement of faecal bile acids in critically ill children [36].

23.8.3 The Promising Effect of Nutrition and Probiotics in Critical Care

EN may be able to help preserve the gut microbiota balance, but this needs to be further investigated in large trials. Prebiotics and probiotics may also play a role to maintain the symbiosis between the microbiota and its host, but there is currently limited evidence. In preterm neonates, a systematic review and meta-analysis including 24 trials concluded that probiotic supplementation prevents severe necrotising enterocolitis (NEC) and reduces all-cause mortality [37]. The ESPGHAN Working Group for Probiotics and Prebiotics published a document using a network meta-analysis approach to identify strains with greatest potential efficacy [37] and a position paper in May 2020 [38]. In critically ill adults, evidence is conflicting. Based on 25 randomised controlled trials, a recent meta-analysis demonstrated a significant reduction in incidence of ventilator-associated pneumonia, sepsis, and ICU-acquired infections in patients receiving symbiotics (combination of probiotics and prebiotics) but not in those receiving only probiotics. No impact was observed on mortality, diarrhoea, or length of ICU stay [39]. In critically ill children, only a few studies have been conducted. Their findings suggest that some specific strains of probiotics may be safe and beneficial to reduce the risk of candidaemia, reduce proinflammatory cytokines and increase anti-inflammatory cytokines [40, 41].

Clostridium difficile colitis is a good example of the importance of the gut microbiota; this disease is usually the consequence of the use of antibiotic, allowing the growth of a pathogenic endogenous colony. This can be treated with antibiotics with an active spectrum on clostridium species, but probiotics and even faecal transplantation are now part of the treatment strategy of severe forms.

The gut microbiota may be altered in critically ill children. The use of probiotics or prebiotics seems promising to reduce infection and inflammation but large trials are needed to identify the optimal strains and their dosage, and to confirm their safety.

Take-Home Messages

The gut is responsible for nutrient absorption and should be used as first line (rather than using parenteral nutrition).

- The gut has also a key role in host immune defence and interacts with other organs through multiple metabolic pathways.
- Gut motility is constantly impacted in critical illness; motility issues should be monitored, prevented and treated proactively to ensure feeding tolerance.
- Gut absorption is altered in case of haemodynamic instability, severe hypoxia and severe overhydration, which, however, are not contraindication per se to enteral feeding.
- New-borns and infants with a history of CHD are at higher risk of NEC, but its occurrence rate remains low and EN should be started in these children with adequate monitoring.
- Intestinal failure is an indication of parenteral nutrition, but its optimal timing remains debated in PICU.
- Enteral feeding intolerance may occur in critically ill children. However, before interrupting EN, it is important to distinguish GI symptoms related to feeds from non-feed-related symptoms.
- The gut microbiota is also involved in multiple interactions with its host. This beneficial symbiosis can be altered in critically ill children.
- Probiotics supplementation seems promising to reduce infection and inflammation during critical illness, but large trials are needed to identify the optimal strains and dosage, and to confirm their safety.

References

1. Kiela PR, Ghishan FK. Physiology of intestinal absorption and secretion. Best Pract Res Clin Gastroenterol. 2016;30(2):145–59.
2. Gropper SAS, Smith JL, Carr TP. Advanced nutrition and human metabolism. 7th ed. Boston: Cengage Learning; 2018.
3. Marieb EN, Hoehn K, Dubé S, Desbiens A, Dupont S, Marieb EN. Anatomie et physiologie humaines, Montréal, Canada. 6th ed; 2019.
4. Chapman MJ, Deane AM. Gastrointestinal dysfunction relating to the provision of nutrition in the critically ill. Curr Opin Clin Nutr Metab Care. 2015;18(2):207–12.
5. Fivez T, Kerklaan D, Mesotten D, Verbruggen S, Wouters PJ, Vanhorebeek I, et al. Early versus Late parenteral nutrition in critically ill children. New Engl J Med. 2016;374(12):1111–22.
6. Vanhorebeek I, Verbruggen S, Casaer MP, Gunst J, Wouters PJ, Hanot J, et al. Effect of early supplemental parenteral nutrition in the paediatric ICU: a preplanned observational study of post-randomisation treatments in the PEPaNIC trial. Lancet Respir Med. 2017;5(6):475–83.
7. Tume LN, Valla FV, Joosten K, Chaparro CJ, Latten L, Marino LV, et al. Nutritional support for children during critical illness: European Society of Pediatric and Neonatal Intensive Care (ESPNIC) metabolism, endocrine and nutrition section position statement and clinical recommendations. Intensive Care Med. 2020;46:411–25.
8. Mehta NM, Skillman HE, Irving SY, Coss-Bu JA, Vermilyea S, Farrington EA, et al. Guidelines for the provision and assessment of nutrition support therapy in the pediatric critically ill patient: Society of Critical Care Medicine and American Society for Parenteral and Enteral Nutrition. Pediatr Crit Care Med. 2017;18(7):675–715.
9. Martinez EE, Douglas K, Nurko S, Mehta NM. Gastric dysmotility in critically ill children: pathophysiology, diagnosis, and management. Pediatr Crit Care Med J Soc Crit Care Med World Fed Pediatr Intensive Crit Care Soc. 2015;16(9):828–36.
10. Zaher S, White D, Ridout J, Branco RG, Meyer R, Pathan N. Effect of nutrition status and inflammatory stimuli on ghrelin and peptide-YY levels among critically ill children: a prospective and observational study. JPEN J Parenter Enteral Nutr. 2022;46(6):1298–306.
11. Havranek T, Madramootoo C, Carver JD. Nasal continuous positive airway pressure affects pre- and postprandial intestinal blood flow velocity in preterm infants. J Perinatol Off J Calif Perinat Assoc. 2007;27(11):704–8.
12. Martinez EE, Zurakowski D, Pereira L, Freire R, Emans JB, Nurko S, et al. Interleukin-10 and Zonulin are associated with post-operative delayed gastric emptying in critically ill surgical pediatric patients—a prospective pilot study. JPEN J Parenter Enteral Nutr. 2020;44(8):1407–16.
13. Lopez J, Botran M, Garcia A, Gonzalez R, Solana MJ, Urbano J, et al. Constipation in the critically iii child: frequency and related factors. J Pediatr. 2015;167(4):857.
14. Lopez-Herce CJ. Nutrition in the critically ill child. Pediatr Barc. 2009;71(1):1–4.
15. Martinez EE, Pereira LM, Gura K, Stenquist N, Ariagno K, Nurko S, et al. Gastric emptying in critically ill children. JPEN J Parenter Enteral Nutr. 2017;41(7):1100–9.
16. Eveleens RD, Joosten KFM, de Koning BAE, Hulst JM, Verbruggen SCAT. Definitions, predictors and outcomes of feeding intolerance in critically ill children: a systematic review. Clin Nutr Edinb Scotl. 2020;39(3):685–93.
17. Tume LN, Valla FV. A review of feeding intolerance in critically ill children. Eur J Pediatr. 2018;177(11):1675–83.
18. Reignier J, Mercier E, Le Gouge A, Boulain T, Desachy A, Bellec F, et al. Effect of not monitoring residual gastric volume on risk of ventilator-associated pneumonia in adults receiving mechanical ventilation and early enteral feeding: a randomized controlled trial. JAMA. 2013;309(3):249–56.
19. Cohen J, Aharon A, Singer P. The paracetamol absorption test: a useful addition to the enteral nutrition algorithm? Clin Nutr Edinb Scotl. 2000;19(4):233–6.
20. Tume LN, Bickerdike A, Latten L, Davies S, Lefèvre MH, Nicolas GW, et al. Routine gastric residual volume measurement and energy target achievement in the PICU: a comparison study. Eur J Pediatr. 2017;176(12):1637–44.
21. Bartlett Ellis RJ, Fuehne J. Examination of accuracy in the assessment of gastric residual volume: a simulated, controlled study. JPEN J Parenter Enteral Nutr. 2015;39(4):434–40.

22. McClave SA, Taylor BE, Martindale RG, Warren MM, Johnson DR, Braunschweig C, et al. Guidelines for the provision and assessment of nutrition support therapy in the adult critically ill patient: Society of Critical Care Medicine (SCCM) and American Society for Parenteral and Enteral Nutrition (A.S.P.E.N.). JPEN J Parenter Enteral Nutr. 2016;40(2):159–211.
23. Kaufman J, Almodovar MC, Zuk J, Friesen RH. Correlation of abdominal site near-infrared spectroscopy with gastric tonometry in infants following surgery for congenital heart disease. Pediatr Crit Care Med J Soc Crit Care Med World Fed Pediatr Intensive Crit Care Soc. 2008;9(1):62–8.
24. Sim JA, Horowitz M, Summers MJ, Trahair LG, Goud RS, Zaknic AV, et al. Mesenteric blood flow, glucose absorption and blood pressure responses to small intestinal glucose in critically ill patients older than 65 years. Intensive Care Med. 2013;39(2):258–66.
25. Sertaridou E, Papaioannou V, Kolios G, Pneumatikos I. Gut failure in critical care: old school versus new school. Ann Gastroenterol. 2015;28(3):309–22.
26. Hehir DA, Easley RB, Byrnes J. Noncardiac challenges in the cardiac ICU: feeding, growth and gastrointestinal complications, anticoagulation, and analgesia. World J Pediatr Congenit Heart Surg. 2016;7(2):199–209.
27. Wong JJM, Cheifetz IM, Ong C, Nakao M, Lee JH. Nutrition support for children undergoing congenital heart surgeries: a narrative review. World J Pediatr Congenit Heart Surg. 2015;6(3):443–54.
28. Typpo KV, Irving SY, Prince JM, Pathan N, Brown AM, Pediatric Organ Dysfunction Information Update Mandate (PODIUM) Collaborative. Gastrointestinal dysfunction criteria in critically ill children: the PODIUM consensus conference. Pediatrics. 2022;149(1 Suppl. 1):S53–8.
29. Fujisaka S, Avila-Pacheco J, Soto M, Kostic A, Dreyfuss JM, Pan H, et al. Diet, genetics, and the gut microbiome drive dynamic changes in plasma metabolites. Cell Rep. 2018;22(11):3072–86.
30. Schuijt TJ, van der Poll T, de Vos WM, Wiersinga WJ. The intestinal microbiota and host immune interactions in the critically ill. Trends Microbiol. 2013;21(5):221–9.
31. Morowitz MJ, Carlisle EM, Alverdy JC. Contributions of intestinal bacteria to nutrition and metabolism in the critically ill. Surg Clin North Am. 2011;91(4):771–85. viii
32. Mittal R, Coopersmith CM. Redefining the gut as the motor of critical illness. Trends Mol Med. 2014;20(4):214–23.
33. Ralls MW, Miyasaka E, Teitelbaum DH. Intestinal microbial diversity and perioperative complications. JPEN J Parenter Enteral Nutr. 2014;38(3):392–9.
34. Lankelma JM, van Vught LA, Belzer C, Schultz MJ, van der Poll T, de Vos WM, et al. Critically ill patients demonstrate large interpersonal variation in intestinal microbiota dysregulation: a pilot study. Intensive Care Med. 2017;43(1):59–68.
35. Wijeyesekera A, Wagner J, De Goffau M, Thurston S, Rodrigues Sabino A, Zaher S, et al. Multi-compartment profiling of bacterial and host metabolites identifies intestinal dysbiosis and its functional consequences in the critically ill child. Crit Care Med. 2019;47(9):e727–34.
36. Kean IRL, Wagner J, Wijeyesekera A, De Goffau M, Thurston S, Clark JA, et al. Profiling gut microbiota and bile acid metabolism in critically ill children. Sci Rep. 2022;12(1):10432.
37. AlFaleh K, Anabrees J. Probiotics for prevention of necrotizing enterocolitis in preterm infants. Cochrane Database Syst Rev. 2014;(4):CD005496.
38. van den Akker CHP, van Goudoever JB, Shamir R, Domellöf M, Embleton ND, Hojsak I, et al. Probiotics and preterm infants: a position paper by the European Society for Paediatric Gastroenterology Hepatology and Nutrition Committee on Nutrition and the European Society for Paediatric Gastroenterology Hepatology and Nutrition Working Group for Probiotics and Prebiotics. J Pediatr Gastroenterol Nutr. 2020;70(5):664–80.
39. Wang K, Zeng Q, Li KX, Wang Y, Wang L, Sun MW, et al. Efficacy of probiotics or synbiotics for critically ill adult patients: a systematic review and meta-analysis of randomized controlled trials. Burns Trauma. 2022;10:tkac004.
40. Kumar S, Bansal A, Chakrabarti A, Singhi S. Evaluation of efficacy of probiotics in prevention of candida colonization in a PICU-a randomized controlled trial. Crit Care Med. 2013;41(2):565–72.
41. Angurana SK, Bansal A, Singhi S, Aggarwal R, Jayashree M, Salaria M, et al. Evaluation of effect of probiotics on cytokine levels in critically ill children with severe sepsis: a double-blind, placebo-controlled trial. Crit Care Med. 2018;46(10):1656–64.

Acute Liver Failure in PICU

Gaurang Upadhyay, Emma C. Alexander, and Akash Deep

Contents

J. Brierley et al. (eds.), *ESPNIC Children's Intensive Care Textbook*,
https://doi.org/10.1007/978-3-031-64762-8_24

Learning Objectives

This chapter will cover the definition of paediatric acute liver failure (PALF), aetiology of PALF and various management options for PALF including management of hepatic encephalopathy (HE). It will also discuss liver supportive therapies and also the management of post-liver transplant patients.

24.1 Introduction

Acute liver failure (ALF) is a clinical syndrome in which abrupt liver injury results in massive necrosis of hepatocytes or severe functional impairment of hepatocytes in a previously healthy individual [1, 2]. It affects the synthetic, excretory, and detoxifying functions of the liver individually to varying extent. In some cases, all functions are severely impaired. A preceding nonspecific prodrome may last days or weeks, but once features of ALF are established, the clinical course is dynamic, unpredictable, and sometimes rapidly progressive. Paediatric acute liver failure (PALF) has a life-threatening prognosis due to the risks of cerebral oedema, sepsis and multi-organ failure. Mortality rates were as high as 72% in the pre-transplant era [3], before research into medical management and extracorporeal therapies began in earnest. At present, mortality is around 5–10%, with 20% of children requiring liver transplantation [4].

24.2 Definition of Paediatric Acute Liver Failure

In an effort to address ambiguity associated with the definition of PALF, the PALF study group was formed in 1999, and consists of a consortium of 24 active paediatric hepatology centres [1]. The aim of the consortium was to create a database of children with PALF. The most widely accepted consensus definition for PALF, established by the study group, is as follows:

1. No known evidence of chronic liver disease.
2. Biochemical evidence of acute liver injury.
3. (a) Coagulopathy with international normalized ratio (INR) >1.5 not corrected by vitamin K in the presence of clinical hepatic encephalopathy, or (b) INR >2 regardless of the presence or absence of clinical hepatic encephalopathy.

Some controversy exists around this definition. Firstly, PALF may be the first presentation of a previously unrecognized autoimmune or metabolic liver disease, e.g., Wilson disease or tyrosinaemia type I. Secondly, many cases of hepatic failure in neonates are secondary to an unknown inborn metabolic error or an intrauterine insult, which would represent a pre-existing disease. Thirdly, some children with acute liver failure develop encephalopathy later than 8 weeks into the course of the illness and are defined as having subacute hepatic failure. Fourthly, encephalopathy may be difficult to detect in infants and small children [5, 6]. It is for this reason that the definition of PALF does not require the diagnosis of encephalopathy, unlike for adults with ALF.

24.3 Aetiology

There are a great many potential causes for PALF. A systematic review and large case series have shown that the most common cause of PALF is indeterminate, with hepatitis A common in developing countries [7–9]. In children under 1, metabolic and infectious diseases are particularly common aetiologies for PALF, with herpes simplex virus (HSV) being the most common infectious aetiology. Paracetamol toxicity is the most common cause of drug-induced ALF, accounting for more than three-quarters of drug-induced cases. Determining the aetiology of PALF through a broad investigative screen is vital to improve outcomes, as many causes have disease-specific therapies. Patients whose aetiology is not determined, namely those with indeterminate PALF, tend to have a worse prognosis, and miss the opportunity to receive targeted therapies [10] (◘ Table 24.1).

◘ Table 24.1 Causes of PALF

Infective	Hepatitis A Hepatitis B Hepatitis C Hepatitis D Hepatitis D Hepatitis E Herpes Simplex virus, Cytomegalovirus Epstein-Barr Virus Varicella Adenovirus Entero virus Parvovirus B19 Dengue fever SARS-CoV-2
Metabolic	Galactosaemia Tyrosinaemia Hemochromatosis (in neonate) Wilson disease, Fructose intolerance Fatty-acid oxidation disorder Mitochondrial cytopathy MCAD deficiency Urea cycle defects Congenital disorders of glycosylation Reye syndrome
Toxic	Acetaminophen, Sulfamide Sodium valproate Sulfasalazine
Autoimmune	Autoimmune Hepatitis (AIH) Autoimmune sclerosing Cholangitis (ASC) De Novo AIH after Liver transplant

(continued)

Table 24.1 (continued)

Haematological	Familial lymphohistiocytosis Macrophage activation syndrome Leukaemia NK cell dysfunction
Vascular	Budd Chiari malformation Heart surgery Myocarditis

24.4 Clinical Manifestation

Children who present with features of PALF should undergo a diagnostic evaluation to ascertain the cause of liver failure and the extent of liver injury. All patients should undergo a complete physical examination, including a thorough assessment of their neurological status.

Clinical symptoms and signs of PALF vary according to the aetiology and the age of the patient. In the newborn, symptoms are nonspecific and related to an altered general well-being/condition including sleepiness, vomiting, and eventual jaundice. In older children, most present with jaundice associated with hepatic encephalopathy. In infective PALF, jaundice is usually associated with fever, myalgia, arthralgia, nausea and abdominal pain. Encephalopathy or bleeding can occur before the occurrence of jaundice in some children after drug-, toxin- or metabolic-induced ALF.

24.5 Hepatic Encephalopathy

Hepatic encephalopathy (HE) is a neuropsychiatric syndrome associated with hepatic dysfunction. It is a reversible metabolic encephalopathy associated with variable degrees of brain oedema [11]. The pathogenesis is multifactorial and incompletely understood. A number of interrelated factors are thought to be responsible. Ammonia (NH_3) plays an important role in the development of HE in PALF. Ammonia, a by-product of nitrogen metabolism, is generated in the enterocytes within the small intestine and the colon by the enzyme glutaminase. Glutaminase breaks down glutamine into ammonia and glutamate, along with urease-producing bacteria that inhabit the gut. The gut-derived ammonia enters the urea cycle and is converted to urea and excreted by the kidneys. Ammonia that bypasses the urea cycle is metabolized by glutamine synthase to glutamine in hepatocytes, skeletal myocytes and astroglial cells [12]. Although ammonia plays a critical role in the pathogenesis of HE, the plasma concentrations of ammonia and the clinical manifestations of HE do not always consistently correlate in patients with HE [13].

Astrocytes are the most abundant cells in the brain and are sensitive to the rapid increase of ammonia. As increasing quantities of ammonia are detoxified to glutamine within the astrocytes, intracellular glutamine concentration increases, raising

24

Table 24.2 HE grading for children under 4 years of age: (modified from [1])

Stage	Clinical	Asterixis/reflexes	Neurological signs	EEG changes
Early (I and II)	Inconsolable crying, sleep reversal, inattention to task	Unreliable/ normal or hyperreflexia	Difficult to test Delayed responses and attention span shortened	Normal or mild slowing
Mid (III)	Somnolence, stupor, combativeness	Unreliable-can be decreased, absent or increased	Difficult to test Progressive decrease in response to external stimuli	Mild or moderate background abnormality with slowing
Late (IV)	Comatose, arouses with painful stimuli, or no response	Unreliable—can be decreased, absent or increased	Decerebrate or decorticate	Severe attenuation or slowing

Table 24.3 Stages of hepatic encephalopathy for children older than 4 years old (modified from [13, 17])

Stage	Clinical (mood and mental status)	Reflexes	Neurological signs	EEG changes
1 (prodromal)	Mood swing; euphoria; depression; mild confusion; slowness of mentation and affect; untidiness; slurred speech; disordered sleep	Normal or hyperreflexia	Tremor, apraxia and impaired handwriting	Normal or diffuse slowing
2	Accentuation of stage 1; lethargy; moderate confusion; inappropriate behaviour; inability to maintain sphincter control	Hyperreflexia	Ataxia, dysarthria	Abnormal generalized slowing
3 (stupor)	Marked confusion, sleepy but arousable, incoherent speech	Hyperreflexia	Rigidity	Abnormal generalized slowing
4 (coma)	Comatose, arouses with painful stimuli (4a), or no response to painful stimuli (4b)	Usually, absent	Decerebrate or decorticate posturing	Abnormal, very slow delta activity

Table 24.4 Potential Investigations in PALF

General	Haematology: Complete blood count, Blood type and screen Direct Antiglobulin test Blood film Prothrombin time/INR, PTT, fibrinogen Coagulation factors: V, VII and VII Biochemistry: Sodium, potassium, chloride, bicarbonate, calcium, magnesium, phosphate Blood glucose AST, ALT, alkaline phosphatase, GGT, total bilirubin, albumin Creatinine, blood urea nitrogen Blood gas (ABG) Arterial lactate Amylase and lipase Arterial ammonia level (avoid venous/capillary samples) Alpha-fetoprotein
Infective	Viral hepatitis serology: Anti-HAV IgM antibody, HBsAg, anti-HBc IgM & IgG, HBeAg, anti-HCV (IgM), anti-HEV antibody (IgM) Virology studies (polymerase chain reaction/antibodies as appropriate): Herpes simplex virus, cytomegalovirus, Epstein-Barr virus, varicella, adenovirus, enterovirus, parvovirus B19, dengue fever, SARS-CoV2 Blood culture Urine culture
Metabolic	Screening investigation: Plasma amino acid profile, urine amino acids and organic acid profile Galactosaemia: Galactose-1-phosphate uridyl transferase Tyrosinaemia: Urinary succinyl acetone Gestational alloimmune liver disease (GALD): Serum ferritin, lip biopsy, MRI of liver and pancreas Wilson disease: Ceruloplasmin level, serum copper, 24 h urine copper, copper pre & post-Penicillamine Fatty-acid oxidation disorder: Lactate, lactate/pyruvate ratio, Mitochondrial cytopathy: Quantitative mitochondrial DNA assay, Mutation analysis, lactate, lactate/pyruvate ratio, CK MCAD deficiency: Plasma acylcarnitine Fructose intolerance: Quantitative enzyme assay, q22.3 band mutation in chr 9 Urea cycle defects: Ammonia, serum amino acid profile Congenital disorders of glycosylation: Transferrin electrophoresis
Immune function	Autoimmune hepatitis serology: Antinuclear antibodies (ANCA), anti-smooth antibodies (anti-SMA abs), immunoglobulin levels (IgG), soluble liver antigen, anti-liver kidney microsomal antibody (anti-LKM abs) NK cell function, granzyme B, perforin, sIL2, triglycerides
Histology/ tissue studies	Liver biopsy Muscle biopsy Bone marrow aspirate
Drugs and toxins	Acetaminophen level Urine toxic screen Salicylate level
Radiological investigations	Hepatic ultrasound with Doppler study 2D ECHO (if necessary) CXR

intracellular osmolarity and generating osmotic stress, which leads to an influx of water into astrocytes and resulting in cerebral oedema (CE).

The other potential contributing factors include serotonin neurotransmission, endogenous opioids, neurosteroids, inflammatory cytokines, and potential manganese toxicity [14–16].

Different grading is used for assessing the severity of HE in children in different age groups. Changes in behaviour, cognition, neurological examination, and electroencephalogram (EEG) are usually assessed to characterize the patient as having one of four clinical Stages of encephalopathy, ranging from stage 0 with minimal or no evidence of neurological dysfunction to stage 4 coma (◘ Tables 24.2, 24.3 and 24.4).

24.6 Management

The early recognition and appropriate management of paediatric patients with hepatic encephalopathy is of paramount importance to reduce the mortality and morbidity associated with cerebral oedema and systemic inflammatory response syndrome (SIRS).

24.6.1 General Supportive Care

1. Children should be kept in a quiet room with minimal stimulation, and unnecessary interventions should be avoided.
2. Frequent neurological examination and assessment of the grade of encephalopathy, however, should be routinely performed. Do not sedate children who are not intubated.
3. Do not correct coagulation unless bleeding actively or before any invasive procedure.

24.6.2 Ventilation Strategies

1. Endotracheal intubation is recommended for airway protection and controlled ventilation in advanced grades of HE. Invasive mechanical ventilation is required in patients who develop grade 3 or 4 encephalopathy.
2. Avoid nasal intubation unless coagulation is corrected.
3. Follow a lung-protective ventilatory strategy to limit tidal volumes to ~6–8 ml/kg and plateau pressure to <30 cm H_20).
4. Permissive hypercapnea is poorly tolerated as any rise in $PaCO_2$ will be associated with a concomitant rise in ICP. Pressures and FiO_2 should be adjusted so as to maintain arterial saturations of more than 96% and $PaCO_2$ between 4.5 and 5.2 kPa.
5. Optimise PEEP to provide maximal recruitment, while reducing alveolar overdistension and guaranteeing optimal oxygen delivery.
6. Hyperventilation ($PaCO_2$ 4.2–4.5 kPa) should be reserved for the emergency treatment of refractory intracranial hypertension.

24.6.3 Neuroprotective Measures

1. Head end elevation to 30° and neutral position to optimize jugular venous outflow and improve CSF drainage.
2. Sedation and analgesia are important components of care for all children with acute liver failure. Pain can result from numerous diagnostic and therapeutic procedures and can aggravate intracranial pressure and contribute to ICH [18]. Cluster nursing care and sedation bolus with each painful procedure (e.g., suctioning, intravenous cannula insertion or any invasive procedure).
3. There is insufficient data to recommend standard agents for sedation and analgesia in patients with PALF, but short-acting agents are preferred. Benzodiazepines and propofol may worsen HE by increasing gamma-aminobutyric acid neurotransmission [19].
4. Strict temperature control aiming for normothermia (36–37 °C). Fever and shivering should be aggressively treated, as these may exacerbate intracranial pressure. A multicentre retrospective study from US ALFSG involving 97 patients found no difference in 21-day mortality and transplant-free survival between those who received therapeutic hypothermia and those who did not [20]. There is no current data in children with PALF to support the routine use of therapeutic hypothermia, although aiming for mild hypothermia (35–36 °C) can be considered in cases of observed intracranial hypertension.
5. Maintain normoglycaemia (4–8 mmol/L). This may require continuous glucose infusions at rates of 10–15 mg/kg/min. However, hypotonic dextrose solutions should be used cautiously due to the risk of hyponatraemia.
6. Continuous EEG should be considered as a screening tool for subclinical seizure activity, especially for children with grade III or IV encephalopathy or if clinically suspected [21]. There is no paediatric data to support the use of prophylactic antiseizure medication in the management of patients with PALF.

24.6.4 Ammonia Scavenging Strategy

1. There is a correlation between arterial ammonia levels, hepatic encephalopathy and intracranial hypertension [22], and hyperammonaemia has been associated with mortality [23, 24]. Hence, ammonia-lowering strategies are considered to be an effective way to treat hepatic encephalopathy. However, there is insufficient evidence to support the use of lactulose or other nonabsorbable antibiotics (rifxaximin, neomycin) to treat HE in patients with PALF [25, 26].
2. Restrict protein intake to 1–2 g/kg/day (with more limited targets in the presence of hyperammonaemia) to limit the production of ammonia.
3. Continuous venovenous haemofiltration should be initiated in patients requiring intubation for encephalopathy to clear ammonia and other neuroactive toxins. In a large cohort of ALF patients, hyperammonaemia was associated with high-grade HE and worse 21-day transplant-free survival. Use of continuous kidney replacement therapy (CKRT) was associated with a reduction in serum ammonia level and improvement of 21-day transplant-free survival [27].

24.6.5 Hemodynamic Monitoring

The early restoration of circulatory volume, systemic perfusion and oxygen delivery is crucial to the successful management of patients with PALF. Many patients with acute liver failure will develop hemodynamic instability independent of infectious complications. Serum cytokine levels likely contribute to systemic vasodilation and cardiac dysfunction. Hypotension can negatively impact cerebral perfusion and should be avoided. Echocardiograms or USCOM ((ultrasound guided cardiac output monitoring) can be helpful in assessing cardiac output, stroke volume, and vascular tone and give information on heart-filling and inotropy. Relative adrenal insufficiency has been described in adults with ALF and should be considered in the setting of refractory hypotension. The incidence of RAI seems to parallel the severity of liver disease [28]. No paediatric-specific data were found to define the incidence or formulate specific recommendations for the diagnosis and management of RAI. In general, additional steroid supplementation should be considered in patients with ALF with fluid refractory, catecholamine-resistant shock [29].

Noradrenaline is the vasopressor of choice. The dose is titrated to maintain the required MAP and cerebral perfusion pressure (CPP).

24.6.6 Fluid Requirement and Nutritional Support

The first choice of fluid is crystalloid (normal saline) with 5% or 10% dextrose, depending upon age and blood glucose level. Colloids (5% human albumin solution) and blood products (FFP, Cryoprecipitate) can be used as volume expanders in the event of abnormal coagulation.

Patients with PALF are likely catabolic and require more calories than resting energy requirements. Enteral feeding is often preferred over total parenteral nutrition (TPN), and both nasogastric or nasojejunal feeds should be considered before TPN. There are no clear guidelines on formula choice [30]. Goals include administration of adequate calories to decrease catabolism, maintaining euglycaemia, and provision of enough protein for metabolic needs without causing hyperammonaemia [30]. TPN may be needed to provide maximal calories with minimal volume, depending on the overall fluid status. For both enteral feed and TPN, protein restriction (1 g/kg protein daily) can be considered if hyperammonaemia is present. Also, lipids should be utilized unless a disorder of fatty acid oxidation or mitochondrial disease is suspected.

24.6.6.1 Role of N-Acetyl Cysteine in Management of Non-acetaminophen (Non-APAP) ALF

N-acetylcysteine (NAC), an antioxidant agent that replenishes mitochondrial and cytosolic glutathione stores, has been used in the treatment of acetaminophen-induced ALF and non-acetaminophen-induced ALF. However, the use of on-acetaminophen-induced ALF is controversial. In a paediatric RCT involving 184 patients, there was no difference in 1-year survival between those who received NAC versus placebo (73% vs. 82%) [31]. The 1-year transplant-free survival was lower in those who received NAC (35%) compared to those who received placebo (53%), especially in children younger than 2 years. Current evidence does not support the use of NAC in children with non-APAP ALF.

24.6.6.2 Antibiotics in PALF

There is a high potential risk of invasive infections in PALF. The development of multi-organ dysfunction secondary to spillover of cytokines and vasoactive mediators from the liver to the systemic circulation leaves patients particularly vulnerable to sepsis, and sepsis is a significant predictor of mortality [32]. For this reason, many centres will commence broad-spectrum prophylactic antibiotics, and antifungals, for patients with PALF from admission. The specialised liver-resident macrophages Kupffer cells are depleted in acute liver injury which enhances susceptibility to infection [33]. In addition, during the process of liver regeneration after injury, there is anti-inflammatory polarisation of macrophages which can also enhance susceptibility to infection.

24.6.7 Neuro-Critical Care Monitoring and Management of Intracranial Hypertension and Cerebral Oedema

The goal in the management of cerebral oedema and increased ICP is to maintain ICP <20 mm Hg while maintaining adequate cerebral perfusion pressure (CPP) [34]. Close clinical monitoring is strongly recommended in children with HE. Clinical monitoring can be very challenging, especially once patients progress to HE Grade 3–4.

1. **Use EEG/Cerebral Function Analysing Monitor (CFAM)** to actively screen for subclinical seizures.
2. **Reverse Jugular Venous Saturation ($SjvO_2$):**
   Sjv02 can be used as a surrogate marker for cerebral metabolism and brain oxy gen consumption [35]. Measuring the oxygen saturation of the jugular vein allows the Arteriovenous Oxygen Difference ($AVDO_2$) to be assessed, which is indicative of metabolic demand compared to oxygenation. Measurement involves placement of a retrograde catheter in the internal jugular vein with the tip at the jugular venous bulb. The normal range for jugular venous oxygen saturation is between 60–75%. High and low absolute jugular venous saturations are equally associated with poor outcomes (Table 24.5) [35]. The $SjvO_2$ –PaO_2 difference can also be interpreted to indicate a number of clinical problems (Table 24.6).

   Limitations of $SjvO_2$ monitoring include inappropriate catheter placement resulting in sampling of blood from outside the brain such as scalp, reducing accuracy. A falsely high $SjvO_2$ may also occur from leftward shift of the oxyhaemoglobin dissociation curve during alkaline conditions [36].

Table 24.5 Clinical significance of absolute $SjVO_2$ value

Low $SjvO_2$ < 55%	High $SjvO_2$ > 80%
Cerebral hypoperfusion due to inadequate CPP Signs of increased cerebral oxygen utilisation as seen with seizure activity or fever Anaemia Hypoxaemia	Cerebral hyperperfusion leading to hyperaemia or inadequate neuronal metabolism and/or neuronal cell death Cerebral vasodilatation

Table 24.6 Clinical implication of $SjVO_2$-PaO_2 ($AVDO_2$) difference

$SjVO_2$-PaO_2 > 40	$SjVO_2$-PaO_2 < 20
Cerebral vasoconstriction (e.g., as a result of hyperventilation and hypocarbia) Hypoxaemia Anaemia Diminished cerebral perfusion pressure Inappropriately high CPP and vasoconstriction induced by exogenous vasoconstrictor Seizures	Hyperaemia Cerebral vasodilatation Brain death

3. **Trans-cranial Doppler (TCD):**
TCD ultrasonography is a non-invasive bedside method that allows estimation of CBF, and has been used in a variety of clinical scenarios [37]. TCD utilises pulsed wave Doppler to image vessels through an acoustic window, of which the trans-temporal window is the most commonly used, allowing flow assessment of the anterior, middle and posterior cerebral arteries. TCD can be used to calculate CBF mean flow velocity and the Pulsatibility index. Flow velocities are age and sex related, and normative data derived by trans cranial Doppler Sonography are lacking in critically ill children. The trend of mean flow velocity is probably the most informative. In small a series of five ALF patients, mean blood flow was reduced in four cases, consistent with a pattern of hypoperfusion [38].
The pulsatility index (PI) = [(systolic velocity – diastolic velocity)/mean velocity] demonstrates a good correlation with ICP. The normal PI value is 0.8–1.2. Low PI indicates increase cerebral blood flow or hypercapnia, and High PI is suggestive of hypocapnia or vasoconstriction or brain death. In a small series of four ALF patients, a PI >1.0 was predictive of a poor outcome [39]. TCD has significant potential, but limitations include inadequacy of transtemporal windows in 10–20% of patients, and it is also highly operator dependent with a long learning curve.
4. **Radiological Monitoring:**
Cerebral imaging with CT is not routinely advocated as moving an unstable child with raised ICP and high INR to the radiology unit might be a challenging task and also is insensitive in detecting elevated ICP [40]; a negative scan does not rule out raised ICP. However, it might be useful to exclude other etiologies such as large bleeds or masses. MRI scanning is more sensitive for cerebral oedema, with a fast diffusion-weighted MRI being preferred due to its accuracy in identifying cytotoxic oedema [41], but overall, the use of MRI is limited by the risks and logistics involved in keeping a critically ill ventilated patient in the MRI scanner for a prolonged period.
Indications for Cerebral CT:
- Unilateral pupillary dilatation.
- Suspected Intracranial bleed.
- Unexplained Prolonged seizures.
- Dilated pupils for more than 6 h not explained by drugs.
- Before Liver transplant (LT) in a child with severely raised ICP after discussion with the multidisciplinary team to determine eligibility for LT.

5. **Invasive ICP monitoring (ICPM):**
   ICPM allows direct, real-time continuous measurements of ICP by placement of a catheter into the cranial cavity, either into the epidural, subdural or ventricular spaces or directly into the brain parenchyma. Although considered the gold-standard, there is a lack of evidence demonstrating a clear survival benefit of ICP monitoring in PALF in children. The multicentre US ALFSG reported no overall improvement in 21-day mortality with ICP monitoring. The study, however, showed increased 21-day mortality in non-acetaminophen (non-APAP) patients with ALF with ICP monitoring [42]. There is no consistent data to demonstrate the benefits of ICP monitoring, and undoubtedly it carries the risk of intracranial bleeding accentuated by the coagulopathy seen in patients with ALF. In one study in PALF, one of 14 children developed a 9 mm intracranial haemorrhage [22]. Therefore, a proper risk assessment must be performed before an ICP bolt is considered, with consideration given to transfusion of blood products pre-insertion if required.

   The goal of invasive method is to maintain age-adequate cerebral perfusion pressure and maintain ICP <20 mmHg. Maintain CPP more than 50 mmHg for children <4 years, more than 55 mmHg for children between 4 and 10 years and > 60 mmHg for children older than 10 years.

24.6.8 Indications

Children >5 years with grade 3 or 4 encephalopathy and ammonia >200 micromoles/litre despite continuous kidney replacement therapy (CKRT), EEG showing focal or subclinical seizures, or neuroimaging showing signs of cerebral oedema should be considered for invasive ICP monitoring.

24.7 Medical Management of ICP

24.7.1 Hypertonic Saline

Hypertonic saline (HTS) decreases ICP by several complex mechanisms. It decreases the brain water content secondary to its osmotic effect. It also improves cerebral blood flow, which in turn causes vasoconstriction and decreases ICP. It stabilizes cerebral endothelial cell volume, which also improves circulation.

In a 2004 RCT from Kings College Hospital, 30 adult patients with ALF with Grade III and IV encephalopathy were randomized to receive 30% HTS and a higher serum sodium target of 145–155 mmol/L, or standard care [43]. The intervention group had significantly lower intracranial pressure over the first 24 h and a significantly lower incidence of intracranial hypertension. The current consensus target is to aim to maintain serum sodium around 145–150 mmol/L in patients with PALF with ICH. HTS is now the standard of care in the treatment of ICH in paediatric patients with traumatic brain injury and some of the management principles of neuromonitoring and neuroprotection are very similar [44].

The potential complications of HTS include hyperchloremic metabolic acidosis, haemorrhages, venous thrombosis, and worsening coagulopathy.

24.7.2 Mannitol

Mannitol is an osmotic diuretic agent used commonly as a first-line therapy to treat increased ICP in adult patients with ALF [25, 29]. Mannitol's main effect manifests through an increase in the serum osmolality, resulting in outward movement of water from brain parenchyma. Mannitol also decreases blood viscosity, which in turn causes vasoconstriction, decreased cerebral blood volume, and ICP. The current recommendation suggests doses of 0.25–1 g/kg/dose [18, 22]. It should be administered to manage an acute rise in ICP with impending brain herniation; prophylactic administration is not recommended. Mannitol is rarely used in clinical practice except in cases of impending herniation. In addition, it is not recommended to use mannitol in the presence of hypovolaemia, renal failure, or a serum osmolality >320 mOsm/L [25, 29].

24.7.3 Thiopentone Sodium

Thiopentone is a short-acting barbiturate. It decreases ICP by decreasing cerebral metabolism, the cerebral metabolic rate for oxygen ($CMRO_2$) and, consequently, cerebral blood flow and cerebral blood volume via flow-metabolism coupling. Barbiturates can lower ICP refractory to all other measures. However, there are no randomised trials examining the effects of barbiturates on outcomes from PALF with raised ICP. A loading dose of 5–10 mg/kg is required, followed by a continuous infusion of 1–5 mg/kg/h. Subsequent doses of thiopentone and the rate of infusion should be titrated to burst suppression on the electroencephalogram (EEG). Further increases in dose are not thought to have additional therapeutic benefit and may increase complications. Thiopentone causes systemic hypotension in a dose-dependent manner through a combination of a negative inotropic effect and a reduction in systemic vascular resistance.

24.7.4 Therapeutic Hypothermia

Hypothermia reduces brain energy metabolism, systemic and neuronal inflammation, and reduces ammonia, while concurrently improving cerebral blood flow and cerebral hemodynamics [45, 46]. Therapeutic hypothermia, however, is associated with side effects such as coagulopathy, cardiac dysrhythmias, increased risk of infection, electrolyte disturbance, hyperglycaemia, and theoretically decreased hepatic regeneration [45, 46].

A multicentre retrospective study from US ALFSG involving 97 patients found no difference in 21-day mortality and transplant-free survival between those who received therapeutic hypothermia and those who did not [20]. There is no data in patients with PALF to support the use of therapeutic hypothermia. At this time, active normothermia (36–37 °C) and avoiding fever may offer the best risk-benefit ratio for patients in standard cases. Mild hypothermia (35–36 °C) can be considered if there is evidence of raised intracranial pressure.

24.7.5 Hyperventilation

Hyperventilation to reduce $PaCO_2$ to 4 kPa is known to quickly lower ICP via decreasing cerebral blood flow and concomitant oxygen delivery. However, it has its own side effects. Temporary hyperventilation is suggested in an attempt to lower ICP in impending herniation. Prolonged hyperventilation is not recommended. It is rarely used in clinical practice. Target $PaCO_2$ levels of between 4.5–5.2 kPa are common.

24.7.6 Coagulation

Coagulopathy is traditionally assessed by measuring prothrombin time (PT) and INR. Measurement of PT/INR, however, reflects a reduction in synthetic function but not necessarily the risk of bleeding. Prolongation of prothrombin time (PT)/INR is universal in children with ALF. However, there is a reduction in both pro- and anti-coagulant factors, because of which patients with ALF have re-balanced haemostasis. In fact, these children tend towards being pro-coagulable due to elevation of endogenous thrombin generation potential. Therefore, these patients with ALF rarely bleed spontaneously. Clinically significant haemorrhage is seen in <5% of patients and <1% have spontaneous intracranial bleeding [47]. Coagulopathy should not be routinely corrected unless one is performing invasive procedures such as inserting a central line or ICP monitoring bolt, or if the patient is actively bleeding.

24.7.7 Acute Kidney Injury

The aetiology for acute kidney injury in PALF is commonly linked to systemic hypotension secondary to SIRS/sepsis, decreased fluid intake or increased losses due to vomiting and diarrhoea or haemorrhage. As PALF generally occurs in children who were thought to be previously healthy, most renal injury is presumed to be acute in nature and otherwise recoverable. Early use of continuous Kidney Replacement Therapy (CKRT) is recommended. Hepatic encephalopathy grade 3–4 and hyperammonaemia are two of the few non-renal indications for the commencement of CKRT. However, it should be emphasised that none of the below indications are considered absolute. The patient's clinical condition and prognosis should be considered in each individual case.

24.7.8 Indication for Starting CKRT in Patients with PALF

1. Metabolic abnormalities (hyperlactataemia, hyperkalaemia, metabolic acidosis resistant to fluid therapy).
2. Hepatic encephalopathy grade 3–4.
3. Ammonia >150 μmol/L.
4. Oliguria.
5. Fluid overload >10%.

Anticoagulation in CKRT for PALF: Since these patients can be functionally prothrombotic, there is a higher chance of circuit/filter clotting when using CKRT. Decreasing downtimes in these patients is of paramount importance as the longer the downtimes, the less effective CKRT will be at removing ammonia and other neurotoxins, and hence, there can be a greater risk of cerebral oedema.

Therefore, it is vital to keep these circuits going by the use of anticoagulants if safe to do so. The choices are unfractionated heparin, regional citrate anticoagulation (with close monitoring for citrate lock and citrate accumulation), platelet inhibitors like prostacyclin, and nafomostat mesylate.

24.7.9 Liver Support Devices

Extracorporeal liver support (ELS) systems have been proposed either as a bridge to liver transplantation or as an assist in recovery from PALF. They are broadly divided into non-biologic and biologic systems. The biological systems use human/non-human cells to detoxify the plasma or blood. The non-biologic system uses a series of filters to detoxify the plasma/blood and these predominate in PALF.

Molecular Adsorbent Recirculating System (MARS) and Prometheus are the two commercially available liver support systems. In adult patients with ALF, MARS has shown improvement in biochemical parameters (including improved ammonia), and hepatic encephalopathy [48]. A recent paediatric case series involving 20 children with PALF who were treated with MARS showed significantly lower levels of serum ammonia, bilirubin, bile acid, and creatinine levels; however, there was no observed survival benefit [49]. However, survival benefit has been been demonstrated.

High-volume CKRT removes cytokines such as TNF-α and IL-1β, which are also implicated in the pathogenesis of ALF and HE. High-volume hemofiltration (HVHF) was used in 22 children with PALF in a single centre in Europe and showed improvements in hemodynamics at 24 h and decreased grade of HE at 48 h [50].

Plasma exchange (PE), a nonselective form of blood purification, is favoured because of its potential to supplement the synthetic function of the liver in addition to the removal of toxins. Plasma exchange has been shown to improve coagulation profile, serum ammonia, encephalopathy, and cerebral perfusion pressure. A randomised controlled trial of high-volume PE in adults with ALF showed that its use was associated with improved survival to hospital discharge [51]. A study of 43 patients with PALF secondary to Wilson's disease showed improved transplant-free survival and median days of survival in patients treated with high-volume PE [52].

Any type of extracorporeal support should be part of multidisciplinary, supportive critical care treatment offered at a liver transplant centre and should not be used as a stand-alone treatment [53]. There is a wide variation from centre to centre in the use of liver support systems in children. Overall, among all ELS, PE shows great promise but more randomised studies are awaited in children with PALF (◘ Table 24.7). Newer blood purification techniques like cytosorbents, Fractionated plasma separation and Adsorption (FPSA), Double Plasma Molecular Adsorption system (DPMAS) have been used with varying success.

Table 24.7 Aetiology-specific treatments for acute liver failure

Aetiology	Treatment
Acetaminophen poisoning	N-acetylcysteine 150 mg/kg IV in 15 min, then maintenance dose 50 mg/kg over 4 h, followed by 100 mg/kg administered over 16 h Or 100 mg/kg/day until INR is normal for at least 48 h or until liver transplantation takes place
Hereditary tyrosinaemia	Nitisinone (NTBC or (2-nitro-4-trifluoromethyl benzoyl—1,3-cyclohexanedione)) (0.5 mg/kg twice a day) + elimination
Neonatal hemochromatosis	N-acetyl cysteine 100–200 mg/kg/day, divided three times daily, by mouth or IV for 17–21 doses Vitamin-E 25 IU/kg/day, divided twice daily, by mouth Selenium 3 microgram/kg/day, IV or PO Prostaglandin E1 0.4 mg/kg/h IV. Desferroxamine 30 mg/kg/day, IV infused over 8 h until the serum ferritin <500 mg/L Double volume exchange transfusion and intravenous immunoglobulin (1 gm/kg)
Herpetic hepatitis	Acyclovir 150 mg/m^2/day IV
Autoimmune hepatitis	Steroids (methylprednisolone—2 mg/kg/day)
Hepatitis B HSV	Lamivudine 4 mg/kg/day once daily orally
Galactosaemia	Galactose and lactose-free diets
Fructose intolerance	Fructose-free diets, avoiding fructose and Sorbitol infusions
Hemophagocytic lymphohistiocytosis	Chemotherapy ± haemotopoietic stem cell transplantation
Mushroom poisoning	Penicillin G 1,000,000 U/kg/day or Thioetic acid (300 mg/kg/day)

24.7.10 Liver Transplant in ALF

Greater experience and accessibility of liver transplantation have improved the survival of patients with PALF [3]. However, it is very challenging to prognosticate these patients and to determine which ones may require or benefit the most from transplantation. Certain aetiologies of PALF (paracetamol toxicity) are more likely to recover spontaneously without transplant, but certain multisystem aetiologies (haemophagocytic lymphohistocytosis, mitochondrial diseases) are less likely to survive or benefit from transplantation [3]. Younger patients and those with indeterminate PALF also tend to have worse prognoses. The best currently known absolute laboratory and clinical indicators of mortality without transplantation in PALF are listed in Table 24.8 [54]. The outcome of liver transplantation following PALF is poorer

Table 24.8 Indicators of Mortality without Transplant in PALF

Non-paracetamol toxicity ALF	Paracetamol toxicity-induced ALF
INR > 4 Factor V concentration of <25%	Arterial pH < 7.3 (after fluid resuscitation) Or The presence of all three of the following criteria: INR >6.5 Serum creatinine >300 μmol per litre (>3.4 mg/dl) Grade III or IV encephalopathy

when compared to liver transplantation done for chronic liver disease, likely due to the high proportion of patients who develop multi-organ dysfunction in association with PALF. In analysis of data from the Studies of Paediatric Liver Transplantation (SPLIT) Registry database from the USA, 1-year patient survival was 74% for PALF compared to 88.2% for other conditions [55]. There are single-centre case series that describe post-liver transplantation survival rates ranging from 55% to 90% [56, 57].

Contraindication for LT: These Are All Relative and Needs to Be Discussed with MDT

- Fixed dilated pupils.
- End-stage intracranial hypertension.
- Uncontrolled multi-organ failure.
- Generalized mitochondrial disease.
- Extra hepatic malignancy.

24.7.10.1 Models to Predict LT

Due to the challenges discussed above, there is no definitive prognostic model in PALF to predict the need for LT. The King's College Hospital criteria, used to predict mortality in adults with ALF, has a lower sensitivity in children [58]. However, the King's College Hospital revised Wilson's Index has been validated with a sensitivity and specificity of 93% and 97% in children presenting with PALF secondary to Wilson's disease [59]. The Pediatric End-Stage Liver Disease (PELD) score is a score designed as a predictor of mortality in children with chronic liver disease listed for liver transplantation, and has 81% specificity and 86% sensitivity for poor outcomes in PALF, which while acceptable remains sub-optimal [60].

The heterogeneity of the cohort of patients with PALF means designing a tailored prognostic model remains an ongoing challenge, and disease-specific models may be more appropriate, although their utility will rely on accurate determination of aetiology which remains difficult in a disease where the highest proportion of patients have an indeterminate cause for their illness [7].

24.7.10.2 Post-Liver Transplant Management

In the early post-transplant period, children with PALF may differ from other children post-liver transplant because of the high incidence of multi-organ involvement at the time of listing for transplant and the greater potential to require multi-organ support in association with transplantation. This is reflected in the lower 5-year patient and graft survival for patients transplanted due to PALF compared to those transplanted due to extrahepatic biliary atresia [61]. Children at highest risk of death post-transplant are those <1 year of age, those with Grade IV encephalopathy, and those who required dialysis pre-operatively [55].

Table 24.9 described post-liver transplant management of these patients. Induction of immunosuppression is most common with high dose IV methylpred-

Table 24.9 Post-Liver transplant management

Laboratory	FBC, U&Es, lactate, glucose, Coagulation screen, ABG Check K—graft necrosis can be associated with rapid onset hyperkalaemia Check Mg—hypo-magnesium occurs post-transplant especially with Tacrolimus Liver enzymes and bilirubin-AST to assess graft function (24 h post-transplant)
Haematology and coagulation anticoagulation	Hb < 10 g/dl at or below 10 g/dl Venesection if Hb is more than >10.5 and replaced with 4.5% human albumin. Do not give blood transfusion unless acute haemorrhage Do not give FFP. Correcting an elevated INR may mask liver dysfunction Low molecular weight to prevent thrombosis of hepatic vessels Dalteparin (low molecular weight) 100 units/kg/day subcutaneous in two divided doses for 10 days When on full oral diet convert to aspirin, after discussion with hepatology and transplant teams
Immunosuppression	Methylprednisolone 2 mg/kg/day IV from day 1 for 3 days and starts reducing after three doses. Tacrolimus (Calcineurin inhibitor - CNI)—Liaise with hepatologist and surgeon dose. Target tacrolimus level of 10-12ug/l target for 3 months Mycophenolate Mofetil is indicated for steroid resistant cellular rejection or to enable the doses of Tacrolimus to be reduced for patients with impaired renal function. Basiliximab in conjunction with a CNI-based immunotherapy.
Gastro intestinal	Monitor Gastric pH 6 hourly (aim to keep pH >4) Nil by mouth for 3–5 days (as per discussion with surgeon) Give Proton Pump inhibitor for gastric protection – Sucralfate (if gastric pH <5)
Fluid management	2/3 normal IV maintenance Preferred fluid 10% dextrose with K+ and Na+ Replace wound losses ml for ml with 4.5% human albumin solution Aim for urine output 1 ml/kg/h, if urine output is <0.5 ml/kg/h Give fluid challenge - 10ml/kg (usually 0.9% saline, occasionally 4.5% albumin) -Do not give diuretic unless advised by senior consultant/surgeon

(continued)

Table 24.9 (continued)

Respiratory support	CXR to confirm ETT position Extubation is usually performed 12–36 h post-operatively after USS Doppler scan confirms good vascular flow
Renal support	If children have raised ICP, sometimes CKRT is continued intra-operatively CKRT is continued post-transplant in these children until the team is sure of the neurologic /fluid volume/AKI status which can be variable

nisolone for a few days alongside a calcineurin inhibitor such as tacrolimus. Many centres will prescribe prophylactic antibiotics and antivirals post-operatively (if not already started pre-operatively) [62].

In the early post-operative period, children will be admitted to the PICU, where surgical complications such as those described in Table 24.10 must be vigilantly watched for. Table 24.10 describes potential post-operative complications for patients after transplant. Hepatic artery and portal vein thrombosis are major causes of graft loss and subsequent mortality and can most easily be detected by Doppler abdominal ultrasound [63]. Treatments include re-transplantation, attempted revascularisation and anticoagulation in some cases [64]. Surgical revascularisation improves survival compared to cases where revascularisation is unsuccessful or not attempted. Bile leak and biliary strictures are other complications and can be treated with percutaneous transhepatic biliary drainage [65]. Developing complications of the graft such as fibrosis, biliary strictures and portal fibrosis can cause late graft loss years later [66].

Patients with PALF are also vulnerable to medical complications post-transplant, which may include SIRS, sepsis [67], primary EBV/CMV, fungal infections, AKI [68], and neurological complications [69]. Regarding AKI, recent studies have suggested there may be an association between preoperative synthetic liver function and intraoperative blood loss [68], and the post-operative likelihood of AKI [70].

If a graft is to be lost, this most commonly occurs in the first 7 days post-operatively [66]. Requiring a ventilator and life support at time of transplant are risk factors for graft failure [61]. Surgical complications such as those described above are common causes of graft failure, as well as primary non-function, and acute rejection. Duration of the anhepatic phase and Child-Pugh score are associated factors with graft loss [66].

24.7.10.3 Long-Term Outcome

Overall survival for patients with PALF has improved in recent years to around 95%, and around 20% of children with PALF will require a liver transplant [3, 4]. As described, of those requiring a transplant, survival rates range between 55% and 90% [56, 57].

For those who are transplanted, they will face a prolonged hospital stay and the prospect of a lifetime of immunosuppression and potential associated complications thereof including risk of infection, post-transplant lymphoproliferative disease, and effects on growth [62]. It is vital that these children have regular follow-up to monitor graft function and also their psychosocial state. There is evidence that these children

Table 24.10 Post-operative complication

Complication	Possible causes	Signs and symptoms	Diagnostic evaluation	Treatment
Post-operative haemorrhage	Anastomotic leak Graft bleeding Cut surface bleeding Coagulopathy	Anaemia Hypotension Tachycardia Irritability Oliguria Increased abdominal girth Sanguineous or frank blood JP drainage	Doppler ultrasound Laboratory monitoring (CBCs, coagulation panel) – Abdominal CT	– PRBC Transfusion Correct coagulopathy Inform surgical team
Hepatic artery thrombosis	Poor arterial flow due to surgical reasons Hypercoaguable state Over transfusion Acute cellular rejection	High fever Abdominal pain and distention Acute elevation in liver chemistries Bacteraemia caused by intra and/or extra hepatic biliary strictures	Doppler abdominal ultrasound Or CT angiogram	Urgent ex-lap to revise artery if liver is non-necrotic Relist status and re-transplantation is indicated if liver develops Necrosis
Portal vein thrombosis	1. Hypercoaguable 2. Portal vein sclerosis or stenosis 3. Over-transfusion 4. Hepatic vein outflow obstruction	Asymptomatic Fever Tachycardia Leucocytosis Elevation in LFTs Ascites Abdominal distension Splenomegaly Portal hypertension, variceal bleeding	Doppler abdominal ultrasound CT or MR Venogram	Surgical re-exploration Surgical shunt Possible re-listing if unable to be revised

(continued)

Table 24.10 (continued)

Complication	Possible causes	Signs and symptoms	Diagnostic evaluation	Treatment
Bile leak	1. Hepatic artery thrombosis with acute bile duct necrosis 2. Bile leak from cut surface	Dark green/Yellowish drain fluid Lower quadrant pain Mental status changes Increase in liver enzymes	Rule out hepatic artery thrombosis, Doppler US ASAP cholangiogram through bile catheter or MRCP	Based on aetiology of the leak and may require surgical intervention
Bile obstruction	Anastomotic stricture	Fever, jaundice, abdominal pain, elevated liver Enzymes especially GGT	MRCP PTC to provide definitive diagnosis of strictures	Treatment with broad-spectrum antibiotics ERCP or IR consult for PTC for stent placement/balloon dilation Surgical revision of anastomosis

may experience some form of neurological impairment and clinicians should proactively engage with schools and social workers to ensure sufficient support is available [71]. Even among all children with PALF (including those who are not transplanted), a recent study there can be an effect on health-related quality of life and executive function, but IQ was not affected [72].

Overall, there have been incredible advances in recent years in the medical and transplant management of PALF. Future research into the role of extracorporeal therapies and models to prognosticate outcomes can further improve morbidity, mortality and quality of life for these young and complex patients.

Take-Home Messages

PALF is a multisystem disease with a dynamic and often unpredictable course.

- The Intensive Care Unit plays a pivotal role in the management of patients with PALF by providing support for failing organs while simultaneously allowing time for hepatic regeneration, as well as the optimisation of clinical status, if liver transplantation is ultimately required. Early transfer to a centre with liver transplant capabilities is of paramount importance.
- Mortality in PALF is predominantly due to raised intracranial pressure, infections and multi-organ failure; therefore, efforts are directed toward the management of these complications while awaiting recovery of liver function, or maintaining stability prior to liver transplantation.

References

1. Squires RH Jr, Shneider BL, Bucuvalas J, Alonso E, Sokol RJ, Narkewicz MR, et al. Acute liver failure in children: the first 348 patients in the pediatric acute liver failure study group. J Pediatr. 2006;148(5):652–8.
2. Ng VL, Li R, Loomes KM, Leonis MA, Rudnick DA, Belle SH, et al. Outcomes of children with and without hepatic encephalopathy from the pediatric acute liver failure study group. J Pediatric Gastroenterol Nutr. 2016;63(3):357–64.
3. Jain V, Dhawan A. Prognostic modeling in pediatric acute liver failure. Liver Transplant. 2016;22(10):1418–30.
4. Kulkarni S, Perez C, Pichardo C, Castillo L, Gagnon M, Beck-Sague C, et al. Use of pediatric health information system database to study the trends in the incidence, management, etiology, and outcomes due to pediatric acute liver failure in the United States from 2008 to 2013. Pediatric Transplant. 2015;19(8):888–95.
5. Alonso EM, Squires RH. Acute liver failure. In: Kelly DA, editor. Diseases of the liver and biliary system in children. 4th ed. Wiley; 2017.
6. Lim YXJ, Kwek SY, How CH, Chan WSD. A clinical approach to encephalopathy in children. Singapore Med J. 2020;61(12):626–32.
7. Berardi G, Tuckfield L, DelVecchio MT, Aronoff S. Differential diagnosis of acute liver failure in children: a systematic review. Pediatr Gastroenterol Hepatol Nutr. 2020;23(6):501–10.
8. Narkewicz MR, Dell Olio D, Karpen SJ, Murray KF, Schwarz K, Yazigi N, et al. Pattern of diagnostic evaluation for the causes of pediatric acute liver failure: an opportunity for quality improvement. J Pediatr. 2009;155(6):801–6.
9. Sundaram SS, Alonso EM, Narkewicz MR, Zhang S, Squires RH. Pediatric acute liver failure study G. Characterization and outcomes of young infants with acute liver failure. J Pediatr. 2011;159(5):813–8.

10. Brennan PN, Donnelly MC, Simpson KJ. Systematic review: non A-E, seronegative or indeterminate hepatitis; what is this deadly disease? Aliment Pharmacol Therapeut. 2018;47(8):1079–91.
11. Abou-Assi S, Vlahcevic ZR. Hepatic encephalopathy. Postgrad Med. 2001;109(2):52–70.
12. Bucuvalas J, Yazigi N, Squires RH. Acute liver failure in children. Clin Liver Dis. 2006;10(1):149–68.
13. Squires RH. Acute liver failure in children. Semin Liver Dis. 2008;28(2):153–66.
14. Ong JP, Aggarwal A, Krieger D, Easley KA, Karafa MT, Van Lente F, et al. Correlation between ammonia levels and the severity of hepatic encephalopathy. Am J Med. 2003;114(3):188–93.
15. Shawcross DL, Davies NA, Williams R, Jalan R. Systemic inflammatory response exacerbates the neuropsychological effects of induced hyperammonemia in cirrhosis. J Hepatol. 2004;40(2):247–54.
16. Kundra A, Jain A, Banga A, Bajaj G, Kar P. Evaluation of plasma ammonia levels in patients with acute liver failure and chronic liver disease and its correlation with the severity of hepatic encephalopathy and clinical features of raised intracranial tension. Clin Biochem. 2005;38(8):696–9.
17. Whitington PF, Alonso EM. Fulminant hepatitis and acute liver failure. In: Kelly DA, editor. Paediatric liver disease. Oxford: Blackwell; 2003.
18. Citerio G, Cormio M. Sedation in neurointensive care: advances in understanding and practice. Curr Opin Crit Care. 2003;9(2):120.
19. Basile AS, Hughes RD, Harrison PM, Murata Y, Pannell L, Jones EA, et al. Elevated brain concentrations of 1,4-benzodiazepines in fulminant hepatic failure. N Engl J Med. 1991;325(7):473–8.
20. Karvellas CJ, Todd Stravitz R, Battenhouse H, Lee WM, Schilsky ML, Group USALFS. Therapeutic hypothermia in acute liver failure: a multicenter retrospective cohort analysis. Liver Transpl. 2015;21(1):4–12.
21. Ellis AJ, Wendon JA, Williams R. Subclinical seizure activity and prophylactic phenytoin infusion in acute liver failure: a controlled clinical trial. Hepatology. 2000;32(3):536–41.
22. Kamat P, Kunde S, Vos M, Vats A, Gupta N, Heffron T, et al. Invasive intracranial pressure monitoring is a useful adjunct in the management of severe hepatic encephalopathy associated with pediatric acute liver failure. Pediatr Crit Care Med. 2012;13(1):e33–e8.
23. Bhatia V, Singh R, Acharya SK. Predictive value of arterial ammonia for complications and outcome in acute liver failure. Gut. 2006;55(1):98–104.
24. Bernal W, Hall C, Karvellas CJ, Auzinger G, Sizer E, Wendon J. Arterial ammonia and clinical risk factors for encephalopathy and intracranial hypertension in acute liver failure. Hepatology. 2007;46(6):1844–52.
25. Polson J, Lee WM. AASLD position paper: the management of acute liver failure. Hepatology. 2005;41(5):1179–97.
26. Dhawan A. Etiology and prognosis of acute liver failure in children. Liver Transplant. 2008;14(S2):S80–S4.
27. Cardoso FS, Gottfried M, Tujios S, Olson JC, Karvellas CJ, Group USALFS. Continuous renal replacement therapy is associated with reduced serum ammonia levels and mortality in acute liver failure. Hepatology. 2018;67(2):711–20.
28. Marik PE, Gayowski T, Starzl TE, Hepatic Cortisol R, Adrenal Pathophysiology Study G. The hepatoadrenal syndrome: a common yet unrecognized clinical condition. Crit Care Med. 2005;33(6):1254–9.
29. Stravitz RT, Kramer AH, Davern T, Shaikh AOS, Caldwell SH, Mehta RL, et al. Intensive care of patients with acute liver failure: recommendations of the U.S. acute liver failure study group. Crit Care Med. 2007;35(11):2498.
30. Plauth M, Cabré E, Riggio O, Assis-Camilo M, Pirlich M, Kondrup J, et al. ESPEN guidelines on enteral nutrition: liver disease. Clin Nutr. 2006;25(2):285–94.
31. Squires RH, Dhawan A, Alonso E, Narkewicz MR, Shneider BL, Rodriguez-Baez N, et al. Intravenous N-acetylcysteine in pediatric patients with nonacetaminophen acute liver failure: a placebo-controlled clinical trial. Hepatology. 2013;57(4):1542–9.
32. Rolando N, Wade J, Davalos M, Wendon J, Philpott-Howard J, Williams R. The systemic inflammatory response syndrome in acute liver failure. Hepatology. 2000;32(4):734–9.
33. Triantafyllou E, Woollard KJ, McPhail MJW, Antoniades CG, Possamai LA. The role of monocytes and macrophages in acute and acute-on-chronic liver failure. Front Immunol. 2018;9:2948.
34. Munoz S, Moritz M, Martin P, Westerberg S, Northrup B, Bell R, et al. Relationship between cerebral perfusion pressure and systemic hemodynamics in fulminant hepatic failure. Transplant Proc. 1993;25:1776–8.

35. Willars C, Auzinger G. Liver transplantation: the patient with severe co-morbidities, CNS disease and increased intracranial pressure. In: Liver anesthesiology and critical care medicine. New York, NY: Springer New York; 2012. p. 267–82.
36. Schell RM, Cole DJ. Cerebral monitoring: jugular venous oximetry. Anesth. Analgesia. 2000;90(3):559.
37. Naqvi J, Yap KH, Ahmad G, Ghosh J. Transcranial Doppler ultrasound: a review of the physical principles and major applications in critical care. Int. J Vasc Med. 2013;2013:629378. 1
38. Abdo A, López O, Fernández A, Santos J, Castillo J, Castellanos R, et al. Transcranial Doppler sonography in fulminant hepatic failure. Transplant Proc. 2003;35(5):1859–60.
39. Kawakami M, Koda M, Murawaki Y. Cerebral pulsatility index by transcranial Doppler sonography predicts the prognosis of patients with fulminant hepatic failure. Clin Imaging. 2010;34(5):327–31.
40. Muñoz SJ, Robinson M, Northrup B, Bell R, Moritz M, Jarrell B, et al. Elevated intracranial pressure and computed tomography of the brain in fulminant hepatocellular failure. Hepatology. 1991;13(2):209–12.
41. Ranjan P, Mishra AM, Kale R, Saraswat VA, Gupta RK. Cytotoxic edema is responsible for raised intracranial pressure in fulminant hepatic failure: in vivo demonstration using diffusion-weighted MRI in human subjects. Metab Brain Dis. 2005;20(3):181–92.
42. Karvellas CJ, Fix OK, Battenhouse H, Durkalski V, Sanders C, Lee WM, et al. Outcomes and complications of intracranial pressure monitoring in acute liver failure: a retrospective cohort study. Crit Care Med. 2014;42(5):1157–67.
43. Murphy N, Auzinger G, Bernel W, Wendon J. The effect of hypertonic sodium chloride on intracranial pressure in patients with acute liver failure. Hepatology. 2004;39(2):464–70.
44. Webster DL, Fei L, Falcone RA, Kaplan JM. Higher-volume hypertonic saline and increased thrombotic risk in pediatric traumatic brain injury. J Crit Care. 2015;30(6):1267–71.
45. Stravitz RT, Larsen FS. Therapeutic hypothermia for acute liver failure. Crit Care Med. 2009;37(7):S258.
46. Vaquero J. Therapeutic hypothermia in the management of acute liver failure. Neurochem Int. 2012;60(7):723–35.
47. Munoz SJ, Stravitz RT, Gabriel DA. Coagulopathy of acute liver failure. Clin Liver Dis. 2009;13(1):95–107.
48. Khuroo MS, Khuroo MS, Farahat KLC. Molecular adsorbent recirculating system for acute and acute-on-chronic liver failure: a meta-analysis. Liver Transpl. 2004;10(9):1099–106.
49. Lexmond WS, Van Dael CML, Scheenstra R, Goorhuis JF, Sieders E, Verkade HJ, et al. Experience with molecular adsorbent recirculating system treatment in 20 children listed for high-urgency liver transplantation. Liver Transpl. 2015;21(3):369–80.
50. Chevret L, Durand P, Lambert J, Essouri S, Balu L, Devictor D, et al. High-volume hemofiltration in children with acute liver failure*. Pediatr Crit Care Med. 2014;15(7).e300.
51. Larsen FS, Schmidt LE, Bernsmeier C, Rasmussen A, Isoniemi H, Patel VC, et al. High-volume plasma exchange in patients with acute liver failure: an open randomised controlled trial. J Hepatol. 2016;64(1):69–78.
52. Pawaria A, Sood V, Lal B, Khanna R, Bajpai M, Alam S. Ninety days transplant free survival with high volume plasma exchange in Wilson disease presenting as acute liver failure. J Clin Apher. 2020;36:109.
53. Wai C-T, Lim S-G, Aung M-O, Lee Y-M, Sutedja DS, Dan Y-Y, et al. MARS®: a futile tool in centres without active liver transplant support. Liver Int. 2007;27(1):69–75.
54. Shanmugam N, Dhawan A. Acute liver failure in children. Pediatric Hepatol. Liver Transplant. 2018:145–53.
55. Baliga P, Alvarez S, Lindblad A, Zeng L. Posttransplant survival in pediatric fulminant hepatic failure: the SPLIT experience. Liver Transpl. 2004;10(11):1364–71.
56. Mahadeb P, Gras J, Sokal E, Otte J-B, Lerut J, Detaille T, et al. Liver transplantation in children with fulminant hepatic failure: the UCL experience. Pediatr Transplant. 2009;13(4):414–20.
57. Centeno MA, Bes DF, Sasbón JS. Mortality risk factors of a pediatric population with fulminant hepatic failure undergoing orthotopic liver transplantation in a pediatric intensive care unit*. Pediatr Crit Care Med. 2002;3(3):227.

58. Sundaram V, Shneider BL, Dhawan A, Ng VL, Im K, Belle S, et al. King's college hospital criteria for non-acetaminophen induced acute liver failure in an international cohort of children. J Pediatr. 2013;162(2):319–23.e1.
59. Dhawan A, Taylor RM, Cheeseman P, De Silva P, Katsiyiannakis L, Mieli-Vergani G. Wilson's disease in children: 37-year experience and revised King's score for liver transplantation. Liver Transpl. 2005;11(4):441–8.
60. Sanchez MC, D'Agostino DE. Pediatric end-stage liver disease score in acute liver failure to assess poor prognosis. J Pediatr Gastroenterol Nutr. 2012;54(2):193.
61. Rhee C, Narsinh K, Venick RS, Molina RA, Nga V, Engelhardt R, et al. Predictors of clinical outcome in children undergoing orthotopic liver transplantation for acute and chronic liver disease. Liver Transpl. 2006;12(9):1347–56.
62. McDiarmid SV. Management of the pediatric liver transplant patient. Liver Transpl. 2001;7(11, Part B):S77-S86:s77.
63. Moreno NF, Hernandez JA, Huang C-S, Desai MS, Haug AB, Cleveland H, et al. Our evolution in the treatment of hepatic artery and portal vein thrombosis in pediatric liver transplantation: success with catheter-directed therapies. Pediatr Transplant. 2022;26:e14306.
64. Ackermann O, Branchereau S, Franchi-Abella S, Pariente D, Chevret L, Debray D, et al. The long-term outcome of hepatic artery thrombosis after liver transplantation in children: role of urgent revascularization. Am J Transplant. 2012;12(6):1496–503.
65. Sanada Y, Katano T, Hirata Y, Yamada N, Okada N, Onishi Y, et al. Long-term outcome of percutaneous transhepatic biliary drainage for biliary strictures following pediatric liver transplantation. Clin Transpl. 2019;33(6):e13570.
66. Sieders E, Peeters PMJG, TenVergert EM, de Jong KP, Porte RJ, Zwaveling JH, et al. Graft loss after pediatric liver transplantation. Ann Surg. 2002;235(1):125–32.
67. Alcamo AM, Alessi LJ, Vehovic SN, Bansal N, Bond GJ, Carcillo JA, et al. Severe sepsis in pediatric liver transplant patients: the emergence of multidrug-resistant organisms. Pediatr Crit Care Med. 2019;20(7):e326–e32.
68. Hamada M, Matsukawa S, Shimizu S, Kai S, Mizota T. Acute kidney injury after pediatric liver transplantation: incidence, risk factors, and association with outcome. J Anesth. 2017;31(5):758–63.
69. Ghosh PS, Hupertz V, Ghosh D. Neurological complications following pediatric liver transplant. J Pediatr Gastroenterol Nutr. 2012;54(4):540.
70. Silver LJ, Pan S, Bucuvalas JC, Reid-Adam JA, Oishi K, Ofori-Amanfo G, et al. Acute kidney injury following pediatric liver transplant. J Intensive Care Med. 2020;37(1):107–13.
71. Ide K, Uchida H, Sakamoto S, Nishimura N, Nakagawa S, Kobayashi T, et al. Neurological impairment in children with acute liver failure following liver transplantation—a single-center experience. Pediatric Transplant. 2022;26(4):e14240.
72. Sorensen LG, Neighbors K, Hardison RM, Loomes KM, Varni JW, Ng VL, et al. Health related quality of life and neurocognitive outcomes in the first year after pediatric acute liver failure. J Pediatr. 2018;196:129–38.

Immunology in Paediatric Intensive Care

Michael J. Carter and Jordi Miatello

Contents

J. Brierley et al. (eds.), *ESPNIC Children's Intensive Care Textbook*,
https://doi.org/10.1007/978-3-031-64762-8_25

Learning Objectives

- To appreciate the development and function of the immune system to maintain health.
- To appreciate the importance of immunity in all children requiring paediatric intensive care.
- To understand the fundamentals of innate immunity for the paediatric intensivist: sensing of pathogen and damaged tissue that induce inflammatory responses.
- To understand the mechanisms of induction of the adaptive immune system in disease.
- To appreciate that dysregulation of immunity is common—if not ubiquitous—in children requiring paediatric critical care and why this is important for your patients.
- To appreciate current and likely future approaches to modulating the immune system in children receiving paediatric critical care, particularly in sepsis.

25.1 Introduction

Physiology should maintain homeostasis and, in children, enable growth. The immune system evolved to protect physiology from external pathogens and cancers and to achieve this without damage to host tissues. However, we shall see that a dysregulated immune response is a major part of some inherited defects of immunity, autoimmune diseases, acquired inflammatory syndromes, and sepsis. In addition, most medical interventions in paediatric critical care also alter immune function: through the removal of mucosal barriers (insertion of venous catheters or endotracheal tubes) or modulation of the hormonal milieu (administration of adrenergic medications or corticosteroids) and microbiota (administration of antibiotics). In brief, the immune system profoundly affects, and is affected by, the trajectory of all children admitted to an intensive care unit.

Here, we briefly review the development and function of the immune system in health and how this is altered in exemplar diseases. We consider the role of innate immunity in early sensing of pathogens, the initiation of inflammation, and the role of vascular endothelium and the coagulation cascade in inflammatory syndromes. We consider the roles of the innate and adaptive immune cells in inflammation and sepsis through the prism of dysregulated immunity. We conclude by offering views on the promise and challenges of personalised immunomodulation in sepsis—and the progress made in this important area during the era of COVID-19. The role of immunity in cancer, and important recent advances (such as the development of monoclonal antibodies and chimeric antigen receptor T cells) are not discussed here.

25.2 Mucosal Immunity

Arthropod-borne diseases, trauma and medical interventions may all bypass mucosal immunity. Nevertheless, the respiratory and gastrointestinal tract and the mucous membranes of mouth, eyes and genitalia are the pre-eminent sites of colonisation for most pathogens. Whether colonisation develops into infection depends upon the effectiveness of the initial mucosal immune response, including aspects of innate and adaptive immunity and specific physical barriers.

In the respiratory tract a pathogen will be met by a thick layer of mucous overlaying epithelial cells, giving a "gel-on-brush" microanatomy. Mucous physically protects epithelial cells from lytic peptides produced by pathogens. It also contains host-derived anti-viral and antibacterial molecules including lysozyme, cathelicidins (that modulate pathogen recognition receptors, PRRs), iron-chelators and nitric oxide [1]. Mucins, particularly MUC5A and MUC5B are components of mucous and enhance phagocytic actions of macrophages and dendritic cells. As we shall see, these cells clear invading pathogens and present antigen to cells of the adaptive immune system. Typically, presentation of antigen will result in the induction of short-lived plasma cells that secrete low affinity IgM to aid clearance of pathogen from the mucous membrane. Activated antigen-presenting cells and plasma cells may also migrate to the follicles of local secondary lymph nodes and initiate the process of somatic hypermutation and affinity maturation of the B cell receptor [2]. This leads to the production of higher affinity immunoglobulins such as IgA (secreted on mucosal surfaces) and IgG (systemic). A subset of long-lived plasma cells (LLPCs) may migrate to bone marrow to maintain basal secretion of immunoglobulin and form a rapid, high-affinity immune response to any immune challenge with the same antigen(s) in future [3].

25.3 Inflammation and Innate Immunity

Evasion of mucosal immunity by pathogen induces inflammation. Circulating peptides and lipids, including complement and eicosanoids, and classical immune cells such as macrophages, neutrophils and dendritic cells are well-recognised mediators of inflammation. However, host epithelial cells adjacent to mucous membranes are likely to be the first targets of invading pathogen. Here, a process of cell autonomous immunity elaborates a complex immune response upon stimulation of PRRs upon or within epithelial cells when ligated by pathogen-associated molecular patterns (PAMPS, ▫ Table 25.1) [4].

25.3.1 Cell Autonomous Immunity

The most well-studied of PRRs are the toll-like receptors. Ligation of TLRs activates a series of complex downstream pathways. When simplified, this leads to either de-repression of nuclear factor κ B (NFκB) and activation of the cell stress response or phosphorylation of interferon regulatory factors (IRF) 3 or 7, leading to secretion of type 1 (anti-viral) interferons (IFN) such as IFNα and IFNβ [5]. The cellular stress response leads to widespread repression of translation—preventing further viral subversion of translation for its own reproduction—but typically leads to cell death. Secretion of interferons leads to upregulation of a complex of more than 200 interferon-stimulated genes that amplify the intrinsic cell immune response [5]. These include increased expression of PRRs, their associated signalling molecules (TRIF and MyD88) and interferon-induced transmembrane (IFITM) pro-

Table 25.1 Key pathogen recognition receptors (PRRs), their ligands, major signalling proteins and (acquired) diseases associated with mutations in the PRR

Pathogen recognition receptor	Ligand	Signalling protein	Polymorphisms associated with disease
RIG I receptors	Double-stranded RNA (viruses)	Mitochondrial anti-viral signalling protein (MAVS)	RNA virus susceptibility
C-type lectin receptors	Carbohydrates on viruses, bacteria and fungi	Spleen tyrosine kinase (SYK)	Severe fungal infections
NOD-like receptors	Peptidoglycans bacterial cell walls	Nuclear factor κ B, inflammasomes	Inflammatory bowel disease, hereditary periodic fever syndromes
Toll-like receptors			
TLR2	Peptidoglycans, bacterial cell walls	MyD88	Mycobacterial infection
TLR3	Double-stranded RNA (viruses)	TRIF	HIV infection, HSV encephalitis
TLR4 (membrane)	Lipopolysaccharide, viruses	MyD88	Crohn's disease, asthma
TLR4 (endosomal)	Lipopolysaccharide, viruses	TRIF	
TLR5	Flagellin	MyD88	Bacterial pneumonia
TLR7	Single-stranded RNA	MyD88	Hepatitis C infection, HIV infection
TLR8	Single-stranded RNA	MyD88/TRIF	Tuberculosis
TLR9	Unmethylated CpR rich DNA	MyD88	Cerebral malaria

teins that inhibit fusion between viral and host cell membranes. PRR activation may also lead to induction of the NLRP3 inflammasome, a recently described complex of proteins that activates caspase-1. This in turn leads to cleavage of pro-IL1β and pro-IL18β to their active forms amplifying the inflammatory cascade. Caspase-1 also induces lytic cell death—a process known as pyroptosis—that damages surrounding cells, but induces widespread inflammation with the aim of controlling an invasive infection [6].

Cell autonomous immunity is a necessary but non-specific response that requires close regulation by specialist immune cells to prevent damage to epithelium that would render the host vulnerable to secondary infection. It is also susceptible to evasion and subversion by pathogens. Respiratory syncytial virus (RSV)—the most prevalent cause of severe respiratory infection globally—initially activates TLR4 via MyD88 and TRIF pathways following F-protein mediated fusion with the host cell membrane. However, early translation of the RSV G protein blocks this signalling cascade, preventing upregulation of NFκB and therefore inhibiting pro-inflammatory pathways. Like TLR4, RIG-I helicases also detect viral RNA and induce cell autonomous immunity via IRF3. This process is subverted by the translation of RSV non-structural proteins, NS1 and NS2, that block signalling downstream of RIG-I, reducing the ability of epithelial cells to upregulate interferon signalling and leading to ongoing infection [7, 8].

25.3.2 Circulating Mediators of Infection

Cell autonomous immunity is more-or-less static, but invasive pathogens circulate. Circulating mediators of inflammation act to spread and amplify inflammation and recruit specialist immune cells to the site of pathogen invasion. Complement proteins are evolutionarily ancient and derived from the same origin as coagulation factors. The central event of complement activation is cleavage of C3. Cleavage of C3 ultimately leads to generation of the membrane attack complex (formed by serial recruitment of later complement proteins that inserts pores to kill infected cells), opsonisation of antigen (improving phagocytosis by macrophages and other antigen-presenting cells), and production of C3a and C3b anaphylatoxin [9].

Initiation of the complement cascade occurs via the classical pathway or via the lectin pathway. In the classical pathway, complement-fixing antibodies such as IgG1 or IgM bind antigens on pathogen surfaces. This enables the C1 complex to stabilise on the constant fragment (Fc) on the tail of the antibody, which cleave C4 and C2 to form the C4bC2a convertase, which in turn leads to C3 cleavage and complement activation. In contrast, the lectin pathway uses less specific circulating PRRs, such as mannose-binding lectin, that form complexes with specific mannose serine proteases (MASP-1 and MASP-2) upon binding of sugar moieties on pathogen surfaces. MASP-1, MASP-2 and MASP-3 cleave C4 and C2 to C4bC2a, leading to C3 cleavage and complement activation [10].

To be effective, the complement cascade needs to be amplified. This is the role of the tightly regulated alternative pathway of activation. During quiescence, C3 spontaneously hydrolyses to C3b at low levels, which in turn binds a specific plasma protein, factor B, which itself is cleaved to form the C3bBb convertase. In the absence of inflammation this is an unstable complex that spontaneously degrades before it contributes to cleavage of C3. However, activated neutrophils release properdin, which stabilises C3bBb, leading to cleavage of C3 to activate complement. In the absence of regulation, the complement cascade is then amplified exponentially. Fortunately, the effect of properdin to stabilise C3bBb is antagonised by factor H, as plasma protein, that promotes degradation of C3b and therefore regulates the alternative pathway of complement activation [11]. Complement is of particular importance for the killing of *Neisseria meningitidis*, the meningococcus, with congenital mutations of complement genes, including properdin, strongly associated with invasive disease. Meningococci are also able to sequester factor H to their cell surface, leaving the regulatory function of complement factor H intact and therefore preventing complement-mediated killing of the bacterium.

An overlooked amplification system for inflammation is mediated by cell membrane-derived lipids: eicosanoids [12]. Inflammation, initiated by cell autonomous immunity, activates lipoxygenases (LOX) and cyclo-oxygenases (COX). These subsequently breakdown arachidonic acid (a metabolite of membrane phospholipids) ultimately to leukotrienes (via LOX) and prostaglandins and thromboxane (COX). Leukotrienes subsequently upregulate inflammation, including recruitment of neutrophils to the site of infection, enhancing nitric oxide and reactive oxygen species generation and enhancing T and dendritic cell recruitment to the site of inflammation. Antagonists of leukotriene effects include corticosteroids that (among other effects) limit the breakdown of arachidonic acid [13], and direct blockade, such as with montelukast. However, there is currently no evidence to support direct modulation of leukotriene activity in severe infection.

The complex relationships between complement, eicosanoids and the coagulation system have been brought into focus by the pandemic of SARS-CoV-2 related disease: COVID-19 and multisystem inflammatory syndrome in children (MIS-C). Injury of alveolar epithelium leads to complement and eicosanoid-mediated damage to vascular endothelium and vasodilatation that positively reinforces further inflammatory damage. This in turn degrades the glycocalyx of the vascular endothelium—a fine layer of protein and sugars extruding into the lumen—to further activate the coagulation cascade [14]. In adults, severe SARS-CoV-2 infection manifested as acute respiratory distress syndrome (ARDS) with associated hyperinflammation and coagulopathy. ARDS is perhaps unsurprising, given the extraordinarily large surface area of the lung [15]. However, it is still uncertain why children—even those with the hyperinflammatory syndrome of MIS-C—rarely developed ARDS.

25.4 Innate Immune Cells

Innate immunity is an evolutionarily ancient system that encompasses the cell autonomous immunity and circulating mediators of inflammation—but also includes an array of diverse cell types (◘ Fig. 25.1). In the round, the goals of professional immune cells are to regulate inflammatory cascades, to remove pathogens and pathogen-infected cells, and to link with the adaptive immune system to induce a more specific immune response capable of providing immune memory [16]. Regulation of inflammation is achieved through the secretion of chemokines (that recruit cells to inflammation, or to other niches within the immune system) and cytokines that directly control the activity of nearby cells. Removal of pathogen is mediated by phagocytosis—typically macrophages and neutrophils—and enhanced by the products of these cells. The link with adaptive immunity is mediated by antigen presentation—typically by dendritic cells and macrophages, but occasionally by other cell types. The creation of a pro-inflammatory milieu also aids the activation of T cells when the T cell receptor (TCR) encounters cognate antigen.

Neutrophils are the most numerous of innate immune cells—and instantly recognisable as pus cells. They circulate through the bloodstream and are typically early arrivals to a site of infection with extracellular pathogen. Their microbiocidal activ-

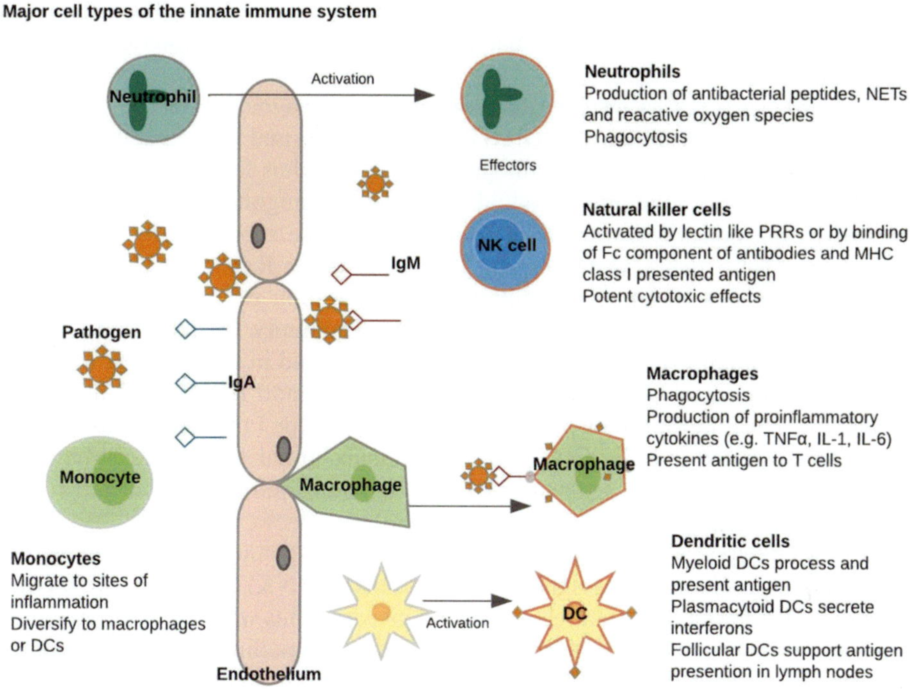

Fig. 25.1 Major cell types of the innate immune system. Schematic shows activation/migration of cells through endothelium from left to right

ity is typically mediated by the generation of reactive oxygen species and the release of antibacterial peptides such as elastase. In a hyperinflammatory state, neutrophils are also capable of releasing neutrophil extracellular traps (NETs) [17]. These consist of DNA, histones and other proteins that are released during apoptosis of highly activated neutrophils. NETs coat pathogens in highly immunogenic material, aiding their phagocytosis by other cells. However, NETS are also pro-coagulant, and increased levels of NETs are highly associated with worse outcomes in both non-COVID-19 and COVID-19 ARDS [18]. Thus, neutrophils provide another link between inflammation and coagulation. There is currently no evidence that extracorporeal removal of NETs may be beneficial in severe ARDS.

Monocytes circulate within the bloodstream along chemokine gradients to sites of inflammation. There is wide functional diversity within these cells, with classical, intermediate and non-classical types described according to the expression of CD16 (a receptor for the Fc portion of immunoglobulin; high in non-classical monocytes) and CD14 (a co-receptor for TLR4; high in classical monocytes) [19]. Further, upon arrival at the site of infection, these cells diversify into macrophages or dendritic cells. Unsurprisingly, macrophages are experts at the removal of pathogens through phagocytosis. This is aided by their expression of Fc gamma receptors, which bind antibodies that have opsonised pathogen antigen—in effect enabling the transfer of specific adaptive immunity (immunoglobulin) to effectors of the innate immune system. Macrophages are also key cells for the presentation of antigens to T cells through their expression of major histocompatibility complex (MHC class II; also known as HLA-DR), and secretion of pro-inflammatory cytokines such as interleukin(IL)-1, IL-6 and TNFα.

Dendritic cells (DCs) are also functionally diverse phagocytes [20]. Myeloid DCs are primarily antigen-presenting cells. They are characterised by their ability to present antigen from phagocytosed pathogens to T cells—thus forming a link between innate and adaptive immunity. Myeloid DCs may also migrate to the germinal centres of lymph nodes where (as follicular DCs) they are supported by T follicular helper cells. Here, they present antigens to B cells via the B cell receptor (BCR) for prolonged periods of time, enabling affinity maturation of the BCR (described below) and the generation of long-lasting specific immunity. Plasmacytoid DCs are another functionally distinct group of cells and are found in low numbers in blood. These cells produce type I interferons (typically IFNα and IFNβ) to counter viral infections. The importance of plasmacytoid DCs and type I interferons has recently been demonstrated in adult COVID-19, with a substantial decline in cell numbers [21] and auto-antibodies against interferon signalling molecules associated with severe disease [22].

But what happens to cells that are infected with viruses and are not killed by cell-autonomous immunity? This is the role of natural killer (NK) cells. These are specialised cells that have PRRs that recognise viral glycoproteins when they are presented on MHC class I proteins. Clustering of PRRs induces signalling via immunoreceptor tyrosine-based activation motifs (ITAMs) within the NK cell membrane that then cascades to activate the NK cell [23]. In turn, cytotoxins are released, pores are inserted into virus infected cell membrane and apoptosis is induced by the binding of Fas ligand. NK cells may also be potent secretors of TNFα. MHC class I receptors also express host antigens. To limit the danger of induction of self-reactivity, NK cells require a second reinforcing signal to mediate cytotoxicity via integrins that bind to activated endothelium (reinforcing the link with cell autonomous immunity). In addition, immunoreceptor tyrosine-based *inhibitory* motifs (ITIMs) downregulate cytotoxicity in the absence of PRR clustering. As with macrophages and monocytes, NK cells also express receptors for the Fc portion of immunoglobulin (CD16)—enabling the transfer of antigen-specific adaptive immunity (opsonisation) to effectors of innate immunity.

25.5 Adaptive Immunity

The importance of adaptive immunity for child health is illustrated by the predisposition of children with antibody defects, cell-mediated immunity, or in severe combined immunodeficiency (SCID) where variable loss of T cell, B cell and NK cell function occur [24]. Tragically, without bone marrow stem cell transplantation, children with SCID typically die within the first year of life from overwhelming infection. Adaptive immunity also offers opportunity to improve child health: vaccination is reliant upon the specific immunity induced by antigen challenge and immune memory.

25.5.1 T-Cell-Mediated Immunity

T cells mature in the thymus. They express a hyper-diverse TCR that is formed from the recombination of variable (V), diversity (D) and junctional (J) segments of typically the α and β chains and more rarely γ and δ chains. Further diversity is ensured by the deletion of intervening gene segments. Both recombination and deletion of gene segments are induced by the recombination activating genes (RAG-1 and RAG-2) [25]. Loss of RAG-1 and RAG-2 function leads to the variable phenotypes of SCID, while self-tolerance is ensured by the deletion of self-reactive TCR-expressing T cells in the thymus during development.

T cells coordinate adaptive immune response and provide support to innate immune cells through secretion of cytokines [26]. Broadly, four groups of T cells are recognised in peripheral blood: CD4+ T helper cells (CD4 T_H cells), CD4+ regulatory T cells (CD4 T_{reg} cells), CD8+ cytotoxic T cells (CD8 T cells) and γδ TCR expressing T cells (γδT cells) [27]. Both CD4 and CD8 are co-receptors for the TCR, with CD4 supporting the detection of pathogen antigen expressed on host cell MHC class II molecules and CD8 supporting the detection of pathogen antigen on host cell MHC class I molecules. This functionally translates to CD4 T_H cells supporting innate immune cells to kill phagocytosed pathogens and CD8 T cells directly killing virus-infected cells.

However, activation of CD4 T_H cells requires two signals. The second signal may be activation by pro-inflammatory cytokines derived from macrophages or CD4 T_H cells themselves. Alternatively, the binding of CTLA-4 on T cells by B7 expressed on antigen-presenting cells may induce T cell activation. Following activation, distinct groups of CD4 T_H cells secrete cytokines: classically, T_{H1} cells secrete IFNγ and IL-2; T_{H17} cells secrete IL-17, which acts as a chemokine for neutrophils and macrophages; and T_{H2} cells secrete IL-4, IL-5, IL-6 and IL-10 and induce activation of B cells—but constrain activation of cytotoxic CD8 T cells. As we shall see, T cells help the activation of B cells, enabling a more specific adaptive immune response.

Activation of CD8 T cells also requires two signals—in this case IL-2 by CD4 T_H cells in the context of restriction of TCR by MHC class I. Thus, the major subsets of T cells work in concert. Like NK cells, CD8 T cells release cytotoxic granules directly into bound virus-infected cells and induce apoptosis of cells that have upregulated Fas ligand in response to type I interferons. The small population of γδT cells also seems able to kill infected cells, but the mechanisms through which these cells are activated remain poorly defined.

In contrast to other groups of T cells, CD4 T_{reg} cells limit inflammation and act as immunosuppressors [28]. As with activated CD8 T cells, they express the IL-2 receptor. Uniquely, they also express the transcription factor FOXP3. As with T_{H1} cells they interact through TCR and CTLA4 with cognate antigen and B7 on the antigen-presenting cell. However, T_{reg} cells secrete IL-10 and TGFβ, which induces anergy and apoptosis in other immune cells. This is likely to be an important physiological response in most cases and contributes to the return of immune homeostasis. However, in a dysfunctional immune response—as seen in sepsis, for example—T_{reg} cell-mediated immunosuppression may lead to failure to clear pathogen or predispose to secondary infection. T_{reg} cells are also targets for immunomodulation in cancer, where their depletion may enable immune reconstitution to enhance the killing of neoplastic cells.

25.5.2 B Cell-Mediated Immunity

B cells mature in the bone marrow. As with T cells, they express a hyper-diverse receptor, the BCR. However, the BCR can also be secreted: a molecule that we call an antibody (or immunoglobulin). Immunoglobulins have classes IgD (important in basophils and mast cells), IgM (non-specific, forms pentamers), IgA (on mucosae, secreted as dimers), IgE (typically found in allergy or anti-parasitic immunity), and IgG (highly specific). BCR and immunoglobulins are formed by RAG-1 and RAG-2 mediated recombination of V, D and J segments that encode the immunoglobulin heavy chain (IGH) and the V and J segments that encode the light chain (IGL) [2]. As with the TCR, this enables an enormous range of cognate antigens to be bound. B cells can be activated without the support of T cells (T cell-independent pathways, ◘ Fig. 25.2). However, the activation of B cells by activated T cells can induce class-switching of antibody and somatic hypermutation and affinity maturation [29], a process through which specific antibody responses are created and where (classically) memory B cell responses are created [30].

25.5.3 T Cell-Independent B Cell Immunity

As we have seen, opsonisation of pathogen antigen with antibody contributes in important ways to innate immunity. Rapid induction of antibody production is therefore important, even at the cost of lower specificity (and potentially the rare risk inducing autoimmunity). B1 cells, the major B cells in peritoneal and pleural cavities, perform this function. These cells are activated by the binding of stereotyped pathogen polysaccharides and RNA to TLRs and other PRRs and produce non-specific IgM to counter an immediate threat. Immunoglobulins from B1 cells do not class-switch.

25.5.4 T Cell-Dependent B Cell Immunity

T cell-dependent B cell immunity requires the migration of B2 cells from the marginal zones of spleen or lymph nodes to upregulate the chemokine receptor CCR7 and migrate to the extrafollicular regions of lymphoid organs. Here, they interact with antigen-presenting cells to internalise foreign antigen, process and present on MHC class II molecules on the surface of the B cell. B cells upregulate CD40 and inducible T cell co-stimulator (ICOS) ligand in the presence of inflammatory cytokines. This enables interaction with follicular T_H cells, with a subset of B cells, then entering the lymph node follicle to form germinal centres. Class-switching and somatic hypermutation are subsequently induced by the activation-induced cytidine-deaminase (AID) that cleaves the genes encoding the Fc portion of IGH (for class-switching) and the V region of IGH (for somatic hypermutation) [31]. These

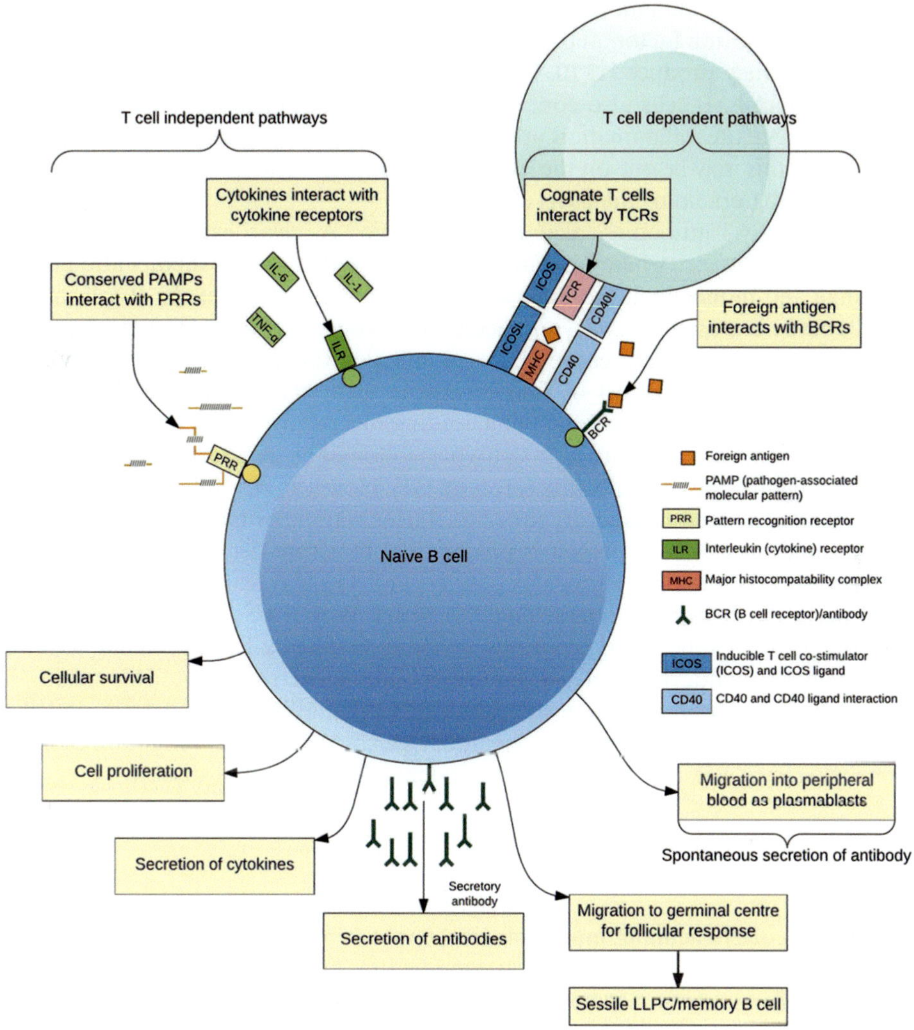

Fig. 25.2 T cell-dependent and independent pathways of activation. From Carter et al. (2017). B cells receive activating signals by T cell-independent or T cell-dependent pathways that predispose the cell to a certain phenotype and antibody production

genomically unstable B cells are selected for survival if their BCR is cognate to the presented antigens in the germinal centre. Affinity maturation of the BCR occurs due to repeated rounds of somatic hypermutation and selection at this stage, with the BCR becoming increasingly specific to the presented antigen. At each stage of selection, there is a small probability that the cell will leave the germinal centre and become either a plasma cell or a memory B cell that will settle in a niche in the bone marrow. Affinity maturation may also be used for therapeutic gain: the SARS-CoV-2 pandemic exploited sequencing of plasma cells to generate therapeutic monoclonal antibodies, and there is every possibility that this technology could be used for other severe infectious diseases [32].

B cells are also immunoregulatory [33]. Unlike T_{reg} cells, they do not express a specific transcription factor, and they are also from diverse B cell lineages. However, functionally, they produce IL-10, IL-25 and TGFβ that mediate anti-inflammatory effects on T cells. B cells also contain ITIMs in the cell membrane that, as in NK cells, downregulate inflammation upon binding of the Fc portion of immunoglobulin. Indeed, this may be one on the (probably multiple) ways that therapeutic intravenous immunoglobulin mediates its effects.

More rarely, antibodies may be pathogenic. A clear example is in autoinflammatory disease, where immunomodulation with steroids, therapeutic plasma exchange and monoclonal antibodies such as rituximab (against the B cell marker CD20) have been used with varying success. From a global perspective, dengue virus disease is a more prevalent cause of severe infection due to antibody-mediated disease. Dengue viruses consist of four serotypes: an initial infection with a dengue virus is typically mild and self-resolving, leading to a relatively short broadly reactive antibody response (against all four serotypes) followed by an effective memory B cell response against the one infecting serotype [34]. However, if a subsequent infection with a second dengue virus serotype occurs during waning of the initial broadly reactive antibody response, a person is predisposed to severe dengue shock syndrome with severe inflammation, glycocalyx damage and vascular leak. A similar phenomenon occurs in infants in dengue-endemic areas. Why is this? In brief, the poorly reactive antibody binds dengue virions, enabling uptake by Fcγ expressing immune cells such as monocytes that are unable to fully clear the virus. This results in extremely high viraemia and a positive cycle of further inflammation and endothelial damage. The shock syndrome and haemorrhage associated with dengue virus infection is therefore a result of antibody-dependent enhancement of disease.

25.6 Sepsis

Sepsis is the overwhelming immunological concern of most paediatric intensivists. The definition of sepsis in adults was modified in 2016 (Sepsis-3) from a focus on systemic inflammatory response syndrome to a *life-threatening organ dysfunction caused by a dysregulated host response to infection* [35]. This was made operational using the sequential (or sepsis-related) organ failure assessment (SOFA) to semi-quantify organ dysfunction, the explicit inclusion of septic shock as part of sepsis. Validation was undertaken in several large (adult) datasets that showed profound circulatory, immunological, and metabolic changes—and an improved sensitivity and specificity for mortality in comparison to previous definitions of sepsis [36]. This approach emphasises the central role of dysregulated immunity in sepsis [37], and by extension, the potential role of immunomodulation in sepsis, in primary infection, to prevent secondary hospital-acquired infections, or subsequently in the SARS-CoV-2 pandemic and severe COVID-19 or MIS-C [38]. An updated version of the paediatric definition of sepsis is keenly awaited [39].

25.6.1 Personalised Immunomodulation in Sepsis?

Following the remarkable work of platform trials, such as the Recovery Trial, corticosteroids have become the first-line treatment for many patients admitted to hospital with COVID-19 [40]. In the original publication, the age-adjusted rate ratio for mortality was 0.83 (95% CI 0.75–0.93) across the cohort of over 2100 adults hospitalised in the United Kingdom. Yet the treatment effect varied considerably by prognosis: among those mechanically ventilated at randomisation the adjusted rate ratio for mortality was 0.64 (95% CI 0.51–0.81) but was 1.19 (95% CI 0.92–1.55) at randomisation. Thus, the guidelines endorsed by the World Health Organisation supported the use of dexamethasone for patients receiving oxygen (or higher-level respiratory support) for COVID-19, but not for other unsupported patients. This process is *prognostic enrichment*, or stratification, of patients.

A slightly different concept is that of *predictive enrichment* of patients based on the biology of disease. This may take the form of simple demographics. For example, patients <70 years of age, males, and Black/Asian/minority ethnic people (in comparison to White ethnic groups) all had lower rate ratios of mortality (age-adjusted where appropriate) than their comparator (older/female/ethnic White) groups in the original Recovery Trial, and this may be related to biology. However, we may be able to go beyond these crude characteristics. Several research groups have analysed the differential regulation of genes (the transcriptome) in sepsis to identify patients who may benefit from immunomodulation [41, 42]. Could these immune signatures be used to stratify patients according to their biology? A secondary analysis of adults with sepsis randomised to receive corticosteroids or placebo (the Vanish Trial) showed that the treatment effect differed based on whether a patient was in the "immunosuppressed" sepsis-response syndrome (SRS)-1 or "immunocompetent" SRS-2 group based on retrospective analysis of the host transcriptome [43]. Unfortunately, in this cohort of adults with sepsis, corticosteroid administration was associated with increased mortality compared with placebo in the SRS-2 group and had no effect on mortality in the SRS-1 group.

Nonetheless, the principle of identifying relevant biology for immunomodulation (or not) of sepsis is becoming established. Key challenges remain, including whether multiple samples are required to assess the trajectory of a patient before administering immunomodulators and whether can tests be simplified (and made quicker) [44]. Only then will we be able to move to randomised controlled trials of immunomodulators stratified on immune phenotype. This may seem problematic, but our colleagues in oncology, rheumatology and infectious diseases have shown that personalised medicine is possible—and we intensivists need to work to join them.

References

1. Zanin M, Baviskar P, Webster R, Webby R. The interaction between respiratory pathogens and mucus. Cell Host Microbe. 2016;19(2):159–68.
2. Rajewsky K. Clonal selection and learning in the antibody system. Nature. 1996;381(6585):751–8.
3. Tarlinton D, Good-Jacobson K. Diversity among memory B cells: origin, consequences, and utility. Science. 2013;341(6151):1205–11.

4. Randow F, MacMicking JD, James LC. Cellular self-defense: how cell-autonomous immunity protects against pathogens. Science. 2013;340(6133):701–6.
5. MacMicking JD. Interferon-inducible effector mechanisms in cell-autonomous immunity. Nat Rev Immunol. 2012;12(5):367–82.
6. Swanson KV, Deng M, Ting JPY. The NLRP3 inflammasome: molecular activation and regulation to therapeutics. Nat Rev Immunol. 2019;19(8):477–89.
7. Chiu C, Openshaw PJ. Antiviral B cell and T cell immunity in the lungs. Nat Immunol. 2015;16(1):18–26.
8. Russell CD, Unger SA, Walton M, Schwarze J. The human immune response to respiratory syncytial virus infection. Clin Microbiol Rev. 2017;30(2):481–502.
9. Walport MJ. Complement. First of two parts. N Engl J Med. 2001;344(14):1058–66.
10. Dunkelberger JR, Song W-C. Complement and its role in innate and adaptive immune responses. Cell Res. 2010;20(1):34–50.
11. Agarwal S, Ferreira VP, Cortes C, Pangburn MK, Rice PA, Ram S. An evaluation of the role of properdin in alternative pathway activation on Neisseria meningitidis and Neisseria gonorrhoeae. J Immunol. 2010;185(1):507–16.
12. Dennis EA, Norris PC. Eicosanoid storm in infection and inflammation. Nat Rev Immunol. 2015;15(8):511–23.
13. Rhen T, Cidlowski JA. Antiinflammatory action of glucocorticoids—new mechanisms for old drugs. N Engl J Med. 2005;353(16):1711–23.
14. Ramlall V, Thangaraj PM, Meydan C, et al. Immune complement and coagulation dysfunction in adverse outcomes of SARS-CoV-2 infection. Nat Med. 2020;26(10):1609–15.
15. Afzali B, Noris M, Lambrecht BN, Kemper C. The state of complement in COVID-19. Nat Rev Immunol. 2022;22(2):77–84.
16. Murphy K. Janeway's immunobiology. 9th ed. New York: Garland Science; 2018.
17. Storisteanu DM, Pocock JM, Cowburn AS, et al. Evasion of neutrophil extracellular traps by respiratory pathogens. Am J Respir Cell Mol Biol. 2017;56(4):423–31.
18. Arcanjo A, Logullo J, Menezes CCB, et al. The emerging role of neutrophil extracellular traps in severe acute respiratory syndrome coronavirus 2 (COVID-19). Sci Rep. 2020;10(1):19630.
19. Cormican S, Griffin MD. Human monocyte subset distinctions and function: insights from gene expression analysis. Front Immunol. 2020;11:1070.
20. Wculek SK, Cueto FJ, Mujal AM, Melero I, Krummel MF, Sancho D. Dendritic cells in cancer immunology and immunotherapy. Nat Rev Immunol. 2020;20(1):7–24.
21. Laing AG, Lorenc A, Del Molino Del Barrio I, et al. A dynamic COVID-19 immune signature includes associations with poor prognosis. Nat Med. 2020;26(10):1623–35.
22. Bastard P, Rosen LB, Zhang Q, et al. Autoantibodies against type I IFNs in patients with life-threatening COVID-19. Science. 2020;370(6515):eabd4585.
23. Bar-Joseph Z, Gerber G, Simon I, Gifford DK, Jaakkola TS. Comparing the continuous representation of time-series expression profiles to identify differentially expressed genes. Proc Natl Acad Sci U S A. 2003;100(18):10146–51.
24. Fischer A, Notarangelo LD, Neven B, Cavazzana M, Puck JM. Severe combined immunodeficiencies and related disorders. Nat Rev Dis Primers. 2015;1(1):15061.
25. Teng G, Maman Y, Resch W, et al. RAG represents a widespread threat to the lymphocyte genome. Cell. 2015;162(4):751–65.
26. Jensen IJ, Sjaastad FV, Griffith TS, Badovinac VP. Sepsis-induced T cell immunoparalysis: the ins and outs of impaired T cell immunity. J Immunol. 2018;200(5):1543–53.
27. Bluestone JA, Mackay CR, O'Shea JJ, Stockinger B. The functional plasticity of T cell subsets. Nat Rev Immunol. 2009;9(11):811–6.
28. Conway Morris A, Datta D, Shankar-Hari M, et al. Cell-surface signatures of immune dysfunction risk-stratify critically ill patients: INFECT study. Intensive Care Med. 2018;44(5):627–35.
29. Carter MJ, Mitchell RM, Meyer Sauteur PM, Kelly DF, Trück J. The antibody-secreting cell response to infection: kinetics and clinical applications. Front Immunol. 2017;8:630.
30. Tonegawa S. Somatic generation of antibody diversity. Nature. 1983;302(5909):575–81.
31. Batista FD, Harwood NE. The who, how and where of antigen presentation to B cells. Nat Rev Immunol. 2009;9(1):15–27.
32. van der Poll T, van de Veerdonk FL, Scicluna BP, Netea MG. The immunopathology of sepsis and potential therapeutic targets. Nat Rev Immunol. 2017;17(7):407–20.

33. Liu J, Zhan W, Kim CJ, et al. IL-10-producing B cells are induced early in HIV-1 infection and suppress HIV-1-specific T cell responses. PLoS One. 2014;9(2):e89236.
34. Whitehorn J, Simmons CP. The pathogenesis of dengue. Vaccine. 2011;29(42):7221–8.
35. Singer M, Deutschman CS, Seymour CW, et al. The third international consensus definitions for sepsis and septic shock (Sepsis-3). JAMA. 2016;315(8):801–10.
36. Shankar-Hari M, Harrison DA, Rubenfeld GD, Rowan K. Epidemiology of sepsis and septic shock in critical care units: comparison between sepsis-2 and sepsis-3 populations using a national critical care database. Br J Anaesth. 2017;119(4):626–36.
37. Hotchkiss RS, Monneret G, Payen D. Sepsis-induced immunosuppression: from cellular dysfunctions to immunotherapy. Nat Rev Immunol. 2013;13(12):862–74.
38. Carter MJ, Fish M, Jennings A, et al. Peripheral immunophenotypes in children with multisystem inflammatory syndrome associated with SARS-CoV-2 infection. Nat Med. 2020;26(11):1701–7.
39. Schlapbach LJ, Javouhey E, Jansen NJG. Paediatric sepsis: old wine in new bottles? Intensive Care Med. 2017;43(11):1686–9.
40. Recovery Collaborative Group, Horby P, Lim WS, et al. Dexamethasone in hospitalized patients with Covid-19. N Engl J Med. 2021;384(8):693–704.
41. Davenport EE, Burnham KL, Radhakrishnan J, et al. Genomic landscape of the individual host response and outcomes in sepsis: a prospective cohort study. Lancet Respir Med. 2016;4(4):259–71.
42. Scicluna BP, van Vught LA, Zwinderman AH, et al. Classification of patients with sepsis according to blood genomic endotype: a prospective cohort study. Lancet Respir Med. 2017;5(10):816–26.
43. Antcliffe DB, Burnham KL, Al-Beidh F, et al. Transcriptomic signatures in sepsis and a differential response to steroids. From the VANISH randomized trial. Am J Respir Crit Care. 2019;199(8):980–6.
44. Rubio I, Osuchowski MF, Shankar-Hari M, et al. Current gaps in sepsis immunology: new opportunities for translational research. Lancet Infect Dis. 2019;19(12):e422–e36.

Metabolic Emergencies in the Paediatric Intensive Care Setting

Thomas Slater and Roshni Vara

Contents

J. Brierley et al. (eds.), *ESPNIC Children's Intensive Care Textbook*,
https://doi.org/10.1007/978-3-031-64762-8_26

Learning Objectives

The chapter aims to provide:

- A basic understanding of common metabolic investigations required in the acute crisis.
- A diagnostic approach to the metabolic emergency.
- Common principles of management.
- Focused management in specific scenarios (hyperammonaemia, glycaemic control, profound metabolic acidosis).

26.1 Introduction

Inborn Errors of Metabolism (IEM) are a rare and heterogeneous group of inherited disorders, some of which have a high risk of metabolic decompensation and early intensive care support in a tertiary setting can significantly improve morbidity and mortality. The majority of IEM's are single gene defects causing an enzyme deficiency which leads to accumulation of toxic substances e.g. ammonia and/or deficiency in essential metabolites e.g. glucose.

The classification of IEMs can be broadly made into intoxication type disorders (e.g. urea cycle defects, organic acidaemias or fatty acid oxidation disorders), disorders of energy metabolism (e.g. glycogen storage disorders, mitochondrial disorders), lysosomal storage disorders (mucopolysaccharidoses, Niemann Pick disease), neurotransmitter disorders and disorders of complex molecules (e.g. peroxisomal disorders).

Often viewed as a challenging group of disorders, these groups of patients are individually rare but collectively common. However, acute presentations can often follow similar themes and therefore a common stepwise approach to diagnosis and management can be appropriate [1].

The clinical features of a metabolic crisis pertaining to an ITU admission can often be very non-specific: lethargy, poor feeding, vomiting, hypotonia and encephalopathy. In the older child, a more insidious course can include developmental delay, behavioural changes and psychosis. Significant red flags in the history such as consanguinity, previously unexplained neonatal deaths and often a symptom-free period can also suggest an IEM [2]. Baseline metabolic tests must include blood glucose, blood gas, lactate, ammonia and ketones.

Identifying the potential metabolic crisis from other more common causes can be complex but the prompt ability to do so can be lifesaving. Whilst the precise diagnosis may come from a specialist metabolic team, having a framework to support and treat these patients is crucial.

26.2 Clinical History and Examination

There can be red flags in the clinical history which suggest an IEM, however, clinical examination can often be non-specific. History-taking is important and may help identify specific toxins or triggers which may have led to acute decompensation. For example, a high protein load in undiagnosed urea cycle defects or fructose ingestion in hereditary fructose intolerance. ◘ Table 26.1 shows red flags which may be useful in identifying IEMs, and ◘ Table 26.2 shows common clinical presentations

Table 26.1 Red flags

Clinical history	Systemic examination
Consanguinity	Dysmorphic features (peroxisomal and lysosomal storage disorders)
Neonatal/infant deaths	Cherry red spot (lysosomal storage disorders)
Acute fatty liver of pregnancy/HELLP syndrome (long-chain fatty acid oxidation defects)	Hypotonia/hypertonia
Symptom-free period Triggers (infection, weaning, fasting)	Hepatomegaly and/or splenomegaly Jaundice
Developmental delay/changes in behaviour	Cataracts (galactosaemia)
Chronic/cyclical vomiting	Odour ('maple syrup', 'sweaty feet')

Table 26.2 Common acute presentations in the acute metabolic patient

Neurological	General
Acute encephalopathy	Poor feeding ± vomiting
Seizures	Lethargy
Stroke-like illness	Rhabdomyolysis
Acute ataxia	Disorders of acid-base balance Sudden collapse
Hepatobiliary	**Cardiac**
Acute liver failure	Myocardial infarction
Chronic liver disease	Cardiomyopathy
Acute pancreatitis	Cardiac arrhythmias
Adapted from [1, 3]	

26.3 Biochemical Investigations

For many, the fear of "metabolic patient" starts with the inevitably long list of laboratory investigations. These tests are often unfamiliar to many and beneficial is an understanding of the rationale of these tests. Close liaison with metabolic and local biochemistry services can reduce sampling error and, in many cases, facilitate more rapid diagnosis. First-line metabolic investigations are summarized in Table 26.3. Second and third-line investigations tend to be more disease-specific and directed by the metabolic specialist. In the current era of genetic diagnosis, it is important to consider gaining consent to store DNA samples early on.

Table 26.3 Summary of common diagnostic investigations in the metabolic emergency

	Notes
Blood glucose	Hypoglycaemia can indicate disorders of carbohydrate metabolism, fatty acid oxidation and energy metabolism
Blood lactate	Primary causes include mitochondrial disorders and glycogen storage disorder type 1 Exclude secondary causes such as sepsis, hypoxia/hypoperfusion, liver dysfunction and cardiac defects
Ketones (3-hydroxybutyrate) and free fatty acids	The presence of ketones in the fed state and in the neonate is normally pathological. The relationship between free fatty acids and ketones can help identify hyperinsulinism and fatty acid oxidation defects Absence of ketones in association with hypoglycaemia can indicate a fatty acid oxidation defect or hyperinsulinaemia *3-Hydroxybutyrate is a ketone body and can confirm ketosis in the bedside or laboratory setting*
Ammonia	This is a mandatory test in all acutely unwell neonates and any child with unexplained encephalopathy. Ammonia is neurotoxic and will detect urea cycle defects and other IEMs *Samples must be sent on ice (to avoid artefactually high readings) and should be analysed immediately* *Normal values are < 50 µmol/L, but mildly raised values up to 80 µmol/L are acceptable in the neonate. >100 µmol/L should be taken seriously. In all cases of a raised ammonia, a repeat sample should be sent as soon as possible and liaison with a metabolic specialist for advice*
Acylcarnitines	These are biological intermediates that play a vital role. They are involved in critical energy production during times of prolonged fasting and increased calorific requirement. Acylcarnitine measurement is used in the diagnosis of fatty acid oxidation disorders and organic acidaemias *Acylcarnitines are usually sent as dried blood spots on a Guthrie card (analysed by tandem mass spectrometry) or can be sent as plasma sample. The analysis of a blood spot sample is more rapid*
Plasma amino acids	These can identify individual deficits or accumulations to isolate the enzymatic defect in a metabolic pathway. They are also sent to monitor specific protein requirements (i.e. in phenylketonuria, maple syrup urine disease) and in conjunction with organic acids can identify specific urea cycle defects
Urine organic acids	These are water-soluble compounds containing one or more carboxyl groups as well as other functional groups (i.e -keto or -hydroxy). They occur as physiologic intermediates in a variety of metabolic pathways The organic acidurias are a group of disorders in which one or more of these pathways are blocked, resulting in a deficiency of normal products and an abnormal accumulation of intermediate metabolites (organic acids) in the body. These excess metabolites are excreted in the urine and can help identify a specific disorder

Adapted from [2, 4–6]

26.4 Management Principles

Approach to the metabolic emergency should be with the normal ABCD resuscitation framework. Dehydration, hypoglycaemia and electrolyte abnormalities should be corrected and seizures should be managed as per national resuscitation protocols. There should be a low threshold to obtain urgent cranial imaging for cerebral oedema.

In intoxication-type disorders, stopping the offending substrate is vital e.g. protein in urea cycle defects and avoiding of catabolism. Adequate calories are crucial to promote anabolism often with high dextrose solutions and/or intravenous nutrition with insulin as advised by a metabolic specialist. In some situations, such as mitochondrial disorders and citrin deficiency, high dextrose-containing fluids can be harmful, and advice should be sought prior to use. Lactate-containing fluids such as Hartmann's are generally avoided due to reduced lactate clearance in many patients. Fasting should be minimized where possible [1]. Early consideration for haemofiltration can be advantageous, and continuous venovenous haemofiltration is normally preferred [7].

In the deteriorating child, early intubation and ventilation should be considered. Propofol, an anaesthetic agent, is best avoided due to potential interference with mitochondrial function.

26.5 Specific Scenarios

26.5.1 Hyperammonaemia

Ammonia, a by-product of protein catabolism (or more precisely, deamination of amino acids), is extremely neurotoxic. Ammonia is detoxified to urea via the urea cycle by a number of enzymatic steps occurring in the hepatocyte. The complete urea cycle is exclusively expressed in the liver. Enzyme deficiencies at any step of the urea cycle can lead to accumulation of ammonia. The most common urea cycle defect is OTC (ornithine transcarbamylase) deficiency. This is an X-linked disorder and the others are all autosomal recessive in inheritance.

Hyperammonaemia is a metabolic emergency. Symptoms can be variable and should always be considered as part of the differential diagnosis in the unwell neonate or child. Prompt management can significantly improve outcome [2]. A number of differential diagnoses should be considered as shown in ◘ Table 26.4. A framework for diagnosis is shown in ◘ Fig. 26.1. Severe urea cycle defects e.g. male infant with OTC deficiency can present within 24 h of birth.

Principles of treatment include ammonia elimination and reduction of ammonia production. Enteral feeds should be withheld and replaced with intravenous dextrose to reduce the protein load. Supportive hydration with intravenous dextrose provides renal protection and improves tissue perfusion. This is summarized in ◘ Fig. 26.2.

Table 26.4 Differentials of hyperammonaemia. Adapted from [5, 7]

Urea cycle defects • N-acetyl glutamate synthetase deficiency (NAGS) deficiency • Carbamyl phosphate synthetase (CPS1) deficiency • Ornithine carbamyltransferase (OTC) deficiency • Argininosuccinate synthetase deficiency (Citrullinaemia) • Argininosuccinate lyase deficiency (Argininosuccinic Aciduria) • Arginase deficiency **Organic acidurias** • Propionic acidaemia • Methylmalonic acidaemia • Isovaleric acidaemia **Disorders of fatty acid oxidation** • Medium-chain acyl CoA dehydrogenase (MCAD) deficiency • Very long-chain acyl CoA dehydrogenase (VLCAD) deficiency • Long-chain hydroxyl acyl CoA dehydrogenase (LCHAD) deficiency	**Acquired** • Transient hyperammonaemia of the newborn • Infections (particularly with urease positive bacteria or Herpes Simplex) • Liver failure • Portosystemic shunting **Others** • Lysinuric protein intolerance • Pyruvate dehydrogenase deficiency • Hyperinsulinaemic hyperammonaemia (HIHA) • Mitochondrial disorders • Citrin deficiency • Ornithine aminotransferase (OAT) deficiency **Artefactual** • Haemolysed specimen • Incorrect transport • Delayed analysis

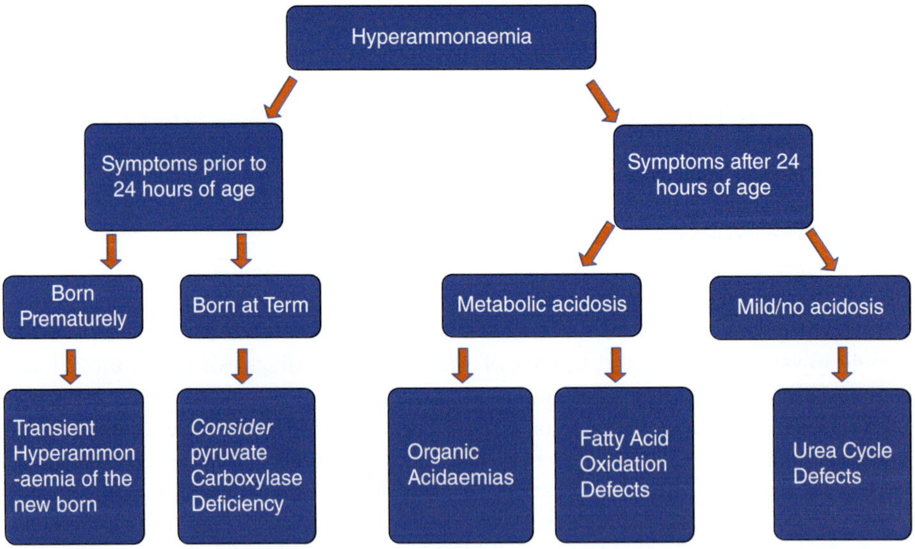

Fig. 26.1 Algorithm for hyperammonaemia in the context of metabolic disorders. Adapted from [3]

- Stop protein intake.
- Promote anabolism with at least 10% dextrose with electrolytes as per table 6.
- Start ammonia lowering agents as per metabolic advice, see table 5.
- Prepare for early CVVH especially if ammonia > 300mmol/L and rising.
- Send plasma and urine samples as soon as possible with EDTA DNA sample for storage.
- Contact metabolic specialist early.

Fig. 26.2 Acute management of hyperammonaemia

Table 26.5 Emergency drug doses for hyperammonaemia

Drug	Loading dose over 90 min	Followed by maintenance dose over 24 h	Maximum daily dose (every 24 h thereafter)
Sodium benzoate	250 mg/kg	250 mg/kg/day	500 mg/kg
Sodium phenylbutyrate	250 mg/kg	250 mg/kg/day	500 mg/kg
L-arginine	200 mg/kg	100–200 mg/kg/day	–

Taken from [5]

Sodium benzoate and sodium phenylbutyrate are ammonia-lowering or alternate pathway medications. They conjugate the amino acids glycine and glutamine, respectively, and divert them away from entering the urea cycle. Arginine can become deficient in some urea cycle defects and cana also be required as an infusion. Loading doses are required in naïve patients. A typical dosing regime is shown in Table 26.5.

Hyperammonaemia requires intensive monitoring and specialist medications. Transfer to intensive care or specialist centre is almost always indicated. Monitoring considerations are shown in Fig. 26.3.

26.5.2 Metabolic Acidosis

Metabolic acidosis is a very non-specific finding. Infection, dehydration and tissue anoxia are all common causes. However an expectedly profound metabolic acidosis can be suggestive of an underlying metabolic disorder. Renal and gastric causes should also be considered but calculating an anion gap can provide useful information:

$$\text{Anion Gap} = \left[Na^{+}\right] - \left[Cl^{-} + HCO_3^{-}\right]$$

- Monitor ammonia at least 4 -6 hourly. Liaise regularly with the specialist metabolic service.
- Monitor electrolytes carefully. Hypokalaemia is common and the sodium content of common infusions is high.
- If the blood glucose exceeds 10mmol/L start an insulin infusion as per local diabetic/neonatal protocols rather than reduce the glucose.
- Treat constipation which can contribute to hyporammonaemia.
- Send plasma and urine samples early with EDTA DNA sample for storage.
- Consider intralipid infusion (discuss with metabolic specialist).

Fig. 26.3 Further considerations when treating the child with a raised ammonia

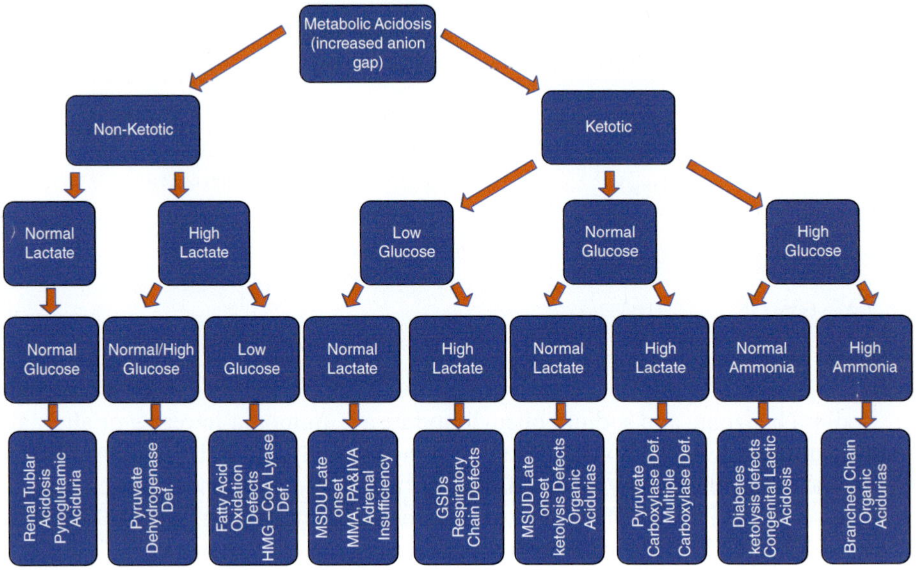

Fig. 26.4 A schematic interpretation of the metabolic acidosis with a raised anion gap. Adapted from [8]

A normal anion gap is <10 mmol/L. A raised anion gap (often >20 mmol/L) suggests a true metabolic acidosis with accumulation of organic acids (i.e. carboxylic acids such as lactate and ketones). A schematic interpretation can be seen in Fig. 26.4.

Ketones, whilst a normal physiological finding of catabolism, can provide clues about the defective metabolic pathway, e.g., they are usually absent in fatty acid oxidation defects.

Lactic acidosis is often much more concerning and one that does not correct after birth in the neonatal period can be highly suggestive of an IEM. An elevated plasma lactate can be secondary to sepsis, cardiac disease, tissue hypoperfusion (i.e. from circulatory failure or hypoxia), liver dysfunction or seizures. Lactate is a weak acid and only begins to contribute to metabolic acidosis when >5 mmol/L.

Table 26.6 IEMs associated with lactic acidosis

Glucose-6-phosphatase deficiency (GSD type 1)
Fructose-1,6-bisphosphatase deficiency
Pyruvate carboxylase deficiency
Pyruvate dehydrogenase deficiency
Organic acidaemias
MELAS syndrome (mitochondrial encephalopathy, lactic acidosis, and stroke-like episodes)
Pyridoxine-dependent epilepsy
Biotinidase deficiency

A primary lactic acidosis may be caused by disorders of pyruvate metabolism or respiratory chain defects, failure of carbohydrate metabolism typically reflects impaired clearance of pyruvate. As such defects in gluconeogenesis, pyruvate dehydrogenase, the tricarboxylic acid TCA cycle or the respiratory chain should be considered [9]. Some IEMs can cause a secondary lactic acidosis (e.g. organic acidaemias and fatty acid oxidation defects). As venous obstruction by tourniquet, crying, or breath holding may increase plasma lactate concentrations by two to threefold, arterial samples are more reliable. Persistent increase of plasma lactate above 3 mmol/l in a neonate without evidence of reduced tissue perfusion and who has no evidence of other organ failure should lead to further investigations for an IEM (Table 26.6).

When compromised, aggressive cardiovascular resuscitation should improve tissue perfusion in the patient with severe metabolic and lactic acidosis. In the acute setting, sodium bicarbonate infusion may support improved intracellular functions, and in conjunction with dialysis, it can also improve the bicarbonate buffer pool without fluid overload [10, 11].

Sodium dichloroacetate may have a role in severe lactic acidosis and is usually only advised by a metabolic specialist. It is an oral agent that stimulates pyruvate dehydrogenase by inhibiting pyruvate dehydrogenase kinase, thereby promoting aerobic oxidation of glucose, pyruvate and lactate. The dose of sodium dichloroacetate can be found in the chapter appendix (Table 26.10).

Ultimately, managing an acidotic patient with an undiagnosed IEM can be troublesome. Careful and structured working between ICU and specialist metabolic teams should allow a considered and individualized approach.

26.5.3 Glycaemic Control

Hypoglycaemia is a common presentation of many IEMs in the setting of a metabolic emergency. Despite the need to correct the low blood sugar, doing so can correct diagnostic and pathological metabolites. A prompt hypoglycaemia screen

Table 26.7 Hypoglycaemia in children

IEM	Hypoglycaemia screen
Glycogen storage diseases	Blood glucose and lactate
Disorders of gluconeogenesis	Insulin, cortisol and growth hormone
Ketotic hypoglycaemia	β-Hydroxybutyrate/blood ketones
Fatty acid oxidation defects	Plasma-free fatty acids
Endocrine causes	Blood spot acylcarnitines
Hypopituitarism	Plasma amino acids
Adrenal insufficiency	Urine organic acids
Hyperinsulinism	Urine toxicology
Other	
Poisoning	

Adapted from [2, 13]

followed by a corrective bolus of glucose (2–3 ml/kg of 10% glucose) is ideal; however, no always possible without sufficient venous access. An important piece of information for the metabolic specialist is the presence or absence of ketones, and this can be measured at the bedside in most centres.

Ketotic hypoglycaemia is by far the most common cause of hypoglycaemia, although admission to intensive care is rarely necessary. Further support and high glucose requirements are more likely to be associated with glycogen storage disorders, neonatal hyperinsulism and fatty acid oxidation defects. A list of causes and essential investigations is shown in Table 26.7. A schematic approach to diagnosis is shown in Fig. 26.5.

Administering IV glucose 10% at maintenance for age and weight is standard and normally supplies sufficient calories to promote anabolism and suppress catabolism [1]. But, calculating the glucose infusion rate (GIR) is essential for understanding the glucose demands of each patient. In the absence of ketones, particularly high glucose demands of >10 mg/kg/min are highly suggestive of hyperinsulinaemia. The GIR is calculated using the following formula:

$$\mathrm{GIR} = \frac{\text{Glucose Concentration}\left(\%\text{or g}/100\ \text{ml}\right)\times \text{Infusion Rate}\left(\text{ml}/\text{h}\right)\times 1000}{\text{Weight}\left(\text{kg}\right)\times 60\left(\text{mins}/\text{h}\right)}$$

Glycaemic control should be strictly regulated (aim blood glucose between 4 to 7 mmol/L). If the blood glucose is persistently elevated, an insulin infusion should be started rather than reducing the glucose concentration in the setting of a possible IEM. Table 26.8 summarizes expected GIR by age and weight which can be useful.

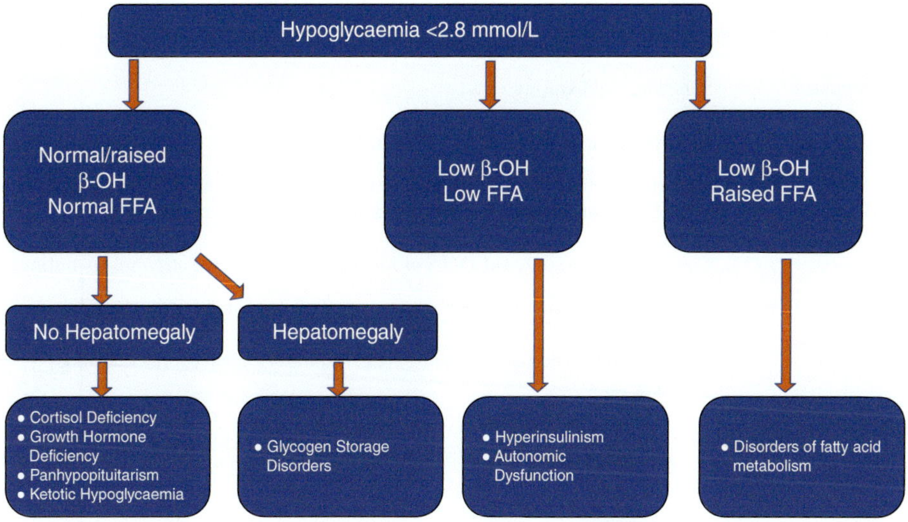

Fig. 26.5 A diagnostic interpretation of the child with hypoglycaemia. *B-OH* beta-hydroxybutyrate, *FFA* free fatty acids. Adapted from [14]

Table 26.8 Glucose infusion rates by age group. For comparison an adult GIR can be as low as 2 mg/kg/min

Age	Glucose infusion rate (GIR) (mg/kg/min)
Up to 2 years	10
2–6 years	8
>6 years and weight < 30 kg	6
>6 years and weight 30–50 kg	4.5

Adapted from [7]

26.6 Peri-Mortem Considerations

IEMs can be fatal at presentation and intensive support may not be successful. Difficult and multi-disciplinary decisions to withdraw care can be required in some situations following discussion with families. In patients for whom the diagnosis is not clear, further investigations can provide conclusive information for families and vital information for future pre-natal counselling. Discussing with parents the need to investigate further before withdrawal of care can be less traumatic than samples being mandatory after death (in the context of a post-mortem investigation). Ensure the basic investigations of Table 26.1 are completed before reviewing the more specialized and recommended investigations in Table 26.9.

Table 26.9 Advised peri/post-mortem investigations in the suspected metabolic child

Sample	Sampling requirements
DNA	EDTA sample. 3–10 ml. Freeze without centrifuging
Skin fibroblast culture	Skin biopsy obtained up to 24 h post-mortem. Stored for up to 2 days in a culture medium or normal saline at ambient/fridge temperature. Not to be frozen Can be used as a source of DNA or for specific and directed enzymology testing
Muscle/liver biopsy	May be obtained up to 1 h post-mortem. Snap frozen on dry ice or liquid nitrogen Can be used for specific enzymology (e.g. respiratory chain complexes) and genetic testing

Adapted from [15]

Take-Home Messages

- Careful review of history baseline investigations performed locally can provide key diagnostic clues and should not be overlooked.
- Early recognition of the metabolic emergency can improve outcomes. Transfer to a specialist intensive care can facilitate rapid specialist management.
- Early liaison with metabolic specialists can support diagnostic pathways and treatment protocols.

Appendix: Other Key Drug Doses in the Intensive Care Setting

See Table 26.10.

Table 26.10 Emergency drug doses of other medications used in hyperammonaemia

Drug	Loading dose over 90 min	Followed by maintenance dose over 24 h	Maximum daily dose (every 24 h thereafter)	Notes
L-carnitine	100 mg/kg	100 mg/kg	300 mg/kg	May have a role in suspected primary and secondary carnitine deficiencies and organic acidaemias Made up to a concentration of 50 mg/ml in 10% dextrose *Not to be given if evidence of cardiomyopathy, cardiac arrythmia or long chain fatty acid oxidation disorders*
Carglumic acid	250 mg/kg	100 mg/kg bd	n/a	Treatment of choice for N-acetylglutamate deficiency and organic acidaemias Specialists advice for maintenance therapy
Sodium dichoroac-etate		50 mg/kg in four divided doses	200 mg/kg in four divided doses	Adjusted to response *Associated with peripheral neuropathy with prolonged use*

Taken from [4, 12]

References

1. Fletcher JM. Metabolic emergencies and the emergency physician. J Ped Child Health. 2016;52:227–30.
2. Ghosh A, Morris AM. Acute presentations of inherited metabolic disorders: investigation and initial management. Paed Child Health. 2019;29:99–104.
3. Leonard JV, Morris AA. Diagnosis and early management of inborn errors of metabolism presenting around the time of birth. Acta Paediatr. 2006;95:6–14.
4. Banta-Wright SA, Steiner RD. Not so rare: errors of metabolism during the neonatal period. Newborn Infant Nurs Rev. 2003;3(4):143–55.
5. British Inherited Metabolic Disease Group. Undiagnosed hyperammonaemia diagnosis and immediate management. Available from: www.bimdg.org.uk/guidelines/guidelines-child.asp
6. Santra S, Hendriksz C. How to use acylcarnitine profiles to help diagnose inborn errors of metabolism. Arch Dis Childhood. 2010;95:151–6.
7. Shanmugam N, Vara R. Acute metabolic decompensation: crisis management. In: Paediatric liver intensive care; 2019. p. 59–64.
8. Saudubray JM, Desguerre I, Sedel F, Charpentier C. Clinical approach to inborn errors of metabolism in children. In: Inborn metabolic diseases; 2016. p. 3–69.
9. Forrest DM, Russell JA. Metabolic acidosis. In: Oxford textbook of critical care; 1999. pp. 573–577.
10. Mathieu D, Neviere R, Billard V, Fleyfel M, Wattel F. Effects of bicarbonate therapy on hemodynamics and tissue oxygenation in patients with lactic acidosis: a prospective, controlled clinical study. Crit Care Med. 1991;19:1352–6.
11. Boyd JH, Walley KR. Is there a role for sodium bicarbonate in treating lactic acidosis from shock? Curr Opin Crit Care. 2008;14:379–83.
12. British Inherited Metabolic Disease Group. National formulary for Inherited Metabolic Diseases (IMDs) 2nd edition—October 2020. Available from: www.bimdg.org.uk/site/formularies.asp
13. Schiff M, Mochel F, Dionisi-Vici. Emergency treatments. In: Inborn metabolic diseases; 2016. p. 109–15.
14. Randell TL. Diagnosis and management of hypoglycaemia beyond the neonatal period. Paed Child Health. 2013;23:152–7.
15. Zschoke J, Hoffman GF. Post mortem investigations. In: Vademecum Metabolicum: diagnosis and treatment of inherited metabolic disorders; 2020. p. 32.

Cardiac Critical Care

Contents

Basics in Cardiac Intensive Care

Iria Duran and Peter Paul Roeleveld

Contents

J. Brierley et al. (eds.), *ESPNIC Children's Intensive Care Textbook*,
https://doi.org/10.1007/978-3-031-64762-8_27

Learning Objectives

- To understand basic cardiac output monitoring and its surrogate markers.
- To understand basic principles of preoperative and post-operative management of patients with congenital heart disease.
- To understand the importance of a lesion-specific physiologic approach.

27.1 Introduction

The main goal of cardiac intensive care is to ensure an adequate cardiac output and oxygen delivery that meets metabolic demands. To achieve this, a comprehensive understanding of the basic principles of oxygen delivery, oxygen consumption, cardiovascular physiology and hemodynamic monitoring is crucial. Clinical management of patients with congenital heart disease also requires understanding the underlying anatomy and lesion-specific (patho)physiology, which allows for anticipating and promptly recognizing complications.

Oxygen delivery is determined by cardiac output and the arterial oxygen content and can be calculated with the following equations:

$$\underline{\text{Arterial oxygen content}}\left(\text{CaO}_2\right):\left(\text{Hb}\left(\text{g/dl}\right)\times 1.39\left(\text{ml/g}\right)\times \text{SaO}_2\right) + \left(\text{PaO}_2\times 0.0031\,\text{ml/mmHg/dl}\right)$$

$$\underline{\text{Oxygen delivery}}\left(\text{DO}_2\right)=\text{CaO}_2\times \text{cardiac output}$$

$$\underline{\text{Cardiac output}}=\text{Heart rate}\times \text{stroke volume}$$

Oxygen consumption (VO_2) is dependent on many factors such as level of sedation/analgesia, physical activity, and temperature. The normal DO_2/VO_2-ratio is 4–5, if it is lower than three oxygen delivery can become inadequate heralding a state of shock.

$DO_2 = CO \times CaO_2$

Heart rate (HR) x Stroke volume (SV) ↵ ↳ (1.39 x Hb X SaO_2) + (0.0031 x PaO_2)

27.2 Hemodynamic Monitoring

27.2.1 Basic Hemodynamic Monitoring

Clinical assessment of cardiac function, cardiac output, and tissue oxygenation based on physical examination only, despite being indispensable, has obvious limitations. Adjunctive hemodynamic monitoring modalities are often needed to achieve objective, accurate and continuous information about the patient's hemodynamic status.

- **Arterial blood pressure monitoring:** Compared to non-invasively measured blood pressure, invasive measurement improves accuracy and allows waveform analysis (◘ Fig. 27.1) as well as arterial blood sampling [1, 2].
- **Central venous pressure monitoring:** Monitoring central venous pressure (◘ Fig. 27.2) provides indirect information on the preload status and right ventricular compliance and permits assessment of response to volume administration. In addition, although not the ideal access for central mixed venous oxygen saturation monitoring (ideally pulmonary artery catheter), sampling offers a good approximation and a valuable trend, especially when using the internal jugular vein. One must be aware of falsely high venous saturation in case of atrial left-to-right shunting.
- **Left atrial pressure monitoring:** After certain surgical repairs in which left ventricular dysfunction is anticipated (e.g., arterial switch operation), a left atrial (LA) line can be left in place, acting as a surrogate for left ventricular function, preload and afterload. Despite providing valuable and accurate hemodynamic information, it is not without risk (bleeding and air embolism) and should be assessed carefully.
- **Capnography:** The graphic display of partial pressure of carbon dioxide (CO_2) in the respiratory gases, measured continuously in both inhaled and exhaled gases and is used to monitor ventilation. The determination of the arterial versus end-tidal CO_2 difference provides information about pulmonary perfusion. Diminished pulmonary flow can lead to impaired CO_2 clearance despite normal minute ventilation indicated by a lower end-tidal CO_2 than the arterial $PaCO_2$. Hence, patients with severe right ventricular dysfunction, CHD with limited pulmonary blood flow (e.g., severe pulmonary stenosis), pulmonary embolism, or severe pulmonary hypertension may have a significant arterial to end-tidal CO_2 gradient. During cardiopulmonary resuscitation (CPR), end-tidal CO_2 should also be used to assess the quality of chest compressions and return to spontaneous circulation [1].

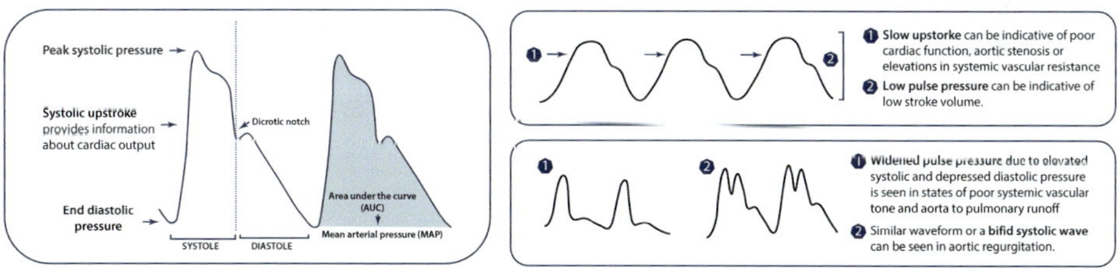

◘ **Fig. 27.1** Arterial pressure waveform analysis

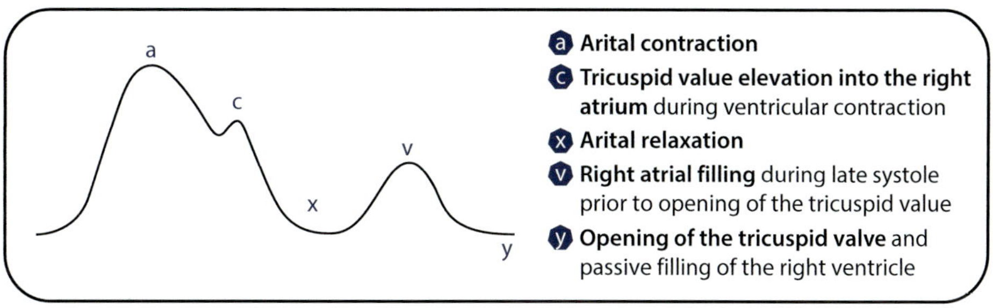

◘ **Fig. 27.2** Venous central pressure waveform analysis

27.2.2 Assessment of Cardiac Output

Cardiac output is a core hemodynamic variable as it is a major determinant of systemic oxygen delivery.

Despite the availability of several different methods, cardiac output is not systematically invasively measured in pediatric practice. This is due to frequent technical difficulties, potential complications, and the common presence of anatomic shunts, which potentially lead to inaccurate measurements [2].

Echocardiography is a widely available, accessible, and non-invasive method which is important in assessing (residual) anatomic lesions and shunts, pericardial effusion, position of central venous lines or ECMO cannulae, and can be used to estimate cardiac function. The presence of pulmonary hypertension can be assessed by indirect signs (septal deviation) or by measuring the pressure in the right ventricle (in the presence of tricuspid regurgitation). Echocardiography can be used to estimate cardiac output by measuring the velocity–time integral (VTI) across the aortic valve by Doppler and by calculating the cross-sectional area measuring the diameter of the aortic valve annulus.

Lactate, acid-basis status, and mixed venous oxygen saturation ($SMvO_2$) are well-known indicators of the balance between tissue oxygen delivery (DO_2) and consumption (VO_2) and, therefore, surrogate markers of cardiac output. Elevated lactate is usually seen when this balance is lost, and the critical oxygen extraction ratio (O_2ER) has been exceeded. However, other causes of high lactate must be also considered, such as regional imbalances of these two variables (such as necrotizing enterocolitis or seizures), impaired utilization of oxygen or impaired metabolic clearance [1].

Near-infrared spectroscopy (NIRS) provides a continuous non-invasive assessment of tissue oxygenation. This technology is based on measuring the relative concentrations of oxy- and deoxy-hemoglobin. Unlike pulse oximetry, NIRS evaluates the non-pulsatile optical component related to the microcirculatory anatomy. Several studies have shown a strong correlation between somatic and cerebral NIRS and venous oximetry and lactate, especially during the immediate post-operative period [3].

27.3 Preoperative Care of Pediatric Cardiac Surgical Patients

Children with CHD may need intensive care support before surgery due to different reasons. Neonates with certain cardiac conditions, such as ductus-dependent circulation, usually require initial stabilization and further intensive care support until surgical repair or palliation. The use of prostaglandins can lead to hypoventilation and/or apnea requiring monitoring in an ICU environment. Decompensated heart failure in the context of the natural progression of CHD or intercurrent illness is another frequent cause of intensive care admission.

27.3.1 Assessment of Patient Status and Predominant Physiology [1, 14]

In order to understand and categorize the often complex congenital heart defects, a physiologic approach is recommended. For that purpose, addressing the following questions may be helpful:

1. How does systemic venous return reach systemic arterial circulation?
2. Is there intracardiac mixing, shunting or outflow obstruction?
3. Is the circulation in series or parallel?
4. Is pulmonary blood flow increased or decreased?
5. Is there a volume load or pressure load on the ventricles?

Congenital heart diseases, despite some of them being extremely complex, can usually be categorized into one or more of the following general physiologies: defects with left-to-right shunts, cyanotic congenital heart defects, obstructive congenital heart defects, or defects characterized by ventricular dysfunction.

27.3.1.1 Defects with Left-to-Right Shunts

Increased pulmonary blood flow is usually the primary problem in this physiology. Eventually, heart cavities dilate as a response to high pulmonary flow. In situations where increased cardiac output is required (e.g., fever, exercise), the heart response can be inefficient as most of the increment in cardiac output is recirculated to the lungs. This clinically results in signs of congestive heart failure, as tachycardia, tachypnoea, increased work of breathing, pulmonary congestion, and liver enlargement. Pulmonary overflow also predisposes to respiratory infections, which is a frequent cause of heart failure decompensation. Some examples of lesions include patent ductus arteriosus, ventricular septal defect (VSD), common atrioventricular canal (AVSD), atrial septal defect (ASD), truncus arteriosus, or aortopulmonary window.

Patients with moderate and severe left-to-right shunts with signs of heart failure are usually on chronic treatment with diuretics and angiotensin-converting enzyme (ACE) inhibitors. Intensive care support in these children is focused on limiting the left-to-right shunt and/or improving systemic cardiac output and typically requires some degree of positive airway pressure, which can be administered non-invasively in more stable patients, and optimizing intravenous diuretic treatment. Milrinone is usually the preferred cardiovascular drug for promoting systemic perfusion via afterload reduction due to its inodilator effect.

27.3.1.2 Cyanotic Congenital Heart Defects

Examples of cyanotic congenital heart defects include transposition of the great arteries (d-TGA), truncus arteriosus (before pulmonary vascular resistance (PVR) drops), tricuspid atresia, and tetralogy of Fallot. Approximately 50% of children with total abnormal pulmonary venous return (TAPVR) present with severe cyanosis. The severity of cyanosis in all these lesions is determined by the presence and severity of associated anatomic lesions, such as pulmonary stenosis, and the changes in PVR, which is high directly after birth and then decreases over time.

Severely cyanotic forms of CHD depend on prostaglandin-E_1 (PGE_1) infusion to maintain pulmonary flow, which may also be required in patients with d-TGA to serve as an additional mixing site if atrial mixing is insufficient. Common side effects of PGE_1 infusion (apnea, hypotension, and fever) are usually well tolerated when administered at normal therapeutic doses. This group of children normally requires surgical repair or palliative procedures (frequently modified Blalock-Taussig (mBT) shunt or patent ductus arteriosus (PDA) stent) within the first weeks of life to establish a stable source of pulmonary flow.

However, some patients with cyanotic congenital heart defects initially present with acceptable pulmonary flow, as is the case in the majority of diagnosis of tetralogy of Fallot. Eventually, fixed stenosis can progress, or dynamic obstruction can become clinically significant, leading to reduced pulmonary blood flow and subsequent cyanosis, requiring additional treatment. When this happens, intensive care support may be necessary until a surgical procedure is performed. Management may include administering beta-blockers (propranolol or esmolol infusion) for dynamic right ventricular tract obstruction, increasing systemic vascular resistance (noradrenaline or phenylephrine), and, in severe cases, intubation and ventilation.

27.3.1.3 Obstructive Congenital Heart Defects

Patients with critical left-sided obstructive lesions may present severely ill with inadequate systemic perfusion and profound metabolic acidosis, especially when the diagnosis is identified postnatally. These lesions include interrupted aortic arch, coarctation of the aorta, critical aortic stenosis or hypoplastic left heart syndrome. Natural ductal closure in neonates with these conditions leads to rapid and severe clinical deterioration and some children may also show post-ductal cyanosis. Indeed, these conditions should always be considered when assessing a neonatal collapse, especially in the absence of femoral pulsations. Management should always include PGE1 to restore ductus-dependent systemic blood flow. In addition, these patients will require adequate resuscitation and stabilization to improve end-organ dysfunction before surgical repair. Some degree of myocardial dysfunction is expected, and inotropic support is usually needed.

27.3.2 Other General Considerations

Intensive care physicians providing care for patients with congenital heart defects should be familiar with common genetic syndromes (◘ Table 27.1) and other co-morbidities associated with certain defects. Ideally, genetic investigations should be conducted before the cardiopulmonary bypass (CPB) (or at least blood samples should be collected) [1, 4, 5]. Some other investigations, such as cranial or abdominal ultrasound, may be required to exclude other malformations prior to surgery.

Table 27.1 Common genetic syndromes associated with congenital heart disease

Down syndrome	ASD, VSD, AVSD, TOF
Turner syndrome	CoA, BAV, AS, HLHS
22q11.2 deletion syndrome	IAA type B, Aortic arch anomalies, TA, TOF
Williams syndrome	SAS, PPS
Noonan syndrome	PS, Hypertrophic cardiomyopathy, ASD
Kabuki syndrome	CoA, ASD, AS, MS, HLHS
Alagille syndrome	PPS, PS, TOF
VACTERL association	VSD, ASD, HLHS, PDA, TGA, TOF, TA
CHARGE	TOF, PDA, DORV, ASD, VSD

ASD atrial septal defect, *VSD* ventricular septal defect, *AVSD* atrioventricular septal defect, *TOF* tetralogy of Fallot, *CoA* coarctation of aorta, *AS* aortic stenosis, *BAV* bicuspid aortic valve, *HLHS* hypoplastic left heart syndrome, *IAA* interrupted aortic arch, *TA* truncus arteriosus, *SAS* supravalvar aortic stenosis, *PPS* peripheral pulmonary stenosis, *PS* pulmonary stenosis, *MS* mitral stenosis, *PDA* patent ductus arteriosus, *TGA* transposition of great arteries, *DORV* double outlet right ventricle

27.4 Post-operative Care of Pediatric Cardiac Patients

27.4.1 Preoperative and Intra-Operative Course Evaluation [6]

The child's preoperative clinical state should be carefully evaluated, considering signs of congestive heart failure (including failure-to-thrive and feeding difficulties), cyanosis, as well as other co-morbidities, such as airway obstruction and other organ abnormalities. It is also important to know about previous procedures, pre-operative tests (chest x-ray, echocardiogram, and ECG) and regular medication.

A comprehensive post-operative handover is crucial to ensure optimal post-operative care. Equally, understanding basic surgical concepts is necessary (Table 27.2). Details regarding surgical procedure, any complications and residual lesions must be verbally reported and documented. Results of invasive hemodynamic measurements and post-operative transoesophageal echocardiography are also relevant. Hemodynamic state since weaning from CPB should be communicated, including heart rate, blood pressure, last blood gases and inotropic support. Many centers use a checklist for a systematic post-operative handover.

27.4.2 General Principles of Post-Operative Care [6, 7, 14]

Understanding each patient's anatomy, physiology and surgical repair is essential to provide optimal post-operative care and to anticipate complications. Initial assessment must include a detailed full physical examination, with a special focus on signs

Table 27.2 Basic concepts in cardiac surgery [6, 7]

Cardiopulmonary bypass (CPB)	Used to replace heart and lung function during surgery. Blood is drained from the right atrium by a single cannula or by bicaval cannulation and returned through a cannula placed in the ascending aorta. The circuit includes a roller pump, an oxygenator and various reservoirs and filters
Hypothermia	Used to minimize venous return to the heart and to reduce cellular metabolism with the objective to preserve organ function
Moderate hypothermia (20–28 °C)	For older children and less demanding cardiac lesions
Deep hypothermia (14–20 °C)	For neonates and infants and complex cardiac repairs Allows to operate with low-flow CPB and nearly bloodless field
Deep hypothermia with circulatory arrest (DHCA)	Allows removing atrial and aortic cannulas. Used, for example, for extensive aortic reconstructions
Cardioplegia	Used to arrest the heart and to preserve the myocardium during ischemia. There are many different solutions but are always high in potassium and are often mixed with oxygenated blood. Can be administered in the aortic root (anterograde), through coronary sinus (retrograde), or both
Modified ultrafiltration (MUF)	The technique of ultrafiltration used after separation from CPB. Removes plasma water and inflammatory mediators (molecular weight lower than 50 kDa) reducing the inflammatory response after CPB

of tissue perfusion, cardiac and pulmonary auscultation (murmurs, rubs and air entry into lung fields) and the presence of hepatomegaly. Despite the fact that a full neurological examination may not be possible initially, pupil response should always be assessed.

An initial chest x-ray is usually needed not only to evaluate lung fields and cardiac silhouette but also to check the position of the several medical devices inserted during the procedure (e.g. endotracheal tube, chest, and mediastinal drains, pacing wires, central venous lines). A baseline 12-lead-ECG is essential and special attention should be paid to dysrhythmias and signs of ischemia. If atrial wires are available, an atrial wire recording can be particularly useful when "p" waves are not clear, which is frequent at faster rates.

Hemodynamic management should be guided by an understanding of the general post-operative issues that may occur (e.g., bleeding, low cardiac output and dysrhythmias, as mentioned below) and a lesion-specific physiology approach (see Table 27.3). Regular revaluation of the child´s condition is essential. This should include physical examination, invasive hemodynamic parameters (arterial and central venous pressure and transthoracic intracardiac lines, if present) and surrogate markers of tissue perfusion (mixed venous saturation, lactate, and urine output).

The optimal time for extubation must be evaluated in every case, considering several factors such as underlying physiology, anticipated complications, and previous co-morbidities. Sedation and mechanical ventilation reduce oxygen demand. In addition, positive pressure ventilation decreases systemic ventricular afterload and counteracts hydrostatic forces that promote pulmonary edema. These effects may

Table 27.3 Lesion-specific management [2, 8, 9]

Lesion	Associated conditions	Presentation	Suggested management
Residual left-to-right shunt	• Unrecognized or untreated septal defects or systemic-to-pulmonary artery shunts	• **Pulmonary overcirculation:** pulmonary edema, pulmonary hypertension, volume overload of systemic ventricle and reduced cardiac output if significant defects • Atrial level shunts are usually well tolerated	• **Optimize balance between pulmonary and systemic resistances** • Positive airway pressure • Afterload reduction • Optimize diuretic treatment • **If clinically significant** despite optimizing medical management, further intervention may be required
Residual systemic ventricular outflow tract obstruction	• Systemic ventricular outflow tract obstruction relief: aortic valvar and supravalvar stenosis • AVSD repair • Surgeries that involve significant volume unloading (Glenn, Fontan)	• Reduced cardiac output if significant obstruction • May associate some degree of dynamic obstruction • Hypertension if frequent, due to hyperdynamic adaptative response	• **Optimize preload** status • After supravalvular obstruction relief, **coronary perfusion** pressure can decrease, and **afterload-increasing agents** may be needed • Careful use of inotropic agents in patients with significant dynamic obstruction • If significant hypertension, vasodilator may be needed to protect surgical repair. However, careful titration is needed in case of fixed obstruction and hypotension should always be avoided

(continued)

Table 27.3 (continued)

Lesion	Associated conditions	Presentation	Suggested management
Tricuspid or mitral valve dysfunction	• After valvar repair or replacement • Occasionally, after closing a shunt lesion valvar dysfunction can be unmasked	• **Left-sided valve**: pulmonary edema, pulmonary hypertension, low cardiac output if severe • **Right-sided valve**: peripheral edema, hepatomegaly, effusions, or high chest losses	• **Left-sided valve**: • Optimize diuretic treatment. • Aggressive treatment of pulmonary hypertension. • After load reduction in regurgitant lesions. • Poor response of stenosis to medical treatment. • **Right-sided valve:** • Optimize diuretic treatment. • Inotropic support if myocardial dysfunction. Given the effect reducing pulmonary vascular resistance, milrinone may be useful
Ventricular diastolic dysfunction	• Cases with significant previous hypertrophy, especially after surgery involving ventriculotomy	• **Left dysfunction**: pulmonary edema, pulmonary hypertension, low cardiac output if severe. • **Right dysfunction**: peripheral edema, hepatomegaly, effusions, or high chest losses. Cyanosis may be present in case of residual atrial shunt	• **Optimize preload** status • Use of milrinone as inodilator • Aggressive treatment of arrhythmias. Both tachycardia and loss of atrioventricular synchrony will be badly tolerated • Gentle diuresis once cardiovascular and fluid shifts have stabilized
Pulmonary hypertension	• Neonates have particularly labile pulmonary resistances and higher risk of PH after bypass • Pulmonary venous obstruction • Mitral valve disease • Severe and prolong left-to-right shunts	• **If present shunt:** cyanosis due to right-to-left shunt • **If no shunt:** signs of right ventricular dysfunction and low cardiac output without significant cyanosis	• **Prevention** by optimizing analgesia (fentanyl boluses may be of help before handling), maintaining pH around 7.4-7.45 and normocapnia and avoiding hypoxemia • **Optimize preload** status • **Nitric oxide** in moderate-severe cases • **If hypotensive/low SVR:** vasopressor support with noradrenaline or vasopressin and inotropic support with adrenaline or milrinone • **Inf normotensive/acceptable SVR:** inodilator support with milrinone

benefit patients with low cardiac output, significant systolic dysfunction, and residual left-to-right shunts. However, the positive intrathoracic pressure can have a negative effect on systemic venous return, decrease RV preload, increase RV afterload thereby decreasing cardiac output. Therefore, some other conditions, especially restrictive right ventricular physiology, and Glenn and Fontan procedures, benefit from early extubation.

Despite advances in intra-operative strategies and the use of modified ultrafiltration (MUF), fluid overload is still a well-known complication after CPB. Fluid restriction is common practice in the immediate post-operative period. Diuretics are usually started once cardiovascular and fluid shifts have stabilized.

27.4.3 Post-operative Complications

Bleeding: Bleeding is one of the most common post-operative complications. Drain output volume and nature should always be carefully evaluated, especially during the immediate post-operative period. Preoperative cyanosis with polycythemia, redo sternotomies and complex surgeries with multiple suture lines are known risk factors for bleeding. Bloody drainage higher than 10 ml/kg/h during first 2 h or 5 ml/kg/h thereafter despite blood products and medical management, may need surgical re-exploration. Full blood count and coagulation parameters should be evaluated and corrected accordingly. In case of excessive bleeding, platelets should be transfused irrespective of absolute platelet count, as CPB leads to platelet dysfunction. Persisting bleeding would require the replacement of losses of red blood cells, platelets, and plasma [6].

Tamponade: A (sudden) drop in chest drain output, followed by tachycardia, increasing central venous pressure and low systemic blood pressure with narrow pulse pressure is highly suggestive of cardiac tamponade. Pulsus paradoxus is often also present. A point-of-care ultrasound (POCUS) should be part of the initial assessment as it can rapidly confirm clinical suspicion. Cardiology and surgical team must be immediately notified. Medical management must include ensuring optimal preload, discontinuing vasodilators, and starting vasopressors if required, while chest re-exploration (or pericardiocentesis, less frequently) is prepared.

Swelling of intrathoracic tissues in response to surgical manipulation and peri-operative systemic inflammatory response can cause a "dry tamponade" with similar clinical presentation. This condition benefits from chest re-opening.

Low cardiac output syndrome (LCOS): LCOS is defined as the inability to provide adequate oxygen delivery to meet tissue demand and can develop in approximately 25% of patients after CPB surgery. It is usually characterized by increased heart rate, metabolic acidosis, poor perfusion on examination and variable degree of organ dysfunction. Hypotension is common, but LCOS can exist in the presence of hypertension [7]. Cardiac output nadir following CPB has been described to occur between 9 and 12 h following surgery, with a return to baseline after 24 h [10].

There are several post-operative conditions which can lead to LCOS, including myocardial dysfunction, arrhythmias, residual lesions, or tamponade. Preload and contractility should be optimized before increasing systemic vascular resistance. The Prophylactic intravenous use of milrinone after cardiac operation in pediatrics (PRIMACORP) study demonstrated that inodilator support with milrinone at 0.75

µg/kg/min reduced LCOS following cardiac surgery in children with biventricular repairs [11].

The inverse relationship between afterload and cardiac function is well-known. However, critically low coronary perfusion should be actively avoided, and vasopressors may be necessary to achieve acceptable blood pressure. In case of catecholamine refractory hypotension, steroids may be used (usually hydrocortisone) for a short period of time. Chest re-opening and extracorporeal life support may be needed for patients not responding to optimized medical treatment. LCOS is discussed separately in ▶ Chap. 29.

Arrhythmias: Post-operative arrhythmias are frequent and characteristic after certain surgical repairs. Volume overload, ventricular hypertrophy, myocardial ischemia, previous ventriculotomy and electrolyte disturbances are common risk factors. Arrhythmias are discussed separately in ▶ Chap. 29. However, some of the most frequent and typical are summarized in ◘ Table 27.4. A detailed understanding of antiarrhythmic therapy and temporary external pacing is essential in managing these post-operative arrhythmias.

Chylothorax [12, 13]: Chylothorax can be caused by direct surgical trauma to the thoracic duct or lymphatic tributary vessels, increased central venous pressure (e.g., right ventricular diastolic disfunction or cavo-pulmonary anastomoses) or central venous thrombosis affecting thoracic duct drainage. Fluid triglyceride level >1.2 mmol/L (110 mg/dl) and total cell count > 1000 cells/µL (predominantly lymphocytes) confirm the diagnosis. Loss of coagulation factors and immunoglobulins should be considering when managing these patients. Conservative management of chylothorax includes treating underlying etiology (central venous thrombi should be actively investigated), dietary modifications (low-fat diet or total parenteral nutrition) and, in persistent cases, octreotide or somatostatin is sometimes used, but often not helpful. Lymphangiography can be helpful in establishing the cause of chyle leak. When medical treatment fails, surgical procedures such as thoracic duct ligation, pleurodesis and pleuroperitoneal shunts can be considered.

Failed extubation and ventilation dependence [2, 9]: Restrictive pulmonary defects can often play a temporary role in the direct post-operative period (e.g. atelectasis, pleural effusions, and edema) but could also be a cause for long-term ventilator dependence (phrenic nerve palsy). Extubation failure is not uncommon after cardiac surgery, especially in younger patients, and has been described up to in 12% of neonates. Used of uncuffed endotracheal tubes and prolonged open sternotomy are independently associated with this complication. Some other frequent causes of failed extubation are summarized in ◘ Table 27.5.

Residual lesions: All operated lesions have an expected post-operative course. Whenever a child is not progressing according to this expected trajectory, one should always consider the possibility of residual cardiac defects, such as intracardiac shunts, obstruction to flow or valve insufficiencies which should be evaluated by echocardiography and/or cardiac catheterization.

Necrotizing enterocolitis: This is relatively common complication after cardiac surgery, especially in neonates, patients with parallel circulation or significant low cardiac output status and should be carefully evaluated.

Table 27.4 Most common arrhythmias after CHD surgery

	ECG findings	Typical surgeries	Management
JET	Narrow complex regular tachycardia with retrograde atrial conduction in 1:1 pattern or AV dissociation with variable conduction (characterized by faster QRS-complexes than *p*-waves)	**Involving ventricular septum:** VSD, TOF, TA, AVSD	Restoring AV synchrony by atrial pacing once lower heart rate is achieved by: • Avoiding hyperthermia. Active hypothermia down to 35 °C can be used in refractory JET • Optimizing sedation • Minimizing beta-adrenergic agents • Amiodarone may be required for rate control • Ivabradine is a newer agent that may be effective Usually resolves within first days post-op
HB	Variable depending on heart block degree. (QRS-complexes typically slower than *p*-waves)	**Around AV node:** VSD, mitral valve replacement, Konno procedure	• First-degree and second-degree type I are usually clinically well tolerated. • Second-degree type II and third-degree block require temporary pacing (ideally DDD, but it is not possible VVI will be needed). Usually due to myocardial edema and resolved within first 7–14 days. If not, a permanent pacemaker is required
ORT	Narrow complex regular tachycardia, with retrograde atrial conduction in 1:1 pattern In the presence of bundle branch block or other interventricular conduction delay, QRS can be broad	**Patients with known accessory pathways** (WPW in Ebstein's anomaly)	• Adenosine • Atrial overdrive pacing • If unstable or refractory – synchronized electrical cardioversion with 0.5–2 J/kg • If recurrent, amiodarone may be needed
VT	Wide complex tachycardia	**Severe myocardial dysfunction:** cardiomyopathy, ventriculotomy, coronary ischemia	• If unstable– electrical cardioversion 2–4 J/kg • Amiodarone may be needed • Avoid low magnesium levels

AV atrioventricular, *AVSD* atrioventricular septal defect, *JET* junctional ectopic tachycardia, *HB* heart block, *ORT* orthodromic reciprocating tachycardia, *VT* ventricular tachycardia, *WPW* Wolf-Parkinson-White, *VSD* ventricular septal defect, *TOF* tetralogy of Fallot, TA *truncus arteriosus*

Table 27.5 Factors that can contribute to the inability to wean from mechanical ventilation

Residual cardiac defects	• Left-to-right shunts • Myocardial dysfunction • Obstruction to flow • Valve incompetencies
Restrictive pulmonary defects	• Pulmonary edema • Pleural effusion • Atelectasias • Chest wall edema • Phrenic nerve palsy
Upper and lower airway problems	• Subglottic edema or stenosis • Vocal cord injury • Extrinsic airway compression • Tracheobronchomalacia
Others	• Inadequate nutrition • Muscular weakness: Critical illness polyneuropathy (CIP) and critical illness myopathy (CIM) • Other neurological co-morbidities: withdrawal, delirium

27.4.4 Discharge from CICU

A comprehensive and well-structured handover is necessary to ensure optimal continuity of care after discharge from intensive care. For that purpose, SBAR communication tool can be useful. Introducing yourself and being aware of who you are transmitting the information to is important. Current problems, active medication and pending investigations should be emphasized.

Case Study

Your patient is a 1-week-old neonate admitted from theater 5 h ago after arterial switch procedure with LeCompte maneuver. She was antenatally diagnosed with transposition of great arteries with intact ventricular septum. She had remained stable before surgery, on low-dose prostaglandin infusion, without requiring balloon atrioseptostomy as atrial communication was large and unrestrictive. Anesthesia and surgical procedure were uneventful. Post-operative echocardiogram showed no residual shunts, mildly impaired left ventricular function, and good coronary flow. She has two atrial and two ventricular pacing wires and one right pleural and one mediastinal drains. Chest is closed and there is no left atrial line. On admission, she is supported on milrinone (0.5 mcg/kg/min) and low dose adrenaline (0.02 mcg/kg/min) and sedated on morphine 20 mcg/kg/h. When you start assessing her, you realize that she is significantly tachycardic (heart rate is around 170 bpm). How would you approach this patient?

27.4.4.1 Proposed Evaluation

1. *Complete a full physical examination and evaluate further clinical hemodynamic parameters:*
   - *Are there clinical signs of poor systemic perfusion? Evaluate peripheral and central temperature, capillary refill time, pulses, and urine output in the last hours.*
   - *Check inotropic support. Confirm doses and exclude delivery issues.*
   - *How much are the chest drain losses?*
   - *Is the patient well sedated?*
   - *How are blood pressure, end-tidal CO2, central venous pressure? Can you see clear sinus rhythm in the monitor trace?*
2. *Collect further information from complementary tests:*
   - *When sinus rhythm is not completely clear in the ECG trace on the monitor, a 12-lead ECG and an atrial wire recording can be particularly useful.*
   - *Perform an arterial and venous blood gas to evaluate signs of low cardiac output. How are mixed venous saturation, lactate, and acid-basis status?*
   - *Are the electrolytes optimized? Electrolyte disturbances are a well-known cause of arrhythmia.*

Causes of tachycardia after cardiac surgery:
Pain, inappropriate sedation, and analgesia
Low cardiac output
Tachyarrhythmia
Pulmonary hypertension
Residual defects
Hypoxia, hypercarbia
Catecholamines and other drugs
Hypoglycemia

After completing your evaluation, you see that your patient is hypotensive (54/26, MAPS 35) and has clinical signs of poor systemic perfusion (she is cold peripherally, with weak femoral pulses and has not passed urine since admission). She has had no drain losses for the last 3 h, despite being around 3–4 ml/kg/h initially. CVP has raised as is now around 20. While you are evaluating your patient, one of your colleagues kindly performs a point-of-care ultrasound (POCUS), showing a significant collection around the heart.

In this situation, optimizing preload by administering volume and starting low-dose noradrenaline infusion in order to ensure coronary perfusion is necessary while awaiting further surgical management. Despite POCUS being of help for initial evaluation with tamponade is suspected, a full echocardiogram is always recommended.

Take-Home Messages

- Cardiac output it is a major determinant of systemic oxygen delivery, together with arterial oxygen content (CaO_2). Optimizing these parameters to meet metabolic demands is the main goal of cardiac intensive care.
- Most patients after congenital cardiac surgery have a predictable post-operative course depending on their underlying condition and operation which the cardiac intensive care team should be aware of.
- Each patient´s underlying anatomy, physiology and surgical repair must be understood in order to provide a tailored, accurate and optimal management and to be able to anticipate and manage possible complications.
- Comprehensive and systematic approach to patient evaluation is always helpful.
- Physiology-guided approach is highly recommended.

Questions

1. In which situations would you expect a widened pulse pressure?
   A. Left ventricular dysfunction with poor contractility
   B. Aortic insufficiency
   C. Large PDA
   D. Aortic stenosis
   E. B and C are correct

2. Which one of the following is not a direct determinant of oxygen delivery?
   A. Heart rate
   B. Stroke volume
   C. Hemoglobin
   D. pCO_2
   E. All of the above are direct determinants

3. Which genetic condition would you suspect in a patient with Tetralogy of Fallot with right aortic arch?
   A. Trisomy 21
   B. 22q11.2 syndrome
   C. Noonan syndrome
   D. Williams syndrome
   E. Having a right aortic arch does not increase the risk of associating a genetic disorder

4. Regarding Deep Hypothermia with Circulatory Arrest (DHCA), which one of the following is false?
   A. It reduces cellular metabolism with the objective to preserve organ function.
   B. It allows removing atrial and aortic cannulas and it is used for extensive aortic reconstructions.
   C. It is systematically used for all type of surgical repairs in neonates.
   D. The patient is actively cooled down to 15 – 20 °C.
   E. All of the above are correct.

5. Which one of the following is not a clinical sign of cardiac tamponade?
   A. Hypotension with narrow pulse pressure
   B. CVP trending down
   C. Tachycardia
   D. Sudden drop in chest drain output
   E. All of the above are correct

Answers

1. **Correct answer is E.** Widened arterial pulse pressure can be seen in patients with significant diastolic aortic runoff as in aortic insufficiency, large PDA (patent ductus arteriosus) or arteriovenous malformations. In situations with low systemic vascular resistance as, for example, in septic shock, a similar waveform can be present.
2. **Correct answer is D.** Oxygen delivery (DO_2) is the product of the cardiac output and arterial oxygen content. At the same time, cardiac output is the product of heart rate and stroke volume. The arterial oxygen content is the amount of oxygen bound to hemoglobin plus the amount of oxygen dissolved in arterial blood (which is minimal).

$$DO_2 = CO \times CaO_2$$

Heart rate (HR) x Stroke volume (SV) ↲ ↳ $(1.39 \times Hb \times SaO_2) + (0.0031 \times PaO_2)$

3. **Correct answer is B.** DiGeorge syndrome (22q11.2 deletion syndrome).
4. **Correct answer is C.** Deep hypothermia with circulatory arrest (DHCA) is a technique to obtain optimal operating conditions while providing cerebral protection, which involves reducing temperature to 15–20 °C and establishing circulatory arrest by discontinuing CPB flow. It is used for extensive aortic reconstructions, but not systematically for all type of neonatal repairs.
5. **Correct answer is B.** Cardiac tamponade classically presents with tachycardia, hypotension with low pulse pressure and increasing central venous pressure after a sudden decrease in mediastinal drainage.

References

1. Bronicki R. Hemodynamic monitoring. Pediatr Crit Care Med. 2016;17:S207–14.
2. Shaffner D, Nichols D. Rogers' textbook of pediatric intensive care; 2016.
3. Ghanayem N, Wernovsky G, Hoffman G. Near-infrared spectroscopy as a hemodynamic monitor in critical illness. Pediatr Crit Care Med. 2011;12:S27–32.
4. Ko J. Genetic syndromes associated with congenital heart disease. Korean Circ J. 2015;45(5):357.
5. Blue G, Kirk E, Sholler G, Harvey R, Winlaw D. Congenital heart disease: current knowledge about causes and inheritance. Med J Aust. 2012;197(3):155–9.
6. Schwartz SM. Cardiac surgery and postoperative management. Multidisciplinary Critical Care Review Course.
7. Shekerdemian L. Perioperative manipulation of the circulation in children with congenital heart disease. Heart. 2009;95(15):1286–96.

8. Ravishankar C, Tabbutt S, Wernovsky G. Critical care in cardiovascular medicine. Curr Opin Pediatr. 2003;15(5):443–53.
9. Dent CL, Schwartz SM. Postoperative care of the pediatric cardiac surgical patient. In: Cardiovascular pediatric critical illness and injury. London: Springer; 2009. https://doi.org/10.1007/978-1-84800-923-3_16.
10. Wernovsky G, Wypij D, Jonas RA, et al. Postoperative course, and hemodynamic profile after the arterial switch operation in neonates and infants. A comparison of low-flow cardiopulmonary bypass and circulatory arrest. Circulation. 1995;92:2226–35.
11. Hoffman T, Wernovsky G, Atz A, Bailey J, Akbary A, Kocsis J, Nelson D, Chang A, Kulik T, Spray T, Wessel D. Prophylactic intravenous use of milrinone after cardiac operation in pediatrics (PRIMACORP) study. Am Heart J. 2002;143(1):15–21.
12. Savla J, Itkin M, Rossano J, Dori Y. Post-operative chylothorax in patients with congenital heart disease. J Am College Cardiol. 2017;69(19):2410–22.
13. Mery C, Moffett B, Khan M, Zhang W, Guzmán-Pruneda F, Fraser C, Cabrera A. Incidence and treatment of chylothorax after cardiac surgery in children: analysis of a large multi-institution database. J Thoracic Cardiovasc Surg. 2014;147(2):678–86.
14. Munoz R, Morell V, Cruz E, Vetterly C, Silva J. Critical care of children with heart disease: basic medical and surgical concepts. London: Springer; 2010.

Further Reading

Haemodynamic Monitoring

Bronicki R. Hemodynamic monitoring. Pediatr Crit Care Med. 2016;17:S207–14. Hemodynamic monitor in critical illness. Pediatr Crit Care Med 12:27–S32

Ghanayem N, Wernovsky G, Hoffman G. Near-infrared spectroscopy as a hemodynamic monitor in critical illness. Pediatr Crit Care Med. 2011;12:S27–32. Comprehensive and detailed review of NIRS technology, including an extensive review of available data in patients with congenital heart disease

Postoperative Care

Shekerdemian L. Perioperative manipulation of the circulation in children with congenital heart disease. Heart. 2009;95(15):1286–96. Excellent review of the management of cardiac patients during the immediate postoperative period, addressing the optimal cardiovascular medical support for different physiologies. ECLS in complex circulations is also discussed

Pre-operative Management of Neonates with Congenital Heart Disease

Alessandra Rizza, Aparna Hoskote, and Angelo Polito

Contents

J. Brierley et al. (eds.), *ESPNIC Children's Intensive Care Textbook*,
https://doi.org/10.1007/978-3-031-64762-8_28

Learning Objectives

- To provide the reader with a basic understanding of the pathophysiology of main neonatal congenital heart disease (CHD):
  - acyanotic and cyanotic CHD
  - critical and non-critical CHD: duct-dependent CHDs (pulmonary and systemic dependence)
- To understand the main physiology underlying the CHD you are dealing with:
  - impaired systemic output?
  - impaired pulmonary blood flow?
  - inadequate central mixing?
  - pulmonary over-circulation?
  - obstructed pulmonary venous obstruction?
- Transition from foetal to neonatal circulation: main changes after birth

Key Points to Understand Pathophysiology of CHD

- **Is the patient cyanotic or acyanotic?**
- **Is the CHD critical or non-critical lesion?**
- A shunt consists of a communication *between two cardiac chambers or two vessels*: Usually the blood goes from higher-pressure to lower-pressure side. Shunting can be left-to-right or right-to-left or bidirectional.
- Prompt recognition and therapy with prostaglandin E1 may be lifesaving in neonatal cardiac emergencies.

- **Acyanotic CHD** includes a spectrum of cardiac defects with variable severity of clinical presentation with:
  (a) left-to-right (L-to-R) shunts (which may be evident after days or weeks after birth) or
  (b) left heart obstructive lesions—may present with acute cardiogenic shock—in case of ductal-dependent lesions—when the ductus closes or asymptomatic.

  According to the clinical presentation, there are critical or non-critical type:
  1. Critical *acyanotic "ductal-dependent" CHD presenting with shock: in this case the normal flow from left ventricle (LV) to systemic circulation is impaired*, because of either stenosis or complete interruption of flow. During the foetal life, patency of ductus arteriosus ensures systemic perfusion; after birth, when ductus closes, the systemic flow will be more reduced, leading to systemic hypoperfusion and shock. The most common acyanotic critical CHD is **neonatal aortic coarctation.**
  2. *Non-critical acyanotic CHD presenting with heart failure*: these lesions are characterized by right to left (R-to-L) shunt, *leading to increased pulmonary blood flow (PBF) and consequently to congestive heart failure*. These CHD include ventricle septal defect (VSD), atrioventricular septal defect (AVSD), patent ductus arteriosus (PDA), and aorto-pulmonary window. High pulmonary vascular resistance (PVR) during neonatal period limits the right-to-left (R-to-L) shunt; as PVRs decrease during the first weeks after birth, the R-to-L shunt will progressively increase, leading to **pulmonary over-circulation and congestive heart failure.**

(continued)

During the pre-operative period, these infants may be seriously ill, due to severe pulmonary over-circulation. These critically ill patients require pre-operative stabilization with mechanical ventilation, diuretics, vasodilatators and inodilators.

The CYANOTIC CHDs include lesions with deoxygenated hemoglobin more than 5g/dL, that can be due to:

INCOMPLETE OXYGENATION of the blood THROUGH THE LUNG, because of lung pathology and intrapulmonary shunt.

- ***INTRACARDIAC shunt from the right to left side of the heart***, due to a cyanotic CHD.

EXTRAPULMONARY SHUNT, at level of PDA or patent foramen ovale (PFO), due to persistent pulmonary hypertension (PPH) needs to be ruled out.

Presence of abnormal hemoglobin (which cannot bind to oxygen) [1].

Neonatal CHD can be classified as:

1. Duct dependent congenital heart disease (CHD)
2. Circulation dependent upon mixing through patent foramen ovale (PFO)
3. Obstructed total anomalous pulmonary venous connection (TAPVC).

1. Duct dependent CHD may be classified as:
   (a) *Pulmonary duct-dependency in right-sided obstructive* lesions - in *cyanotic* CHD, such as:
      - Pulmonary atresia with intact ventricular septum (PA-IVS) or with ventricular septal defect (PA-VSD)
      - Critical pulmonary stenosis (PS)
      - Tricuspid atresia (TA) with pulmonary atresia (PA) or pulmonary stenosis (PS)
      - Univentricular heart with pulmonary atresia (PA)
      - Severe Ebstein anomaly
   (b) Systemic duct-dependency in left-sided obstructive lesions - in acyanotic CHD, such as:
      - Hypoplastic left heart syndrome (HLHS)
      - Critical aortic stenosis/atresia (AS)
      - Severe coarctation of aorta (CoAo)
      - Interrupted aortic arch (IAA)
      - Single ventricle with severe aortic stenosis/coarctation
   (c) CHD with parallel circulation requiring adequate central mixing as
      - Transposition of great vessels with intact ventricular septum (TGA-IVS)
2. CHD dependent on central mixing at PFO (requiring urgent intervention if is restricted to maintain haemodynamic stability)
   (a) to maintain systemic blood flow (Tricuspid atresia, PA-IVS, TAPVC)
   (b) to reduce pulmonary congestion (HLHS, mitral stenosis/atresia)
   (c) to permit adequate mixing of deoxygenated and oxygenated blood (TGA-IVS)

(continued)

3. Obstructed total anomalous pulmonary venous connection (TAPVC) described later.

Which Are the Changes in the Circulation After Birth?

1. During foetal life, the presence of shunts is essential.
2. During foetal development, pulmonary blood flow (PBF) is restricted due to high pulmonary vascular resistance (PVR) and right-to-left shunts through the patent foramen ovale (PFO) and patent ductus arteriosus (PDA). However, upon birth, ventilation and oxygenation cause a rapid drop in PVR, redirecting right ventricular output to the lungs. Simultaneously, systemic vascular resistance (SVR) increases after cord clamping. This shift in SVR and PBF results in left atrial pressure exceeding right atrial pressure, leading to the closure of the foramen ovale. Shortly after ventilation begins, left-to-right flow commences. With the closure of the ductus venosus (typically within the first 7 days) and the PDA (usually within 12–72 h), foetal circulation transitions to the postnatal series circulation [1].
3. A shunt consists of a communication *between two cardiac chambers or two vessels*: in this case the blood goes from higher-pressure to the lower-pressure side. Shunting can be left-to-right or right-to-left or bidirectional [2].

Differential Diagnosis Between CHD and Other Diseases

- It is important to rule out persistent **Pulmonary hypertension of newborn (PPHN),** rare causes of methaemoglobinaemia and metabolic disorders, cerebral diseases, hypoglycaemia and hypocalcaemia, mediated via respiratory or pulmonary vascular derangement.
- *Cyanosis may be due to incomplete oxygenation of the blood through the lung,* because of lung pathology and intrapulmonary shunt: thus, it is important to rule out lung disease in cyanotic neonates.
- Clinical differences between PPHN and *duct dependent pulmonary circulation* is extremely difficult: echocardiography is essential.
- Infants with persistent foetal circulation have a R-to-L shunt at intracardiac and ductal levels, oligaemic lung fields, such as in cyanotic neonates. A prostaglandin infusion usually is effective only in infants with a duct dependent CHD. However, for treating “persistent foetal circulation” a trial with inhaled nitric oxide (iNO) is indicated: iNO will improve oxygen saturation in case of transient pulmonary hypertension!
- Neonatal sepsis is an important cause of cardiovascular collapse and has to be considered in the differential in case of CHD with systemic obstruction flow. The differential diagnosis between *aortic coarctation/critical aortic stenosis* and septic shock is challenging, because a murmur or weak pulses could be present or absent in both cases. Thus, echocardiography is mandatory.
- Neonatal bradyarrhythmia or tachyarrhythmia may be present both in the case of septic shock and structurally normal heart, and in the case of critically obstructed systemic circulation. All neonates with suspected or confirmed CHD need to have ECG performed.

28.1 Lesion-Specific Management

In this section, the main critical CHD presenting in neonatal period will be discussed:

28.2 Duct Dependent Systemic Lesions

28.2.1 Coarctation of Aorta

Coarctation of the aorta (CoAo) represents about 5–8% of all CHD [3, 4]. It is defined as a narrowing of the aortic lumen by a ridge, usually located opposite to the insertion of the PDA.

28.2.1.1 Pathophysiology

Coarctation of the aorta (CoAo) is generally well-tolerated in utero because the narrowing of the aorta doesn't significantly affect blood flow to the lower body. However, it is frequently missed during prenatal screening, with over 60% of cases being diagnosed after birth [5]. This delayed diagnosis can lead to an increased risk of mortality and morbidity. Once the PDA closes after birth, CoAo can result in aortic obstruction, leading to decreased blood flow to the lower body, kidney dysfunction, and metabolic acidosis. Additionally, the increased workload on the LV, can lead to heart failure, potentially progressing to acute cardiogenic shock.

28.2.1.2 Clinical Signs

Classical clinical findings

- reduced peripheral pulses
- a supine arm-leg blood pressure gradient >20 mmHg
- a murmur due to rapid blood flow across the CoAo
- signs of systemic hypoperfusion (acidosis, hypotension, end-organ impairment) [6].

28.2.1.3 Pre-operative Management

The fundamental principles in case of systemic perfusion obstruction are:

- **P*rostaglandin* E1 (PGE) INFUSION must be titrated at a rate sufficient to maintain patency of ductus arteriosus, because ductal patency is crucial to provide systemic perfusion.** Apnoea is the main adverse effect, and it may be an indication to intubate the patient.
- After establishing of ductal patency, **the balance between systemic and pulmonary blood flows is crucial,** because **the pulmonary, systemic and myocardial blood flow are in continuous and dynamic competition.**
- **Pulmonary over-circulation related to PDA can be managed by mechanical ventilation, FiO_2 adjustment and diuretics**: ventilatory parameters should be regulated to manipulate pulmonary vascular resistance.

- **Vasoactive agents:** the vasoactive support must be also considered in case of signs of low cardiac output syndrome, or if the **diastolic blood pressure falls below acceptable ranges secondary to diastolic 'runoff' through the PDA.** It should be considered that this 'runoff' may decrease the coronary artery perfusion and compromise myocardial oxygen delivery. A low-to-moderate dose of dopamine or adrenaline, higher FiO_2, and Hb level optimization could be useful in these patients [1].

28.2.2 Critical Aortic Stenosis

Critical neonatal aortic stenosis (AS) can be valvular, subvalvular or supravalvular. Valvular AS is commonly caused by bicuspid aortic valve, rarely by unicuspid valve. Subvalvular form of AS is usually associated to other lesions, such as VSD or PDA or to left-ventricular outflow tract (these forms are commonly associated to "Shone complex syndrome").

28.2.2.1 Pre-operative Management

Severe AS in neonatal is a critical left heart obstructive lesion and PGE are essential to ensure PDA and systemic perfusion. Inotropic agents may be required to treat LV dysfunction.

To treat the critical AS—percutaneous balloon valvuloplasty has become the treatment of choice in neonatal age and it should be performed as soon as possible [7].

28.2.3 Hypoplastic Left Heart Syndrome (HLHS)

28.2.3.1 Pathophysiology

HLHS is a spectrum with severe underdevelopment of the left heart-aorta complex, consisting of aortic and/or mitral valve atresia, stenosis, or hypoplasia; with marked hypoplasia or absence of the LV and hypoplasia of the ascending aorta and of the aortic arch. It is characterized by:

- Functional single right ventricle (RV)
- Severe systemic outflow obstruction
- Intracardiac mixing of deoxygenated systemic venous and oxygenated pulmonary venous blood
- Systemic output maintained through a PDA [8].

The systemic and pulmonary circulations run parallel to each other instead of in series. This creates a delicate balance among systemic, pulmonary, and coronary blood flows (◘ Fig. 28.1).

28.2.3.2 Main risk Factors for Postnatal Survival in HLHS Include

- a highly restrictive or intact atrial septum [8]
- tricuspid valve regurgitation
- genetic or syndromic or extracardiac-associated anomalies

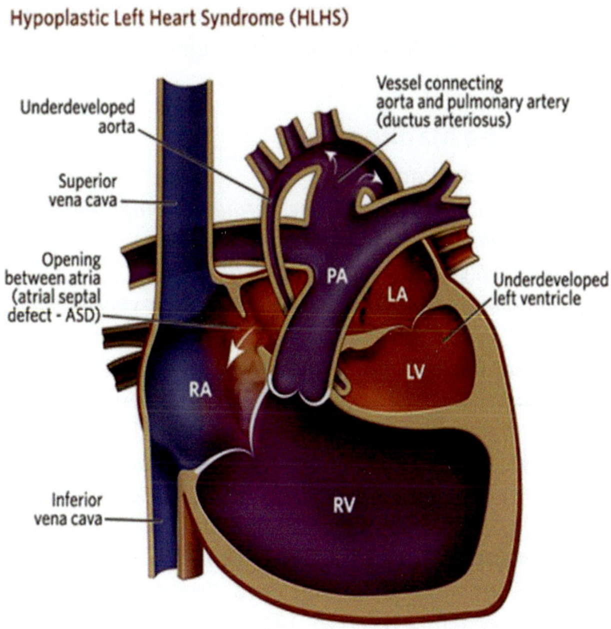

Fig. 28.1 HLHS with mitral-aortic hypoplasia and small LV *(from Metcalf MK, Rychik J. Outcomes in Hypoplastic Left Heart Syndrome Pediatr Clin N Am 2020;67: 945–962)*

- prematurity
- pulmonary venous obstruction [9]

28.2.3.3 Clinical Signs

The stability of a newborn with HLHS depends on:

- the natural patency of the ductus arteriosus (PDA)
- the pulmonary vascular resistance (PVR)
- the size of the atrial communication
- the intrinsic cardiac structure and function
- Following birth, infants may appear to have a normal physical examination as PVR remains high and the ductus arteriosus remains open. However, in the first days of life, PVR decreases physiologically, leading to increased blood flow across the pulmonary vascular bed. This imbalance in circulation can result in various clinical manifestations:
  - Feeding difficulties
  - Respiratory distress
  - Metabolic/lactic acidosis, myocardial dysfunction, peripheral tissue ischaemia, and shock
  - Restrictive atrial communication can cause inadequate mixing, leading to left atrial hypertension, pulmonary venous congestion, and rapid cardiac decompensation.

The prognosis for infants with HLHS and an intact or highly restrictive atrial septum remains poor due to irreversible pulmonary vascular damage that likely occurred during foetal life [10–12].

28.2.3.4 Pre-operative Management

Treatment is generally focused on:

1. *Ensuring patency of the systemic outflow, through prompt administration of PGE*
2. *Assuring open communication at the atrial level*
3. *Balancing the pulmonary and systemic blood flows*
4. *Sustaining the function of the single RV to maximize* ***oxygen delivery (DO_2)***

Standard pre-operative monitoring is based on: **systemic oxygen saturation (SaO_2)**, systemic blood pressure, mixed venous oxygen saturation, if a venous catheter is placed in the SVC.

In the case of single ventricle physiology, **direct measurement of cardiac output (CO) and systemic DO_2 is particularly challenging,** especially in the pre-operative setting.

A **systemic oxygen saturation (SaO_2), between 75% and 85%,** is the most used surrogate parameter of an adequate Qp/Qs ratio, however, this value may be considered a poor measure of systemic **DO_2** [13, 14].

Qp/Qs ratio in a single-ventricle heart with parallel circulation can be expressed as:

$$Qp / Qs = \frac{SaO_2 - SvO_2}{SpvO_2 - SaO_2}$$

where

- SaO_2 is the systemic arterial oxygen saturation
- $SpvO_2$ is pulmonary venous oxygen saturation
- SvO_2 is the systemic venous oxygen saturation

SaO_2 and SvO_2 values can be measured, but $SpvO_2$ is difficult to measure invasively and is generally estimated [15]. Before or after palliative surgery $SpvO_2$ is often assumed to be normal (>96%). However, pulmonary venous desaturation occurs frequently, especially on inspired room air [16].

- *In the single ventricle physiology*:
  - **SaO_2 correlates poorly with Qp/Qs** and mixed venous oxygen saturation (SvO_2) significantly improves the ability to estimate Qp/Qs.
  - **Low values of SvO_2 may indicate low DO_2.**
  - High values of Qp/Qs are related to low DO_2, which only partially are counterbalanced by increasing CO.
  - SaO_2 showed no significant relationship to anaerobic metabolism.
  - **SvO_2 is a better indicator of systemic DO_2 than SaO_2** [14], **reflects the adequacy of end-organ oxygenation and can detect if anaerobic metabolism occurs.** Low SvO_2 can predict poor outcome after Norwood procedure for HLHS [17].
  - Near-infrared spectroscopy (NIRS) is a continuous non-invasive measurement of cerebral and somatic oxygenation index provides an estimation of regional tissue and venous oxygen saturation. Although the NIRS and mixed

venous saturation are not interchangeable, it may be useful in following changes in systemic oxygen consumption [18].
  - The therapeutic PGE dosing range is 10–60 ng/kg/min. Intravenous PGE is an effective vasodilator, that can induce hypotension. Due to its proinflammatory effect, collateral effects such as fever, leucocytosis and tissue oedema are extremely frequent. Another point of a long-lasting PGE1 infusion is the risk of necrotizing enterocolitis associated with enteral feeding. While the nutritional beneficial effects of early enteral feeding in pre-term and critically ill term newborns have been still confirmed, concerns remain about intestinal hypoperfusion due to the risk of ductal splanchnic steal phenomenon [19].

Actually, children with CHD and necrotizing enterocolitis are noted to have a major prevalence of retrograde diastolic flow patterns in the descending aorta [20].
  - Pre-operative nutritional practices vary widely among institutions [21]. However, data from recent studies suggested that enteral feeding is well-tolerated in ductus-dependent CHD [22–24]. Only a minority of teams base their enteral feeding strategies on the ductal flow direction [22].
- *Pre-operative management of* PVR and SVR:
  - Pre-operative sedation and paralysis may be necessary to decrease oxygen consumption in critically ill neonates.
  - Pulmonary over-circulation due to the physiologically raised PVR decreasing after birth, may require mechanical ventilation, manipulation of $PaCO_2$, and maintaining high haematocrit. Factors influencing PVR are shown in Table 28.1 [25–28].
  - Newborns with HLHS rarely require pulmonary vasodilators.
  - Pre-operative systemic vascular resistance optimization may improve systemic perfusion.

Table 28.1 Factors influencing pulmonary vascular resistance (PVR)

Increased PVR	Decreased PVR
Acidosis	Alkalosis
Mechanical hypoventilation	Mechanical hyperventilation
Inspired carbon dioxide	Sodium bicarbonate
Alveolar hypoxia	Avoid hypoxia
Inspired nitrogen	Oxygen
Endogenous sympatheitc stimulation	Sedation or paralysis
Elevated haematocrit	Low haematocrit
Vasoconstrictors	Vasodilators
Catecholamines	Phosphodiesterase inhibitors
Pleural effusion, atelectasis	Nitric oxide, sidenafil
Elevated airway pressure	Decreased airway pressure

Adapted from Graham and Bradley [18]

- Managing haemodynamics in parallel circulation remains challenging due to dynamic changes in PVR and limited monitoring of SVR. Thus, pre-operative use of vasoactive drugs in parallel circulation varies, depending on the institution, with limited evidence available for their effects on haemodynamics and systemic oxygen delivery.
- Surgical palliation for HLHS should ideally not be delayed beyond the first week of life unless other vital organs require stabilization.

28.3 Duct Dependent Pulmonary Lesions

28.3.1 Critical Pulmonary Stenosis

Pulmonary stenosis can be anatomically due to a pulmonary valvular dysplasia (with thickened leaflets and variable hypoplastic anulus) or to fusion of the thin leaflets with underdeveloped/absent commissures leading to narrowed orifice.

28.3.1.1 Pathophysiology and Clinical Signs

Clinical presentation depends on the severity of the stenosis. Critical PS with ductal-dependency of pulmonary flow presents with severe tachypnea, decreased cardiac output and cyanosis due to right-to left shunt at the atrial level. RV hypertension, hepatomegaly and peripheral vasoconstriction are related to RV inability to maintain adequate cardiac output [29].

28.3.1.2 Pre-operative Management

Neonatal PS require emergency intervention.

- PGE infusion are essential to maintain PDA and improve the pulmonary blood flow (PBF).
- After stabilization, the gold standard procedure is the percutaneous pulmonary valve balloon dilatation.
- After percutaneous valvuloplasty PGE may be discontinued.
- However, some newborns, even after successful intervention, need additional PBF because RV stiffness, with abnormal diastolic function and/or infundibular muscular hypertrophy prevents an adequate anterograde PBF.
- The additional source of PBF can be a stenting of PDA or a surgical systemic-pulmonary shunt [30].

28.3.2 Pulmonary Atresia with Intact Ventricular Septum

Pulmonary atresia with intact ventricular septum (PA-IVS) is anatomically characterized by:

- Complete pulmonary valvular obstruction
- Intact interventricular septum
- Tricuspid valve and RV abnormalities (varying from mild to severe tricuspid hypoplasia with mild/severe ventricular dilatation)

- Communications between the RV and epicardial coronary arteries (so-called sinusoids) may be present in the most severe lesions.

28.3.2.1 Pathophysiology and Clinical Signs

- Cyanosis is the typical sign, due to right-to-left shunting at atrial level.
- A large PFO is present.
- Tricuspid valve (TV) may be abnormal (ranging from mild to severe annular hypoplasia or with significant regurgitation as in Ebstein anomaly).
- TV annular size is strongly correlated to RV dimension: TV may be normal or severely hypoplastic in case of small RV, or severely dilated in case of Ebstein-like features.
- In case of complete pulmonary valve obstruction and competent TV, RV has suprasystemic pressure.
- PV atresia may be **functional** and not anatomical: in this case pulmonary artery has three sinuses, PV has three thin leaflets but an hypoplastic annulus.
- RV can be defined as tripartite (if the three portions inlet, trabecular and infundibular portions are present), or bipartite (if only inlet and infundibular are present) or unipartite (if just the inlet portion developed).
- The presence of communications between RV and coronary circulation, so-called "coronary sinusoids" is commonly correlated to TV hypoplasia and may involve both the right and left coronary circulation. These RV-to-coronary fistulae may have variable degrees of stenosis at proximal or distal levels: in case of proximal coronary stenosis, myocardial perfusion is dependent on sinusoids' desaturated blood; this condition is called "RV-dependent coronary circulation".
- Cardiac catheterization is recommended to evaluate the coronary circulation and the possibility of RV decompression [31].

28.3.2.2 Pre-operative Management

- Firstly, newborns with PA-IVS require PGE1 infusion to ensure PBF through PDA.
- Secondly, cardiac catheterization is essential for evaluating RV decompression suitability: in case of wide RV-dependence coronary circulation, RV decompression is not feasible.

If RV decompression is suitable, it can be performed by catheter-based radiofrequency perforation of the pulmonary valve, followed by valvar balloon dilation [32, 33]

- RV diastolic dysfunction is commonly present, associated with RV hypertrophy/hypoplasia: in these cases, RV decompression may not immediately provide adequate PBF and an oxygen saturation level >75%. As described in PS, an additional source of PBF may be required, consisting of either a surgical *modified Blalock-Taussig shunt* (mBTS) or percutaneous arterial duct stenting.

- In general, a surgical mBTS or percutaneous PDA stent implantation are recommended when RV decompression is not suitable at the initial cardiac catheterization.

A restrictive interatrial shunt is extremely rare in PA-IVS and may require balloon atrial septostomy, at the time of cardiac catheterization [34].

28.3.3 Tetralogy of Fallot

Tetralogy of Fallot (TOF) is the most common cyanotic CHD [35].

The classic TOF includes:

1. a perimembranous, large and unrestrictive VSD
2. the rightward shifting ("override") of the aorta, directly above the ventricular septum (leading to a biventricular origin of aortic flow with an enlarged aorta and smaller pulmonary artery)
3. the right ventricular outflow tract obstruction (RVOTO) at the subvalvular, valvular, or supravalvular levels
4. right ventricular hypertrophy

28.3.3.1 Pathophysiology and Clinical Signs

The pulmonary blood flow obstruction in TOF is due to "fixed obstruction" elements of pulmonary valve/artery stenosis and the dynamic element of increasing RVOT hypertrophy prior to surgical correction.

After birth, right ventricular hypertrophy increases over time due to pulmonary stenosis and exposure of the RV to systemic pressures because of the VSD.

In the case of the sudden increase of circulating catecholamines, with a consequent increase in cardiac contractility, an R-to-L shunting across the VSD induces a bypass of the blood flow through the lungs, leading to severe cyanosis (a "tet spell") [36].

28.3.3.2 Pre-operative Management

The treatment of *pre-operative acute cyanotic spells* include:

- blood volume optimization (infusion of *volume to increase the preload*)
- the raise of SVR, e.g. through the phenylephrine
- promoting more pulmonary blood flow into the RVOT, through the relaxation of the muscular infundibulum (morphine, benzodiazepines, and dexmedetomidine may be rapidly effective in decreasing the stress-related infundibulum spasm in awake patients)
- treatment of metabolic acidosis (with sodium bicarbonate)
- beta-blocker agents, such as esmolol
- **in any case of neonatal cyanosis waiting for a definitive diagnosis, PGE infusion is recommended** [37].

28.4 Common Mixing Lesion

28.4.1 Transposition of Great Arteries

Transposition of the great arteries (TGA) is the one of most common form of cyanotic CHD, accounting for 5–9% of all CHD [37]. It is determined by the presence of **concordant atrioventricular connections but ventriculoarterial discordance,** with the aorta arising anteriorly from the morphologic RV and the pulmonary artery arising posteriorly from the morphologic LV (◘ Fig. 28.2). This discordant relationship creates parallel systemic and pulmonary circulations, resulting in systemic hypoxaemia due to ineffective delivery of blood to the pulmonary circulation.

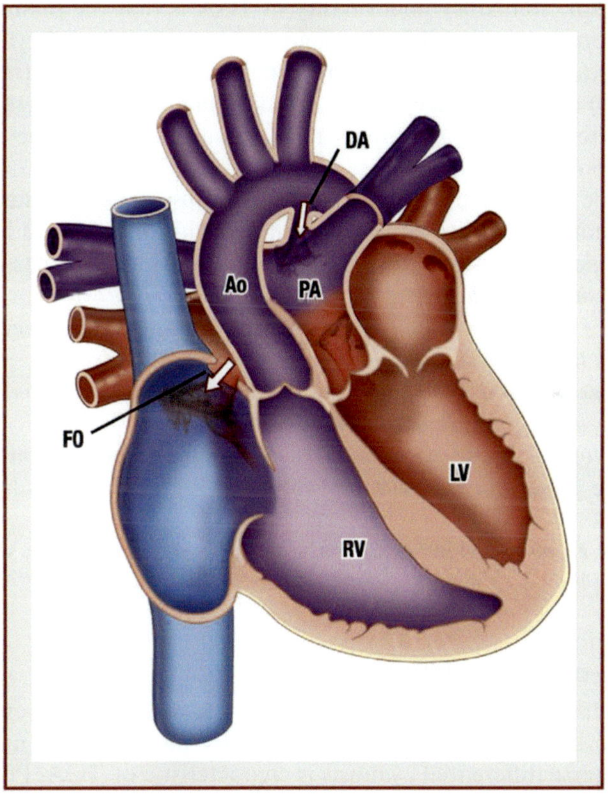

◘ **Fig. 28.2** Transposition of the great arteries with an intact ventricular septum at birth. The aorta arises from the right ventricle and the pulmonary artery arises from the left ventricle. Thus, aortic blood saturation is poor and newborns become cyanotic. At birth two foetal communications exist concomitantly: the foramen ovale and the ductus arteriosus. Ao: aorta; DA: ductus arteriosus; FO: foramen ovale; LV: left ventricle; PA: pulmonary artery; RV: right ventricle *(from Séguéla PE, Roubertie F, Kreitmann B Transposition of the great arteries: Rationale for tailored pre-operative management. Archives of Cardiovascular Disease (2017) 110, 124—134)*

Current pre-operative and surgical advances have favourably changed patient outcomes, with long-term survival approaching 97% [38]. PDA minimizes infant risks, improves outcomes [39, 40] and may predict the need for emergent postnatal intervention, such as balloon atrial septostomy (BAS) [41]. However, as prenatal prediction of the adequacy of the interatrial communication is imperfect, it is recommended that neonates with TGA be delivered in a BAS performing centre [42, 43].

In the normal foetal circulation, the most oxygen-rich and glucose-rich blood is delivered to the ascending aorta and subsequently to the brain. With TGA, the blood delivered to the brain has a lower saturation, and cerebral autoregulation must account for this reduced oxygen delivery [44, 45]. Current data suggests that delivery at 39–40 weeks might improve neurodevelopmental outcome [46–48].

28.4.1.1 Pathophysiology

The fundamental circulatory abnormality in TGA is that the pulmonary and systemic circulations run in parallel. The degree of hypoxaemia and cyanosis is dependent on the presence and patency of mixing sites, that may be **intracardiac (PFO, ASD and VSD)** or **extracardiac—(PDA, bronchopulmonary collaterals).**

Shunting sites allow oxygen supply to the tissues, as well as the oxygenation of desaturated blood in the lungs.

In TGA, the typically used terms such as *left-to-right shunt* must be used with caution, and more descriptive terms are used to avoid confusion (◘ Fig. 28.3):

- The ***anatomical left-to-right shunt*** refers to all the blood that passes ***from the left to the right side of the heart.***
- The ***effective pulmonary blood flow*** represents ***desaturated systemic venous blood that reaches the pulmonary vascular bed.***
- The ***effective systemic blood flow*** represents *the* ***oxygen-rich pulmonary venous blood that reaches the systemic circulation.***
- The ***physiological left-to-right shunt*** involves all the blood that is recirculated through the pulmonary circulation (volume of recirculating pulmonary venous blood flow).
- **Physiologic right-to-left shunting** is the volume of recirculating systemic venous blood flow [49].

28.4.1.2 Pre-operative Management

Without prenatal diagnosis, suspicion of TGA is warranted if cyanosis persists despite oxygen supplementation, with respiratory distress being uncommon. The presence of reverse differential cyanosis is characteristic of TGA. Prompt initiation of prostaglandin E1 (PGE) and urgent transfer to a specialized centre are essential. Most hypoxemic neonates with TGA benefit from early PGE administration, but those with a restrictive PFO may experience complications such as left atrial hypertension and low cardiac output, necessitating urgent balloon atrial septostomy (BAS). Despite apparently adequate oxygen saturation with PGE, neonates are at risk of complications such as apnoea, hypotension, and fever, especially those with lower birth weights. Mechanical ventilation, infection, and other complications may

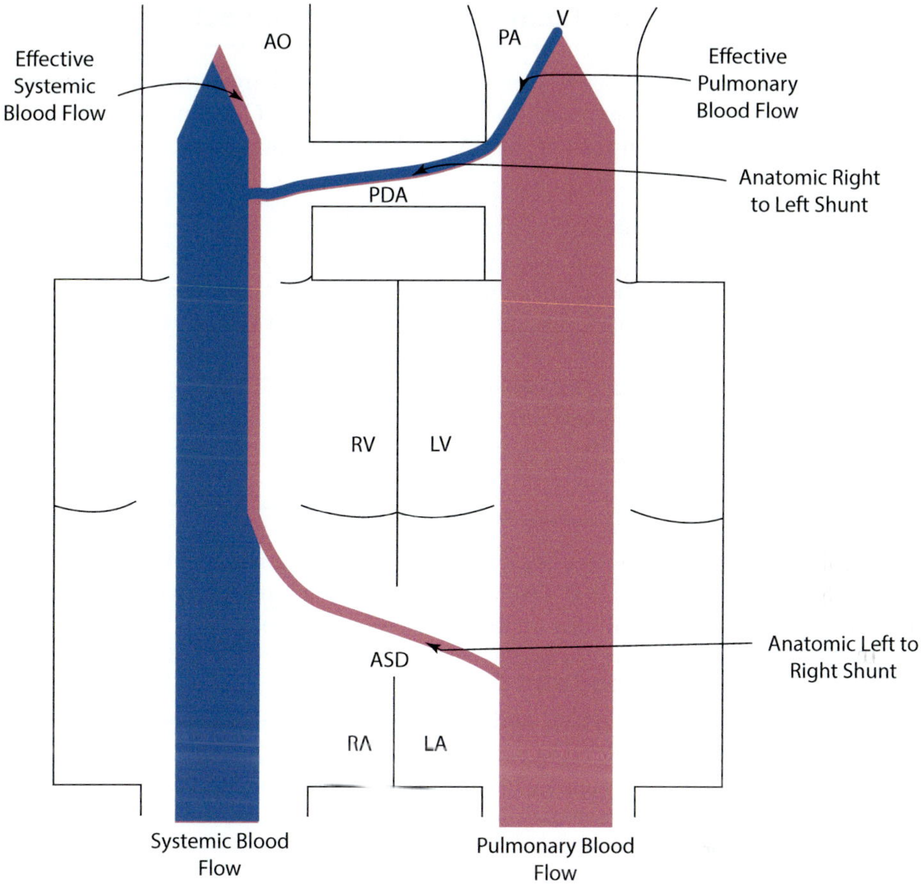

Fig. 28.3 Circulation of TGA with intact ventricular septum. The majority of the systemic and pulmonary blood flow recirculates within the parallel circulation and itis ineffective. At the ATRIAL LEVEL there is an anatomical left to-right shunt, that is directed into the systemic circulation as **oxygenated effective systemic blood flow**. At the LEVEL OF PDA there is an equal volume of blood that passes from the aorta to the pulmonary artery as **deoxygenated effective pulmonary blood** flow. As seen in the shunt at the PDA, a small portion of the anatomical shunt is derived from the pulmonary circulation; thus, the anatomical shunt may be greater than the effective pulmonary blood flow. This concept is important when understanding bidirectional shunting (from *Files MD, Arya B. Pre-operative Physiology, Imaging, and Management of Transposition of the Great Arteries Seminars in Cardiothoracic and Vascular Anesthesia. 2015, Vol. 19(3) 210–222)*

occur while awaiting surgery. Attempting to wean off PGE after BAS is recommended, although predictors of successful withdrawal are lacking, and PGE may need to be restarted in approximately half of cases. Currently, scheduling arterial switch operation (ASO) within 2–4 days of diagnosis is increasingly common, but decisions regarding BAS and PGE discontinuation vary by centre [49, 50].

28.4.2 Total Anomalous Pulmonary Venous Connection

Total anomalous pulmonary venous connection (TAPVC) is characterized by an anomalous connection among some (partial) or all (in case of TAPVC) pulmonary veins, that drain directly into the RA instead of the LA, or through one/more systemic veins.

The abnormal site of connection of the pulmonary veins to the systemic circulation can be:

1. **Supracardiac** (the pulmonary veins drain to a confluence behind the LA, which is connected via an ascending vertical vein to the SVC or left innominate or the azygous vein).
2. **Cardiac** (the veins drain to the coronary sinus or directly into the RA).
3. **Infracardiac** (the vertical vein descends to join the portal vein or the ductus venosus).
4. **Mixed** [51, 52]

The Scimitar syndrome is a peculiar form of infradiaphragmatic PAPVC, associated with right lung hypoplasia [53]. If TAPVC is obstructed, it represents a life-threatening neonatal emergency, that calls for an immediate surgical repair [54].

28.4.2.1 Pathophysiology and Clinical Signs

The prenatal diagnosis of TAPVC and PAPVC remains challenging due to the scarcity of pulmonary venous blood in utero [55].

Postnatally diagnosed patients with obstructed TAPVC exhibit marked cyanosis, while those without obstruction may show signs of pulmonary overflow, such as mild cyanosis and dyspnoea. Pulmonary hypertension is always present due to chronic obstruction of pulmonary blood flow, leading to muscularization of pulmonary vessels. LV mass remains normal, but filling is reduced, and RV hypertension causes leftward displacement of the IVS, distorting LV morphology [56].

Prompt corrective surgery is necessary to prevent irreversible LV structural alterations. Newborns with obstructed TAPVC experience severe acidosis and cyanosis immediately after birth. There are two bidirectional cardiac shunts: a left to-right shunt via the pulmonary veins draining into the systemic venous system, and a right-to-left shunt across the atrial communication, resulting in severe and unresponsive cyanosis. Preductal and postductal oxygen saturations are usually similar, but differential cyanosis may occur in infracardiac and supracardiac TAPVC cases. In these patients, PGE induce PBF augmentation, without clinical improvement [56].

The optimal surgical timing for TAPVC without obstruction is still debated, but earlier repair is associated with shorter pre-operative mechanical ventilation, postoperative support, and lower severity of LV structural alterations. In conclusion, newborns with congenital heart disease exhibit significant heterogeneity and require personalized treatment based on a comprehensive understanding of their pathophysiology [57–61].

Key Messages: Use of Prostaglandin and Differential Diagnosis

CHD with left outflow obstruction—defined as duct-dependent systemic lesions (including coarctation of Aorta, Aortic Stenosis, Interrupted Aortic Arch, HLHS).

CHD with right outflow obstruction—defined as duct dependent pulmonary lesions (including critical Pulmonary Stenosis, Tricuspid Atresia, Pulmonary Atresia + Intact Ventricular Septum, tetralogy of Fallot).

TGA, TAPVC, DILV, Truncus Arteriosus, are characterized by common mixing.

Who should be given Prostaglandin?

All symptomatic neonates with suspected CHD should have prostaglandin infusion commenced until full evaluation by cardiology specialists. However, it is important to remember that there are some caveats to prostaglandin administration, where it may not be beneficial.

The two examples include:

(1) the newborn with TAPVC and obstructed pulmonary venous return, where prostaglandin increases the pulmonary blood flow and the pulmonary congestion.

(2) the newborn with TGA with intact ventricular septum, who needs atrial septostomy because patent ductus arteriosus does not provide adequate mixing

References

1. Singh Y, Lakshminrusimha S. Perinatal cardiovascular physiology and recognition of critical congenital heart defects. Clin Perinatol. 2021;48:573–94.
2. Anderson RH, Baker EJ, Penny D, et al. Paediatric cardiology. 3rd ed. Philadelphia: Elsevier; 2009.
3. Baumgartner H, Bonhoeffer P, De Groot NM, et al. Task Force on the Management of Grown-up Congenital Heart Disease of the European Society of Cardiology (ESC); Association for European Paediatric Cardiology (AEPC); ESC Committee for Practice Guidelines (CPG). ESC guidelines for the management of grown-up congenital heart disease (new version 2010). Eur Heart J. 2010;31:2915–57.
4. Singh S, Hakim FA, Sharma A, et al. Hypoplasia, pseudocoarctation and coarctation of the aorta—a systematic review. Heart Lung Circ. 2015;24:110–8.
5. Liberman RF, Getz KD, Lin AE, et al. Delayed diagnosis of critical congenital heart defects. trends and associated factors. Pediatrics. 2014;134:e373–81.
6. Bayer ML, Frommelt PC, Blei F, et al. Congenital cardiac, aortic arch, and vascular bed anomalies in PHACE syndrome (from the international PHACE syndrome registry). Am J Cardiol. 2013;112:1948–52.
7. Maskatia SA, Ing FF, Justino H, et al. Twenty-five year experience with balloon aortic valvuloplasty for congenital aortic stenosis. Am J Cardiol. 2011;108:1024–8.
8. Feinstein JA, Benson DW, Dubin AM, et al. Hypoplastic left heart syndrome: current considerations and expectations. J Am Coll Cardiol. 2012;59:S1–42.
9. Glatz JA, Tabbutt S, Gaynor JW, et al. Hypoplastic left heart syndrome with atrial level restriction in the era of prenatal diagnosis. Ann Thorac Surg. 2007;84:1633–8.
10. Rychik J, Szwast A, Natarajan S, et al. Perinatal and early surgical outcome for the fetus with hypoplastic left heart syndrome: a 5-year single institutional experience. Ultrasound Obstet Gynecol. 2010;36:465–70.
11. Friedman KG, Sleeper LA, Freud LR. Improved technical success, postnatal outcome and refined predictors of outcome for fetal aortic valvuloplasty. Ultrasound Obstetr Gynecol. 2018;52(2):212–20.

12. Beatti MJ, Friedman KG, Sleeper LA. Late gestation predictors of a postnatal biventricular circulation after fetal aortic valvuloplasty. Prenatal Diagn. 2021;41(4):479–85.
13. Barnea O, Austin EH, Santamore WP. Balancing the circulation: theoretic optimization of pulmonary/systemic flow ratio in hypoplastic left heart syndrome. J Am Coll Cardiol. 1994;24:1376–81.
14. Barnea O, Santamore WP, Rossi A, et al. Estimation of oxygen delivery in newborns with a univentricular circulation. Circulation. 1998;98:1407–13.
15. Whyte RK. Mixed venous oxygen saturation in the newborn: can we and should we measure it? Scand J Clin Lab Invest Suppl. 1990;203:203–11.
16. Taeed R, Schwartz SM, Pearl JM, et al. Unrecognized pulmonary venous desaturation early after Norwood palliation confounds Qp:Qs assessment and compromises oxygen delivery. Circulation. 2001;103:2699–704.
17. Hoffman GM, Ghanayem NS, Kampine JM, et al. Venous saturation and the anaerobic threshold in neonates after the Norwood procedure for hypoplastic left heart syndrome. Ann Thorac Surg. 2000;70:1515–21.
18. Graham EM, Bradley SM, Atz AM. Preoperative management of hypoplastic left heart syndrome. Expert Opin Pharmacother. 2005;6(5):687–93.
19. Howley LW, Kaufman J, Wymore E, et al. Enteral feeding in neonates with prostaglandin-dependent congenital cardiac disease: international survey on current trends and variations in practice. Cardiol Young. 2012;22:121–7.
20. McElhinney DB, Hedrick HL, Bush DM, et al. Necrotizing enterocolitis in neonates with congenital heart disease: risk factors and outcomes. Pediatrics. 2000;106:1080.
21. Talosi G, Katona M, Turi S. Side-effects of long-term prostaglandin E(1) treatment in neonates. Pediatr Int. 2007;49:335–40.
22. Willis L, Thureen P, Kaufman J, Wymore E, Skillman H, da Cruz E. Enteral feeding in prostaglandin-dependent neonates: is it a safe practice? J Pediatr. 2008;153:867–9.
23. Iannucci GJ, Oster ME, Mahle WT. Necrotising enterocolitis in infants with congenital heart disease: the role of en teral feeds. Cardiol Young. 2013;23:553–9.
24. Becker KC, Hornik CP, Cotten CM, et al. Necrotizing enterocolitis in infants with ductal-dependent congenital heart disease. Am J Perinatol. 2015;32:633–8.
25. Riordan CJ, Randsbaek F, Storey JH, Montgomery WD, Santamore WP, Austin EH. Inotropes in the hypoplastic left heart syndrome: effects in an animal model. Ann Thorac Surg. 1996;62:83–90.
26. Shime N, Hashimoto S, Hiramatsu N, et al. Hypoxic gas therapy using nitrogen in the preoperative management of neonates with hypoplastic left heart syndrome. Pediatr Crit Care Med. 2000;1:38–41.
27. Chang AC, Zucker HA, Hickey PR, et al. Pulmonary vascular resistance in infants after cardiac surgery: role of carbon dioxide and hydrogen ion. Crit. Care Med. 1995;23:568–75.
28. Bradley SM, Simsic JM, Atz AM. Hemodynamic effects of inspired carbon dioxide after the Norwood procedure. Ann Thorac Surg. 2001;72:2088–94.
29. Stamm C, Anderson RH, Ho SY. (1998) Clinical anatomy of the normal pulmonary root compared with that in isolated pulmonary valvular stenosis. J Am Coll Cardiol. 1998;31(6):1420–5.
30. Holzer RJ, Gauvreau K, Kreutzer J, et al. Safety and efficacy of balloon pulmonary valvuloplasty: a multicentre experience. Catheter Cardiovasc Interv. 2012;80:663–72.
31. Bull C, de Leval MR, Mercanti C, et al. Pulmonary atresia and intact ventricular septum: a revised classification. Circulation. 1982;66:266–80.
32. Justo RN, Nykanen DG, Williams WG, et al. Transcatheter perforation of the right ventricular outflow tract as initial therapy for pulmonary valve atresia and intact ventricular septum in the newborn. Catheter Cardiovasc Diagn. 1997;40(4):408–13.
33. Humpl T, Soderberg B, McCrindle BW, et al. Percutaneous balloon valvotomy in pulmonary atresia with intact ventricular septum: impact on patient care. Circulation. 2003;108:826–32.
34. Gewillig M, Boshoff DE, Dens J, et al. Stenting the neonatal arterial duct in duct-dependent pulmonary circulation; new techniques, better results. J Am Coll Cardiol. 2004;43:107–12.
35. Triedman JK, Newburger JW. Trends in congenital heart disease: the next decade. Circulation. 2016;133(25):2716–33.
36. Montero JV, Nieto EM, Vallejo IR, et al. Intranasal midazolam for the emergency management of hypercyanotic spells in tetralogy of Fallot. Pediatr Emerg Care. 2015;31:269–71.
37. Tomar M. Neonatal cardiac emergencies: evaluation and management. J Intensive Crit Care. 2016;2:1–12.

38. Oster ME, Lee KA, Honein MA, Riehle-Colarusso T, Shin M, Correa A. Temporal trends in survival among infants with critical congenital heart defects. Pediatrics. 2013;131:e1502–8.
39. Fricke TA, d'Udekem Y, Richardson M, et al. Outcomes of the arterial switch operation for transposition of the great arteries: 25 years of experience. Ann Thorac Surg. 2012;94:139–45.
40. Oda S, Nakano T, Sugiura J, et al. Twenty-eight years'experienceof arterial switch operation for transposition of the great arteries in a single institution. Eur J Cardiothorac Surg. 2012;42:674–9.
41. Calderon J, Angeard N, Moutier S, et al. Impact of prenatal diagnosis on neurocognitive outcomes in children with transposition of the great arteries. J Pediatr. 2012;161(1):94–8.
42. Bonnet D, Coltri A, Butera G, Fermont L, Le Bidois J, Kachaner J, Sidi D. Detection of transposition of the great arteries in fetuses reduces neonatal morbidity and mortality. Circulation. 1999;99:916–8.
43. Punn R, Silverman NH. Fetal predictors of urgent balloon atrial septostomy in neonates with complete transposition. J Am Soc Echocardiogr. 2011;24:425–30.
44. Punn R, Silverman NH. Fetal predictors of urgent balloon atrial septostomy in neonates with complete transposition. J Am Soc Echocardiogr. 2011;24(4):425–30.
45. Turah S, Turan O, Hussein M, et al. Patterns of compromised fetal brain growth in congenital heart disease. Am J Obstet Gynecol. 2012;206:S176–7.
46. Jouannic JM, Benachi A, Bonnet D, et al. Middle cerebral artery Doppler in fetuses with transposition of the great arteries. Ultrasound Obstet Gynecol. 2002;20:122–4.
47. Manzar S, Nair AK, Pai MG, Al-Khusaiby SM. Head size at birth in neonates with transposition of great arteries and hypoplastic left heart syndrome. Saudi Med J. 2005;26:453–6.
48. Limperopoulos C, Tworetzky W, McElhinney DB, et al. Brain volume and metabolism in fetuses with congenital heart disease: evaluation with quantitative mag- netic resonance imaging and spectroscopy. Circulation. 2010;121:26–33.
49. Wernovsky G. Transposition of the great arteries. In: Allen HD, Shaddy R, Feltes T, editors. Moss and Adams' heart disease in infants, children, and adolescents: including the fetus and Young adult. Philadelphia: Wolters Kluwer Health/Lippincott Williams & Wilkins; 2008. p. 1027–84.
50. Rudolph AM. Congenital diseases of the heart: clinical-physiological considerations. Chichester, UK: Wiley-Blackwell; 2009.
51. Padalino MA, Cavalli G, De Franceschi M, et al. Surgical outcomes of total anomalous pulmonary venous connection repair: a 22-year experience. J Card Surg. 2014;29:678–85.
52. Hines MH, Hammon JW. Anatomy of total anomalous pulmonary venous connection. Oper Tech Thorac Cardiovasc Surg. 2001;6:2–7.
53. Musewe NN, Smallhorn JF, Freedom RM. Anomalies of pulmonary venous connections including cor triatriatum and stenosis of individual pulmonary veins. In: Freedom RM, Benson LN, Smallhorn JF, editors. Neonatal heart disease. Springer-Verlag: London; 1992. p. 309–31.
54. Hyde JAJ, Stumper O, Barth M-J, Wright JGC, Silove ED, de Giovanni JV, Brawn WJ, Sethia B. Total anomalous pulmonary venous connection: outcome of surgical correction and management of recurrent venous obstruction. Eur J Cardiothorac.
55. Allan LD, Sharland GK. The echocardiographic diagnosis of totally anomalous pulmonary venous connection in the fetus. Heart. 2001;85:433–7.
56. Haworth SG, Reid L. Structural study of pulmonary circulation and of heart in total anomalous pulmonary venous return in early infancy. Br Heart J. 1977;39:80–92.
57. Yap SH, Anania N, Alboliras ET, Lilien LD. Reversed differential cyanosis in the newborn: a clinical finding in the supracardiac total anomalous pulmonary venous connection. Pediatr Cardiol. 2009;30:359–62.
58. Chowdhury UK, Airan B, Malhotra A, et al. Mixed total anomalous pulmonary venous connection: anatomic variations, surgical approach, techniques, and results. J Thorac Cardiovasc Surg. 2008;135:106–16.
59. Scott JP, Hoffman GM. Near-infrared spectroscopy: exposing the dark (venous) side of the circulation. Paediatr Anaesth. 2014;24:74–88.
60. Sinzobahamvya N, Arenz C, Brecher AM, Blaschczok HC, Urban AE. Early and long-term results for correction of total anomalous pulmonary venous drainage (TAPVD) in neonates and infants. Eur J Cardiothorac Surg. 1996;10:433–8.
61. Frommelt PC, Sheridan DC, Deatsman S, et al. Unobstructive total anomalous pulmonary venous return: impact of early elective repair on the need for prolonged mechanical ventilatory support. Pediatr Cardiol. 2010;31:1191–7.

Further Reading

Baumgartner H, Bonhoeffer P, De Groot NM, et al. Task Force on the Management of Grown-up Congenital Heart Disease of the European Society of Cardiology (ESC); Association for European Paediatric Cardiology (AEPC); ESC Committee for Practice Guidelines (CPG). ESC guidelines for the management of grown-up congenital heart disease (new version 2010). Eur Heart J. 2010;31:2915–57.

Donofrio MT, Levy RJ, Schuette JJ, et al. Specialized delivery room planning for fetuses with critical congenital heart disease. Am J Cardiol. 2013,111:737–47.

Donofrio MT, Skurow-Todd K, Berger JT, et al. Risk-stratified postnatal care of newborns with congenital heart disease determined by fetal echocardiography. J Am Soc Echocardiogr. 2015;28(11):1339–49.

Donofrio MT, Moon-Grady AJ, Hornberger LK. Diagnosis and treatment of fetal cardiac disease a scientific statement from the American Heart Association. Circulation. 2014;129:2183–242.

Donofrio MT, Moon-Grady AJ, Hornberger LK, et al. American Heart Association Adults With Congenital Heart Disease Joint Committee of the Council on Cardio- vascular Disease in the Young and Council on Clinical Cardiology, Council on Cardiovascular Surgery and Anesthesia, and Council on Cardiovascular and Stroke Nursing. Diagnosis and treatment of fetal cardiac disease: a scientific statement from the American Heart Association. Circulation. 2014;129:2183–24.

Feinstein JA, Benson DW, Dubin AM, et al. Hypoplastic left heart syndrome: current considerations and expectations. J Am Coll Cardiol. 2012;59:S1–42.

Finnemore A, Groves A. Physiology of the fetal and transitional circulation. Semin Fetal Neonatal Med. 2015;44:1–7.

Morton S, Brodsky D. Fetal physiology and the transition to extrauterine life. Clin Perinatol. 2016;43(3):395–407.

Rudolph AM. Congenital diseases of the heart: clinical-physiological considerations. Chichester, UK: Wiley- Blackwell; 2009.

Sanapo L, Moon-Grady A, Donofrio MT. Perinatal and delivery management of infants with congenital heart disease. Clin Perinatol. 2016;43:55–71.

Singh S, Hakim FA, Sharma A, et al. Hypoplasia, pseudocoarctation and coarctation of the aorta—a systematic review. Heart Lung Circ. 2015;24:110–8.

Wernovsky G. Transposition of the great arteries. In: Allen HD, Shaddy R, Feltes T, editors. Moss and Adams' heart disease in infants, children, and adolescents: including the fetus and young adult. Philadelphia: Wolters Kluwer Health/Lippincott Williams & Wilkins; 2008. p. 1027–84.

Principles of Postoperative Management in the Paediatric Cardiac Intensive Care: Low Cardiac Output State (LCOS) and Lesion-Specific Management

Y. Feinstein, Aparna Hoskote, and Uri Pollak

Contents

J. Brierley et al. (eds.), *ESPNIC Children's Intensive Care Textbook*,
https://doi.org/10.1007/978-3-031-64762-8_29

Learning Objects

Low Cardiac Output State

- Learn what LCOS is, the challenges in defining the syndrome, and how we can diagnose it.
- Learn what measures we have to prevent and predict LCOS:
  - Milrinone—get familiar with the PRIMACORP study
  - LCOS scores—get familiar with the challenge of definition and prediction of LCOS
- Learn how to treat LCOS physiologically
  - Reducing oxygen consumption
  - Optimising preload
  - Improving myocardial function—systolic and diastolic function
  - Manipulating afterload
  - Role of cardiopulmonary interactions
  - Role of corticosteroids
  - Role of non-pharmacologic interventions—systemic hypothermia
  - Mechanical circulatory support

Lesion-Specific Postoperative Management for Children After Cardiac Surgery

- Understand that management should be tailored to the pathophysiology and clinical condition
- Learn about the common concerns and complications in the postoperative management of different defects

29.1 Introduction

The long-term survival of neonates, infants and children with congenital heart defects has significantly improved in the last four decades due to the major advances in the diagnosis, operative capabilities, peri-operative management and long-term follow-up [1–3]. Advances in understanding the physiology and haemodynamics in the hours post complex cardiopulmonary bypass (CPB) surgery have helped progress the safe management of children in the postoperative period in the cardiac intensive care unit (CICU).

In this chapter, we focus on the Low Cardiac Output State (LCOS), a common and important haemodynamic state seen in the postoperative period in children who have undergone complex open-heart surgery. Early identification and timely appropriate management are of utmost importance as otherwise, it can lead to significant morbidity and mortality. In addition, we will review the postoperative management of certain specific lesions according to their different pathophysiology patterns and predicted complications. The review will include a discussion of specific clinical scenarios.

29.2 Low Cardiac Output State (LCOS)

29.2.1 Definition

LCOS is a temporary fall in the tissue oxygen delivery in the immediate postoperative period after congenital heart surgery, resulting in inadequate oxygen delivery to match the oxygen demands. The causes for this LCOS are multifactorial and include myocardial dysfunction seen after surgery involving cardiopulmonary bypass. LCOS remains a significant postoperative complication and is adversely related to morbidity and mortality [4, 5].

Several studies have described LCOS in children undergoing congenital heart surgery. Parr et al. [6], back in 1975, reported an acute fall in cardiac index in nearly 25% of young children postoperatively measured by dye dilution, which was related to acute cardiac death. Some 20 years later, Wernovsky et al. [4] reported that 25% of neonates who underwent an arterial switch operation for transposition of the great arteries had a decline in cardiac index, mostly noticed between 6 and 18 h after surgery. Both reports showed an associated increase in systemic vascular resistance (SVR) and pulmonary vascular resistance (PVR) from baseline values. Similar findings have been reported in recent studies as well [5, 7]. This transient decrease in cardiac function usually improves within 24 h from surgery [4, 8].

Although LCOS is a well-known and well-described phenomenon, there is no clear definition, and different criteria are used in clinical and research [9–13] publications. Furthermore, clinicians vary considerably in the definition and diagnosis of LCOS [14, 15]. Due to these variabilities, recent attempts have been made to develop and validate scoring systems to diagnose probable LCOS. These scores incorporate the Vasoactive-Inotropic Score (VIS). A strong association has been described between the peak VIS in the first 24 h and morbidity and mortality for infants [7, 8, 16, 17]. The VIS is a simple calculation of the dosage of vasoactive agents given to a patient; it is a measure of pharmacological support and does not necessarily reflect the inadequate delivery of oxygen to the issues, which is the mainstay of LCOS. Ulate et al. [11] developed the LCOS Score (LCOSS), a composite of clinical characteristics and pharmacologic cardiovascular support, trying to improve the 'VIS's relevance to the clinical syndrome. The score includes the following components: (1) heart rate, (2) urine output, (3) peripheral temperature, (4) volume administration requirements, (5) near-infrared spectroscopy (NIRS) measurements, (6) levels of arterial lactate and (7) use of vasoactive-inotropic infusions other than milrinone. This score is also based on therapeutic measures, which have the same limitations as the VIS. Other scoring systems like the inadequate oxygen delivery index (IDO_2), an etiometry-based score that includes vital signs and laboratory results monitoring, have failed to predict LCOS or its adverse sequelae [12]. To conclude, more work is needed to find a better definition of LCOS that can be used in research studies.

A pragmatic definition would be a clinical syndrome based on a constellation of clinical signs and laboratory values characterising poor systemic perfusion such as low pulse volumes, prolonged capillary refill time, low blood pressure, poor urine output, rising metabolic and lactic acidosis, reduced mixed venous oxygen saturation, rising arterio-venous oxygen saturation difference and signs of end-organ dysfunction.

Table 29.1 Contributing factors to the development of LCOS

Contributing factors to the development of LCOS:
Haemodynamic alterations:
Postoperative acute changes in ventricular loading conditions: • Volume load—e.g. PDA or intracardiac shunt • Pressure load—e.g. obstructions, valve stenosis, conduits stenosis • Alterations in SVR or PVR—e.g. vasoplegia, pulmonary vascular reactivity
Direct myocardial trauma
CPB-Related alterations: • SIRS • Myocardial reperfusion injury
Pulmonary reperfusion injury
Increase in total body oxygen demand: • Bleeding • SIRS • Arrhythmias • Fever
LCOS low cardiac output state, *PDA* patent ductus arteriosus, *SVR* systemic vascular resistance, *PVR* pulmonary vascular resistance, *SIRS* systemic inflammatory response syndrome

29.2.2 Pathophysiology and Aetiology

The aetiology of LCOS after congenital heart surgery is multifactorial, ranging from the effects of cardiopulmonary bypass (CPB) and resultant systemic inflammation, myocardial protection from the aortic cross-clamp, the haemodynamic changes following repair to increased oxygen demand or oxygen consumption (Table 29.1). Cardiac dysfunction may result from either systolic, diastolic function impairment or both, and it can involve the right, left or systemic ventricle.

29.2.3 Diagnosis

The mainstay of managing LCOS involves early diagnosis and timely interventions before end-organ dysfunction or cardiac arrest ensues. As discussed before, there is no validated standardised definition of LCOS. In the CICU, infants and children are monitored for many physiologic, clinical and laboratory variables, thus helping the bedside clinician to appropriately assess the condition and commence the necessary treatment. Unfortunately, the clinical assessment of cardiac function, organ perfusion and tissue oxygenation does not necessarily correlate with the measured values obtained by invasive and non-invasive modalities (such as dye dilution, thermodilution, echocardiographic parameters such as ejection fraction; ultrasonic cardiac output monitoring (USCOM) and NIRS [18, 19]) [20]. Therefore, multi-modality monitoring complements each other to facilitate diagnosis and management. The modalities are listed in Table 29.2.

Table 29.2 Clinical assessment of LCOS

Monitored variables for early diagnosis of LCOS
Vital signs—heart rate and rhythm; blood pressure and pulse pressure; peripheral oxygen saturation; temperature—core to peripheral temperature gradient; central venous pressure (when available); atrial pressures (when available); respiratory rate
Physical examination—the level of consciousness, pupillary response, capillary refill time, heart sounds, auscultation, liver span, lung auscultation, physical tests for fluid responsiveness, and urine output
Metabolic biomarkers: lactate, troponin, mixed venous saturation, pH, bicarbonate
Tissue oxygen delivery monitoring—e.g. Near Infra-Red Spectroscopy (NIRS)

29.2.4 Prevention

As LCOS is associated with significant morbidity and even mortality, anticipation and prevention of LCOS are the key to managing children daily in the cardiac intensive care unit (CICU). Preventing LCOS may reduce mortality and hospital and intensive care length of stay, thus lowering the risk for end-organ dysfunction with a beneficial impact on costs, resources and patient experience [13, 21]. Therefore, the prevention of LCOS remains the focus of many studies, mostly using inotropic and vasodilator agents to improve tissue perfusion and reduce the mismatch between oxygen delivery and oxygen consumption. As catecholamines may be arrhythmogenic and result in tachycardia, an increase in afterload and myocardial oxygen consumption, phosphodiesterase 3 (PDE3) inhibitors such as milrinone have been extensively studied. They are advantageous as they provide an inotropic effect combined with afterload reduction to improve tissue perfusion. See ► Box 29.1 for details on the PRIMACORP study. In addition, several centres have studied the use of levosimendan, a calcium sensitiser, which acts as an inodilator with lusitropic properties that improve haemodynamics with no significant increase in myocardial oxygen consumption [10, 11, 14–18].

Nearly 20 years after the PRIMACORP study, milrinone remains the standard of care for children perceived to have a high chance of developing LCOS [14]. In 2015, Burkhardt et al. [22] conducted a Cochrane systematic review of the prophylactic use of milrinone to prevent LCOS. Although the meta-analysis confirmed the efficacy of prophylactic milrinone in reducing LCOS incidence, the conclusion was that there is insufficient evidence of effectiveness in preventing death compared to placebo due to the small trials and their risk of bias. Two years later, levosimendan was reviewed as well for the Cochrane library by Hummel et al. [23], and a similar conclusion was drawn. Further research is needed to achieve more high-quality evidence.

29.2.5 Treatment

The treatment of LCOS aims to ensure adequate oxygen delivery to the tissues by reducing the delivery and demand mismatch at the cellular level. See ▶ Box 29.2 for calculations of oxygen variables. Cardiac output is influenced and determined by several physiological variables and their interactions. Hence, optimising cardiac out put encompasses a combination of therapeutic strategies, including (1) controlling heart rate and rhythm, (2) maintaining adequate ventricular preload, (3) improving cardiac contractility with the use of inotropic agents, (4) manipulating ventricular afterload, (5) optimising cardiopulmonary interactions and (6) mechanical circulatory support. ◘ Figure 29.1 is a schematic illustration of the physiological variables that determine the cardiac output: preload, contractility, afterload and heart rate. Targeted interventions using these variables can help achieve better cardiac output.

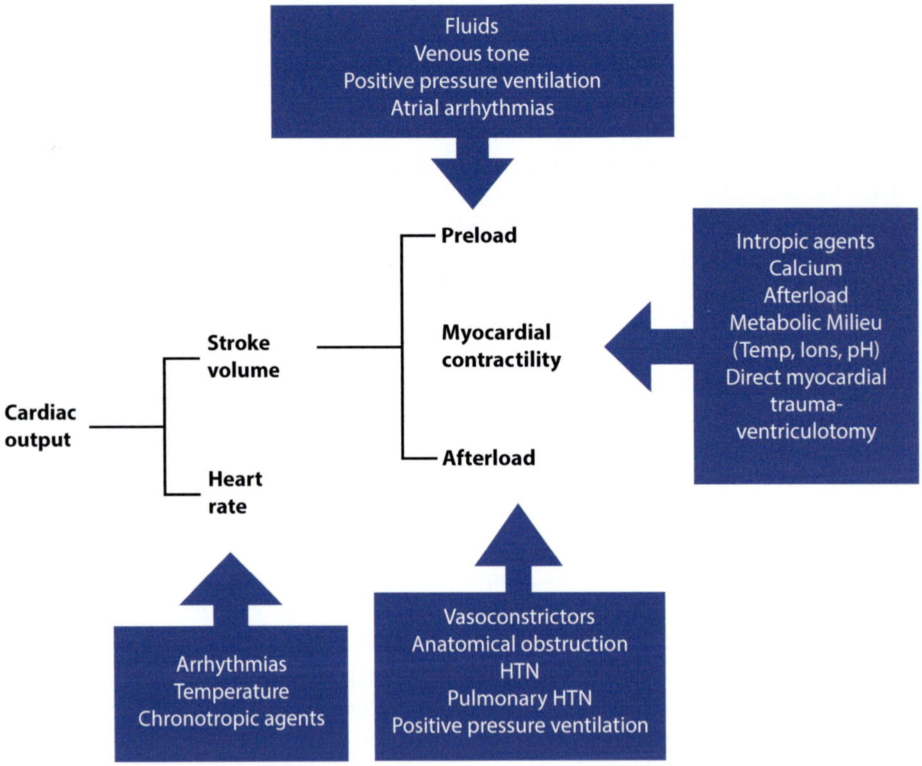

◘ **Fig. 29.1** Physiological variables that determine the cardiac output: cardiac output is determined by several physiological variables, including filling pressures (preload), the myocardium's ability to create force (contractility) and the ventricles' afterload. There is a complex relationship between these variables, and their product will determine the stroke volume. The heart rate will also influence cardiac output, and children can change their heart rate significantly. Many factors can change these variables and influence cardiac output

Reducing metabolic demands by ensuring adequate sedation and analgesia, as well as maintaining normothermia, further helps reduce oxygen consumption. In addition, monitoring the cardiac rhythm and treating dysrhythmias is important. Maintaining the haemoglobin level at an adequate level is also essential to optimise oxygen delivery.

29.2.5.1 Optimising Preload

One of the most critical and easily remedial therapies in the management of LCOS is correcting hypovolaemia as determined by tachycardia, low central venous pressure (CVP) and poor peripheral perfusion. Determination of optimal ventricular filling pressures for a given physiology in the postoperative period begins with assessing where the ventricle is situated on its pressure-volume curve. Understanding this will direct the appropriate management of preload. However, a few challenges should be borne in mind, especially in the population treated for LCOS. Ventricular compliance may vary and influence the relationship between atrial pressure and stroke volume. Also, the correlations between the left and right atrial pressures and the left ventricle may be altered in the post-repair physiology. Administration of fluids and assessment of the response can guide the treatment. The response to fluids includes monitoring the change in vital signs (e.g. heart rate and blood pressure), CVP, atrial pressures and perfusion markers such as lactate and mixed venous oxygen saturation. Consideration should be taken that the response may be confounded by the presence of positive pressure ventilation that alters the afterload of the ventricles.

A few considerations of note:

- Watch out for occult bleeding
- Determine the adequate preload for the patient and understand what the filling pressure represents in the individual patient
- Post right heart surgery, higher right-sided filling pressures may be needed in RV diastolic dysfunction, for example, Tetralogy of Fallot repair, Glenn and Fontan
- Remember, ventricular compliance is variable, e.g., using only smaller aliquots of fluid following a late arterial switch surgery.

29.2.5.2 Improving Myocardial Function

Systolic function is generated by a myocardium that can contract synchronously and efficiently to provide stroke volume and cardiac output. Once the ventricular loading conditions are optimised, inotropic support may be needed. The choice of the specific vasoactive 'agents' combination depends on the anatomical substrate and is specific to the lesion and resultant physiology. For example, a patient with Tetralogy of Fallot who underwent full repair may require high filling pressures and the use of noradrenaline to maintain adequate stroke volume due to a non-compliant hypertrophic right ventricle. As opposed to this patient, a patient with aberrant origin of the left coronary artery from the pulmonary artery (ALCAPA) will have persistent, significant left ventricle dysfunction even after repair and will not tolerate high fluid volumes and vasoconstrictors that may increase the afterload.

There are many possible vasoactive agents with different haemodynamic effects that are also dose-dependent, and each has different side effects. See ◘ Table 29.3 for

Table 29.3 Common vasoactive agents for the treatment of LCOS

Agent	Mechanism of action	Dose (mcg/kg/min)	Effect
Dopamine	Dopaminergic	0.5–4	Modest inotrope Increase heart rate
	β adrenergic	4–10	Modest inotrope Increase heart rate Peripheral vasoconstriction
	α > β adrenergic	11–20	Increase Pulmonary Vascular Resistance (PVR) Dysrhythmias
Dobutamine	β_1 and β_2 adrenergic	1–20	Modest inotrope Vasodilation (β_2) of venous and arterial vessels May reduce ventricular filling pressures Decreases PVR Increase heart rate and extrasystoles
Epinephrine	β > α adrenergic	0.01–1.0	Strong Inotrope Increase heart rate Decreased renal flow Dysrhythmias Vasodilator in low doses <0.1 mcg/kg/min (β_2 activity) Vasoconstrictor in high doses (α activity)
Norepinephrine	α > β adrenergic	0.05–1.0	Potent vasoconstrictor—arterial and venous Inotrope Increase Systemic Vascular Resistance (SVR) and PVR
Vasopressin	V1 receptors	0.0003–0.002 unit/kg/min	Potent vasoconstrictor Increase SVR No chronotropic effect
Sodium Nitroprusside	Nitric oxide donor	0.5–10	Vasodilator: Arterial greater than venous Cyanide toxicity
Nitroglycerin	Nitric oxide donor	1–20	Vasodilator: Venous greater than arterial At low doses (<3 mcg/kg/min)—increases venous capacitance High doses—decrease SVR Increase methemoglobin
Milrinone	PDE3 inhibitor	0.2–1	Inotrope Chronotrope Vasodilation
Levosimendan	Calcium sensitiser	0.1–0.2	Inotrope No increase in myocardial oxygen demand Vasodilation of venous capacitance and arterial resistance vessels

29

a general review of the existing agents. It is essential to perform an echocardiogram to assess ventricular function and rule out other factors, for example, pericardial effusion, that may affect the function.

Another non-classic inotrope in the treatment of LCOS is the calcium ion (Ca^{2+}). Calcium is essential for myocardial contraction. Myocardial contraction begins with an increase in cytoplasmic calcium concentration. The Ca^{2+} binds to the troponin C, enabling the sliding of the actin and myosin that will result in myocardium cell shortening and an increase in systolic pressure with forwarding ejection of blood. The amount of Ca^{2+} bound to the troponin C will determine the force created in the ventricle. Furthermore, the neonatal heart is known to be sensitive to changes in the serum Ca^{2+} levels since the sarcoplasmic reticulum is not fully developed and has limited storage capacity [24]. Therefore, maintaining adequate levels of ionised calcium is vital, especially in neonates and intravenous Ca^{2+} administration can be used to increase myocardial contractility. There are reports that Ca^{2+} administration in the paediatric CICU population with LCOS improves haemodynamics regardless of the baseline Ca^{2+} level [5, 24, 25].

After cardiac surgery, changes in ventricular relaxation may reduce ventricular compliance resulting in diastolic dysfunction. Patients with "restrictive physiology"—when there is preoperative hypertrophy of the ventricle that is aggravated by postoperative myocardial oedema—are more prone to develop diastolic dysfunction. Diastolic dysfunction is common in patients with tetralogy of Fallot, whose ventricular cavity volume is small, and the stroke volume may be compromised. Managing this can be challenging as inotropic agents may decrease the ventricular volume further, and the chronotropic effect can also decrease the ventricular filling time. On the other hand, using ß Adrenergic antagonists and calcium channel blockers may cause myocardial depression and decrease arterial blood pressure. Therapeutic strategies should avoid tachycardia to optimise the diastolic ventricular filling time and reduce the myocardial oxygen demands. A combination of low-dose inotropic agents with the administration of small aliquots of fluids to increase the intravascular volume can improve ventricular capacity and diastolic function. The second line of treatment can be using vasodilators to alter the ventricular afterload and improve stroke volume [26]. Use of vasodilators increases the capacity of the vascular bed, and therefore fluid replacement should be given simultaneously.

A few considerations of note:

- The left ventricular function can be ascertained more easily than the right ventricular function
- Assessing LV function can be problematic in the context of a large VSD patch or when temporary pacing is in use

29.2.5.3 Manipulating Afterload

Vasodilators

The nadir in cardiac output seen in the postoperative period is accompanied by an increase in systemic SVR and PVR from baseline values, resulting in increased ventricular afterload [4, 6]. Therapy aimed to reduce the afterload can improve cardiac output, which becomes more significant when there is systolic dysfunction. Management may be targeted to reduce SVR, PVR or both dependent on anatomical substrate, baseline pathology and postoperative physiology.

SVR Reduction

Systemic vasodilators offer afterload reduction and improve ventriculoarterial coupling [27]. Phosphodiesterase (PDE) type 3 inhibitors, like milrinone, inhibit the breakdown of cyclic adenosine monophosphate (cAMP) and its accumulation in vascular smooth muscle cells, thus resulting in vasodilation and improved myocyte contractility. Hence, these agents can provide PVR and SVR reduction as well as inotropic support. They also have less effect on heart rate and are less arrhythmogenic than catecholamines. Hence, milrinone is more frequently used to treat LCOS [11, 14, 28]. Other vasodilators are nitric oxide (NO) donors, nitroprusside and nitroglycerin, which work via cyclic guanyl monophosphate (cGMP) pathway to release NO from vascular endothelium, resulting in vascular smooth muscle cell relaxation. Nitroprusside is a short-acting but potent vasodilator that affects venous capacitance and arterial resistance vessels. Nitroglycerin vasodilates venous capacitance vessels when used in low doses and vasodilates arterial resistance vessels in higher doses. Both agents are in use in the treatment of LCOS in various indications.

29

A few considerations of note

- Important to consider whether additional afterload reduction would be more helpful than increased inotropy
- Important to bear in mind that vasodilatation in the context of hypovolaemia may be detrimental
- As the capacity of the vascular bed increases after vasodilatation, simultaneous volume replacement may be indicated

PVR Reduction

Pulmonary hypertension (PH) is one of the many factors that may contribute to the development of LCOS. When there is a fall in cardiac output, even a mild increase in pulmonary pressures will significantly reduce the right ventricle cardiac output, which may not be tolerable. Therefore, pharmacological manipulation of the PVR is frequently required using agents such as inhaled NO (iNO), sildenafil and rarely prostacyclin. iNO is a selective pulmonary vasodilator that decreases PVR with minimal effect on SVR. Sildenafil, a PDE type 5 inhibitor, enhances NO-mediated pulmonary vasodilatation through the cGMP pathway and is also used for this purpose. Prostacyclin is a metabolite of arachidonic acid via cyclo-oxygenase synthesis and is a potent vasodilator and inhibitor of platelet activation. Limited by its effect on systemic vasodilation, prostacyclin is not usually used to address PH in the setting of LCOS, and its use is preserved for cases not responsive to iNO. In a systematic review, Avila-Alvarez et al. [29] reported several reports supporting the use of these agents in LCOS treatment, but further research is needed to provide strong evidence of its safety and efficacy.

A few considerations of note:

- iNO causes a reduction in RV afterload.
- iNO should be used with caution in patients with severe left ventricular dysfunction.
- Withdrawal of iNO may result in rebound pulmonary hypertension.

29.2.6 Vasoconstrictors

Some patients presented with LCOS may experience changes in the vasomotor response after cardiac surgery. Vasoplegia syndrome is characterised as a pathological fall in vascular tone, increased venous capacity and low SVR, resulting in significant hypotension and reduced perfusion to vital organs. Vasoconstrictors are used to restore the impaired vascular tone. Vasopressin is a hormone synthesised in the hypothalamus. It acts as a potent vasoconstrictor by activating the arginine vasopressin receptor 1A (AVPR1A) in the arterioles, which causes activation of protein kinase C to cause vasoconstriction. It has been used in the setting of septic shock after demonstrating low vasopressin levels in adults [30]. It has been employed for children following cardiac surgery with favourable results of a decrease in fluids and catecholamines requirements [31, 32]. Increasing SVR could also cause a fall in cardiac output due to an increase in the ventricular afterload, especially in situations of impaired systolic function.

Noradrenaline is also a potent vasoconstrictor which has an inotropic effect. See Table 29.3 for details.

In single ventricle physiology, in the presence of complete mixing, LCOS can result from an imbalance of systemic and pulmonary flow. Therefore, a specific therapeutic approach directed to increase the systemic flow and provide adequate cardiac output is necessary.

29.2.6.1 The Role of Positive Pressure Ventilation (PPV)

Most patients with LCOS will still be ventilated at the time of identification. However, PPV influences cardiac output, and this cardiopulmonary interaction can be used as part of the treatment of LCOS. The heart is located inside the thoracic cavity and is subjected to intrathoracic pressure's effects. PPV increases the intrathoracic pressure, thus decreasing the transmural pressure of the systemic ventricle and reducing the systemic ventricular afterload. This reduction is especially significant in patients with systemic ventricular systolic dysfunction. Therefore, alterations of the Positive End-Expiratory Pressure may improve cardiac output in the failing systemic heart by lowering the transmural pressure [33]. Another advantage of mechanical ventilation is the decrease in the patient's work of breathing and reduction in the respiratory muscles' blood perfusion, which reduces the tissue oxygen demands [34].

29.2.6.2 The Role of Corticosteroids

The use of corticosteroids to prevent LCOS in managing children undergoing cardiac surgery remains debatable. Studies showed conflicting results ranging from association with better outcomes to a possible harmful effect [35]. In practice, Flores et al. [36] reported a large variability regarding the use of corticosteroids in an international survey. The rationale for using corticosteroids is based on the role of corticosteroids in cardiovascular tone, fluid distribution and vascular permeability, as well as their anti-inflammatory effect of attenuating the systemic inflammatory response incited by cardiopulmonary bypass. However, despite a few reports showing an improvement in haemodynamics and inflammatory markers [37–39], no study has demonstrated an improvement in actual outcomes. Moreover, an association with increased morbidity, particularly in lower-surgical risk groups, was also reported [37]. Hydrocortisone is reported to be the most used agent to treat LCOS. There is also variability regarding the dosage to be used, with regiments of 50 mg/m^2/day, 100 mg/m^2/day, 2 mg/kg/day, and 1 mg/kg/day being used in different centres. In summary, according to the evidence available, postoperative corticosteroids should be used selectively for patients with refractory LCOS and not preemptively.

29.2.6.3 Mechanical Circulatory Support (MCS)

When maximal medical therapy fails to achieve adequate cardiac output and any residual anatomical lesions have been ruled out, MCS should be considered. Patients may be placed onto Veno-Arterial Extracorporeal life support (V-A ECLS) via central cannulation (to the right atrium and aorta) or neck cannulation (to the right carotid artery and right internal jugular vein). Refractory LCOS is one of the most common indications for MCS after a cardiac operation and accounts for 36% of cases [40–42]. Outcomes were strongly associated with the patient's condition at the time of cannulation; hence it should be aimed to be initiated before established organ injury occurs [40]. Mortality rates of patients on ECLS post-cardiac operation are high, and rates of 29–61% have been reported [42–44]. Risk factors for mortality were duration of ECLS support, peak serum lactate level on the first day after initiation of ECLS, renal failure required renal replacement therapy, sepsis, and high volumes of blood products transfusions needed [41–43]. Treatment of LCOS is illustrated in ◘ Fig. 29.2.

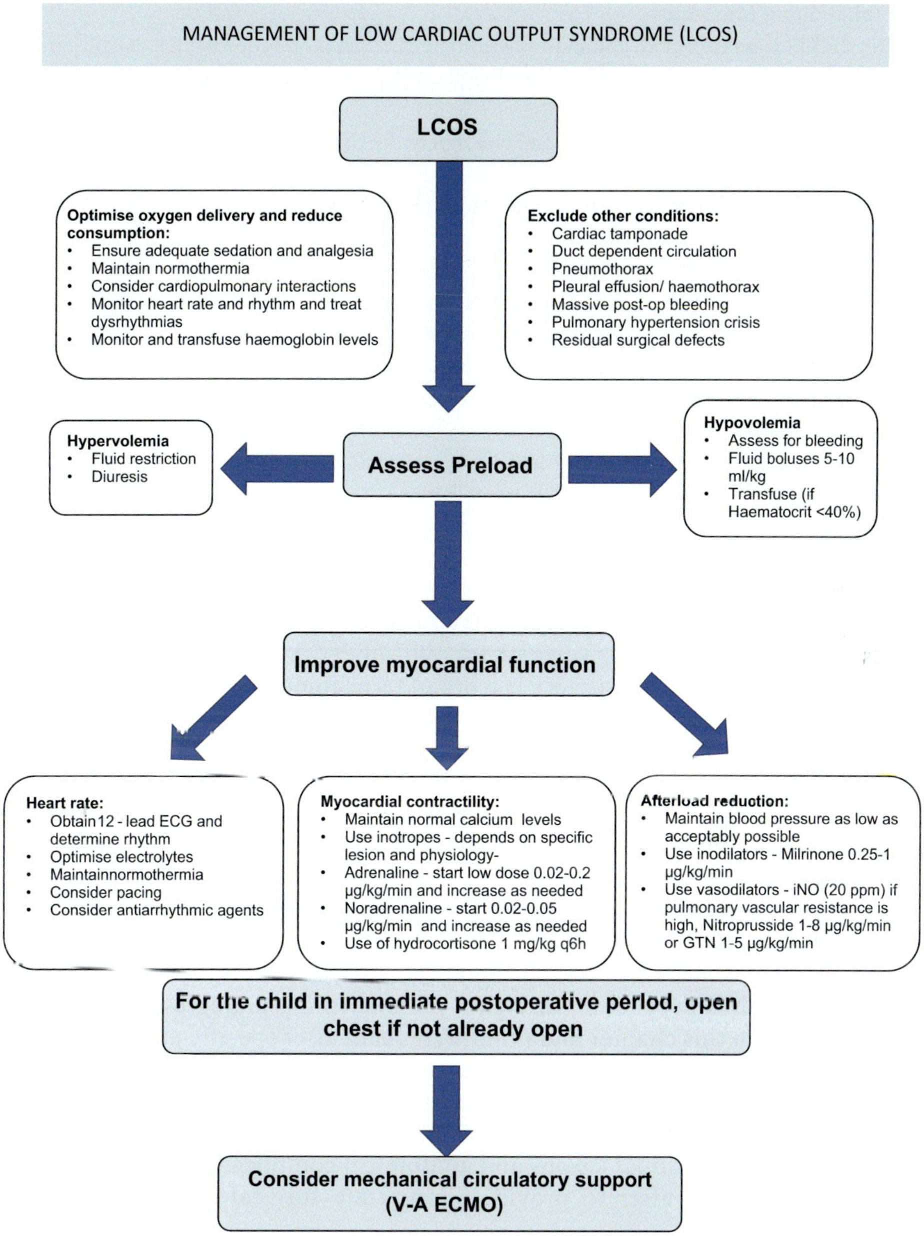

Fig. 29.2 Comprehensive Management Approach for Low Cardiac Output Syndrome (LCOS) in Pediatric Patients: A structured flowchart outlining the management of Low Cardiac Output Syndrome (LCOS), focusing on optimizing oxygen delivery, assessing preload, and improving myocardial function. It also outlines postoperative care with key interventions such as fluid management, myocardial contractility support with inotropes, heart rate optimization, afterload reduction strategies, and the potential need for mechanical circulatory support (V-A ECMO) in severe cases

Take-Home Messages

- LCOS is an expected, common physiologic phenomenon following paediatric cardiac surgery that requires close and vigilant bedside monitoring with timely intervention.
- A physician caring for infants and children in the CICU should be familiar with the syndrome and its management.
- Therapeutic strategies aim to improve the balance between oxygen demands and oxygen supply.
- Maximising cardiac output and improving end-organ perfusion and oxygen capacity may be achieved using inotropes, corticosteroids, lusiotropes, vasodilators, afterload-reducing agents, and appropriate mechanical ventilation.
- Residual surgical lesions that can impair cardiac function and will not necessarily respond to medical treatment must be diagnosed and addressed.
- Mechanical circulatory support should be considered when medical therapeutic measures fail to ensure end-organ perfusion while allowing for myocardial recovery.

29.3 Lesion-Specific Postoperative Management

Cardiac congenital defect surgery is a broad term composed of a wide spectrum of pathologies presenting various physiological patterns, clinical features and sequelae. There are many considerations when caring for children undergoing interventions for congenital defects. Identifying the lesion and the child's physiology, alongside the familiarity with the surgery performed, would be crucial in delivering the appropriate management in the CICU. ◘ Table 29.4 provides a schematic view of the different lesions and complications anticipated post-op. For example, children with acyanotic lesions with increased pulmonary circulation are prone to have pulmonary hypertension that might need treatment. Cyanotic lesions with RVH can be complicated with diastolic dysfunction and a ventricle, which is dependent on higher preload filling pressures. LCOS is discussed earlier in this chapter and is more frequent after specific procedures such as post-arterial switch operation for transposition of the great arteries, post-Aorto-Pulmonary window repair and post-total anomalous pulmonary venous drainage repair. Arrhythmias can result from direct injury by sutures or automaticity activity. Residual lesions and anatomical complications should be considered and sought after to provide appropriate surgical management when needed.

Table 29.4 Lesion-specific postoperative management of children and infants after cardiac surgery

Pathophysiology	Defect	LCOS	Common postoperative considerations	Longer-term complications
Acyanotic lesions increased pulmonary circulation	Patent ductus arteriosus	Off-pump, usually no LCOS	Diuresis for pulmonary congestion Early extubation	Stent migration Pulmonary arteries stenosis Pneumothorax
	Aorto-Pulmonary window	Yes	Diuresis for pulmonary congestion Pulmonary HTN	
	Atrial septal defect	Older patients may have LCOS	Atrial/junctional arrhythmias (not frequent) Early extubation	Postcardiotomy syndrome Occlusion of PV or SVC
	Ventricular septal defect	Yes	Diuresis for pulmonary congestion Early extubation Pulmonary hypertension Arrhythmias—JET/AVB May have AR and MR	Residual AVV and AV regurgitation
	Atrioventricular septal defect	Yes	Pulmonary HTN Arrhythmias—JET and AVB May have AVVR	Atrio ventricular valve regurgitation
	Truncus Arteriusus	LCOS—frequent, mainly RV dysfunction. May have LV dysfunction d/t coronary ischaemia. Delayed chest closure is common	Significant Pulmonary HTN Arrhythmias—JET and AVB Anatomical complications—Truncal valve insufficiency, pulmonary arteries malformations, conduit malfunction	

(continued)

Table 29.4 (continued)

Pathophysiology	Defect	LCOS	Common postoperative considerations	Longer-term complications
Acyanotic lesions normal pulmonary circulation	Aortic Stenosis	LCOS d/t LVH	Treat HTN—maintain BP as low as sufficient Arrhythmias—LBBB, AVB MR Residual MS	Anticoagulation for mechanical valve Coronary insufficiency MR
	Coarctation of Aorta		Treat HTN—maintain BP as low as sufficient Residual VSD, CoA Post coarcectomy syndrome: • intestinal ischaemia • intractable HTN Monitor Injury to adjacent structures- • Thoracic duct injury → chylothorax • Recurrent laryngeal nerve injury → vocal cord palsy • Phrenic nerve injury → diaphragm palsy • Spinal cord ischaemia → acute paraplegia	Vocal cords palsy Diaphragm palsy Necrotising Enterocolitis
	Interrupted Aortic arch	Yes	Pulmonary HTN in some cases Arrhythmias-AVB common Anatomical complications—Residual CoA, LVOTO, bronchial/LPA obstruction	Vocal cords palsy Diaphragm palsy Hypocalcaemia
	Mitral Valve Stenosis	May have LCOS (if preop MR) Ensure sufficient LV preload and LAP in early-stage then diuresis	Pulmonary HTN Arrhythmias—Atrial and AVB May need prolonged ventilation	Anticoagulation for mechanical valves
	Cor triatriatum	Yes	Pulmonary HTN Atrial Arrhythmias	

Cyanotic lesions	Pulmonic stenosis	LCOS—RV Dysfunction can be severe with Suicide RV—severe RV dysfunction d/t sub valvar obstruction with muscular bundles that become significant after the major stenosis resolved	Avoid hypovolemia, keep adequate preload AT JET VT d/t VSD closure and RT myectomies Residual PI/PS	Cyanosis d/t non-compliant RV with Rt to Lt shunt
	Tetralogy of Fallot (TOF)	LCOS—RV diastolic dysfunction. Maintain RV preload to ensure good CO, but after stabilisation, start gentle diuresis	Arrhythmias—JET, AVB Residual RVOTO Residual VSD	
	TOF/pulmonary atresia	Yes RV Dysfunction-requires high CVP fluids, Avoid tachycardia	Pulmonary HTN Arrhythmias—JET AVB Extubation as soon as possible for afterload reduction of the RV	
	TOF/Absent Pulmonic Valve	RV Dysfunction and diastolic dysfunction needs high CVPs May require delayed sternal closure	May need delayed sternal closure for cardiac and due to bronchomalacia	PI RV Dilation d/t PI bronchomalacia
	Pulmonary atresia/intact ventricular septum	RV dysfunction d/t ventriculostomy	Depends on the pathway taken—two/single ventricles. Cyanosis d/t RV dys, atrial Rt → Lt If RV Dependent Coronary Circulation—monitor for arrhythmias	Coronaries insufficiency Circular shunt
	Ebstein's Anomaly	Yes	Pulmonary HTN—Maintain well-sedated and adequate analgesia May require prolonged diuresis Lung hypoplasia/malacia requires good ventilatory volumes Extubation as soon as possible for afterload reduction of the RV, though, may be challenging given respiratory dysfunction Frequent arrhythmias—atrial and ventricular	Airway malacia
	Total anomalous pulmonary venous drainage	In non-obstructed cases—early extubation, LCOS is rare. In obstructed cases—LCOS is common and may require delayed sternal closure and ECMO support	Pulmonary HTN Arrhythmias—supraventricular Residual venous obstruction	
	Transposition of great arteries	LCOS d/t deconditioning	Try to avoid arterial HTN to reduce bleeding Pulmonary HTN Arrhythmias d/t coronaries insufficiency	Coronary insufficiency

(continued)

Table 29.4 (continued)

Pathophysiology	Defect	LCOS	Common postoperative considerations	Longer-term complications
Single Ventricle	Pulmonary artery banding		Maintain a balance of Qp/Qs May have Pul THN if the band is too tight or cyanosis if the band is too loose	Migration of the band to the main PA
	Aorto—Pulmonary Shunts		Maintain a balance of Qp/Qs Monitor flow in shunts	Shunt obstruction/thrombosis Necrotising Entero colitis
	Norwood	Yes Employ Cardiac assessment with echo/cath to demonstrate anatomic complications	Maintain a balance of Qp/Qs Treat arrhythmias early as not tolerated Look for Aortic obstruction, Shunt obstruction/thrombosis Watch for NEC	Shunt obstruction/thrombosis Aortic obstruction/stenosis
	Hybrid		Preop physiology not changed Maintain Qp/Qs May have Pulmonary HTN if the band is too tight or cyanosis if the band is too loose	PDA obstruction, stent migration PA Bands too loose/tight Restrictive VSD
Cavo-pulmonary connections	Glenn		Treat HTN—good analgesia and sedation, Maintain head in elevated mid-position. Monitor Transpulmonary Pressure CVP-Common AP) and treat it accordingly Early extubation is recommended Drainage of pleural effusions, improve lung volume Treat arrhythmias early as not well tolerated Avoid thrombosis—take out CVL ASAP	Anticoagulation treatment SVC Syndrome Monitor the Transpulmonary Pressure (CVP-Common Atrial pressure)
	Fontan	LCOS with high PA and LA pressure suggest ventricular dysfunction, severe Atrioventricular regurgitation, or systemic outflow obstruction	Monitor Transpulmonary Pressure CVP-Common AP) and treat it accordingly Systolic impairment is not common; Diastolic impairment can happen and will need volume Treat arrhythmias early as not well tolerated If cyanosis persists—look for collaterals Early extubation is recommended Drainage of pleural effusions, improve lung volume	Ascites Chylothorax Protein-losing enteropathy Hypercoagulability anticoagulation

Myocardial ischaemia	Abbarent origin of the left coronary artery from the pulmonary artery	LCOS can be severe and may need ECMO/VAD Avoid excessive volume administrations and catecholamines May requires prolonged ventilation d/t cardiac dysfunction	Ventricular arrhythmias Coronaries spasm May need nitroglycerine to maintain coronary perfusion	Coronaries spasm MR
Airway and oesophagus stenosis	Vascular rings	LCOS may occur as post CPB effect unless done off-pump	Usually early extubation Will require O_2 Airway Malacia—Stridor	Diaphragm palsy Chylothorax d/t thoracic duct injury Airway malacia
Broad-spectrum from a-cyanotic with increased pulmonary circulation to single ventricle	Double outlet right ventricle	Depends on specific lesions	Depends on specific lesions—If preop increased pulmonary circulation: pulmonary HTN is common Look for residual lesions—VSD Obstruction/stenosis of large arteries Arrhythmias—AVB	

Box 29.1

The Prophylactic intravenous use of milrinone after cardiac operation in paediatrics (PRIMACORP) study was a multicentre, randomised, double-blind, placebo-controlled trial with three parallel treatment groups (low-dose milrinone; high-dose milrinone; placebo) of paediatric patients undergoing cardiac surgery ($N = 238$). The primary endpoint was a composite of death or the development of LCOS requiring treatment during 36 h of drug administration. As no patients died during the study drug administration, the primary endpoint was only the occurrence of LCOS, which required treatment. The use of high-dose milrinone significantly reduced the risk of LCOS compared with that of placebo (relative risk reduction of 55% $P = 0.023$), with a statistically insignificant beneficial trend in the low-dose milrinone group. Furthermore, at the follow-up visit (up to 30 days after randomisation), there was a significant risk reduction in the composite endpoint (death or the development of LCOS) in the high-dose milrinone group of 48% ($P = 0.049$) [21].

There are several limitations to the study: the 'patients' population included only patients who underwent biventricular repair; the diagnosis of LCOS was at the clinician's discretion; there was no formal CO measurement; patients who received milrinone in the operating room were excluded from the study. Hence, the patients at the highest risk might have been excluded, creating a selection bias.

Box 29.2 Oxygen Variables Calculations

$$\textit{Oxygen content}: \mathrm{CaO_2} = \left(\mathrm{SaO_2} \times \mathrm{Hb} \times 1.34^{*}\right) + \left(0.003 \times \mathrm{PaO_2}\right) \text{ normal range} = 17 - 20\ \mathrm{ml/dl}$$

$$\textit{Oxygen delivery}: \mathrm{DO_2} = \mathrm{CaO_2} \times \mathrm{CO} \text{ normal range} = 570 - 670\ \mathrm{ml/min/m^2}$$

$$\textit{Oxygen consumption}: \mathrm{VO_2} = \mathrm{DO_2} \times \mathrm{O_2ER} = \mathrm{CO} \times \left(\mathrm{CaO_2} - \mathrm{CvO_2}\right) \text{ normal range} = 120 - 200\ \mathrm{ml/min/m^2}$$

O_2 oxygen, *SaO_2* O_2 arterial saturation, *Hb* Haemoglobin, *PaO_2* O_2 arterial partial pressure, *CO* cardiac output, *O_2ER* O_2 extraction rate, CvO_2 = mixed venous blood oxygen content; CaO_2 = arterial blood oxygen content

*Differ in different measurements due to the number of different forms of haemoglobin

References

1. van der Bom T, Zomer AC, Zwinderman AH, Meijboom FJ, Bouma BJ, Mulder BJM. The changing epidemiology of congenital heart disease. Nat Rev Cardiol. 2011;8(1):50–60.
2. Checchia PA, Brown KL, Wernovsky G, Penny DJ, Bronicki RA. The evolution of pediatric cardiac critical care. Crit Care Med. 2021;49(4):545–57.
3. Horak RV, Alexander PM, Amirnovin R, Klein MJ, Bronicki RA, Markovitz BP, et al. Pediatric cardiac intensive care distribution, service delivery, and staffing in the United States in 2018. Pediatr Crit care Med a J Soc Crit Care Med World Fed Pediatr Intensive Crit Care Soc. 2020;21(9):797–803.

4. Wernovsky G, Wypij D, Jonas RA, Mayer JEJ, Hanley FL, Hickey PR, et al. Postoperative course and hemodynamic profile after the arterial switch operation in neonates and infants. A comparison of low-flow cardiopulmonary bypass and circulatory arrest. Circulation. 1995;92(8):2226–35.
5. Chandler HK, Kirsch R. Management of the low cardiac output syndrome following surgery for congenital heart disease. Curr Cardiol Rev. 2016;12(2):107–11.
6. Parr GV, Blackstone EH, Kirklin JW. Cardiac performance and mortality early after intracardiac surgery in infants and young children. Circulation. 1975;51(5):867–74.
7. Du X, Chen H, Song X, Wang S, Hao Z, Yin L, et al. Risk factors for low cardiac output syndrome in children with congenital heart disease undergoing cardiac surgery: a retrospective cohort study. BMC Pediatr. 2020;20(1):87.
8. Ungerleider RM, Meliones JN, McMillan KN, Cooper DSJJ. Critical heart disease in infants and children. 3rd ed. Elsevier; 2019. 933 p
9. Pérez-Navero JL, Merino-Cejas C, Ibarra de la Rosa I, Jaraba-Caballero S, Frias-Perez M, Gómez-Guzmán E, et al. Evaluation of the vasoactive-inotropic score, mid-regional pro-adrenomedullin and cardiac troponin I as predictors of low cardiac output syndrome in children after congenital heart disease surgery. Med Intensiva. 2019;43(6):329–36.
10. Pérez-Navero JL, de la Torre-Aguilar MJ, Ibarra de la Rosa I, Gil-Campos M, Gómez-Guzmán E, Merino-Cejas C, et al. Cardiac biomarkers of low cardiac output syndrome in the postoperative period after congenital heart disease surgery in children. Rev Esp Cardiol (Engl Ed). 2017;70(4):267–74.
11. Ulate KP, Yanay O, Jeffries H, Baden H, Di Gennaro JL, Zimmerman J. An elevated low cardiac output syndrome score is associated with morbidity in infants after congenital heart surgery. Pediatr Crit Care Med a J Soc Crit Care Med World Fed Pediatr Intensive Crit Care Soc. 2017;18(1):26–33.
12. Rogers L, Ray S, Johnson M, Feinstein Y, Dominguez TE, Peters MJ, et al. The inadequate oxygen delivery index and low cardiac output syndrome score as predictors of adverse events associated with low cardiac output syndrome early after cardiac bypass. Pediatr Crit care Med A J Soc Crit Care Med World Fed Pediatr Intensive Crit Care Soc. 2019;20(8):737–43.
13. Hoffman TM, Wernovsky G, Atz AM, Kulik TJ, Nelson DP, Chang AC, et al. Efficacy and safety of milrinone in preventing low cardiac output syndrome in infants and children after corrective surgery for congenital heart disease. Circulation. 2003;107(7):996–1002.
14. Roeleveld PP, de Klerk JCA. The perspective of the intensivist on inotropes and postoperative care following pediatric heart surgery: an international survey and systematic review of the literature. World J Pediatr Congenit Heart Surg. 2018;9(1):10–21.
15. Tibby SM, Hatherill M, Marsh MJ, Murdoch IA. 'Clinicians' abilities to estimate cardiac index in ventilated children and infants. Arch Dis Child. 1997;77(6):516–8.
16. Gaies MG, Jeffries HE, Niebler RA, Pasquali SK, Donohue JE, Yu S, et al. Vasoactive-inotropic score is associated with outcome after infant cardiac surgery: an analysis from the Pediatric Cardiac Critical Care Consortium and Virtual PICU System Registries. Pediatr Crit care Med a J Soc Crit Care Med World Fed Pediatr Intensive Crit Care Soc. 2014;15(6):529–37.
17. Gaies MG, Gurney JG, Yen AH, Napoli ML, Gajarski RJ, Ohye RG, et al. Vasoactive-inotropic score as a predictor of morbidity and mortality in infants after cardiopulmonary bypass. Pediatr Crit care Med a J Soc Crit Care Med World Fed Pediatr Intensive Crit Care Soc. 2010;11(2):234–8.
18. Phelps HM, Mahle WT, Kim D, Simsic JM, Kirshbom PM, Kanter KR, et al. Postoperative cerebral oxygenation in hypoplastic left heart syndrome after the Norwood procedure. Ann Thorac Surg. 2009;87(5):1490–4.
19. Yu P, Esangbedo I, Li X, Wolovits J, Thiagarajan R, Raman L. Early changes in near-infrared spectroscopy are associated with cardiac arrest in children with congenital heart disease. Front Pediatr. 2022;10:894125.
20. Lobos A-T, Lee S, Menon K. Capillary refill time and cardiac output in children undergoing cardiac catheterisation. Pediatr Crit care Med a J Soc Crit Care Med World Fed Pediatr Intensive Crit Care Soc. 2012;13(2):136–40.
21. Hoffman TM, Wernovsky G, Atz AM, Bailey JM, Akbary A, Kocsis JF, et al. Prophylactic intravenous use of milrinone after cardiac operation in pediatrics (PRIMACORP) study. Prophylactic intravenous use of milrinone after cardiac operation in pediatrics. Am Heart J. 2002;143(1):15–21.
22. Beu B, Rücker G, Stiller B. Prophylactic milrinone for the prevention of LCOS and mortality in paediatric patients undergoing surgery for CHD. Cochrane Database Syst Rev. 2015;2015(3):CD009515.

23. Hummel J, Rücker G, Stiller B. Prophylactic levosimendan for the prevention of low cardiac output syndrome and mortality in paediatric patients undergoing surgery for congenital heart disease. Cochrane Database Syst Rev. 2017;8(8):CD011312.
24. Tume SC, Goldberg J, Molossi S, Bronicki RA. Pharmacologic approach to heart failure in children. Curr Cardiol Rev. 2016;12(2):117–20.
25. Averin K, Villa C, Krawczeski CD, Pratt J, King E, Jefferies JL, et al. Initial observations of the effects of calcium chloride infusions in pediatric patients with low cardiac output. Pediatr Cardiol. 2016;37(3):610–7.
26. Friedman WF, George BL. Treatment of congestive heart failure by altering loading conditions of the heart. J Pediatr. 1985;106(5):697–706.
27. Mills KI, Costello JM, Almodovar MC. A review of systemic vasodilators in low cardiac output syndrome following pediatric cardiac surgery. Curr Vasc Pharmacol. 2016;14(1):29–36.
28. Wright EM, Skoyles J, Sherry KM. Milrinone in the treatment of low output states following cardiac surgery. Eur J Anaesthesiol Suppl. 1992;5:21–6.
29. Avila-Alvarez A, Del Cerro Marin MJ, Bautista-Hernandez V. Pulmonary vasodilators in the management of low cardiac output syndrome after pediatric cardiac surgery. Curr Vasc Pharmacol. 2016;14(1):37–47.
30. Landry DW, Oliver JA. The pathogenesis of vasodilatory shock. N Engl J Med. 2001;345(8):588–95.
31. Mastropietro CW, Davalos MC, Seshadri S, Walters HL 3rd, Delius RE. Clinical response to arginine vasopressin therapy after paediatric cardiac surgery. Cardiol Young. 2013;23(3):387–93.
32. Alten JA, Borasino S, Toms R, Law MA, Moellinger A, Dabal RJ. Early initiation of arginine vasopressin infusion in neonates after complex cardiac surgery. Pediatr Crit care Med a J Soc Crit Care Med World Fed Pediatr Intensive Crit Care Soc. 2012;13(3):300–4.
33. Mitaka C, Nagura T, Sakanishi N, Tsunoda Y, Amaha K. Two-dimensional echocardiographic evaluation of inferior vena cava, right ventricle, and left ventricle during positive-pressure ventilation with varying levels of positive end-expiratory pressure. Crit Care Med. 1989;17(3):205–10.
34. Hussain SN, Roussos C. Distribution of respiratory muscle and organ blood flow during endotoxic shock in dogs. J Appl Physiol. 1985;59(6):1802–8.
35. Amirnovin R, Markovitz B. A tale of two controversies: low cardiac output syndrome and corticosteroids. Pediatr Crit Care Med. 2017;18:719–20.
36. Flores S, FitzGerald MR, Iliopoulos I, Daily JA, Rodriguez M, Nelson DP, et al. An international survey of corticosteroid use for the management of low cardiac output syndrome. Pediatr Crit care Med a J Soc Crit Care Med World Fed Pediatr Intensive Crit Care Soc. 2017;18(7):630–7.
37. Graham EM. The role of prophylactic postoperative steroids in pediatric cardiac operations. Pediatr Crit Care Med. 2015;16:676–7.
38. Graham EM, Martin RH, Buckley JR, Zyblewski SC, Kavarana MN, Bradley SM, et al. Corticosteroid therapy in neonates undergoing cardiopulmonary bypass: randomized controlled trial. J Am Coll Cardiol. 2019;74(5):659–68.
39. Robert SM, Borasino S, Dabal RJ, Cleveland DC, Hock KM, Alten JA. Postoperative hydrocortisone infusion reduces the prevalence of low cardiac output syndrome after neonatal cardiopulmonary bypass. Pediatr Crit Care Med a J Soc Crit Care Med World Fed Pediatr Intensive Crit Care Soc. 2015;16(7):629–36.
40. Joffe AR, Lequier L, Robertson CMT. Pediatric outcomes after extracorporeal membrane oxygenation for cardiac disease and for cardiac arrest: a review. ASAIO J. 2012;58(4):297–310.
41. Chai PJ, Jacobs JP, Dalton HJ, Costello JM, Cooper DS, Kirsch R, et al. Extracorporeal cardiopulmonary resuscitation for post-operative cardiac arrest: indications, techniques, controversies, and early results--what is known (and unknown). Cardiol Young. 2011;21(Suppl. 2):109–17.
42. Kumar TKS, Zurakowski D, Dalton H, Talwar S, Allard-Picou A, Duebener LF, et al. Extracorporeal membrane oxygenation in postcardiotomy patients: factors influencing outcome. J Thorac Cardiovasc Surg. 2010;140(2):330–6.
43. Hoskote A, Bohn D, Gruenwald C, Edgell D, Cai S, Adatia I, et al. Extracorporeal life support after staged palliation of a functional single ventricle: subsequent morbidity and survival. J Thorac Cardiovasc Surg. 2006;131(5):1114–21.
44. Walters HL 3rd, Hakimi M, Rice MD, Lyons JM, Whittlesey GC, Klein MD. Pediatric cardiac surgical ECMO: multivariate analysis of risk factors for hospital death. Ann Thorac Surg. 1995;60(2):327–9.

ECMO in Children with Cardiac Failure

Susana Abreu and Uri Pollak

Contents

J. Brierley et al. (eds.), *ESPNIC Children's Intensive Care Textbook*,
https://doi.org/10.1007/978-3-031-64762-8_30

Learning Objectives
To Understand
- History of cardiac ECMO in children.
- Description and indications for cardiac ECMO in children.
- Cannulation process and the ECMO circuit.
- How to manage and monitor a patient on ECMO.
- Troubleshooting on ECMO.
- Weaning process.
- Cardiac ECMO outcomes and survival.
- The future of cardiac ECMO support.

30.1 History of Cardiac ECMO

The first heart-lung machine used for extracorporeal support in humans was developed by Dr. JH Gibbon and was used for the first time in the operating room in 1953 to assist in the repair of an atrial septal defect in an 18-year-old patient [1, 2]. Improvements in circuitry, particularly, oxygenators, and the use of anticoagulation allowed application for cardiac surgery in infants for the first time in 1970 [3].

These successful results prompted the use of extracorporeal support outside the operating room with Dr. JD Hill in 1972 reporting the first cannulation and prolonged use in the intensive care unit (ICU) setting [4].

The use of ECMO has expanded progressively across the world, and so have the indications for its use over the years. The development of a standardized international patient database to track results greatly contributed to improvement in care and outcomes. This database transitioned into the ELSO Registry, which is now the largest repository of extracorporeal support data in the world producing annual reports on ECMO outcomes ► https://www.elso.org/.

From a total of nearly 200,000 ECMO runs registered, approximately 85,000 are pediatric or neonatal [5]. While pulmonary ECMO is the predominant subgroup in neonates, in the pediatric group, it is the cardiac ECMO [5]. However, the trend over the years has been a decline in the number of respiratory ECMOs in neonates due to the advances in conventional therapies. In contrast, there has been a notable increase in the number of cardiac ECMOs in children, especially in neonates, reflecting the advances in complex neonatal cardiac surgery.

30.2 Cardiac ECMO: Description and Indications

Veno-arterial (V-A) ECMO is a type of mechanical circulatory support (MCS) in which a membrane oxygenator is incorporated into the circuit, providing not only forward systemic flow but also oxygenation of the blood. The venous systemic blood is drained from the body, propelled by the pump into a membrane oxygenator where it is oxygenated, and then returned to the systemic arterial vasculature (◘ Fig. 30.1). Hence, V-A ECMO provides full cardiac and respiratory support. A great proportion of cardiac ECMO in children is noted to be needed after cardiac surgery for congenital heart disease (nearly 50% in neonates and around 30% in the pediatric group)

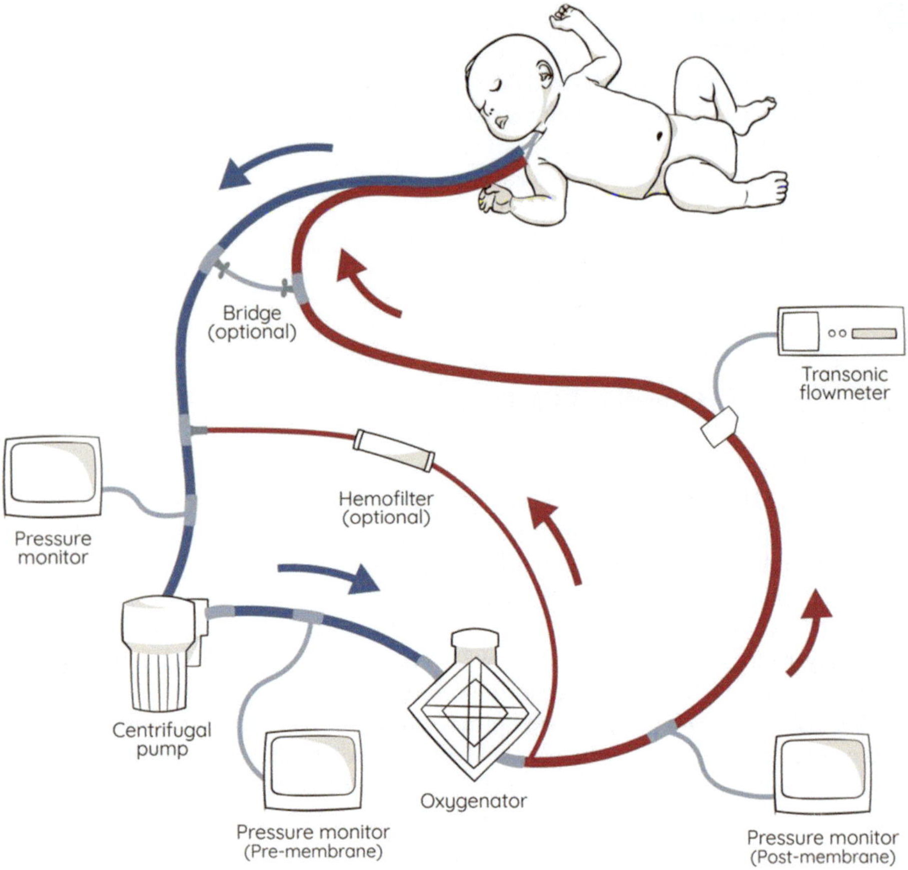

Fig. 30.1 Example of a veno-arterial ECMO circuit

[5]. ECMO should be considered for children with evidence of inadequate end-organ perfusion and oxygen delivery resulting from the inadequate native cardiac output as evidenced by hypotension, persistent oliguria and diminished pulses, persistent low mixed venous saturation (<60%) and lactic acidosis despite optimal medical management [6].

The indications for cardiac ECMO and the specifications for each indication are described in Table 30.1.

Table 30.1 Indications for cardiac ECMO

Indications for ECMO	Aim	Incidence	Comments
Preoperative stabilization	To optimize oxygen delivery, minimize end-organ failure before surgery	Rare. Most patients can be stabilized medically before surgery [7]	Can be challenging in uncorrected CHD (e.g. HLHS)
Post-cardiotomy	To ensure myocardial recovery, time to exclude residual lesions	Incidence up to 6% [8] Post-Norwood procedure—17% [8]	Bleeding, if SV physiology—careful shunt management
ECPR	To provide cardio-pulmonary support when conventional CPR fails to achieve ROSC or within 20 min after ROSC	18% and 5% of all pediatric and neonatal ECMO cannulations [5] More frequent in post-cardiotomy patients (59% of ECPR cases) [9] Post-Norwood up to 8% [10]	Higher % of neurologic complications (4.4–17.7%) [11]
Acute HF in myocarditis and cardiomyopathy	To provide cardio-pulmonary support for recovery or bridge to transplant/durable device	6–20% of myocarditis patients will need ECMO [12] 1.4% of pediatric cardiac ECMO runs (2017–2021) were in cardiomyopathy patients [5]	Highest survival for myocarditis patients (72%) [12]
Posttransplantation	To provide time to recovery or re-transplant in patients who fail to come off bypass, develop LCOS, primary graft dysfunction, acute rejection and graft vasculopathy	17% need V-A ECMO after heart transplant for early and/or late graft failure [13]	Lower survival for patients who need ECMO posttransplantation (40% vs 80%) [14]
Intractable arrhythmias	To provide cardiovascular support during medical management or before the ablation attempt	Infrequent <1% [15]	In the post-cardiotomy setting, residual lesions and coronary ischemia should be ruled out
Septic shock	To provide cardiovascular support in refractory septic shock	1.6% of pediatric septic shock patients need V-A ECMO [16]	Very low survival for herpes septic shock [17]

CHD congenital heart disease, *HLHS* hypoplastic left heart syndrome, *SV* single ventricle, *ECPR* extracorporeal cardiopulmonary resuscitation, *CPR* cardiopulmonary resuscitation, *ROSC* return of spontaneous circulation, *HF* heart failure, *LCOS* low cardiac output syndrome

30.3 Use and Strategy

The strategy for ECMO use is related to the patient's characteristics and underlying diagnosis, but irrespective of the indication, V-A ECMO is considered as a temporary form of support, which can be used as (1) bridge to recovery, (2) bridge to durable ventricular assist device (VAD), (3) bridge to transplantation and finally (4) as a bridge to decision. The majority of patients have reversible disease/myocardial dysfunction and receive this support as a bridge to recovery. For children with cardiomyopathy, it can be used as a bridge to transplantation although outcomes are worse when compared to patients bridged with a VAD [6, 18–20]. In most cases, the patient is bridged with ECMO to a more durable VAD while waiting for the transplant (bridge-to-bridge strategy). The timing for transition is critical as prolonged ECMO support (>14 days) results in inferior posttransplant survival [6, 18]. The potential for myocardial recovery may be unknown at the time of cannulation and a bridge-to-decision strategy can be used. During this period, transplant candidacy, neurologic status and end-organ recovery can be assessed to aid the decision-making process.

30.4 Contraindications

Contraindications have decreased over the years, and conditions that were regarded as absolute contraindications, are now considered relative contraindications. Overall, ECMO is inappropriate if the underlying condition is irreversible and/or no timely, reasonable therapeutic option is available or if the probability of poor neurological outcome is high. For pediatric cardiac failure, it is generally agreed that absolute contraindications are extreme prematurity or low birth weight, lethal chromosomal abnormalities (trisomy 13 or 18), uncontrollable hemorrhage and irreversible brain damage [21].

30.5 Cannulation and ECMO Circuit

Before initiating ECMO, it is important to prepare and anticipate any problems that can occur. An example of a checklist prior to ECMO initiation is shown in ◘ Table 30.2.

30.5.1 Cannulation Technique

The type and method of cannulation depend on the patient's size, context of cannulation and underlying diagnosis.

There are two methods for accessing the vessels and cannulating. The direct "cut down" technique consists of cannulation under direct visualization of the vessels and is preferred in small children, especially in neck cannulation. The disadvantages are being more time-consuming and needing ligation of the vessels afterward.

Percutaneous cannulation can be achieved through the Seldinger technique under ultrasound guidance. Its use is limited by the size of the patient's vessels.

Table 30.2 Checklist prior to ECMO initiation

ECMO initiation checklist	✓
Staff	
– Surgeon	
– Cardiac theaters scrub staff	
– Consultant intensivist and medical team	
– ECMO coordinator/nurse specialist/intensive care nurse	
– Perfusionist	
Equipment	
– ECMO cannulae	
– ECMO circuit	
– Surgical instruments	
Blood products	
– Blood red cells	
– Platelets	
– Fresh frozen plasma ± cryoprecipitate	
Drugs	
– Sedation (for example, fentanyl, ketamine) – Paralysis (for example, vecuronium)	
– Resuscitation drugs (adrenaline, bicarbonate and calcium gluconate)	
– Heparin—bolus dose (to be given immediately prior to cannulation of the vessel)	
– Fluid bolus	
– Prophylactic antibiotics	
– Anti-arrhythmic drugs	
Venous access – Central access needed. Ensure enough lumens and adequacy of access	
Pacing	
– If patient has pacing wires, test sensitivity and output before procedure	
– Temporary pacing system should be accessible during procedure	
Parental consent: an informed consent after explaining procedure, benefits and risks and ECMO information leaflet	
Surgical time-out and safety checklist	

30.5.2 Site of Cannulation

There are essentially two types of cannulation: peripheral and central. For peripheral cannulation, there are mainly two options, the use of cervical or femoral vessels. The choice of the type of cannulation depends on the size of the patient, size of the vessels, underlying diagnosis and anatomy and indication for cannulation. The size of the vessels must be adequate to accommodate a cannula large enough to supply adequate flow to and from the circuit. A hybrid type of cannulation might be required if venous drainage, systemic perfusion or oxygenation is insufficient. The patient's clinical condition and needs may change over time and prompt a change in the ECMO configuration:

1. Cervical cannulation: cannulation of the internal jugular vein and right common carotid artery. Preferred for small children (<15 kg) due to the small size of femoral vessels.
2. Femoral cannulation: cannulation of femoral vein and artery. Generally used for adults and potentially larger children (>30 kg). The main disadvantage is the risk of inadequate arterial perfusion due to significant occlusion of the artery by the cannula, so close monitoring of distal pulses is warranted. If the cannulas are placed by cut down, a distal perfusion catheter or a graft with end-to-side anastomosis can be placed in order to improve distal limb perfusion [22]. Other possible disadvantages are the development of Harlequin syndrome [23] and insufficient venous drainage (due to the smaller size of the vessel) that can result in insufficient cardiac support. In these cases, a hybrid cannulation might be needed. The differential perfusion of the upper and lower body also known as Harlequin syndrome occurs when the lung function is poor and native cardiac output is preserved. To overcome this complication, a venous-arteriovenous (V-AV) cannulation strategy with the placement of an additional internal jugular vein return cannula allows the delivery of oxygenated blood to the upper body (◘ Fig. 30.2). In the case of insufficient venous drainage, the use of a venous-venous-arterial cannulation (VV-A) with the placement of an additional internal jugular venous drainage cannula increases the venous drainage and allows better cardiac support (◘ Fig. 30.2) [24, 25].
3. Transthoracic or central cannulation is used in patients who are unable to come off cardiopulmonary bypass in the operating room, when urgent initiation on

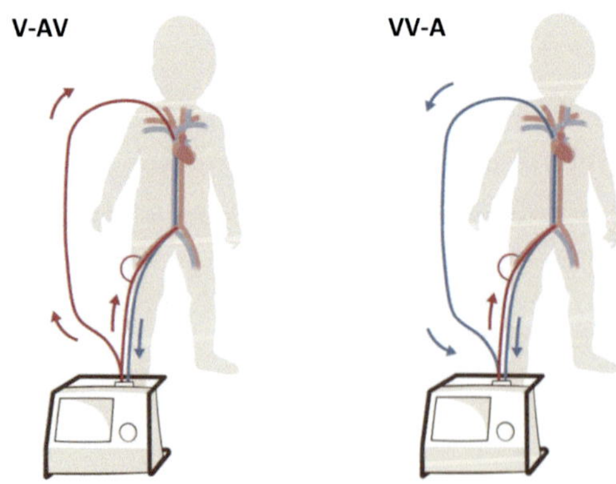

◘ **Fig. 30.2** Venous-arteriovenous (V-AV) and venovenous-arterial (VV-A) cannulation strategies

ECMO is needed, if larger cannulas are needed to achieve target blood flow rates or in case peripheral cannulation is not possible or contraindicated. It is achieved by cannulation of the right atrial appendage and the ascending aorta via sternotomy. The main disadvantages are increased risk of bleeding and mediastinitis [22].

30.5.3 Additional Cannulas

The addition of a further cannula may be required for optimizing venous drainage, as mentioned before, or for efficient left ventricular (LV) decompression. The left atrium (LA) can be decompressed through the placement of an LA vent that will be connected to the venous limb of the ECMO circuit. The vent can be placed via sternotomy or percutaneously. The placement of the vent through the LV apex is also possible, especially if the mitral valve is competent.

30.5.4 Circuit

The ECMO circuit consists of drainage and infusion cannulas, tubing, a mechanical blood pump, a membrane oxygenator, a heat exchanger and a pressurized gas source. The cannulas and the tubing are adjusted to the size/weight of the patient and site of cannulation. The aim should be to have the biggest cannula/tube with the shortest length to allow optimal venous drainage and avoid high resistance pressure drop on the blood return side.

1. The blood pump directs the venous drainage through the membrane lung and returns it to the patient. There are two types: roller and centrifugal. Roller pumps deliver a fixed output by using sequential compression of the circuit tubing, while in centrifugal pumps, the flow is variable as it is preload dependent and afterload sensitive. Overall, there has been an increase in centrifugal pump use in pediatric patients in view of its potential benefits such as the ability to use smaller circuits and decrease the activation of inflammatory factors. However, its use is still variable, and some centers prefer the use of roller pumps for small children due to higher rates of hemolysis and other complications associated with centrifugal pumps in this population. A large and recent meta-analysis comparing centrifugal and roller pumps points to lower mortality and fewer complications associated with the use of roller pumps [26]. Rupture of the circuit can happen when the post-pump pressure exceeds 300 mmHg. Centrifugal pumps create suction and negative pressure which can lead to hemolysis and cavitation, so pressures should be targeted to no more negative than −50 mmHg [1].
2. The membrane lung (oxygenator) achieves gas exchange through the perfusion of venous blood through a network of small hollow fibers. The tubes are filled with gas (the "sweep gas"), and the blood flows exterior to the fibers and diffusion of O_2 and CO_2 occurs across the membrane. The CO_2 clearance is determined by the sweep gas flow rate; the higher the flow, the higher the CO_2 clearance. Oxygen delivery from the circuit should allow adequate systemic saturation at low ventilation settings and an AVO2 difference of <20–30%. As for CO_2 clearance, as a general guide, a sweep gas flow rate less than the blood flow rate can be used at the beginning and adjusted later according to arterial gas monitoring [6].

Monitoring is vital during ECMO and most circuits include monitoring of blood flow, pre- and post-membrane lung blood pressure measurements, pre-pump venous drainage line pressure and pre- and post-membrane lung oxyhemoglobin saturation. The blood gases are measured from the pre-oxygenator site to assess perfusion and oxygen delivery of the patient and from the post-oxygenator site to assess membrane efficiency (post-membrane PaO_2 should be 25–35 kPa).

30.6 ECMO Run: Management, Monitoring and Complications

30.6.1 Goals and Principles of Cardiac ECMO

The medical management is directed at ensuring myocardial recovery by maximizing myocardial perfusion and adequate decompression of the heart, improving or maintaining end-organ perfusion and preventing and mitigating any ECMO-related risks and complications. One must remain vigilant for patient-related (bleeding, neurologic injury infection and renal failure) and circuit-related (air in the circuit, thrombosis, unplanned decannulation and hemolysis) complications.

The ECMO flow should be calculated according to age and weight (cardiac index of 2.5–3 L/min/m^2 or 100–150 ml/kg/min in infants/70–100 ml/kg/min in larger children) and should be sufficient to ensure good systemic perfusion, as monitored from markers of systemic perfusion (lactate clearance, mixed venous oxygen saturation and end-organ function) [6]. Additionally, the pulse pressure should be at least 10 mmHg, as this is an indication of ventricular ejection which decompresses the heart and reduces the risk of systemic ventricular thrombosis [6].

There are some important aspects unique to cardiac ECMO that should be considered while managing the patient and circuit such as myocardial stun, LV distention, postsurgical bleeding or supporting a patient with single ventricle physiology. During the management, it is important to keep in mind that the centrifugal circuit is preload dependent and afterload sensitive.

30.6.2 Myocardial Stun

After the initiation of full ECMO flows, there is a sudden decrease in preload but most importantly a significant increase in afterload. These changes, in a poorly functioning heart, can induce a period of worsened cardiac function with minimal to no pulse pressure. The expected time to recovery is 3–7 days and responds to good afterload reduction and adequate decompression of the heart.

30.6.3 Ventricular Decompression

There is no direct decompression of the LA or the LV during cardiac ECMO unless there is the presence of an LA vent or interatrial communication. Even on full ECMO support, LA receives returning blood from the bronchial and Thebesian veins and from the right side of the heart. In the presence of poor myocardial function and increased afterload, the ventricle may not be able to empty adequately and thus become increasingly distended, resulting in high left atrial and pulmonary venous pressures and pulmonary edema. Elevated end-diastolic pressures may also compromise coronary perfusion and cause subendocardial ischemia, further damaging myocardial function. Additionally, the stagnant intracavitary blood increases the risk of clot formation. Signs of inadequate decompression include pulmonary vein congestion, loss of arterial ejection and pulse pressure on the arterial trace, finally leading to pink frothy secretions from the endotracheal tube and pulmonary edema noted on the chest radiograph—both relatively late signs (◘ Fig. 30.3). On echocardiogram signs of inadequate decompression are distension of the LV and LA with no/minimal opening of the aortic valve, spontaneous contrast in LV and mitral regurgitation.

Early decompression is associated with a shorter ECMO course and improved LV recovery [27, 28] and can be achieved by the insertion of an LA vent (post-cardiotomy ECMO) or by performing balloon septostomy or atrial septal defect balloon dilatation (◘ Fig. 30.4).

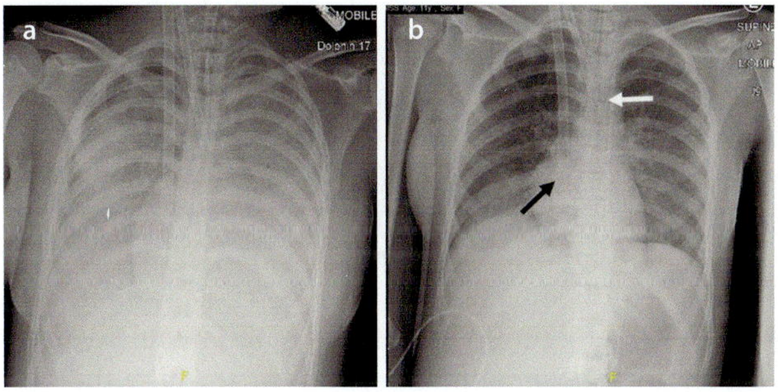

◘ **Fig. 30.3** Chest X ray in patient on VA ECMO before **a** and after **b** balloon atrial septostomy for LA decompression. Severe pulmonary edema in **a** and significant improvement after the procedure. Black arrow: venous cannula, white arrow: arterial cannula

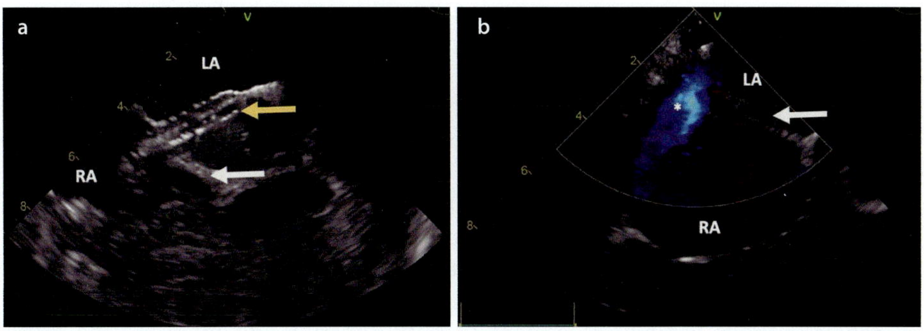

◘ **Fig. 30.4** Transesophageal images of balloon septostomy performed in patient on ECMO. **a** balloon (orange arrow) crossing interatrial septum (white arrow). **b** after septostomy flow (asterisk) from the LA to RA. *LA* Left atrium, *RA* right atrium, white arrow—interatrial septum, orange arrow—balloon; *flow from LA to RA

30.6.4 Residual Lesions

In postoperative cardiac patients needing ECMO, residual lesions must be carefully considered and excluded, especially if the patient is not following an anticipated trajectory or is unable to wean from ECMO support. Residual lesions such as valvar regurgitation, outflow tract obstruction, coronary abnormalities and refractory arrhythmias need to be appropriately investigated with echocardiography, chest ultrasound, cardiac catheterization and electrophysiology studies. However, some lesions can only be detected by cardiac catheterization [29]. Cardiac catheterization can be safely performed while on ECMO and should be considered promptly as early detection and intervention for residual lesions is associated with a higher rate of successful decannulation and better survival to hospital discharge [30].

30.6.5 Single Ventricle Physiology

The main indications for ECMO in single-ventricle patients include the inability to separate from cardiopulmonary bypass, refractory low cardiac output syndrome, cardiopulmonary arrest, thrombosis of the shunt and elective support for procedures such as therapeutic cardiac catheterization in high-risk patients [31]

1. Stage 1 palliation (Norwood procedure): about 16% need postoperative ECMO and survival to discharge is 35%, with lower survival outcomes (16%) for patients palliated with a hybrid procedure [32, 33]. Patients cannulated for hypoxemia, particularly with thrombosis of the shunt, have significantly improved survival compared with those supported for hypotension or cardiovascular collapse [34]. When patients have a Blalock Thomas Taussig (BTT) shunt, higher flows might be required (150–200 ml/kg/min) in order to maintain adequate systemic circulation and compensate for the pulmonary run-off through the shunt. If high pulmonary flow becomes problematic or if systemic perfusion is inadequate even with higher flows, then surgical shunt constriction may be required. Shunt occlusion during ECMO is not recommended as it results in higher mortality [24, 35]. Slippage of the cannula in the carotid artery into the shunt can result in loss of all cardiac output, so the cannula position should be monitored closely.
2. Bidirectional cavopulmonary anastomosis (Glenn shunt): cannulation and ECMO management can be challenging as there are two separate sources of systemic venous return. Monitoring for superior vena cava syndrome and/or venous congestion is important as failure of flow through the pulmonary bed can be difficult to recognize while oxygenation is maintained by the ECMO support. Cannulation of both SVC and common atrium might be required to achieve adequate venous decompression and systemic perfusion [36].
3. Total cavopulmonary connection (Fontan): adequate venous drainage might not be achieved with a single cannula, especially if peripheral and some patients require venous cannula placement in both superior and inferior vena cavae. Venous decompression is particularly important in Fontan patients as they usually have elevated transpulmonary gradient and minimal native cardiac output. Therefore, high ECMO flows might be required to decompress and provide adequate circulatory support [37]. Overall, CPR in Fontan patients is inefficient, and

ECMO should be deployed before cardiac arrest. The largest series points to a survival of 35% in Fontan patients requiring ECMO [36].

30.7 Cardiovascular Management and Monitoring

Blood pressure while on ECMO is determined by blood flow (pump flow and native cardiac output) and vascular resistance. The adequacy of perfusion and oxygenation is assessed by clinical parameters such as capillary refill time, warmth and color of extremities, urine output and neurological monitoring. One can indirectly assess native cardiac output by evaluating pulse pressure, as an increase in pulse pressure is seen when myocardial function and ejection return. Dysrhythmias do not usually cause hemodynamic instability but should be treated, as they increase myocardial demands [38].

ECMO is dependent on adequate preload, and inadequate preload will result in impaired flows. The trend of central venous pressure (CVP) should be monitored rather than the absolute number. If device flow is impaired and CVP is low, volume expansion might be required. If device flow is low and CVP is high, tamponade or tension pneumothorax should be sought as well as mechanical problems such as cannula displacement and clotting. If device flow is maintained and CVP is high, hypervolemia may be present.

30.7.1 Inotropes and Vasoactive Drugs

Although full support is achieved by ECMO, a low dose of inotropes (adrenaline and/or milrinone) might be required in order to promote native cardiac function and prevent ventricular distention.

Vasoactive drugs help control vessel reactivity and device flow. Increased afterload (hypertension) results in decreased flow and a vasodilator agent (phentolamine and nitroprusside) will reduce afterload and improve flow. Due to low cardiac output prior to cannulation, post-cannulation patients might experience high systemic vascular resistance (SVR) due to high plasma renin activity. Additionally, high ECMO flows, suboptimal sedation, hypothermia, hypervolemia and seizures can also contribute to hypertension and high SVR. On the contrary, a vasoconstrictor agent (noradrenaline and vasopressin) may be required if flow is adequate and the patient remains hypotensive. Hypotension requiring inotropes while on ECMO may be due to sepsis, hypovolemia and hyperthermia.

30.7.2 Respiratory Management and Monitoring

The aim of invasive ventilation should be to maintain lung volume and prevent atelectasis. Cardiac patients are usually submitted to cardiac surgery under cardiopulmonary bypass (CPB) and/or large volumes of blood product administration prior to ECMO cannulation which puts them at risk of developing lung edema. For this reason, a common ventilation strategy is to keep high PEEP (10 cm H_20), low tidal volume (6–8 ml/kg), respiratory rate (10 bpm) and peak inspiratory pressures (18–20 cm H_20). The FiO_2 is usually kept at 40% in order to oxygenate the blood coming from the right side, as this blood, in the presence of ejection will perfuse the coronary arteries and should be well oxygenated.

If the patient is peripherally cannulated and has no lung pathology, spontaneous breathing or extubation might be considered. Gas exchange is managed through the circuit by titrating the sweep gas and FiO_2. Oxygen delivery from the circuit should be adequate and achieve a systemic saturation >95%. The venous saturation should be around 20–30% less than the arterial, indicating that systemic oxygen delivery is 3–5 times oxygen consumption. CO2 clearance is managed by titrating the sweep gas flow rate, and normal values should be targeted.

30.7.3 Anticoagulation

ECMO requires full anticoagulation, and unfractionated heparin (UNFH) has been the anticoagulant of choice due to the familiarity with its use, availability and low price. Maintaining adequate anticoagulation and monitoring the effect of UNFH can be challenging. Monitoring for the drug-specific effect might not be enough, as other factors such as endothelial responses, inflammatory state and end-organ dysfunction influence anticoagulation. A tailored strategy for each patient is advised. There are several blood tests and essays to assess coagulation which are limited by the lack of standardization [39]. The different tests are specified in ◘ Table 30.3.

30.7.4 Bleeding Management

Bleeding is a common complication in ECMO patients, especially after cardiac surgery, and is associated with increased mortality [39]. Risk factors are mediastinal exploration prior to ECMO, greater surgical complexity, early postoperative cannulation and longer bypass time [40]. Significant bleeding can impair circuit function by decreasing the preload or by causing tamponade physiology.

Preventing bleeding is important and simple procedures such as venipuncture, endotracheal suctioning and passage of urinary or nasogastric catheter can result in bleeding. Thus, all these procedures should only be done after assuring that the anticoagulation status is optimal. If bleeding ensues, the first step is to treat correctable causes and identify/exclude surgically correctable ones. If bleeding persists, anticoagulation can be stopped. However, this increases the risk of clot formation, and a primed circuit should be available [39].

30.7.5 Blood Product Administration

Blood product requirement is high during ECMO due to the need for circuit priming, increasing oxygen delivery, maintenance of hemostatic balance and treatment of hemorrhagic complications. While optimizing oxygen delivery for ECMO patients, it

Table 30.3 Coagulation tests used for heparin effect control during ECMO

Test	What it tests	Non-heparin interference	Target values	Advantages/ disadvantages	How/when
ACT	Whole blood test	↑With anemia, thrombocytopenia or coagulation factor deficiency	180–220 seconds	Quick, bedside test Not specific to heparin effect	Standard measurement in most centers to control UNFH effect
aPTT	Intrinsic and final common pathway	Influenced by coagulation factors, heparin and antithrombin ↑ With acute phase reactants	Usually 60–80	Infants have baseline prolonged values—not reliable Poor correlation with anti-Xa levels and UNFH	Additional exam to asses clotting
Anti-factor Xa activity	UNFH activity	↓ If hyperbilirubinemia or hemolysis	0.3–0.7 IU/ml	Not affected by coagulopathy, thrombocytopenia or dilution	Evaluation of UNFH effect if other coagulation tests deranged
TEG	Multiple phases of clot formation	Whole blood test. Influenced by clotting factors, platelets and fibrinolysis	–	Heparin effect evaluated if heparinase added	Excessive bleeding or clotting
AT 3	Antithrombin III activity	No	>30–80%	Specific test	Escalating UNFH requirements (>35–40 units/kg/h) Clinically subtherapeutic anticoagulation

ACT activated clotting time, *aPTT* activated partial thromboplastin time, *UNFH* unfractionated heparin, *TEG* thromboelastography; *AT 3* antithrombin III

is important to note that high requirements of red blood cell transfusion are associated with increased mortality in ECMO patients [41].

With an increasing understanding of the adverse effects related to blood product transfusion, the risk/benefit equipoise rapidly changes, and the practitioners are more cautious with liberal thresholds for transfusion guided by the patient's clinical status and institutional protocols.

30.7.6 Renal Function

Renal dysfunction is common in cardiac patients, and it can be precipitated by impaired renal blood flow prior to ECMO deployment and the use of nephrotoxic drugs. Fluid overload is also frequent and associated with worse cardiac, pulmonary, gastrointestinal and renal function and prolongs time on ECMO. Renal failure is associated with lower survival in ECMO patients and should be avoided [42]. Renal replacement therapy is feasible while on ECMO and might be needed to address renal failure or fluid overload. Evidence shows that ECMO patients requiring hemofiltration have worse outcomes, but it is not clear if this is related to the hemofiltration itself or if it is a reflection of a more severe underlying disease [43].

30.7.7 Neurology and Sedation

Neurologic injury is common in ECMO patients, especially in the congenital heart disease population and is associated with poorer outcomes [44]. Comprehensive neurological assessments should be performed frequently and should include pupillary size and response to light, response to pain or assessment of signs of embolic or hemorrhagic stroke. Cranial ultrasound should be performed within the first 24 hours and repeated depending on clinical evolution, and EEG can detect subclinical seizures that might warrant treatment. The trend of near infrared spectroscopy (NIRS) monitoring can be helpful in high-risk patients, especially during manipulations of circuits or weaning of the flows. Overall, there should be a high index of suspicion for neurologic events and a low threshold for performing further imaging exams. Regarding sedation and analgesia, the goal should be to keep the patient comfortable. There has been a growing trend toward minimizing the use of sedation to allow the patient to breathe spontaneously, participate in care and interact with healthcare and family members. The benefits include better neurologic assessment and possibly decreased long-term muscle weakness [45].

30.7.8 Infection

The most important risk factor seems to be the duration of support, but cardiac disease and the presence of an open chest can also predispose to infection [46]. Bloodstream infections are the most common, but diagnosing infection can be difficult as temperature is controlled in the ECMO circuit, and patients might not display fever; the white blood cell count can be low secondary to large volume transfusion of blood products, not reflecting the presence or absence of infection and inflammatory markers can be increased due to systemic inflammation. Additional attention is required in patients with prosthetic valves or shunts who are at risk of developing endocarditis.

30.8 Weaning and Decannulation

Successful ECMO weaning is defined as survival after discontinuation of ECMO without the need for re-initiation of mechanical support for the next 48 hours. For postoperative patients, rapid recovery is expected, whereas, on primary myocardial dysfunction, recovery occurs over days to months.

Readiness to be weaned is assessed by evidence of myocardial recoveries such as an increase in pulse pressure, increase in systolic pressure, rising end-tidal CO_2 (in children without systemic to pulmonary shunts) and improving function on echocardiography [47, 48]. In patients with LA vent or atrial septostomy, lower left atrial vent flows and a drop in circuit mixed venous oxygen saturations are signs of recovery.

Preparation for the weaning trial includes starting a low dose of inotropes, confirming endotracheal tube position, resuming conventional ventilation and if there is a risk of pulmonary hypertension initiating inhaled nitric oxide. Pacemaker wires should be tested and connected to the pacemaker box, and metabolic and coagulation abnormalities should be corrected.

The weaning trial consists of reducing the contribution of ECMO and assesses suitability for decannulation by monitoring cardiac function on echocardiography, cardiac output, oxygenation and ventilation. It can be achieved by incremental decrease in the flows with concomitant administration of fluid and titration of ventilation and inotropes, by clamping the cannula proximal to the patient and circulating the circuit through the AV bridge or by pump-controlled retrograde trial (◘ Table 30.4). If the myocardial function is judged sufficient, the patient can be decannulated. However, before that, it is vital to anticipate and establish a plan for managing complications that may arise (low cardiac output, pulmonary hypertension and bleeding) and define candidacy for re-initiation of ECMO. The timing of decannulation should take into consideration the availability of resources (material and human) should the patient need ECMO re-initiation. If the patient fails to wean from ECMO, residual lesions or factors preventing myocardial recovery should be sought aggressively.

Table 30.4 ECMO weaning checklist

ECMO weaning checklist	✓
Staff	
– Surgeon	
– Nursing staff from cardiac theaters	
– Consultant intensivist	
– ECMO nurse specialist/intensive care nurse	
– Perfusionist	
– Cardiologist	
Exams review	
– Chest XR	
– Echocardiogram	
– FBC, coagulation and ABG	
Drugs	
– Patient must be sedated and paralyzed	
– Low dose of inotropes should be started before the procedure	
– Resuscitation drugs (adrenaline, bicarbonate and calcium gluconate)	
– Fluid bolus	
– Prophylactic antibiotic for the procedure	
Reduction of flow	
– Reduce flows progressively (by 10% at the time) and monitor vital signs, gas exchange and lactate clearance	
– Adjust ventilation and inotropes if needed during weaning	
– When at 70% flow, repeat ABG, reduce sweep flow to 0.1 L/min and adjust ventilation as needed and repeat echocardiogram	
Clamping off	
– When flows 50%, clamp cannulas off	
– Clamp off all Y connectors	
– Maintain circuit heparin infusion (5 units/kg/h) aiming ACT> 150	
– Flush cannulas/bridge/vent frequently to prevent clotting	
Decannulation	
– If patient considered apt to decannulation, surgeons can proceed	

30.9 Outcomes

Outcomes of ECMO for children with cardiac indication are worse than for respiratory indication [49]. This can be explained by the higher rate of complications associated with poorer outcomes in the cardiac ECMO population such as infection, bleeding, thrombosis, renal failure and neurologic events [44, 50–52]. In addition, younger age, presence of congenital abnormalities and comorbidities, complex cardiac surgery requiring longer cardiopulmonary bypass and longer duration on ECMO increase the mortality risk [53].

The overall survival to hospital discharge for cardiac ECMO is 52% and 43% for the pediatric and neonatal groups, respectively. As for long-term outcomes, reports show an additional late mortality of 4–12% related to the severity of the underlying cardiac disease and the presence of comorbidities [54, 55].

Acute neurological events are the most feared complication as they impact not only early mortality but also later survival, neurodevelopment and quality of life. Its reported incidence is 14%, and prematurity, low weight, severe acidosis and prior cardiac arrest are factors associated with a higher risk [44].

For cardiac ECMO survivors, in particular, studies show a decreased IQ with 50–67% of patients having some degree of mental delay and a high risk for gross motor issues (25–40%) [56, 57]. Some of these neurodevelopmental abnormalities only manifest later in life and neuro-imaging exam findings seem to not correlate with early neurodevelopmental outcome [58] which highlights the importance of surveillance and follow-up for ECMO survivors and further studies in this area.

30.10 Future of Cardiac ECMO

Despite an increased use of cardiac ECMO in neonatal and pediatric patients, the survival rates have not changed significantly in the past decade (◘ Fig. 30.5). Anticoagulation remains the main challenge in neonatal and pediatric ECMO due to the developing hemostasis and poor correlation of coagulation tests and the level of anticoagulant in this age group. There are different bioactive and biopassive surfaces being developed for the circuit coating, aiming for less thrombogenic/inflammatory effects, namely nitric oxide coating or more recently endothelialized surfaces [59].

Another developing area is the use of direct thrombin inhibitors. These are especially appealing to the neonatal and pediatric groups as their action is independent of antithrombin III levels, which are frequently low in infants and critically ill children. Bivalirubin is already used in adult ECMO and pediatric VAD patients with good outcomes [60]. Finally, patient candidacy continues to be an important issue. There are still no prediction scores for cardiac ECMO in children, and candidacy remains a local team decision.

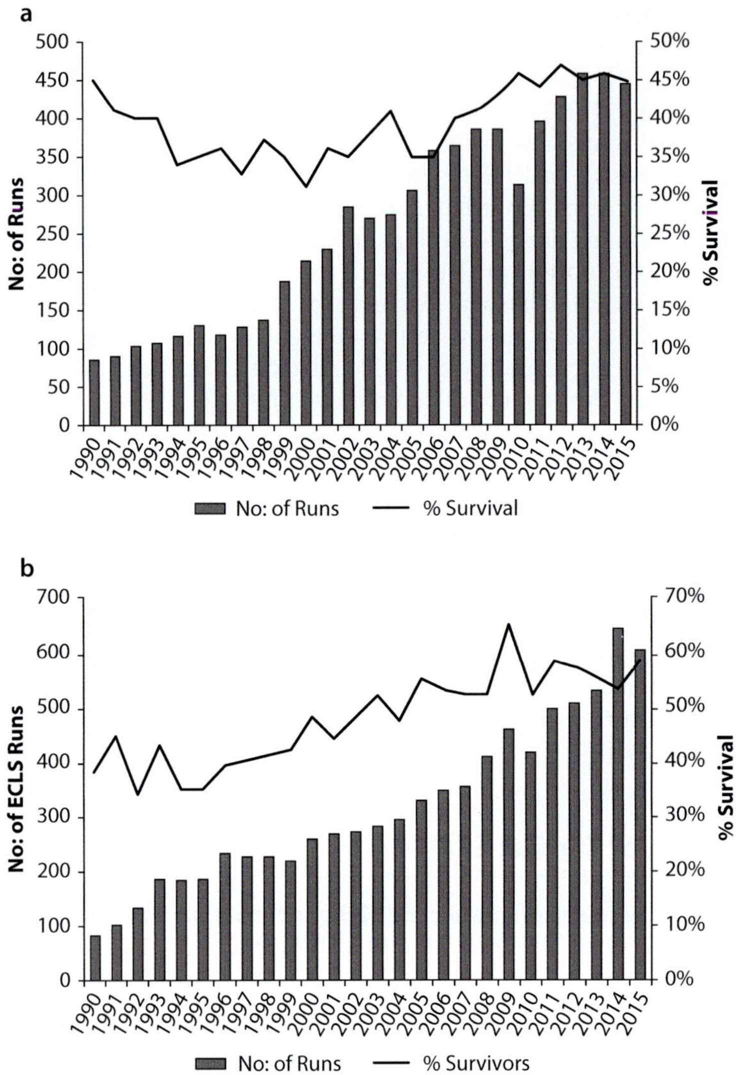

Fig. 30.5 Extracorporeal life support use and survival in cardiac disease. **a** Neonates; **b** pediatric patients. Adapted from Extracorporeal Life Support Organization Registry International Report 2016, R.R Thiagarajan et al, 2016, ASAIO

Take-Home Messages

- The number of cardiac neonatal and pediatric ECMO runs is increasing.
- Candidacy and patient selection are of paramount importance.
- Cardiac ECMO serves as a temporary treatment to bridge the patient to recovery, decision, another device or transplant.
- Bleeding and neurologic events are the major complications associated with cardiac ECMO.
- Preparation and anticipation of complications is key.
- Outcomes depend on the patient's characteristics and underlying disease.
- Addressing new anticoagulation strategies and patient selection score systems will be the upcoming challenges.

References

1. Maclaren G, et al. Extracorporeal life support: the ELSO red book. 6th ed. Extracorporeal Life Support Organization; 2022.
2. Lim MW. The history of extracorporeal oxygenators. Anaesthesia. 2006;61(10):984–95.
3. Baffes TG, Fridman JL, Bicoff JP, Whitehill JL. Extracorporeal circulation for support of palliative cardiac surgery in infants. Ann Thorac Surg. 1970;10(4):354–63. https://doi.org/10.1016/s0003-4975(10)65613-5.
4. Hil JD, et al. Prolonged extracorporeal oxygenation for acute post-traumatic respiratory failure (shock-lung syndrome). Use of the Bramson membrane lung. N Engl J Med. 1972;286(12):629–34. https://doi.org/10.1056/NEJM197203232861204.
5. Extracorporeal Life Support Organization, ECLS Registry Report, International Summary, October 2022, Extracorporeal Life Support Organization, November 2022. Available: https://www.elso.org/Portals/0/Files/Reports/2022_October/International%20Report%20October.pdf
6. Brown G, et al. Extracorporeal Life Support Organization (ELSO): guidelines for pediatric cardiac failure. ASAIO J (1992). 2021;67(5):463–475. doi: https://doi.org/10.1097/MAT.0000000000001431.
7. Bautista-Hernandez V, et al. Preoperative extracorporeal membrane oxygenation as a bridge to cardiac surgery in children with congenital heart disease. Ann Thorac Surg. 2009;88(4):1306–11. https://doi.org/10.1016/j.athoracsur.2009.06.074.
8. Lorusso R, et al. Structured review of post-cardiotomy extracorporeal membrane oxygenation: Part 2—Pediatric patients. J Heart Lung Transplant. 2019;38(11):1144–61.
9. Lasa JJ, et al. Extracorporeal Cardiopulmonary resuscitation (E-CPR) during pediatric in-Hospital Cardiopulmonary arrest is associated with improved survival to discharge. Circulation. 2016;133:165–76.
10. Alsoufi B, et al. Late outcomes of infants supported by extracorporeal membrane oxygenation following the Norwood operation. World J Pediatr Congenit Heart Surg. 2015;6(1):9–17. https://doi.org/10.1177/2150135114558072.
11. Said AS, et al. Neurological monitoring and complications of pediatric extracorporeal membrane oxygenation support. Pediatr Neurol. 2020;108:31–9.
12. Gutierres ME, et al. extracorporeal membrane oxygenation cannulation timing in the pediatric myocarditis population: an exploratory analysis from the extracorporeal life support organization registry. Crit Care Explor. 2023;5(1):e0826.
13. Nair AG, et al. Extracorporeal membrane oxygenation support after heart transplantation in children—outcomes of a single center cohort. Pediatr Crit Care Med. 2020;21(4):332–9.
14. Kaushal S, et al. A multicenter study of primary graft failure after infant heart transplantation: impact of extracorporeal membrane oxygenation on outcomes. Pediatr Transplant. 2014;18(1):72–8. https://doi.org/10.1111/petr.12181.
15. Well A, et al. Arrhythmias requiring ECMO in infants without structural congenital heart disease. Pediatr Cardiol. 2022;43(4):914–21.

16. Schlapbach LJ, et al. Defining benefit threshold for extracorporeal membrane oxygenation in children with sepsis—a binational multicenter cohort study. Crit Care Lond Engl. 2019;23(1):429. https://doi.org/10.1186/s13054-019-2685-1.
17. Butt WW, Chiletti R. ECMO for neonatal sepsis in 2019. Front Pediatr. 2000:8. https://doi.org/10.3389/fped.2020.00050.
18. Almond CS, et al. Berlin Heart EXCOR pediatric ventricular assist device for bridge to heart transplantation in US children. Circulation. 2013;127(16):1702–11. https://doi.org/10.1161/CIRCULATIONAHA.112.000685.
19. Fraser CD, et al. Prospective trial of a pediatric ventricular assist device. N Engl J Med. 2012;367(6):532–41. https://doi.org/10.1056/NEJMoa1014164.(19).
20. Conway J, Cantor R, Koehl D, et al. Survival after transplant listing for infants on mechanical circulatory support. J Am Heart Assoc. 2020;9(21):e011890.
21. Di Nardo M, et al. ECLS in pediatric cardiac patients. Front Pediatr. 2016;4:109. https://doi.org/10.3389/fped.2016.00109.
22. Harvey C. Cannulation for neonatal and pediatric extracorporeal membrane oxygenation for cardiac support. Front Pediatr. 2018;6 https://doi.org/10.3389/fped.2018.00017.
23. Rao P, Khalpey Z, Smith R, Burkhoff D, Kociol RD. Venoarterial extracorporeal membrane oxygenation for cardiogenic shock and cardiac arrest. Circ Heart Fail. 2018;11(9):e004905. https://doi.org/10.1161/CIRCHEARTFAILURE.118.004905.
24. Finck C. Cannulation for ECLS. Am Pediatr Surg Assoc. 2021; https://www.pedsurglibrary.com/apsa/view/Pediatric-Surgery-NaT/829154/all/Cannulation_for_ECLS
25. Napp LC, et al. Cannulation strategies for percutaneous extracorporeal membrane oxygenation in adults. Clin Res Cardiol. 105(4):283–96. https://doi.org/10.1007/s00392-015-0941-1.
26. Papadimas E. Centrifugal and Roller pumps in neonatal and pediatric extracorporeal membrane oxygenation: a systematic review and meta-analysis of clinical outcomes. ASAIO J. 2022;68(3):311–7. https://doi.org/10.1097/MAT.0000000000001475.
27. Hacking DF, et al. Elective decompression of the left ventricle in pediatric patients may reduce the duration of venoarterial extracorporeal membrane oxygenation. Artif Organs. 2015;39(4):319–26. https://doi.org/10.1111/aor.12390.
28. Sperotto F, Polito A, Amigoni A, Maschietto N, Thiagarajan RR. Left atrial decompression in pediatric patients supported with extracorporeal membrane oxygenation for failure to wean from cardiopulmonary bypass: a propensity-weighted analysis. J Am Heart Assoc. 2022;11(23):e023963. https://doi.org/10.1161/JAHA.121.023963.
29. Agarwal HS, et al. Residual lesions in postoperative pediatric cardiac surgery patients receiving extracorporeal membrane oxygenation support. J Thorac Cardiovasc Surg. 2014;147(1):434–41. https://doi.org/10.1016/j.jtcvs.2013.03.021.
30. Boscamp NS, Turner ME, Crystal M, Anderson B, Vincent JA, Torres AJ. Cardiac catheterization in pediatric patients supported by extracorporeal membrane oxygenation: a 15-year experience. Pediatr Cardiol. 2017;38(2):332–7. https://doi.org/10.1007/s00246-016-1518-0.
31. Friedland-Little JM, et al. Risk factors for requiring extracorporeal membrane oxygenation support after a Norwood operation. J Thorac Cardiovasc Surg. 2014;148(1):266–72. https://doi.org/10.1016/j.jtcvs.2013.08.051.
32. Mayr B, et al. Single centre outcome of extracorporeal membrane oxygenation after neonatal Norwood procedure. Eur J Cardiothorac Surg. 2022;62(3):ezac129.
33. Roeleveld PP, de Wilde R, Hazekamp M, Rycus PT, Thiagarajan RR. Extracorporeal membrane oxygenation in single ventricle lesions palliated via the hybrid approach. World J Pediatr Congenit Heart Surg. 2014;5(3):393–7. https://doi.org/10.1177/2150135114526420.
34. Allan CK, Thiagarajan RR, del Nido PJ, Roth SJ, Almodovar MC, Laussen PC. Indication for initiation of mechanical circulatory support impacts survival of infants with shunted single-ventricle circulation supported with extracorporeal membrane oxygenation. J Thorac Cardiovasc Surg. 2007;133(3):660–7. https://doi.org/10.1016/j.jtcvs.2006.11.013.
35. Misfeldt AM, et al. Outcomes of single-ventricle patients supported with extracorporeal membrane oxygenation. Pediatr Crit Care Med J Soc Crit Care Med World Fed Pediatr Intensive Crit Care Soc. 2016;17(3):194–202. https://doi.org/10.1097/PCC.0000000000000616.
36. Booth KL, Roth SJ, Thiagarajan RR, Almodovar MC, del Nido PJ, Laussen PC. Extracorporeal membrane oxygenation support of the Fontan and bidirectional Glenn circulations. Ann Thorac Surg. 2004;77(4):1341–8. https://doi.org/10.1016/j.athoracsur.2003.09.042.

37. Bacon MK, Gray SB, Schwartz SM, Cooper DS. Extracorporeal Membrane Oxygenation (ECMO) support in special patient populations—the bidirectional Glenn and Fontan circulations. Front Pediatr. 2018;6:299. https://doi.org/10.3389/fped.2018.00299.
38. Schwartz M, Schmidt A. Medical and nursing care of the child on mechanical circulatory support. Pediatr Crit Care Med J Soc Crit Care Med World Fed Pediatr Intensive Crit Care Soc. 2013;14(5 Suppl. 1):S43–50. https://doi.org/10.1097/PCC.0b013e318292dfdc.
39. McMichael AB, Ryerson LM, Ratano D, Fan E, Faraoni D, Annich GM. 2021 ELSO adult and pediatric anticoagulation guidelines. ASAIO J. 2022;68(3):303–10. https://doi.org/10.1097/MAT.0000000000001652.
40. Werho DK, et al. Hemorrhagic complications in pediatric cardiac patients on extracorporeal membrane oxygenation: an analysis of the Extracorporeal Life Support Organization Registry. Pediatr Crit Care Med. 2015;16(3):276–88.
41. Keene SD, et al. Blood product transfusion and mortality in neonatal extracorporeal membrane oxygenation. Transfusion. 2020;60(2):262–8.
42. Askenazi DJ, et al. Acute kidney injury and renal replacement therapy independently predict mortality in neonatal and pediatric noncardiac patients on extracorporeal membrane oxygenation. Pediatr Crit Care Med. 2011;12(1):e1–6.
43. Paden ML, et al. Recovery of renal function and survival after continuous renal replacement therapy during extracorporeal membrane oxygenation. Pediatr Crit Care Med. 2011;12(2):153–8.
44. Polito A, et al. Neurologic injury in neonates with congenital heart disease during extracorporeal membrane oxygenation: an analysis of extracorporeal life support organization registry data. ASAIO J. 2015;61(1):43–8.
45. Nichols DG. Roger's textbook of pediatric intensive care. 4th ed. Lippincott, Williams & Wilkins; 2008.
46. Cashen K, et al. Acquired infection during neonatal and pediatric extracorporeal membrane oxygeantion. Perfusion. 2018;33(6):472–82.
47. Naruke T, et al. End-tidal carbon dioxide concentration can estimate the appropriate timing for weaning off from extracorporeal membrane oxygenation for refractory circulatory failure. Int Heart J. 2010;51(2):116–20.
48. Park BW, et al. Pulse pressure as a prognostic marker in patients receiving extracorporeal life support. Resuscitation. 2013;84(10):1404–8.
49. Barbaro RP, et al. Pediatric extracorporeal life support organization registry international report 2016. ASAIO J Am Soc Artif Intern Organs. 2017;63(4):456–63. https://doi.org/10.1097/MAT.0000000000000603.
50. Brown KL, et al. Healthcare-associated infection in pediatric patients on extracorporeal life support: the role of multidisciplinary surveillance. Pediatr Crit Care Med. 2006;7(6):546–50.
51. Dalton HJ, et al. Association of bleeding and thrombosis with outcome in extracorporeal life support. Pediatr Crit Care Med. 2015;16(2):167–74.
52. Gupta P, Beam B, Schmitz ML. Outcomes associated with the use of renal replacement therapy in children receiving extracorporeal membrane oxygenation after heart surgery: a multi-institutional analysis. Pediatr Nephrol. 2015;30(6):1019–26.
53. Sperotto F, et al. Extracorporeal membrane oxygenation support for failure to wean from cardiopulmonary bypass after pediatric cardiac surgery: analysis of extracorporeal life support organization registry data. Crit Care Explor. 2020;2(9):e0183.
54. Iguchi A, et al. Long-term survival outcomes and causes of late death in neonates, infants, and children treated with extracorporeal life support. Pediatr Crit Care Med. 2013;14(6):580–6.
55. Bahr V, et al. Long term survival and causes of late death in children treated with extracorporeal membrane oxygenatio. Pediatr Crit Care Med. 2017;18(3):272–80.
56. Wagner K, et al. Clinical and psychosocial follow-up study of children treated with extracorporeal membrane oxygenation. Ann Thorac Surg. 2007;84(4):1349–55.
57. Chow G, et al. Predictors of mortality and neurological morbidity in children undergoing extracorporeal life support for cardiac disease. Eur J Cardiothorac Surg. 2004;26(1):38–43.
58. Rollins MD, et al. Utility of neuroradiographic imaging in predicting outcomes after neonatal extracorporeal membrane oxygenation. J Pediatr Surg. 2012;47(1):76–80.
59. Canjunga D, et al. Improving hemocompatibility of artificial lungs by clik conjugation of glycoengineered endothelial cells onto blood-contacting surfaces. Biomater Adv. 2022;137:212824.
60. Valdes CA, et al. Heparine-based versus bivalirudin-based anticoagulation in pediatric extracorporeal membrane oxygenation: a systematic review. Front Med. 2023;10:137134.

Extracorporeal Cardiopulmonary Resuscitation in Pediatric Age

Francesca Sperotto and Matteo Di Nardo

Contents

J. Brierley et al. (eds.), *ESPNIC Children's Intensive Care Textbook*,
https://doi.org/10.1007/978-3-031-64762-8_31

Learning Objectives

After reading this chapter, the reader will be able to:

- Define ECPR.
- Define the main ECPR objective and its current indications within the pediatric population.
- Describe current ECPR epidemiology and outcomes in pediatric age.
- Define the most important ECPR peculiarities for specific pediatric subpopulations.
- Describe the most frequent cannulation strategies and the other components needed for a successful ECPR.
- Describe current ECPR algorithms and team organization.
- Describe features of optimal post-ECPR care.

31.1 Introduction

Survival after in-hospital cardiac arrest (CA) in children has improved significantly in the last decades [1–3]. In the intensive care units, current survival rates for pulseless and bradycardic arrests are 38% and 66%, respectively, and survival among pediatric patients with cardiac disease is around 50% [1–3]. Different factors have contributed to this trend, including the standardization and optimization of cardiopulmonary resuscitation (CPR) approaches and the improvement of postarrest care protocols [4, 5]. In parallel, the use of extracorporeal membrane oxygenation (ECMO) as a resuscitation strategy following conventional CPR (ECPR) has increased over time worldwide [6–9], likely contributing to the increased survival trend. In a nationwide study comparing cardiac patients who did or did not undergo ECPR, Lasa et al. demonstrated that patients receiving ECPR had higher odds of survival to discharge (odds ratio [OR] 2.80; 95% CI 2.13–3.69) and survival with favorable neurological outcome (OR 2.64; 95% CI 1.91–3.64) than patients who received only CPR [10]. This association persisted when the cohorts were analyzed using propensity-matching to adjust for baseline differences [10]. In the 2015 update of the pediatric resuscitation guidelines, the American Heart Association supported ECMO consideration as part of the resuscitation strategy, particularly in cardiac patients, when expertise and equipment are available [5].

In this chapter, we aim to review the ECPR definition, its objectives and indications, its epidemiology and outcomes, the main ECPR techniques including cannulation strategies, the most important peculiarities for specific ECMO populations, and details of post-ECPR care.

31.2 Definition of ECPR, Objective, and Indications

Extracorporeal cardiopulmonary resuscitation is defined as the rapid deployment of veno-arterial (V-A) ECMO or cardiopulmonary bypass (CPB) as a resuscitation strategy to provide oxygenation and cardiopulmonary support during or immediately following a CA when conventional CPR is unsuccessful in achieving a sustained return to spontaneous circulation (ROSC) [8, 11, 12]. Sustained ROSC is defined as the presence of a stable circulation for at least 20 min, with no need to restart chest compressions [13]. In 2018, ELSO additionally defined EPCR as the rapid deployment of V-A ECMO even within 20 min of ROSC without ongoing compressions [8].

The main objectives of ECPR are to provide an artificial return of circulation and adequate gas exchange—i.e., oxygenation and carbon dioxide removal—with the final aim of reducing ischemic injury to organs, especially the brain and the heart. In fact, while conventional CPR is able to provide only partial flow to organs, ECMO is usually able to provide a better flow similar to a normal cardiac output [14]. In this context, ECMO, in the form of ECPR, may provide:

- A bridge to recovery, as in the case of fulminant myocarditis.
- A bridge to therapy and recovery together, as in the case of sepsis, intoxications, or rewarming.
- A bridge to diagnostics and intervention, as in the case of the presence of significant residual lesions in post-cardiac surgery patients.
- A bridge to organ transplant, including heart and lung transplant.
- A bridge to placement of a ventricular assistance device (VAD), as in the case of cardiomyopathies or severe heart failure in congenital heart diseases.
- A bridge for transport.
- Less frequently, a bridge to palliative care or organ donation.

31.3 Epidemiology of ECPR

Since first reported in children by del Nido and Dalton in 1992 for the support of a patient with cardiac disease who experienced CA after pediatric cardiac surgery [11], the use of ECPR has continued to increase over time worldwide [6–8, 15]. According to the most recent ELSO Registry report, a total of 2261 neonatal and 5682 pediatric ECPR runs have been reported from 1992 to 2020, with a steady increase in number over time as depicted in ◘ Fig. 31.1 [8, 15]. In a recent study including all pediatric CPR events from 2000 to 2018 in the US reported to the Get With The Guidelines Resuscitation (GWTG-R) Registry, 9% of the pulseless CA cases and 4% of the non-pulseless CA cases were supported with ECMO [1]. A recent meta-analysis assessing trends of cardiac arrests among patients with cardiac disease admitted to the ICU showed that about 22% of the CA cases (95% confidence interval [CI], 14–33%) were supported with ECPR [3].

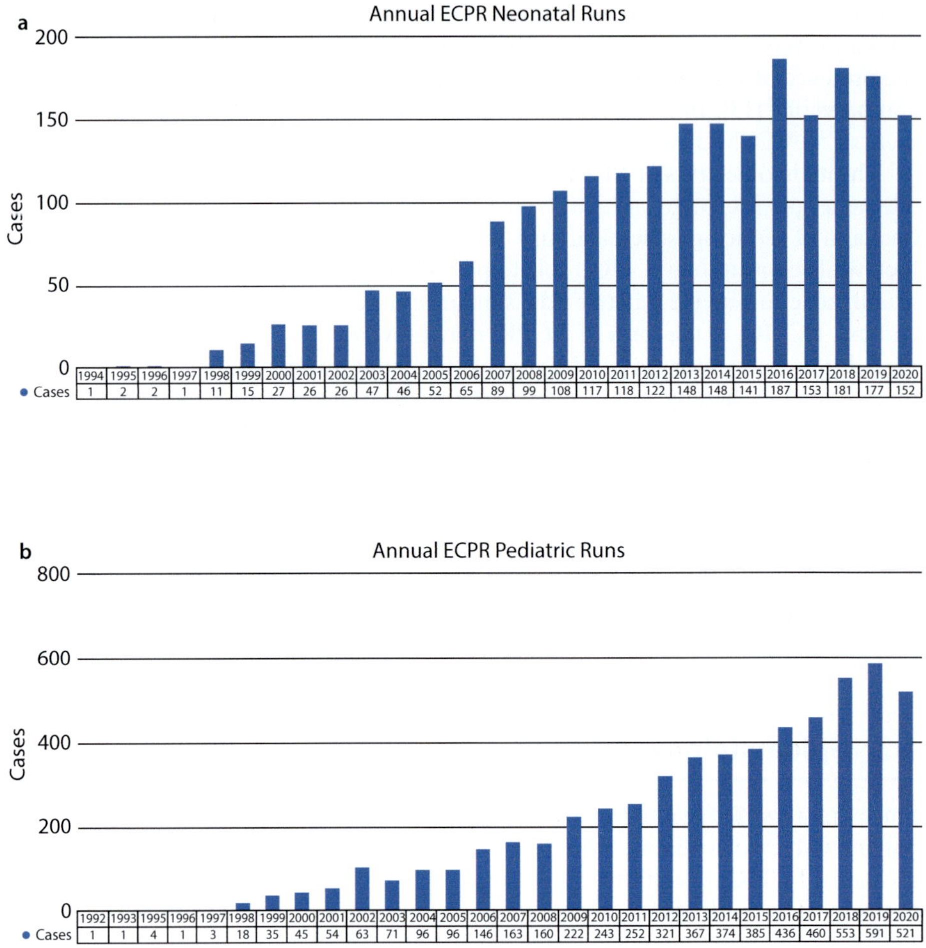

Fig. 31.1 Number of annual neonatal **a** and pediatric **b** ECPR runs reported to the ELSO International Registry from 1992 to 2020 (▶ https://www.elso.org/registry/internationalsummaryandreports.aspx)

31.4 Outcomes

Although outcomes after ECPR are still suboptimal compared to the outcomes of ECMO used for pediatric cardiac failure, data analyses have shown that ECPR may improve survival in refractory cardiac arrest compared to conventional CPR [10]. A large multicenter study summarizing data on ECPR events entered to the ELSO Registry from 1992 to 2005 reported a survival rate at hospital discharge of 38% [16]; 52% of the non-survivors died within 72 hours of ECMO initiation [16]. Data from the most recent ELSO Registry report (2021) showed that 70% of the reported neonatal cases from 1992 to 2020 survived at the time of decannulation and 42% at discharge; among the pediatric cases reported within the same period, 59% survived at the time of decannulation and 42% at the time of discharge [15]. Among neonates, survival at hospital discharge between 1998 and 2010 was 39% [17]. Similar results were found in a more recent study that combined data from the ELSO Registry and the AHA GWTW-R Registry (2010–2014), which showed a 41% survival rate at discharge. A recent meta-analysis that pooled data from 30 EPCR pediatric studies reported a pooled survival at hospital discharge of 44% (95% CI 40–47%). More recent data from the Asia Pacific ELSO Registry indicated an overall 51% survival rate although this does not show a clear increased trend of survival over time [18].

The main factors associated with increased mortality risk were low birth weight and prematurity [17], noncardiac diagnosis [19], pre-existing renal insufficiency [19, 20], sepsis [20, 21], low pH before cannulation [20–22], longer CPR duration before cannulation [19, 20], multiorgan failure [20, 23], and ECMO-related complications [6, 18, 20, 22, 24].

31.4.1 Neurologic Outcomes

Only a few studies have reported on neurologic outcomes following ECPR in pediatric age to date. A study investigating the prevalence and risk factors of severe acute neurologic injury among 682 EPCR pediatric patients found that 22% of them had brain death (11%), cerebral infarction (45%), or intracranial hemorrhage (7%). ECMO complications including pulmonary hemorrhage, use of dialysis, and CPR during ECMO support were all factors associated with an increased risk of acute neurologic injury [24]. Among patients with acute neurologic injury, the hospital mortality rate was 89%. A more recent single-center study investigating detailed neuroimaging data showed that, among patients who underwent at least one brain computed tomography (CT) or magnetic resonance imaging (MRI), 74% demonstrated at least one pathologic finding including hypoxic-ischemic injury in 47% and brain hemorrhage in 45% [23]. The degree of neurologic injury assessed by the modified Alberta Stroke Program Early Computed Tomography Score (mASPECTS) or its corresponding version for MRI was directly associated with in-hospital mortality or severe neurologic and functional outcome (functional status score (FSS)) at discharge [23]. Other factors associated with neurologic and functional outcome at discharge, when adjusting for baseline FSS, were single ventricle physiology, ECMO duration, and the mean Pediatric Logistic Organ Dysfunction-2 (PELOD-2) score in the first 28 days or up to the day of death when death occurred sooner [23]. A recent study using ELSO Registry data showed that factors associated with brain death were age >1 year, arterial blood carbon dioxide tension (PaCO2) value greater than 82 mmHg, and lactate greater than 15 mmol/L before ECMO cannulation, as well as persistence of lactate >3.9 mmol/L after ECMO cannulation [25]. Among survivors at hospital discharge, outcomes were described to be generally good, with 84% of patients being discharged home rather than to inpatient rehabilitation service in the first study [25], and a median functional status score (FSS) at discharge of 8 (interquartile range 6–8; with optimal FSS = 6) [23].

31.4.2 Medium and Long-Term Outcomes

Data on medium and long-term outcomes for pediatric ECPR patients are limited. A recent single-center study on pediatric cardiac patients showed that the survival rate at 6 months was 43%, with very good neurologic and functional outcomes described as an FSS equal to 6 (interquartile range 6–8, with optimal FSS = 6) [23]. Secondary analyses of the THAPCA trial showed that 41% of patients survived at 12 months.

Among these, 30% survived with a very good functional/behavioral status at 12 months (Vineland Adaptive Behavior Scale, second edition >70; with 100 = optimal), and 22% survived with a functional status similar to the pre-ECPR one (with ≤15 points variation) [26]. This demonstrated that, while many patients had favorable outcomes at 12 months, there was also a decline in some domains compared to pre-arrest baseline, with neurocognitive outcome scores lower than population means [26]. A call for a longitudinal ECMO-related functional follow-up has been raised recently and should apply to the ECPR population as well [27].

31.5 ECPR Peculiarities in Specific Populations

31.5.1 ECPR in Children with Cardiac Disease

Cardiac patients are at high risk of hemodynamic failure compared to healthy children [28, 29, 30] as a result of their propensity for myocardial dysfunction, arrhythmias, and hemodynamic instability. Children with congenital heart diseases often have circulation abnormalities, which include outflow tract obstructions, common mixing lesions, and intracardiac shunts; these lesions often lead to abnormal pressure or volume loading conditions, cyanosis, or congestive heart failure. Taken together, these factors increase the risk of CA, especially in the postoperative period after surgical correction or palliation. Additionally, the anatomical and physiological substrates of congenital heart disease can also influence the effectiveness and success of the conventional CPR strategy itself, especially in single ventricle patients and neonates [3, 29, 30]. For this reason, ECMO may be considered early for these patients, either in the pre-arrest phase, shortly during a CA, or shortly after ROSC if the risk of recurrent CA is particularly high [3, 29, 30]. In fact, as previously mentioned, in 2015 the American Heart Association advised consideration of EPCR in cardiac patients when expertise and equipment are available [5]. Recently pooled data showed that, in centers with ECMO expertise, up to a quarter of patients with cardiac disease in the ICU are supported with ECPR [3].

31.5.2 ECPR in Children with Noncardiac Disease

Among children with structurally normal hearts receiving EPCR, acute respiratory failure, sepsis, and pneumonia were found to be the most common baseline noncardiac diagnoses [21]. Overall, outcomes for ECPR were found to be worse in children with noncardiac diagnosis compared to those with cardiac disease, with a 31% in-hospital survival among medical noncardiac patients and a 20% survival among those with a surgical noncardiac diagnosis [6].

For some categories of patients with noncardiac diagnosis, ECPR may not be effective due to the baseline disease, such as pulmonary embolism, severe irreversible respiratory failure which impacts the likelihood of weaning from ECMO, severe forms of pulmonary hypertension, heart rhythm instability due to refractory severe hyperkalemia as in the case of tumor lysis syndrome or severe rhabdomyolysis, and certain types of drug overdose as calcium channel blockers. ECMO support should be considered early in the care plan for these cases [15].

31.5.3 Out-of-Hospital ECPR and ECPR for Deep Hypothermia

There is currently very limited data to support the use of ECPR in out-of-hospital cardiac arrest in children. Additionally, data in adults show inconsistent results in terms of increased survival compared to conventional CPR [31]. Therefore, EPCR for out-of-hospital cardiac arrest is not currently recommended in pediatric patients. Limited data exist also for pediatric ECPR in case of severe hypothermia (core temperature < 28 °C) as in cases of drowning, snow burial, or cold outdoor exposure, for which ECMO may serve as EPCR or as a rewarming strategy [32]. Survival rates of adult and pediatric patients supported with ECMO after drowning were reported to be around 23% in a study from the ELSO Registry, with worse outcomes for those who experienced pre-ECLS cardiac arrest [32]. However, pediatric-specific guidelines on this topic are currently missing.

31.6 Patient Selection and Factors Influencing EPCR Decision

Overall, high-quality ECPR is a complex intervention that is best suited for selected patient populations and should be delivered by organized systems with ECMO expertise [8]. ECMO deployment prior to CA may also be considered in high-risk populations, such as in patients with significant hemodynamic instability and in those for which chest compression will be unlikely successful, as patients with single ventricle physiology, significant systemic or pulmonary obstructive lesions, refractory ventricular fibrillation, or certain poisoning [8].

Patient selection should include a careful consideration of the following factors:

- Low birth weight: although it may be able to cannulate patients weighing <2 kg, the likelihood of survival is significantly lower for this category of patients [8, 17].
- Baseline diagnosis, particularly cardiac or noncardiac (the least having lower likelihood of survival [19]).
- Presence of pathologic parameters that may limit the effectiveness of conventional CPR (e.g., limited stroke volume with chest compressions, limited effective pulmonary blood flow and oxygenation with compressions, and limited cerebral perfusion). In the presence of any of these conditions, EPCR should be considered early [8, 12].
- Main indication: bridge to recovery, therapy, diagnostics or intervention, transplant, VAD, transport, palliative care, and organ donation.
- Presence of pathologic states that can limit the effectiveness of ECMO support such as significant aortic regurgitation, the presence of a large ductus arteriosus, or systemic to pulmonary shunts. In these cases, the risk/benefit of ECPR should be weighted very carefully, and strategies to address these lesions should be considered shortly after ECMO deployment.

The decision to offer or initiate ECPR should be based on the following:

- The expertise of the center.
- The availability of a trained team with adequate resources.
- The time needed to gather people, resources, and equipment at the bedside, with a suggested benchmark time being <30 or < 40 min [10, 12, 19].

31.7 Team and Algorithm

A highly coordinated team of expert-trained professionals remains one of the key elements to ensure rapid and successful deployment of ECMO for cardiopulmonary resuscitation. In ECPR institutions, a dedicated ECPR algorithm should summarize roles and collaborative interactions among team members with different expertise to facilitate the delivery of optimal ECPR care [8, 12].

Conventional resuscitation measures should be initiated by the first-line providers who should focus on delivering high-quality CPR [5], with minimal interruptions before and during ECMO deployment. A team calling system is usually used to efficiently mobilize a second team of individuals, who are skilled providers with rapid cannulation and preparation of the ECMO circuit (ECPR team). This team may vary in composition across systems and settings. Once the ECMO is deployed, care will be split among the patient—with particular attention to post-arrest care strategies [5]—and the circuit, to maintain adequate flow and avoid circuit and equipment-related complications [8, 12].

Given that ECPR is a low-volume high-risk event, simulation may be a useful strategy to maintain team efficiency [8, 12, 33]. Simulation may also be of help in optimizing institutional ECPR algorithm, with the inclusion of safety checklists, space maps for the organization of the location of the team and ECMO equipment, and specific institution-related features [8].

31.8 Cannulation Strategies and Equipment

Cannulation must be achieved rapidly and executed by a highly skilled team with expertise. Based on the patient's characteristics and setting, it may be achieved either peripherally or centrally. During cardiac compressions, peripheral cannulation is often associated with less frequent interruptions compared with central cannulation; however, to date, no evidence exists to support one approach over the other in pediatrics. Smaller patients, especially those with postsurgical correction/palliation with an open chest or a relatively fresh wound, are elected to be cannulated centrally [8, 12]. In patients with congenital heart diseases, cannulation strategies should be tailored to the baseline anatomy and physiology, as depicted in ◘ Fig. 31.2 [12].

a, **b**, and **c** show strategies for structurally normal hearts or biventricular circulation. **a** Central cannulation with venous access in the right atrium and arterial access in the aorta. **b** Peripheral cervical cannulation with venous access in the internal jugular vein and arterial access in the common carotid artery. **c** Peripheral femoral cannulation with venous access in the femoral vein and arterial access in the femoral artery. **d** and **e** show strategies for single ventricle patients after Stage 1 palliation: **d**. Stage 1 with central cannulation with venous access in the common atrium and arterial access in the aorta. **e** Stage 1 with peripheral cannulation with venous access in the internal jugular vein and arterial access in the common carotid artery. **f** and **g** show strategies for single ventricle patients after Stage 2 palliation: **f**. Stage 2 with central cannulation with venous access in the superior vena cava or in the common atrium and arterial access in the aorta. **g**. Stage 2 with peripheral cannulation with venous access with the internal jugular vein or femoral vein and arterial access with the common carotid

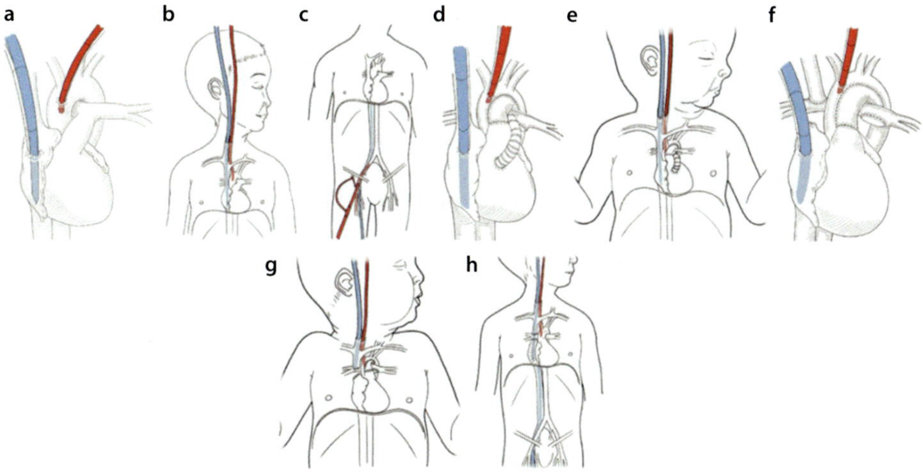

Fig. 31.2 ECMO cannulation strategies based on patient's cardiac physiology. (Pediatric Extracorporeal Cardiopulmonary Resuscitation ELSO Guidelines, ▶ https://www.elso.org/ecmo-resources/elso-ecmo-guidelines.aspx)

artery. **h** shows a potential strategy for cannulation of single ventricle patients after Fontan palliation: **h**. Peripheral cannulation with venous access in the internal jugular vein and or femoral vein with arterial access in the common carotid artery

31.9 Post-ECPR Care

Post-arrest care initiates immediately after the return of circulation and adequate gas exchange are achieved. Initially, the target pump blood flow is set by estimating the theoretical cardiac output for age and by the physiologic needs based on the underlying disease. The ECMO flow is then titrated to optimize end-organ perfusion and oxygen delivery and should therefore be followed by clinical observation of improvement of perfusion and neurologic function, by resolution of laboratory markers of acidosis and/or ischemia, as well as restoration of adequate urine output [8, 12]. Inotropic and vasoactive support should be weaned as tolerated. Post-arrest care should then mirror the current post-arrest guidelines [5], with attention to normoxemia (or appropriate oxygen saturation based on baseline heart disease), target temperature management (avoid fever), and hypoglycemia. Given that deep sedation is often required in pediatric patients on ECMO and neurologic clinical observation is often not possible, neuromonitoring should be considered in the post-arrest phase with continuous electroencephalogram [5, 8, 12].

Take Home Messages

- ECPR is defined as the rapid deployment of V-A ECMO or cardiopulmonary bypass as a resuscitation strategy to provide oxygenation and cardiopulmonary support during or immediately following a CA when conventional CPR is unsuccessful.

(continued)

- The main objectives of ECPR are to provide an artificial return of circulation and adequate gas exchange, with the final aim of reducing ischemic injury to organs.
- The use of ECPR has continued to increase over time worldwide, with various indications including the bridge to recovery, therapy, diagnosis, intervention, transplant, VAD, transport, palliative care, and organ donation.
- Survival of pediatric patients who underwent ECPR remains suboptimal, with survival rates ranging from 38% to 51%.
- ECPR peculiarities for different subpopulations exist and should be considered at the time of ECPR consideration. Data on these different subpopulations may also help prognostication.
- Cannulation strategies vary based on the baseline cardiac physiology.
- ECPR is a low-volume high-risk event that requires a highly coordinated team of experts and an institutional organization. Simulation may be a useful strategy to maintain the efficiency of high-performing teams.
- Post-ECPR care should target the optimization of end-organ perfusion, oxygen delivery, and restoration of organ function. Post-ECPR care should mirror the post-arrest guideline algorithms.

References

1. Holmberg MJ, Wiberg S, Ross CE, et al. Trends in survival after pediatric in-hospital cardiac arrest in the United States. Circulation. 2019;140:1398–408.
2. Berg RA, Nadkarni VM, Clark AE, et al. Incidence and outcomes of cardiopulmonary resuscitation in PICUs. Crit Care Med. 2016;44:798–808.
3. Sperotto F, Daverio M, Amigoni A, Gregori D, Dorste A, Allan C, Thiagarajan RR. Trends in In-Hospital Cardiac Arrest and Mortality Among Children With Cardiac Disease in the Intensive Care Unit: A Systematic Review and Meta-analysis. JAMA Netw Open. 2023;6(2):e2256178.
4. Kleinman ME, Chameides L, Schexnayder SM, et al. Part 14: Pediatric advanced life support: 2010 American Heart Association Guidelines for Cardiopulmonary Resuscitation and Emergency Cardiovascular Care. Circulation. 2010;122:876–908.
5. De Caen AR, Berg MD, Chameides L, et al. PALS pediatric resuscitation AHA 2015. Circulation. 2015;132:526–43.
6. Bembea MM, Ng DK, Rizkalla N, et al. Outcomes after extracorporeal cardiopulmonary resuscitation of pediatric in-hospital cardiac arrest. Crit Care Med. 2019;47:1.
7. Barbaro RP, Paden ML, Guner YS, et al. Pediatric extracorporeal life support organization registry international report 2016. ASAIO J. 2017;63:456–63.
8. Guerguerian A-M, Jacobs J, Laussen P, Thiagarajan R (2023) Extracorporeal cardiopulmonary resuscitation in children. In: ELSO red book, 6th ed. pp. 283–297.
9. Sperotto F, Daverio M, Amigoni A, Gregori D, Dorste A, Kobayashi RL, Thiagarajan RR, Maschietto N, Alexander PM. Extracorporeal Cardiopulmonary Resuscitation Use Among Children With Cardiac Disease in the ICU: A Meta-Analysis and Meta-Regression of Data Through March 2024. Pediatr Crit Care Med. 2024;25(10):e410–e417.
10. Lasa JJ, Rogers RS, Localio R, et al. Extracorporeal Cardiopulmonary Resuscitation (E-CPR) during pediatric in-hospital cardiopulmonary arrest is associated with improved survival to discharge. Circulation. 2016;133:165–76.
11. Del Nido PJ, Dalton HJ, Thompson AE, Siewers RD. Extracorporeal membrane oxygenator rescue in children during cardiac arrest after cardiac surgery. Circulation. 1992;86:300–4.
12. Guerguerian AM, Sano M, Todd M, et al. Pediatric extracorporeal cardiopulmonary resuscitation ELSO guidelines. ASAIO J. 2021;67:229–37.
13. Jacobs I, Nadkarni V, Bahr J, et al. Cardiac arrest and cardiopulmonary resuscitation outcome reports: Update and simplification of the Utstein templates for resuscitation registries. A state-

ment for healthcare professionals from a task force of the international liaison committee on resusci. Resuscitation. 2004;63:233–49.
14. Topjian AA, Berg RA, Nadkarni VM. Pediatric cardiopulmonary resuscitation: advances in science, techniques, and outcomes. Pediatrics. 2008;122:1086–98.
15. Extracorporeal Life Support Organization. ELSO Registry Report. October. 2021;2021:1–40.
16. Thiagarajan RR, Laussen PC, Rycus PT, Bartlett RH, Bratton SL. Extracorporeal membrane oxygenation to aid cardiopulmonary resuscitation in infants and children. Circulation. 2007;116:1693–700.
17. Mcmullan DM, Thiagarajan RR, Smith KM, Rycus PT, Brogan TV. Extracorporeal cardiopulmonary resuscitation outcomes in term and premature. Neonates. 2010:9–16.
18. Chen GL, Qiao YR, Ma JH, Wang JX, Hei FL, Yu J. Extracorporeal cardiopulmonary resuscitation in children of Asia Pacific: a retrospective analysis of extracorporeal life support organization registry. Chinese Med J. 2018;131(12):1436–43. https://doi.org/10.4103/0366-6999.233946.
19. Bembea MM, Ng DK, Rizkalla N, Rycus P, Lasa JJ, Dalton H, et al. Outcomes after extracorporeal cardiopulmonary resuscitation of pediatric in-hospital cardiac arrest: a report from the get with the guidelines-resuscitation and the extracorporeal life support organization registries. Crit Care Med. 2019;47:E278–85.
20. Sood N, Sangari A, Goyal A, Conway JAS. Predictors of survival for pediatric extracorporeal cardiopulmonary resuscitation: a systematic review and meta-analysis. Medicine (United States). 2022;101:E30860.
21. Conrad S, Bridges N, Kalra Y, Pietsch J, Smith A. Extracorporeal cardiopulmonary resuscitation among patients with structurally normal hearts. ASAIO J. 2017;63:781–6.
22. Melvan JN, Davis J, Heard M, et al. Factors associated with survival following extracorporeal cardiopulmonary resuscitation in children. World J Pediatric Cong Heart Surg. 2020;11:265–74.
23. Sperotto F, Saengsin K, Danehy A, et al. Modeling severe functional impairment or death following ECPR in pediatric cardiac patients: planning for an interventional trial. Resuscitation. 2021;167:12–21.
24. Barrett CS, Bratton SL, Salvin JW, Laussen PC, Rycus PT, Thiagarajan RR. Neurological injury after extracorporeal membrane oxygenation use to aid pediatric cardiopulmonary resuscitation. Pediatric Crit Care Med. 2009;10(4):445–51. https://doi.org/10.1097/PCC.0b013e318198bd85.
25. Joye R, Cousin VL, Wacker J, et al. Death by neurologic criteria in children undergoing extracorporeal cardiopulmonary resuscitation: retrospective extracorporeal life support organization registry study, 2017–2021. Pediatr Crit Care Med. 2024;25(3):e149–57.
26. Meert K, Guerguerian A, Barbaro R, et al. Therapeutic Hypothermia After Pediatric Cardiac Arrest (THAPCA) Trial Investigators: extracorporeal cardiopulmonary resuscitation: one-year survival and neurobehavioral outcome among infants and children with in-hospital cardiac Arrest. Crit Care Med. 2019;47:393–402.
27. Wray J, Kakat S, Brown K, Callaghan MO, Thiruchelvam T, Hoskote A. Childhood extracorporeal membrane oxygenation survivors: parents highlight need for structured follow-up and support after hospital discharge. Pediatric Crit Care Med. 2020;21(5):461–8.
28. Lowry AW, Knudson JD, Cabrera AG, Graves DE, Morales DLS, Rossano JW. Cardiopulmonary resuscitation in hospitalized children with cardiovascular disease: Estimated prevalence and outcomes from the Kids' Inpatient database. Pediatr Crit Care Med. 2013;14:248–55.
29. Marino BS, Tabbutt S, MacLaren G, et al. Cardiopulmonary resuscitation in infants and children with cardiac disease. Circulation. 2018;137:691–782.
30. Sperotto F, Gearhart A, Hoskote A, et al. Cardiac arrest and cardiopulmonary resuscitation in pediatric patients with cardiac disease: a narrative review. Eur J Pediatr. 2023;182(10):4289–308.
31. Holmberg MJ, Geri G, Wiberg SG, et al. Extracorporeal cardiopulmonary resuscitation for cardiac arrest: a systematic review. Resuscitation. 2018;131:91–100.
32. Burke CR, Chan T, Brogan TV, et al. Extracorporeal life support for victims of drowning. Resuscitation. 2016;104:19–23.
33. Sawyer T, Burke C, Mcmullan DM, et al. Impacts of a Pediatric Extracorporeal Cardiopulmonary Resuscitation (ECPR) simulation training program. Acad Pediatr. 2019;19:566–71.

Mechanical Circulatory Support in Paediatric Heart Failure

Emma Simpson, Teresa Chila', and Aparna Hoskote

Contents

J. Brierley et al. (eds.), *ESPNIC Children's Intensive Care Textbook*,
https://doi.org/10.1007/978-3-031-64762-8_32

Learning Objectives

- To know the role of mechanical circulatory support (ventricular assist device) and the indications for use in the paediatric population.
- To know the complications of VAD therapy and how these are prevented and managed.
- To know the principles of the management of anticoagulation on VAD.
- To have an awareness of the multidisciplinary care of a child on VAD.
- To know the issues surrounding the home discharge of a child on VAD.
- To know the outcomes for a child on VAD and to define high-risk populations.

32.1 Introduction

The first successful paediatric ventricular assist device (VAD) implantation occurred in 1989 when a 9-year-old boy underwent successful heart transplantation after 12 h of support with a Biomedicus™ centrifugal pump [2].

The introduction of pneumatic extracorporeal devices for paediatric patients into routine clinical practice began in 1991 when an 8-year-old child was supported with an adult-sized VAD until successful transplantation at the Deutsches Herzzentrum in Berlin [3].

Subsequently, miniaturised paracorporeal (outside the body) pumps and cannulae for long-term support of small children and infants became available. Progressively better outcomes were demonstrated as experience grew within Europe. FDA approval for the US market occurred in December 2011, following the publication of the multicentre compassionate use North American experience with Berlin Heart EXCOR™ study [4]. Off-label application and compassionate use of support devices still play a crucial role in paediatric VAD practice.

Paediatric VADs are now an established therapy for end-stage heart failure, improving the condition and survival of children awaiting heart transplantation. Despite a limited range of pumps, it is possible to provide support for months and years.

VAD support is considered in any child with end-stage acute or chronic cardiac failure inadequately managed by medicines. The pathology may be inherited, acquired and idiopathic cardiomyopathy, myocarditis or congenital heart disease. Myocarditis has a greater likelihood of cardiac recovery, thus avoiding transplant, but the diagnosis can only be confirmed on cardiac muscle biopsy (usually taken at the time of VAD implantation). Heart transplants can be done in all age groups, but waiting times can be long due to low donation rates, matching an individual's blood group, tissue typing and size. If a patient accumulates morbidity during the VAD course, the transplant may no longer be an option.

The timing of implantation is crucial. Early VAD implantation, performed before the establishment of multiple organ impairment, offers survival benefits. However, premature VAD insertion can be seen as exposing the child for longer to the risk of device-related morbidity, but restoring adequate circulation is fundamental to improving long-term outcomes.

32.2 Part 1: VAD Support

32.2.1 Choice of Support Strategy: ECMO versus VAD

ECMO is available in many paediatric institutions to manage cardiac and respiratory failure, via peripheral or central cannulation. Unless there is an impending risk of cardiac arrest, ECMO is not the best option to support a child with progressive or acute heart failure in the medium or long-term. Patients placed on ECMO will initially demonstrate a stunned left ventricle with no effective ejection, leading to the need for decompression of the left chambers via the surgical vent, atrial septostomy or Impella™ device in as many as 30% of cases [5], to avoid pulmonary venous hypertension and pulmonary haemorrhage.

VAD therapy facilitates effective ventricular unloading and, compared to ECMO, causes less thrombogenic/inflammatory stimulation due to the absence of the oxygenator. Due to secure cannulation, durable VADs offer better patient mobility and comfort. VAD can therefore be used more successfully for cardiac support that is required for longer than a couple of weeks.

32.2.2 Types of VAD

VADs relevant to the paediatric population are summarised in ▫ Table 32.1. Images are seen in ▫ Fig. 32.1.

Paracorporeal (outside the body) continuous flow VAD is currently the most widely adopted option for short-term support, (e.g. in the context of myocarditis, acute graft failure or infants with single ventricle lesions) or as a bridge to durable support if the suitability and/or duration of support is unclear. A myocardial biopsy can be obtained at implantation to guide the decision-making progress.

Intracorporeal (inside the body) continuous flow VAD (e.g. HeartMate 3) and paracorporeal pulsatile flow (e.g. Berlin Heart EXCOR TM - Figure 32.1a and intracorporeal (inside the body) continuous flow VAD (e.g. HeartMate 3) Fig 32.1b are most widely used for long-term support in children.

32.2.3 Selecting the Right Type of VAD

Durable intracorporeal devices, e.g. HeartMate 3 carry the lowest risk of stroke; however, in addition, the choice of the type of device depends upon the following:

Patient-related factors: body surface area (therefore, blood flow need), anatomy, urgency (INTERMACS profile), the prospect of recovery/transplantation, expected time on support and LVAD or BIVAD.

Centre experience: PICU and surgeon expertise, availability and technical support.

Short-term devices are often used for stabilisation of deteriorating patients (INTERMACS 1 or 2), as a bridge to long-term device, decision or recovery. This is due to ease of implant and cost. Other advantages are fine-tuning of flow and the

Table 32.1 Ventricular assist devices currently in use in paediatric populations

Short-term device	Centrimag™
	Impella® (Abiomed, Danvers, Massachusetts)
	TandemLife Protek Duo (TPD; TandemLife, Pittsburgh, PA)
Long-term	Berlın Heart EXCOR®
	Jarvik 2000 infant Jarvik 2015
	HeartWare[a]
	HeartMate 3 (Abbott Corporation, Abbott Park, IL)
	Syncardia TAH

[a]HeartWare device was withdrawn from open market in June 2021

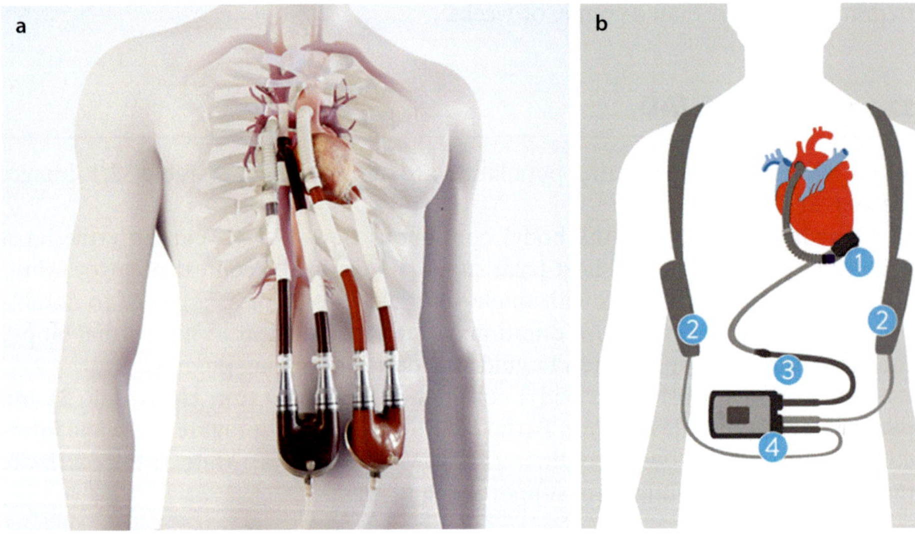

Fig. 32.1 **a** Berlin Heart EXCOR BIVAD. **b** HeartMate 3

opportunity to temporarily add an oxygenator. The duration can be stretched longer than 6 weeks (if required by the clinical setting), and these devices can be used as a bridge to transplant. The off-label use of tunnelled, durable cannulae combined with a paracorporeal continuous flow pump (e.g. Levitronix Centrimag™ pump with Berlin Heart cannulae) is a possible way of managing children with challenging anatomy [6].

32.3 Part 2: Devices/Strategies LVAD, BiVAD and UVAD

32.3.1 Strategies and Applications

Most paediatric VAD implants are performed when heart failure causes end-organ dysfunction (renal, gastro or hepatic) despite inotropic support or following ECMO. The pre-implant profile of the patient can be described by the INTERMACS classification: (1) critical cardiogenic shock; (2) progressive decline; (3) stable but inotrope dependent and (4) resting symptoms or less sick [7].

32.3.2 Right Ventricular Dysfunction

The decision to support only the left ventricle (LVAD) or both ventricles (BiVAD) begins in the preoperative setting using echocardiography, with a qualitative assessment of the RV function.

The provisional plan of LVAD-only support can change at the following times:

- At implant in theatre, if the child fails to wean from CPB.
- In the early postoperative course, if the child remains unstable despite medical optimisation, including high inotropic support and afterload reduction for the RV.
- In the late postoperative course, if the child remains on inotropic support.

Approximately, 40% of LVAD recipients develop RVD and need inotropic RV support and a longer intensive care admission. RV dysfunction is defined as the use of an LVAD with an elevated central venous pressure (>16 mm Hg) with inotropic therapy and/or inhaled nitric oxide for longer than 96 hours or the need for a BIVAD [8]. This can be caused by the effect of the CPB on the RV, the increase in RV preload following LV implant, higher pulmonary vascular resistance in patients with restrictive physiology or suboptimal decompression of the LV. Refractory RVD can require an RVAD implant at the second stage. If BIVAD is used as a rescue therapy, this leads to the poorest outcomes. Having two pumps increases the risk of infection and clot formation, and two periods of CPB increases postoperative bleeding [8].

32.3.3 Single-Ventricle Anatomy

Univentricular VAD (UVAD) is a VAD that supports the systemic ventricle in a functionally single-ventricle circulation. Single-ventricle circulation compared with biventricular physiology does not increase the risk of death before transplant or before hospital discharge [9]. However, the use of MCS in single-ventricle patients remains a challenge due to complex anatomy and abnormal physiology.

32.3.4 Recovery and Explant

About 10-15% of children supported with VAD recover and undergo VAD explants. This depends on the underlying aetiology, with the infant age group and myocarditis or repaired coronary artery anomalies having a better chance of recovery [10].

Anti-failure treatment is started (ACE inhibitor; angiotensin II receptor blocker; angiotensin receptor/neprilysin inhibitor; carvedilol; spironolactone), and ventricular function is monitored. If improvement in ventricular performance is noted, the child undergoes a clinical and echocardiographic assessment while progressively decreasing VAD support. A cardiac catheterisation study may also be performed. After a successful stress test, decommissioning or explant of VAD occurs as soon as possible.

32.3.5 Destination Therapy

DT is the use of a VAD to prolong life and allow discharge home when heart transplantation is contraindicated or not desired [11]. Suitable patients include those with Duchenne muscular dystrophy, children with chemotoxicity-induced cardiomyopathy with ongoing malignancy, those with re-transplantation graft dysfunction in the setting of noncompliance and children with neurological impairment and uncertain outcome [11].

32.4 Part 3: Anticoagulation

32

One of the most critical aspects of VAD therapy is the management of bleeding and the prophylaxis and treatment of thrombosis.

Similar to ECMO, there exists a wide variation in anticoagulation protocols across different VAD centres. Manufacturers' recommendations are often extrapolated from adult experience, and most of the paediatric studies are observational in design [12, 13].

Despite the differences between centres in terms of the primary anticoagulant, the antiplatelet agent(s), the method of monitoring and therapeutic range targeted, the threshold for intervention on a clot and the way that bleeding is managed, there are several principles of good management which are almost universally agreed.

Principles of Anticoagulation Management

1. Ensure excellent surgical haemostasis [14, 15].
2. Correct coagulopathy and address bleeding before starting anticoagulants [15].
3. Proactive surveillance for thromboses in the VAD system, particularly in the initial phase [16].
4. Minimise blood trauma by using well-designed systems and avoid excessive shear and turbulence [15].
5. Consider patient factors which would confer high bleeding/thrombosis risk and tailor the anticoagulation plan in the light of this [15].
6. Ensure adequate platelet numbers before starting an antiplatelet agent [15].
7. Monitor and treat hypertension [17].
8. Increase vigilance during and after febrile illness, which is a high-risk time for both bleeding and thrombosis [15, 16].

Many centres historically used heparin (unfractionated or low-molecular-weight) and are now using direct thrombin inhibitors, which are potentially superior, to establish initial anticoagulation and thereafter switch to an oral vitamin K antagonist when feeding is established [13, 18]. Usually, antiplatelet agent(s) will be used and monitored using platelet mapping or specialised thromboelastography, e.g. Multiplate™.

32.4.1 Detection of Thrombosis

In the Berlin Heart EXCOR™ pump, thrombotic deposits are most often directly visualised at the artificial valves of the pump (see ◘ Image 32.1) [19]. In the intracorporeal devices, elevated lactate dehydrogenase, increased plasma free haemoglobin, decreased haptoglobin, increased unconjugated bilirubin and haematuria strongly suggest LVAD thrombosis, and these usually occur before device changes such as increased power consumption, altered flow and low pulsatility index or the nonspecific signs on echocardiography are seen [20]. Management includes increasing anticoagulation, tissue plasminogen activator or device exchange, depending on the situation.

32.5 Part 4: Patient Management and Outcomes

One of the goals of VAD therapy is to improve end-organ function prior to transplant. The early timing of VAD implantation is important since pre-implant cardiogenic shock, mechanical ventilation, liver congestion and renal dysfunction are independently associated with mortality but can be difficult to achieve in the paediatric age group where patients frequently present in a perilous state [21–24]. In one large study of paediatric patients on the EXCOR device, 24% had suffered a recent cardiac arrest and 40% had VAD implantation following ECMO [24]. Survival outcomes have improved in recent years for children <10 kg, but those weighing <5 kg remain at higher risk of mortality [24–26] (◘ Fig. 32.2). Children who have VAD following surgery for CHD then ECMO are an especially high-risk group, because of a poor pre-implant state and the technical challenges [23].

32.5.1 Thrombotic and Bleeding Complications

Cardiopulmonary bypass, surgical incisions and exposure of blood components to artificial surfaces activate the coagulation and complement systems [27]. Embolic and haemorrhagic strokes occur despite biocompatible pump components and 'optimal management' of anticoagulation. One-third of children having an embolic stroke on VAD sustain a severe or fatal brain injury. Others can show significant recovery or only mild disability [28, 29]. Uncommonly, infarcted areas of the brain can undergo a haemorrhagic transformation; see ◘ Image 32.2.

Bleeding can occur at other sites, commonly the mediastinum (potentially causing tamponade), nasopharynx and gastrointestinal (GI) tract. Nasopharyngeal bleeding may require cautery and/or nasal packing. Gastrointestinal bleeding can result from upper GI stress ulceration, intestinal ischaemia and reperfusion injury. Patients on con-

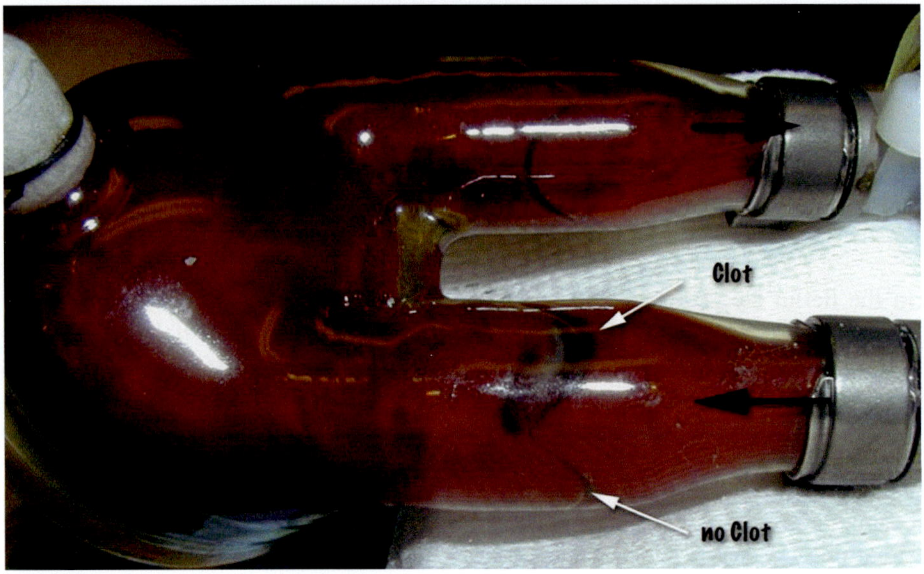

Image 32.1 Clot in Berlin Heart ventricle

tinuous flow (cfVAD) devices are at risk of gastrointestinal angiodysplasia and acquired Von Willebrand syndrome [30]. Angiodysplasia affects 28–40% of adults with long-term cfVAD and is less likely with greater pulse pressure and aortic valve opening [31].

32.5.2 Optimising Haemodynamics

32

VAD settings should be adjusted to achieve decompression of the ventricles, neutral interventricular septum and minimal mitral regurgitation [32]. In a borderline patient, fluid overload or sepsis can precipitate RV decompensation [8]. Regular echocardiography informs that atria are not dilated, valves are competent, pericardial fluid collections are resolving and cannula position is such that the likelihood of damage to valve apparatus, suctioning and stasis are minimised. Intermittent opening of the aortic valve will reduce the risk of thromboembolism. To maximise chances of recovery, ventricles should be unloaded, interventricular septum normally positioned, cardiac arrhythmias treated, blood pressure controlled and oral anti-failure drug treatments established. Adjustments to settings ensure support keeps up with the needs of growth and activity.

32.5.3 Nursing and Multi-professional Care

Meticulous care must be taken of the driveline or cannula exit site(s). Dressings and fixation devices must secure the cannula/driveline to the abdominal skin to prevent movement which would irritate the tissues and promote infection [33]. Image 32.3 shows the grades of cannula site infection which can be seen [34]. Capable parents can be trained to do their own child's dressings very competently and to a high standard of asepsis.

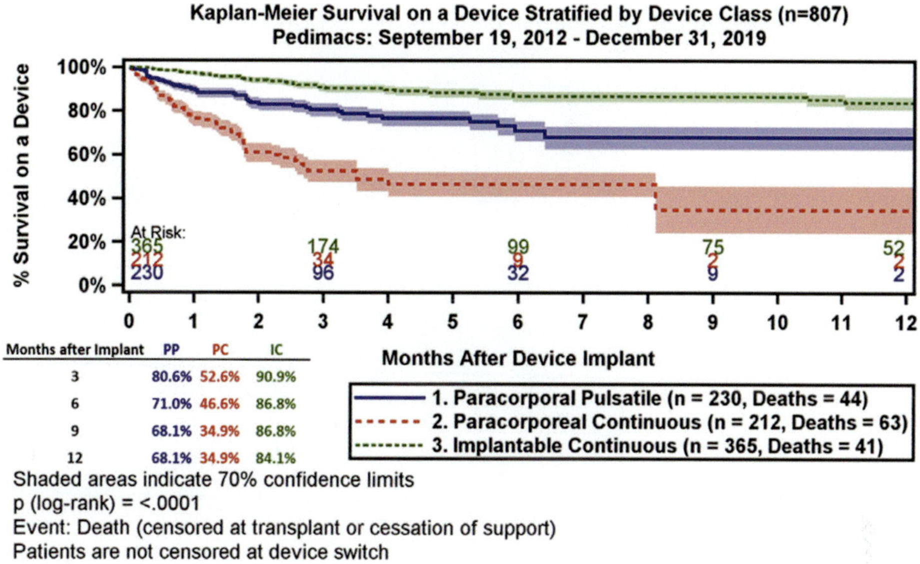

Fig. 32.2 Survival according to Patient Weight

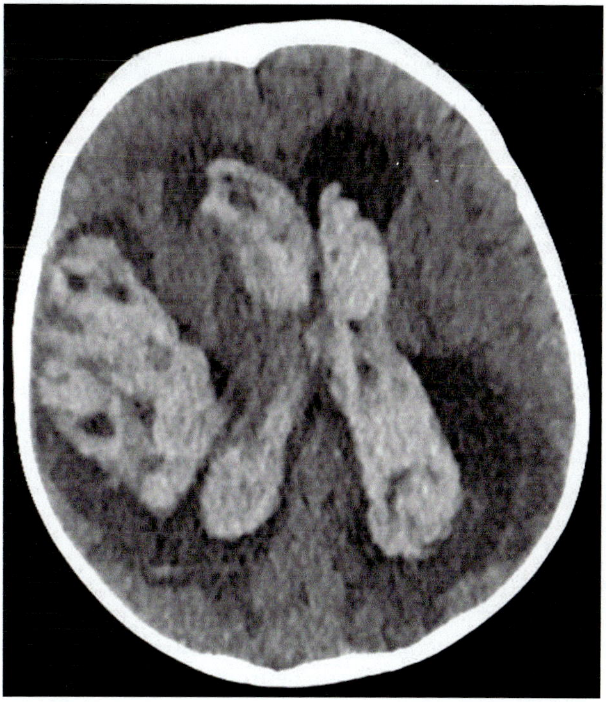

Image 32.2 Fatal cerebral bleed

Wound Classification of VAD-specific Berlin Heart® EXCOR BIVAD Cannula Infection
Grade 0 No signs of skin irriation. No fluid drainage. No tenderness.
Grade 1 Slight skin irritation with redness. Beginning of tenderness and slight wound drainage.
Grade 2 Early skin retraction. Wound drainage. Extension of hyperthermic redness around the cannulas.
Grade 3 Hypertrophic granulation/ granuloma pyogenicum. Sever wound drainage. Skin tenderness and pain around the cannula exit sites
Grade 4 Extensive wound granulation with subsequent skin arosion. Open wounds around the cannulas. Extreme tenderness and pain.

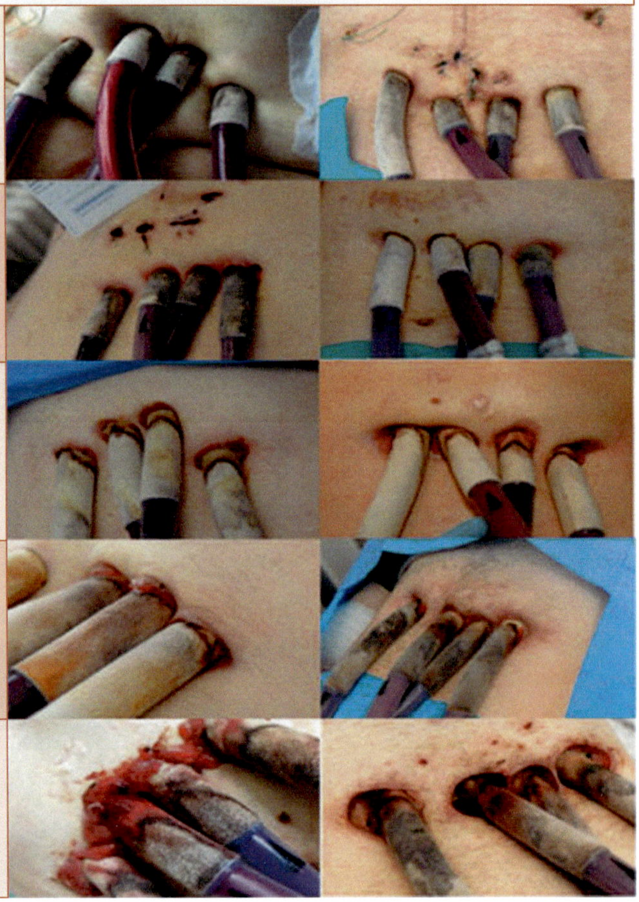

Image 32.3 Classifications of wound infection

Physical rehabilitation should begin as early as possible by a specialist therapy team to ensure safe mobility and graded exercise for these deconditioned children, who may also require support with nutrition, psychological help and specialist seating and adaptations.

32.5.4 Outcomes

Mortality and morbidity outcomes depend on device and patient factors. Although many problems can be overcome, severe neurological injury or multi-organ failure can occur such that successful transplantation is not possible. Cerebrovascular events are less frequent with intracorporeal durable continuous flow devices (8.9% incidence at 6 months) compared to paracorporeal continuous flow devices (30.5%) or paracorporeal pulsatile devices (17.2%) [35]. A low stroke rate makes survival to transplant more likely (see Fig. 32.3), and the overall risk profile is

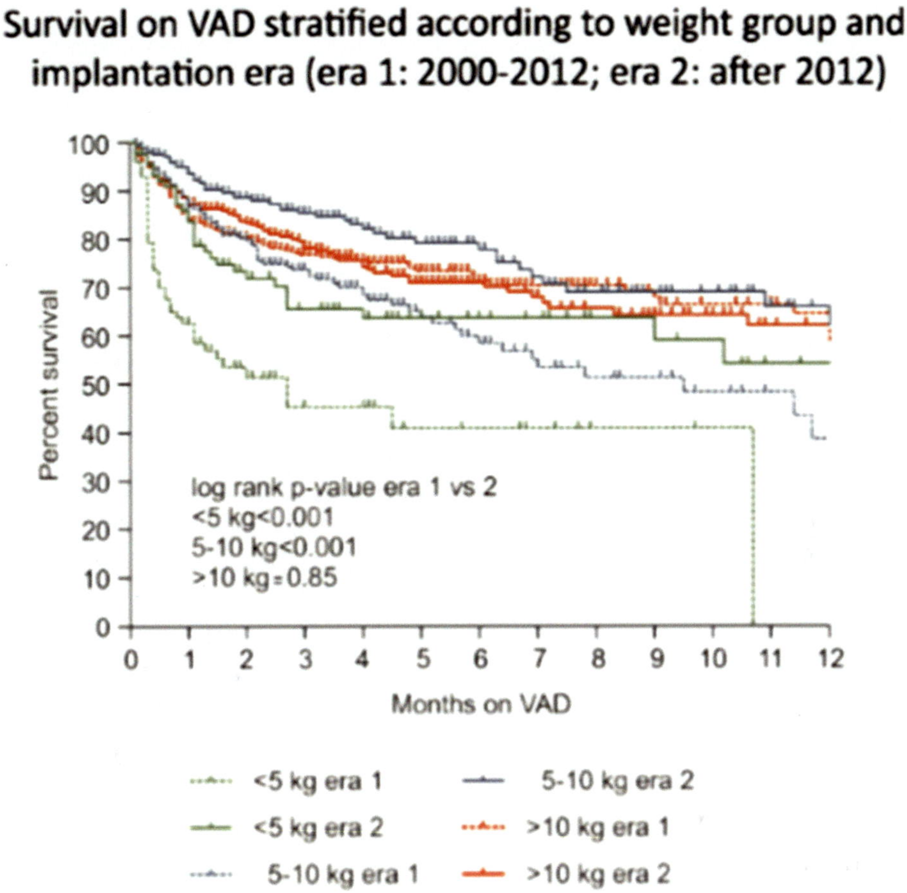

Fig. 32.3 Survival Curve for Different Types of VAD

usually more favourable in this older age group. Longer support time awaiting an organ increases the period of risk.

Case Studies

Case 1

A previously well 13-month-old girl presented with cardiac failure and was stabilised with ventilation and inotropes, avoiding end-organ dysfunction. The initial support strategy was tracheostomy, ventilation and milrinone. She deteriorated further with lung congestion so durable LVAD cannulas were implanted in the LV apex and aorta and were attached to the Levitronix Centrimag™ pump.

Endocardial biopsy showed moderate endocardial fibroelastosis and mild interstitial fibrosis with mild inflammation suggestive of active mild lymphocytic myocarditis. Anticoagulation was challenging due to inflammation and recurrent thrombotic

(continued)

deposits in the circuit despite heparin, aspirin and clopidogrel. She required nasojejunal feeding and had recurrent Gram-positive infection.

After 3 weeks, a stress test showed that her heart function had recovered enough to support her circulation without VAD, and the LVAD was explanted. Heart function showed continued improvement, and over the next few months, she began feeding normally and her tracheostomy was removed.

Myocarditis is an inflammatory disease of the myocardium diagnosed by endomyocardial biopsy (EMB) using established histological, immunological and immunohistochemical criteria [41].

The causes of myocarditis are heterogeneous (mostly viral in children). The course and outcome of the illness in the paediatric population represent a complex interaction between etiologic agents and the immune system, which is still not fully understood.

The clinical presentation and course vary widely from mild illness to acute refractory heart failure, arrhythmia, chest pain and sudden death [42].

The incidence of adverse events including death and heart transplantation is about 13%. Therapeutic options are antiarrhythmic, immunosuppression, circulatory support, intravenous immunoglobulin and antivirals. ECMO support is necessary in about 7% and VAD in 1.5% of the children with myocarditis [42].

Case 2

A 16-year-old boy with Becker muscular dystrophy presents with dilated cardiomyopathy and vitamin D deficiency. His chest pain and fatigue progressed despite digoxin, lisinopril and diuretics, and he was listed for heart transplantation. He was subsequently admitted with abdominal pain, lethargy and poor perfusion. The echocardiogram showed bi-atrial enlargement and severely impaired biventricular function. There was a clot at the LV apex, and he was started on unfractionated heparin (Platelet count 300,000).

32

Despite inotropes, he had further deterioration, so he underwent evacuation of LV clot and implantation of a Heartware™ LVAD. Heartware™ data showed a flow of 3.5–5.2 L/min (CI 2–3), 2400 RPM and power 2.8 W. The bleeding settled and he was restarted on unfractionated heparin. The following day, the platelet count fell from 100,000 to 61,000. On POD #2, he was extubated and had a platelet transfusion (platelet count 75,000). The following day, there were subtle signs of left-sided weakness and improving drowsiness. Prothrombin time was 17 s, activated partial thromboplastin time was 183 s, normal serum fibrinogen and anti-factor Xa was 0.18, so fresh frozen plasma was given.

On POD #4, there was a sudden increase in power to 5.7 W lasting 5 h. Six hours later, the flow increased to 9 and then remained at >10 (power 5 W). Heparin was changed to bivalirudin while awaiting the results of a HIT screen (subsequently positive). Haemolysis was evident and D dimers 2351. On the echocardiogram, a laminar thrombus was seen in the apex. He became drowsy and developed a haemothorax. A pump exchange was planned pending normal CT of the brain. Sadly, this showed a large right parieto-occipital infarct with oedema and a small left frontal haemorrhage. Despite therapeutic bivalirudin (APTT 70-100), there was a rapid power rise to 25 W, and suddenly, the Heartware stopped. During CPR, he was cannulated for V-A ECMO

(continued)

and taken for LA decompression (LAP 50). Unfortunately, he sustained severe end-organ damage, and intensive care was subsequently withdrawn.

This case highlights catastrophic bleeding and thrombotic consequences of heparin-induced thrombocytopenia in the early postoperative period of implantable ventricular assist device ◘ Image 32.4.

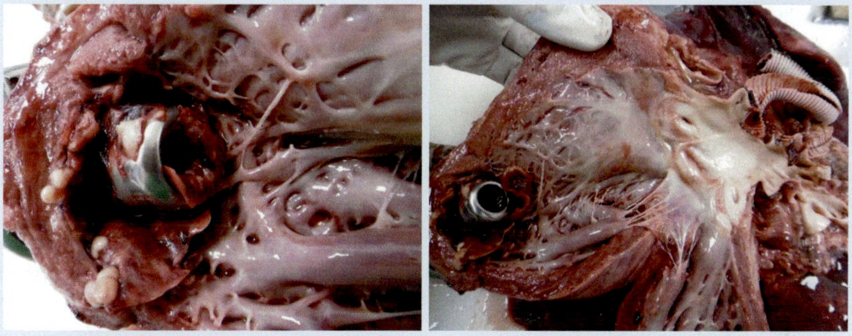

◘ **Image 32.4** Post-mortem photograph of thrombosed HeartWare outflow graft

Case 3

A 14-year-old boy presented to his local hospital with 1 weak history of palpitation, vomiting and diarrhoea, initially managed as acute abdomen. He was found to have cardiomyopathy and on arrival at the tertiary paediatric hospital, he was in cardiogenic shock. Atrial tachyarrhythmia was suspected as a cause of the cardiomyopathy. He was cannulated for V-A ECMO and underwent an electrophysiology study and ablation. He was listed for a heart transplant. While on ECMO, the end-organ function improved, but his left ventricular function did not improve despite the return of sinus rhythm. A week later, he underwent an LVAD Heartmate 3™ implant. After a month of recovery and parent training on Heartmate 3™ management, he was transferred first to the hospital accommodation and then home. He was readmitted to hospital twice over a year due to drive line infection and also treated for depression [43]. After 14 months, he successfully underwent a heart transplant.

Case 4

A 1-year-old girl presented to her local hospital with 2 weeks history of cough, lethargy and diarrhoea. On examination, she was found *in extremis*, pale, with cold peripheries and increased work of breathing. A chest XR revealed cardiomegaly. She was started on nasal CPAP and milrinone infusion. She was transferred to a tertiary paediatric hospital where MCS was available. On arrival at the cardiac PICU, she was intubated with the ECMO team on standby. She was started on adrenaline infusion, sedated, muscle relaxed and kept nil by mouth. Her echocardiogram showed severe biventricular impairment. She had liver and renal impairment. The following morning, she underwent a BiVAD Berlin Heart EXCOR™ implant and was listed for a heart transplant. She was weak and cachectic, so underwent a tracheostomy 2 weeks after

(continued)

the implant. This facilitated sedation and ventilation weaning. She was transferred to the cardiology ward on a mobile ventilator and established on warfarin and aspirin. She was able to attend physiotherapy and engage in developmental play. She could leave the ward in a pram and go to the hospital Café with her parents.

About 3 months after the VAD implant, she was successfully transplanted. During the transplant, she was nasally intubated to allow a clean surgical field and extubated within a few days.

Summary

Paediatric ventricular assist devices are an essential component of heart failure management for children who require bridging to heart transplant or recovery. Well-timed implantation occurs before there is substantial end-organ damage, using a device strategy tailored to the patient's condition and postoperative care by an expert and multidisciplinary team. Good outcomes can be achieved as long as serious complications are avoided, and holistic care is important for families since VAD therapy can entail months in the hospital or discharge home on the device.

32.6 Part 5: Palliative and Holistic Care

Many programmes have professionals supporting the family, and engaging a palliative care team early can have advantages such as future care planning and a greater degree of psychological and family support [36]. The approach taken is 'parallel planning', in which the patient undergoes full active treatment without limitations, and at the same time, palliative care principles are employed such as symptom management, enabling the fulfilment of life experiences, and if appropriate, the family is supported to have an open discussion of their wishes if the worst should happen [37]. The key principles of full disclosure and open and honest communication of the risks of embarking on mechanical support and the path to transplant are essential so that families are fully informed and have realistic expectations. This, in turn, increases the likelihood that they will accept the support they need through this difficult journey.

32.6.1 Home Discharge

Stress and lifestyle restrictions are huge drivers to designing VADs that are portable and enable children who are stable to be discharged home. In doing so, parents and carers take on responsibility for the technology keeping their child alive, and they are likely to need psychological, social and practical support to be able to do this. Some families are unable to cope with the responsibility, for a variety of reasons, despite it seeming like the obvious solution to the problem of a prolonged hospital stay [38]. But for the majority of children and young people, home discharge allows participation in their usual social and educational life [39].

Take-Home Messages

- *Timing of Support Affects Outcome.*
  The outcome is better if VAD implantation occurs before organ failure becomes established. Converting from ECMO to VAD support can only be done if lung function is good enough.
- *Optimise Settings.*
  Settings are adjusted so good cardiac output is provided, without pulmonary oedema, stasis or haemolysis and with left ventricular offloading to encourage recovery of native function.
- *Stroke Risk-Reduction Measures Are Crucial.*
  Reducing the risk of stroke while on VAD requires meticulous attention to anticoagulation, infection prevention and blood pressure control.
- *Holistic Care of the Patient, Education and Rehabilitation Are Important.*
  The care of a VAD patient requires a multidisciplinary approach involving various professionals: intensivist, microbiologist, haematologist, cardiologist, physiotherapist, play therapist, psychologist, occupational therapist, teacher, community teams and a palliative care team for parallel planning.
- *Home Discharge Is Possible.*
  It is possible to discharge home a patient on intracorporeal VAD. This requires education and technical training of the patient and his/her carers with a comprehensive care package and close monitoring.

Questions

1. True or false—bowel ischaemia is unlikely after VAD insertion?
2. How is VAD cannulation different from ECMO cannulation?
3. True or false: the number of blood transfusions a patient has during the VAD course can limit their opportunities for heart transplants.
4. How do I know if the heart has recovered function and no longer needs VAD?
5. Can a patient have a cardiac arrest while on LVAD?

Answers

1. False. Bowel ischaemia may happen due to thromboembolism from the LVAD device or ischaemia-reperfusion. Sedation-related gastroparesis and high venous pressure due to RV failure are also a cause of bowel dysfunction, slow transit and feed intolerance in the postoperative period.
2. ECMO cannula takes blood from the RA (or SVC/IVC) and returns it to the aorta. In contrast, a left-sided VAD takes blood from the LV (or LA, in selected cases) and returns it to the aorta. Right-sided VAD takes blood from the RA and returns it to the main pulmonary artery. This means that pulmonary vascular resistance and the ability of the lungs to perform gas exchange are important in VAD. In addition, VAD is better at decompressing the left heart.
3. True. Exposure to multiple blood donors and homografts used in the repair of congenital heart lesions can cause HLA sensitisation, and this can limit the number of suitable organs. Addressing bleeding and haemolysis promptly and help-

ing the patient to increase their own red cell population will reduce the need for blood products. Desensitisation is a possibility for some patients.

4. A stress test is an evaluation of the ventricular function that can be performed while on VAD to assess the recovery and the likelihood of a successful VAD explantation. Protocols vary according to the type of VAD. Multiple echocardiograms are performed while reducing/pausing the VAD for a specified time period. To prevent clots, anticoagulation may be increased while the VAD flow is stopped or decreased. The VAD can be explanted or decommissioned (turned off while remaining inside the patient).
5. Acute mechanical failure or obstructive thrombosis can stop LVAD. Aside from this, the LVAD relies on the RV for preload. A patient on LVAD can suffer cardiac arrest if, following an acute deterioration of the RV function or a pulmonary hypertensive crisis, the LVAD preload has a sudden decrease. Optimisation of the RV starts preoperatively with the reduction of RV dilatation and optimisation of preload (diuretics), afterload (iNO and sildenafil), contractility (inotropic support) and rhythm control. Then, in the peri-implantation phase, a 'normal', rather than an excessive, LVAD output will ensure decompression of the left ventricle and prevent an acute increase in RV preload [30]. If cardiac output cannot be restored, VAD patients should have chest compressions performed despite a risk of bleeding, cannula/device displacement and major vessel rupture [40].

References

1. Stein ML, Dao DT, Doan LN. Ventricular assist devices in a contemporary pediatric cohort: Morbidity, functional recovery, and survival. J Heart Lung Transplant. 2016;35(1):92–8.
2. Frazier DH, Bricker JT, Macris MP, Cooley DA. Use of a left ventricular assist device as a bridge to transplantation in a pediatric patient. Tex Heart Inst J. 1989;16(1):46.
3. Warnecke H, et al. Mechanical left ventricular support as a bridge to cardiac transplantation in childhood. Eur J Cardiothorac Surg. 1991;5:330–3.
4. Morales DL, Almond CS, Jaquiss RD. Bridging children of all sizes to cardiac transplantation: the initial multicentre North American experience with the Berlin Heart EXCOR ventricular assist device. J Heart Lung Transplant. 2011;30(1):1–8.
5. Canter CE, Simpson KE. Diagnosis and treatment of myocarditis in children in the current era. Circulation. 2014;129(1):115–28.
6. Chen PC, Zea-Vera R, Burgman C, McKenzie ED, Elias B, Adachi I. Use of an extracorporeal centrifugal pump with the Berlin cannulas. ASAIO J. 2019;65(5):527–9.
7. Stevenson LW, Pagani FD, Young JB. INTERMACS profiles of advanced heart failure: the current picture. J Heart Lung Transplant. 2009;28(6):535–41.
8. Karimova A, Pockett CR, Lasuen N. Right ventricular dysfunction in children supported with pulsatile ventricular assist devices. J Thorac Cardiovasc Surg. 2014;147:1691–7.
9. De Rita F, Hasan A, Haynes S. Mechanical cardiac support in children with congenital heart disease with intention to bridge to heart transplantation. Eur J Cardiothorac Surg. 2014;46:656–62.
10. Tominaga Y, Ueno T, Kido T, Kanaya T, Narita J, Ishida H, Toda K, Kuratani T, Sawa Y. Bridge to recovery with Berlin Heart EXCOR in children <10 kg with dilated cardiomyopathy: a histological analysis. Eur J Cardiothorac Surg. 2020;58(2):253–60.
11. VanderPluym CJ, Fynn-Thompson F, Blume ED. Ventricular assist devices in children progress: with an orphan device application. Circulation. 2014;129:1530–7.
12. May LJ, Lorts A, VanderPluym CJ. Marked practice variation in antithrombotic care with the Berlin heart excor pediatric ventricular assist device. ASAIO J. 2019;65(7):731–7.
13. Miera O, Schmitt KL, Akintuerk H. Antithrombotic therapy in pediatric ventricular assist devices: multicenter survey of the European EXCOR Pediatric Investigator Group. Int J Artif Org. 2018;41(7):385–92.

14. Eckman PM, John R. Bleeding and thrombosis in patients with continuous-flow ventricular assist devices. Circulation. 2012;125:3038–47.
15. Leebeek FWG, Muslem R. Bleeding in critical care associated with left ventricular assist devices: pathophysiology, symptoms, and management. Hematol Am Soc Hematol Educ Program. 2019;2019(1):88–96.
16. Maeda K, Almond C, Hollander SA. Characteristics of deposits and pump exchange in the Berlin Heart EXCOR ventricular assist device: experience with 67 cases. Pediatr Transplant. 2018;2018:e13181.
17. Villa CR, VanderPluym CJ. ABCs of stroke prevention. Circ Cardiovasc Qual Outcomes. 2020;13:e006663.
18. Zafar F, Conway J, Bleiweis MS, Al-Aklabi M, Ameduri R, Barnes A, Bearl DW, Buchholz H, Church S, Do NL, Duffy V, Dykes JC, Eghtesady P, Fisher L, Friedland-Little J, Fuller S, Fynn-Thompson F, George K, Gossett JG, Griffiths ER, Griselli M, Hawkins B, Honjo O, Jeewa A, Joong A, Kindel S, Kouretas P, Lorts A, Machado D, Maeda K, Maurich A, May LJ, McConnell P, Mehegan M, Mongé M, Morales DLS, Murray J, Niebler RA, O'Connor M, Peng DM, Phelps C, Philip J, Ploutz M, Profsky M, Reichhold A, Rosenthal DN, Said AS, Schumacher KR, Si MS, Simpson KE, Sparks J, Louis JS, Steiner ME, VanderPluym C, Villa C, ACTION Learning Network Investigators. Berlin Heart EXCOR and ACTION post-approval surveillance study report. J Heart Lung Transplant. 2021;40(4):251–9.
19. Maeda K, Almond C, Hollander SA. Characteristics of deposits and pump exchange in the Berlin Heart EXCOR ventricular assist device: experience with 67 cases. Pediatr Transplant. 2018;22(4):e13181.
20. Bartoli CR, Ghotra AS, Pachika AR, Birks EJ, McCants KC. Hematologic markers better predict left ventricular assist device thrombosis than echocardiography or pump parameters. Thorac Cardiovasc Surg. 2014;62(05):414–8.
21. Almond CS, Morales DL, Blackstone EH. Berlin Heart EXCOR pediatric ventricular assist device for bridge to heart transplantation in US children. Circulation. 2013;127:1702–11.
22. Zhigalov K, Van den Eynde J, Chrosch T. Outcomes of left ventricular assist device implantation for advanced heart failure in critically ill patients (INTERMACS 1 and 2): a retrospective study. Artif Org. 2021;45(7):706–16.
23. Morales DLS, Zafar F, Almond CS. Berlin Heart EXCOR use in patients with congenital heart disease. J Heart Lung Transplant. 2017;36(11):1209–16.
24. Morales DLS, Rossano JW, VanderPluym C. Third annual pediatric interagency registry for mechanical circulatory support (pedimacs) report: preimplant characteristics and outcomes. Ann Thorac Surg. 2019;107(4):993–1004.
25. Miera O, Morales DL, Thul J. Improvement of survival in low-weight children on the Berlin Heart EXCOR ventricular assist device support. Eur J Cardiothorac Surg. 2019;55(5):913–9.
26. Fouilloux V, El Louali F, Gran C, Henaine R, Roubertie F, Chenu C, Fiorini M, Le Bel S, Mauriat P, Neidecker J, Macé L, Kreitmann B, Ovaert C. Berlin Heart EXCOR paediatric ventricular assist device: does weight matter? Heart Lung Circ. 2021;30(4):585–91.
27. Yeh T, Kavarana MN. Cardiopulmonary bypass and the coagulation system. Prog Pediatr Cardiol. 2005;21(1):87–115.
28. Jordan LC, Ichord RN, Reinhartz O. Neurological complications and outcomes in the Berlin Heart EXCOR® pediatric investigational device exemption trial. J Am Heart Assoc. 2015;4(1):e001429.
29. Rohde S, Sandica E, Veen K, Miera O, Amodeo A, Napoleone CP, Özbaran M, Sliwka J, Thiruchelvam T, Zimpfer D, Schubert S. Cerebrovascular accidents in paediatric patients supported by the Berlin Heart EXCOR. Eur J Cardiothorac Surg. 2022;62(3):ezac381.
30. Uriel N, Pak SW, Jorde UP. Acquired von Willebrand syndrome after continuous-flow mechanical device support contributes to a high prevalence of bleeding during long-term support and at the time of transplantation. J Am Coll Cardiol. 2010;56(15):1207–13.
31. Crow S, John R, Boyle AM. Gastrointestinal bleeding rates in recipients of nonpulsatile and pulsatile left ventricular assist devices. J Thorac Cardiovasc Surg. 2009;137(1):208–15.
32. Hayashi H, Naka Y, Sanchez J. Consequences of functional mitral regurgitation and atrial fibrillation in patients with left ventricular assist devices. J Heart Lung Transplant. 2020;39(12):1398–407.
33. Zinoviev R, Lippincott CK, Keller SC. In full flow: left ventricular assist device infections in the modern era. Open Forum Infect Dis. 2020;7(5):ofaa124.

34. Kremer J, El-Dor A, Rivinius R, Schlegel P, Sommer W, Warnecke G, Karck M, Ruhparwar A, Meyer AL. Wound infections in adult patients after Berlin Heart® EXCOR biventricular assist device implantation. Life. 2022;12:1550.
35. Ashfaq A, Lorts A, Rosenthal D, Adachi I. Predicting Stroke for Pediatric Patients Supported with Ventricular Assist Devices: A Pedimacs Report. Ann Thorac Surg. 2024;118(4):889-897.
36. McKenna M, Clark SC. Palliative care in cardiopulmonary transplantation. BMJ Support Palliat Care. 2015;5(1):427–34.
37. Sidgwick P, Fraser J, Fortune P. Parallel planning and the paediatric critical care patient. Arch Dis Child. 2019;104:994–7.
38. Crowe L, Simpson E, Reinhardt Z. Parental responsibility for pediatric ventricular assist devices: views of families on the acceptability of hospital discharge. Pediatr Transplant. 2020;24(1):e13636.
39. Petruik C, Mack C, Conway J. Talking with caregivers of children living in the community with ventricular assist devices. Pediatric Transplant. 2017;2017:e13049.
40. Esangbedo ID, Yu P. Chest compressions in pediatric patients with continuous flow ventricular assist devices: case series and proposed algorithm. Front Pediatr. 2022;10:883320.
41. Richardson P, McKenna RW, Bristow M. Report of the 1995 World Health Organization/International Society and Federation of Cardiology Task Force on the definition and classification of cardiomyopathies. Circulation. 1996;93:841–2.
42. Pomiato E, Perrone MA, Palmieri R. Pediatric myocarditis: what have we learnt so far? J Cardiovasc Dev Dis. 2022;9(1):143.
43. Diaz I, Thurm C, Hall M, Auerbach S, Bearl DW, Dodd DA, Mettler BA, Smith AH, Fuchs DC, Godown J. Disorders of adjustment, mood, and anxiety in children and adolescents undergoing heart transplantation and the association of ventricular assist device support. J Pediatr. 2020;217:20–4.

Cardiac Arrhythmias: Diagnosis and Management for the Paediatric Intensivist

Angela Aramburo and Leonie Wong

Contents

J. Brierley et al. (eds.), *ESPNIC Children's Intensive Care Textbook*,
https://doi.org/10.1007/978-3-031-64762-8_33

Learning Objectives

- Understand the normal cardiac conduction system
- Structured approach to the electrocardiogram
- Recognise the substrate and risk factors for arrhythmias
- Understand the mechanism of common paediatric arrhythmias
- Appropriate initial management of common paediatric arrhythmias in the paediatric intensive care unit (PICU)

Cardiac arrhythmias may pose a significant haemodynamic threat to the paediatric patient. Not only extremes in heart rates and/or the loss of atrioventricular (AV) synchrony can greatly compromise the cardiac output, but sustained tachycardias can also lead to heart failure and cardiomyopathy in an otherwise healthy child. The immediate postoperative period is an especially vulnerable time for the development of arrhythmias, and therefore, the paediatric intensivist should be comfortable in their recognition and initial management. This chapter will offer a general approach to the diagnosis and treatment of the most commonly seen cardiac arrhythmias in the PICU.

33.1 Normal Cardiac Conduction

33.1.1 Electrical Anatomy of the Heart

To understand cardiac arrhythmias, it is often helpful to first appreciate the basic electrical anatomy of the heart and how the normal sinus rhythm is generated (Fig. 33.1). The physical contraction of the heart results from the coordinated electrical activation of myocardial cells in the atria and ventricles. The atria and ventricles are electrically separated by the fibrous rings of the mitral and tricuspid valves, and

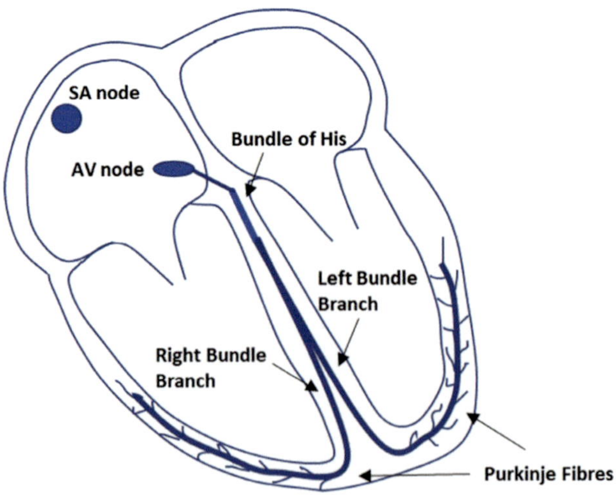

Fig. 33.1 Anatomy of the cardiac conduction system. *SA node* sino-atrial node, *AV node* atrioventricular node

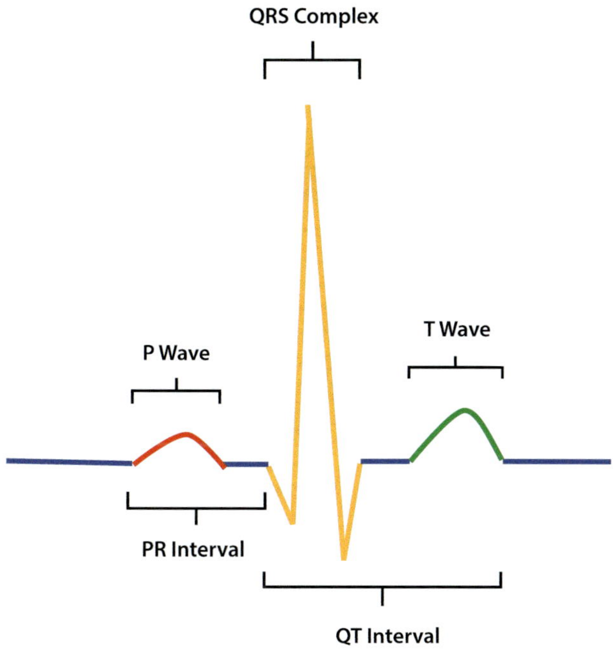

Fig. 33.2 Components of the surface ECG

usually, the only pathway for atrioventricular (AV) conduction is via the AV node. The electrical impulse originates at the sinoatrial (SA) node and initially propagates through the atria, resulting in atrial contraction. This is visualised as the P wave on a surface electrocardiogram (ECG) (Fig. 33.2). The electrical impulse is then transmitted through the AV node which accounts for the AV nodal conduction delay, reflected as the isoelectric PR interval on the ECG. The electrical impulse is then conducted to both ventricles via specialised fast-conducting tissue comprising the Bundle of His, left and right bundle branches and Purkinje fibres. This causes near simultaneous contraction of both ventricles, represented as the QRS complex on the ECG. The subsequent relaxation of the ventricles is seen on the ECG as the T wave.

33.1.2 ECG Recording in PICU

The *12-lead ECG* is the conventional way of recording the electrical activity of the heart. A standard 12-lead ECG comprises three standard limb leads (I, II and III), three augmented limb leads (aVL, aVR and aVF) and six precordial (or chest) leads (V1–V6). The limb electrodes are placed on the right upper and lower limbs, respectively. The precordial electrodes are positioned as shown in Fig. 33.3. V1 and V2 are positioned right and left parasternal in the 4th intercostal space. V4 is in the 5th intercostal space in the midclavicular line, and V5 and V6 are in line with V4 in the anterior and mid-axillary lines, respectively. The 12-lead ECG is normally recorded at a speed of 25 mm/s with a voltage gain of 10 mm/mV (i.e. 1 mm square represents 40 ms (0.04 s) on the horizontal axis and 0.1 mV on the vertical axis).

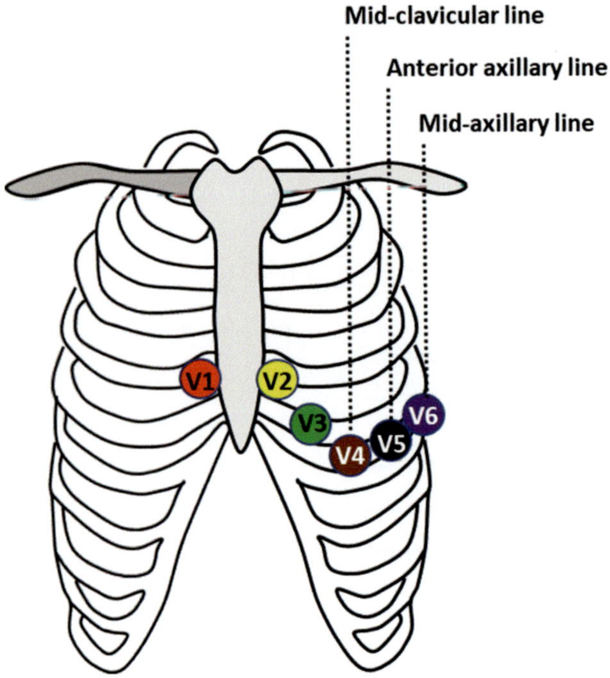

Fig. 33.3 Precordial electrode positioning for a 12-lead ECG

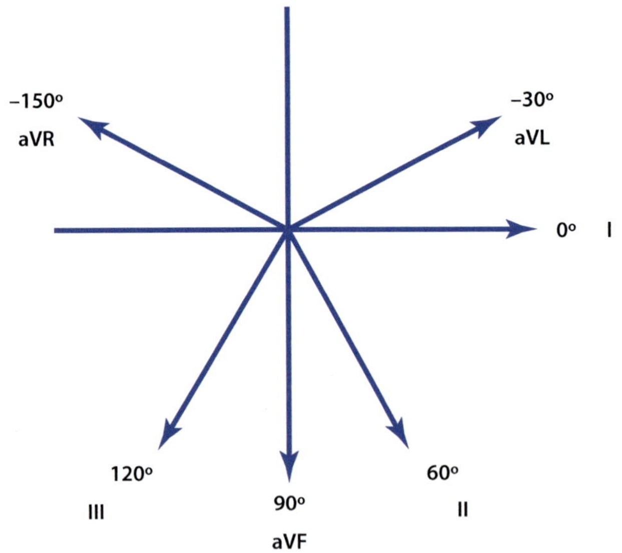

Fig. 33.4 Relationship of the limb leads to the cardiac axis

Analysis of the 12-lead ECG consists of a structured approach, with an initial assessment of the rate, rhythm and axis (Fig. 33.4). The heart rate should be determined to either be appropriate for age and clinical status or inappropriately fast or slow. It is helpful to identify if the rhythm is regular or irregular. The amplitude, duration and axis of the P wave, QRS complex and T wave should be evaluated. A sinus P wave should have an axis of 0–90°, reflected as positive deflections in leads I and aVF. QRS duration can be used to classify the rhythm as narrow or broad complex, while a deviated QRS axis can be secondary to ventricular hypertrophy or fascicular block. Inverted T waves can be a sign of ischaemia or strain. The measurement of the PR, QRS and QT intervals can also identify the presence of conduction or repolarisation abnormalities. Normal age-related values for ECG measurements in the paediatric population have been published in the literature [1–3].

There are other specific considerations with regard to ECG recording in cardiac patients in PICU. A 12-lead ECG should be performed prior to any cardiac intervention which would provide a baseline comparison for future ECGs. Postoperatively, a 12-lead ECG is needed to document the heart rhythm and any changes in cardiac conduction. For example, there may be evidence of AV block or a new bundle branch block after cardiac surgery. For patients with temporary cardiac pacing wires, an atrial wire study (or 12-lead ECG with atrial electrograms) should be performed. This 12-lead ECG recording is done by connecting the temporary atrial pacing wire(s) to the limb leads or precordial leads, thus augmenting the P wave and identifying the relationship between atrial and ventricular depolarisation. We would recommend obtaining a unipolar atrial electrogram by connecting the atrial pacing wire to lead V1 (or arm lead) and recording a 3-lead or 12-lead rhythm strip to allow simultaneous display of both the atrial electrogram and surface ECG, which helps to discriminate atrial from ventricular activity. This is particularly useful when P waves are not clearly visible on the standard 12-lead ECG and can help differentiate between different forms of tachyarrhythmias, particularly junctional ectopic tachycardia (JET) which is commonly seen in the postoperative period following cardiac surgery. An example of a rhythm strip showing a unipolar atrial electrogram is shown in ◘ Fig. 33.5.

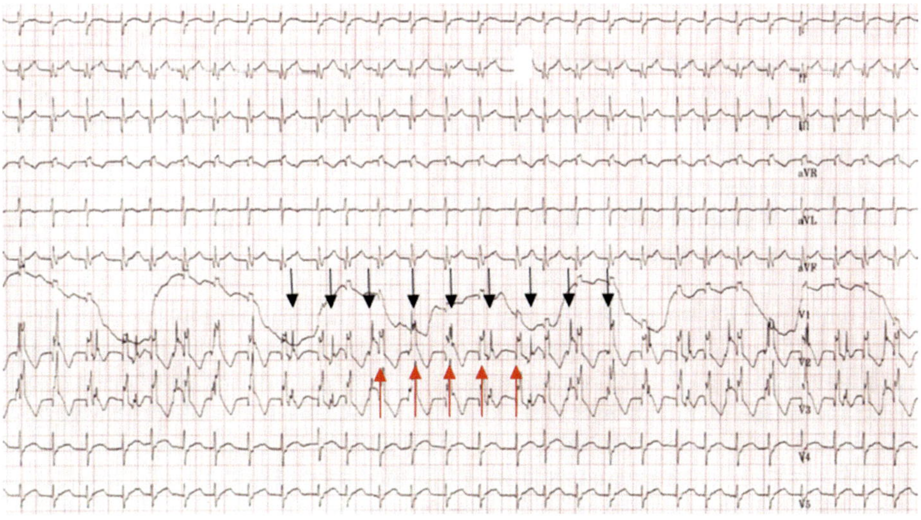

◘ **Fig. 33.5** 12-lead rhythm strip with atrial electrograms (lead V2 and V3) showing junctional ectopic tachycardia. Narrow complex tachycardia with VA dissociation. Faster ventricular activity is denoted by red arrows and atrial activity by black arrows

Cardiac telemetry is a 3-lead ECG that enables continuous real-time monitoring of the cardiac rate and rhythm both at the bedside and remotely. It is an essential tool in PICU patients as it not only allows the heart rate profile to be visualised over a defined time period but also captures any episode of paroxysmal arrhythmia that may be short-lived or asymptomatic and hence, less amenable to being documented with a standard 12-lead ECG. Telemetry can be individually set up with specific heart rate limits and rhythm criteria to alert the clinical team to significant episodes of arrhythmia relevant to the clinical situation, and it should always be reviewed as part of the investigations of a child with arrhythmia.

33.2 Mechanism of Cardiac Arrhythmias

Within the PICU setting, there are several factors which may contribute to the development of cardiac arrhythmias:

1. Direct trauma from surgery
2. Myocardial oedema and inflammation
3. Mechanical irritation from indwelling cardiac catheters or wires
4. Increased sympathetic tone
5. Use of adrenergic or arrhythmogenic drugs
6. Electrolyte disturbances
7. Hypoxaemia and acidosis
8. Haemodynamic instability
9. Structural substrate—i.e. cardiomyopathy and fibrosis

Understanding the underlying mechanism of a cardiac arrhythmia not only leads to a more definitive diagnosis but also guides the ongoing management of the patient as it allows more specific and targeted treatment. Most tachycardias are due to re-entry or abnormal automaticity. Less commonly, tachycardias can be secondary to triggered activity.

Re-entry tachycardias account for most of the tachycardias seen in the paediatric population. It results from and continues to be maintained by the propagation of an excitation wave-front around a distinct circuit. The requirements for re-entry include the following:

1. An anatomical circuit
2. An area of unidirectional block
3. An area of slow conduction

Different cardiac cells within the circuit conduct electrical impulses with different velocities. There is, however, a duration of time after a cardiac cell is excited when it cannot be re-excited. This is termed the refractory period. The ability of a circuit to sustain a re-entrant tachycardia depends on the relative conduction velocities and refractory periods of the different components. Re-entry is usually initiated by an atrial or ventricular premature beat which then propagates around the circuit in one direction and arrives back at the point of origin after its refractory period to re-excite those cells, setting up a self-propagating excitation wave-front that continuously goes around the same circuit in a loop. Interruption of the re-entry circuit should terminate the tachycardia by disrupting the continued propagation of the depolarising wave-front. An example of re-entry tachycardia is atrioventricular re-entry tachycardia (AVRT) which is secondary to the presence of an accessory pathway. In orthodromic AVRT, which is the most common form of supraventricular tachycardia in children, the anatomical circuit comprises the atrium, AV node, ventricle and accessory pathway. The area of slow conduction is in the AV node, and the area of unidirectional block can occur in the accessory pathway. An atrial premature beat propagates anterogradely from the atrium to the ventricle across the AV node and then retrogradely across the accessory pathway from the ventricle to the atrium, setting up the re-entry circuit (◘ Fig. 33.6). Other tachyarrhythmias resulting from a re-entry mechanism include AV nodal re-entry tachycardia (AVNRT), atrial flutter, macroreentrant atrial tachycardias and some forms of ventricular tachycardias. Re-entry tachycardias can be terminated by pacing or direct current (DC) cardioversion. Re-entry tachycardia involving the AV node as part of the circuit can be terminated by momentarily blocking the AV node with adenosine.

Automaticity refers to the ability of a cardiac cell to spontaneously depolarise and initiate an electrical impulse. All cardiac cells can initiate an electrical impulse, but only a few specialised cells do so spontaneously on a 'routine' basis and act as pacemakers. In the normal heart, the sinus node is the main cardiac pacemaker with the highest intrinsic rate of depolarisation and is thus the main determinant of the heart rate. Abnormal automaticity results in ectopic foci of tachycardia and can be secondary to myocardial ischaemia, electrolyte disturbances, hypoxia or sympathetic stimulation. Automatic (or ectopic) tachycardias include atrial ectopic tachycardia,

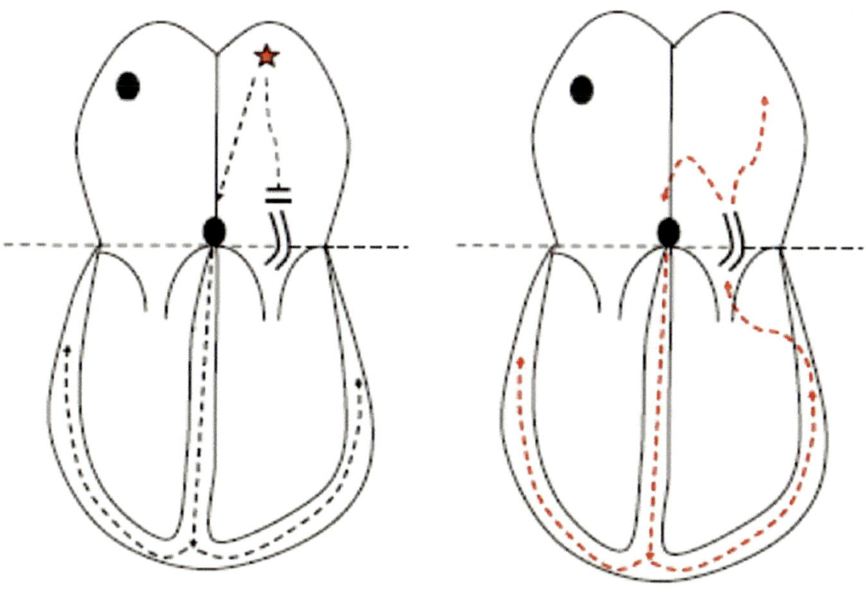

◘ **Fig. 33.6** Orthodromic AVRT. An atrial ectopic (denoted by star) initiates re-entry tachycardia with antegrade conduction down the AV node and retrograde conduction via the accessory pathway

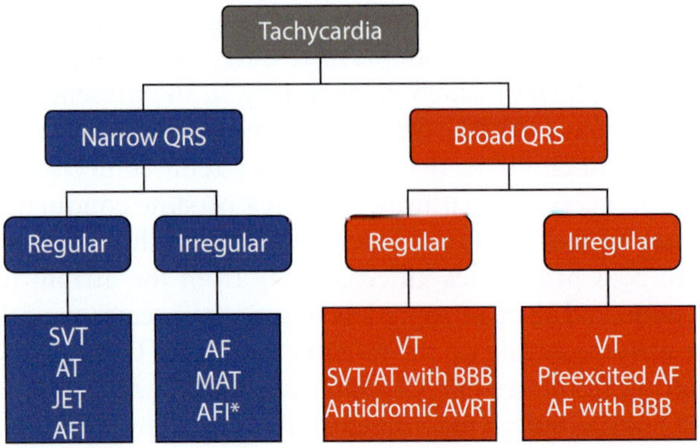

Fig. 33.7 Differential diagnosis of tachyarrhythmias. *SVT* supraventricular tachycardia, *AT* atrial tachycardia, *JET* junctional ectopic tachycardia, *AFl* atrial flutter, *MAT* multifocal atrial tachycardia, *AF* atrial fibrillation, *VT* ventricular tachycardia, *BBB* bundle branch block, *AVRT* atrioventricular re-entry tachycardia. *Atrial flutter can result in an irregular rhythm due to variable AV conduction

junctional ectopic tachycardia and some forms of ventricular tachycardia. Unlike re-entry tachycardias, automatic tachycardias cannot be terminated with pacing or DC cardioversion but can be suppressed with overdrive pacing.

Triggered activity is the least common mechanism for tachyarrhythmias. Depolarisation of a cardiac cell can be triggered by an early (EAD) or delayed (DAD) after-depolarisation, which is depolarisation occurring during or after the repolarisation phase. The after-depolarisation may then generate an action potential, giving rise to premature beats that can trigger tachyarrhythmias. This is often seen in the context of ventricular tachyarrhythmias associated with channelopathies such as long QT syndrome (LQTS) and catecholaminergic polymorphic ventricular tachycardia (CPVT).

33

Bradyarrhythmias are usually due to a failure either of impulse generation (secondary to reduced automaticity) or appropriate conduction. The most common bradyarrhythmias in the PICU setting result from sinus node dysfunction and complete atrioventricular (AV) block.

An approach to the diagnosis of common tachyarrhythmias is summarised in Fig. 33.7.

33.3 Management

33.3.1 General Considerations

The spectrum of cardiac arrhythmias encountered in the PICU range from life-threatening events to rhythm disturbances with little or no haemodynamic consequences [4, 5]. Rhythm disturbances that may be well-tolerated in a normal heart may lead to haemodynamic compromise when occurring in the immediate postoperative period [6]. Therefore, the first consideration is to determine the impact of the rhythm on the patient's haemodynamics and whether immediate intervention is required. If the cardiac arrhythmia is accompanied by signs of haemodynamic compromise, immediate action must be taken. This should be prioritised over a precise diagnosis and may imply electrical cardioversion, defibrillation or pacing. Otherwise, diagnostic studies including a 12-lead ECG and atrial electrogram if available should be performed first. Echocardiography is also indicated in the initial evaluation of the child to assess the cardiac function and rule out congenital heart disease (CHD). For certain forms of tachyarrhythmias, the administration of adenosine with concomitant ECG recording can be diagnostic and/or therapeutic. Cardiac telemetry should always be reviewed, and all rhythm disturbances must be fully assessed as they have an impact on postoperative morbidity and mortality [7, 8].

A key aspect in the management of cardiac arrhythmias in PICU is to identify, avoid and treat possible triggers, especially in the vulnerable early postoperative period following cardiac surgery. This includes keeping appropriate electrolyte levels (i.e. potassium 4.5–5 mM, magnesium >1 mM and ionised calcium >1 mM), correcting hypoxaemia and acidosis, maintaining normothermia, maintaining good pain and anxiety relief, minimising exogenous catecholamine administration whenever possible and treating myocardial dysfunction and ischaemia. In addition, discontinuation of arrhythmogenic drugs should be considered, and the QT interval should be monitored with drugs at risk of prolonging it (e.g. macrolides, amiodarone and sotalol).

The risk of thromboembolism should also be considered before electrical or pharmacologic cardioversion of sustained atrial arrhythmias such as atrial fibrillation or flutter, especially in the setting of repaired CHD, such as patients with a univentricular circulation or with impaired ventricular function. Appropriate anticoagulation should be considered and administered.

33.3.2 Antiarrhythmics

Medical therapy plays an important role in the acute and chronic management of arrhythmias in children. Antiarrhythmic drugs are often used in the first-line management of arrhythmias, particularly in the PICU setting. The primary goal of antiarrhythmic drugs is to achieve rhythm control by terminating the tachycardia and maintaining normal sinus rhythm. If rhythm control is not possible, then the next best option would be to aim for adequate rate control. The overall purpose of this is to achieve an appropriate heart rate to maintain haemodynamic stability. The following is a brief summary of the commonly used antiarrhythmic drugs used in the paediatric population, but referring to a paediatric formulary is recommended for more detailed information.

Adenosine exerts its main electrophysiological effects on the SA node and AV node. It reduces SA node automaticity and slows/blocks AV nodal conduction. It also reduces atrial refractory periods but has little effect on ventricular myocardium. The primary use of adenosine is in the diagnosis and treatment of sustained regular tachycardias through its effect on the AV node. Adenosine can terminate a re-entry tachycardia involving the AV node as part of its circuit (i.e. AVRT and AVNRT) (◘ Fig. 33.8) and is very useful for unmasking the underlying mechanisms for other tachyarrhythmias such as atrial flutter and atrial tachycardias (◘ Fig. 33.9). In ventricular tachycardias, adenosine administration rarely disrupts the tachycardia, but careful analysis of the ECG may identify momentary retrograde block causing VA dissociation. Adenosine is metabolised by red blood cells and has a very short half-life, thus to have any effect on

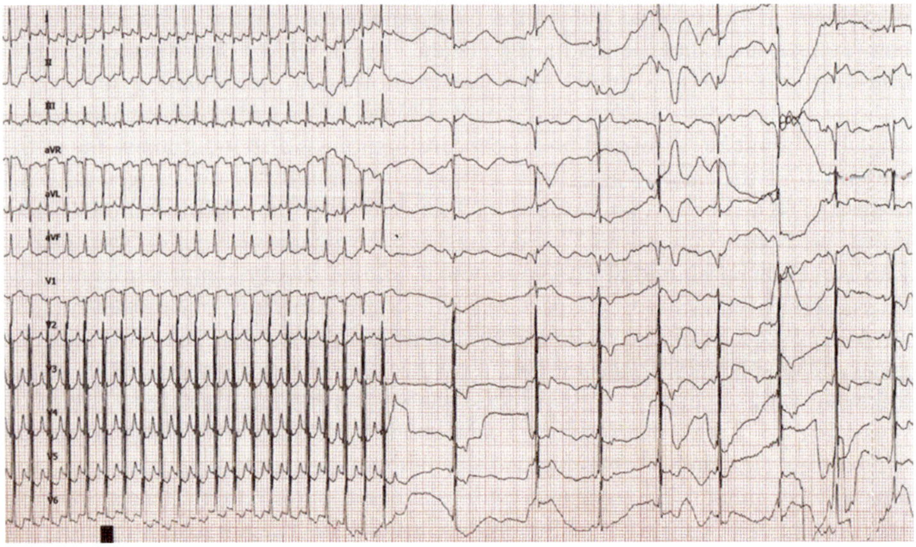

Fig. 33.8 Adenosine administration resulting in termination of tachycardia in AVRT. Note the appearance of ventricular pre-excitation (delta wave) during sinus rhythm suggesting the presence of an accessory pathway

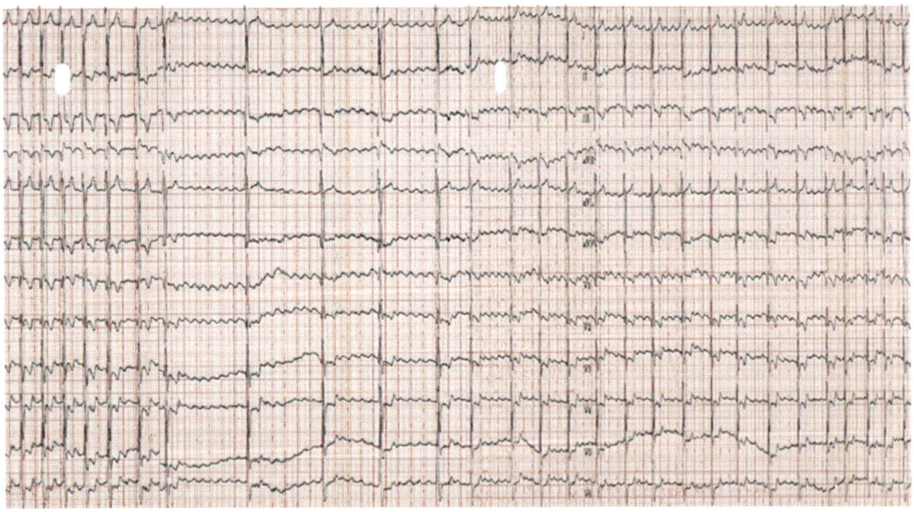

Fig. 33.9 Adenosine administration unmasking flutter waves in atrial flutter

the heart, it needs to be given as a rapid intravenous bolus when administered via a peripheral injection. A rhythm strip should be kept running during adenosine administration to capture the momentary ECG changes that occur. This is often crucial to the identification of the underlying mechanism and diagnosis of the arrhythmia.

Beta-blockers are commonly used in the treatment of paediatric arrhythmias, the more common examples being oral propranolol, atenolol, nadolol and intravenous esmolol. Beta-blockers are Class II agents in the Vaughan-Williams classification [9].

They work by binding to beta-adrenoreceptors and counteracting the action of adrenaline. This results in reduced automaticity of the SA node and other ectopic foci, as well as decreased cardiac conduction velocity, particularly in the AV node. Beta-blockade can affect cardiac contractility due to its effects on calcium haemostasis. Intravenous esmolol can be very useful in the PICU setting as it has a very short half-life and any negative effects of beta-blockade are not persistent once the infusion is discontinued.

Amiodarone is primarily a Class III antiarrhythmic. It works mainly by blocking potassium currents responsible for cardiac repolarisation during Phase 3 of the action potential. This results in an increased action potential duration and prolonged refractory period of cardiac cells. Amiodarone also blocks beta-adrenoreceptors, sodium and calcium channels. The combined effect of its pharmacological action leads to decreased automaticity and cardiac conduction velocity. Amiodarone is particularly useful in PICU due to its wide-ranging effects on the cardiac conduction system and thus its ability to effectively treat a variety of tachyarrhythmias regardless of the underlying mechanism. It is the least negatively inotropic antiarrhythmic drug, and hence, it is relatively safe to use especially in the context of myocardial dysfunction. Amiodarone, when given intravenously, can result in significant hypotension with a rapid infusion, hence it is important to infuse it slowly, with the loading dose usually given over 4 h. Regular ECG monitoring should be performed to assess for QT prolongation, particularly during intravenous administration. Thyroid and liver function should be regularly monitored (at least every 6 months) on chronic amiodarone therapy.

Digoxin has little direct antiarrhythmic effect on the heart. Its antiarrhythmic effect indirectly results from its parasympathomimetic action which causes sinoatrial slowing and conduction delay across the AV node. It may be useful in treating re-entry tachyarrhythmias where the AV node is an essential part of the circuit; or in cases where rhythm control is not possible, it helps to achieve rate control by limiting the ventricular response. In addition, digoxin exerts a positive inotropic through its inhibitory action on the cellular Na/K ATPase, which may be helpful in the setting of myocardial dysfunction in the PICU. Digoxin levels need to be monitored due to a relatively narrow therapeutic safety window. The dose of digoxin should also be halved with concurrent use of amiodarone.

Ivabradine is an emerging option in the management of postoperative junctional ectopic tachycardia (JET) [10]. Ivabradine selectively inhibits the If ("funny") current in the sinoatrial node, reducing heart rate without affecting myocardial contractility. Interestingly, although JET arises from ectopic automaticity in the AV junction, ivabradine still appears to have an effect by reducing the rate of automatic depolarization in these cells [11].

33.3.3 Cardioversion and Defibrillation

Direct current (DC) cardioversion delivers a low-energy shock (1–2 J/kg) synchronised with the R wave of the ECG. Synchronisation minimises the risk of inducing ventricular fibrillation (VF) with a shock delivered during ventricular repolarisation ('R-on-T' phenomenon). Cardioversion is indicated in any tachyarrhythmia with haemodynamic compromise. The use of vagal manoeuvres or adenosine can be attempted as long as they do not delay cardioversion. Cardioversion is also the treatment of choice for neonatal flutter.

Immediate defibrillation, delivering an asynchronous high-energy shock (4 J/kg), should be performed in any wide QRS (or broad complex) tachycardia without a pulse and in ventricular fibrillation as per current resuscitation guidelines [12].

33.3.4 Temporary Cardiac Pacing

Temporary cardiac pacing is frequently used in the postoperative care of cardiac patients in the PICU. In the management of tachyarrhythmias, cardiac pacing can either terminate re-entry tachycardias or maintain AV synchrony through overdrive pacing of automatic tachycardias. Cardiac pacing is also indicated in the management of bradyarrhythmias with haemodynamic compromise or to optimise the cardiac output (e.g. postoperative heart block and sinus bradycardia coming off cardio-pulmonary bypass). Lastly, cardiac pacing can also be useful to maintain a regular rhythm in the setting of frequent premature beats.

The most common and reliable temporary pacing method in PICU is through pairs of bipolar epicardial atrial (A) and/or ventricular (V) leads placed during cardiac surgery. By convention, the A wires are brought out through the skin on the right of the sternum and the V wires on the left. Chest radiographs and electrograms can be used to confirm the lead/chamber relationships if uncertain. Alternative temporary pacing methods include transvenous endocardial pacing, or for shorter periods of time, transoesophageal atrial pacing and transcutaneous ventricular pacing via multifunction self-adhesive pads or external paddles.

Cardiac pacing modes are classified by the first three letters of the NBG generic code [13]: P (the chamber paced), S (the chamber sensed) and R (response to sensing). The chamber paced or sensed can either take the letter A(trium), V(entricle), D(ual) or O(none); the response to sensing can either be I(nhibit), T(rigger), D(ual) or O(no response, asynchronous pacing). Common pacing modes include:

- *AAI*. The pacemaker senses the atrium and paces the atrium if the sensed rate falls below the set lower rate. It is indicated in sinus bradycardia, sick sinus syndrome or JET. For AAI to be effective, AV conduction must be intact.
- *VVI*. The pacemaker senses the ventricle and paces the ventricle if the sensed rate falls below the set lower rate. It is commonly used as a ventricular backup for sinus rhythm with unreliable AV conduction (e.g. at risk of or recovering from heart block) or for sudden unexpected bradycardia.
- *DDD*. The pacemaker senses both the atrium and the ventricle as well as paces the atrium and/or ventricle when rates fall below the set lower rate. It can be used for all indications, including heart block, but caution must be taken with atrial tachyarrhythmias due to the risk of fast ventricular rate due to atrial tracking.
- *VOO*. Asynchronous ventricular pacing can used in instances such as emergent transcutaneous pacing.

Three essential variables must be programmed for single-chamber pacemakers: lower rate limit, current output and sensitivity. The *lower rate limit* is the rate at which the pacemaker will pace if no intrinsic event is sensed, expressed in pulses per minute (ppm). It should be individualised, aiming to optimise cardiac output or set up as a 'backup' (60–100 ppm, depending on age) to minimise pacing and allow the patient to remain in their intrinsic rhythm until the occurrence of significant bradycardia. The *output* and *sensitivity* are configured according to their respective capture and sensing thresholds.

The *capture threshold* is the minimum amount of energy (measured in millivolts, mV) required to stimulate the cardiac chamber consistently. To check the capture threshold, one should first set the pacing rate above the patient's intrinsic rate so consistent pacing is achieved and then progressively reduce the pacemaker output until capture is lost. The output is then set at least twice this threshold. Note that the capture threshold can increase with acidosis, potentially leading to a sudden loss of capture if unrecognised.

The *sensing threshold* is the highest programmable voltage level at which the pacemaker still detects intrinsic cardiac activity. It is determined in AAI, VVI or DDD modes by first slowly decreasing the pacing rate below the patient's intrinsic rate (if present) so that no pacing occurs. Then, the sensitivity (in mV) on the pacemaker generator is slowly increased (making the pacemaker less sensitive) until the sensing indicator stops flashing and asynchronous pacing occurs. At this point, the sensitivity is reduced again until adequate sensing is regained. Sensitivity should then be programmed to one-half of the sensing threshold. Setting the sensitivity too low can result in the pacemaker over-sensing noise and inappropriately inhibiting cardiac pacing. If rapid or progressive increases in thresholds are observed (common after a few days), new pacing wires or a permanent pacemaker should be considered.

The capture and sensing thresholds should be checked regularly as any metabolic derangement or administration of certain medications (such as sodium channel blockers) may alter these measurements.

Additional adjustable variables exist for dual chamber pacing:

1. The *upper rate limit* is the fastest ventricular pacing rate allowed in response to a sensed atrial event. It needs to be sufficiently high (usually above 200 beats per minute in paediatrics) to allow appropriate tracking of atrial activity.
2. The *AV interval* (or AV delay), reflected on an ECG as the PR interval, is usually set at a physiologic length. Longer AV intervals will allow intrinsic AV conduction to occur and may also be beneficial in ventricles with restrictive filling patterns.
3. The *post-ventricular atrial refractory period* (PVARP) is the time following a ventricular event (paced or sensed) during which an atrial sensed event does not trigger a response. The purpose of PVARP is to prevent pacemaker-mediated tachycardia in the event of atrial activation via retrograde VA conduction triggering a ventricular response and setting up a re-entrant loop.

Lastly, when the pacemaker is in use, the underlying rhythm and need for ongoing pacing need to be assessed regularly. The safest way to do so is to reduce the pacemaker rate. This should be done gradually as the intrinsic activity may be absent or not emerge rapidly after an abrupt interruption of pacing. Also, it is not recommended to reduce the output current until capture is lost, as the subsequent recapture threshold may increase or be impossible to be re-established.

33.4 Individual Arrhythmias

33.4.1 Premature Atrial and Ventricular Complexes

Premature atrial complexes (PAC) are common in the first few months of life. The QRS is preceded by a P wave and can be broad and complex, reflecting rate-related aberrant conduction. The ectopic beat is sometimes so premature that no AV conduction occurs (isolated P wave) resulting in intermittent pauses. PACs do not require treatment unless they precipitate runs of sustained tachycardia.

Premature ventricular complexes (PVC) are characterised by a broad complex QRS without a typical bundle branch block pattern, absent P wave and a fully compensatory pause (not seen if underlying sinus arrhythmia). They do not require antiarrhythmic therapy unless very frequent or if there are runs of sustained tachycardia.

33.4.2 Tachyarrhythmias

33.4.2.1 Junctional Ectopic Tachycardia (JET)

JET is usually a transient postoperative arrhythmia related to increased automaticity of the AV junction. It is usually associated with VA dissociation with faster ventricular rates (> 170 bpm) and can result in significant postoperative haemodynamic instability and increased mortality [14]. The incidence of JET varies but has been associated with younger age, complex surgical repairs (including Tetralogy of Fallot), long cardiopulmonary bypass time, hypomagnesaemia and high-dose inotropic support, among others [15]. To diagnose JET, an atrial electrogram is helpful to demonstrate sinus P waves 'marching through' narrow QRS complexes to demonstrate VA dissociation (◘ Fig. 33.5). Occasionally, 1:1 VA conduction can occur resulting in the ECG appearance of a narrow complex QRS with a retrograde P wave.

As an automatic tachycardia, JET does not respond to adenosine or cardioversion. Treatment aims to either restore sinus rhythm or to slow the tachycardia to a rate where AV synchrony can be regained by overdrive atrial pacing (AAI or DDD). Management includes optimising preload, normalising electrolytes and blood gases, avoiding hyperthermia and minimising endogenous and exogenous catecholamines. If this is not sufficient, intravenous antiarrhythmics (amiodarone infusion is usually the first line) and/or moderate cooling to 34–36 °C can be considered. Digoxin, betablockers and flecainide have also been used. More recently, dexmedetomidine and ivabradine have been proposed as potential useful therapies, but further studies are needed [16, 17].

33.4.2.2 Atrial Ectopic Tachycardia (AET)

AET is an automatic tachycardia secondary to an ectopic atrial focus. It may present with incessant tachycardia at 180–200 bpm leading to dilated cardiomyopathy (usually in the neonatal period or early infancy), or it can occur transiently following cardiac surgery. It is characterised by abnormal P wave morphology and a typical warm-up and slow-down pattern (◘ Fig. 33.10). If multiple P wave morphologies

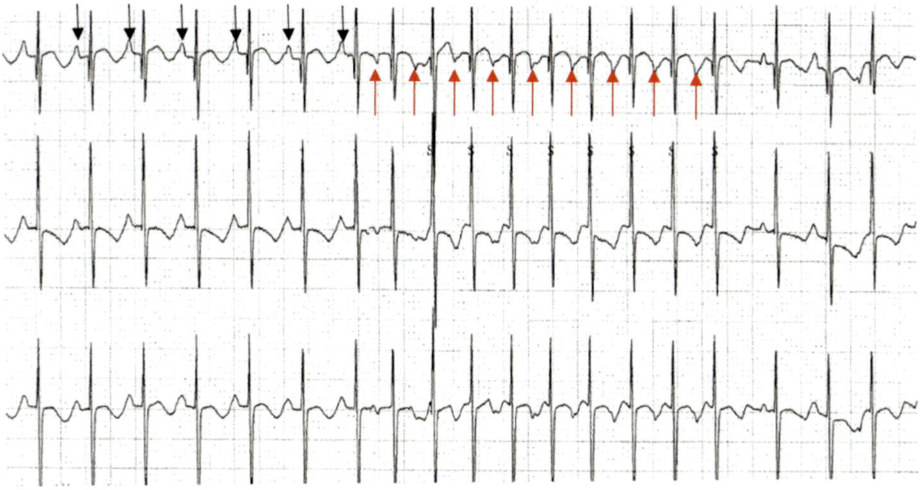

Fig. 33.10 Rhythm strip showing a short run of atrial ectopic tachycardia. Sinus P wave is denoted by black arrows and the ectopic atrial P wave by red arrows

are identified with short non-sustained bursts of tachycardia and irregularly irregular QRS complexes, it is known as multifocal atrial tachycardia (MAT). Although it may respond to cardioversion, it usually requires anti-arrhythmic treatment (amiodarone or flecainide) to suppress it. AV nodal blocking agents (e.g. digoxin and beta-blockers) may also be used to decrease the ventricular response rate and improve a patient's haemodynamics.

33.4.2.3 Supraventricular Tachycardia (SVT)

SVT is a re-entry tachycardia involving the AV node. Its onset is abrupt, and heart rates usually reach 180–300 bpm. Although it is sometimes associated with CHD, SVT is mostly seen in children without underlying structural heart disease. Neonates and young infants can present to PICU with acute heart failure after a period of unrecognised sustained SVT.

The re-entry circuit is mediated either through an accessory pathway at the AV annulus (AVRT) or through dual AV node pathways (AVNRT). AVRT is more common in younger children, and AVNRT is more prevalent in children above 10 years of age. An RP interval >80 ms with retrograde P waves in the ST segment during SVT usually indicates AV re-entry, whereas a very short RP interval with the P wave concealed within or seen immediately after the QRS is more suggestive of AV nodal re-entry.

Accessory pathways that only conduct retrogradely (VA) are 'concealed' in sinus rhythm. Some accessory pathways can also conduct anterogradely, resulting in pre-excitation and a characteristic delta wave in sinus rhythm (Wolf-Parkinson-White syndrome).

The QRS complex in SVT is usually narrow, as the ventricles are depolarised via the normal AV conduction system. However, the QRS complex in SVT can be broad if there is a pre-existing conduction delay (e.g. repaired tetralogy of Fallot with residual right bundle branch block) or if there is rate-related aberrancy. In these cases, the QRS will usually have a typical right or left bundle branch block morphology. A broad complex QRS is also seen in antidromic AVRT, i.e. antegrade conduction down the accessory pathway and retrograde conduction via the AV node.

Irrespective of the mechanism, SVT responds to manoeuvres or drugs that block AV nodal conduction. If there is a haemodynamic compromise, immediate synchronised cardioversion (or rapid overdrive pacing if available) should be performed. Otherwise, vagal manoeuvres or adenosine can be tried, which is often diagnostic and therapeutic. In patients with recurrent SVT, regular anti-arrhythmic medications such as beta-blockers, flecainide or amiodarone may be required.

33.4.2.4 Atrial Flutter and Intra-atrial Re-entry Tachycardia (IART)

Atrial flutter results from a macroreentrant circuit within the right atrium. Typical atrial flutter occurs with rates around 300 bpm with 1:1 but more commonly 2:1 or 3:1 conduction to the ventricle (◘ Fig. 33.11). The wave-front travels along a circuit around the tricuspid annulus. It is a known cause of fetal hydrops and is rarely seen in paediatrics outside the fetal and neonatal periods. Adenosine administration reveals the typical 'saw tooth' appearance on ECG but does not terminate the tachycardia. The treatment of choice is synchronised DC cardioversion after which it rarely recurs.

Atypical flutter includes a broad range of macroreentrant atrial tachycardias where the wave-front does not travel around the tricuspid annulus, resulting in a less characteristic P wave appearance (◘ Fig. 33.12). It can be seen in adolescents and adults with repaired CHD, especially after Mustard or Senning and Fontan procedures [18]. This scar-related re-entry atrial arrhythmia is frequently referred to as intra-atrial re-entry tachycardia (IART) to distinguish it from typical flutter.

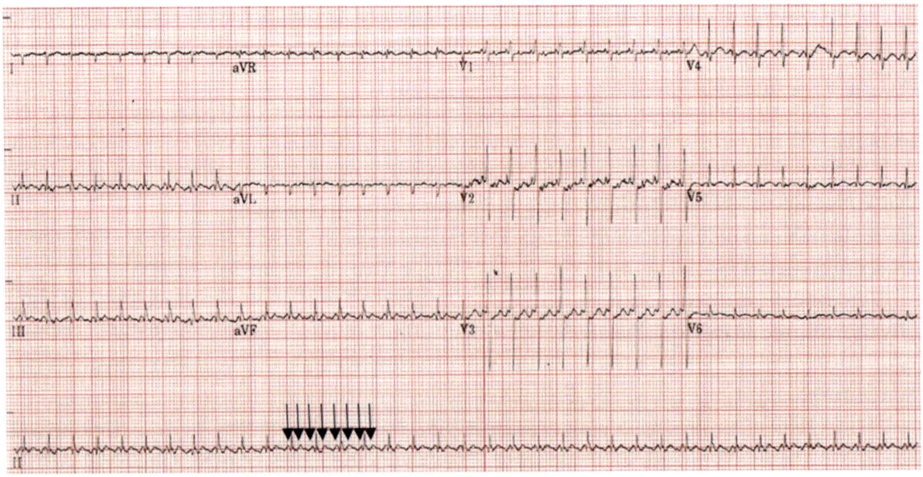

◘ **Fig. 33.11** 12-lead ECG demonstrating atrial flutter with 2:1 conduction in a neonate with a structurally and functionally normal heart. Flutter waves are denoted by black arrows

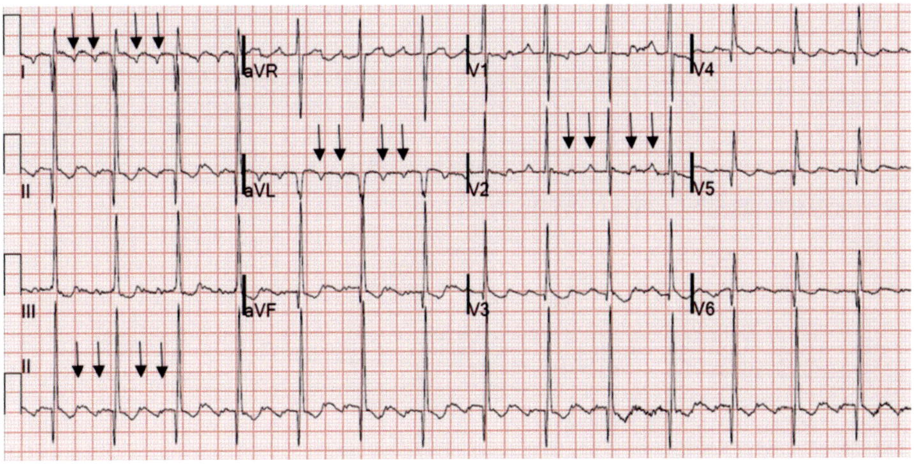

Fig. 33.12 12-lead ECG demonstrating macroreentrant atrial tachycardia with 3:1 conduction in a univentricular heart following a bidirectional Glenn procedure. Atrial beats are denoted by black arrows

ECG demonstrates an ectopic P-wave morphology, but unlike AET, IART has a more abrupt onset and offset. AV block is variable, and 2:1 block may make the diagnosis difficult. Treatment can be challenging but includes cardioversion, anti-arrhythmic medications, ablation, right-sided maze procedure or pacemaker implantation if associated with sinus node dysfunction.

33.4.2.5 Ventricular Tachycardia (VT)

Non-sustained VT is defined as a run of three or more consecutive ventricular ectopics that self-corrects to sinus rhythm within 30 s. Sustained VT lasts greater than 30 s and can lead to haemodynamic compromise. VT can be monomorphic or polymorphic.

Monomorphic VT can be secondary to a focal scar in the myocardium due to underlying cardiac disease or prior cardiac surgery. The main differential diagnosis is SVT with aberrancy or antidromic AVRT. A trial of adenosine can thus be helpful in the diagnosis. On ECG, there can be 1:1 VA conduction or VA dissociation (Fig. 33.13). The demonstration of VA dissociation (with the persistence of the tachycardia after adenosine administration), as well as the presence of capture and/or fusion beats, suggest a ventricular origin. An irregularly irregular broad complex tachycardia could be due to pre-excited atrial fibrillation (AF), i.e. AF in the presence of an accessory pathway.

Polymorphic VT is generally associated with acute myocardial ischaemia or an underlying channelopathy, such as long QT syndrome or catecholaminergic polymorphic VT, presenting as Torsade de Pointes, with the characteristic twisting of QRS complexes around an isoelectric line.

Treatment will depend on the patient's cardiovascular stability. In an unstable patient with a palpable pulse, immediate synchronised DC cardioversion should be performed. Defibrillation should be performed if there is no palpable pulse. More

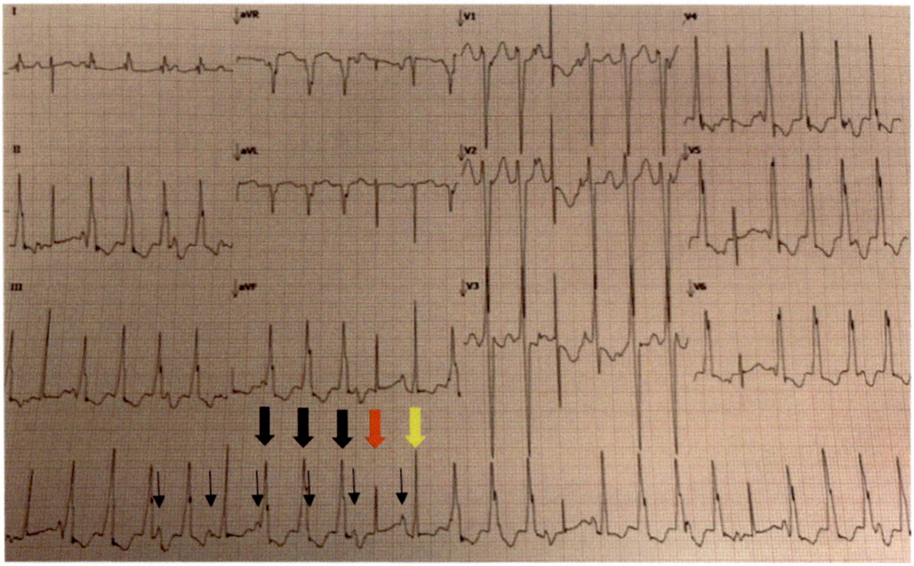

Fig. 33.13 12-lead ECG demonstrating ventricular tachycardia. Regular broad complex tachycardia with AV dissociation (atrial beats—thin black arrows, ventricular beats—thick black arrows) capture beats (red arrow) and fusion beats (yellow arrow)

stable patients can be treated pharmacologically, with medications such as beta-blockers, flecainide, amiodarone or lidocaine. Magnesium can also be helpful in the treatment of Torsade de Pointes.

33.4.3 Bradyarrhythmias

33.4.3.1 Sinus Node Dysfunction

Sinus node dysfunction results from abnormal automaticity of the sinus node. In children, it is most commonly seen following cardiac interventions that involve manipulation of the right atrium (e.g. sinus venosus atrial septal defect repair, Fontan procedure and heart transplantation). It results in a slow sinus rhythm, sinus pauses or complete absence of sinus activity, often accompanied by an atrial or junctional escape (Fig. 33.14). Treatment involves temporary or permanent atrial pacing.

33.4.3.2 Atrioventricular (AV) Block

AV block is the failure of 1:1 conduction from the atrium to the ventricle and can result from a conduction abnormality along the AV node or further downstream in the His-Purkinje system. In *first-degree AV block*, all atrial impulses are conducted to the ventricle but with a prolonged PR interval. In *second-degree AV block*, not all atrial impulses are conducted. It can take two major forms: Mobitz type I (or Wenckebach), where there is a progressive lengthening of the PR interval until one P

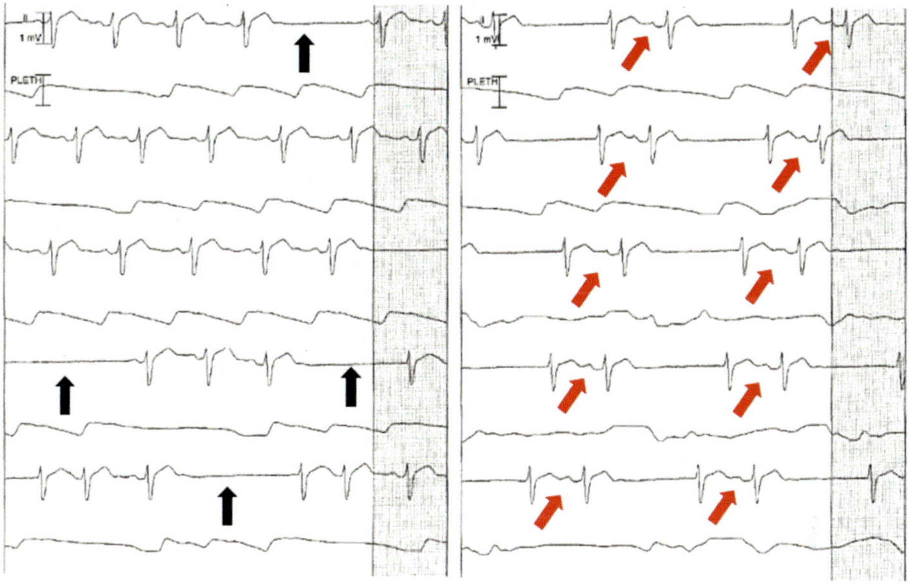

Fig. 33.14 Cardiac telemetry demonstrating signs of sinus node dysfunction—sinus bradycardia, sinus pauses (black arrows) and escape capture bigeminy (red arrows)

wave is not conducted; or Mobitz type II, where there is a constant PR interval for conducted P wave prior to a blocked P wave; and a consistent ratio of conducted to non-conducted P waves, i.e. 2:1 or 3:1 AV block. Whereas Mobitz type I does not usually require treatment as the conduction abnormality is within the AV node, in Mobitz type II, the block is more commonly in the His-Purkinje conduction system and potentially carries a higher risk of evolving and progressing to a more advanced AV block. Mobitz type II block can be related to direct surgical damage, ischaemia or diffuse myocardial disease and can be treated by cardiac pacing. *Third-degree AV block* is secondary to complete AV dissociation with faster atrial compared to ventricular rates (Fig. 33.15). There is usually an escape rhythm from a subsidiary pacemaker along the conduction system. It may be congenital or acquired (e.g. surgical injury, myocarditis and rheumatic fever). The surgical procedures at greater risk for postoperative complete heart block are left ventricular outflow tract obstruction relief, followed by VSD closure and TOF repair [19]. Patients with L-transposition of the great arteries have a higher incidence of spontaneous as well as postoperative heart block. Treatment involves temporary or permanent cardiac pacing. Of note, postoperative AV block can be transient, so unless there is clear evidence of permanent damage to the conduction system, it is worth waiting 7–10 days before implanting a permanent pacemaker [19, 20]. Extended follow-up is recommended as there is a risk of heart block recurring within the first postoperative year [21].

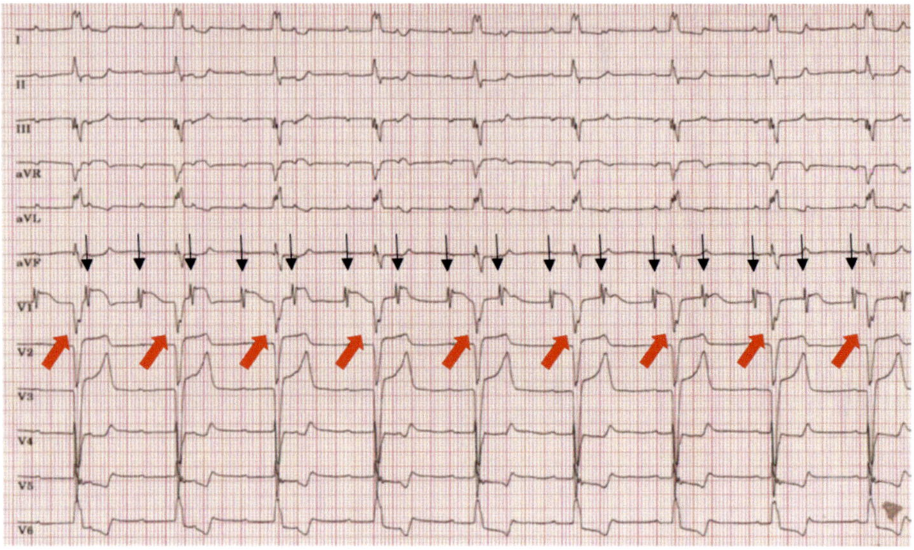

Fig. 33.15 12-lead rhythm strip with atrial electrogram (lead V1) showing complete heart block. Complete AV dissociation with faster atrial activity is denoted by black arrows and ventricular escape by red arrows

References

1. Davignon A, Rautaharju P, Boisselle E, et al. Normal ECG standards for infants and children. Pediatr Cardiol. 1979;1:123–31.
2. Rijnbeek PR, Witsenburg M, Schrama E, et al. New normal limits for the paediatric electrocardiogram. Eur Heart J. 2001;22:702–11.
3. Macfarlane PW, Coleman EN, Pomphrey EO, et al. Normal limits of the high fidelity pediatric ECG. Preliminary observations. J Electrocardiol. 1989;22(suppl):162–8.
4. Cooper DS, Knilans TK. Arrhythmias. In: Wheeler DS, Wong HR, Shanley TP, editors. Pediatric critical care medicine, vol. 2. London: Springer; 2014. p. 451–66.
5. Reinelt P, Karth GD, Geppert A, Heinz G. Incidence and type of cardiac arrhythmias in critically ill patients: a single center experience in a medical-cardiological ICU. Intensive Care Med. 2001;27(9):1466–73.
6. Lan YT, Lee JC, Wetzel G. Postoperative arrhythmia. Curr Opin Cardiol. 2003;18:73–8.
7. Balaji S, Ellenby M, McNames J, Goldstein B. Update on intensive care ECG and cardiac event monitoring. Card Electrophysiol Rev. 2002;6(3):190–5.
8. Brown KL, Ridout DA, Goldman AP, Hoskote A, Penny DJ. Risk factors for long intensive care unit stay after cardiopulmonary bypass in children. Crit Care Med. 2003;31(1):28–33.
9. Lei M, Wu L, Terrar DA, Huang CL. Modernized classification of cardiac antiarrhythmic drugs. Circulation. 2018;138(17):1879–96.
10. Ivabradine in Post-operative Junctional Ectopic Tachycardia (JET): Breaking New Ground. Krishna MR, Kunde MF, Kumar RK, Balaji S. Pediatr Cardiol. 2019;40(6):1284–1288. https://doi.org/10.1007/s00246-019-02149-5. Epub 2019 Jul 18. PMID: 31317219.
11. Ivabradine Versus Amiodarone in the Management of Postoperative Junctional Ectopic Tachycardia: A Randomized, Open-Label, Noninferiority Study.Arvind B, Kothari SS, Juneja R, et al. JACC Clin Electrophysiol. 2021;7(8):1052-1060. https://doi.org/10.1016/j.jacep.2021.01.020. Epub 2021 Mar 31. PMID: 33812837.

12. Maconochie IK, Bingham R, Eich C, Lopez-Herce J, Rodriguez-Nunez A, Rajka T, et al. European resuscitation council guidelines for resuscitation 2015: section 6. Paediatric life support. Resuscitation. 2015;95:223–48.
13. Bernstein AD, Daubert JC, Fletcher RD, Hayes DL, Luderitz B, Reynolds DW, et al. The revised NASPE/BPEG generic code for antibradycardia, adaptive-rate, and multisite pacing. North American Society of Pacing and Electrophysiology/British Pacing and Electrophysiology Group. Pacing Clin Electrophysiol. 2002;25(2):260–4.
14. Hoffman TM, Bush DM, Wernovsky G, Cohen MI, Wieand TS, Gaynor JW, et al. Postoperative junctional ectopic tachycardia in children: incidence, risk factors, and treatment. Ann Thorac Surg. 2002;74(5):1607–11.
15. Dodge-Khatami A, Miller OI, Anderson RH, Gil-Jaurena JM, Goldman AP, de Leval MR. Impact of junctional ectopic tachycardia on postoperative morbidity following repair of congenital heart defects. Eur J Cardiothorac Surg. 2002;21(2):255–9.
16. Chrysostomou C, Beerman L, Shiderly D, Berry D, Morell VO, Munoz R. Dexmedetomidine: a novel drug for the treatment of atrial and junctional tachyarrhythmias during the perioperative period for congenital cardiac surgery: a preliminary study. Anesth Analg. 2008;107(5):1514–22.
17. Kumar V, Kumar G, Joshi S, Sharma V. Ivabradine for junctional ectopic tachycardia in post congenital heart surgery. Indian Heart J. 2017;69(5):666–7.
18. Li W, Somerville J. Atrial flutter in grown-up congenital heart (GUCH) patients. Clinical characteristics of affected population. Int J Cardiol. 2000;75(2–3):129–37; discussion 38–9
19. Weindling SN, Saul JP, Gamble WJ, Mayer JE, Wessel D, Walsh EP. Duration of complete atrioventricular block after congenital heart disease surgery. Am J Cardiol. 1998;82(4):525–7.
20. Gregoratos G, Abrams J, Epstein AE, Freedman RA, Hayes DL, Hlatky MA, et al. ACC/AHA/NASPE 2002 guideline update for implantation of cardiac pacemakers and antiarrhythmia devices: summary article. A report of the American College of Cardiology/American Heart Association Task Force on Practice Guidelines (ACC/AHA/NASPE Committee to Update the 1998 Pacemaker Guidelines). J Cardiovasc Electrophysiol. 2002;13(11):1183–99.
21. Bonatti V, Agnetti A, Squarcia U. Early and late postoperative complete heart block in pediatric patients submitted to open-heart surgery for congenital heart disease. Pediatr Med Chir. 1998;20(3):181–6.

Further Reading

Cooper DS, Knilans TK. Arrhythmias. In: Wheeler DS, Wong HR, Shanley TP, editors. Pediatric critical care medicine, vol. 2. London: Springer; 2014. p. 451–66.

Kothari DS, Skinner JR. Neonatal tachycardias: an update. Arch Dis Child Fetal Neonatal Ed. 2006;91(2):F136–44.

Lee Beerman GA, Park SC. Arrhythmias in the intensive care unit. In: Muñoz VOM RA, da Cruz EM, Vetterly CG, editors. Critical care of children with heart disease: basic medical and surgical concepts. London: Springer; 2010. p. 619–363.

Outcomes of Paediatric Cardiac Intensive Care

Katherine L. Brown

Contents

J. Brierley et al. (eds.), *ESPNIC Children's Intensive Care Textbook*,
https://doi.org/10.1007/978-3-031-64762-8_34

Learning Objectives

- Identify the important outcome measures for cardiac intensive care.
  This section will discuss how outcomes are defined including the outcomes of early mortality, critical care morbidities or complications and long-term outcomes such as quality of life and neurodevelopment.
- Explain how these outcomes are evaluated locally, nationally and internationally.
  This section will review local, national and international audit processes and analysis methods that are used for monitoring outcomes. This section will cover the role of case mix or case complexity in determining outcomes and how this can be considered.
- Describe the challenges in monitoring the outcomes of cardiac intensive care and the solutions that have been found.
  This section will discuss the challenges of measuring increasingly complex types of outcomes, the difficulties in conveying outcome data to stakeholders and cover solutions that have been deployed to address these challenges.

34.1 Introduction

Due to improvements in the intensive care and surgical management of children with heart disease over the last three decades, early operative mortality for paediatric cardiac surgery is now very low: the raw 30-day mortality rate from Registry data is 2–4%. As operative survival has increased, the current expectation is that most children with heart disease will survive admission to an intensive care unit and grow into adulthood. There are an increasing number of survivors with congenital heart disease (CHD) of greater complexity as well as children with associated comorbidities and those who require serial interventions. More complex patients spend longer periods in the hospital and are exposed to a greater risk of complications, which may include renal and liver injury, myocardial injury and long-term myocardial failure, brain hypo-perfusion, stroke and other thromboembolic complications, seizures and neurodevelopmental (ND) delays. Any or all of these complications impact long-term patient quality of life. It has been argued that intense scrutiny and reflection on outcomes leads to healthcare improvements, which are clearly of great importance for the overall well-being of patients and their families. Local, national and international efforts have explored new ways to evaluate outcomes, analyse the data and share results with stakeholders.

34.2 Outcome Measures

Early postoperative mortality is historically a vital measure of outcome and is considered an important safety metric that underpins many outcome reports, including those of the Society for Thoracic Surgery (STS) Registry in North America, the European Association of Cardiothoracic Surgery (EACTS) in Europe and the National Congenital Heart Diseases Audit (NCHDA) in the UK. This has been defined as mortality within 30 days of an index operation and or mortality within a hospital after an index operation. A very important issue to consider in the current era is that mortality is very low [1] and has been improving in multiple registry-based reports from different regions. For example, more than 98% of children operated in the UK now survive at least 30 days after surgery [2] although operative mortality is higher for complex CHD [3, 4]. Therefore, to leverage further improvements, we need to look beyond this relatively crude metric.

Morbidities and complications: Outcomes that go beyond early operative mortality include complications or morbidities such as postoperative extracorporeal membrane oxygenation (ECMO), unplanned reoperations or acute neurological events. In recent years, these have started to feature within national and international audits and registries. The evaluation of complications or morbidity measures requires clear definitions and the resources to undertake consistent data collection because these are more complex than survival [5]. If morbidity monitoring is achieved, it adds considerably to the key safety metric of 30-day or in-hospital survival. A recent multicentre prospective study found excellent outcomes in children who had no morbidities: their survival at 6 months post-operation was 99·3%, and their median length of stay was 8 days [6]. In contrast, among just over 20% of children who experienced one or more morbidity or complication, the survival at 6 months post-operation was much lower at 81.5%. The children with morbidities spent more time in the hospital and had worse quality of life in the first few months after surgery, and their care was more costly. The occurrence of postoperative ECMO and multiple morbidities are particularly important adverse outcomes, associated with high mortality, high resource use and lower quality of life for surviving patients over 6 months after surgery [7] (◘ Fig. 34.1).

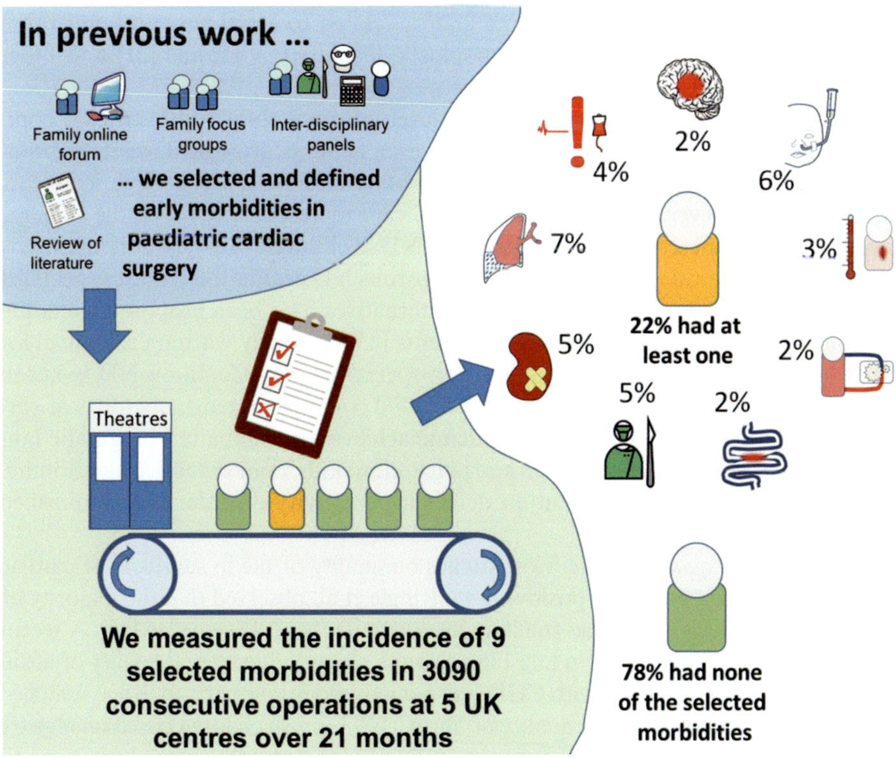

◘ **Fig. 34.1** Important early morbidities with paediatric cardiac surgery. Adapted from [6]

Derived metrics: Cardiac intensive care teams have used a range of ways to measure outcomes with derived metrics, designed to judge the care provided. An example of this is the concept of 'failure to rescue,' which represents the mortality rate specifically among patients who experience complications. The success with which teams are able to 'rescue a patient with complications' such that the patient survives has been viewed as an important safety measure, and researchers have shown that better rates of rescue are found in high-volume centres [8, 9]. There have been attempts at reporting morbidity after paediatric cardiac surgery using methods to combine outcomes to form metrics. Two single-centre studies generated an aggregate 'morbidity index' by assigning subjective weights to postoperative complications [10, 11]. The STS in North America, developed a 'morbidity score,' based on data from their multicentre registry to judge inter-centre differences in outcomes [12]. Whilst helpful to track overall outcomes, one problem with this approach is that condensing diverse morbidities into a single score may lead to a loss of information, which might make it harder for clinicians to learn from the data.

Post-discharge survival: An important outcome measure that is not routinely audited but is very important to consider is long-term survival; however, these data are frequently unavailable. In the USA, evaluation of long-term survival in registries is challenging because of legal [13] and logistic [14] barriers. A systematic review of long-term survival in CHD identified a total of only 16 population-based studies of long-term survival worldwide [15]; however, most studies incorporated patients born before many currently available treatments existed, and hence are now out of date. One reason that these outcomes have been collected within specific collaborative efforts is that late deaths are common among children with CHD, especially over the first year of life, either post-discharge and/or related to serial surgeries and other health issues [16–20], especially in hypoplastic left heart syndrome [21] and other complex CHDs [19].

Measures of neurodevelopment: Neurodevelopmental (ND) problems are common in children with heart disease [22]; however, acute neurological events are routinely detected following only a small minority of admissions [6]. Therefore, it appears that neurological events detected in intensive care represent the 'tip of the iceberg,' and hence, the ideal scope of surveillance for ND in children with heart disease needs to extend well beyond hospital discharge. Rigorous ND evaluation requires specialist resources, which are not always available. Alternatives have been proposed including screening questionnaires completed by parents [23] and early warning measures for child development that are suitable for non-specialists [24]. Common ND issues in child and adolescent CHD survivors include mild cognitive impairment (30% of survivors will have a lower IQ), lower academic achievement, impaired pragmatic language, decreased visual construction and perception skills, poor executive functioning, an increased prevalence of attention deficit hyperactivity disorder and diminished fine and gross motor skills [22].

Health-related quality of life: Most studies on quality of life in survivors of cardiac intensive care report relatively positive data. Ringle et al. observed that the majority of children operated for CHD lead fulfilling lives with limited ND sequelae [25]. A recent meta-analysis of 18 studies, including 1786 patients, showed that overall quality of life in adolescents and young adults with CHD was not reduced in comparison to age-matched controls [26]. Kyosti studied the quality of life in 1109 Finnish children based on registry data, 6 years after intensive care admission, and found that children with chronic conditions such as heart disease, ND problems and greater use of health services had poorer quality of life [27]. A controversy in quality of life measurement for critically ill children is that baseline values are commonly missing, so changes linked to critical illness may be difficult to quantify. Moreover, the young ages of many children mean that quality of life is reported based on parent perception rather than directly from the child.

34.3 Outcome Evaluation

34.3.1 Registries and Multi-Institutional Collaborations

Recent decades have seen the creation of high-quality patient registries that have been extremely important in enabling audit and research related to patient outcomes and quality assurance. For example, the STS database, established in 1989, contains detailed data related to several million paediatric cardiac procedures from North America and Europe. Data science enables the linkage of registries with a range of other patient datasets such as the Pediatric Health Information System (PHIS) for hospital episodes in the USA and the Office of National Statistics (ONS) for independent verification of vital status in the UK. These data linkages and analyses have facilitated the understanding of population trends, risk factors for outcomes and patient trajectories [28].

Contributions, based on observational data, have been made by associations consisting of multiple institutions joined together, for a particular purpose, referred to as consortia. The Pediatric Cardiac Critical Care Consortium (PC^4) was set up in 2009 and provides partner sites with access to real-time, reliable and actionable data to be used for local quality improvements [29–32]. However, membership of PC^4 is voluntary for institutions on a subscription basis; the reported measures have been selected by clinicians, the reporting of outcomes is accessible only to subscribing member institutions and these are limited to in-hospital measures. More recently, other collectives have emerged such as the National Pediatric Cardiac-Quality Improvement Collaborative (NPCQIC) in the USA, which is dedicated to measuring a range of outcomes within the hypoplastic left heart syndrome (HLHS) population, the Cardiac Neurodevelopmental Outcome Collaborative (CNOC), which is an international collaborative focussed on long-term ND outcomes and the International Quality Improvement Collaborative (IQIC), which is an international collaborative including mainly low and middle-income countries, focusing on evaluating postoperative survival and complications of heart surgery.

Describing case mix complexity: A historic barrier to the analysis of outcomes in CHD is the great variability diversity and complexity of the disease types in the patient population, which involves not only the primary CHD diagnoses and operation types but also noncardiac comorbidities and weight or size differences [33–35]. CHD is served by a specific coding scheme called the International Pediatric Congenital Cardiac Code (IPCCC) [36]: a child's condition may incorporate several individual IPCCC atomic codes, which together in particular combinations represent a specific primary CHD diagnosis and or a specific type of operation. Patient complexity and risk are also determined by comorbidities, which again are diverse. Over the last 10–15 years, informed by an accruing mass of data in registries, researchers have learned how to group and organise these codes in order to account for many aspects of case mix, but no method will ever be perfect (◘ Fig. 34.2).

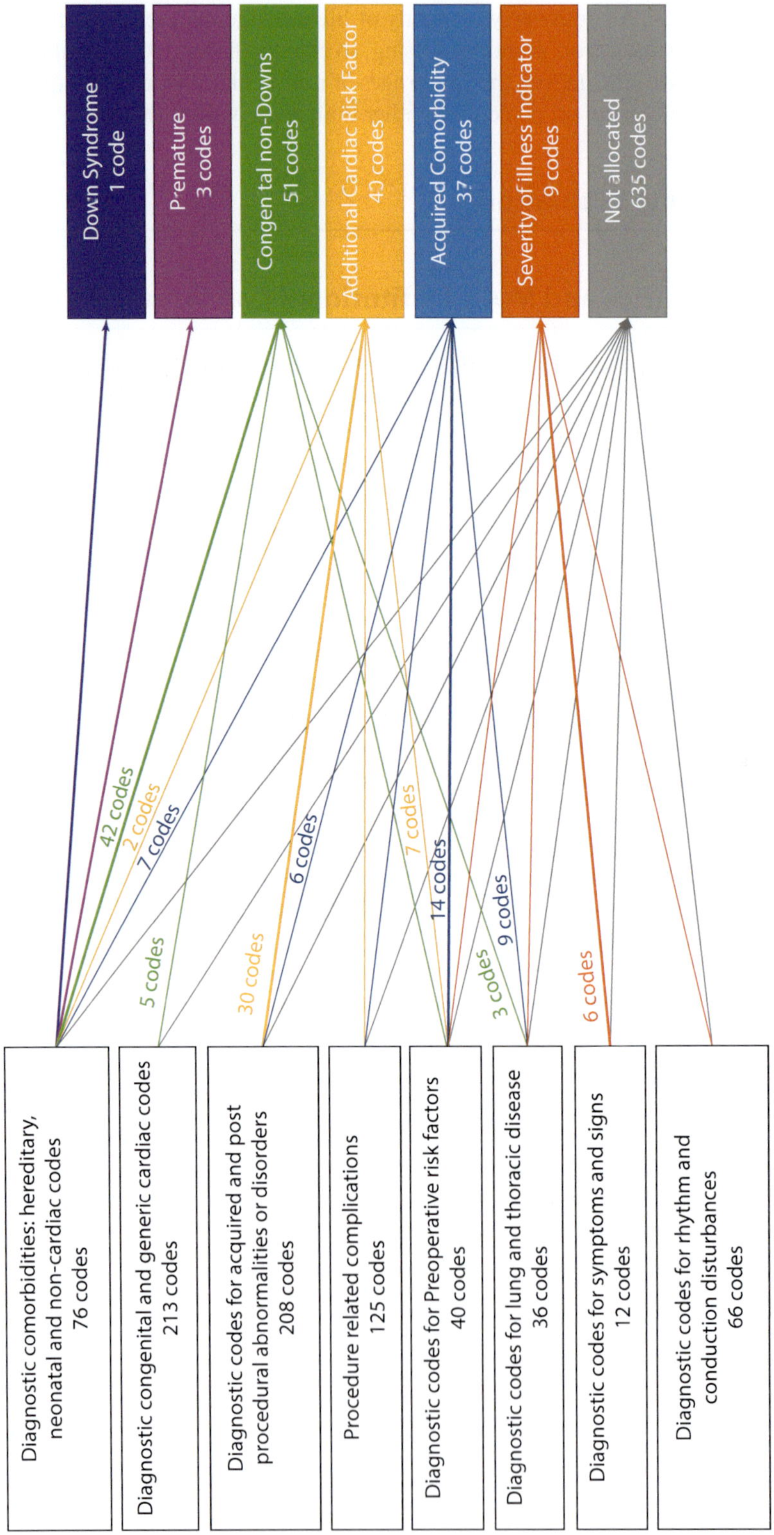

Fig. 34.2 Comorbidity groups for risk adjustment in paediatric cardiac surgery. Adpated from [37]

34.3.2 Relationship Between Case Mix Complexity and Outcomes

Early mortality: Risk adjustment methods to predict early mortality have been developed and validated, by teams working within major registries where the necessary data have accrued, including STS, EACTS and NCHDA [38–41]. The various patient factors that account for case complexity are included, such as CHD type, operation type or comorbidity.

Complications of surgery: When exploring the relationship between case mix and the occurrence of postoperative complications or morbidities, risk factors have many parallels with those implicated in early mortality. Important risk factors for morbidity are neonatal age, complex CHD, increased preoperative severity of illness and prolonged cardiopulmonary bypass [6].

Neurodevelopmental outcome: Procedure-specific risk factors (cardiopulmonary bypass with risks such as embolisation and systemic inflammatory response) are relatively weak predictors of ND outcome. However, postoperative factors (prolonged hospital length of stay, cardiopulmonary arrest and extracorporeal membrane oxygenation) significantly influence ND outcomes; as do patient-specific risk factors (severity of CHD, genetic or syndromic abnormalities, prematurity and low birth weight). Cerebral hypo-perfusion, hypoxia and cyanosis contribute to pre-, peri-, and postoperative ischemic brain injury, resulting in an increased risk of stroke and white matter injury [42].

Health-related quality of life: Quality of life may be adversely influenced by disease-related factors (CHD complexity and increased medical care utilisation), neurologic injury, educational impairment, poor self-esteem, anxiety and patient or parent post-traumatic stress [43].

Sociodemographic and ethnic risk: Healthcare access and socioeconomic deprivation are important issues that may influence the outcomes of cardiac intensive care. Children who are from families in the most deprived sociodemographic sector of society are more likely than the general population to suffer from CHD and are more likely to be admitted to cardiac intensive care. Several studies from the USA indicate that outcomes are worse among Black children, followed by Hispanic children with the best outcomes in White children [44]. These findings relate at least in part to socioeconomic deprivation and impaired access to care. In the UK, South Asian children account for 12% of cardiac surgeries, which is a higher proportion than would be expected [45], and severe CHDs are more common in the most deprived quintile of the population [46]. British children of South Asian ethnicity experience a higher incidence of more severe CHD types [16], and they experience higher risk-adjusted operative mortality than White British children [45, 47]. The reasons for this are unclear but may relate in part to aspects of case complexity that are poorly addressed by the risk adjustment model.

34.4 Solutions and Future Directions

Health informatics and graphical displays of outcome: A very positive development in recent years that has accompanied a wider 'transparency agenda' has been the use of health informatics to share information about outcomes with stakeholders. Graphical methods may display trends in hospital outcomes for review; one common approach is the variable life-adjusted display chart (VLAD). As shown in the ◘ Fig. 34.3, each point on the VLAD chart represents an episode of care. If the outcome is survival, then the VLAD plot goes up, and if death, the VLAD plot goes down. The vertical axis shows the total number of (predicted minus actual) deaths. When this is positive, there have been fewer than predicted deaths; when this is negative, there have been more than predicted deaths. Over time, if outcomes are as expected by the risk model, the end of the VLAD plot will tend to be close to zero. The risk model essentially benchmarks the unit's outcomes against recent national outcomes in paediatric heart surgery. Despite this being one of the most complex areas of surgery and lifesaving for the children involved, the UK has excellent outcomes with very low mortality rates. Since the estimated risk of death for a patient is small, this means that the VLAD will rise much more slowly for a run of survivors than it will fall for a run of deaths.

Recent work on using graphical methods to routinely monitor a range of morbidities [49] highlighted the complexity of graphically summarising multiple morbidities [50]. Nonetheless, graphical summaries of complications and morbidities have been developed and are shared in the form of 'dashboards.' Clinical teams, engaged in quality assurance, then review and discuss the dashboard, looking for shared learning (◘ Fig. 34.4).

Audit data have been used to co-develop parent and carer information resources, showing what the morbidities are and how their incidence and the length of stay may vary based on the complexity of the child's condition. Parents stated that it helps to know; first, they are not alone in facing a morbidity, second, clinical teams have seen morbidities before and know how to deal with them and third, that it is better as a parent to 'be prepared' [52].

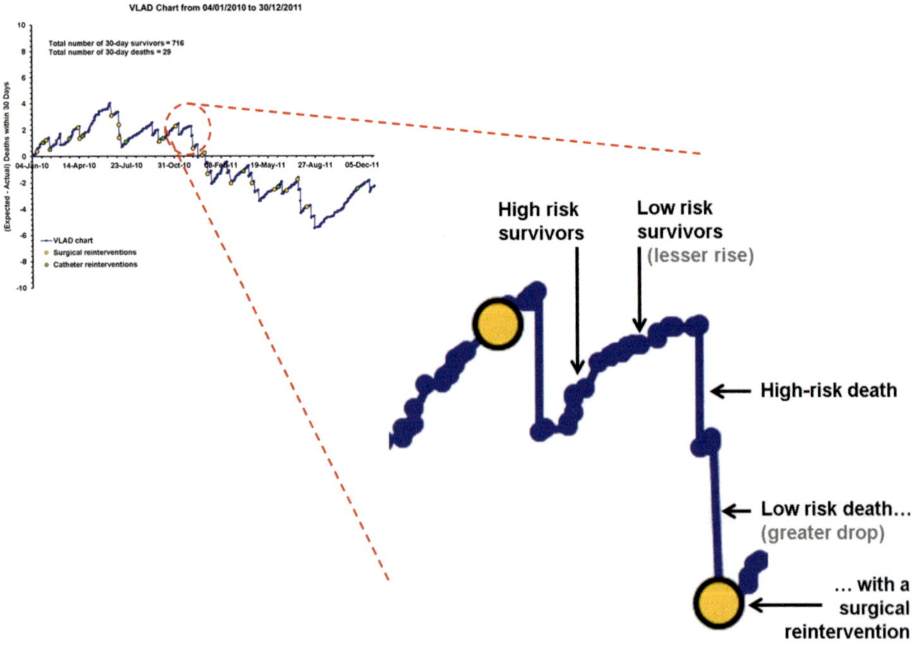

◘ **Fig. 34.3** VLAD chart and detail to show VLAD trend. Reproduced from [48]

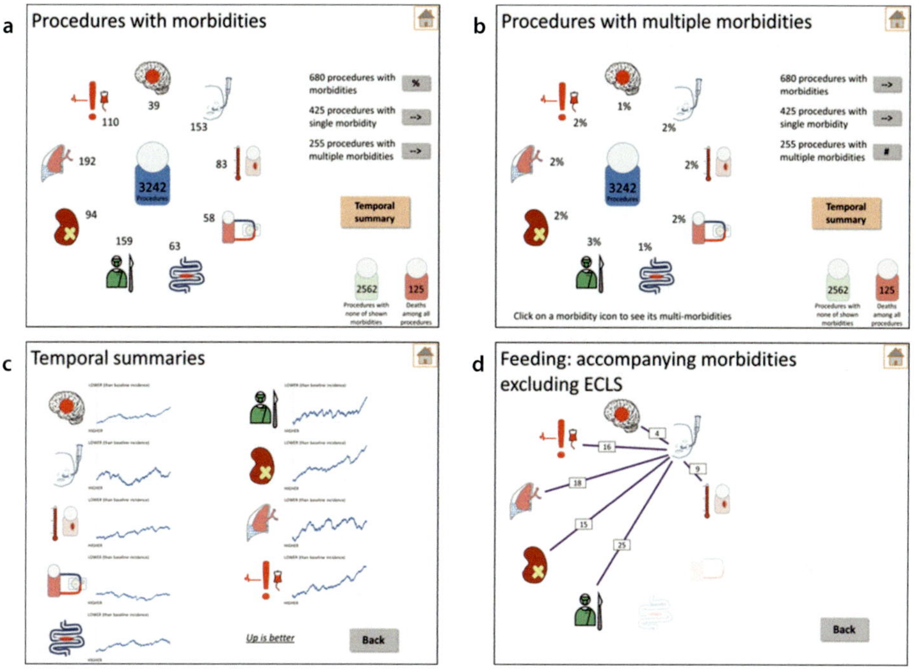

Fig. 34.4 Postoperative complication dashboard example. Reproduced from [51]

Long-term follow-up after intensive care admission: There is an increasing awareness as to the need for long-term follow-up of outcomes after intensive care admission, among an increasingly large number of survivors. A population-based study by Gilboa et al. estimated there were 2.4 million patients with CHD in the USA of whom 60% or 1.4 million were adults [20]. Psychosocial issues, for which support might be needed, include impaired social, behavioural and emotional function, anxiety and depression and impaired communication skills with increased incidence of autism spectrum disorders and psychiatric disorders [53]. For high-risk children, the American Heart Association (AHA) and the American Academy of Pediatrics (AAP) recommend [22] the following:

1. Referral to formal developmental and medical evaluation.
2. Referral to early intervention services or early childhood special education services prior to confirmation of a specific developmental diagnosis.
3. Periodic re-evaluations at 12–24 months, 3–5 years and 11–12 years of age.
4. Referral of young adults for higher education and/or vocational counselling.

In settings, where it is not feasible to deploy the AHA/AAP Guidelines, parental questionnaires about ND may provide an alternative, given that an awareness of ND issues should be maintained over the long-term by both parents and clinicians.

Interventions targeting functional outcome: There is an increasing interest and awareness that interventions directed at function may improve outcomes in survivors of cardiac intensive. Examples include pipeline studies of early rehabilitation; a positive trial of a psychosocial intervention for parents of infants with CHD developed in Northern Ireland; [54] Internet-based cognitive behavioural therapies to reduce internalizing symptoms for adolescents with psychiatric and somatic conditions; [55] evidence-based online information portal to smooth adolescent transition to adult services [56] and interventions promoting a healthy lifestyle both for parents and children [57].

Take-Home Messages

- Important early outcomes are mortality and complications of surgery and critical illness.
- Long-term outcomes are very important and include neurodevelopmental and psychological problems.
- Population-based registries and multi-institutional collaborations have been a 'game changer' in propelling outcome analysis forward.
- Scrutiny of outcomes by stakeholders is vital to the transparency agenda and has leveraged some of the key improvements in outcomes over the last decade.

References

1. Brown KL, Crowe S, Franklin R, McLean A, Cunningham D, Barron D, et al. Trends in 30-day mortality rate and case mix for paediatric cardiac surgery in the UK between 2000 and 2010. Open Heart. 2015;2(1):e000157.
2. NICOR. NICOR: National Institute for Cardiovascular Outcomes Research: Congenital Heart Diseases. London: University College London; 2017. www.nicor4.nicor.org.uk/CHD
3. Crowe S, Brown KL, Pagel C, Muthialu N, Cunningham D, Gibbs J, et al. Development of a diagnosis- and procedure-based risk model for 30-day outcome after pediatric cardiac surgery. J Thorac Cardiovasc Surg. 2013;145(5):1270–8.
4. Jacobs JP, O'Brien SM, Pasquali SK, Jacobs ML, Lacour-Gayet FG, Tchervenkov CI, et al. Variation in outcomes for risk-stratified pediatric cardiac surgical operations: an analysis of the STS congenital heart surgery database. Ann Thorac Surg. 2012;94(2):564–71. discussion 71-2
5. Brown KL, Pagel C, Brimmell R, Bull K, Davis P, Franklin RC, et al. Definition of important early morbidities related to paediatric cardiac surgery. Cardiol Young. 2017;27(4):747–56.
6. Brown KL, Ridout D, Pagel C, Wray J, Anderson D, Barron DJ, et al. Incidence and risk factors for important early morbidities associated with pediatric cardiac surgery in a UK population. J Thorac Cardiovasc Surg. 2019;158(4):1185–96 e7.
7. Brown KL, Pagel C, Ridout D, Wray J, Anderson D, Barron DJ, et al. What are the important morbidities associated with paediatric cardiac surgery? A mixed methods study. BMJ Open. 2019;9(9):e028533.
8. Pasquali SK, He X, Jacobs JP, Jacobs ML, O'Brien SM, Gaynor JW. Evaluation of failure to rescue as a quality metric in pediatric heart surgery: an analysis of the STS congenital heart surgery database. Ann Thorac Surg. 2012;94(2):573–9; discussion 9–80
9. Pasquali SK, Li JS, Burstein DS, Sheng S, O'Brien SM, Jacobs ML, et al. Association of center volume with mortality and complications in pediatric heart surgery. Pediatrics. 2012;129(2):e370–6.
10. Bojan M, Gerelli S, Gioanni S, Pouard P, Vouhe P. Evaluation of a new tool for morbidity assessment in congenital cardiac surgery. Ann Thorac Surg. 2011;92(6):2200–4.
11. Costello JM, Cooper DS, Jacobs JP, Chai PJ, Kirsch R, Rosenthal T, et al. Intermediate-term outcomes after paediatric cardiac extracorporeal membrane oxygenation-what is known (and unknown). Cardiol Young. 2011;21(Suppl 2):118–23.
12. Jacobs ML, O'Brien SM, Jacobs JP, Mavroudis C, Lacour-Gayet F, Pasquali SK, et al. An empirically based tool for analyzing morbidity associated with operations for congenital heart disease. J Thorac Cardiovasc Surg. 2013;145(4):1046–57.
13. Health Insurance Portability and Accountability Act (HIPAA), 1996.

14. Shahian DM, He X, Jacobs JP, Rankin JS, Peterson ED, Welke KF, et al. Issues in quality measurement: target population, risk adjustment, and ratings. Ann Thorac Surg. 2013;96(2):718–26.
15. Best KE, Rankin J. Long-term survival of individuals born with congenital heart disease: a systematic review and meta-analysis. J Am Heart Assoc. 2016;5(6)
16. Brown KL, Wray J, Knowles RL, Crowe S, Tregay J, Ridout D, et al. Infant deaths in the UK community following successful cardiac surgery: building the evidence base for optimal surveillance, a mixed-methods study. Southampton: Health Services and Delivery Research; 2016.
17. Crowe S, Ridout DA, Knowles R, Tregay J, Wray J, Barron DJ, et al. Death and emergency readmission of infants discharged after interventions for congenital heart disease: a National Study of 7643 infants to inform service improvement. J Am Heart Assoc. 2016;5(5):e003369.
18. Billett J, Majeed A, Gatzoulis M, Cowie M. Trends in hospital admissions, in-hospital case fatality and population mortality from congenital heart disease in England, 1994 to 2004. Heart. 2008;94(3):342–8.
19. Knowles RL, Bull C, Wren C, Dezateux C. Mortality with congenital heart defects in England and Wales, 1959–2009: exploring technological change through period and birth cohort analysis. Arch Dis Child. 2012;97(10):861–5.
20. Gilboa SM, Salemi JL, Nembhard WN, Fixler DE, Correa A. Mortality resulting from congenital heart disease among children and adults in the United States, 1999 to 2006. Circulation. 2010;122(22):2254–63.
21. Ghanayem NS, Allen KR, Tabbutt S, Atz AM, Clabby ML, Cooper DS, et al. Interstage mortality after the Norwood procedure: results of the multicenter single ventricle reconstruction trial. J Thorac Cardiovasc Surg. 2012;144(4):896–906.
22. Marino BS, Lipkin PH, Newburger JW, Peacock G, Gerdes M, Gaynor JW, et al. Neurodevelopmental outcomes in children with congenital heart disease: evaluation and management: a scientific statement from the American Heart Association. Circulation. 2012;126(9):1143–72.
23. Squires J. The ages and stages questionnaire. 3rd ed. Baltimore, MD; 2006
24. Brown KL, Ridout DA, Pagel C, Lakhanpaul M, Kakat S, Banks V, et al. Validation of the brief developmental assessment in pre-school children with heart disease. Cardiol Young. 2018;28(4):571–81.
25. Ringle ML, Wernovsky G. Functional, quality of life, and neurodevelopmental outcomes after congenital cardiac surgery. Semin Perinatol. 2016;40(8):556–70.
26. Schroder M, Boisen KA, Reimers J, Teilmann G, Brok J. Quality of life in adolescents and young adults with CHD is not reduced: a systematic review and meta-analysis. Cardiol Young. 2016;26(3):415–25.
27. Kyosti E, Ala-Kokko TI, Ohtonen P, Peltoniemi O, Rautiainen P, Kataja J, et al. Factors associated with health-related quality of life 6 years after ICU discharge in a Finnish paediatric population: a cohort study. Intensive Care Med. 2018;44(9):1378–87.
28. Riehle-Colarusso TJ, Bergersen L, Broberg CS, Cassell CH, Gray DT, Grosse SD, et al. Databases for congenital heart defect public health studies across the lifespan. J Am Heart Assoc. 2016;5(11):e004148.
29. Alten JA, Rahman AF, Zaccagni HJ, Shin A, Cooper DS, Blinder JJ, et al. The epidemiology of health-care associated infections in pediatric cardiac intensive care units. Pediatr Infect Dis J. 2017;37:768.
30. Hickey PA, Connor JA, Cherian KM, Jenkins K, Doherty K, Zhang H, et al. International quality improvement initiatives. Cardiol Young. 2017;27(S6):S61–S8.
31. Gaies M, Werho DK, Zhang W, Donohue JE, Tabbutt S, Ghanayem NS, et al. Duration of postoperative mechanical ventilation as a quality metric for pediatric cardiac surgical programs. Ann Thorac Surg. 2018;105(2):615–21.
32. Buckley JR, Graham EM, Gaies M, Alten JA, Cooper DS, Costello JM, et al. Clinical epidemiology and centre variation in chylothorax rates after cardiac surgery in children: a report from the pediatric cardiac critical care consortium. Cardiol Young. 2017;1-8:1678.
33. Jacobs JP, Jacobs ML, Mavroudis C, Backer CL, Lacour-Gayet FG, Tchervenkov CI, et al. Nomenclature and databases for the surgical treatment of congenital cardiac disease—an updated primer and an analysis of opportunities for improvement. Cardiol Young. 2008;18(Suppl 2):38–62.

34. Franklin RC, Jacobs JP, Tchervenkov CI, Beland MJ. Bidirectional crossmap of the short lists of the European paediatric cardiac code and the international congenital heart surgery nomenclature and database project. Cardiol Young. 2002;12(5):431–5.
35. Franklin RC. The European paediatric cardiac code long list: structure and function. Cardiol Young. 2000;10(Suppl 1):27–146.
36. Franklin RC, Jacobs JP, Krogmann ON, Beland MJ, Aiello VD, Colan SD, et al. Nomenclature for congenital and paediatric cardiac disease: historical perspectives and the international pediatric and congenital cardiac code. Cardiol Young. 2008;18(Suppl 2):70–80.
37. Rogers L, Brown KL, Franklin RC, Ambler G, Anderson D, Barron DJ, et al. Improving risk adjustment for mortality after pediatric cardiac surgery: the UK PRAiS2 model. Ann Thorac Surg. 2017;104(1):211–9.
38. O'Brien SM, Clarke DR, Jacobs JP, Jacobs ML, Lacour-Gayet FG, Pizarro C, et al. An empirically based tool for analyzing mortality associated with congenital heart surgery. J Thorac Cardiovasc Surg. 2009;138(5):1139–53.
39. Jenkins KJ, Gauvreau K, Newburger JW, Spray TL, Moller JH, Iezzoni LI. Consensus-based method for risk adjustment for surgery for congenital heart disease. J Thorac Cardiovasc Surg. 2002;123(1):110–8.
40. Lacour-Gayet F, Clarke D, Jacobs J, Gaynor W, Hamilton L, Jacobs M, et al. The Aristotle score for congenital heart surgery. Semin Thorac Cardiovasc Surg Pediatr Card Surg Annu. 2004;7:185–91.
41. Leegaard M, Watt-Watson J, McGillion M, Costello J, Elgie-Watson J, Partridge K. Nurses' educational needs for pain management of post-cardiac surgery patients: a qualitative study. J Cardiovasc Nurs. 2011;26(4):312–20.
42. Hovels-Gurich HH. Factors influencing neurodevelopment after cardiac surgery during infancy. Front Pediatr. 2016;4:137.
43. Ernst MM, Marino BS, Cassedy A, Piazza-Waggoner C, Franklin RC, Brown K, et al. Biopsychosocial predictors of quality of life outcomes in pediatric congenital heart disease. Pediatr Cardiol. 2018;39(1):79–88.
44. Nembhard WN, Salemi JL, Ethen MK, Fixler DE, Dimaggio A, Canfield MA. Racial/ethnic disparities in risk of early childhood mortality among children with congenital heart defects. Pediatrics. 2011;127(5):e1128–38.
45. Nicholas OCD, Brown K, Franklin D, on behalf of the Steering and Research Committees of NCHDA at NICOR. Analysis of candidate risk factors in paediatric cardiac surgery 30-day risk modelling: ethnicity, deprivation, sex, year, volume, distance from home, weekday or weekend. NICOR UCL: University College London; 2015.
46. Knowles RL, Ridout D, Crowe S, Bull C, Wray J, Tregay J, et al. Ethnic and socioeconomic variation in incidence of congenital heart defects. Arch Dis Child. 2016;102:496–502.
47. Parslow RC, Tasker RC, Draper ES, Parry GJ, Jones S, Chater T, et al. Epidemiology of critically ill children in England and Wales: incidence, mortality, deprivation and ethnicity. Arch Dis Child. 2009;94(3):210–5.
48. Pagel C, Utley M, Crowe S, Witter T, Anderson D, Samson R, et al. Real time monitoring of risk-adjusted paediatric cardiac surgery outcomes using variable life-adjusted display: implementation in three UK centres. Heart. 2013;99(19):1445–50.
49. Salvin JW, Scheurer MA, Laussen PC, Wypij D, Polito A, Bacha EA, et al. Blood transfusion after pediatric cardiac surgery is associated with prolonged hospital stay. Ann Thorac Surg. 2011;91(1):204–10.
50. Utley M, Brown K, Tsang V. Invited commentary. Ann Thorac Surg. 2012;94(5):1602–3.
51. Grieco L, Pagel C, Utley M, Barron DJ, Stoica S, Tibby S, et al. A tool for routine monitoring and feedback of morbidities following paediatric cardiac surgery. Cardiol Young. 2020;30(1):28–33.
52. Rajagopal VB, Brown K, Pagel C, Wray J. Parental understanding of health professional communication about paediatric cardiac surgical morbidity: a qualitative study. BMJ Open Paediatr. 2019; In press
53. Karsdorp PA, Everaerd W, Kindt M, Mulder BJ. Psychological and cognitive functioning in children and adolescents with congenital heart disease: a meta-analysis. J Pediatr Psychol. 2007;32(5):527–41.

54. McCrossan B, Morgan G, Grant B, Sands AJ, Craig BG, Doherty NN, et al. A randomised trial of a remote home support programme for infants with major congenital heart disease. Heart. 2012;98(20):1523–8.
55. Vigerland S, Lenhard F, Bonnert M, Lalouni M, Hedman E, Ahlen J, et al. Internet-delivered cognitive behavior therapy for children and adolescents: a systematic review and meta-analysis. Clin Psychol Rev. 2016;50:1–10.
56. Etnel JRG, van Dijk APJ, Kluin J, Bertels RA, Utens E, van Galen E, et al. Development of an online, evidence-based patient information portal for congenital heart disease: a pilot study. Front Cardiovasc Med. 2017;4:25.
57. Morrison ML, Sands AJ, McCusker CG, McKeown PP, McMahon M, Gordon J, et al. Exercise training improves activity in adolescents with congenital heart disease. Heart. 2013;99(15):1122–8.

Neurocritical Care

Contents

IX

Paediatric Major Trauma in Context for the PICU Clinician

Matt Edwards, Tom Breen, and Bogdana Zoica

Contents

J. Brierley et al. (eds.), *ESPNIC Children's Intensive Care Textbook*,
https://doi.org/10.1007/978-3-031-64762-8_35

35.1 What Is Major Trauma?

Learning Objectives

By the end of this section, PICU clinicians will be able to:
- Describe the observed patterns of paediatric trauma across various age groups
- Understand how paediatric major trauma cases present to hospital
- Describe the principle of centralised trauma care within a trauma network

Injury produces a significant health burden for children, being a leading cause of both death and disability. While the majority of the annual four million paediatric injury presentations to emergency departments in the UK are not life-threatening, there is a significant proportion of trauma that will require the skills and expertise of PICU clinicians and nurses.

The national database of trauma cases, Trauma Audit Research Network (TARN), is an invaluable resource and produces specific reports for injured children in the UK [1]. Of all the significantly injured children recorded on the TARN database, approximately 50% are admitted to HDU/ITU environments.

Children suffer injury in relatively predictable patterns in developed countries. The patterns of injury are aligned with the child's stage of development and along stereotypical gender-based behavioural tendencies for risk-taking [1].

- There is a peak in childhood major trauma in those under 2 years of age. Being less independently mobile, they are either injured by falls or by non-accidental injury (NAI). It is also extremely common in NAI cases for children to not present as trauma and not to present to major trauma centres. There are particular injury patterns associated with NAI in small children and infants, but the initial approach will be the same as in other causes of accidental injury.
- As children become more mobile, falls from height start to predominate as a cause of significant injury, peaking between 3 and 8.
- Increasingly from about the age of 3, children are involved in more road traffic incidents, normally as pedestrians or cyclists, peaking in early adolescence.
- In later adolescence, the incidence of major trauma due to assault starts to increase, as does the incidence of self-harm. Self-harm mechanisms leading to significant physical injury are relatively evenly split between falls from height and asphyxia.
- The proportion of males to females injured is similar under 2 years of age. After that, males predominate as victims in most cases, particularly in assault and self-harm scenarios.

35.1.1 Paediatric Major Trauma Networks

Many developed nations have moved to centralise care for traumatically injured patients utilising a 'hub and spoke' model [2]. At the centre of these trauma networks are major trauma centres, where all the intensive care, surgical and rehabilitation specialists should be available and the peripheral trauma units that feed into them. Prehospital services have criteria for bypassing trauma units when they are managing patients who have suffered major trauma and that includes paediatrics [3]. It has been found that there is variability in triage tools from one prehospital service to the next, and in paediatrics, there is relatively poor sensitivity and specificity for major trauma (as defined by ISS > 15) [4].

Two issues make the provision of paediatric major trauma care over large geographical areas more challenging.

- The first is that not all major trauma centres are paediatric major trauma centres. Paediatric MTCs require key paediatric surgical trauma specialists and a PICU. Conversely, some of the larger PICUs are not based within an MTC.
- Second, approximately 25% of paediatric major trauma cases are brought by private vehicles to the nearest hospital which is unlikely to be a paediatric MTC [1].

If a patient needs urgent transfer to the MTC, it won't normally be appropriate to wait for critical care retrieval services. Unless there are dedicated prehospital trauma teams available, the trauma unit will need to formulate a team of critical care seniors to transfer the injured child [5]. This has implications for training and preparedness at trauma units.

For the reasons above, it is strongly advised for all emergency departments, whether they are an MTC or not, to train for the child who is severely injured and arrives unannounced by a private vehicle.

35.2 Paediatric 'Trauma Call'

Learning Objectives

By the end of this section, PICU clinicians will be able to:

- Describe the standard sequence of a 'trauma call' and understand their role.
- Appreciate the leadership challenges characteristic in paediatric trauma calls.

Despite a huge variety of possible clinical scenarios, a trauma call should have a standardised approach that the team are expecting to follow. Trauma training courses such as ATLS [6], APLS [7] and ETC [8] utilise a similar structure. Described below are the eight suggested steps that a trauma call will progress through:

- Pre-alert*
- Team preparation*
- Transfer from prehospital transport equipment*
- Handover/initial information from the patient or person bringing the patient
- Primary survey
- Decisions
- Transfer
- Secondary survey

*These steps will obviously not occur if the trauma case arrives unannounced or is a delayed recognition of major trauma. Classic examples of delayed trauma calls would be those with abdominal bicycle handlebar injuries [9] and infants having suffered NAI. Once major trauma has been recognised and the trauma call put out, team members will arrive in a staggered fashion. After immediate tasks are initiated, there should be an early attempt to pause and silence the team to establish a shared mental model and communicate a plan.

35.2.1 Pre-alerts

It is standard practice for ambulance services to give a 'pre-alert' to give some basic information to the receiving hospital so they can prepare the space and the team for the patient. The short time given to prepare allows the team to establish the names of the team members, identify roles and allocate key rate-limiting steps.

35.2.2 Role of the PICU Doctor in a Trauma Call

Given the broad range of critical care skills that a PICU doctor will bring to a trauma call, they can theoretically occupy many key roles in the team. It will generally depend on local protocols and the availability of other staff as to which role they play. To illustrate, while they may be able to lead the advanced airway management, if there is also a consultant anaesthetist present, their skills may be better directed towards intravenous access or placing chest drains. In other situations, where there is a big team available, their primary role may be the organisation and preparation of the bed space in the PICU. As explained above, the majority of paediatric trauma calls do not require critical care, and in these cases, the PICU team can expect to be released early by the team leader.

35.2.3 Team Preparation and 'Crowd Control'

Effective communication and leadership in paediatric trauma care are often challenging due to the large number of staff that can attend. There are often lots of senior team members involved in these cases. Dividing staff into three groups: those to remain in the cubicle, those outside but available and those to be sent away helps streamline the response. Large crowds and lots of noise in the cubicle are not only riskier and more chaotic; it is also intimidating for the child and their parent.

35.2.4 Parents

Evidence supports the presence of a parent during the resuscitation of critically unwell or injured children [10]. It is common for an experienced staff member to be allocated to support them.

35.2.5 Handover

During the handover in paediatric trauma care, vital information is transferred, including the child's age and mechanism of injury. Immediate life-threatening concerns, e.g. airway obstruction, must be quickly identified and addressed rather than awaiting the full handover. Once urgent issues are handled, the team leader can take a moment to process information and then bring the team together to clarify the situation and devise a plan.

If there are no immediate concerns or they have been swiftly resolved, a concise handover with the prehospital team should take place. This provides an opportunity to share the mental model, gain clarification and avoid repetition. The whole team should listen to the information from the prehospital care team, and an introduction to the parent helps involve them in the process. The child may be terrified, screaming and squirming, and so a staff member may need to devote their time to consoling the child while the rest of the team gets handover.

35.3 Assessing the Paediatric Trauma Patient aka 'The Primary Survey'

Learning Objectives

By the end of this section, PICU clinicians will be able to:

- Perform a sequential primary survey to identify and treat key life-threatening injuries
- Appreciate the age-specific challenges in assessing and treating injuries found at each step during the primary survey

The primary survey in paediatric trauma care follows the C-ABCDE approach [11]. Its purpose is to identify and treat life-threatening injuries as they are found in order of priority.

Adaptations may be needed based on the child's age and the nature of the trauma. The next paragraph will explore these aspects of the primary survey and any differences in paediatric trauma patients compared to adults (Table 35.1).

35.3.1 Catastrophic Haemorrhage

Catastrophic haemorrhage from a major artery is rapidly fatal. Managing external bleeding remains crucial for trauma clinicians as re-bleeding can occur even in the resuscitation room. Direct pressure or pressure applied to a compressible site of the

Table 35.1 Meaning of the C-ABCDE acronym

C	Catastrophic haemorrhage	Torrential external haemorrhage, normally from a major artery
A	Airway issues	Obstructed or unable to maintain their own airway
B	Breathing issues	Failure to ventilate or oxygenate adequately
C	Circulatory collapse	All causes of hypoperfusion. This should include an examination of sites of internal blood loss
D	'Disability'	Recognition and addressing signs of neurological deficit resulting from spinal and brain injury
E	'Exposure'	Ensuring that areas of major injury have been identified. Identification of hidden sites of penetrating trauma. Identification of contributory factors such as hypothermia and hypoglycaemia

supplying artery is effective and superior to simply applying layers of dressings. Haemostatic agents can be used with direct pressure for cavities. Windlass tourniquets designed for adults may still be applied for arterial bleeding from children's limbs [12]. Once bleeding is controlled, the exact time of application should be noted, and surgical intervention should be arranged immediately.

Although uncommon in small children, life-threatening injuries can occur from collisions with sharp objects such as broken glass. Even blood loss from less typical areas, such as the scalp from a dog bite, can result in catastrophic haemorrhage in small children [13]. Estimating external blood loss is difficult, but any obvious blood loss in a small child is likely significant, and ongoing bleeding must be immediately addressed.

35.3.2 Airway Issues

Airway issues and injuries in paediatric trauma care can be critical and require prompt attention. The most common airway problem in injured children is reduced consciousness. The initial interventions for maintaining the airway include proper head positioning, airway opening manoeuvres, simple adjuncts and suctioning. Nasopharyngeal airways (NPAs) can be useful for children with a low consciousness level and airway obstruction risk. They are, however, considered contraindicated in severe head and facial injuries due to the rare risk of inadvertent intracranial insertion [14]. Obtaining correctly sized NPAs can be challenging in smaller children, but using adapted endotracheal tubes for this purpose is possible.

Oropharyngeal and supraglottic airways are helpful adjuncts, but they should be carefully sized and placed gently to avoid stimulating laryngospasm in smaller children.

Direct laryngeal injuries in children are rare but pose significant challenges. From asymptomatic to complete laryngeal disruption, the presentation can vary. The small airway in children can be more severely compromised by subsequent oedema. Children with signs of direct laryngeal trauma should be allowed to adopt a comfortable position despite concerns about cervical spinal injury.

Formulating a plan promptly with senior staff, including anaesthesia and, ideally, ENT/otolaryngology surgeons, is essential. It is best to execute the plan calmly and in a controlled environment, preferably in the theatre. In cases of actual or impending airway obstruction, clinicians must proceed to endotracheal intubation as quickly as possible. If there are surgical skills immediately available, primary tracheotomy could be considered [15].

35.3.3 Breathing (Thoracic Injury)

35.3.3.1 Blunt Injuries

As a general rule, when a child reaches skeletal maturity, the injuries of the chest can be considered analogous to those in the adult trauma literature [16]. Prior to this age, the compliance of the chest wall means that force can be transmitted across the lungs and mediastinum without ribs fracturing or providing the same protection. It is more common therefore for pulmonary contusions to exist without overlying rib fracture. Fortunately, the mediastinum is also relatively compliant to sheer forces, so cardiac and large vessel injuries are rare. A few key concepts are important for the PICU clinician to appreciate:

- Clinical signs of chest injury can be subtle. Any persistent minor drop in oxygen saturation in an otherwise healthy child should be considered significant. A simple chest X-ray is likely adequate to investigate low-risk cases yet CT remains the golden standard to investigate concurrent thoracic trauma [17]. Point-of-care lung ultrasound has an emerging role in the identification of injuries usually difficult to exclude clinically: pneumothorax, haemothorax and contusions [18].
- Pulmonary contusions can be severe and necessitate invasive ventilation. There may be a delayed deterioration as pulmonary contusions can worsen. The ventilation strategy will be protective and similar to that employed in acute respiratory distress syndrome (ARDS). In head injury patients, this can result in a challenging battle of priorities between neuroprotection and pulmonary protection [19]. With advancing ECMO technologies, there may be options for supporting damaged lungs and hearts in the PICU while waiting for them to recover [20].
- Diaphragmatic injury [21] and cardiac injury are easily missed and are more common in cases of significant pulmonary contusions. Blunt cardiac contusions can be effectively excluded with ECG and troponin tests [22]. Cardiac tamponade due to haemopericardium in blunt trauma in children is extremely rare.
- Tension pneumothorax is more likely to occur when a simple pneumothorax is positive pressure ventilated than in those breathing for themselves. The decision to prophylactically decompress a simple pneumothorax when a child is ventilated is debatable. Many small pneumothoraxes can be closely observed even on mechanical ventilation [23], and ultrasound may have a useful role in monitoring progression [24].
- Subtle and small haemothoraxes are relatively common in significant blunt thoracic trauma, and conservative treatment is more commonplace [25]. The rare large haemothorax has the potential for both rapid haemodynamic and respiratory compromise with associated significant mortality. While this may be challenging, there should be aggressive but careful blood and clotting factor replacement prior to emergency anaesthesia followed by immediate chest drainage. If the chest drain output is severe and ongoing, proceeding to thoracotomy may be required [26]. This is incredibly rare in blunt trauma, but the more common possibility in penetrating trauma is outlined in the next paragraph.
- Placing chest drains in smaller children is challenging, likely requiring general anaesthesia. This clearly comes with its own risks and a plan should be made for decompensation when switching to positive-pressure ventilation. More details of the variations in the procedure can be found in Teague et al. (2019) [27]. While decompression of the chest using needles has fallen out of favour in adults and large teenagers, needles may still have a place in the emergency in a smaller child [28]. It should be noted, however, that many modern 'closed system safety' cannulas have valves that make chest decompression impossible, so it is important to know which type is being used [29].
- Large amounts of air swallowing are common in injured small children, so an NG tube should be considered as part of the ventilation strategy.

35.3.4 Penetrating Injuries

Tragically, interpersonal violence does not exclude children, and a proportion of paediatric thoracic injuries will be caused by knives and guns. The path and depth of such injuries are often difficult to predict and therefore an abdominal wound, for example, could potentially cross the diaphragm. In the UK, penetrating trauma is almost exclusively caused by knife stab wounds. In comparison to blunt trauma, operative management is more common. Given the older age of these patients, many can be operatively managed by adult trauma surgeons. Reassuringly, even in moderately sized heamopneumothoraces, the vast majority can be managed with a surgical chest drain, normally placed under procedural sedation in conjunction with local anaesthesia [30].

35.3.4.1 Thoracotomy

In cases of chest drain loss exceeding 2–3 mL/kg for consecutive hours or ongoing blood loss of 10–15 mL/kg over 24 h, serious consideration should be given to interventional radiology and/or thoracic surgery [7]. Blunt trauma rarely requires such intervention, and decisions may be more challenging based on the child's age, equipment availability and surgical team familiarity. Ultrasound can aid in identifying these injuries. If time permits and the child can reach the operating room, a limited left-sided thoracotomy or midline sternotomy is the preferred option. Needle pericardiocentesis is no longer recommended for haemorrhagic pericardial tamponade. If the child loses cardiac output due to penetrating torso trauma, an immediate clamshell thoracotomy (resuscitative thoracotomy) is indicated to access the pericardium, release the pericardial haematoma and identify the bleeding site. This procedure, performed by prehospital trauma clinicians in some cases, allows for open heart massage and aortic compression to improve brain and coronary perfusion [31].

35.3.5 Circulation (Haemorrhage)

35.3.5.1 Challenge of the Bleeding Child

Assessing significant blood loss in children can be challenging. The volume of external bleeding is difficult to assess, and physiological parameters may not be helpful. Clinical signs mimicking hypovolaemia can be caused by various factors such as pain, distress, hypothermia and other types of shock. Traumatic brain injury can also cause cardiovascular instability [32]. Younger children have additional challenges as they can compensate for marked blood loss, making it difficult to assess their condition accurately.

In the very early management of adolescents with penetrating trauma, there is a role for 'permissive hypotension' to reduce clot disruption. However, this strategy is not supported beyond the first hour of resuscitation and lacks evidence in bleeding small children [33] whose baseline blood pressure is close to the limits of cerebral autoregulation [34].

Relying solely on blood gas analysis triggers to justify or avoid transfusion should be avoided. Normal haemoglobin or lactate levels do not necessarily indicate the absence of significant blood loss.

In critically injured and potentially hypovolemic children, simultaneous optimisation for all possible causes is crucial. This includes addressing external haemorrhage, providing oxygen, analgesia and antiemetics and administering warmed blood products if blood loss is felt to be the cause. Frequent reassessment is essential to monitor the response and stabilise the child.

Rapidly anaesthetising shocked patients should be delayed until oxygenation, and haemodynamics are optimised whenever possible. Positive pressure ventilation in critically hypovolemic patients is high-risk, potentially precipitating cardiovascular collapse [35].

In cases of less obvious injuries, there should be consideration for significant blood loss, and a high-dependency environment may be required, even for those who do not require immediate surgery. Non-operative management can be suitable for most bleeding from solid organs [36]. Supportive treatment in a critical care environment would include blood product replacement, coagulopathy correction and regular surgical review.

35.3.5.2 'One on the Floor and Four More'

A simple aide memoire for the areas to consider in the assessment of potentially life-threatening blood loss is 'one on the floor and four more.' This often-taught phrase refers to the large volumes of blood that can be lost into the chest, the abdomen, the pelvis and the femurs in addition to external haemorrhage. This may apply in the skeletally mature child, but in the younger child, the locations of significant bleeding are different. To illustrate, smaller children are highly unlikely to lose significant blood volume from pelvic [37] or femoral fractures [38], whereas areas such as haematomas of the scalp or even intracranially in infants may hold larger volumes. It may be that, in polytrauma patients, there is simply a combined burden of small bleeds rather than one large source. All bleeding, even seemingly minor venous oozing, needs attention and urgent haemostasis.

35.3.5.3 Blood Products or Crystalloid

It seems sensible to state that 'like should be replaced with like,' and so bleeding should be treated with warmed blood products administered in ratios that best replicate what the child has lost. In principle, this is difficult to argue against; however, diagnostically there can be uncertainty (as described above) and logistically this is not always possible. Crystalloids may be used in the initial phase when blood is not available or haemorrhage is uncertain, acknowledging that there are risks of haemodilution and potentially worsening coagulopathy. There are risks to over-transfusion [39] in these critically unwell children. A sensible strategy is to use blood product bolus doses of 5 mL/kg, followed by a pause and reassessment.

Debate exists surrounding the most appropriate ratio of blood products. There is variation in local policies and availability, but a ratio of approximately 1:1 PRBCs: Plasma is reasonable [40] with early consideration of platelets and cryoprecipitate if bleeding continues. Where available, TEG studies can provide a tailored transfusion strategy for the patient far faster than lab coagulation results. The aim of providing balanced ratios of blood products to the patient is to address hypovolaemia and oxygen delivery to tissues and to avoid coagulopathy associated with major trauma and haemorrhage.

35.3.5.4 'Code Red' Care in Children

Significant haemorrhage requiring massive transfusion in injured non-adolescent children is not common [41]. The most pragmatic recent definition of massive transfusion is defined as >40 mL/kg of blood products [42] analogous to approximately 50% of the child's circulating volume in 24 h. Clearly, this is a retrospective definition, and many centres have adopted the concept of a 'Code Red' trauma patient to describe a patient who is early in their resuscitation but is clinically predicted to require significant transfusion.

Coordination of this Code Red response alongside the leadership of a paediatric trauma call is challenging and often requires a specific senior team member in the role. Code Red care should involve most of the following:

- Deciding on a definitive plan for haemorrhage control. As soon as a child is declared 'Code Red,' theatres and the surgical team should be informed.
- Coordination of the staff involved—administering and checking the blood, hospital porter, those running samples and those in the lab.
- Gaining IV access that is adequate to deliver blood as quickly as is necessary.
- Ensuring balanced ratios of products are delivered by keeping accurate records.
- Including associated infusions, specifically calcium supplementation and tranexamic acid.
- Ensuring that temperature control is maintained.
- Ensuring that early samples are sent to monitor for coagulopathy. Depending on availability, this would include 'point-of-care' thromboelastogram (TEG) or rotational thromboelastometry (ROTEM) samples to guide transfusion ratios.
- Monitoring closely that units of blood products are not wasted and that the response in the lab is stood down as soon as possible.

This response and coordination of the balanced responsive transfusion should continue through to the theatre or the critical care environment. In true massive transfusion cases, blood product requirements and ongoing treatment of coagulopathy will often continue beyond theatre to the PICU. In the PICU, the cycle of replacement and testing for coagulopathy and ongoing losses continues alongside the surgical teams assessing whether the patient needs operative management.

35.3.6 Disability (Traumatic Brain Injury and Spinal Injury)

As part of the primary survey, the patient's consciousness level and the movements in the limbs will be assessed. Traumatic brain injury and its management are discussed in other chapters.

Spinal trauma is a rare but potentially devastating injury in paediatric trauma patients. For the PICU clinician, it is helpful to consider it from the perspective of two scenarios: the confirmed spinal injury and the more common issue of the 'potential' spinal injury.

35.3.6.1 Potential Spinal Injury and Immobilisation

Spinal trauma in children is rare; however, among children who have suffered significant blunt trauma requiring PICU, that rate will be far higher [43]. The high energy patterns required to cause spinal trauma may also result in concomitant severe TBI and haemorrhage. In these scenarios, the presence of spinal injury will be difficult to exclude clinically, and therefore a policy of 'assuming there is a spinal injury' is appropriate in PICU. This will involve full spinal precaution until the child can be adequately assessed or the child has had adequate imaging. Those precautions would consist of the patient lying supine with tape and blocks holding the head in a normal position, team log rolling for transfer and nursing care and potentially a well-fitting semi-rigid collar. In smaller children, semi-rigid collars are difficult to fit, hard to tolerate when awake and may cause increased intracranial pressure [8] and are no longer routinely recommended. It should be noted that immobilisation is meant to hold the child's neck in a neutral anatomical position, so the shoulders of the small child should be carefully raised to avoid abnormal neck flexion.

It is a very reasonable trauma principle that the movement of any unstable injury should be minimised. There is also understandable clinical concern regarding any movement of the neck for fear that it may cause further spinal cord damage. All efforts should be made to minimise movement of the injured spine, but there is little evidence that small, brief and low-energy movements of the spine necessary for laryngoscopy will have a detrimental effect [44]. Manual inline stabilisation has little evidence that it reduces the neck movement [45] so if the child's airway is at risk, securing the airway with a good view is always the priority.

CT scans are not adequate to exclude spinal injury in children who have not reached skeletal maturity [46]. Considerable shearing forces across the spinal cord can cause spinal cord injury without radiological abnormality (SCIWORA) in the absence of fractures. This is of concern in children with high-speed deceleration injuries and mechanisms of axial loading, i.e. landing directly on the head from a fall. With the new MRI protocols for trauma, it may be that brain and spine MRI may be the most appropriate investigation but are practically more challenging than CT in the immediate phase.

A common PICU scenario is for a child with severe TBI in whom spinal injury cannot be excluded. Unless the child can be extubated quickly, spinal precautions could remain in place for an extended period. This is not without risks [47]. 'Log rolling' requires more staff, collars create pressure sores and may lead to increased intra cranial pressure (ICP). In recognition of the harm of unnecessary spinal precautions, early MRI is advocated by many centres for intubated children who cannot be clinically assessed in 72 h [48]. Although there are extremely rare cases of persistent neurological deficit despite a normal MRI, the normal MRI, alongside senior spinal/neurosurgical and neuroradiology support, can still reasonably reassure clinicians that the spine itself is stable enough to care for the patient in the PICU without strict immobilisation [49, 50].

35.3.6.2 Confirmed Spinal Injury

The immobilisation techniques described above would apply for the child with a confirmed injury but only temporarily. A definitive plan for surgery and/or external forms of stabilisation should be gained quickly. A child with an obvious neurological deficit has a high risk of pressure sores and will need nursing on an appropriate mattress immediately.

Different age groups exhibit different injury patterns. The smallest children sustain high spinal injuries such as atlantoaxial dislocation due to forces on their flexible, weak necks during high-speed car accidents or shaking. This can be fatal due to spinal cord and brain stem disruption. Intubation and ventilation are common due to associated traumatic brain injury, and ventilatory support is necessary for high spinal injuries due to diaphragm nerve supply loss.

In older children with mature skeletons, different mechanisms and injuries occur further down the spine. Spinal injury above T6 may lead to cardiovascular instability with relative euvolaemia or distributive shock. It is a preferred strategy in these cases to utilise vasopressors such as noradrenaline in order to avoid fluid overload [51].

The key principle in managing neurological injuries in the PICU is to deliver enhanced supportive care that confers the best chance of avoiding secondary neurological injury. This is achieved by avoiding hypoxia and hypotension, maintaining normal $PaCO_2$ levels, proactively managing any autonomic derangement and controlling any temperature and glucose fluctuations. Surgical management options may be considered based on injury type and severity. More specialist advice should be gained early from dedicated spinal units.

Some cervical spine injuries may also involve intimal damage to neck vessels, potentially leading to carotid artery dissection and stroke risk [52]. Vascular imaging in cases of high-energy cervical spine injury and skull base fractures would be reasonable.

35.3.7 Exposure

It is important that the child has full exposure to look for signs of life-threatening trauma. This is distinct from the secondary survey, where the patient is carefully examined from top to toe for any minor injuries. Once exposed, the patient should be warmed and covered again to minimise further thermal losses. A log roll to expose the back is not strictly necessary before imaging but ensure the patient's back has been visualised at some point of the initial assessment.

For physiologically stable penetrating trauma with less concern for unstable spinal injury, a 'stab check' can be conducted during the exposure part of the primary survey. The 'stab check' involves examining specific hidden areas for wounds: neck, axillae, back, buttocks, groin, perineum and thighs.

Given the rapid availability in most centres, many consider a venous blood gas result part of the primary survey. Most can give a blood glucose level and other important information that assists with subsequent decisions.

35.4 Decision-Making After the Primary Survey

Learning Objectives

By the end of this section, PICU clinicians will be able to:

- Understand some of the key decisions required after the primary survey
- Describe common rate-limiting steps in the initial management of paediatric major trauma cases

As described in ▶ Sect. 35.2, the initial handover combined with the primary survey will give the trauma team leader the information required for the patient's next steps towards definitive management. Various life-threatening injuries may have already been found in the primary survey as described in ▶ Sect. 35.3, and decisions will have been made to initiate treatment. Depending on the problems found and the stability of the patient after the primary survey, the team leader will make the decision of what to do next. The options are:

- The patient requires no more intervention or investigation and can proceed to the secondary survey. This decision is probably more common in paediatric trauma calls as the mechanism of injury may have concerned prehospital teams enough to trigger a trauma call, but once there has been an opportunity for a longer period of observation and a more comprehensive assessment, there is no longer concern for severe injuries. Clearly at this point the PICU team is unlikely to have any further involvement in the case.
- The patient is stable and requires advanced targeted imaging to further delineate injuries. The type and extent of that imaging will be dictated by the paediatric trauma imaging decision aids such as The Royal College of Radiologists Paediatric trauma protocols.
- The patient is unstable but the benefit of imaging outweighs the risk of the transfer to CT. Advanced imaging is often vital to the optimal management of the child, especially given the non-operative or interventional radiology options available in many traumatic injuries. Resuscitation will need to continue en route and in the CT room. There must always be a plan to abort the attempt at imaging and move directly to the theatre if required.
- The patient is so unstable that the only option is emergency surgery. Resuscitation room emergency thoracotomy is a possible but rarely required intervention as described in ▶ Sect. 35.6. With ongoing resuscitation and liaison with the surgical teams, a plan and path to damage control surgery should be made. Any child in this category is highly likely to need a PICU bed postoperatively.

Most of the decisions above will require a rapid safe transfer from the resuscitation area. PICU clinicians will be well-versed in critical transfers and will be vital in this process. Emergency departments should be well-stocked with immediately available transfer equipment such as dedicated transfer bags, portable suction units and ventilators. Maintaining rapidly warmed blood transfusion on the route can be extremely challenging as the infusers are often bulky, on their own set of wheels and precariously tethered to precious intravenous access. It is rare that there is such a need for nonstop transfusion that it outweighs the logistics and risks of continuing while on the move for short periods.

35.5 Burns and Blasts

Learning Objectives

By the end of this section, PICU clinicians will be able to:

- Describe the common burns scenarios where PICU may be required

- Appreciate some of the common concerns and pitfalls in burns management including electrical burns
- Understand the multiple potential mechanisms of injury that occur during a significant blast injury and the key principles of managing them in PICU

In developed countries and outside war zones, the predominant cause of burns in small children is scald injuries. PICU clinicians are involved due to the facial burns and the large body surface area affected. However, in most cases, simple measures of care—listed below—are sufficient.

- Strong analgesia such as intranasal fentanyl
- 20 min of running room-temperature tap water within 3 h of the injury
- Debridement of dead skin and blisters
- Dressing of the burns

Ironically, one of the major iatrogenic sequelae of thermal injury is hypothermia. So as soon as the 20 min of cooling have been completed, the child must be insulated from further heat loss and warmed [53].

PICU clinicians may be consulted because of concerns of impending airway swelling, but the risk of airway compromise should not delay first aid measures. It is extremelu unlikely that a common scalp affects the airway. There are case reports of burns to the anterior neck leading to laryngeal oedema, however, so airway concerns cannot be entirely discounted [54].

Simple scalds generally do not require intensive care unless >20%BSA is involved. In such cases, large fluid shifts and systemic inflammation warrant high dependency admission. Balancing fluid responsiveness against fluid tolerance is a challenging quest. Widespread oedema and fluid requirements will often result in respiratory distress, and so many severely burned children will need early intubation. Where possible, vasopressors should be avoided to preserve blood flow to the injured skin. Ensure that the burns have been debrided of devitalised skin, photographed for the receiving unit and dressed with a non-adherent dressing. PICU teams may be involved in the initial stabilisation and transfer to a specialist burns unit.

Less commonly, small children may have sustained burns at the hands of their carers, but the pattern tends to be more specific and associated with other indicators of child abuse.

Thermal burns due to fire commonly involve older children:

- Patients with burns from fire are more likely to suffer from thermal inhalation and progressive airway oedema, making early intubation a crucial consideration for any child showing signs of airway burns. Post-intubation, facial swelling can be significant, and caution must be exercised not to damage the tube. Alternative methods of securing the tube, such as suturing, may be necessary.
- The burns sustained from fire are often deeper due to prolonged exposure to higher temperatures, leading to a higher likelihood of eschar formation. The tight and inelastic eschar can cause compartment syndromes and restrict chest expansion, requiring emergency escharotomies prior to transfer. Collaboration with paediatric or adult surgeons should be based on local protocols and age cut-offs.
- Burn injuries from explosions or fires may be associated with blunt trauma, but this can be overlooked due to the absence of an injury history and the focus on burn injuries. Conducting a ‘whole body CT’ is recommended in cases where

there is a possibility of serious associated injuries. Additionally, a detailed 'secondary survey' should not be neglected to identify other injuries before the patient is transferred.

- Inhalation of the gases and smoke emitted from a fire may cause severe lung inflammation and toxicity.
  - Carbon monoxide and cyanide are common inhalant toxins and should be considered in all smoke inhalation. COHb is normally measured as 'point of care testing' and is treated with high FiO_2. Hyperbaric treatment for levels >20% has some evidence for benefit, but the risks and logistics of the transfer of critically unwell patients into a hyperbaric chamber make this option generally unrealistic.
  - Cyanide can be suspected if there is high or refractory lactic acidosis [55]. The treatment is hydroxycobalamin 70 mg/kg IV up to a maximum dose of 5 g [56].

35.5.1 Electric Burns

Electric burns in paediatric patients are relatively uncommon for PICU teams. Most cases involve domestic current and cause minimal injury, but young children may experience more severe burns due to lower skin resistance. Burns may be deep and small, typically found on hands or feet as entrance and exit paths for the current. Nerves and muscles, being the most conductive tissues, tend to suffer the most damage.

PICU clinicians may be involved if a patient experiences respiratory arrest, arrhythmias or muscle injury, leading to rhabdomyolysis. Preschool children who sustain oral electric burns, often from chewing on cables, face a unique concern: delayed severe bleeding of the labial artery, which can occur around 1 week after the injury [57]. Management is akin to treating severe post-tonsillectomy bleeding [58], requiring controlled yet rapid intubation to protect the airway and control the haemorrhage.

35.5.2 Blast Injuries

35

In civilian situations, blast injuries can occur accidentally due to domestic gas ignition or fireworks [59] and then rarely due to terrorist activity where the mortality is far higher [60]. Incidents such as the Manchester Arena bombing in 2017 [61] have demonstrated that such multi-casualty events can predominantly involve children. PICU services are generally in short supply and so, in that eventuality, creative solutions incorporating adult critical care services would inevitably be required. All PICU departments should be familiar with their local and regional major incident policy for the unlikely yet devastating situation of a paediatric-predominant mass casualty event.

Virtually all civilian practice is informed from military experience. It is therefore advisable to get advice from military healthcare staff if possible and reference the international Paediatric Blast Injury Field Manual [62] when these events occur.

Blast trauma involves multiple types of trauma across the whole body, according to different stages of the explosion [63]:

- Primary injury: the 'blast wave' causes extreme pressure differential leading to extremity amputations and immediate fatalities. Any air-filled spaces are susceptible to barotrauma resulting in pneumothorax, bowel perforation, tympanic membrane rupture and the infamous 'blast lung'. Blast lung is a common cause of death and can present in a delayed fashion as worsening dyspnoea, possibly haemoptysis culminating in apnoea, bradycardia and cardiovascular collapse. In PICU, 'blast lung' should be managed similarly to severe ARDS (field manual).

- Secondary injury: 'blast wind,' consists of intense heat and flying projectiles, resulting in burns and penetrating trauma.
- Tertiary injury: the body may be launched by the blast wind causing impact injuries with immovable objects.
- Quaternary injuries: immediate after the blast wind injuries depending on blast environment and type, including burns, chemical contact, radiation exposure, entrapment and crush injuries.

Following the prioritisation principles of C-ABCDE is crucial, as there might be visually striking limb injuries and burns that could distract from life-saving priorities. Other specific considerations for the PICU clinician regarding blast injury:

- Emergency anaesthesia is frequently required for children significantly affected by a blast, due to various injuries but also as a humanitarian act in severe cases such as limb amputations that may occur in the blast wave.
- A thorough secondary survey is always important but in blast injuries, there is potential for an almost unlimited collection of 'minor' injuries. The child will need an early log roll to fully examine their back for burns, wounds and foreign bodies. Ocular injuries can be easily missed in intubated patients as can tympanic rupture, which has a high specificity for concomitant blast lung [64].
- Projectiles causing penetrating injuries are frequently heavily contaminated including human bone leading to a high risk of infection. Early administration of antibiotics, tetanus and human virus prophylaxis is essential. Combine this risk with the areas of devitalised tissue, and sepsis is highly likely. Sepsis is likely due to the combination of contamination and devitalised tissue, often requiring extensive debridements and amputations.

35.6 Traumatic Cardiac Arrest

Learning Objectives

By the end of this section, PICU clinicians will be able to:

- Appreciate the types of patients that may survive traumatic cardiac arrest
- Describe the algorithm of concurrent activity that should be used to optimise chances of survival
- Understand when attempts of resuscitation can stop
- Appreciate the necessity of debriefing the teams in these situations

Injured children who lose cardiac output have an extremely poor prognosis [65]. If the treating prehospital teams are unable to achieve the return of spontaneous circulation (ROSC), before reaching the hospital, injured children almost never survive to discharge and if they do, there is a high risk of profound neurological disability. Historically, the situation was similar for traumatic cardiac arrest (TCA) in adults.

More recently, a strategy of immediately, aggressively and concurrently addressing reversible causes of cardiac arrest has yielded better outcomes [66, 67]. These benefits do appear to be limited to the prehospital arena in those patients, of any age, who have had a minimum of 'downtime'. This is irrespective of whether there has been bystander basic life support (BLS) or not. Attempts have been made to gain consensus in formulating a TCA management algorithm in children specifically; however, many aspects remain controversial [68].

It is important for the PICU clinician to understand the current concepts surrounding TCA because:

- Rare survivors of TCA would require intensive care regardless of neurological outcome.
- Knowledge of managing TCA and its differences from medical cardiac arrest benefits PICU doctors in peri-arrest situations.
- Most children with resuscitation attempts initiated are transported to the hospital, and PICU clinicians are part of receiving trauma teams.
- Small children in arrest may not initially appear to have suffered trauma, but it could be due to non-accidental injury.
- Understanding when further interventions are futile allows the focus of cardiac arrest management to shift to care for the parent and the team.

35.6.1 Which Children Survive TCA?

The key two elements for a child to survive TCA are first, for it to be caused by a reversible pathology and second, for that pathology to be addressed extremely quickly. The reversible causes of TCA can be remembered by the acronym 'HOT' and are as follows:

1. H—hypovolaemia/exsanguination
2. O—oxygenation/hypoxia
3. T—tension pathology—pneumothorax and, rarely, cardiac tamponade

For a chance of meaningful survival, every second is important. To address these causes with the speed required, other common aspects of cardiac arrest care are de-emphasised, specifically, chest compressions, adrenaline and rhythm analysis.

35.6.2 Logistics of Running the Arrest

The reversible causes need to be addressed concurrently. With a team member or two focused on restoring circulating volume, ventilating with 100% oxygen and decompressing the chest, this necessitates a very busy cubicle. Strict marshalling of the space will be vital and no team member without a direct role should be permitted. There will likely need to be prioritisation of the most likely cause.

35.6.3 H: Addressing Hypovolaemia

Exsanguination is an uncommon cause of death in blunt trauma of the small child and is most common in penetrating trauma in adolescents. The rate-limiting step in many cases, especially in the small child, is gaining working IV access. Intraosseous (IO) access may be viewed as the solution but it must be noted that, in the arrest situation, many intraosseous needles have been found to be incorrectly placed [69]. An experienced PICU clinician may be able to swiftly perform ultrasound-guided vascular access in the largest available vessel of a non-injured limb. A bolus of warmed fluid (preferably PRBCs if the patient has lost blood) should be administered quickly. Warming fluids may not be possible. Measures should be taken to apply tourniquets where bleeding had occurred, pelvic binders in the older child and femur fracture reduction. These would assist in preventing blood loss in the event of ROSC. A plan for theatre should be considered if ROSC is gained.

35.6.4 O: Addressing Hypoxia

While endotracheal intubation is considered the gold standard, a well-fitting and functioning supraglottic airway can suffice in the initial phases. $ETCO_2$ monitoring is vital to confirm ETT placement, detect possible ROSC and aid in decision-making on futility. In arrest situations, ETTs are often placed too deep, and ventilation may occur too rapidly and with excessive pressure and volume. Monitoring chest movement and any airway leaks is essential to identify potential issues such as pneumothorax or endobronchial placement.

35.6.5 T: Addressing Tension Pathology

In arrest situations, this is challenging due to the limited reliability of clinical examination to rule out pneumothorax. Needle decompression of the chest is no longer the preferred method, and open thoracostomies are recommended. If the treating team lacks the competencies for thoracostomy and the cannulas lack valves, needle decompression may be used as an alternative. In cases of penetrating torso trauma, a clamshell thoracotomy should be considered to address cardiac tamponade.

35.6.6 Non Accidental Injury or Suspected Physical Abuse

In the unexpected cardiac arrest of infants or small children, trauma should be considered as a possible cause, even if external signs are not evident. Cardiac arrest management follows initial BLS principles and potential traumatic causes are addressed within the '4H and 4T' framework in the 'non-shockable' pathway. In cases of non-ambulant children who have suffered NAI, severe TBI is the predominant cause of cardiac arrest. The decision to administer blood and perform thoracostomies to treat potential exsanguination and tension pneumothorax may need to be carefully considered in prolonged arrest without ROSC.

35.6.7 Rational Prioritisation

In managing severe paediatric trauma, interventions may vary based on the specific cause. Some aspects of the algorithm may not be applicable in certain situations, such as RTC or fall from height, but it is essential to consider all options. Prioritisation depends on the mechanism of injury, with the entire algorithm typically applied in cases of blunt force or penetrating trauma.

35.6.8 Recognition of Futility

In cases where there are injuries incompatible with life or obvious rigor mortis, children will be declared 'life extinct' in the community. If resuscitation attempts are initiated and the child does not achieve ROSC before transport to the hospital, neurologically intact survival is virtually never seen.

On arrival at the hospital, efforts may be made to address reversible causes of the TCA. Once these causes have been addressed, further attempts at resuscitation become futile. Signs such as a broad, agonal or asystolic rhythm on a cardiac trace sustained low $ETCO_2$ value, and no cardiac activity on basic cardiac ultrasound can support this decision.

Once futility is recognised, multiple rounds of CPR and adrenaline should be avoided. The focus of care shifts from attempting to save the child's life to providing compassionate care for the parents, and the members of the medical team. CPR may continue temporarily to facilitate effective and empathetic communication that everything appropriate has been done, and the child has died.

35.6.9 Debrief

Debriefing is essential for severe paediatric trauma and traumatic cardiac arrest situations, which are uncommon and emotionally challenging for most clinicians. Conducting both a 'hot' debrief immediately after the arrest and a 'cold' debrief at a later date, possibly after postmortem results, is considered good practice. Despite the pressures of the health service, making time for debriefs should be a standard part of the process. Colleagues covering the PICU should be aware that a debrief will take place, and the involved PICU clinician should be encouraged to attend if possible.

35.7 Traumatic Asphyxia—Hanging and Drowning

Learning Objectives

By the end of this section, PICU clinicians will be able to:

- Appreciate that hanging and drowning are classified as major traumas, but there are important differences in approach and decision-making
- Understand the key principles in early management when drowning and hanging patients arrive with and without a pulse
- Appreciate the challenges with prognostication for these patients in PICU

35.7.1 Hanging and Near Hanging

Hanging is defined as 'suspension by the neck resulting in asphyxia and death' [70] if the patient survives or at least, does not die immediately, the term is 'near hanging'. While the absolute numbers are thankfully small, hanging, as an injury mechanism, is one of the most likely to result in childhood death in the UK alongside drowning and traumatic brain injury [1]. It again tends to fit a bimodal distribution of ages—it occurs by accident in small ambulatory children, and then later in adolescence, it is the most common method of completed suicide. Hanging can be divided into 'judicial,' i.e. it involves a drop and sudden stop, or 'non-judicial' where the patient is merely suspended or partially suspended by the neck. It is useful to understand the differences in these mechanisms as they affect management and may assist in understanding the devastating neurological sequelae. Hanging with a drop may cause immediate death by high cervical spine injury, but in simple suspension, the mechanism of death is a little more complex. In simple suspension, cervical spine injuries are rare, as are injuries of the neck vessels and death was thought to occur due to simple asphyxia. Hanging appears to cause unconsciousness and cardiac arrest faster than simple obstruction of the airway and hypoxia would [71], suggesting that other mechanisms such as complete obstruction of cerebral venous outflow and early cardiac arrythmia may play a significant role.

Advanced airway management in near-hanging patients is frequently required, and there are specific challenges to prepare for:

- Agitation
  - Near-hanging patients may present with very low glascow coma score (GCS), but a proportion will be simply profoundly agitated as a consequence of the brain injury and adrenergic drive. Similarly, to those agitated head injury patients requiring intubation, a strategy of 'delayed sequence intubation' could be considered. In this technique, sedating medication is used early to facilitate preoxygenation and other optimisation [72, 73].
- Laryngeal injury
  - Injury is clearly more likely in a judicial hanging as it transfers considerable force across the larynx. The adolescent cohort of paediatric hangings do occasionally suffer from fractures or ruptures of laryngeal structures. Those injuries are even less likely in preschool children as they have more flexible structures and less force applied. There can, however, be swelling and haematoma in the narrow airways of small children making securing the airway and, later, the extubation more challenging [74].
- Ventilation
  - Due to the high negative thoracic pressure generated against the airway obstruction, near-hanging patients often develop pulmonary oedema. This will result in a more precipitous drop in saturations when securing the airway and occasionally even florid oedema obstructing the view of the cords. Clinicians should expect this and have suction immediately available. It could also make video laryngoscopy impossible. Following intubation, ventilation may be challenging and require more positive end expiratory pressure (PEEP) and very frequent suctioning to address the oedema.
- Potential cervical spine injury

- As described earlier, securing the airway should proceed with manual in line stabilisation (MILS), but if MILS causes challenges with gaining the airway, it should be released. Securing the airway takes priority over the concerns of cervical spine injury.

While the available evidence suggests that cervical spine injury in non-judicial hanging is rare [75], it is not impossible. It is however impossible to clinically assess for spinal injury when the patients are unconscious. This leaves the PICU clinician with a difficult decision. The clinician must decide whether to consider the patient as having a 'potential injury,' ultimately resulting in an MRI to exclude it or they decide that sufficient force has not been applied across the cervical spine and therefore no further imaging or immobilisation is required. Discussion and agreement will need to be made among senior team members on a case-by-case basis.

Arrhythmias are common in near hanging [76] and cardiac arrest, despite it being a 'traumatic cardiac arrest,' should be managed as a normal medical arrest, prioritising ventilation, chest compressions and identification of shockable rhythms [77]. Post return of spontaneous circulation (ROSC) therapeutic hypothermia down to 32–34°C in hanging cases is debated [78], but targeted temperature management and avoiding hyperthermia is still recommended [79].

Only about half of near-hanging paediatric cases, i.e. those found with a cardiac output, will go on to have good neurological recovery [80]. GCS seems to be less predictive than in adults for whether the child will have permanent ischaemic encephalopathy. Prognostication can therefore be challenging despite the use of MRI and EEG, and the evidence is generally weak [81]. Virtually none of those found pulseless will survive with a good neurological outcome [81].

35.7.2 Drowning

Worldwide, drowning is the third leading cause of injury death in children [82], and for those drowning cases that arrive at the hospital, the mortality is around 50% (1). The available evidence to inform practice is limited, however [83]. The situation of how children become submerged or immersed will differ with age, but classically babies will slip under water when unsupervised, inquisitive preschool children fall into water, and then in adolescents, there is increased risk-taking and substance misuse around water. Epilepsy is the most common comorbidity in drowning cases [84].

35

The causes of death for a drowning patient are asphyxia with hypoxic brain injury, aspiration pneumonia and hypothermia. Four critical questions in paediatric drowning are:

- What was the state of the child when they were rescued? The mortality for drowning cases unsurprisingly follows the severity of initial clinical symptoms and signs specifically the presence of a pulse, hypotension and any signs of pulmonary oedema. As a rule of thumb, a minimum of an high dependency unit (HDU) environment is recommended for a child rescued with signs of significant pulmonary oedema and/or cardiovascular compromise [85]. The child may seem to have improved on arrival at the hospital, but pulmonary oedema can recur. Pulmonary oedema can be treated with similar ventilation protocols to ARDS and tends to resolve faster. Non-invasive ventilation seems to be of benefit in mild-moderate

cases. In extreme cases where even mechanical ventilation is inadequate, extracorporeal life support is a viable option with reasonable survival rates [86]. Discuss challenging cases with the nearest ECMO centre as soon as the severity is recognised.
- Has the child sustained trauma or just immersion? Trauma and cervical spinal injury need to be considered, but unless the child has fallen from height into water, there tends to be no other injury. Drowning is classified as a traumatic mechanism of injury, but resuscitation has been shown to have similar outcomes whether patients are brought to an MTC or local hospital [87]. Without evidence of other trauma, cardiac arrest algorithms should follow standard medical algorithms (Vasello).
- How long has the child been immersed? While submersion duration can be used as a prognostic indicator when making prehospital search and rescue decisions, the evidence is not robust when the child reaches the hospital. Observational studies do demonstrate a significant drop off in survival in any patient known to have been immersed for more than 10 min [88].
- If the child is hypothermic, was the child hypothermic before drowning? Based on physiological principles and case reports of survival in hypothermic drowning cases, the size of the child and the core temperature at the point of drowning should impact on potential for neurological recovery. If a small child whose brain temperature should drop faster falls into cold water (<6°C) or an adolescent who becomes hypothermic from swimming in cold water and subsequently drowns, then the core temperature at the point of drowning is protective to the brain. Studies investigating this, however, have not shown good evidence that the age of the patient or the temperature of the water has a bearing on neurological recovery [89].

Despite case reports demonstrating the potential for survival in child drownings in the extremes of immersion times and resuscitation duration, recent ILCOR guidance recommends 'against the use of age, EMS response time, water type (fresh or salt), water temperature and witness status when making prognostic decisions' [89]. ILCOR case-by-case decisions with seniors will need to be made.

35.8 Deterioration in PICU

Learning Objectives

By the end of this section, PICU clinicians will be able to:

- Describe the basic principles of the pathologies that cause children to deteriorate after major trauma in the PICU
- Predict which types of patients and injuries are likely to get worse before they get better
- Understand in what situations significant injuries can be missed and when to have a high index of suspicion for them

Although the actual trauma epidemiology has changed [89], it is still a useful principle to consider those who die from trauma to follow a trimodal pattern—the first group are those who die immediately or very soon after the injury, and the second are those who die from severe injuries within the first 24 h in the hospital and then the third group are those who suffer delayed deterioration on the ward or in PICU [90]. A cohort of these late deaths will be largely unpreventable, i.e. severe brain trauma and/or hypoxic brain injuries making further recovery impossible. Preventing mortality for the rest of the patients in that third group relies on excellent initial management and then on clinicians predicting and responding to complications such as:

- Inflammation
- Sepsis
- ARDS
- Coagulopathy
- Rebleed
- Ischaemia
- Rhabdomyolysis
- Compartment syndrome
- Missed/occult injuries

Following major trauma, especially in blunt trauma where there have been more widespread forces and damage across the body, a series of inflammatory processes have been found to occur [91]. Patients are more at risk when this occurs systemically, leading to systemic inflammatory response syndrome (SIRS) concomitant infection in sepsis and ultimately multi-organ failure [92]. Significant local areas of contusion are almost likely to get worse, e.g. pulmonary contusions, as the classic inflammatory process of swelling and capillary leak proceeds over the first few days. Combining SIRS systemically and direct contusions of the lungs locally tends to a high risk of acute respiratory distress syndrome (ARDS). These widespread inflammatory complications are more likely to occur as the burden of injury increases, and therefore they are common sequelae for injured children taken directly to the PICU. Knowing this potential for deterioration, however, allows the PICU clinician to be proactive in the review of trauma patients, even if the child does not require an intensive care bed on admission.

Coagulopathy following trauma is a complex and evolving area of understanding, involving both an early deranged response to bleeding and a later constituent of multi-organ failure [93]. It may be observed as early as the prehospital phase, may be independent of actual blood loss [94] and is even a recognised phenomenon in isolated head injuries [95]. As general principles, alongside the surgical plan for bleeding control, the trauma and PICU clinician should pay close attention to balanced blood product transfusion, frequently test and respond to haematology testing (as often as every 30 min in severe cases (BSH)) and be scrupulous with temperature control.

There are a number of factors that may contribute to a child's bleeding again after initial haemostasis. In the hyperacute phase, the patient may theoretically rebleed as the blood pressure is restored before the controlling clot is stable [96]; young arteries are also more liable to go into a protective spasm which could rebleed slightly later [97], then there may be the issue of coagulopathy as described above and then there is the late phenomenon of pseudoaneurysm formation. These late sequelae tend to occur days after liver and splenic injury in particular, hence the common practice of ultrasound follow-up 5–10 days after injury [98].

Shearing forces, compression and vasospasm all contribute to impaired vascular supply and the potential for ischaemic tissue. Supportive care gives 'at risk' tissues the best chance of survival. This would involve optimising oxygen delivery and tissue perfusion, and conversely avoiding hyperoxia and high doses of vasopressors. It is an important and ancient trauma principle that devitalised tissue be debrided or resected as soon as it is identified. Rising lactate and refractory sepsis may indicate the presence of ischaemic tissue; however, it is clearly better to recognise and target threatened organs such as the bowel, before these deleterious effects take hold.

Skeletal muscle damage is common in trauma with rhabdomyolysis being most commonly associated with crush injuries [99]. This may result in acute kidney injury. Children's kidneys cope better than adults with myoglobinaemia after muscle damage and chronic renal impairment is extremely rare. That notwithstanding, in cases of severe crush injury, electrical injury, blast injury and polytrauma, serial creatinine kinase levels are recommended [100]. Optimising renal perfusion is the mainstay of treatment with there being little evidence for diuretic or steroid therapy. Early haemofiltration is controversial [101] but may be considered in severe cases.

Mechanisms described above may contribute to acute swelling within poorly compliant fascial compartments resulting in increased pressure and subsequent ischaemia. Compartment syndrome is actually very rare in children despite their higher normal compartment pressures [102]. Examination of limbs looking for signs suggestive of compartment syndrome should still be a necessary part of the review of polytrauma patients in PICU. Awake smaller children may simply be agitated and anxious with escalating analgesic requirements. It should be noted that there is a concern that lower limb regional anaesthesia may mask the pain of early compartment syndrome. The evidence suggests single nerve blocks are safe as long there is a regular review of the limb at risk [103].

Early CT scans are not 100% sensitive or specific for certain subtle injuries that may become more evident with time in the PICU. A high index of suspicion is required, taking the mechanism of injury into account [104]. Classic injuries to be suspicious of would be diaphragmatic, pancreatic and mesenteric injuries in blunt abdominal trauma, subtle rib fractures and cardiac injury in thoracic trauma, vascular injury at any junctional region of sheer stress and rectal and urological and gynaecological injury in pelvic trauma. SCIWORA and subtle spinal injuries would be included in this list and have been discussed previously. To illustrate, if a child restrained by a lap belt in a road traffic accident has sustained a lumbar vertebral fracture, it is almost impossible for this to occur without some intrabdominal injury [105]. Musculoskeletal injuries are the most common missed injuries for the critically unwell trauma patient [106] along with commonly forgotten areas such as the eyes and the back. Hence, the importance of a detailed secondary survey of critically injured children. This includes patients who have suffered critical penetrating trauma. It is not uncommon, in the rush to the theatre, for other more minor wounds to be missed or for concomitant blunt trauma sustained during assault or running away (e.g. calcaneal fractures), to get missed.

References

1. The Trauma Audit and Research Network (TARN) Severe Injury in Children (January 2019–December 2020). www.tarn.ac.uk. Accessed Feb 2023.
2. Lendrum RA, Lockey DJ. Trauma system development. Anaesthesia. 2013;68(Suppl 1):30–9.

3. Moran CG, Lecky F, Bouamra O, Lawrence T, Edwards A, Woodford M, Willett K, Coats TJ. Changing the system—major trauma patients and their outcomes in the NHS (England) 2008-17. EClinicalMedicine. 2018;2-3:13–21.
4. Gianola S, Castellini G, Biffi A, Porcu G, Fabbri A, Ruggieri MP, Stocchetti N, Napoletano A, Coclite D, D'Angelo D, Fauci AJ, Iacorossi L, Latina R, Salomone K, Gupta S, Iannone P, Chiara O, Italian National Institute of Health guideline working group. Accuracy of pre-hospital triage tools for major trauma: a systematic review with meta-analysis and net clinical benefit. World J Emerg Surg. 2021;16(1):31.
5. South Thames Retrieval Service Clinical Guidelines: Time Critical Neurosurgical Transfer. STRS London UK 2019. https://www.evelinalondon.nhs.uk/resources/our-services/hospital/south-thames-retrieval-service/neurosurgical-transfer-mar-2018.pdf. Accessed 26 Dec 2022.
6. ATLS Subcommittee; American College of Surgeons' Committee on Trauma; International ATLS Working Group. Advanced trauma life support (ATLS®): the ninth edition. J Trauma Acute Care Surg. 2013;74(5):1363–6.
7. Advanced Life Support Group M. Advanced paediatric life support. 6th ed. Wiley Blackwell; 2016.
8. Thies K, Gwinnutt C, Driscoll P, et al. The European Trauma Course—from concept to course. Resuscitation. 2007;74:135–41.
9. Cheung R, Shukla M, Akers KG, Farooqi A, Sethuraman U. Bicycle handlebar injuries—a systematic review of pediatric chest and abdominal injuries. Am J Emerg Med. 2022;51:13–21.
10. Mark K. Family presence during paediatric resuscitation and invasive procedures: the parental experience: an integrative review. Scand J Caring Sci. 2020;35(1):20–36.
11. Hodgetts TJ, Mahoney PF, Russell MQ, et al. ABC to <C>ABC: redefining the military trauma paradigm. Emergency Medicine Journal. 2006;23:745–6.
12. Harcke HT, Lawrence LL, Gripp EW, Kecskemethy HH, Kruse RW, Murphy SG. Adult tourniquet for use in school-age emergencies. Pediatrics. 2019;143(6):e20183447.
13. Jakeman M, Oxley JA, Owczarczak-Garstecka SC, Westgarth C. Pet dog bites in children: management and prevention. BMJ Paediatr Open. 2020;4(1):e000726.
14. Roberts K, Whalley H, Bleetman A. The nasopharyngeal airway: dispelling myths and establishing the facts. Emerg Med J. 2005;22(6):394–6.
15. Oosthuizen JC. Paediatric blunt laryngeal trauma: a review. Int J Otolaryngol. 2011;2011:183047.
16. Peterson RJ, Tepas JJ 3rd, Edwards FH, Kissoon N, Pieper P, Ceithaml EL. Pediatric and adult thoracic trauma: age-related impact on presentation and outcome. Ann Thorac Surg. 1994;58(1):14–8.
17. The Royal College of Radiologists. Paediatric trauma protocols. London: The Royal College of Radiologists; 2014. https://www.rcr.ac.uk/system/files/publication/field_publication_files/BFCR(14)8_paeds_trauma.pdf. Accessed Jan 2023
18. Rovida S, Orso D, Naeem S, Vetrugno L, Volpicelli G. Lung ultrasound in blunt chest trauma: a clinical review. Ultrasound. 2022;30(1):72–9.
19. Goedeke J, Boehm R, Dietz HG. Multiply trauma in children: pulmonary contusion does not necessarily lead to a worsening of the treatment success. Eur J Pediatr Surg. 2014;24(6):508–13.
20. Wen PH, et al. Non-heparinized ECMO serves a rescue method in a multitrauma patient combining pulmonary contusion and nonoperative internal bleeding: a case report and literature review. World J Emerg Surg. 2015;10:15.
21. Elkbuli E, Meneses A, Shepherd M, McKenney M, Boneva D. Traumatic diaphragmatic rupture successfully managed in 4-year-old patient: case report and literature review. Int J Surg Case Rep. 2020;72:237–40.
22. Emigh B, Grigorian A, Dilday J, Condon F, Nahmias J, Schellenberg M, Martin M, Matsushima K, Inaba K. Risk factors and outcomes in pediatric blunt cardiac injuries. Pediatr Surg Int. 2023;39(1):195.
23. Barrios C, Tran T, Malinoski D, et al. Successful management of occult pneumothorax without tube thoracostomy despite positive pressure ventilation. Am Surg. 2008;74(10):958–96.
24. Oveland NP, Lossius HM, Wemmelund K, Stokkeland PJ, Knudsen L, Sloth E. Using thoracic ultrasonography to accurately assess pneumothorax progression during positive pressure ventilation: a comparison with CT scanning. Chest. 2013;143(2):415–22.
25. Choi PM, Farmakis S, Desmarais TJ, Keller MS. Management and outcomes of traumatic hemothorax in children. J Emerg Trauma Shock. 2015;8(2):83–7.

26. Wyrick DL, Dassinger MS, Bozeman AP, Porter A, Maxson RT. Hemodynamic variables predict outcome of emergency thoracotomy in the pediatric trauma population. J Pediatr Surg. 2014;49(9):1382–4.
27. Teague WJ, Amarakone KV, Quinn N. Rule of 4's: Safe and effective pleural decompression and chest drain insertion in severely injured children. Emerg Med Australas. 2019;31(4):683–7.
28. Leonhard G, Overhoff D, Wessel L, et al. Determining optimal needle size for decompression of tension pneumothorax in children—a CT-based study. Scand J Trauma Resusc Emerg Med. 2019;27:90.
29. National Patient Safety Alert: Blood control safety cannula and needle thoracostomy for tension pneumothorax. NHS England. 02 April 2020. https://www.england.nhs.uk/wp-content/uploads/2020/04/NatPSA-Blood-control-safety-cannula-needle-thoracostomy-for-tension-pneumothorax-April-2020.pdf. Accessed 4 Feb 2023.
30. Havelock T, Teoh R, Laws D, Gleeson F, BTS Pleural Disease Guideline Group. Pleural procedures and thoracic ultrasound: British Thoracic Society Pleural Disease Guideline 2010. Thorax. 2010;65(Suppl 2):ii61–76.
31. Wise D, et al. Emergency thoracotomy: "how to do it". Emerg Med J. 2005;22(1):22–4.
32. Gavrilovski M, El-Zanfaly M, Lyon RM. Isolated traumatic brain injury results in significant pre-hospital derangement of cardiovascular physiology. Injury. 2018;49(9):1675–9.
33. Hughes NT, Burd RS, Teach SJ. Damage control resuscitation: permissive hypotension and massive transfusion protocols. Pediatr Emerg Care. 2014;30(9):651–6.
34. Clebone A. Pediatric trauma transfusion and cognitive aids. Curr Opin Anaesthesiol. 2018;31(2):201–6.
35. Crewdson K, Rehn M, Brohi K, Lockey DJ. Pre-hospital emergency anaesthesia in awake hypotensive trauma patients: beneficial or detrimental? Acta Anaesthesiol Scand. 2018;62(4):504–14.
36. Notrica DM, Eubanks JW 3rd, Tuggle DW, Maxson RT, Letton RW, Garcia NM, Alder AC, Lawson KA, St Peter SD, Megison S, Garcia-Filion P. Nonoperative management of blunt liver and spleen injury in children: evaluation of the ATOMAC guideline using GRADE. J Trauma Acute Care Surg. 2015;79(4):683–93.
37. Ciarallo L, Fleisher G. Femoral fractures: are children at risk for significant blood loss? Pediatr Emerg Care. 1996;12(5):343–6.
38. Hermans E, et al. Paediatric pelvic fractures: how do they differ from adults? J Child Orthop. 2017;11(1):49–56.
39. Hussmann B, Lefering R, Kauther MD, Ruchholtz S, Moldzio P, Lendemans S, Trauma Register DGU®. Influence of prehospital volume replacement on outcome in polytraumatized children. Crit Care. 2012;16(5):R201.
40. Akl M, Anand T, Reina R, El-Qawaqzeh K, Ditillo M, Hosseinpour H, Nelson A, Obaid O, Friese R, Joseph B. Balanced hemostatic resuscitation for bleeding pediatric trauma patients: a nationwide quantitative analysis of outcomes. J Pediatr Surg. 2022;57(12):986–93.
41. Shroyer MC, Griffin RL, Mortellaro VE, Russell RT. Massive transfusion in pediatric trauma: analysis of the National Trauma Databank. J Surg Res. 2017;208:166–72.
42. Neff LP, et al. Clearly defining pediatric massive transfusion: cutting through the fog and friction with combat data. J Trauma Acute Care Surg. 2015;78:22.
43. Lemley K, Bauer P. Pediatric spinal cord injury: recognition of injury and initial resuscitation, in hospital management, and coordination of care. J Pediatr Intensive Care. 2015;4(1):27–34.
44. Wiles MD. Airway management in patients with suspected or confirmed traumatic spinal cord injury: a narrative review of current evidence. Anaesthesia. 2022;77(10):1120–8.
45. Lennarson PJ, Smith DW, Sawin PD, Todd MM, Sato Y, TraynelisVC. Cervical spinal motion during intubation: efficacy of stabilization maneuvers in the setting of complete segmental instability. J Neurosurg. 2001;94:265–70.
46. Expert Panel on Pediatric Imaging, Kadom N, Palasis S, Pruthi S, Biffl WL, Booth TN, Desai NK, Falcone RA Jr, Jones JY, Joseph MM, Kulkarni AV, Marin JR, Milla SS, Mirsky DM, Myseros JS, Reitman C, Robertson RL, Ryan ME, Saigal G, Schulz J, Soares BP, Tekes A, Trout AT, Whitehead MT, Karmazyn B. ACR Appropriateness Criteria® Suspected Spine Trauma-Child. J Am Coll Radiol. 2019;16(5S):S286–99.
47. Chan M, Al-Buali W, Charyk Stewart T, et al. Cervical spine injuries and collar complications in severely injured paediatric trauma patients. Spinal Cord. 2013;51:360–4.

48. Booth TN. Cervical spine evaluation in paediatric trauma. AJR Am J Roentgenol. 2012;198(5):W417–25.
49. Freigang V, Butz K, Seebauer CT, Karnosky J, Lang S, Alt V, Baumann F. Management and mid-term outcome after "Real SCIWORA" in children and adolescents. Global Spine J. 2022;12(6):1208–13.
50. Brauge D, Plas B, Vinchon M, Charni S, Di Rocco F, Sacko O, Mrozek S, Sales de Gauzy J. Multicenter study of 37 pediatric patients with SCIWORA or other spinal cord injury without associated bone lesion. Orthop Traumatol Surg Res. 2020;106(1):167–71.
51. Ploumis A, Yadlapalli N, Fehlings MG, Kwon BK, Vaccaro AR. A systematic review of the evidence supporting a role for vasopressor support in acute SCI. Spinal Cord. 2010;48(5):356–62.
52. Orman G, Tekes A, Poretti A, Robertson C, Huisman TA. Posttraumatic carotid artery dissection in children: not to be missed! J Neuroimaging. 2014;24(5):467–72.
53. London and South England Burn Network guidance 2020. https://www.mysurgerywebsite.co.uk/page1.aspx?p=16&pr=X13911&t=2
54. Verhees V, Ketharanathan N, Oen IMMH, Baartmans MGA, Koopman JSHA. Beware of thermal epiglottis! A case report describing 'teapot syndrome'. BMC Anesthesiol. 2018;18(1):203.
55. Parker-Cote JL, Rizer J, Vakkalanka JP, Rege SV, Holstege CP. Challenges in the diagnosis of acute cyanide poisoning. Clin Toxicol (Phila). 2018;56(7):609–17.
56. Graham J, Traylor J. Cyanide toxicity. [Updated 2023 Feb 13]. In: StatPearls [Internet]. Treasure Island, FL: StatPearls Publishing; 2023. https://www.ncbi.nlm.nih.gov/books/NBK507796.
57. Hoffman KA, Trigger CC. Pediatric oral commissure burn. Clin Pract Cases Emerg Med. 2017;1(1):59–60.
58. Windfuhr JP, Schloendorff G, Baburi D, Kremer B. Lethal outcome of post-tonsillectomy hemorrhage. Eur Arch Otorhinolaryngol. 2008;265(12):1527–34.
59. Nunziato CA, Riley CJ, Johnson AE. How common are civilian blast injuries in the national trauma databank, and what are the most common mechanisms and characteristics of associated injuries? Clin Orthop Relat Res. 2021;479(4):683–91.
60. Tovar MA, Pilkington RA, Goodwin T, Root JM. Pediatric blast trauma: a systematic review and meta-analysis of factors associated with mortality and description of injury profiles. Prehosp Disaster Med. 2022;37(4):492–501.
61. Deeming H. The Kerslake report: an independent review into the preparedness for, and emergency response to, the Manchester Arena attack on 22nd May 2017, 2018.
62. Reavley P, Bree S, Horne S, Mayhew E. The paediatric blast injury field manual. The Paediatric Blast Injury Partnership. 2019. https://www.imperial.ac.uk/media/imperial-college/research-centres-and-groups/centre-for-blast-injury-studies/PBIP-BlastInjuryManual2019_I_web.pdf. Accessed 2 July 2023.
63. DePalma RG, Burris DG, Champion HR, Hodgson MJ. Blast injuries. N Engl J Med. 2005;352(13):1335–42.
64. Peters P. Primary blast injury: an intact tympanic membrane does not indicate the lack of a pulmonary blast injury. Mil Med. 2011;176(1):110–4.
65. Alqudah Z, Nehme Z, Williams B, Oteir A, Bernard S, Smith K. A descriptive analysis of the epidemiology and management of paediatric traumatic out-of-hospital cardiac arrest. Resuscitation. 2019;140:127–34.
66. Lockey DJ, Lyon RM, Davies GE. Development of a simple algorithm to guide the effective management of traumatic cardiac arrest. Resuscitation. 2013;84(6):738–42.
67. Barnard EBG, Hunt PAF, Lewis PEH, Smith JE. The outcome of patients in traumatic cardiac arrest presenting to deployed military medical treatment facilities: data from the UK Joint Theatre Trauma Registry. J R Army Med Corps. 2018;164(3):150–4.
68. Vassallo J, Webster M, Barnard EBG, On behalf of PERUKI (Paediatric Emergency Research in the UK and Ireland), et al. Epidemiology and aetiology of paediatric traumatic cardiac arrest in England and Wales. Arch Dis Child. 2019;104:437–43.
69. Harcke HT, Curtin RN, Harty MP, Gould SW, Vershvovsky J, Collins GL, Murphy S. Tibial intraosseous insertion in pediatric emergency care: a review based upon postmortem computed tomography. Prehosp Emerg Care. 2020;24(5):665–71.
70. Van Hasselt TJ, Hartshorn S. Hanging and near hanging in children: injury patterns and a clinical approach to early management. Arch Dis Child Educ Pract Ed. 2019;104(2):84–7.

71. Sauvageau A, Laharpe R, King D, Dowling G, Andrews S, Kelly S, Ambrosi C, Guay JP, Geberth VJ, Working Group on Human Asphyxia. Agonal sequences in 14 filmed hangings with comments on the role of the type of suspension, ischemic habituation, and ethanol intoxication on the timing of agonal responses. Am J Forensic Med Pathol. 2011;32(2):104–7.
72. Weingart SD, Trueger NS, Wong N, Scofi J, Singh N, Rudolph SS. Delayed sequence intubation: a prospective observational study. Ann Emerg Med. 2015;65(4):349–55.
73. Miescier MJ, Bryant RJ, Nelson DS. Delayed sequence intubation with ketamine in 2 critically ill children. Am J Emerg Med. 2016;34(6):1190.e1–2.
74. Hackett AM, Kitsko DJ. Evaluation and management of pediatric near-hanging injury. Int J Pediatr Otorhinolaryngol. 2013;77(11):1899–901.
75. Salim A, Martin M, Sangthong B, Brown C, Rhee P, Demetriades D. Near-hanging injuries: a 10-year experience. Injury. 2006;37(5):435–9.
76. Wagner J, Reiter K, Schön C, Keil J, Strobelt M, Olivieri M, Hoffmann F. Ventricular fibrillation as initial rhythm in pediatric cardiac arrest by suicidal hanging. Resuscitation. 2017;117:e9–e10.
77. Vassallo J, Nutbeam T, Rickard AC, Lyttle MD, Scholefield B, Maconochie IK, Smith JE. Paediatric traumatic cardiac arrest: the development of an algorithm to guide recognition, management and decisions to terminate resuscitation. Emerg Med J. 2018;35(11):669–74.
78. Harhay MO, Blette BS, Granholm A, Moler FW, Zampieri FG, Goligher EC, Gardner MM, Topjian AA, Yehya N. A Bayesian interpretation of a pediatric cardiac arrest trial (THAPCA-OH). NEJM Evid. 2022;2(1):EVIDoa2200196.
79. Nolan JP, Sandroni C, Böttiger BW, Cariou A, Cronberg T, Friberg H, Genbrugge C, Haywood K, Lilja G, Moulaert VRM, Nikolaou N, Olasveengen TM, Skrifvars MB, Taccone F, Soar J. European Resuscitation Council and European Society of Intensive Care Medicine guidelines 2021: post-resuscitation care. Intensive Care Med. 2021;47(4):369–421.
80. Kleinman ME, Perkins GD, Bhanji F, Billi JE, Bray JE, Callaway CW, de Caen A, Finn JC, Hazinski MF, Lim SH, Maconochie I. ILCOR scientific knowledge gaps and clinical research priorities for cardiopulmonary resuscitation and emergency cardiovascular care: a consensus statement. Circulation. 2018;137(22):e802–19.
81. Davies D, Lang M, Watts R. Paediatric hanging and strangulation injuries: A 10-year retrospective description of clinical factors and outcomes. Paediatr Child Health. 2011;16(10):e78–81.
82. Pellegrino F, Raffaldi I, Rossi R, De Vito B, Pagano M, Garelli D, Bondone C. Epidemiology, clinical aspects, and management of pediatric drowning. Ital J Pediatr. 2023;49(1):74.
83. Bierens J, Abelairas-Gomez C, Furelos RB, Beerman S, Claesson A, Dunne C, Elsenga HE, Morgan P, Mecrow T, Pereira JC, Scapigliati A. Resuscitation and emergency care in drowning: a scoping review. Resuscitation. 2021;162:205–17.
84. Peri F, De Nardi L, Canuto A, Gaiero A, Noli S, Ferretti M, Vergine G, Falcioni A, Copponi E, Tagliabue B, Massart F. Drowning in children and predictive parameters: a 15-year multicenter retrospective analysis. Pediatr Emerg Care. 2023,39:516–23.
85. Szpilman D, Bierens JJ, Handley AJ, Orlowski JP. Drowning. N Engl J Med. 2012;366(22):2102–10.
86. Thom O, Roberts K, Devine S, Leggat PA, Franklin RC. Treatment of the lung injury of drowning: a systematic review. Crit Care. 2021;25(1):253.
87. Dakessian A, Bachir R, El Sayed M. Impact of trauma designation levels on survival of drowning victims: an observational study from trauma centers in the United States. Medicine (Baltimore). 2019;98(43):e17721.
88. Perkins GD, Olasveengen TM, Mancini MB, Chung S, Considine J, Kudenchuck P, Semeraro F, Smith C, Morley PT, on behalf of the International Liaison Committee on Resuscitation Basic Life Support Task Force. Drowning Consensus on Science with Treatment Recommendations [Internet]. Brussels: International Liaison Committee on Resuscitation (ILCOR) Advanced Life Support Task Force; 2020. http://ilcor.org
89. Demetriades D, Kimbrell B, Salim A, Velmahos G, Rhee P, Preston C, Gruzinski G, Chan L. Trauma deaths in a mature urban trauma system: is "trimodal" distribution a valid concept? J Am Coll Surg. 2005;201(3):343–8.
90. Trunkey DD. Trauma. Accidental and intentional injuries account for more years of life lost in the U.S. than cancer and heart disease. Among the prescribed remedies are improved preventive efforts, speedier surgery and further research. Sci Am. 1983;249(2):28–35.
91. Rai V, Mathews G, Agrawal DK. Translational and clinical significance of DAMPs, PAMPs, and PRRs in trauma-induced Inflammation. Arch Clin Biomed Res. 2022;6(5):673–85.

92. Ertel W, Friedl HP, Trentz O. Multiple organ dysfunction syndrome (MODS) following multiple trauma: rationale and concept of therapeutic approach. Eur J Pediatr Surg. 1994;4(4):243–8.
93. Morton AP, Moore EE, Wohlauer MV, Lo K, Silliman CC, Burlew CC, Banerjee A. Revisiting early postinjury mortality: are they bleeding because they are dying or dying because they are bleeding? J Surg Res. 2013;179(1):5–9.
94. Chang R, Fox EE, Greene TJ, Swartz MD, SM DS, Stein DM, Bulger EM, Melton SM, Goodman MD, Schreiber MA, Zielinski MD, O'Keeffe T, Inaba K, Tomasek JS, Podbielski JM, Appana S, Yi M, Johansson PI, Henriksen HH, Stensballe J, Steinmetz J, Wade CE, Holcomb JB, PROHS Study Group. Abnormalities of laboratory coagulation tests versus clinically evident coagulopathic bleeding: results from the prehospital resuscitation on helicopters study (PROHS). Surgery. 2018;163(4):819–26.
95. Webb AJ, Brown CS, Naylor RM, Rabinstein AA, Mara KC, Nei AM. Thromboelastography is a marker for clinically significant progressive hemorrhagic injury in severe traumatic brain injury. Neurocrit Care. 2021;35(3):738–46.
96. Stern SA, Dronen SC, Birrer P, Wang X. Effect of blood pressure on hemorrhage volume and survival in a near-fatal hemorrhage model incorporating a vascular injury. Ann Emerg Med. 1993;22(2):155–63.
97. Wahlgren CM, Kragsterman B. Management and outcome of pediatric vascular injuries. J Trauma Acute Care Surg. 2015;79(4):563–7.
98. Martin K, Vanhouwelingen L, Bütter A. The significance of pseudoaneurysms in the nonoperative management of pediatric blunt splenic trauma. J Pediatr Surg. 2011;46(5):933–7.
99. Kodadek L, Carmichael SP, Seshadri A, et al. Rhabdomyolysis: an American Association for the Surgery of Trauma Critical Care Committee Clinical Consensus Document. Trauma Surg Acute Care Open. 2022;7:e000836.
100. Szugye HS. Pediatric rhabdomyolysis. Pediatr Rev. 2020;41(6):265–75.
101. Zeng X, Zhang L, Wu T, et al. Continuous renal replacement therapy (CRRT) for rhabdomyolysis. Cochrane Database Syst Rev. 2014;6:CD008566.
102. Erdos J, Dlaska C, Szatmary P, Humenberger M, Vecsei V, Hajdu S. Acute compartment syndrome in children: a case series in 24 patients and review of the literature. Int Orthop. 2011;35:569–75.
103. Nathanson MH, Harrop-Griffiths W, Aldington DJ, Forward D, Mannion S, Kinnear-Mellor RGM, Miller KL, Ratnayake B, Wiles MD, Wolmarans MR. Regional analgesia for lower leg trauma and the risk of acute compartment syndrome. Anaesthesia. 2021;76:1518–25.
104. Didion P, Crombé A, Dabadie A, Hassid S, Seux M, Gorincour G, Banaste N. Emergency whole-body CT scans in pediatric patients with trauma: patterns of injuries, yield of dual-phase scanning, and influence of second read on detection of injuries. Eur Radiol. 2022;32(12):8473–84.
105. Hazen BJ, Keane OA, Vandewalle RJ, Grady Z, Wetzel M, Chern JJ, Santore MT. Difference in presentation and concomitant intra-abdominal injury with chance fracture in pediatric and adult populations. Am Surg. 2023;89(6):2486–91.
106. Buduhan G, McRitchie DI. Missed injuries in patients with multiple trauma. J Trauma. 2000;49(4):600–5.

Traumatic Brain Injury

Helen Ord and Hari Krishnan

Contents

J. Brierley et al. (eds.), *ESPNIC Children's Intensive Care Textbook*,
https://doi.org/10.1007/978-3-031-64762-8_36

Learning Objectives

- Have an understanding of the causes and epidemiology of traumatic brain injury (TBI) in the paediatric population
- Have an understanding of the basic concepts of paediatric TBI including cerebral autoregulation, and pressure-volume relationships
- Understand what is meant by traumatic brain injury and how it is acutely assessed and managed
- Have a broad understanding of the mechanisms of secondary injury caused by trauma to the brain
- Have a framework for managing paediatric patients with severe TBI in the intensive care environment and understand the evidence base behind this
- Understand what is meant by multimodal neuromonitoring, its current and potential future role in TBI management
- Consider late effects of TBI and outcomes
- Summary of paediatric TBI trials in over the last 20 years

36.1 Introduction

Traumatic brain injury (TBI) is a leading cause of morbidity and mortality in children worldwide [1]. While reported numbers of TBI vary greatly across countries, in part due to reporting differences, there are a number of common findings. Road traffic accidents (RTA) are overall the most common cause of injury in those requiring admission to the paediatric intensive care unit (PICU), and of those, 60% have identifiable abnormalities on CT brain [2]. A bimodal distribution is seen where children under the age of 2 years are more commonly affected by inflicted injury, whereas school-aged children and adolescents are more commonly involved in RTAs [3].

TBI is particularly challenging to manage because it is a heterogeneous disease entity. It encompasses a wide range of aetiological, anatomical, pathophysiological, functional and temporal variability. It is usually categorised according to Glasgow Coma Scale (GCS) as follows: mild (GCS 13–15), moderate (GCS 9–12) and severe (GCS 3–8). Prevention of secondary insults, extension of primary injury sustained at the time of the event and optimising conditions for recovery are the main focus of management of any head injury.

Management of TBI in the PICU requires clinicians to have a good understanding of physiological principles, access to multidisciplinary resources, adherence to standardised algorithms, as well as need for individualised patient-specific decision-making. Unfortunately, high-quality evidence to guide such management is lacking. While differences in admission criteria for TBI patients to PICU may exist, children with severe TBI are typically admitted and managed in the PICU. Hence, this will be the focus of this chapter.

36.2 Basic Concepts

36.2.1 Cerebral Blood Flow, Perfusion Pressure, Autoregulation

Adequate cerebral blood flow (CBF) is required for neuronal cell homeostasis. In order to maintain adequate CBF, there must be a careful balance of cerebral blood volume, cerebrospinal fluid (CSF) and brain tissue. Due to fixed volume within the skull, as described by the Monro-Kellie doctrine, there is limited ability to accommodate changes in volume of any of these components. For example, any increase in brain tissue volume due to vasogenic oedema must be compensated for either by a reduction in CSF volume or a reduction of cerebral blood volume in order to balance the sum of volumes within the cranial vault.

While such compensatory mechanisms are intact, the ICP is barely affected by cerebral blood volume changes. However, when compensatory mechanisms are overwhelmed due to a significant increase in volume of contents inside the skull, the intracranial pressure-volume relationship becomes linear, perhaps up to the point of herniation.

Cerebral perfusion pressure (CPP) is the difference between mean arterial blood pressure (MAP) and intracranial pressure (ICP) as summarised in the equation below:

- CPP = MAP – ICP

The MAP is measured at the level of the heart and the ICP usually at the level of the tragus. The differences due to this disparity are typically ignored as much of the literature generated includes this disparity and the individual trends over time are usually apparent so long as there is consistency in the site of measurement for the duration of patient care.

Cerebrovascular autoregulation is the ability of cerebral circulation to maintain constant CBF despite changes in MAP or CPP. Although a myogenic response of increasing tone with higher pressure is commonly implied as an underlying explanation, autoregulation is much more complex and includes metabolic, neural and endothelial components.

- CBF = CPP/CVR = (MAP-ICP)/CVR

As shown in ◘ Fig. 36.1, over a range of MAP, CBF remains constant due to increasing cerebral vascular resistance (CVR). At the extreme ends, the ability to autoregulate is lost and this leads to either hypoperfusion or hyperaemia. The tolerable range of MAP varies with age. Newborn infants, more so those who are premature, have a much narrower perfusion window than adults and this, in part, explains their vulnerability to acute changes in perfusion pressure [1].

There is evidence that the ability to autoregulate CBF is impaired after TBI, as there is uncoupling of the normal flow-metabolism relationship. Particularly acutely, TBI leads to increased metabolic demand which coupled with impaired ability to autoregulate, renders already damaged brain tissue even more vulnerable to ischaemia and hypoxia [4].

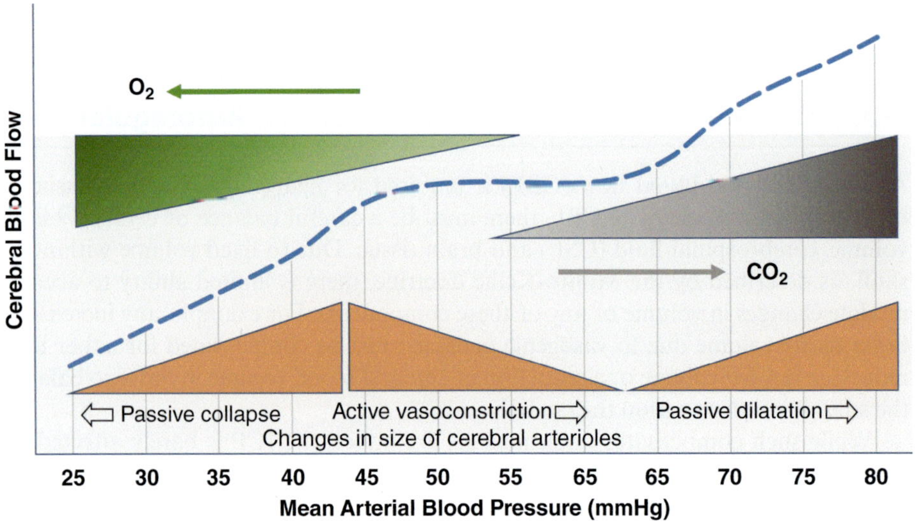

Fig. 36.1 Response of CBF to changes in MAP, arterial oxygen and carbon dioxide content

As well as responding to changes in BP, cerebral vasculature also has the ability to alter tone relative to carbon dioxide and oxygen tension. Hypoxia leads to vasodilatation of cerebral vasculature, in an effort to maximise oxygen delivery, in contrast to hyperoxia which leads to vasoconstriction. These responses have the overall aim of keeping CBF constant. Hypercapnia leads to vasodilatation, and hypocapnia leads to vasoconstriction. This relationship is linear, which explains why the use of hyperventilation in the management of critical intracranial hypertension can produce noteworthy changes in CBF and therefore ICP, with only small changes in $PaCO_2$ [1, 5].

In addition, CBF is also affected by temporal trends after TBI. It has been suggested there are three phases in CBF after TBI, moving from poor perfusion in the first 12 h post-injury, to a phase of 'luxury perfusion', followed by an increased risk of vasospasm [4].

In clinical practice, CPP is used as a surrogate for CBF. Optimal CPP targets are currently estimated according to the age of the child and have been made largely by extrapolation from adult data and a few paediatric studies. Manipulation of cerebral blood flow to optimise CPP and prevent cerebral ischaemia, while avoiding hyperaemia, is a core principle in management of severe TBI.

36.2.1.1 ICP Waveforms

The normal ICP waveform is synchronous with the arterial pulse, and there are three distinct peaks (Fig. 36.2). P1 is known as the percussion wave and correlates with the transmission of the arterial pulse through the choroid plexus. P2 is known as the tidal wave and roughly represents cerebral compliance. P3 is known as the dicrotic wave and correlates with closure of the aortic valve.

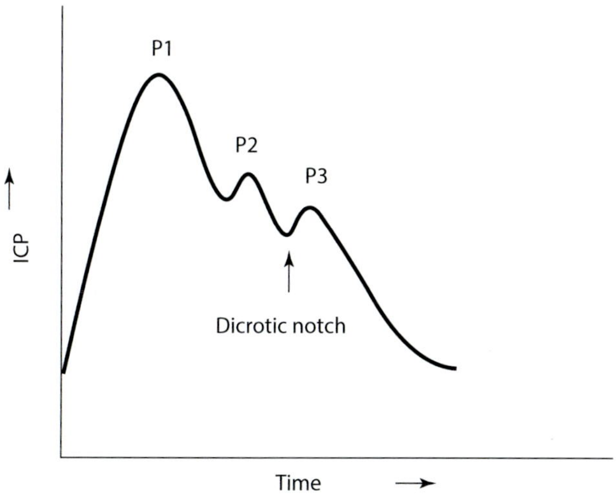

Fig. 36.2 Characteristics of intracranial pressure waveform

Changes in the ICP waveform can indicate changes in ICP and therefore cerebral blood flow and 'brain compliance'. For example, the pulse amplitude of the ICP waveform increases linearly with the ICP when compensatory reserve is poor. Similarly, P2 may be higher than P1 indicating poor brain compliance [6].

Other trends in ICP can be visualised when plotted over longer periods of time. When plotted over several seconds, respiratory variation can also be seen and is synchronous with respiratory variation in central venous pressure [7, 8]. When plotted over several minutes, the Lundberg B-wave, which occur at a frequency of 0.5–2 waves per minute can be observed as small fluctuations (10–20 mmHg) in baseline ICP. Although exact origins are unclear, they are often thought to be vasogenic in nature and perhaps related to a neural pacemaker system. Some of the smaller fluctuations may not always be pathological. When plotted over an hour or longer, the ICP A-waves, also known as plateau waves, may be visible. Plateau waves are pathological increases of ICP that are steeper than B-waves (>20 mmHg) and may persist for 5–20 min. They may lead to significant secondary brain insult and may even lead to herniation. C-waves are rhythmic, relatively small physiological oscillations synchronous with arterial blood pressure variations that occur every 4–8 min.

36.2.1.2 The Pressure-Time Burden

We now know that it is not only the severity of intracranial hypertension, in terms of peak measured ICP values which impacts the outcome, but also the duration of intracranial hypertension, and the cumulative effect of these episodes. There is some evidence to suggest that children have a poorer tolerance for prolonged periods of raised ICP than adults [9, 10]. Concurrent reduction in CPP is also likely to have an additive effect with duration and depth of reduction both having an impact.

36.2.2 Concepts Behind Brain Injury

36.2.2.1 Primary Brain Injury

The primary brain injury is sustained during or immediately after the event. The exact type of insult is determined by the mechanism of injury, and in many cases, there will be multiple forms. For example, a skull fracture with an associated contusion and a bleed.

Blunt injury, such as in a pedestrian vs car RTA, causes the skull to flatten at the point of contact and the injury dissipates outwards from that point. There will be a direct contusion injury at the point of contact, and depending on the degree of deceleration, there may also be a contrecoup injury to the other side of the brain.

Axonal injury results from shearing of the axons secondary to acceleration-deceleration movement, for example due to an inflicted shaking injury. Infants are at a greater risk of rotational and acceleration-deceleration type injuries due to their relatively large head and weak neck muscles. Diffuse axonal injury (DAI) is associated with significant morbidity and mortality.

All mechanisms of injury leading to TBI may be associated with intracranial bleeding. ◘ Table 36.1 summarises the principal types of intracranial haemorrhage associated with TBI.

36.2.2.2 Secondary Injury

The focus of PIC management is minimising secondary insult, or extension of the primary injury sustained at the event. While some of the finer molecular pathways remain unclear, there are a number of processes which we know promote secondary injury:

- Ischaemia
- Excitotoxicity and inflammation
- Oxidative stress
- Cortical spreading depolarisation
- Impaired glymphatic circulation
- Energy failure

◘ **Table 36.1** Types and mechanism of intracranial bleeding

Intracranial bleed	Mechanism	Vessel involved
Subdural	Abrupt deceleration Acceleration-deceleration	Bridging dural veins
Extradural	Direct/blunt injury	Middle meningeal artery, emissary veins [11]
Subarachnoid	More common in inflicted injury than accidental trauma	Microvascular rupture

Ischaemia

Reduced cerebral blood flow especially around the regions of contusions—the penumbra, the area of potentially salvageable brain tissue—results in secondary extension of the primary brain injury. It is not uncommon for CBF to reduce from a baseline of ~50 mL/100 g/min to <30 mL/100 g/min. Once the CBF reduction worsens to <20 mL/100 g/min, anaerobic metabolism and other ischaemic injury processes are triggered. Disruption in blood-brain barrier, vasogenic, cytotoxic oedema and disrupted flow-metabolism coupling all result in micro- and macrovascular disruption of blood supply to the neurons exacerbating the ischaemic injury. Periods of hypotension with associated reduction in cerebral perfusion pressure or hyperventilation may worsen any ischaemic injury. Intracranial hypertension can trigger a vicious cycle that perpetuates further ischaemic injury which in turn may worsen intracranial hypertension. The reversibility of ischaemia depends on its severity and duration.

Excitotoxicity and Inflammation

Damaged neurones release excitatory and inflammatory neurotransmitters contribute to ongoing damage and repair. Glutamate is the main excitatory neurotransmitter released by damaged neurones into the extracellular space. Excess glutamate leads to overstimulation of post-synaptic receptors (NMDA, amino-3-hydroxy-5-methylisoxazole-4-proprionic acid) which leads to an influx of calcium and sodium. This, in turn, leads to fragmentation of cell membranes and intracellular structures [12].

Cellular stress or damage also causes release of molecules called damage-associated molecular patterns (DAMPS), which initiate the innate immune response via interaction with pattern recognition receptors (PPRs). They form a multi-protein complex called an inflammasome which triggers further release of inflammatory cytokines such as IL-6 and IL-10. Further secondary tissue damage ensues [1]. This process is of course not unique to TBI. Influx of pro-inflammatory cells and release of proteinaceous material on cell injury also add to the oncotic load and increase cerebral oedema. The role of anti-inflammatory therapy in TBI has been suggested, but may increase the risk of infection and the inflammatory process also plays a role in regeneration.

Oxidative Stress

Oxidative stress is caused by free radicals which can be grouped into reactive oxygen species (ROS; e.g. hydrogen peroxide and superoxide anion) and reactive nitrogen species (RNS; e.g. nitric oxide). They are produced in excess following insults such as TBI via various mechanisms. In health and in moderate quantities, they are used as signalling mechanism. However, excessive quantities of oxidative molecules cause alteration of cellular macromolecules including DNA, proteins, lipids and wreaking havoc on various cellular processes.

Cortical Spreading Depolarisation

Following acute ischaemia, there is loss of ion homeostasis and persistent depolarisation ensues. Further pathophysiological changes such as rise in excitatory neurotransmitters, increased intracellular calcium and cytotoxic oedema propagate cortical injury.

There is evidence that these waves of persistent depolarisation, sometimes referred to as brain tsunamis, then extend from the penumbra and lead to structural cortical lesions that can be seen on MRI. Even early lesions at the site of injury can be seen as diffusion restriction [13].

Impaired Glymphatic Drainage

The glymphatic system is an exchange portal and waste clearance system unique to the CNS, with a similar role to the lymphatic system in peripheral tissues [14]. There is emerging evidence that TBI impairs function of the glymphatic system. Biomarkers such as C-tau and B-amyloid are released after TBI and have also been linked to neurodegenerative disease. Impaired glymphatic clearance of these markers may in part explain the increased risk of later neurodegenerative disease in some patients following TBI.

Energy Failure

Energy failure may be caused by ischaemia, mechanical disruption of blood flow or metabolic demand in excess of resources. Cerebral metabolic demand is described as $CMRO_2$ (cerebral metabolic rate for oxygen) and, in a healthy brain, is directly coupled with CBF. As metabolic demand increases, so does blood flow to meet this. There is evidence to suggest TBI can cause flow-metabolism uncoupling which can lead to either ischaemia or hyperaemia [4]. The brain relies heavily on oxygen-dependant metabolism of glucose for energy and hence is particularly sensitive to disruption of this. This is one of the reasons a considerable part of our management in the PICU is aimed at minimising brain tissue metabolic demand. Energy failure is probably part of the final common pathway resulting in neuronal cell death.

36.2.2.3 Herniation Syndromes

With rising ICP, the risk of herniation increases. Herniation may occur due to cerebral oedema or mass effect secondary to haemorrhage or hydrocephalus. The specific location of herniation can be estimated by clinical signs, and ◘ Table 36.2 below summarises this.

◘ Table 36.2 Features of herniation syndromes

Syndrome	Mechanism	Clinical signs
Tonsillar	Downward displacement of cerebellar tonsils through foramen magnum	Ataxic breathing Hypertension, bradycardia (late sign) Extensor/opisthotonic posturing
Cingulate	Cingulate gyrus herniates under anterior falx, risk to anterior cerebral artery	Contralateral lower extremity paresis
Uncal	Medial tentorial lobe displaced inferiorly Risk to midbrain + posterior cerebral artery	Contralateral hemiparesis Ipsilateral dilated pupil + ptosis (CN III palsy)
Central trans-tentorial	Downward displacement of one or both cerebral hemispheres	Bilateral decorticate/ decerebrate posturing

36.3 Management

36.3.1 Pre-Hospital Management

Time is of the essence in management of a child with severe head injury. Immediate resuscitation, if appropriate, stabilisation and transfer of a child to a major trauma centre, if feasible, are the immediate goals. Immediate actions required often include C-spine protection, and some form of immediate support of the airway, breathing and circulation. GCS on arrival to an emergency department and occurrence of secondary insults such as hypoxia and hypotension have been identified as independent predictors of poor prognosis [2].

36.3.2 Emergency Room

Within the hospital, a trauma team-based management strategy utilising life support or other trauma algorithms is recommended. This typically consists of stepwise but simultaneous assessment and interventions using a C-ABCDE (catastrophic external haemorrhage, airway, breathing, circulation, disability, exposure) or similar approach.

During the golden hour, a child with head injury should undergo primary assessment, treatment of any potentially life-threatening injury and undergo a CT scan of the head ± neck, with other areas as relevant to mechanism of injury and clinical assessment. Typically, patients with suspected or confirmed severe head injury will require intubation and mechanical ventilation prior to transfer to radiology, if not already performed by the pre-hospital team.

While there is no ideal induction medication, the goal, as in most other critically ill children, is to maintain haemodynamic stability during intubation and transfer. Strict avoidance of hypotension, and thereby avoiding secondary ischaemic brain injury, should be a key consideration. Ketamine, despite theoretical concerns related to intracranial pressure, has been used extensively in children with head injury as well as in multi-trauma settings. Hypotension or massive blood loss causing haemorrhagic shock are indicators of injury to other organ systems, rather than traumatic brain injury per se.

Various decision support rules for identification of patients with head injury who require a CT brain, such as CHALICE, PECARN and CATCH, exist. However, any child with suspected severe head injury being discussed in this chapter is likely to need one. CT scan without contrast is the most common radiological investigation in acute TBI and offers a number of advantages over other modalities. It enables identification of skull and facial fractures, significant parenchymal injuries alongside intracranial haemorrhage, for which it is more sensitive than MRI in the acute phase. Practically, it is also quicker and more readily available than MRI in most settings.

Invariably, cervical spine immobilisation will also be required in such patients either because of altered level of consciousness, or due to signs and symptoms consistent with a C-spine injury. Manual in-line stabilisation should be maintained at all times, unless either a well-fitting hard collar or blocks with tape are in situ. In most patients, a cervical spine injury cannot be definitively ruled out from CT alone, until either the patient is conscious and a clinical examination can be performed or a spinal MRI is performed.

There is currently no clear evidence for benefit of using tranexamic acid acutely in severe paediatric TBI. However, the CRASH-3 trial in adults did find a statistically significant reduction in head injury related deaths when tranexamic acid was used within 3 h in mild to moderate head injury [11].

36.3.3 PICU Management

Children with severe TBI may require neurosurgery and/or neuroprotection in PICU. The most appropriate strategy will be based on combination of history, clinical findings, neuroimaging and need for mechanical ventilation for injuries sustained elsewhere. An expanding mass lesion, or a mass lesion with signs of raised intracranial pressure or midline shift requires urgent neurosurgical intervention prior to PICU admission. This may encompass evacuation of haematoma, and/or decompressive craniectomy, with or without an insertion of an external ventricular drain (EVD) or an ICP monitoring catheter. In patients who require a period of neuroprotection in the PICU, ICP monitoring as part of multimodal neuromonitoring may be helpful.

36.3.3.1 ICP Monitoring

Given the weight of evidence that intracranial hypertension in the context of TBI is harmful, it might be assumed that monitoring and management of ICP would be underpinned by robust evidence base. Unfortunately, there continues to be uncertainty about the merits of ICP monitoring in TBI whether to use one at all, and appropriate patient selection if used. The BEST:TRIP trial that included some teenagers with TBI in Latin America, and a propensity-weighted effectiveness analysis of a large paediatric dataset from North America, failed to identify a clinical benefit. In centres that routinely use ICP monitoring, patients expected to have catastrophic brain damage (e.g. bilateral unreactive pupils or additional severe hypoxic ischaemic injury) or those reclassified as having moderate rather than severe head injury are often not monitored. As with many aspects of management of the TBI patient, this signifies its complexity and the need to make management decisions based on the specific patient, understanding the risk—benefit balance of every intervention. It must be recognised that ICP is merely a monitoring modality, with the measurement reflecting severity of injury and is a guide to aid timing and choice of the management strategies.

While various options exist, the commonest choices are either a parenchymal fibre-optic catheter inserted through a 'bolt' or an external ventricular drain placed within the ventricular system, usually the lateral ventricles. Given that the EVD provides a therapeutic option in the form of CSF drainage, it remains the preferred option [8]. However, it is not often feasible to either insert or maintain within the ventricular system in a considerably swollen brain. It also carries a small infection risk especially when used beyond a few days. The fibre-optic micro-transducers, on the other hand, carry less infection and secondary haemorrhage risk, but do not have the ability to drain CSF, and cannot be recalibrated after insertion [1].

The decision to insert an ICP monitoring device will often be made jointly by the local neurosurgical team and PICU. We would recommend insertion of an ICP monitor in patients with severe TBI with an abnormal admission CT scan, and mild/moderate TBI with a mass lesion that requires the child to be sedated. Some children with extra-axial haemorrhage without any parenchymal abnormalities may only require surgical intervention rather than neuroprotection in the ICU. Similarly, others who are deemed not to need an intracranial bolt device may be woken up for assessment in the ICU. All others with an ICP monitoring device are typically managed with neuroprotection bundle, monitoring, management of intracranial hypertension and maintenance of CPP.

36.3.4 Post-TBI Neuroprotection Bundle

The foundation of PICU management of severe TBI is prevention of secondary injury through maintenance of homeostasis in order to optimise cerebral perfusion and reduction of raised intracranial pressure to subsequently improve outcomes. A protocolised bundle-based care, which also allows for flexibility to provide individualised care, is recommended (Table 36.3).

Table 36.3 Suggested components of a neuroprotection bundle

Neuroprotection bundle element	Target	Comment
Sedation, analgesia	Target deep sedation	Monitor using sedation and/or pain score(s). (e.g. COMFORT score) Typically benzodiazepine-opiate combination used
Neuromuscular blockade	Minimise cough, shivering, muscular activity and maintain alignment	Further reduction in metabolic demand, some additive effect in lowering ICP, better synchrony with mechanical ventilation postulated, but unproven. Additional monitoring for non-convulsive seizures may be required
Oxygen	SpO_2: 92–99 PaO_2: 12–14 kPa, 90–100 mmHg	Aim normoxia. Role of conservative O_2 saturation targets (e.g. 88–92) is unclear, and not widely used
Carbon dioxide	4.5–5.3 kPa 35–40 mmHg	Monitor tidal/minute volume and $ETCO_2$
Mechanical ventilation	PEEP 4–8 cmH_2O Vt 4–7 mL/kg FiO_2: <0.60	Theoretical concerns are as follows: High PEEP impeding cerebral venous return. Higher PEEPs may be required if atelectasis, ARDS related to multi-trauma, TRALI or ventilator-associated pneumonia present. Aim lowest possible PEEP required where possible

(continued)

Table 36.3 (continued)

Neuroprotection bundle element	Target	Comment
Temperature	36.5–37.6 °C	External cooling devices may be required to prevent/treat pyrexia Hypothermia for ICP reduction discussed elsewhere
Glucose	4–10 mmol/L 72–180 mg/dL	Insulin recommended if blood glucose in excess of 12 mmol/L (200 mg/dL)
Haemoglobin	>70 g/L	Many institutions recommend a higher haemoglobin target of 90–100 g/L
Volume status, fluids	Euvolaemia, 75–100% enteral nutrition or maintenance intravenous fluids. Target Na ≥140 mmol/L	Combination of clinical examination, urine output, central venous pressure monitoring (e.g. 4–10 mmHg) based on local practices
Nutrition	Early enteral nutrition, ideally within 72 h of injury unless contra-indication	Delayed gastric emptying may require post-pyloric feeds with an oro- or nasojejunal feeding tube
Position	Supine, head midline Elevation at head end of bed to 30	Skin care and periodic log-roll may be required to prevent pressure ulcers
Lines, catheters	Arterial, central venous and urinary catheters Oral (or nasal- if base of skull fracture excluded) gastric or post-pyloric feeding tubes	To continuously monitor and calculate CPP. CVC for hyperosmolar therapies, CVP monitoring and vasopressor infusion to achieve CPP targets. Prevent urinary retention
Seizure prophylaxis	Phenytoin or levetiracetam commonly used Monitoring with cEEG or qEEG recommended especially is neuromuscular blockade used	Reduces early post-traumatic seizure prevalence
Other supportive therapies	DVT prophylaxis especially in post-pubertal children who are immobilised for several days Stress ulcer prophylaxis Tetanus prophylaxis Pneumococcal vaccination if CSF leak Antibiotics for ventilator-associated pneumonia	Mechanical devices such as stockings or pneumatic compression devices, if size appropriate. Pharmacologic prophylaxis with LMWH may also be required on a case-by-case basis

Table 36.4 Suggested minimum CPP threshold ranges

Age (years)	Range of minimum CPP (mmHg)
<1	40
1–5	40–50
6–10	50–60
>11	60–70

36.3.4.1 Managing CPP

Maintaining CPP is paramount to the care of patients following severe TBI and is achieved through a balance of ICP and MAP. While there is not a robust evidence for precise CPP targets, there is some evidence to suggest age-appropriate paediatric targets. The most recent iteration of the brain trauma foundation guidelines recommends a minimum CPP target of at least 40–50 mmHg [15]. However, many institutions across the world routinely recommend higher CPP thresholds as part of their management guidelines [10]. We recommend age-based minimum CPP threshold in the ranges as shown in Table 36.4.

If the CPP is below minimum threshold value and the circulating volume is felt to be adequate, the patient may require an inotropic or vasopressor support depending on the cardiac function and the likely cause of hypotension. Myocardial depression may occur as a consequence of large doses of sedatives for instance. Noradrenaline infusion remains the first-choice medication. With episodes of intracranial hypertension, CPP may drift below the minimum threshold because of high ICP rather than because of hypotension. We recommend concurrent management of raised ICP, while simultaneously titrating arterial BP using vasopressors to maintain CPP in the interim.

36.3.5 Multimodal Neuromonitoring

The aim of neuromonitoring is to detect changes which may cause or worsen secondary injury, thereby enabling early intervention. Given the inadequacies of individual monitoring methods, multimodal monitoring is recommended to provide a more comprehensive assessment of the health of the brain.

Pros and cons of several multimodal neuromonitoring methods are summarised in Table 36.5, and specific details related to certain monitoring methods are discussed further.

36.3.5.1 Quantitative EEG

Seizures may occur in patients following TBI, and prompt management aims to halt the increased metabolic demand they cause. It is particularly important in those who are muscle relaxed as any seizure will be non-convulsive. Delivery of continuous

Table 36.5 Benefits and limitations of neuromonitoring methods

Modality	Uses	Limitations
Continuous EEG	Non-invasive Continuous Detect real-time electrical seizure activity Prognostic information Ease of comparison over time	Resource-intensive Requires neurophysiology, neurology input Affected by sedative + AEDs
Quantitative EEG (aEEG, CDSA, etc.)	Ease of application and real-time seizure detection by bedside PICU team Prognostic information Can be implemented with fewer resources than cEEG	Typically fewer channels, may miss focal seizures (Multi-channel possible) Sensitivity/specificity lower than cEEG Continuing education required to maintain expertise
NIRS	Non-invasive Bedside Continuous May identify major sentinel events promptly Can be used to derive autoregulation indices	Regional (frontal) measure of cerebral oxygenation—Poor correlation with global oxygenation measures Ischaemic thresholds not defined Treatment algorithms unclear Limited validation outside of neonates
TCD	Non-invasive Repeated measurements to derive trends possible Relative global perfusion (not absolute) Various indicators of autoregulation can be measured Non-invasive ICP estimation May be used as an adjunct in brain death diagnosis in some countries	Requires expertise, experience Absent acoustic window in some patients Continuous monitoring methods for children under development Treatment algorithms and thresholds unclear Poor accuracy of non-invasive ICP estimation
Partial pressure of oxygen in the brain tissue ($PbtO_2$)	Real time Continuous Accurate reflection of local milieu	Invasive Larger sized ICP bolt required Local not global measure of oxygen tension Thresholds and treatment algorithms unclear Unproven effect on outcomes in children
Intracranial pressure	Good worldwide experience Well described treatment algorithms Continuous Reasonably safe Provides information for estimates of autoregulation	Invasive Increased risk of infection (particularly with EVD) Insufficient evidence base to indicate improved outcomes

(continued)

■ **Table 36.5** (continued)

Modality	Uses	Limitations
Autoregulation indices (e.g. PRx)	Measure of autoregulation May provide individualised optimum-CPP targets based on zone of intact autoregulation Prognostic information	Not proven to improve outcomes in prospective studies or clinical trials yet
Microdialysis	Real-time chemical evidence of energy failure	Invasive Low-level evidence of correlation with patient outcome Remains confined as a research tool not used in routine clinical practice yet
Optic nerve sheath diameter (ONSD)	Non-invasive Non-radiating, bedside surrogate monitor of ICP Evidence in adult population that changes in ICP quickly reflected in ONSD Repeated assessments can provide trends	Intermittent Lack of normative data for various age-ranges Correlation may not be as good as other techniques, also unclear whether changes reflect acutely ongoing intracranial hypertension or a historical (but recent) increase Limited evidence in paediatric population [16]
Tympanic membrane displacement	Non-invasive bedside surrogate monitor of ICP Bedside No radiation Repeated assessment can provide trends Objective	Intermittent Correlation may not be as good as other techniques Also unclear whether changes reflect acutely ongoing intracranial hypertension or a historical (but recent) increase Limited evidence of accuracy in clinical practice base [17]
Automated infrared pupillometry	Detailed information: Individual components of pupillary light reflex (latency, constriction velocity, % change in pupil size) Accuracy (even <0.1 mm) Objective compared to manual pen-torch test	May be affected by medications May not provide temporal trends Normal values possible in moderate to severe injuries Lack of sensitivity Intermittent
Jugular bulb oximetry	Usually intermittent; although continuous oximetry possible Global, although unilateral, indicator of $CMRO_2$ and may provide information re: CBF	Interventions targeted at SjO_2 have not shown to improve outcomes Limited correlation with other markers of brain injury Infrequently used Thrombosis or obstruction of venous return may cause increased ICP

multi-channel EEG is resource-intensive and requires round-the-clock expertise to detect changes. Even in PICUs with such capability, most are reviewed only several times a day. Therefore, real-time display of changes or seizures remains challenging. Quantitative EEG is a technique of displaying processed EEG that makes detection of changes over longer periods of time easier. Real-time seizure detection is possible by the PICU team at the bedside. While several automated seizure detection algorithms have been developed, their accuracy is not yet sufficient to recommend routinely. Several techniques of qEEG such as amplitude-integrated EEG (aEEG), density spectral array (DSA), envelope trends, etc. exist. We recommend a combination of techniques such as aEEG and DSA. Typical qEEG set-up includes limited channels compared to multi-channel cEEG. So spatial resolution may be relatively limited and small focal changes may not be visualised. Improved accuracy of seizure detection with qEEG requires a continuing education package aimed at PICU clinicians [18]. The 2019 brain trauma foundation guidelines for management of paediatric severe TBI guidelines also support its use but recognise there is currently insufficient evidence to confirm seizure treatment actually improves outcomes [19]. qEEG can also offer key prognostic information.

36.3.5.2 Near-Infrared Spectroscopy (NIRS)

NIRS is a method of non-invasive regional (superficial brain tissue) saturation (rSO_2) monitoring. It uses a similar principle to standard oxygen saturation monitoring, but does not rely on a pulse. It relies on the principle of the Beer-Lambert law which describes the relationship between absorption of light with path length, concentration and absorptivity of the substance [20]. The absorption spectra for oxy- and deoxygenated haemoglobin differ, and the relative proportion of oxyhaemoglobin can be calculated.

While NIRS is commonly used in neonatology and in infants undergoing cardiac surgery, there is currently little evidence to support good correlation with global or other regional cerebral oxygenation measures, such as invasively monitored cortical brain tissue oxygenation ($PbtO_2$) [1]. However, it may be a helpful adjunct to other monitoring and clinical information. Furthermore, it may be that the trend rather than an isolated value which is particularly informative for the individual patient and use of a combination of modalities which gives the greatest value. Caution is required in clinical practice as the interventions aimed at improving the rSO_2 value, such as increasing FiO_2, CO_2 and haemoglobin, may paradoxically worsen brain ischaemia or increase ICP further. Further prospective validation of its use, interpretation and treatment algorithms based on NIRS monitoring in TBI is required.

36.3.5.3 $PbtO_2$ (Brain Tissue Oxygen Monitoring)

In patients who have a parenchymal ICP monitor placed, an additional oxygen sensing probe can be inserted to measure partial pressure of oxygen in brain tissue ($PbtO_2$). It can then be used to detect cerebral hypoxia, particularly alongside measurement and management of ICP and CPP [21, 22]. Low $PbtO_2$ has been associated with poor outcomes after TBI [22].

When monitored, a minimum target value of 10 mmHg is recommended by the 2019 brain trauma foundation consensus guidelines [19]. Some institutions use higher

$PbtO_2$ thresholds for intervention (e.g. 15–20 mmHg). However, some specific interventions to increase $PbtO_2$ such as increasing FiO_2, increasing haemoglobin with a blood transfusion, allowing mild hypercarbia, or increased cerebral perfusion pressure beyond minimum thresholds to increase cerebral blood flow have not been shown to improve outcomes, and may paradoxically contribute to increased ICP. The optimal placement of the probe is considered to be in at risk, but viable tissue. However, there is some argument that placing it in normal tissue may be more reflective of global brain oxygenation [22].

36.3.5.4 Transcranial Doppler (TCD)

TCD is a non-invasive technique using ultrasound waves to measure velocity within vessels of the circle of Willis, with the middle cerebral and basilar arteries being the most commonly used. It provides real-time evaluation, which can be repeated with ease at the bedside. It is well established in adult neurocritical care both in TBI and in assessment of vasospasm following aneurysmal subarachnoid haemorrhage. Its use in children is a little more challenging given different absolute values of flow velocity varies with age, gender and with angle of insonation. Also, the vessels themselves are identified at different depths which vary with head size. Despite differences in absolute flow velocities, comparable resistive (RI) and pulsatility (PI) indices may be derived. TCD-derived PI is sometimes used to generate non-invasive ICP. Various autoregulation indices can be derived using TCD-generated values. Continuous estimation of TCD in PICU shows theoretical promise but requires feasibility assessment and prospective clinical validation.

36.3.5.5 Pressure Reactivity Index (PRx)

PRx is one of the several different proxy-measures of autoregulation which can be calculated, but is perhaps the most widely used in ongoing clinical research [10]. PRx is calculated as a moving, linear correlation between ICP and MAP over time and provides a value between −1 and 1. A negative value or values lower than +0.25 or 0.30 (i.e. an inverse correlation between ICP and MAP) are considered to indicate intact cerebral autoregulation, whereas higher values closer to 1 are indicative of impaired cerebral autoregulation. By plotting PRx values against CPP, upper and lower limits of autoregulation and 'optimal' CPP may be identified. In theory, this may provide an amenable therapeutic target, provided results of ongoing prospective studies are supportive.

36.3.5.6 ICP Treatment Thresholds

It is not only the actual value of ICP, but the rate of rise, duration at high levels and whether CPP is maintained above the threshold levels are also important. It is widely accepted ICP should be maintained below 20 mmHg and that treatment should be initiated when the value is above or equal to 20 mmHg for 5 min or over or more than 25 mmHg for any period of time [1]. That said research priorities for the future include considerations around the need for age-based ICP thresholds. Depending on the degree and duration of the ICP rise it may be these interventions can be initiated in a stepwise manner, or a number should be initiated in parallel. This must be judged by the bedside clinician and every intervention assessed for its impact.

36.3.6 ICP Reduction Strategies

The 2019 brain trauma foundation guidelines for the management of paediatric severe traumatic brain injury provide management algorithms for tiered therapies [19]. When ICP exceeds the treatment thresholds described above, first-tier therapies are started, often using an algorithm-based approach (◘ Table 36.6). An algorithm-based care offers structure and consistency in management of paediatric TBI [19].

36.3.6.1 Hyperosmolar Therapy

Hyperosmolar therapy is the most common first-line therapy used in the management of raised ICP. About 2.7 or 3% hypertonic saline and 10 or 20% mannitol are the commonly used medications. While there is no robust evidence to choose between the two, hypertonic saline has theoretical advantages. Due to a higher capillary reflection coefficient, it is able to generate a stronger osmotic gradient across the BBB than mannitol, allowing greater movement of water out of neuronal cells. Additional anti-inflammatory, membrane stabilising properties have also been proposed. Hypertonic saline also has the benefit of increasing intravascular volume, which may in turn increase MAP and enhance CPP [23]. Hypertonic saline (2.7/3%) can be given either as a bolus (1–5 mL/kg), or as an infusion (1 mL/kg/h or 1 mmol/kg/h). It is preferable to administer via a central venous catheter given its tonicity, though peripheral use in an emergency while central access is not available is acceptable. Care must be taken with both bolus dosing and infusions, that sodium is carefully monitored as a rapid rise (or fall) can precipitate seizure activity. Serum sodium should be maintained between 145 and 155 mEq/L, and should not exceed 160 mEq/L where possible. Acute kidney injury, possibly related to hyperchloraemia and coagulopathy, especially when higher sodium values (155–160) are required/targeted are potential adverse events that require monitoring.

Other more concentrated solutions of sodium chloride may also be used. In particular, 23.4% hypertonic saline has been recommended as a second-tier option in refractory raised ICP. When used it is typically administered as an infusion over 10 min via a central venous catheter at a dose of 0.5 mL/kg (sodium load of 2 mmoL/

◘ Table 36.6 Tiered therapies for ICP control

First-tier therapies	Second-tier therapies
Optimisation of neuroprotection bundle elements	Infusion of hyperosmolar solutions or the use of more concentrated hyperosmolar solutions
Neuromuscular blockade in addition to optimal sedation, if not already done so	Mild hyperventilation (3.8–4.5 kPa/28–34 mmHg)
CSF drainage (if EVD present)	Titrated hypothermia (lowest 32–33 C)
Hyperosmolar therapy (2.7–5% saline or 10–20% mannitol) boluses	Barbiturate infusion
	Decompressive craniectomy

kg) up to a maximum of 30 mL. While the sodium load is similar, the smaller volumes used may confer some advantage in minimising fluid overload.

Mannitol is used in doses of 0.25–1 g/kg. Monitoring serum osmolality (aim <320 mOsm/L) is recommended to prevent nephrotoxicity. Large volume osmotic diuresis may cause, and administration may need to be followed by further volume expansion. It may also cause a rebound increase in ICP on termination of an infusion [24].

Use of other combinations including 10% mannitol with 10% glycerol and hypertonic sodium lactate have been described but there is limited experience or evidence base to recommend these [19].

36.3.6.2 CSF Drainage

If an external ventricular drain is available, then draining 5–10 mL of CSF in response to episodes of raised ICP is often effective and safe.

36.3.6.3 Tier 2 Therapies

Typically, requirement of second-tier therapies implies a more severe injury and refractory intracranial hypertension [19]. Of note, prior to initiation of tier 2 therapy, one must assess whether it is in the best interests of the individual patient to undergo further management of refractory intracranial hypertension. The term 'refractory' here means raised ICP despite management according to tier 1 therapy [19].

36.3.6.4 Hyperventilation

Hyperventilation results in cerebral vasoconstriction thereby reducing CBF, hence volume and consequently ICP. Given the sensitivity of cerebral vasculature to carbon dioxide, this effect can be seen rapidly and is relatively transient for a given change in $PaCO_2$ [1].

The risk of relative ischaemia increases proportionate to degree of hyperventilation, and the risk is likely to be greatest in the first 24 h post-injury when a reduction in CBF is poorly tolerated. Manual hand ventilation of a patient to rapidly lower CO_2 is sometimes used in emergency situations such as impending herniation syndromes. For intracranial hypertension refractory to hyperosmolar therapy, mild hyperventilation ($PaCO_2$ 28–34 mmHg or 3.8–4.5 kPa) is sometimes used [19]. Advanced neuromonitoring to detect worsening cerebral ischaemia is recommended in such patients. Wherever possible, aim to limit the degree and duration of hyperventilation titrated to reduction in ICP. Moderate hyperventilation (pCO_2 < 3.8 kPa/28 mmHg) is not recommended.

36.3.6.5 Hypothermia

Multiple trials have failed to demonstrate improved outcomes following use of hypothermia in TBI in various settings. Prophylactic hypothermia to prevent intracranial hypertension is not recommended. However, late use of hypothermia to reduce ICP refractory to first-tier therapies still remains an option [19]. The potential deleterious effects of shivering (causing increased metabolic demand), abnormal coagulation and reduced cerebral blood flow secondary to vasoconstriction must be considered. If used, the temperature should be titrated to effect, in steps of 0.5 °C intervals down to 32–34 °C as the lowest range, rather than a fixed target temperature as in therapeutic hypothermia in neonatal hypoxic ischaemic encephalopathy. Neuromuscular blockade is often employed to prevent problems associated with shivering. When used successfully, temperature is maintained for 12- to 24-h period for stability, followed by slow rewarming at rate of 0.5C every 2 h so long as ICP remains acceptable.

36.3.6.6 Barbiturate Infusion

The most commonly used barbiturates are phenobarbital and thiopental. The choice will depend upon familiarity within the individual unit. Given the short duration of onset, thiopental may be used as either an infusion or bolus dosing to manage intracranial hypertension. Continuous EEG or qEEG monitoring to prevent excessive suppression of cerebral activity is recommended. Care must be taken to mitigate against common and often troublesome side effects of hypotension and withdrawal. Particular attention to the patient's volume status and CVP is required [19]. Development of fixed dilated pupils may also be related to thiopentone toxicity.

36.3.6.7 Decompressive Craniectomy

Decompressive craniectomy undoubtedly reduces ICP by expanding the skull volume. However, evidence to support a beneficial effect on outcomes in TBI remains unclear.

In patients with ICP refractory to other medical management strategies, often a repeat CT scan is warranted to detect either a new or an expanding mass lesion [10]. If a new or expanding mass lesion is found, removal with or without a decompressive craniectomy offers a rapid reduction in ICP and can potentially prevent herniation. Where there are no mass lesions to evacuate, decompressive craniectomy may still be performed. But appropriate counselling of parents with information about high probability of poor outcomes despite slightly better chances of survival. While surgical technique will often vary, either unilateral or bilateral fronto-temporo-parietal craniectomy with wide dural opening is recommended.

36.3.7 The Lund Concept

The Lund concept, in existence since the early 90 s, is an approach to the management of severe TBI based on reduction of cerebral oedema by reducing trans-capillary leak due to imbalance of Starling forces. The Lund concept aims to improve cerebral microcirculation by avoidance of vasoconstrictors, prevention and management of cerebral oedema by maintaining oncotic pressure and reducing hydrostatic pressure [23]. Management strategies used as part of the Lund concept include red cell, albumin transfusions, metoprolol, clonidine, steroids and dihydroergotamine, with the latter being used infrequently or not at all recently.

36.4 Rehabilitation and Outcomes

36.4.1 Step-Down from PICU

After a period of stability of ICP and reduction in therapies to control intracranial hypertension, the ICP bolt is removed and children are weaned off sedation. There is wide variability in the practice of timing and practice of step-down from PICU. Step-down may follow extubation of a patient who attained reasonable recovery of brain function, or alternatively a tracheostomy with or without continuing ventilatory support in others who do not achieve good recovery. Further recovery of cognitive and physical function is possible up to several months to 2 years after TBI. However, with variable trajectories dependent on multitude of factors, individualised decision-making is required.

Survivors of severe paediatric TBI often suffer neuro-cognitive, behavioural and social functioning difficulties, which pose a significant burden upon families, relationships and education. Outcome from paediatric TBI has also been linked to the environment within which the child recovers. Children from a low socio-economic background, with family dysfunction, have worse outcomes compared to those without these risk factors [25, 26]. As with all complex injury and illness in children, a multidisciplinary family-centred approach yields optimal outcomes. A comprehensive rehabilitation programme requires elements of physiotherapy, occupational therapy, speech, language, psychology, family support and social care support, in addition to multidisciplinary medical and nursing support.

36.4.2 Outcomes and Prognostication

Worldwide mortality secondary to severe TBI in paediatric patients is around 15–25%, and those presenting with a GCS of less than 5 are the most likely to die [2, 11, 12, 27]. There are a number of indicators associated with a poor prognosis. They include low presenting GCS (<5), mechanism of injury (inflicted injury), especially if associated with an abnormal pupillary response [1, 2, 28]. Inflicted TBI may be associated with increased mortality and morbidity due to delay in presentation or identification of trauma as the cause of symptoms after presentation and often multiple layers of maltreatment [1].

Hypotension, hypoxia, prophylactic hypothermia, severity and duration of intracranial hypertension have also been demonstrated by a large number of studies to be associated with worse outcome [10, 11]. These factors are not only associated with survival data, but short- and long-term neurocognitive outcomes too [28]. Even in those presenting with mild TBI, around 10% are reported to have emotional, memory and behavioural difficulties [29].

Alongside the presence or absence of factors known to be associated with outcome, there are methods of risk stratification. In adult practice, characteristics of the acute CT scan are used in risk stratification using composite scores such as the Rotterdam CT score, which has been shown to correlate well with later neurological outcomes and mortality or using the individual variables—petechial haemorrhages, obliteration of the third ventricle or basal cisterns, subarachnoid bleeding, midline shift, non-evacuated haematoma—as in the CRASH trial-based prognostic calculator [30]. When used to assess paediatric TBI, however, a CT scan-based score is likely to underestimate mortality at the lower score range but over-estimate at the higher score range [27].

A health system that is able to deliver all elements of the TBI chain of survival maximises the probability of good outcomes in TBI (◘ Fig. 36.3).

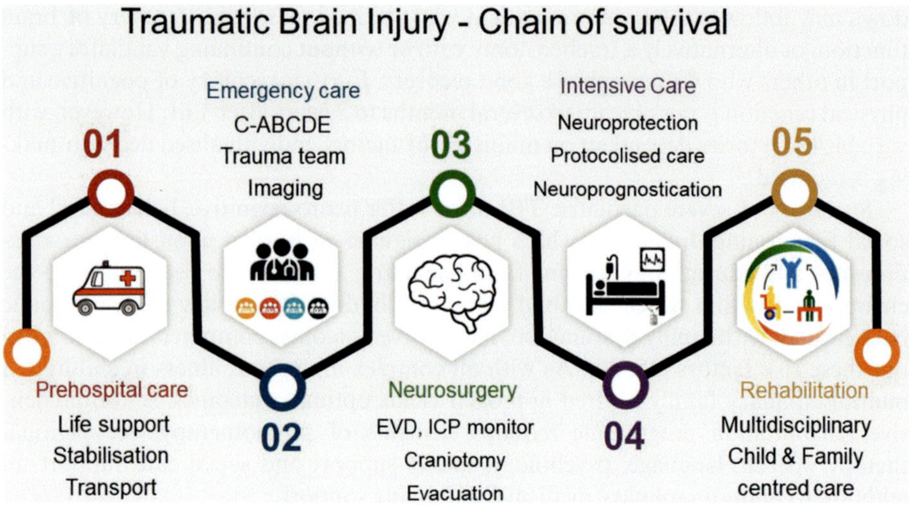

Fig. 36.3 Traumatic Brain Injury: Chain of survival

36.4.3 Biomarkers

There is growing interest in protein biomarkers to aid prognostication. The hope is that they may be used in conjunction with imaging, risk factors and clinical trajectory to predict outcomes after TBI. Levels of particular acute-phase markers have been shown to correlate with poor prognosis in some pre-clinical studies. For example, S100B (an astroglial calcium-binding protein), in pre-clinical animal studies, has been shown to correlate with GCS at 6 months post-injury [32]. Similarly, GFAP (glial fibrillary acidic protein) is released following damage to brain tissue and plasma levels may correlate with injury severity and patient outcome [32]. Neuron-specific enolase (NSE), neurofilament light polypeptide (NFL) and cleaved tau protein (C-tau) may also play a role pending further evaluation in paediatric TBI in the future. While a number of other biomarkers are under review, micro-RNA appears to be at the forefront of ongoing research including concussion in contact sports-related injury.

36.4.4 Late Effects of Paediatric TBI

The late effects of paediatric TBI are vast and are summarised in Fig. 36.4. There is emerging evidence that even mild TBI risks psychosocial deficits and disorders of hyperactivity and inattention [33]. There is evidence that children who have suffered TBI are at increased risk of communication difficulties, sleep disorders, anxiety and reduced quality of life compared to peers. The frequency of hypothalamic-pituitary injury is high, and is quoted in the region of 25–65%. Factors related to TBI which are associated with dysfunction include loss of consciousness at presentation, skull fracture and subdural haemorrhage [1].

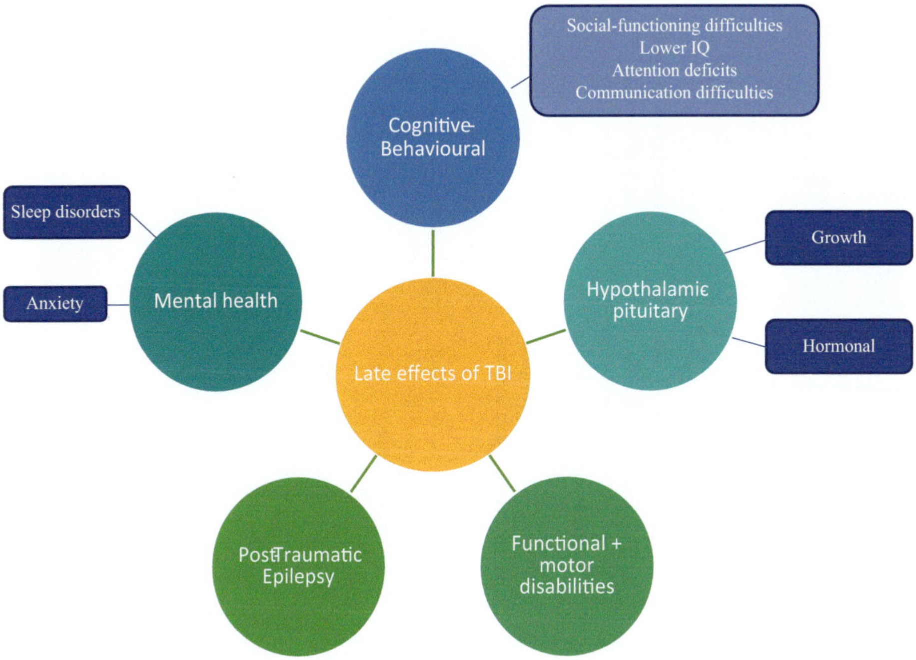

Fig. 36.4 Late effects of paediatric TBI

The effects of hypopituitarism most commonly include growth hormone deficiency, hypogonadism and thyroid dysfunction. Posterior pituitary dysfunction (SIADH, diabetes insipidus) appears to be a more transient phenomenon than anterior pituitary dysfunction.

The incidence of post-traumatic seizures following paediatric TBI is somewhere between 5 and 20% and increases in likelihood as the severity of TBI increases [14]. It is, however, still a risk even with mild TBI.

36.5 Clinical Trials in Paediatric TBI

Contrary to very large trials in adults such as CRASH with over 10,000 participants, the largest paediatric TBI trial had just over 200 patients recruited (Table 36.7). Despite the promise of many trials over the last two decades, few have yielded positive evidence to improve outcomes. That said, they have helped us understand the pathophysiology of secondary injury better and dismissed ineffective therapies. ADAPT study, a relatively large observational comparative effectiveness research project, is expected to recruit over 1000 children and provide insights into intracranial hypertension treatment strategies.

Table 36.7 Summary of paediatric TBI trials

Trial (or) publication	Intervention	Comparison	Outcome	Comment
Clark et al., PLoS One (2017) NCT01322009	*N*-acetylcysteine and probenecid	Placebo	Intervention appeared safe. Probenecid and NAC concentrations were detectable in CSF (EVD)	$N = 14$ Phase I trial to inform pharmacokinetics
RESCUE-ICP; NEJM (2016)	Decompressive craniectomy	Medical therapy including barbiturates	Decompressive craniectomy in patients with TBI and refractory intracranial hypertension resulted in lower mortality, but higher rates of poor functional outcomes than medical care	Not a paediatric trial per se, but included some children >10 years of age
Hypothermia in Traumatic Brain Injury (HiTBIC) pilot RCT NCT00282269 (2015)	Early (<6 h) prophylactic hypothermia to a temperature of 32–33 °C for 72 h followed by slow rewarming	Normothermia 36–37 °C for 72 h	No evidence of benefit with early therapeutic hypothermia	$N = 55$ Pilot multi-centre study
Cool Kids Phase 3 NCT00222742 (2013)	Early (<6 h) hypothermia 32–33 °C for 48–72 h, then rewarmed by 0·5–1·0 °C every 12–24 h	Normothermia 36·5–37·5 °C	No benefit on mortality or functional outcomes	$N = 77$ Terminated early for futility
Li et al., J Neurotrauma (2009)	Selective head cooling with target 34.3–34.7 °C	Normothermia 37.5–38.5 °C	Improved biomarker profile; safe	$N = 22$ Long-term outcomes not studied
HyP-HIT NEJM (2008)	Hypothermia 32.5 °C for 24 hinitiated <8 h	Normothermia 37 °C	Trend towards worse outcome with hypothermia	$N = 225$ Multi-centre, international study

Natale JE et al., PCCM (2007)	Magnesium sulphate (50 mg/kg) bolus followed by (8.3 mg/kg/h) infusion for 24 h	Placebo	$MgSO_4$ did not decrease mean BP or CPP	*N* = 6 (4 = $MgSO_4$; 2 = placebo)
Sakellaris et al., J Trauma (2006)	Creatine 0.4 g/kg mixed with juice for 6 months	Nothing	Significant improvement in functional outcomes	*N* = 39
Adelson et al., Neurosurgery (2005)	Hypothermia 33–33 °C < 6 h for 48 h; rewarming 1 °C q3–4 h, with slower rates for high ICP	Normothermia	Safe; trend towards better outcomes and more arrhythmias with hypothermia but did not reach significance	*N* = 75 Of these, 27 were delayed recruits or other exclusion criteria
Prabhakaran et al., J Neurosurgery (2004)	CPP >70 mmHg if >2 years old and >60 mmHg for patients <2	ICP < 20 and CPP > 50 mmHg	Safe, feasible but differences unclear	*N* = 17 (12 = CPP arm; 5 = ICP arm)
Biswas et al., Crit Care Med (2002)	Hypothermia 32–34 °C maintained for 48 h. Rewarming over 12 h	Normothermia 36.5–37.5 °C	Safe, potentially reduced ICP	*N* = 21
Taylor et al., Childs Nerv Sys (2001)	Very early decompressive craniectomy	Conventional medical management	Trend towards improved outcome with decompressive craniectomy	*N* = 27 in 7 years Bitemporal craniotomy without dural opening

Take-Home Messages

- Paediatric TBI poses a significant burden to society in terms of mortality and morbidity.
- Key indicators of poor prognosis include GCS on arrival, pupillary reaction, intracranial hypertension, hypotension and hypoxia.
- The foundation of management in PIC is prevention of secondary injury through maintenance of homeostasis, efficient and effective management of raised intracranial pressure.
- The 2019 PCCM consensus guidelines for the management of severe traumatic brain injury in children provide concise, evidence-based algorithms for management.
- Multimodal neuromonitoring provides supplementary information about cerebral perfusion pressure, oxygenation and ICP which in conjunction with more standard bedside monitoring, allow the bedside clinician to identify evolving changes which may cause or worsen secondary injury enabling early intervention.
- The consequences of paediatric TBI are substantial and include poor mental health, schooling and language difficulties, hypopituitarism causing growth and pubertal failure and post-traumatic epilepsy.
- It is hoped in the future, further research and advances in multimodal neuromonitoring will allow us to identify CPP and ICP targets that are relative to both the individual patient and their disease course and there will be robust biomarkers of disease stratification.

References

1. Morrison EW, Nelson McMillan LK, Shaffner HD. Rogers' Handbook of Pediatric Intensive Care. 5th ed. Lippincott: Williams and Wilkins; 2016. p. 205–54.
2. Riemann L, Zweckberger K, Unterberg A, el Damaty A, Younsi A. Injury causes and severity in pediatric traumatic brain injury patients admitted to the Ward or intensive care unit: a collaborative European neurotrauma effectiveness research in traumatic brain injury (CENTER-TBI) study. Front Neurol. 2020;11:345.
3. Parslow RC, Morris KP, Tasker RC, Forsyth RJ, Hawley CA. Epidemiology of traumatic brain injury in children receiving intensive care in the UK. Arch Dis Child. 2005;90(11):1182–87.
4. Udomphorn Y, Armstead WM, Vavilala MS. Cerebral blood flow and autoregulation after pediatric traumatic brain injury. Pediatr Neurol. 2008;38(4):225–34.
5. Bennett TD, Marsh R, Maertens JA, Rutebemberwa A, Morris MA, Hankinson TC, et al. Decision-making about intracranial pressure monitor placement in children with traumatic brain injury. Pediatr Crit Care Med. 2019;20(7):645–51.
6. Kawoos U, McCarron R, Auker C, Chavko M. Advances in intracranial pressure monitoring and its significance in managing traumatic brain injury. Int J Mol Sci. 2015;16(12):28979–97.
7. Nag DS, Sahu S, Swain A, Kant S. Intracranial pressure monitoring: gold standard and recent innovations. World J Clin Cases. 2019;7(13):1535–53.
8. Czosnyka M, Pickard JD. Monitoring and interpretation of intracranial pressure. J Neurol Neurosurg Psychiatry. 2004;75(6):813–21.
9. Güiza F, Depreitere B, Piper I, Citerio G, Chambers I, Jones PA, et al. Visualizing the pressure and time burden of intracranial hypertension in adult and paediatric traumatic brain injury. Intensive Care Med. 2015;41(6):1067–76.
10. Young AMH, Guilfoyle MR, Donnelly J, Smielewski P, Agarwal S, Czosnyka M, et al. Multimodality neuromonitoring in severe pediatric traumatic brain injury. Pediatr Res. 2018;83:41–9.

11. Araki T, Yokota H, Morita A. Pediatric traumatic brain injury: characteristic features, diagnosis, and management. Neurol Med Chir. 2017;57:82–93.
12. Schimmel S, Acosta S, Lozano D. Neuroinflammation in traumatic brain injury: a chronic response to an acute injury. Brain Circ. 2017;3(3):135–42.
13. Hartings JA, Shuttleworth CW, Kirov SA, Ayata C, Hinzman JM, Foreman B, et al. The continuum of spreading depolarizations in acute cortical lesion development: examining Leão's legacy. J Cereb Blood Flow Metab. 2017;37(5):1571–94.
14. Jessen NA, Munk ASF, Lundgaard I, Nedergaard M. The glymphatic system: a Beginner's guide. Neurochem Res. 2015;40(12):2583–99.
15. Kochanek PM, Tasker RC, Carney N, Totten AM, Adelson PD, Selden NR, et al. Guidelines for the management of pediatric severe traumatic brain injury, third edition. Pediatr Crit Care Med. 2019;20:S1–82.
16. Lin J-J, Chen AE, Lin EE, Hsia S-H, Chiang M-C, Lin K-L. Point-of-care ultrasound of optic nerve sheath diameter to detect intracranial pressure in neurocritically ill children - a narrative review. Biomed J. 2020;43(3):231–9.
17. Gwer S, Sheward V, Birch A, Marchbanks R, Idro R, Newton CR, et al. The tympanic membrane displacement analyser for monitoring intracranial pressure in children. Child's Nerv Syst. 2013;29(6):927–33.
18. Rowberry T, Kanthimathinathan HK, George F, Notghi L, Gupta R, Bill P, et al. Implementation and early evaluation of a quantitative electroencephalography program for seizure detection in the PICU. Pediatr Crit Care Med. 2020;21(6):543–9.
19. Kochanek PM, Tasker RC, Bell MJ, Adelson PD, Carney N, Vavilala MS, et al. Management of Pediatric Severe Traumatic Brain Injury: 2019 Consensus and Guidelines-Based Algorithm for First and Second Tier Therapies. Pediatr Crit Care Med. 2019;20(3):269–279.
20. Tosh W, Patteril M. Cerebral oximetry. BJA Educ. 2016;16(12):417–21.
21. Zoerle T, Carbonara M, Zanier ER, Ortolano F, Bertani G, Magnoni S, et al. Rethinking neuroprotection in severe traumatic brain injury: toward neuroprotection. Front Neurol. 2017;8:354.
22. Smith M. Multimodality neuromonitoring in adult traumatic brain injury: a narrative review. Anesthesiology. 2018;128:401–15.
23. Grande PO. Critical evaluation of the Lund concept for treatment of severe traumatic head injury, 25 years after its introduction. Front Neurol. 2017;8:315.
24. Shawkat H, Westwood M-M, Mortimer A. Mannitol: a review of its clinical uses. Contin Educ Anaesth Crit Care Pain. 2012;12(2):82–5.
25. Li L, Liu J. The effect of pediatric traumatic brain injury on behavioral outcomes: a systematic review. Dev Med Child Neurol. 2013;55(1):37–45.
26. Crowe LM, Catroppa C, Babl FE, Rosenfeld J, v., Anderson V. Timing of traumatic brain injury in childhood and intellectual outcome. J Pediatr Psychol. 2012;37(7):745–54.
27. Liesemer K, Riva-Cambrin J, Bennett KS, Bratton SL, Tran H, Metzger RR, et al. Use of Rotterdam CT scores for mortality risk stratification in children with traumatic brain injury. Pediatr Crit Care Med. 2014;15(6):554–62.
28. Fulkerson DH, White IK, Rees JM, Baumanis MM, Smith JL, Ackerman LL, et al. Analysis of long-term (median 10.5 years) outcomes in children presenting with traumatic brain injury and an initial Glasgow Coma Scale score of 3 or 4. J Neurosurg Pediatr. 2015;16(4):410–9.
29. Hawley CA, Ward AB, Magnay AR, Long J. Outcomes following childhood head injury: a population study. J Neurol Neurosurg Psychiatry. 2004;75(5):737–42.
30. Tasker RC. CT characteristics, risk stratification, and prediction models in traumatic brain injury. Pediatr Crit Care Med. 2014;15(6):569–570.
31. Wang KK, Yang Z, Zhu T, Shi Y, Rubenstein R, Tyndall JA, et al. An update on diagnostic and prognostic biomarkers for traumatic brain injury. Expert Rev Mol Diagn. 2018;18(2):165–80.
32. McKinlay A, Dalrymple-Alford JC, Horwood LJ, Fergusson DM. Long term psychosocial outcomes after mild head injury in early childhood. J Neurol Neurosurg Psychiatry. 2002;73(3):281–8.
33. Petridis AK, Doukas A, Maslehaty H, Mehdorn HM. Predictors and incidence of posttraumatic seizures in children and adolescents after brain injury. Clin Pract. 2012;2(3):e66.

Monitoring the Brain

Karl Reiter

Contents

J. Brierley et al. (eds.), *ESPNIC Children's Intensive Care Textbook*,
https://doi.org/10.1007/978-3-031-64762-8_37

Learning Objectives

- To improve outcomes after acute brain injury, it is essential to avoid or at least decrease secondary injury in the days after the insult.
- To detect and diagnose secondary injurious processes, neuromonitoring is essential. Neurological examination is indispensable but misses important processes (e.g. non-convulsive status epilepticus).
- An array of neuromonitoring modalities has been developed in recent years regarding different aspects of potential pathology (intracranial pressure, brain oxygenation, cerebral haemodynamics, continuous EEG and others).
- As no single modality maps all relevant processes multi-modality neuromonitoring is most promising although paediatric evidence is still developing.

37.1 Introduction

A majority of children in the PICU have some degree of neurological involvement in various types and prognoses. This may range from transient delirium to status epilepticus, brain edema or severe injury including brain death among others. If untreated, many of these can result in permanent neurologic disability which may be prevented by early and specific diagnosis.

Clearly, neurological examination is of major importance in determining a diagnostic plan and monitoring a patient's clinical course. Advanced neuromonitoring modalities are indispensable in defining the pathogenic process, following a treatment response and allowing prognostication. An array of neuromonitoring devices is available, each covering different aspects of pathological processes. In many circumstances, a combination of neuromonitoring modalities, so-called multimodal neuromonitoring, will map complex pathology best [1–3].

37.2 Neuromonitoring Techniques

37.2.1 EEG

One of the mainstays of neuromonitoring is the detection of seizure activity by EEG. In at least half of encephalopathic PICU patients, seizures are clinically silent or show only unspecific symptoms (e.g. instability of vital signs and prolonged coma), and non-convulsive status epilepticus occurs in 10–40% of these patients [4, 5]. In addition, clinically terminated convulsive status epilepticus often persists in the form of non-convulsive status [6]. In one study, 33% of children had ongoing electrographic seizures after clinically terminated generalized convulsive status epilepticus [7]. The risk for non-convulsive status epilepticus is higher in the paediatric age group compared to adults [8] and has been reported to be up to 33% in infants after abusive head trauma [9]. If untreated, seizures have been shown to impair short and long-term outcomes [10]. A multiplicity of pathologic EEG patterns with various prognostic utility are well-known after cardiac arrest in children [11]. ECMO is another reported risk factor for pathologic EEG patterns which may be associated with outcomes [12].

The indications for performing EEG studies therefore are relatively broad and encompass encephalopathic children with or without apparent seizures [13, 14]. Of note, specific ischaemia detection by EEG is relatively poor. Clearly, patients receiving muscle relaxants should be monitored by EEG if risk factors for neurological impairment are present.

There is a lack of a uniform classification of EEG characteristics which includes seizure classification and background pathology. In order to improve comparability and thus bring the field forward, EEG nomenclature and reporting should be standardized [15]. Standards have been developed by the American Clinical Neurophysiology Society [13, 14, 16].

The gold standard for the detection of epileptic seizures in the PICU is continuous 16-channel EEG using the 10–20 system. In unselected acutely encephalopathic PICU patients, about half of electrographic seizures will be missed, when EEG is restricted to 1 h [5, 17]. Most experts recommend applying continuous EEG monitoring for at least 24 h after the last registered seizure or up to 72 h after hypoxic-ischemic injury.

Therefore, continuous EEG monitoring is regarded as the standard of care in post-hypoxic-ischemic injury and status epilepticus as well as encephalopathic patients with high risk of seizures. Nevertheless, prompt availability of expert reading of EEG tracings by neurophysiologists is rarely achievable in most institutions, and EEG interpretation is suboptimal even by trained PICU physicians. In particular, a high rate of false positive seizure diagnoses has been found, which in one report amounted to 52% [17].

To facilitate seizure pattern recognition and cope with the massive data accumulation produced by continuous EEG, various simplification strategies and signal processing software have been developed (quantitative electroencephalography: qEEG). Amplitude-integrated EEG (aEEG) uses only two channels and visualizes the EEG signal after several filtering and processing steps in a time-compressed scale. aEEG has an established role in the treatment of hypoxic-ischemic encephalopathy in newborns; fewer data are available on the paediatric patient [18, 19]. Seizures as well as background activity can be discerned relatively easily by non-epileptologists. Sensitivity for seizure detection was in the range of 80% by PICU personnel [20] and probably can be increased by using a combination of methods. Already under clinical evaluation is a colour density spectral array (CDSA) [17, 19]. This method uses a time-compressed and colour-coded display of the power of EEG (amplitude2/Hz) at frequencies between 0 and 30 Hz after a fast Fourier transformation of the raw EEG. Colour coding of power spectra which differ between seizure activity and low-amplitude background leads to more intuitive visualization.

Several other algorithms have been developed to help clinicians in the identification of seizure activity where clinical validation has to be awaited [21, 22]. Of major importance, regular training and audits have to be implemented for a PICU-led EEG-monitoring programme to be successful [17].

Apart from seizure detection, investigators have tried to correlate EEG patterns and certain characteristics with prognosis in paediatric cardiac arrest patients [2, 23–25]. EEG background categories portending a poor outcome have included discontinuous EEG, discontinuous burst suppression, attenuated flat EEG and absent EEG reactivity to stimuli (albeit with high inter-rater variability) [26]. The presence of sleep spindles within 24 h after cardiac arrest was associated with a good outcome

[27]. Prognostication by EEG is best performed 12–24 h after ROSC but has to be integrated into a multimodal concept due to insufficient specificity.

37.2.2 Imaging

Neuroimaging is indispensable in neurocritical care although the choice of modality (CT, MRI and ultrasonography) has to account for several factors including sensitivity regarding specific pathologies, limitations and potential to harm a patient.

Bedside cerebral ultrasound will be the first choice in neonatology and infants with sufficiently open anterior fontanella. Intracerebral/intraventricular haemorrhage and hydrocephalus can readily be diagnosed. Sensitivity for hypoxic-ischaemic encephalopathy is lower, and detection of parietal haemorrhage or pathology of the posterior fossa may be difficult to diagnose, especially in older infants. There is a growing interest in developing transcranial Doppler applications in paediatric and adult neurointensive care (see below).

Cranial CT is the imaging modality of choice when urgent treatment decisions are required due to its general availability, speed of data acquisition and sensitivity regarding most acute disease processes. Non-contrast CT is invaluable in diagnosing fractures and acute cerebral haemorrhage as well as hydrocephalus (or slit ventricles) in ventricular shunt dysfunction or herniation syndromes. Contrast-enhanced CT (and delivering) will delineate venous sinus thrombosis and larger thrombi in cerebral arteries including the basilar artery. Ischaemia and brain oedema will often not be discernible until 4–6 h and cannot be excluded by CT. Perfusion contrast CT delivers much better detail and blood flow data but with much larger radiation exposure. Infectious processes that can be easily detected by contrast-enhanced CT are brain abscesses and meningitis.

Much progress has been made in neuroimaging by MRI technology and specifics of many newly developed sequences tend to get puzzling at least for non-neuroradiologists. The most important drawback of MRI is the need for transport entailing safety issues and long data acquisition times. With the exception of neonates and small infants, most children will therefore need prolonged anaesthesia.

The basic sequences comprise T1, T2, fluid-attenuated inversion recovery (FLAIR), DWI and ADC. These may be supplemented by sequences sensitive to extravascular blood (T2* and SWI). Anatomic detail is better displayed in T1-weighted images, whereas T2 sequences are better suited to imaging tissue oedema. FLAIR sequences improve the detection of grey and white matter abnormalities, e.g. contusions and diffuse axonal injury.

37

Often, the most critical questions asked in neurointensive care are: is there brain oedema, and if yes, of what type? Is there acute ischaemia?

DWI will show ischemic lesions as bright signals within minutes after injury. These appear dark in the ADC map, which needs to be obtained to confirm acute ischaemia. This type of induced tissue oedema constitutes cytotoxic oedema, characterized by an increase in intracellular water content due to energy depletion. It is most commonly caused by ischaemia and severe metabolic derangements and involves both grey and white matter. On the other hand, vasogenic oedema, resulting from blood-brain barrier disruption leading to extravascular and extracellular oedema shows dark or grey signal intensity in DWI and high signal intensity on the

ADC map. This may be a common pattern of trauma, tumours and inflammatory lesions. White matter is predominantly involved. A third type of oedema, interstitial oedema, may be seen in obstructive hydrocephalus.

However, lesion patterns may differ according to maturational age and mechanism of ischaemia, and different cerebral regions may be targeted at different time periods due to age-dependent vulnerability [28–33].

It is important to keep in mind the dynamic evolution of MRI abnormalities after insult. DWI abnormalities typically peak at 3–5 days post-injury and show the phenomenon of "pseudonormalization"by about the end of the first week.

Several investigations have shown the prognostic value of MRI performed within the first week after injury, specifically cardiac arrest [16, 33]. In an adult series, it was suggested that the ideal time window for prognostication using DWI was between 49 and 108 h after cardiac arrest [34].

Cerebral blood flow can be measured by an MRI technique called arterial spin labeling. Still, an investigational procedure requires transport and time exceptional detail can be gained. Regional disturbances in cerebral blood flow have been demonstrated in a preliminary study in paediatric TBI [35].

37.2.3 Increased Intracranial Pressure (ICP) and Advanced Cerebral Monitoring

Increased intracranial pressure can lead to reduced cerebral blood flow, irreversible injury even when brief [36] and devastating herniation syndromes. Therefore, ICP is the target of many treatment approaches in neurointensive care. Invasive measurement using an epidural, subdural, intraparenchymal or intraventricular probe is a critical tool, whereas noninvasive modalities, e.g. TCD, measurement of tympanic membrane displacement or optic nerve sheath diameter have limited reliability [37]. Fundoscopy looking for papilloedema will not be of help in the acute case as it usually takes at least 48 h to develop after increases in ICP. CT should not be regarded as a modality to exclude raised ICP.

Although the intraventricular catheter is regarded as the gold standard for ICP measurement and allows CSF drainage to reduce ICP, there are still caveats to consider: in many children, ventricles are quite narrow which is much pronounced with brain oedema, and placement may be difficult or impossible. With continuous drainage of CSF, measurements are erroneous, so ICP can be determined only intermittently when draining is stopped. Catheters may become occluded by blood or high protein levels in the CSF.

All invasively placed catheters have inherent risks of causing haemorrhage or infection which may significantly be reduced by correcting coagulation disturbances and adhering to meticulous hygiene. In a meta-analysis of haemorrhagic complications of intraventricular catheters placed by neurosurgeons in adult patients, significant bleeding occurred in 0.8% of patients [38]. Device-related infections have been reported in up to 9% of adult patients [39]. Antibiotic-coated catheters have no clear advantage.

Intraparenchymal probes have been shown to give ICP values that correlate well with the gold standard of intraventricular measurements and in modern transducers may be combined with further measurements (temperature, brain tissue pO_2 and microdialysis). Recalibration is impossible after placement, but transducers using strain gauge technology appear to have negligible zero drift.

Invasive measurement of ICP is recommended in adult and paediatric severe TBI [40, 41] although treatment targeting ICP has not been proven to affect the outcome [42, 43]. Up to 80% of paediatric patients with severe TBI will have increased ICP initially or during the first several days, and raised ICP has been shown to be injurious [36]. Treatment should be initiated when ICP rises above 20 mmHg over more than 5 min. An approach without using ICP measurement would necessitate frequent CT procedures with inherent transport and radiation risks and does not allow for continuous and extended (multimodality) monitoring. Intermittent but still injurious increases in ICP cannot be detected, and treatment response cannot be followed in a timely fashion.

Much less evidence is available to lead decisions to place invasive ICP probes in other disease processes where elevated ICP is regularly encountered, e.g. post-cardiac arrest or severe hepatic encephalopathy [44]. Deranged coagulation is a contraindication, and outcome improvement has not been shown. Therefore, noninvasive methods to measure ICP have been sought. Principally, these rely on correlation analysis of TCD with ICP waveforms [37, 45].

The placement of an intracerebral probe for ICP measurement allows more physiological insight than raw ICP data. Cerebral perfusion pressure (CPP) is the difference between ICP and mean ABP and is regarded as an essential parameter in neuromonitoring. Although both are not exclusive, the relative value of ICP-targeted vs. CPP-targeted treatments (using CPP as the primary treatment target) is still a matter of debate. In the calculation of CPP, it has to be accounted for that usually ABP is zeroed to the level of the right atrium, whereas the external auditory canal makes more physiological sense.

Cerebral autoregulation is the process of physiological adaptation of cerebral blood flow to metabolic demands and is mainly regulated by arterial vascular resistance [46–48]. Several mechanisms are at play. For example, increases in blood pressure elicit arterial vasoconstriction which counters the increase in cerebral blood volume which would ensue without vasoconstriction. In the majority of severe TBI cases, cerebral autoregulation has been shown to be disturbed at least in blood pressure (or CPP) ranges, currently recommended as standard (40 mmHg for infants, 50 mmHg for children and 60 mmHg for CPP in older children and adolescents) [47].

Sophisticated algorithms have been developed to detect disturbed cerebral autoregulation by analyzing the correlation of ICP and ABP pressure curves over short-time domains [49–52]. A commercially available software (ICM+ software (Cambridge Enterprise, Cambridge, United Kingdom)) may allow the identification of CPP ranges where autoregulation may be achieved at least to a certain extent (so-called optimal CPP). Preliminary studies demonstrate a possible effect on outcomes in severe paediatric TBI by this approach although patient numbers are small and the used algorithm may have some drawbacks [48]. Another approach to evaluate for disturbed cerebral autoregulation is looking at changes in blood flow velocity by TCD (assumed to mirror the vascular tone of cerebral vessels) with variations in arterial blood pressure or pCO_2. Near-infrared spectroscopy has been used in an analogous manner. In this method, brain oxygenation is the read-out parameter. Both techniques have not been evaluated sufficiently to diagnose or exclude intact cerebral autoregulation.

Another recent approach in characterizing the risk of detrimental ICP increases is the estimation of dynamic intracerebral compliance by correlating end-tidal CO_2 values with ICP variation. Increases in CO_2 entail increases in cerebral blood volume. If ICP remains stable with such increases, this would signify the maintained capacity of the brain to tolerate abrupt physiologic changes [53].

37.2.4 Brain Oxygenation and Metabolism

Physiologically, the metabolic state of injured brain tissue is an appropriate target for treatment. Newer intracranial probes allow the combined measurement of ICP, brain tissue oxygenation ($p_{bt}O_2$) and several substances characterizing metabolism in the brain extracellular fluid, e.g. pH, lactate and glucose by using microdialysis. These devices are about the same size as ICP probes and usually are required to be introduced to a depth of more than 2 cm.

Tissue oxygenation is measured with the use of Clark-type cells. In diffuse cerebral injury, the probe is usually placed in the frontal subcortical white matter. Measurement results depend on the relationship between arterial and venous vessels surrounding the probe which may vary. Generally, more than 70% of the cortical microvasculature consists of venous vessels, but even in normal tissue, a wide range of pO_2 values may be seen. Misleading values will result when probes are placed into haemorrhage or infarcted tissue.

The 2019 BTF guideline on paediatric severe TBI suggests $p_{bt}O_2$-measurement to fine-tune CBF when $p_{bt}O_2$ values are below 20 mmHg [40]. Evidence for outcome improvement when incorporating $p_{bt}O_2$ is still insufficient for a general recommendation.

Both ICP and $p_{bt}O_2$ are associated with outcomes although there is only a poor correlation between the two. Interfering factors may be the type of brain oedema, the metabolic state of brain tissue or if hyperaemia is present. Supplemental O_2 will affect $p_{bt}O_2$ directly but not ICP.

Noninvasive determination of brain oxygenation can be achieved by near-infrared spectroscopy (NIRS) which has been in use for more than 3 decades [54]. Most reported applications are in cardiac surgery patients, and few reports are available regarding neuromonitoring in PICU patients. NIRS technology is based on the transmission and absorption of near-infrared light by electrodes placed on the forehead. Brain tissue up to about 2 cm in depth from the scalp surface is reached for measurement. A normal range for NIRS-derived cerebral oxygen saturation values is usually assumed to be 60–75% due to the predominance of cerebral venous vessels. A major drawback of this monitoring technique is the lack of normal values or accepted threshold values for treatment. Nevertheless, NIRS may have value for detecting trends and has been used for the determination of autoregulation.

Microdialysis is a technique that allows the measurement of metabolic or inflammatory substances in the brain tissue extracellular fluid. The catheter is composed of concentric tubes allowing the permanent perfusion of a dialysis fluid along a semipermeable membrane at the tip of the probe. Several recently developed catheters combine ICP, $p_{bt}O_2$ and microdialysis. Glucose, lactate/pyruvate and markers of tissue damage are measured routinely, but the method has great potential for various omics studies in the future [55, 56]. A clear drawback is the restricted area of brain tissue accessed, so the choice of catheter placement is critical.

37.2.5 Transcranial Doppler (TCD)

TCD has a long history of application in neurointensive care, and although established in adult NCC, particularly for the detection of vasospasm in subarachnoidal haemorrhage, it is not widely used in paediatric NCC. This is due in major part to technical issues, especially the prominent operator-dependency of measurements among several other factors that physiologically influence blood flow velocity in the brain.

Basal cerebral arteries in the vicinity of the circle of Willis are interrogated for blood flow velocity using Doppler technology. Importantly, it has to be kept in mind that this is not a measure of cerebral blood flow and therefore, conclusions if the provision of brain tissue with metabolic substrates is sufficient cannot be drawn directly. For example, high blood flow velocity may indicate vasospasm and ischaemia or intact cerebral autoregulation in arterial hypertension without brain ischaemia. Further factors that have an effect on blood flow velocity are haematocrit and partial pressure of CO_2 in the blood.

Patterns in the raw TCD signal that are clearly helpful are absent flow in an intracerebral artery as in embolic closure or very low or reverse diastolic flow as seen in severely increased ICP. In addition, oscillating flow around the zero line with low amplitude is demonstrable in brain death.

The most common parameter used in TCD is the pulsatility index (systolic minus diastolic divided by diastolic flow). Several reports have investigated the correlation of this index with ICP and CPP with inconsistent results [45, 57–60]. Nevertheless, in clinical practice, a highly abnormal pulsatility index should elicit further investigation.

In a survey of American Neuro-PICUs, TCD was in variable use to guide clinical decisions on when to obtain a neuroimaging study; how to manipulate cerebral perfusion pressure with fluids/vasopressors; and whether to perform a surgical intervention [61].

Due to the ease of application at the bedside, TCD can be regarded as a useful screening and monitoring tool when used by experienced examiners.

37.2.6 Key Points

- Imaging, optimally by MRI, continuous EEG, transcranial Doppler and invasive ICP-monitoring are the mainstay of neuromonitoring in severe brain insults.
- Multimodality neuromonitoring (i.e. the combination of monitoring techniques) captures different aspects of focal or generalized pathology, functional state and treatment response and has the potential to allow better-informed treatment modifications.
- Recent additions in advanced neuromonitoring are quantitative EEG, noninvasive techniques of ICP estimation and measurement of brain tissue oxygenation and metabolism. More evidence is needed if outcomes can be improved by using these technologies.

References

1. Young AM, Donnelly J, Czosnyka M, Jalloh I, Liu X, Aries MJ, Fernandes HM, Garnett MR, Smielewski P, Hutchinson PJ, Agrawal S. Continuous multimodality monitoring in children after traumatic brain injury-preliminary experience. PLoS One. 2016;11:e0148817.
2. Hunfeld M, Ketharanathan N, Catsman C, Straver DCG, Dremmen MHG, Bramer W, Wildschut E, Tibboel D, Buysse C. A systematic review of neuromonitoring modalities in children beyond neonatal period after cardiac arrest. Pediatr Crit Care Med. 2020;21(10):e927–33. https://doi.org/10.1097/PCC.0000000000002415.
3. Topjian AA, Zhang B, Xiao R, Fung FW, Berg RA, Graham K, Abend NS. Multimodal monitoring including early EEG improves stratification of brain injury severity after pediatric cardiac arrest. Resuscitation. 2021;167:282–8. https://doi.org/10.1016/j.resuscitation.2021.06.020.
4. Abend NS. Electrographic status epilepticus in children with critical illness: epidemiology and outcome. Epilepsy Behav. 2015;49:223–7.
5. Abend NS, Gutierrez-Colina AM, Topjian AA, Zhao H, Guo R, Donnelly M, Clancy RR, Dlugos DJ. Nonconvulsive seizures are common in critically ill children. Neurology. 2011;76(12):1071–7.
6. Yuliati A, Weber ARB. Use of continuous EEG monitoring in children presenting with encephalopathy following convulsive status epilepticus. J Clin Neurophysiol. 2019;36(3):181–5.
7. Sánchez Fernández I, Abend NS, Arndt DH, Carpenter JL, Chapman KE, Cornett KM, Dlugos DJ, Gallentine WB, Giza CC, Goldstein JL, Hahn CD, Lerner JT, Matsumoto JH, McBain K, Nash KB, Payne E, Sánchez SM, Williams K, Loddenkemper T. Electrographic seizures after convulsive status epilepticus in children and young adults: a retrospective multicenter study. J Pediatr. 2014;164(2):339–46.
8. Abend NS, Wusthoff CJ, Goldberg EM, Dlugos DJ. Electrographic seizures and status epilepticus in critically ill children and neonates with encephalopathy. Lancet Neurol. 2013;12(12):1170–9.
9. Hasbani DM, Topjian AA, Friess SH, Kilbaugh TJ, Berg RA, Christian CW, Dlugos DJ, Huh J, Abend NS. Nonconvulsive electrographic seizures are common in children with abusive head trauma. Pediatr Crit Care Med. 2013 Sep;14(7):709–15.
10. Payne ET, Zhao XY, Frndova H, McBain K, Sharma R, Hutchison JS, Hahn CD. Seizure burden is independently associated with short term outcome in critically ill children. Brain. 2014;137:1429–38.
11. Fung FW, Topjian AA, Xiao R, Abend NS. Early EEG features for outcome prediction after cardiac arrest in children. J Clin Neurophysiol. 2019;36(5):349–57.
12. Sansevere AJ, DiBacco ML, Akhondi-Asl A, LaRovere K, Loddenkemper T, Rivkin MJ, Thiagarajan RR, Pearl PL, Libenson MH, Tasker RC. EEG features of brain injury during extracorporeal membrane oxygenation in children. Neurology. 2020;95(10):e1372–80.
13. Herman ST, Abend NS, Bleck TP, Chapman KE, Drislane FW, Emerson RG, Gerard EE, Hahn CD, Husain AM, Kaplan PW, LaRoche SM, Nuwer MR, Quigg M, Riviello JJ, Schmitt SE, Simmons LA, Tsuchida TN, Hirsch LJ, Critical Care Continuous EEG Task Force of the American Clinical Neurophysiology Society. Consensus statement on continuous EEG in critically ill adults and children, part I: indications. J Clin Neurophysiol. 2015;32(2):87–95.
14. Herman ST, Abend NS, Bleck TP, Chapman KE, Drislane FW, Emerson RG, Gerard EE, Hahn CD, Husain AM, Kaplan PW, LaRoche SM, Nuwer MR, Quigg M, Riviello JJ, Schmitt SE, Simmons LA, Tsuchida TN, Hirsch LJ, Critical Care Continuous EEG Task Force of the American Clinical Neurophysiology Society. Consensus statement on continuous EEG in critically ill adults and children, part II: personnel, technical specifications, and clinical practice. J Clin Neurophysiol. 2015;32(2):96–108.
15. Sansevere AJ, Arya R, Sánchez Fernández I, Gaillard WD, Tasker RC, Lai YC, Anderson AE, Tchapyjnikov D, Chapman KE, Brenton JN, Carpenter JL, Gaínza-Lein M, Goldstein JL, Goodkin HP, Jackson MC, Kapur K, Mikati MA, Peariso K, Glauser TA, Topjian AA, Wainwright M, Wilfong AA, Williams KL, Loddenkemper T, Abend NS, Pediatric Status Epilepticus Research Group (pSERG). Electroencephalographic reporting for refractory status epilepticus. J Clin Neurophysiol. 2019;36(5):365–70.
16. Hirsch LJ, LaRoche SM, Gaspard N, et al. American Clinical Neurophysiology Society's standardized critical care EEG terminology: 2012 version. J Clin Neurophysiol. 2013;30:1–27.

17. Rowberry T, Kanthimathinathan HK, George F, Notghi L, Gupta R, Bill P, Wassmer E, Duncan HP, Morris KP, Scholefield BR. Implementation and early evaluation of a quantitative electroencephalography program for seizure detection in the PICU. Pediatr Crit Care Med. 2020;21(6):543–9.
18. Bruns N, Sanchez-Albisua I, Weiß C, Tschiedel E, Dohna-Schwake C, Felderhoff-Müser U, Müller H. Amplitude-integrated EEG for neurological assessment and seizure detection in a German pediatric intensive care unit. Front Pediatr. 2019;7:358.
19. Du Pont-Thibodeau G, Sanchez SM, Jawad AF, Nadkarni VM, Berg RA, Abend NS, Topjian AA. Seizure detection by critical care providers using amplitude-integrated electroencephalography and color density spectral array in pediatric cardiac arrest patients. Pediatr Crit Care Med. 2017;18:363–9.
20. Lalgudi Ganesan S, Stewart CP, Atenafu EG, Sharma R, Guerguerian A, Hutchison JS, Hahn CD. Seizure identification by critical care providers using quantitative electroencephalography. Crit Care Med. 2018;46:e1105–11.
21. Amorim E, van der Stoel M, Nagaraj SB, et al. Quantitative EEG reactivity and machine learning for prognostication in hypoxic-ischemic brain injury. Clin Neurophysiol. 2019;130:1908–16.
22. Jonas S, Rossetti AO, Oddo M, Jenni S, Favaro P, Zubler F. EEG-based outcome prediction after cardiac arrest with convolutional neural networks: performance and visualization of discriminative features. Hum Brain Mapp. 2019;40:4606–17.
23. Brooks GA, Park JT. Clinical and electroencephalographic correlates in pediatric cardiac arrest: experience at a tertiary care center. Neuropediatrics. 2018;49:324–9.
24. Topjian AA, Sánchez SM, Shults J, Berg RA, Dlugos DJ, Abend NS. Early electroencephalographic background features predict outcomes in children resuscitated from cardiac arrest. Pediatr Crit Care Med. 2016;17(6):547–57. https://doi.org/10.1097/PCC.0000000000000740.
25. Ostendorf AP, Hartman ME, Friess SH. Early electroencephalographic findings correlate with neurologic outcome in children following cardiac arrest. Pediatr Crit Care Med. 2016;17(7):667–76. https://doi.org/10.1097/PCC.0000000000000791.
26. Duez CHV, Ebbesen MQ, Benedek K, Fabricius M, Atkins MD, Beniczky S, Kjaer TW, Kirkegaard H, Johnsen B. Large inter-rater variability on EEG-reactivity is improved by a novel quantitative method. Clin Neurophysiol. 2018;129:724–30.
27. Ducharme-Crevier L, Press CA, Kurz JE, Mills MG, Goldstein JL, Wainwright MS. Early presence of sleep spindles on electroencephalography is associated with good outcome after pediatric cardiac arrest. Pediatr Crit Care Med. 2017;18:452–60.
28. Weiss N, Galanaud D, Carpentier A, Naccache L, Puybasset L. Clinical review: prognostic value of magnetic resonance imaging in acute brain injury and coma. Crit Care. 2007;11(5):230.
29. Gutierrez LG, Rovira A, Portela LA, Leite Cda C, Lucato LT. CT and MR in non-neonatal hypoxic-ischemic encephalopathy: radiological findings with pathophysiological correlations. Neuroradiology. 2010;52:949–76.
30. Barkovich AJ. MR and CT evaluation of profound neonatal and infantile asphyxia. Am J Neuroradiol. 1992;13:959–72.
31. Cervos-Navarro J, Diemer NH. Selective vulnerability in brain hypoxia. Crit Rev Neurobiol. 1991;6:149–82.
32. Huang BY, Castillo M. Hypoxic ischemic brain injury: imaging findings from birth to adulthood. Radiographics. 2008;28:417–39.
33. Oualha M, Gatterre P, Boddaert N, Dupic L, De Saint BL, Hubert P, Lesage F, Desguerre I. Early diffusion-weighted magnetic resonance imaging in children after cardiac arrest may provide valuable prognostic information on clinical outcome. Intensive Care Med. 2013;39(7):1306–12.
34. Yacoub M, Birchansky B, Mlynash M, Berg M, Knight L, Hirsch KG, Su F. Revive initiative at Stanford Children's Health. The prognostic value of quantitative diffusion-weighted MRI after pediatric cardiopulmonary arrest. Resuscitation. 2019;135:103–9. https://doi.org/10.1016/j.resuscitation.2018.11.003.
35. Manchester LC, Lee V, Schmithorst V, Kochanek PM, Panigrahy A, Fink EL. Global and regional derangements of cerebral blood flow and diffusion magnetic resonance imaging after pediatric cardiac arrest. J Pediatr. 2016;169:28–35.e1.
36. Stein DM, Hu PF, Brenner M, Sheth KN, Liu KH, Xiong W, Aarabi B, Scalea TM. Brief episodes of intracranial hypertension and cerebral hypoperfusion are associated with poor functional outcome after severe traumatic brain injury. J Trauma. 2011;71:364–73.

37. Robba C, Cardim D, Czosnyka M, Abecasis F, Pezzato S, Buratti S, Moscatelli A, Sortica C, Racca F, Pelosi P, Rasulo F. Ultrasound non-invasive intracranial pressure assessment in paediatric neurocritical care: a pilot study. Childs Nerv Syst. 2020;36(1):117–24.
38. Bauer DF, Razdan SN, Bartolucci AA, Markert JM. Meta-analysis of hemorrhagic complications from ventriculostomy placement by neurosurgeons. Neurosurgery. 2011;69(2):255–60.
39. Bota DP, Lefranc F, Vilallobos HR, Brimioulle S, Vincent JL. Ventriculostomy-related infections in critically ill patients: a 6-year experience. J Neurosurg. 2005;103(3):468–72.
40. Kochanek PM, Tasker RC, Carney N, Totten AM, Adelson PD, Selden NR, Davis-O'Reilly C, Hart EL, Bell MJ, Bratton SL, Grant GA, Kissoon N, Reuter-Rice KE, Vavilala MS, Wainwright MS. Guidelines for the management of pediatric severe traumatic brain injury, third edition: update of the brain trauma foundation guidelines. Pediatr Crit Care Med. 2019;20(3S Suppl 1):S1–S82.
41. Le Roux P, Menon DK, Citerio G, Vespa P, Bader MK, Brophy GM, Diringer MN, Stocchetti N, Videtta W, Armonda R, Badjatia N, Böesel J, Chesnut R, Chou S, Claassen J, Czosnyka M, De Georgia M, Figaji A, Fugate J, Helbok R, Horowitz D, Hutchinson P, Kumar M, McNett M, Miller C, Naidech A, Oddo M, Olson D, O'Phelan K, Provencio JJ, Puppo C, Riker R, Robertson C, Schmidt M, Taccone F. Consensus summary statement of the International Multidisciplinary Consensus Conference on Multimodality Monitoring in Neurocritical Care: a statement for healthcare professionals from the Neurocritical Care Society and the European Society of Intensive Care Medicine. Neurocrit Care. 2014;21(Suppl 2):S1–S26.
42. Bennett TD, DeWitt PE, Greene TH, Srivastava R, Riva-Cambrin J, Nance ML, Bratton SL, Runyan DK, Dean JM, Keenan HT. Functional outcome after intracranial pressure monitoring for children with severe traumatic brain injury. JAMA Pediatr. 2017;171(10):965–71.
43. Chesnut RM, Temkin N, Carney N, Dikmen S, Rondina C, Videtta W, Petroni G, Lujan S, Pridgeon J, Barber J, Machamer J, Chaddock K, Celix JM, Cherner M, Hendrix T. A trial of intracranial-pressure monitoring in traumatic brain injury. N Engl J Med. 2012;367(26):2471–81.
44. Hunt A, Tasker RC, Deep A. Neurocritical care monitoring of encephalopathic children with acute liver failure: a systematic review. Pediatr Transplant. 2019;23(7):e13556.
45. Fanelli A, Vonberg FW, LaRovere KL, Walsh BK, Smith ER, Robinson S, Tasker RC, Heldt T. Fully automated, real-time, calibration-free, continuous noninvasive estimation of intracranial pressure in children. J Neurosurg Pediatr. 2019;23:1–11.
46. Vavilala MS, Lee LA, Lam AM. The lower limit of cerebral autoregulation in children during sevoflurane anesthesia. J Neurosurg Anesthesiol. 2003;15:307–12.
47. Lewis PM, Czosnyka M, Carter BG, Rosenfeld JV, Paul E, Singhal N, Butt W. Cerebrovascular pressure reactivity in children with traumatic brain injury. Pediatr Crit Care Med. 2015;16(8):739–49.
48. Akhondi-Asl A, Vonberg FW, Au CC, Tasker RC. Meaning of intracranial pressure-to-blood pressure fisher-transformed Pearson correlation-derived optimal cerebral perfusion pressure: testing empiric utility in a mechanistic model. Crit Care Med. 2018;46(12):e1160–6.
49. Alali AS, Gomez D, Sathya C, Burd RS, Mainprize TG, Moulton R, Falcone RA Jr, de Mestral C, Nathens A. Intracranial pressure monitoring among children with severe traumatic brain injury. J Neurosurg Pediatr. 2015;16(5):523–32.
50. Güiza F, Depreitere B, Piper I, Citerio G, Jorens PG, Maas A, Schuhmann MU, Lo TM, Donald R, Jones P, Maier G, Van den Berghe G, Meyfroidt G. Early detection of increased intracranial pressure episodes in traumatic brain injury: external validation in an adult and in a pediatric cohort. Crit Care Med. 2017;45:e316–20.
51. Calviello L, Donnelly J, Cardim D, Robba C, Zeiler FA, Smielewski P, Czosnyka M. Compensatory-reserve-weighted intracranial pressure and its association with outcome after traumatic brain injury. Neurocrit Care. 2018;28(2):212–20.
52. Young AMH, Guilfoyle MR, Donnelly J, Smielewski P, Agarwal S, Czosnyka M, Hutchinson PJ. Multimodality neuromonitoring in severe pediatric traumatic brain injury. Pediatr Res. 2018 Jan;83(1–1):41–9.
53. Wolf MS, Rakkar J, Horvat CM, Simon DW, Kochanek PM, Clermont G, Clark RSB. Assessment of dynamic intracranial compliance in children with severe traumatic brain injury: proof-of-concept. Neurocrit Care. 2020;15:1–9.
54. Adelson PD, Nemoto E, Colak A, Painter M. The use of near infrared spectroscopy (NIRS) in children after traumatic brain injury. A preliminary report. Acta Neurochir Suppl. 1998;71:250–4.

55. Hutchinson PJ, Jalloh I, Helmy A, Carpenter KLH, Rostami E, Bellander B-M, Boutelle MG, Chen JW, Claassen I, Dahyot-Fizelier C, Enblad P, Gallagher CN, Helbok R, Hillered L, Le Roux PD, Magnoni S, Mangat HS, Menon DK, Nordström CH, O'Phelan KH, Oddo M, Perez Barcena J, Robertson C, Ronne-Engström E, Sahuquillo J, Smith M, Stocchetti N, Belli A, Carpenter TA, Coles JP, Czosnyka M, Dizdar N, Goodman JC, Gupta AK, Nielsen TH, Marklund N, Montcriol A, O'Connell MT, Poca MA, Sarrafzadeh A, Shannon RJ, Skjøth-Rasmussen J, Smielewski P, Stover JF, Timofeev I, Vespa P, Zavala E, Ungerstedt U. Consensus statement from the 2014 international microdialysis forum. Intensive Care Med. 2015;41:1517–28.
56. Ercole A, Magnoni S, Vegliante G, Pastorelli R, Surmacki J, Bohndiek SE, Zanier ER. Current and emerging technologies for probing molecular signatures of traumatic brain injury. Front Neurol. 2017;8:450.
57. Figaji AA, Zwane E, Fieggen AG, Argent AC, Le Roux PD, Siesjo P, Peter JC. Pressure autoregulation, intracranial pressure, and brain tissue oxygenation in children with severe traumatic brain injury. J Neurosurg Pediatr. 2009;4:420–8.
58. Figaji AA, Zwane E, Thompson C, Fieggen AG, Argent AC, Le Roux PD, Peter JC. Brain tissue oxygen tension monitoring in pediatric severe traumatic brain injury. Part 1: relationship with outcome. Childs Nerv Syst. 2009;25(10):1325–33.
59. Abecasis F, Cardim D, Czosnyka M, Robba C, Agrawal S. Transcranial Doppler as a non-invasive method to estimate cerebral perfusion pressure in children with severe traumatic brain injury. Childs Nerv Syst. 2020;36:125–31.
60. Figaji AA, Zwane E, Fieggen AG, Siesjo P, Peter JC. Transcranial Doppler pulsatility index is not a reliable indicator of intracranial pressure in children with severe traumatic brain injury. Surg Neurol. 2009;72:389–94.
61. LaRovere KL, Tasker RC, Wainwright M, Reuter-Rice K, Appavu B, Miles D, Lidsky K, Vittner P, Gundersen D, O'Brien NF, Pediatric Neurocritical Care Research Group (PNCRG). Transcranial doppler ultrasound during critical illness in children: survey of practices in pediatric neurocritical care centers. Pediatr Crit Care Med. 2020;21(1):67–74.

Management of Seizures and Refractory Status Epilepticus in Critically Ill Children

Sonia Khamis, Rahul Raman Singh, Suresh Pujar, and Shruti Agrawal

Contents

J. Brierley et al. (eds.), *ESPNIC Children's Intensive Care Textbook*,
https://doi.org/10.1007/978-3-031-64762-8_38

Learning Objectives

- Define status epilepticus
- Understand different seizure terminologies and their definitions
- Possible aetiologies for each seizure category
- Investigations
- Pharmacology and mechanism of action of anti-seizure medications
- Stepwise treatment approach for seizures

38.1 Introduction

Status epilepticus (SE) is the most common medical neurological emergency affecting approximately 15–20 per 100,000 children annually [1] with the highest incidence in children under the age of 4 years. It is the commonest neurological diagnosis requiring paediatric intensive care (PICU) admission. The aetiology for SE is varied and differs in different paediatric age groups. Despite various algorithms defining prompt diagnosis and management, SE carries significant morbidity and mortality burden. Delay in treatment can lead to significant systemic and neuro-morbidity with some patients progressing to refractory SE.

Apart from the children with admission diagnosis of SE, seizures are common in children admitted to PICU with a primary neurological insult such as traumatic or hypoxic-ischaemic brain injury (TBI and HIBI, respectively), central nervous system (CNS) infectious and inflammatory conditions, toxin exposure, electrolyte imbalance, and fever, which can worsen the secondary brain injury and neurodevelopmental outcomes. These seizures can be difficult to diagnose clinically as these patients would usually be heavily sedated and/or paralyzed as a part of neuroprotection and require vigilance for prompt detection and treatment.

The majority of seizures terminate spontaneously with a few progressing to SE and warranting time-critical interventions. Most of the SE episodes also terminate after anaesthesia induction and intubation; however, a small proportion would continue for a longer duration becoming refractory status epilepticus (RSE) and super-refractory status epilepticus (SRSE) with considerable mortality and morbidity. Approximately 23–48% of the stabilized patients with SE will progress to RSE, while 22% of patients with RSE further transition to SRSE [2]. Prompt recognition and aggressive treatment are crucial to decrease morbidity and improve outcomes.

38.1.1 Definitions

Status epilepticus (SE): Traditionally, it was defined as "a condition characterized by an epileptic seizure that is sufficiently prolonged or repeated at sufficiently brief intervals so as to produce an unvarying and enduring epileptic condition" [3, 4]. In clinical practice, SE is defined as either a single seizure lasting >5 min or frequent

◘ **Table 38.1** Operational dimensions with t1 indicating the time that emergency treatment of SE should be started and t2 indicating the time at which long-term consequences may be expected

Types of SE	t1 (when a seizure is likely to become prolonged leading to continuous activity)	t2 (when a seizure may cause long-term sequelae)
Tonic-clonic SE	5 min	30 min
Focal SE with impaired awareness	10 min	>60 min
Absence SE	10–15 min	Unknown

clinical seizures without an interictal return to the baseline clinical state. The 5-min window corresponds to the time at which urgent treatment should be initiated.[1]

The International League Against Epilepsy (ILAE) defines SE as a condition resulting either from the failure of the mechanisms responsible for seizure termination or activation of mechanisms that lead to abnormally prolonged seizures (after time point t1); and a condition that can have long-term consequences (after time point t2), including neuronal injury, neuronal death, and alteration of neuronal networks, depending on the type and duration of seizures (◘ Table 38.1) [5].

For generalized convulsive SE, the ILAE definition stipulates that t1 and t2 are 5 and 30 min, respectively. For other types of SE, the most appropriate time intervals for t1 and t2 are not well-defined. The ILAE suggests using a t1 and t2 of 10 and >60 min for focal SE with impaired consciousness and a t1 of 10–15 min for absence SE [5].

Refractory SE (RSE): It is defined as ongoing clinical seizures despite two appropriately selected and appropriately dosed anti-seizure medications (ASM)—an adequate dose of benzodiazepine and a second-line ASM such as levetiracetam, phenytoin, or valproic acid. The duration of the seizures does not remain a defining criterion for RSE.

Super-refractory status epilepticus (SRSE): It is defined as continuous or recurrent seizure activity lasting 24 h or more following initiation of anaesthetic medications. This includes cases in which seizure control is attained after induction of anaesthetic drugs but recurs on weaning the patient off the anaesthetic agent [6].

New-onset RSE (NORSE): It is a clinical presentation in patients without epilepsy or pre-existing neurological disorder, who present with RSE without a clear acute or active structural, toxic, or metabolic cause [7].

Febrile infection-related epilepsy syndrome (FIRES): It is a subcategory of NORSE that requires a preceding febrile illness starting between 2 weeks and 24 h prior to the onset of refractory status epilepticus. Fever may be absent at the onset of RSE [7].

1 The 5-min window corresponds with the time at which urgent treatment should be initiated. At least one study has found that a convulsive seizure lasting more than 5 min has a high risk of lasting 30 min or more . Also, treatment delay is associated with delayed treatment response.

38.1.2 Epidemiology: Incidence of Each Including Morbidity and Mortality

The annual incidence of paediatric SE with the latest definition is not known at present; it was estimated to be 17–23 episodes per 100,000 children with a mortality rate of 2–7% as per the previous definition of SE [1]. The highest incidence is in children below 2 years of age, with the greatest peak in the first year of life [8]. Approximately, 23–48% of patients with SE progress to RSE with a mortality rate of 16–43.5% [9, 10], and 22% of patients with RSE transition to SRSE which has significant morbidity and mortality if not recognized early [2].

38.1.3 Aetiology

Different aetiologies are responsible for the development of RSE and SRSE (◘ Table 38.2).

They can be categorized as follows:

- *Acute symptomatic:* Triggered by an acute neurological insult such as CNS infections (herpes simplex virus (HSV), HIV, malaria, tuberculosis, viral/autoimmune encephalitis, and meningitis), immune-mediated encephalitis, traumatic brain injury (TBI), hypoxic-Ischaemic brain injury (HIBI), sepsis, metabolic or toxic disturbance, low levels of antiepileptic drugs, and acute brain ischaemia (cerebrovascular disease including cerebral venous sinus thrombosis).
- *Remote symptomatic:* Secondary to a previous neurological abnormality with an acute precipitant such as cerebral palsy or hydrocephalus with VP shunt with fever, hypoxic-ischaemic encephalopathy, and post-transplant CNS lymphoproliferative disorder.
- *Progressive encephalopathy*: RSE in epilepsy secondary to a progressive neurodegenerative disease sub-sclerosing panencephalitis (SSPE), CNS tumours, metabolic diseases, and epileptic encephalopathies.
- *Prolonged febrile SE:* It is triggered by an acute febrile illness (excluding CNS infections).

Studies show that aetiology varies according to age groups and geographic location. The most common aetiology in children under 1 year of age is acute symptomatic (28.5%); prolonged febrile convulsions are seen commonly in children of 1–5 years (33.8%); and remote symptomatic aetiologies are seen in 40% of children between 5 and 10 years, and in 36.8% of patients between 10 and 16 years old [11]. In developing countries, acute symptomatic aetiology remains the most frequent aetiology in children, followed by remote symptomatic and unknown aetiologies [12].

In SRSE, the most common aetiologies include encephalitis, FIRES, and epileptic encephalopathy [13]. Immune-mediated encephalitis was found in 40% of patients with SRSE in one study, and these included post-infectious mycoplasma encephalitis, anti-*N*-methyl-D-aspartate (NMDA) receptor encephalitis, and Rasmussen's

Table 38.2 Causes of refractory and super-refractory status epilepticus

Aetiology of RSE, SRSE, NORSE, and FIRES
Acute symptomatic
– Cerebrovascular disease (stroke, CVST, subarachnoid haemorrhage, intracerebral haemorrhage)
– CNS infection (HSV, HIV, malaria, TB, viral, meningitis, abscess)
– Immune-mediated encephalitis (anti-*N*-methyl-D-aspartate (NMDA) receptor encephalitis, anti–GABA receptor, anti-GAD, anti-glycine receptor encephalitis, Rasmussen's encephalitis, anti-VGKC complex antibodies, paraneoplastic syndromes)
– Sepsis
– Electrolyte imbalance (hypoglycaemia, hyperammonaemia, renal failure)
– Hypertensive encephalopathy, posterior reversible encephalopathy syndrome
– Low levels of anti-seizure medications/withdrawal syndromes
– Drugs and toxins
– Traumatic brain injury
– Hypoxic-ischaemic brain injury
Remote symptomatic
– Previous neurological pathology (cortical dysplasia, hypoxic-ischaemic encephalopathy)
– Hydrocephalus with blocked VP shunt
– Post-stroke/post-traumatic brain injury
– Post-transplant CNS lymphoproliferative disease
Genetic epilepsy syndromes
– SCN1A, SCN2A, CACNA1A [57–59]
– Ring chromosome 20
Progressive encephalopathy
– Progressive neurodegenerative disease—Sub-sclerosing panencephalitis (SSPE), CNS tumours, epileptic encephalopathies including genetic epilepsies, progressive myoclonic epilepsy (PME)
– Metabolic/mitochondrial disorders (mutations in POLG1, D1MNL)
Unknown (cryptogenic)

CVST central venous sinus thrombosis, *VGKC* voltage-gated potassium channel-complex, *GABA* gamma aminobutyric acid, *GAD* glutamic acid decarboxylase, *HSV* herpes simplex virus, *CNS* central nervous system, *SCN* neuronal voltage-gated sodium channel, *POLG1* mitochondrial DNA polymerase gamma, *D1MNL* dynamin1-like, *CACNA* calcium channel-L subtype

encephalitis. Genetic epilepsies (PCDH19 and GABRG2 mutations) were diagnosed in 20% of children followed by epilepsy of a known metabolic etiology and NORSE in 10% [14].

38.1.4 Pathophysiology

Seizures are sustained by either an imbalance of neuronal excitation and inhibition or failure of normal inhibitory mechanisms [15]. Glutamate is an excitatory neurotransmitter that mediates excess excitation via the *N*-methyl-D-aspartate (NMDA) receptor, and γ-aminobutyric acid (GABA) is an inhibitory neurotransmitter preventing neurons from excess excitation by activation of the GABA receptor.

During uncontrolled seizure activity, NMDA receptors are upregulated, resulting in a glutamate-mediated increase in intracellular calcium which in turn leads to increased excitation, apoptosis, and necrosis of neurons. Moreover, GABA receptors are internalized from the extracellular membrane to the cytosol, thus leading to a reduction in the number of GABA receptors [16]. This mechanism along with an increase in glutaminergic receptors at the cell surface reduces the overall GABAergic activity, thus reducing the effectiveness of GABA agonists such as benzodiazepines and barbiturates that target them [17]. However, NMDA receptor blockers such as ketamine may remain effective late in the course of SE [18].

In RSE and SRSE, other mechanisms are likely to be responsible for the persistence of seizures. Some of the reported mechanisms include (a) mitochondrial failure or insufficiency [19], (b) neuro-inflammation (i.e., pro-inflammatory cytokines and autoantibodies to neural elements) [20] resulting in decreased integrity of the blood-brain barrier and higher potassium levels [21, 22], (c) sensitivity to NMDA-mediated neuronal stimulation [23], and (d) changes in gene expression [24].

The resulting excitotoxicity [25] causes calcium influx into the cells triggering a cascade of harmful processes leading to neuronal injury and cell loss [26]. The cerebral damage that ensues includes neuronal cell necrosis, gliosis, and network reorganization contributing to increased morbidity.

38.2 Investigations and Diagnosis

The aims of evaluation in RSE/SRSE include early recognition and rapid diagnostic evaluation of underlying aetiology and treatment to prevent poor outcomes and long-term sequelae.

Most patients presenting with SE undergo routine initial investigations as outlined in ◘ Table 38.3. In children with RSE/SRSE, identifying the underlying aetiology remains paramount, and targeted investigations are required based on clinical background, disease phenotype, and age of the patient.

Brain imaging such as MRI, MRA, MRV, or CT scan is indicated in all patients presenting with a suspicion of cerebrovascular insult, or brain injury, and in children with no known aetiology. MR spectroscopy is indicated in children with a suspicion of inborn error of metabolism (IEM).

Lumbar puncture and CSF analysis should be performed after initial stabilization to evaluate for underlying infection, immune-mediated pathology, and IEM.

EEG is vital for the diagnosis and ongoing management of RSE/SRSE. It is also useful in monitoring the achievement of burst suppression and identification of subsequent electrographic seizures after induction with anaesthetic agents.

Table 38.3 List of investigations

Investigations

Urgent investigations

- Finger prick blood glucose
- Laboratory tests: Full blood count, C-reactive protein, electrolytes, creatinine, calcium (total and ionized), magnesium, serum anti-convulsant levels
- Ammonia if neonate/suspect inborn error of metabolism
- Consider toxicology screen (especially teenagers)
- Blood pressure (exclude malignant hypertension)
- Head CT if focal signs/new focal seizure, trauma, possible VP shunt complication, or space-occupying lesion
- EEG, ECG, and CXR as available depending on individual cases

Individualized investigations

- Liver function tests
- Coagulation profile
- *Infection screen (serum)*
  - Viral serology—HIV, HSV1, HSV2, VZV, EBV, enterovirus
  - Blood culture for bacteria and fungi
  - Respiratory panel PCR
- *CSF analysis*
  - Opening pressure
  - CSF biochemistry (cell count, protein level, glucose, lactate, cytology)
  - Bacterial stains and culture including *mycobacteria tuberculosis*
  - Viral PCR—HSV 1/2, VZV, EBV, Parechovirus (if <3 years), mycoplasma serology
  - Neurotransmitters, amino acids, oligoclonal bands (paired with serum)
  - Cytokine analysis (paired with serum) in FIRES
- *Brain MRI/MR spectroscopy*
- *Autoimmune screening*
  - ANA, ANCA, Ro, La, dsDNA, anti-phospholipid, C3, C4, anti-thyroid, anti-neuronal surface antigens
  - Antibody panel—NMDAR, AMPAR, GABAR, LGI1, Caspr2, GlyR, anti-Hu, anti-MOG
- *Metabolic screening*
  - Plasma ammonia, lactate, pyruvate, acylcarnitine profile, plasma amino acids, urine organic acids, VLCFA, LDH
- Muscle biopsy
- *Genetic tests*
  - CGH array, whole genome sequencing, rapid trio exome sequencing
  - Mitochondrial genetics

ECG electrocardiogram, *EEG* electroencephalogram, *CXR* chest X-ray, *CT* computerized tomography, *CSF* cerebral spinal fluid, *HSV* herpes simplex virus, *VZV* Varicella Zoster virus, *EBV* Ebstein-Barr virus, *ANA* antinuclear antibody, *ANCA* anti-neutrophil cytoplasmic antibody, *AMPAR* α-amino-3-hydroxy-5-methyl-4-isoxazolepropionic acid receptor, *GABAR* gamma-aminobutyric acid receptor, *LGI1* leucine-rich glioma-inactivated1, *CASPR2* anti-contactin-associated protein-like 2 antibody, *GlyR* glycine receptor, *VLFCA* very long-chain fatty acid, *LDH* lactate dehydrogenase, *CGH* comparative genomic hybridization

38.3 Treatment

38.3.1 Stabilization

The primary aim of treatment is to stop clinical seizures with the objective to prevent initial excitotoxicity, provide neuroprotection, and prevent systemic complications [6].

In the initial stabilization of a child with SE, assessment, and management of airway, breathing, and haemodynamic resuscitation alongside simultaneous administration of anti-seizure medication is important. Other aspects of acute management include bedside evaluation and screening for a possible aetiology as well as identifying areas for urgent intervention such as trauma, sepsis-meningitis/encephalitis, cerebral oedema, and other possible acute intracranial pathologies (e.g., bleeds, abscesses, and space-occupying lesions).

Airway protection is required in any child with ongoing seizures to avoid the risk of aspiration as well as provide adequate oxygenation, ventilation, and tissue perfusion. This can be carried out with 100% supplemental oxygen along with positioning—jaw thrust and use of non-invasive methods such as airway adjuncts—nasopharyngeal/oropharyngeal airways or bag-mask-assisted ventilation. However, early intubation is recommended in SE and RSE as they are at risk of seizure and medication-associated hypoventilation, especially with the use of multiple ASMs.

Vascular access, circulatory support, and treatment of emergent electrolyte imbalances including hypoglycaemia need to be addressed as outlined in ◘ Fig. 38.1. Temperature control is important in children who present with fever as this lowers the seizure threshold. In addition, hyperthermia may be caused by ongoing seizures and muscle activity which can also lead to rhabdomyolysis and end-organ damage. In these circumstances, antipyretics are of no benefit, and the child will require rapid sequence intubation (RSI) and paralysis along with active cooling.

All patients presenting with SE will need *emergent initial therapy* with a first-line ASM followed by *urgent control therapy* with a second-line ASM. This is often combined with an ASM *maintenance therapy*.

38.3.2 First-Line Therapy

Benzodiazepines are the drug of choice for emergent initial treatment of seizures that persist for >5 mins. The intravascular (IV) route is preferred; however, they can also be administered via intramuscular (IM), intranasal, buccal, or rectal route if there is a delay in obtaining IV access (◘ Table 38.4).

38

The first dose of benzodiazepine must be administered within 5 mins, and if seizures persist, a second dose of benzodiazepine may be administered at 10 mins [27]. Care must be taken as repeated doses of benzodiazepines may result in respiratory depression and hypotension.

Benzodiazepines: Gamma-aminobutyric acid (GABA) is a neurotransmitter that is widely distributed throughout the central nervous system and exerts postsynaptic inhibition. The GABA (A) receptor complex has binding sites for GABA, benzodi-

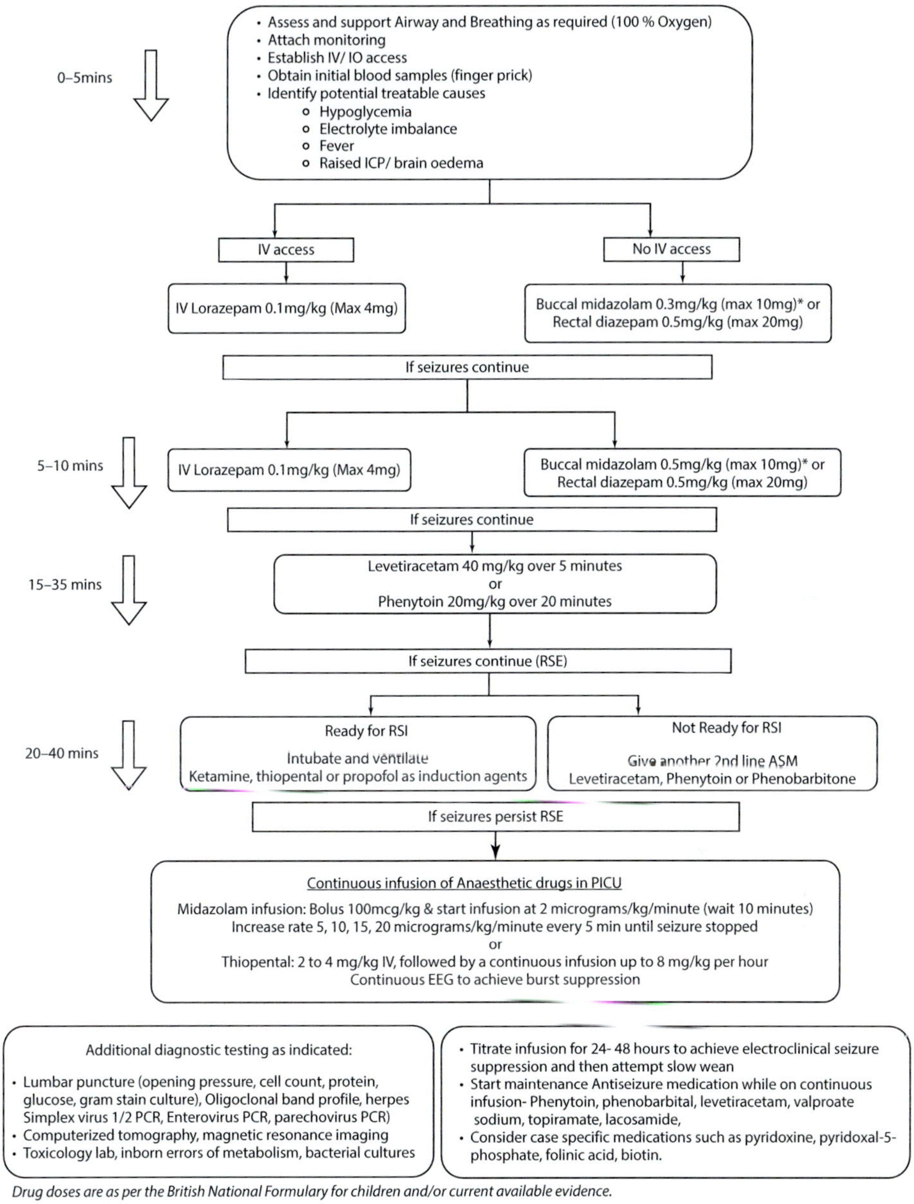

Fig. 38.1 Proposed algorithm for managing SE. Adapted from APLS guidelines [27, 60] Drug doses are as per the British National Formulary for children and/or current available evidence

azepines, and phenobarbital. Benzodiazepines act by binding to the GABA (A) receptor and facilitate the attachment of GABA to its binding site on the receptor. The inhibitory action of endogenous GABA is magnified because benzodiazepines increase the chloride channel openings. The three most used benzodiazepines are lorazepam, midazolam, and diazepam. Lorazepam IV is preferred in view of its longer duration of action compared to IV diazepam.

Table 38.4 Medications used in SE

	Medications used in SE	Dosing	Precautions
Emergent initial therapy	Lorazepam	IV: 0.1 mg/kg (max 4 mg), may repeat in 5–10mins	Respiratory depression
	Diazepam	IV: 0.3 mg–0.4 mg/kg (max 10 mg) Rectal: 0.5 mg/kg *(max 20 mg), may repeat in 5 mins – <1 month: 1.25–2.5 mg – 1 month–1 year: 5 mg – 2–11 years: 5–10 mg – 12–17 years: 10-20 mg	Respiratory depression
	Midazolam	Buccal: 0.3 mg/kg (max 10 mg) – <2 months: 0.3 mg/kg – 3–11 months: 2.5 mg – 1–4 years: 5 mg – 5–9 years: 7.5 mg – 10–17 years: 10 mg	Respiratory depression
Urgent control therapy	Levetiracetam	IV: 40 mg/kg (max 3 g)	Behavioural changes
	Phenytoin	IV: 20 mg/kg (max 2 g), may give additional 5–10 mg/kg	Arrhythmias Hypotension
	Phenobarbitone	IV: 20 mg/kg (max 1 g), may give additional 5–10 mg/kg	Respiratory depression Hypotension
	Valproate	IV: 20 mg/kg, may give additional 20 mg/kg	Thrombocytopenia Hyperammonaemia Pancreatitis, hepatotoxicity

Lorazepam: Lorazepam is less lipid-soluble and has less pronounced redistribution into adipose tissue giving it a longer duration of action. For this reason, it provides continued seizure control until the loading dose of a second agent can be completed.

Diazepam: Diazepam is highly lipid-soluble and rapidly crosses the blood-brain barrier. However, it is also rapidly redistributed from the adipose tissue leading to a short distribution half-life. Repeated doses may compensate for this but can lead to saturation of the peripheral compartments and unpredictable sudden rises in serum levels.

Midazolam: Midazolam is very effective in acutely terminating seizures, especially when IV access cannot be established. However, it has a short half-life in the central nervous system. It is most commonly used in buccal routes in the community and can also be administered by IM or intranasal routes.

38.3.3 Second-Line Therapy

For patients who fail emergent initial therapy with two doses of benzodiazepines, a second therapy with a long-acting ASM is indicated. The goal of urgent control therapy is to administer a drug that will reach rapid therapeutic levels in order to stop

SE. There is some evidence to suggest that early aggressive control and prompt start of non-benzodiazepine ASM may lead to fewer medical complications, less progression to SRSE, and improved neurobehavioural outcomes [28].

ASM used for urgent control is influenced by patient-specific conditions like the aetiology of seizures, previous response to ASM, and local drug availability. For example, in patients with established epilepsy, it might be worth considering the administration of an IV bolus of the ASM the child is already taking to target higher than normal concentrations of the ASM for seizure control, prior to initiating an additional agent [29].

The most common drugs previously used as second-line agents included phenytoin/fosphenytoin, phenobarbitone, and valproate. However, IV levetiracetam is now recommended as a second-line drug in view of fewer adverse reactions and ease of administration [30].

Levetiracetam: The exact mechanism of action of levetiracetam is unclear. However, it is known to bind to synaptic vesicle protein SV2A[2] [29, 31] modulating synaptic transmission through alteration of vesicle fusion. Levetiracetam also indirectly modulates gamma-aminobutyric acid (GABA) [32].

Its metabolism is independent of the cytochrome P450 (CYP) system, limiting the potential for pharmacokinetic interaction with other anti-seizure medications and it can safely be used in children with underlying hepatic or metabolic conditions.

Levetiracetam is relatively well-tolerated; however, increased agitation and aggression have been reported particularly in children with intellectual disability and behavioural problems [33].

Phenytoin: Phenytoin blocks voltage-dependent neuronal sodium channels and acts by diminishing synaptic transmission, limiting fluctuation of neuronal ionic gradients via sodium-potassium ATPase, and affecting second messenger systems by inhibiting calcium-calmodulin protein phosphorylation. It is metabolized in the liver and is an inducer of CYP. Several anti-seizure medications and other drugs can influence the serum concentration of phenytoin, including renal and hepatic failure.

Side effects of phenytoin include hypotension and cardiac arrhythmias and must be administered under close cardiac monitoring. Phenytoin can exacerbate myoclonic and absence seizures and therefore must be avoided in those children with known juvenile myoclonic epilepsy. Although contraindicated in Dravet's syndrome, it can sometimes be effective in the emergency management of SE in these children and must not be used without neurological consultation.

Phenobarbitone: ► Phenobarbital is a long-acting anti-seizure medication that works by binding to the GABA(A) receptor, thus improving the effect of GABA by extending the duration of GABA-mediated chloride channel openings. This process permits an increasing flow of chloride ions across the membrane, causing neuronal hyperpolarization. Like phenytoin, phenobarbitone is also an inducer of the CYP system and may interact with other drugs.

In view of its sedative side effects and respiratory depression and apnoea, phenobarbitone is reserved for use when initial treatment with levetiracetam and phenytoin fails. The risk of prolonged sedation with phenobarbital is greater than the

---

2 SV2A is a synaptic vesicle membrane protein expressed in neurons and endocrine cells and involved in the regulation of neurotransmitter release. It has been identified as a specific binding site for levetiracetam.

other anticonvulsants because its half-life is 87–100 h and often longer in newborns [34].

Valproate: Valproic acid has several mechanisms of action in controlling seizures. It blocks voltage-dependent sodium channels, thus reducing repetitive neuronal firing and increasing brain GABA concentrations. GABA concentrations are increased by the presynaptic effect of valproate on GABA (B) receptors, inhibition of nerve terminal GABA transaminase (GABA-T),[3] and by increasing GABA synthesis by activating glutamic acid decarboxylase (GAD). Because it has other mechanisms independent of GABA receptors, valproate may be effective later in RSE once GABA receptors have been expended by other anti-seizure medications.

Although valproate is well-tolerated, it is extensively metabolized in the liver and must be avoided in hepatic impairment. It is contraindicated in children with known metabolic disorders (e.g., urea cycle disorder and mitochondrial disorders) or in children <2 years of age with a suspicion of an underlying metabolic disorder. Rarely, valproate is known to cause hypotension [35].

38.3.4 Anaesthetic Drugs: Refractory and Super Refractory SE

If seizure activity persists after both first and second-line treatments have been given, the child is in RSE. As per definition, no specific time must elapse, hence emphasizing the importance of inducing pharmacological coma with third-line medications with continuous infusion of anaesthetic agents and proceeding with rapid sequence induction (RSI). While preparing for RSI, intermittent boluses of second-line medications (phenytoin, valproate, and levetiracetam) can be used if not previously given, especially in children who are haemodynamically stable [27]. The primary goal of therapy is to stop both clinical and electrographic seizures or achieve burst suppression. This should be maintained for a minimum of 24–48 h before withdrawal of continuous infusions. The management should continue with close input from paediatric neurologists. If seizures persist despite 24 h of continuous infusion or recur immediately after weaning off anaesthetic drugs, it indicates that the child has progressed to SRSE. In these cases, the continuous infusions are gradually up-titrated until seizure cessation is achieved. In some specific conditions, other therapies such as ketogenic diet, immunomodulation, vagus nerve stimulation, and epilepsy surgery may be considered. If <2 years, pyridoxine (100 mg IV) should be considered.

The most commonly used agents for coma induction are midazolam, barbiturates, and propofol, ideally with continuous EEG monitoring to titrate therapy (◘ Table 38.5).

38.3.4.1 Midazolam

Midazolam is given by intravenous (IV) infusion and rapidly penetrates the blood-brain barrier. It is given as an initial bolus infusion of 0.1 mg/kg IV followed by a continuous infusion of 0.05–2 mg/kg per hour. Additional boluses of 0.1–0.2 mg/kg can be given for breakthrough seizures,[4] for immediate control of seizures; this is fol-

38

3 GABA is mainly degraded to succinic semialdehyde in a reaction catalyzed by the enzyme GABA-transaminase (GABA-T). Inhibition of this enzyme produces considerable elevation of GABA.

4 Increasing the infusion rate without bolus dosing would lead to a very slow increase in serum levels and will not help in terminating the seizures; hence, bolus doses are indicated for breakthrough seizures.

Table 38.5 Medication recommendations for RSE/SRSE

Drug	Loading dose	Infusion rates	Precautions
Midazolam	0.2 mg/kg	0.05-2 mg/kg/h **Breakthrough SE**: 0.1–0.2 mg/kg bolus followed by an increase in infusion by 0.05–0.1 mg/kg/h every 3–4 h	Respiratory depression, hypotension, metabolic acidosis
Thiopental	2–7 mg/kg	0.5–5 mg/kg/h **Breakthrough SE**: 1–2 mg/kg bolus followed by increasing infusion by 0.5–1 mg/kg/h q 12 h	Hypotension Cardiorespiratory depression, prolonged recovery, toxicity
Propofol	1–2 mg/kg	20 mcg/kg/min titrated by 5–10 mcg/kg/min **Breakthrough SE**: Increase infusion rate by 5–10 mcg/kg/min every 5 min (Caution not to exceed 65 mcg/kg/min)	PRIS Hypotension Cardiorespiratory depression
Ketamine	0.5–3 mg/kg	1-10 mg/kg/h	Tachycardia, hypertension Raised ICP, neurotoxicity
Immunomodulatory medications			
Methylprednisolone	30 mg/kg/day (max 1 g/d)	Given for 3 days	Hyperglycaemia Hypertension Altered immunity Psychiatric disturbances Adrenal suppression
IVIG[a]	0.4 g/kg/day over 5d or 2 g/kg over 2 days		Hypersensitivity reactions Coagulation disturbances Hypertension Aseptic meningitis
Plasmapheresis		5 exchanges on alternate days over 10 days	

[a] All diagnostic serum antibody tests should be sent prior to initiating treatment as IVIG can alter future results

lowed by a subsequent increase in infusion rate by 0.05–0.1 mg/kg per hour, every 3–4 h [34] titrated to achieve cessation of clinical or electrographic seizure suppression or EEG burst suppression.

Cardiorespiratory depression and hypotension occur at higher doses of midazolam, and tachyphylaxis occurs mostly after prolonged use. Due to its short half-life, the anticonvulsant effects of midazolam can cease rapidly when it is stopped, hence leading to withdrawal seizures.

38.3.4.2 Thiopental/Pentobarbital

Thiopental and its metabolite pentobarbital act by enhancing the action of the GABA (A) receptor and also exhibit neuroprotective properties such as hypothermia which are beneficial in SE. It is given as an initial bolus infusion of 2–4 mg/kg IV followed by a continuous infusion of up to 8 mg/kg per hour. Owing to their long half-life, the effect of this anaesthetic agent leads to a long recovery time that can persist for days. Significant side effects include respiratory depression, hypotension, myocardial depression, and reduced cardiac output requiring the use of vasopressors. The continuous infusion should be used under continuous EEG monitoring to achieve burst suppression and avoid complete electric silence so as to minimize the side effects.

38.3.4.3 Propofol

Propofol works in a similar way to barbiturates by acting on GABA (A) receptors. As a continuous infusion, it may rapidly treat seizures and induce burst suppression, but it is usually avoided in the paediatric population due to propofol infusion syndrome that consists of severe lactic acidosis, rhabdomyolysis, hyperkalaemia, bradycardia, cardiac dysfunction, and multi-organ failure with a high risk of death. Propofol infusion syndrome often occurs at high infusion doses (>67 mcg/kg per minute or >4 mg/kg per hour), prolonged administration (>48 h), or if administered to children on corticosteroids, catecholamines, or the ketogenic diet [36]. Lower doses (5 mg/kg per hour), if given under careful monitoring, reduce the adverse effects of propofol but may not be effective in controlling seizures [37]. Another disadvantage of propofol is drug-induced involuntary movements (myoclonic appearance) that may resemble seizures. It has been suggested that the propofol-induced movements are of the peripheral origin or due to the lack of cortical inhibition, a small dose of muscle relaxant such as vecuronium, may help distinguish myoclonus of peripheral and central origin [38].

38.3.4.4 Ketamine

Ketamine is a potent *N*-methyl-D-aspartate (NMDA) receptor antagonist and has evidence of efficacy in advanced stages of RSE/SRSE. This mechanism of action helps to reduce epileptiform burst discharges and prevent glutamate-mediated neurotoxicity [39, 40]. It is the only anaesthetic agent that is not associated with cardiorespiratory depression and hypotension.

38.3.5 Special Considerations for Seizures in Critically Ill Children with Acute Neurological Conditions

Children admitted to PICU with acute neurologic conditions are at a high risk of both convulsive and non-convulsive seizures with the potential to degenerate to SE. Increasing the use of continuous EEG in this patient cohort is improving our understanding of these seizures. The evidence supports using continuous EEG in monitoring these children to assess neurological status and the presence of seizures and ES; electrical SE (ESE) is associated with poor outcomes and it should be treated effectively [41]. Whether treating sub-clinical seizures improves outcomes is still to be proven [42].

38.3.5.1 Post-traumatic Seizures and Status Epilepticus

Seizures are common after traumatic brain injury (TBI) both in the early acute phase (<7 days) and late seizures (>7 days) with an estimated incidence of 12–43% [43–45]. Clinical seizures in patients undergoing neuroprotection in PICU are difficult to diagnose; increasing use of continuous EEG monitoring shows that electrographic seizures are common, can lead to increased length of hospital stay, and affect the neurodevelopmental outcome [46]. This finding is also corroborated by small studies using intracranial electroencephalography in children with TBI [43, 47]. Some of the risk factors for early seizures include children below the age of 5, acute intracerebral haematoma, acute subdural haematoma, diffuse cerebral oedema, focal neurologic deficits, skull fractures, loss of consciousness or amnesia lasting over 30 min, and non-accidental injury [48]. There is some evidence to support that early seizure prophylaxis with phenytoin and levetiracetam may reduce the incidence of early seizures [49].

There is as yet no effective treatment against post-traumatic epileptogenesis and no reliable biomarker that can allow clinicians to predict patient susceptibility to post-traumatic epilepsy [50].

38.3.5.2 Post-anoxic Seizures

Seizures are common in children with hypoxic-ischaemic brain damage, and RSE can occur in comatose patients following cardiac arrest; the presence of seizures or SE both predict poor neurological outcomes [51]. They are often diagnosed with continuous EEG monitoring and can be non-convulsive in nature. Clinical motor seizures (myoclonic, clonic, or tonic-clonic) [52] have also been reported, and these are generally resistant to treatment. Seizure prophylaxis is not recommended unless confirmed via EEG or the presence of clinical seizures [53].

Treatment of seizures, SE, or RSE in post-anoxic patients remains controversial. Recommendations are to treat SE in the presence of clinical features such as the return of brain-stem reflexes or preserved cortical somatosensory evoked responses upon sedation weaning and achieving normothermia [54].

38.3.6 Other Agents to Consider

38.3.6.1 Anti-Seizure Medications

Anti-seizure medications (ASM) are often used concurrently with anaesthetic agents. The efficacy of their use in RSE/SRSE is unclear; however, their role is vital during the weaning of anaesthetic agents to prevent the recurrence of seizures. Some of the commonly used ASMs are levetiracetam, phenobarbital, topiramate, lacosamide, and phenytoin.

38.3.6.2 Pyridoxine, Pyridoxal-5-Phosphate, Folinic Acid, and Biotin

Pyridoxine: It is useful for pyridoxine-responsive super-refractory status epilepticus in children with ALDH7A1 mutations, pyridoxine 5-phosphate oxidase deficiency, hypophosphatasia, and nutritional pyridoxine deficiency. Owing to its safety, it is routinely used in infants and younger children in SRSE where a suspicion of inborn error of metabolism is high. IV Pyridoxine is administered as a 100 mg injection, and seizure termination is often achieved after 1–5 doses. However, in about 20% of infants with pyridoxine-dependent epilepsy, the first dose of pyridoxine can also cause cerebral depression, which is more likely if the infant is receiving anti-convulsant drugs.

Pyridoxal-5-phosphate: The active form of pyridoxine, pyridoxal-5-phosphate (PLP) is used in infants who present with pyridoxal phosphate-dependent neonatal epileptic encephalopathy or pyridoxine phosphate oxidase (PNPO) deficiency. The dose used is 30–60 mg/kg/d in 4–6 divided doses. Doses are gradually increased if seizures recur.

Folinic acid: Folinic acid-responsive seizures are caused by alpha-AASA dehydrogenase deficiency and mutations in the ALDH7A1 gene and are identical to pyridoxine-dependant epilepsy. The seizures promptly respond to folinic acid at a dose of 15 mg once daily. However, if seizures recur, doses (up to 8 mg/kg/day) are used alongside anti-convulsant therapy.

Biotin: Biotin is used in children who present with RSE and have neurological features consistent with biotinidase deficiency (hypotonia, seizures, ataxia, and alopecia). Treatment includes biotin 5 mg BD.

38.3.6.3 Steroids and Immunotherapy

Steroids and immunotherapy are used in RSE/SRSE and cryptogenic status epilepticus with a confirmed or postulated inflammatory/immunological aetiology. Some of these disorders include Rasmussen encephalitis, central nervous system vasculitis, NMDAR encephalitis, and limbic encephalitis.

Steroids are often used as first line immunomodulatory therapy with a standard dose of IV methylprednisolone 30 mg/kg/day (maximum 1 g/day) for 3 days. Caution needs to be taken in children with presumed infectious aetiology where appropriate antiviral and antimicrobial cover is required.

If there is inadequate response or contraindication to steroids, IVIG is recommended as second-line immunotherapy. This is administered as 2gm/kg given over 2–5 days.

Plasma exchange is reserved for those children who continue to be symptomatic and show little or no response to IVIG. A course of plasma exchange includes 5 exchange cycles on alternate days. Drug levels of anti-seizure medication (where applicable) should be monitored/adjusted in order to remain within therapeutic range as they can be altered with plasma exchange.

Finally, rituximab and cyclophosphamide may be used in children with a confirmed autoimmune or paraneoplastic aetiology.

38.3.6.4 Ketogenic Diet

The ketogenic diet (KD), a high-fat, low carbohydrate diet, as an emergency treatment has been shown to be effective in children with SRSE [55, 56]. Some epileptic syndromes that respond well to KD include: Doose syndrome (epilepsy with myoclonic-atonic seizure), Dravet syndrome (SCN1A mutation), GLUT-1 deficiency syndrome (SLC2A1 mutation), and Pyruvate dehydrogenase deficiency. It has also shown efficacy in children with febrile infection-related refractory epileptic encephalopathy (FIRES) [55].

KD is contraindicated in children with inborn errors of metabolism that involve the transport or oxidation of long-chain fatty acids as well as porphyria. It should not be used alongside propofol as it increases the risk of propofol infusion syndrome.

38.3.6.5 Epilepsy Surgery

In patients with a potentially epileptogenic brain lesion and concordant neurophysiology, urgent epilepsy surgery may be considered. Surgeries include lesionectomy, corpus callosotomy, and hemispherectomy.

Other treatment interventions such as therapeutic hypothermia and vagal nerve stimulation (VNS) may also be considered.

Take-Home Messages

- Early aggressive management of status epilepticus (SE) can help reduce complications.
- Latest evidence supports reducing the interval between two doses of benzodiazepines and early use of anaesthetic drugs to control SE.
- Resuscitation of the child should continue following the ABC approach while controlling SE.
- It is important to identify the underlying cause of seizures to help control ongoing SE.
- Follow a stepwise treatment approach for effective control and minimum side effects.

References

1. Chin RF, Neville BG, Peckham C, Bedford H, Wade A, Scott RC. Incidence, cause, and short-term outcome of convulsive status epilepticus in childhood: prospective population-based study. Lancet. 2006;368(9531):222–9.
2. Dubey D, Kalita J, Misra UK. Status epilepticus: refractory and super-refractory. Neurol India. 2017;65(Supplement):S12–S7.
3. Gastaut H. Dictionary of epilepsy. 1973.
4. Roger J. Status epilepticus. Handbook Clin Neurol. 1974;15:145–88.
5. Trinka E, Cock H, Hesdorffer D, Rossetti AO, Scheffer IE, Shinnar S, et al. A definition and classification of status epilepticus–report of the ILAE task force on classification of status epilepticus. Epilepsia. 2015;56(10):1515–23.
6. Shorvon S, Ferlisi M. The treatment of super-refractory status epilepticus: a critical review of available therapies and a clinical treatment protocol. Brain. 2011;134(10):2802–18.
7. Hirsch LJ, Gaspard N, van Baalen A, Nabbout R, Demeret S, Loddenkemper T, et al. Proposed consensus definitions for new-onset refractory status epilepticus (NORSE), febrile infection-related epilepsy syndrome (FIRES), and related conditions. Epilepsia. 2018;59(4):739–44.
8. Kumar UA. Study of comparing the efficacy of intravenous levetiracetam versus intravenous valproate in the management of refractory status epilepticus in children. Eur J Mol Clin Med. 2022;9(3):1766–78.

9. Sahin M, Menache CC, Holmes GL, Riviello JJ Jr. Outcome of severe refractory status epilepticus in children. Epilepsia. 2001;42(11):1461–7.
10. Gilbert DL, Gartside PS, Glauser TA. Efficacy and mortality in treatment of refractory generalized convulsive status epilepticus in children: a meta-analysis. J Child Neurol. 1999;14(9):602–9.
11. Tully I, Draper E, Lamming C, Mattison D, Thomas C, Martland T, et al. Admissions to paediatric intensive care units (PICU) with refractory convulsive status epilepticus (RCSE): a two-year multi-centre study. Seizure. 2015;29:153–61.
12. Lingappa L, Konanki R, Patel R, Vooturi S, Jayalakshmi S. Clinical profile and outcome of refractory convulsive status epilepticus in older children from a developing country. Seizure. 2016;36:31–5.
13. Farias-Moeller R, Bartolini L, Pasupuleti A, Brittany Cines R, Kao A, Carpenter JL. A practical approach to ketogenic diet in the pediatric intensive care unit for super-refractory status epilepticus. Neurocrit Care. 2017;26(2):267–72.
14. Appavu B, Vanatta L, Condie J, Kerrigan JF, Jarrar R. Ketogenic diet treatment for pediatric super-refractory status epilepticus. Seizure. 2016;41:62–5.
15. Fountain NB, Lothman EW. Pathophysiology of status epilepticus. J Clin Neurophysiol. 1995;12(4):326–42.
16. Arancibia-Cárcamo IL, Kittler JT. Regulation of GABAA receptor membrane trafficking and synaptic localization. Pharmacol Ther. 2009;123(1):17–31.
17. Bayrlee A, Ganeshalingam N, Kurczewski L, Brophy GM. Treatment of super-refractory status epilepticus. Curr Neurol Neurosci Rep. 2015;15(10):1–9.
18. Mazarati AM, Wasterlain CG. N-methyl-D-asparate receptor antagonists abolish the maintenance phase of self-sustaining status epilepticus in rat. Neurosci Lett. 1999;265(3):187–90.
19. Cock HR, Tong X, Hargreaves IP, Heales SJ, Clark JB, Patsalos PN, et al. Mitochondrial dysfunction associated with neuronal death following status epilepticus in rat. Epilepsy Res. 2002;48(3):157–68.
20. Shorvon S. Super-refractory status epilepticus: an approach to therapy in this difficult clinical situation. Epilepsia. 2011;52:53–6.
21. David Y, Cacheaux LP, Ivens S, Lapilover E, Heinemann U, Kaufer D, et al. Astrocytic dysfunction in epileptogenesis: consequence of altered potassium and glutamate homeostasis? J Neurosci. 2009;29(34):10588–99.
22. Friedman A, Dingledine R. Molecular cascades that mediate the influence of inflammation on epilepsy. Epilepsia. 2011;52:33–9.
23. Borris DJ, Bertram EH, Kapur J. Ketamine controls prolonged status epilepticus. Epilepsy Res. 2000;42(2–3):117–22.
24. Henshall DC. MicroRNAs in the pathophysiology and treatment of status epilepticus. Front Mol Neurosci. 2013;6:37.
25. Fujikawa DG. Prolonged seizures and cellular injury: understanding the connection. Epilepsy Behav. 2005;7:3–11.
26. Meldrum B. 9. Excitotoxicity and epileptic brain damage. Epilepsy Res. 1991;10(1):55–61.
27. Bacon M, Appleton R, Bangalore H, Brand C, Browning J, Chin RF, et al. Review of the new APLS guideline (2022): management of the convulsing child. Arch Dis Child Educ Pract. 2023;08(1):43–8.
28. Vasquez A, Farias-Moeller R, Sanchez-Fernandez U, Abend NS, Amengual-Gual M, Anderson A, Arya R, et al. Super-refractory status epilepticus in children: a retrospective cohort study. PCCM. 2021;22(12):e613–25.
29. Brophy GM, Bell R, Claassen J, Alldredge B, Bleck TP, Glauser T, et al. Guidelines for the evaluation and management of status epilepticus. Neurocrit Care. 2012;17(1):3–23.
30. Lyttle MD, Rainford NE, Gamble C, Messahel S, Humphreys A, Hickey H, Woolfall K, Roper L, Noblet J, Lee ED, Potter S, Tate P, Iyer A, Evans V, Appleton RE. Paediatric emergency research in the United Kingdom & Ireland (PERUKI) collaborative. Levetiracetam versus phenytoin for second-line treatment of paediatric convulsive status epilepticus (EcLiPSE): a multicentre, open-label, randomised trial. Lancet. 2019;25(10186):2125–34.
31. Custer KL, Austin NS, Sullivan JM, Bajjalieh SM. Synaptic vesicle protein 2 enhances release probability at quiescent synapses. J Neurosci. 2006;26(4):1303–13.

32. Doelken MT, Hammen T, Bogner W, Mennecke A, Stadlbauer A, Boettcher U, et al. Alterations of intracerebral γ-aminobutyric acid (GABA) levels by titration with levetiracetam in patients with focal epilepsies. Epilepsia. 2010;51(8):1477–82.
33. Hurtado B, Koepp MJ, Sander JW, Thompson PJ. The impact of levetiracetam on challenging behavior. Epilepsy Behav. 2006;8(3):588–92.
34. Donn SM, Grasela TH, Goldstein GW. Safety of a higher loading dose of phenobarbital in the term newborn. Pediatrics. 1985;75(6):1061–4.
35. White JR, Santos CS. Intravenous valproate associated with significant hypotension in the treatment of status epilepticus. J Child Neurol. 1999;14(12):822–3.
36. Baumeister F, Oberhoffer R, Liebhaber G, Kunkel J, Eberhardt J, Holthausen H, et al. Fatal propofol infusion syndrome in association with ketogenic diet. Neuropediatrics. 2004;35(04):250–2.
37. van Gestel JJ, Blusse van Oud-Alblas H, Malingre M, Ververs FT, Braun KJ, van Nieuwenhuizen O. HIGH Propofol and thiopental for refractory status epilepticus in children. Neurology. 2005;65(4):591–2.
38. Voss LJ, Sleigh JW, Barnard JP, Kirsch HE. The howling cortex: seizures and general anesthetic drugs. Anesth Analg. 2008;107(5):1689–703.
39. Wasterlain CG, Chen JW. Mechanistic and pharmacologic aspects of status epilepticus and its treatment with new antiepileptic drugs. Epilepsia. 2008;49:63–73.
40. Aram J, Martin D, Tomczyk M, Zeman S, Millar J, Pohler G, et al. Neocortical epileptogenesis in vitro: studies with N-methyl-D-aspartate, phencyclidine, sigma and dextromethorphan receptor ligands. J Pharmacol Exp Ther. 1989;248(1):320–8.
41. Abend NSSS, Berg RA, Dlugos DJ, Topjian AA. Current treatment of elcetrographic seizures and status epilepticus in critically ill children: a single center experience. Seizure. 2013;22(6):467–71.
42. Holleville MJG, Perier F, Fontaine C, Legriel S. Epileptic seizures in critically ill patients: diagnosis, managemengt and outcomes. J Clin Med. 2020;9:2218.
43. Arndt DHLJ, Matsumoto JH, Madikians A, Yudovin S, Valino H, et al. Subclinical early post-traumatic seizures detected by continuous eEG monitoring in a consecutive pediatric cohort. Epilepsia. 2013;54:1780–8.
44. Emanuelson I, Uvebrant P. Occurrence of epilepsy during the first 10 years after traumatic brain injury acquired in childhood up to the age of 18 years in the south western swedish population-based series. Brain Inj. 2009;23:612–6.
45. Liesemer KBS, Zebrack CM, Brockmeyer D, Statler KD. Early post-traumatic seizures in moderate to severe pediatric traumatic brain injury: rates, risk factors, and clinical features. J Neurotrauma. 2011;28:755–62.
46. Snooks KCYK, Farias-Moeller R, Fink EL, Hanson SJ. Continuous EEG and antiseizure medication use in an international pediatric traumatic brain injury population. Neurocrit Care. 2022;36:573–83.
47. Appavu BFS, Temkit M, Jacobson A, Burrows BT, Brown D, Boerwinkle V, Marku I, Adelson PD. Electroencephalography in pediatric severe traumatic brain injury. PCCM. 2020;21(3):240–7.
48. Elsamadicy AAKA, David WB, Lee V, Zogg CK, Kundishora AJ, Hong C, Reeves BC, Sarkozy M, Kahle KT, DiLuna M. Post-traumatic seizures following pediatric traumatic brain injury. Clin Neurol Neurosurg. 2021;203:106556.
49. Kochanek PM, Tasker RC, Carney N, Totten AM, Adelson PD, Selden NR, et al. Guidelines for the management of pediatric severe traumatic brain injury, third edition: update of the brain trauma foundation guidelines. Pediatr Crit Care Med. 2019;20(3S Suppl 1):S1–S82.
50. Lowenstein DH. Epilepsy after head injury: an overview. Epilepsia. 2009;50:4–9.
51. Muhlhofer WSJ. Prognostic value of EEG in patients after cardiac arrest-an updated review. Curr Neurol Neurosci Rep. 2018;18(4):16.
52. Lybeck A, Friberg H, Aneman A, Hassager C, Horn J, Kjaergaard J, et al. Prognostic significance of clinical seizures after cardiac arrest and target temperature management. Resuscitation. 2017;114:146–51.
53. Topjian AA, de Caen A, Wainwright MS, Abella BS, Abend NS, Atkins DL, et al. Pediatric post-cardiac arrest care: a scientific statement from the American Heart Association. Circulation. 2019;140(6):e194–233.
54. Rossetti AO. Should postanoxic status epilepticus be treated aggressively?-no! J Clin Neurophysiol. 2015;32(6):447–8.

55. François LL, Manel V, Rousselle C, David M. Ketogenic regime as anti-epileptic treatment: its use in 29 epileptic children. Arch Pediatrie. 2003;10(4):300–6.
56. Nabbout R, Mazzuca M, Hubert P, Peudennier S, Allaire C, Flurin V, et al. Efficacy of ketogenic diet in severe refractory status epilepticus initiating fever induced refractory epileptic encephalopathy in school age children (FIRES). Epilepsia. 2010;51(10):2033–7.
57. Kobayashi K, Ouchida M, Okumura A, Maegaki Y, Nishiyama I, Matsui H, et al. Genetic seizure susceptibility underlying acute encephalopathies in childhood. Epilepsy Res. 2010;91(2–3):143–52.
58. Jafarpour S, Hodgeman RM, Capeletto CDM, de Lima MTA, Kapur K, Tasker RC, et al. New-onset status epilepticus in pediatric patients: causes, characteristics, and outcomes. Pediatr Neurol. 2018;80:61–9.
59. Gugger JJ, Husari K, Probasco JC, Cervenka MC. New-onset refractory status epilepticus: a retrospective cohort study. Seizure. 2020;74:41–8.
60. Advanced Paediatric Life Support: A practical guide. 6th ed. Australia/New Zealand: Wiley Blackwell; 2017.

Hematological Issues in PICU

Contents

Haemoglobinopathies and Haemostatic Disorders in the PICU

Nadirah El-Amin and Oliver Karam

Contents

J. Brierley et al. (eds.), *ESPNIC Children's Intensive Care Textbook*,
https://doi.org/10.1007/978-3-031-64762-8_39

Learning Objectives

- To identify and treat the multiple life-threatening complications encountered in patients with sickle cell disease and to differentiate between the different types of transfusions used to treat sickle cell patients
- To recognize the importance of factor infusions in patients with haemophilia
- To identify and treat sepsis in patients with thalassaemia
- To recognize the catastrophic antiphospholipid syndrome and when to initiate certain treatment options
- To treat simple and refractory immune thrombocytopenia
- To identify the various presentations of thrombotic thrombocytopenic purpura and to recognize the importance of therapeutic plasma exchange
- To recognize that heparin is the only evidence-based treatment for disseminated intravascular coagulation

39.1 Introduction

There are multiple complex disorders that result from abnormalities in the blood and its components. Because of its numerous functions, including regulating the clotting cascade, carrying oxygen and nutrients to tissues and supporting the immune system, there is potential for significant morbidity and mortality when any one of these functions is abnormal or dysregulated.

In this chapter, we will address three haemoglobinopathies (sickle cell disease, thalassaemia and haemophilia) and four acute haemostatic disorders (antiphospholipid syndrome, immune thrombocytopenia, thrombotic thrombocytopenic purpura and disseminated intravascular coagulation) and discuss the proper management of these disorders in an intensive care unit.

39.2 Sickle Cell Disease

Sickle cell disease (SCD) is a clinically heterogeneous genetic condition that is characterized by the polymerization of haemoglobin S (HbS) [1]. This polymerization leads to multiple cellular interactions that result in haemolysis, vaso-occlusion, inflammation and RBC membrane damage [2]. The clinical effects of these changes are vast and can impact almost every organ system in patients with sickle cell disease. The most common clinical complications include vaso-occlusive episodes or acute pain crises, acute chest syndrome (ACS), haemolysis leading to significant anaemia, renal impairment, cardiomyopathy, venous thromboembolism and stroke. Acute chest syndrome, multi-organ dysfunction syndrome (MODS) and acute ischaemic stroke are the most commonly encountered complications in the ICU. The cornerstone of management for most sickle cell emergencies is a red blood cell transfusion.

39.2.1 Multi-System Organ Failure

This is a life-threatening complication of SCD in which multiple organ systems are affected by ischaemia or infarction. The most common organs affected include the liver, lungs and kidneys, and it is typically seen in the setting of an acute painful episode in a patient who has otherwise mild disease [3]. The onset of symptoms includes fever, rapid fall in haemoglobin level and platelet count, non-focal encephalopathy, and rhabdomyolysis [3]. Rapid reversal of this process can been achieved with prompt and aggressive exchange transfusion therapy as well as supportive care [4].

39.2.2 Acute Chest Syndrome

ACS is a syndrome defined by a new radiodensity on the chest radiograph, fever and/or respiratory symptoms (cough, shortness of breath and chest pain). It is an acute complication of SCD that often leads to significant morbidity and mortality if not promptly managed. It is thought that vaso-occlusion within the pulmonary microvasculature is the main driver of this clinical syndrome. This vaso-occlusion is thought to be triggered by several inciting events including infection, asthma, hypoventilation secondary to pain or fat embolism [5–7]. Management of ACS involves several interventions:

- Aggressive respiratory support with supplemental oxygen, non-invasive ventilation or intubation and mechanical ventilation.
- Pain control with parenteral analgesia, preferably via patient-controlled analgesia (PCA).
- Bronchodilators if there is an element of reactive airway disease.
- Initiation of broad-spectrum antibiotics. The most common antibiotic regimen includes a third-generation cephalosporin and a macrolide [8, 9]; however, antibiotic coverage should be tailored for clinical severity or for a specific organism.
- Blood transfusions should be considered for any patient with rapidly dropping haemoglobin or signs of clinical deterioration. This should be initiated promptly to reduce morbidity and mortality [10].

39.2.3 Stroke

Patients with SCD are at an increased risk of ischaemic and haemorrhagic stroke. Prompt clinical assessment and neuroimaging are necessary to determine the type of stroke and initiate management. Patients should be managed with standard stroke protocols including airway protection, blood pressure management, close attention to oxygenation, management of seizures if present and maintenance of hydration. Furthermore, laboratory workup should include a complete blood count, reticulocyte count, type and crossmatch, haemoglobin electrophoresis to assess for the percentage of foetal haemoglobin, prothrombin time, activated partial thromboplastin time and a basic metabolic panel [11].

All patients should receive a transfusion within 2 h of onset of neurological symptoms, ideally with an exchange transfusion [12]. However, if there is no capability to perform an exchange transfusion or it would not be available within 2 h, then a simple transfusion should be initiated assuming that the haemoglobin level is ≤8.5 g/dL, to avoid hyper-viscosity [12].

39.2.4 Transfusions for Sickle Cell Disease

The goal of transfusions in sickle cell disease is to increase oxygen-carrying capacity and to decrease the amount of HbS. Caution should be taken to avoid hyperviscosity by over-transfusing above a patient's baseline haemoglobin. Generally, haemoglobin levels should not be raised above 100 g/L [13].

A simple transfusion is usually the quickest and easiest method of transfusion. It involves only transfusing packed red blood cells (PRBCs). These transfusions are best for symptomatic anaemia, an uncomplicated pain crisis or splenic sequestration. However, these carry a risk for hyperviscosity and iron overload and do not provide the best control of HbS. It is recommended to transfuse PRBCs until the Hb level is 100 g/L [13].

The 2018 Transfusion and Anemia Expertise Initiative guidelines recommend that SCD patients with life-threatening complications, such as stroke or acute chest, should get an exchange transfusion over a simple (non-exchange) transfusion if the child's condition is deteriorating [13]. Manual exchange transfusions or modified exchange transfusions involve first phlebotomizing the patient followed by a transfusion of packed red blood cells and/or fluids. This method allows for better control of haemoglobin levels, slightly better control of HbS and helps to reduce iron overload. However, it is time-consuming and requires more skilled nursing. Automated red cell exchange transfusion involves using a pheresis machine to remove the patient's RBCs and replace them with donor PRBCs. This results in significantly better control of HbS without increasing viscosity (since the overall blood volume and haematocrit remain constant) and can be done rapidly [14]. Additionally, it allows for the best control of iron overload. In general, this is considered the gold standard for transfusion therapy in patients with life-threatening complications from their sickle cell disease [15]. Disadvantages include limited availability in resource-poor areas, significant staff training and the need for central access.

39.3 Haemophilia

Haemophilia A and B refer to factor VIII and factor IX deficiency, respectively, and are caused by pathogenic variants in the *F8* or *F9* gene [16, 17]. They are X-linked bleeding disorders that predominantly affect males [17]. Patients with haemophilia are at risk of developing life- and limb-threatening bleeding that often requires emergency care. Laboratory analysis of a patient with haemophilia would demonstrate a normal PT, prolonged aPTT, normal platelet count, bleeding time and INR. The cornerstone of management is the replacement of the deficient factor. Serious or life-threatening bleeds include central nervous system bleeds, iliopsoas bleeds, ocular bleeds, deep muscle bleeding with neurovascular compromise, bleeding into the airway, and intra-abdominal and GI bleeds [18]. The basic tenet of management for severe or life-threatening bleeds is to treat immediately with factor, preferably within an hour of presentation, even if a full diagnostic assessment has not been completed [18]. Factor administration should not be delayed for imaging studies.

39.3.1 Haemophilia A

Patients should be given an initial dose of factor VIII 50 IU/kg to raise the factor VIII level to approximately 100% [19]. A factor level should be checked approximately 15 min post-infusion to help determine future dosing needs. The subsequent doses should be given at approximately one half-life of the factor product infused, typically every 8–12 h as needed to maintain factor VIII levels above 50%. Another option is to give the initial dose of factor followed by a continuous infusion [20] at a dose of approximately 4 IU/kg/h of standard half-life factor VIII products. This method decreases the need for frequent monitoring and ensures a steady delivery of factors. If factor VIII is unavailable, cryoprecipitate can be used as it has abundant amounts of factor VIII. In children, up to 1 unit (bag) can be administered per 6 kg of body weight every 12 h [21].

39.3.2 Haemophilia B

Factor dosing for haemophilia B patients tends to be more product-specific. However, in general, patients should be given an initial dose of factor IX of 100–120 IU/kg to raise the factor IX level to 100% [19]. A factor level should be checked approximately 15 min after the infusion to help determine future doses. Subsequent doses should be given based on the half-life of the product, approximately every 18–24 h as needed to maintain levels above 50%. Patients can also be maintained on a continuous infusion at an approximate dose of 6 IU/kg/h [20].

Experts agree that the duration of factor replacement for severe bleeding is individualized based upon a variety of issues including surgical management, extent and site of bleeding, and response to factor replacement.

39.4 Thalassaemia

Thalassaemias constitute a variable group of anaemias characterized by a defect in the synthesis of one or more of the globin subunits of haemoglobin [22]. Common manifestations of thalassaemias include an imbalance in the α/β-globin chain ratio, ineffective erythropoiesis, chronic haemolytic anaemia and iron overload [23]. Currently, the mainstay of treatment is the initiation of chronic transfusion programmes and chelation protocols in childhood. As a result, these patients are living longer and are now presenting with more complications from their treatment later in life.

Sepsis is one of the leading causes of mortality in patients with thalassaemia [24], secondary to risk factors such as splenectomy, transfusions and iron overload [25]. Oftentimes, patients with thalassaemia will have a splenectomy due to its role in clearing defective red blood cells and the subsequent effect of worsened anaemia. *Klebsiella pneumoniae*, *Escherichia coli*, *Streptococcus pneumoniae*, *Salmonella typhi*, *Yersinia enterocolitica* and other Gram-negative bacteria are the main culprits of bacterial infections [25, 26]. Prompt initiation of fluid resuscitation and initiation of broad-spectrum antibiotics are crucial to increasing survival. Antibiotics should be tailored once a specific bug is identified. Fluid resuscitation should be monitored closely in any patient who has cardiomyopathy or cardiovascular disease from their thalassaemia.

39.5 Catastrophic Antiphospholipid Syndrome (CAPS)

Antiphospholipid syndrome (APS) is an autoimmune disorder characterized by an increased risk of venous, arterial and small vessel thrombosis and pregnancy loss, secondary to persistent antiphospholipid antibodies [27]. Approximately, 1% of those with APS will develop a more severe presentation of APS called catastrophic antiphospholipid syndrome [27]. CAPS is characterized by a widespread thrombosis usually in the small vessels, multiple organ failure, rapid decline in clinical picture and very elevated antibody titres [28, 29]. Laboratory values are often suggestive of microangiopathic vasculitis, with elevated lactate dehydrogenase, low platelet count, schistocytes on a blood smear and elevated markers of haemolysis [30].

Despite evolving treatment, the mortality associated with CAPS remains high. Thus, it is important for prompt evaluation and recognition of the disease. The current management for CAPS includes anticoagulation, usually with heparin and pulse glucocorticoids as the first-line treatment. If the patient has life-threatening CAPS, then IVIG [31], rituximab [32] and plasma exchange [31] therapy should also be considered. Triple therapy with anticoagulation, glucocorticoids and plasma exchange and/or IVIG has been shown to confer the highest rates of survival [31]. It is also the most cost-effective [33].

39.6 Immune Thrombocytopenia

Immune thrombocytopenia (ITP), previously known as idiopathic thrombocytopenic purpura, is a haematological disease characterized by isolated thrombocytopenia (platelet count <100,000 × 10^9/L) with normal haemoglobin and white blood cell count. The pathophysiology involves autoantibodies in about 60% of the cases, most frequently immunoglobulin G which are directed against platelet antigens (e.g. glycoprotein IIb/IIIa complex) [34]. ITP can be either primary, i.e. in the absence of other causes, or secondary, when it is associated with an underlying condition such as immune deficiency, a viral infection or a systemic disease.

In the absence of clinically significant manifestations, most clinicians will observe only. However, most will initiate treatment when the platelet count falls below 10,000 × 10^9/L or when the patient has active bleeding [35]. For typical acute ITP with minor bleeding, front-line management includes a short course of corticosteroids (usually for less than 1 week) or intravenous immunoglobulin (IVIG); in Rh(D)-positive children, anti-D therapy should be considered [35]. In patients with ITP refractory to first-line treatments and who have non-life-threatening mucosal bleeding, the latest American Society of Hematology recommends the use of thrombopoietin receptor agonist (TPO-RA, either romiplostim or eltrombopag) over rituximab or splenectomy [36]. Platelet transfusions are to be avoided unless severe bleeding is present.

Life-threatening bleeding occurs in less than 1 of children with ITP. In those situations, experts will usually administer all the following therapies at the same time: methylprednisone 30 mg/kg (up to 1 g) per day for 3–4 days, IVIG 1 g/kg per day for 1–3 days and TPO-RA, as well as larger-than-normal platelet transfusion doses (up to 30 mL/kg) to correct platelet counts as quickly as possible [37].

39.7 Thrombotic Thrombocytopenic Purpura

Thrombotic thrombocytopenic purpura (TTP) is a clinical syndrome that combines fever, thrombocytopenia, microangiopathic haemolytic anaemia and disseminated microvascular thrombi. These lead to organ dysfunction, most importantly the brain and kidneys, although microthrombi can be found in other organs, such as in the heart, gastrointestinal tract and liver. Fewer than half of patients present with the full pentad of symptoms (fever, microangiopathic haemolytic anaemia, thrombocytopenia, central nervous system symptoms and renal failure), but three-fourths manifest a triad of microangiopathic haemolytic anaemia, neurologic symptoms and thrombocytopenia.

The pathophysiology is a deficiency in ADAMTS-13, a metalloprotease that normally cleaves von Willebrand factor (vWF). In acquired forms, the deficit is often associated with anti-ADAMTS-13 autoantibodies, which are sometimes linked to systemic infections, bone marrow transplantation or autoimmune diseases [38]. The deficit in ADAMTS-13 leads to ultra-large von Willebrand factor (ULVWF) multimers that can trigger platelet adhesion to the endothelium. Platelet consumption in thrombi leads to thrombocytopenia and consequently to haemorrhage, microvascular hypoperfusion and organ dysfunction [39].

Left untreated, TTP has a mortality of up to 90% [39]. The first successful treatments of TTP involving the use of therapeutic plasma exchange (TPE) were published in 1959 [40], decades before the ADAMTS-13 was characterized in 2001 [41]. Over the years, TPE has become a standard therapy for patients with TTP because it replaces ADAMTS-13 and removes both ULVWF and ADAMTS-13 inhibitors. TPE has been shown to be more effective than plasma transfusion alone [42]. A retrospective study of 108 patients showed an association between TPE and improved survival [43]. TTP should be started as soon as the diagnosis of TTP is established or even suspected (i.e. thrombocytopenia, anaemia and altered mental status) and is usually prescribed as 1.5 × plasma volume exchange for the first run, followed by 1.0 × patient plasma volume for subsequent runs [44]. TPE is performed daily until organ involvements have resolved (cerebral manifestations, renal failure, etc.), platelet count has recovered and haemolysis has ceased.

Although there is a theoretical rationale for the use of steroids in TTP, there is a lack of high-quality studies. Some experts suggest systematically associating steroids (methylprednisolone1.5 mg/kg/d for 3 weeks) with TPE, once obvious contraindications have been ruled out.

Rituximab, an anti-CD20 monoclonal antibody, may also be beneficial in patients who have unsatisfactory responses to TPE (± steroids). Two prospective studies and a small randomized controlled trial [45] have suggested that rituximab (375 mg/m^2 weekly for 4 weeks), in addition to TPE and steroids, is associated with high rates of response and low rates of relapse.

Platelet transfusions are generally not recommended in patients with TTP because of increased thrombotic risk. However, some observational studies have suggested transfusing platelets which might be appropriate in situations of life-threatening bleeding [46].

39.8 Disseminated Intravascular Coagulation

Disseminated intravascular coagulation (DIC) is a syndrome characterized by excessive activation of coagulation, resulting in both haemorrhage and thrombosis. DIC can be triggered by a variety of clinical conditions, such as sepsis (the most frequent cause), trauma, malignancy, liver failure, envenomation or even acute haemolytic transfusion reactions [47]. These situations will lead to intravascular deposition of fibrine, which will lead to thrombi of small and mid-size vessels, and to consumption of coagulation factors and platelets. This will lead to bleeding, which will further trigger the coagulation. In addition, both bleeding and microcirculation clots will lead to cellular hypoperfusion (due to decreased oxygen delivery), which will cause organ failure.

There is no single laboratory assay that can confirm or rule out the diagnosis of DIC. Therefore, most definitions will rely on a combination of diagnostic tests. The International Society of Thrombosis and Haemostasis (ISTH) uses four items: platelet counts, elevated fibrin-related markers (such as d-dimers), prolonged prothrombin time and hypofibrinogenaemia [48]. The Japanese Association for Acute Medicine (JAAM) definition is based on systemic inflammatory response syndrome (SIRS) criteria, thrombocytopenia, prolonged prothrombin time and hypofibrinogenaemia [49]. A revised definition, where the SIRS score is replaced with antithrombin activity, has been shown to have a similar accuracy in predicting mortality [50].

In a meta-analysis of adults with severe sepsis, heparin has been shown to decrease mortality [51].

Other therapies have also been evaluated. The administration of antithrombin to patients with severe sepsis led to more bleeding without improving mortality [52]. Although the initial trial of activated protein C (drotrecogin alfa activated) seemed to suggest a benefit [53], future studies failed to demonstrate improved survival but showed increased bleeding [54], which led to the medication being withdrawn. Tifacogin, a recombinant tissue factor pathway inhibitor, was also shown not to decrease mortality in adults with severe sepsis with an abnormal international normalized ratio (INR > 1.1) but significantly increased bleeding events [55]. Similarly, thrombomodulin also failed to decrease mortality [56]. Therefore, besides heparin, there does not seem to be any effective drug to treat DIC.

Since there is a paucity of pharmacological options, some researchers have evaluated therapeutic plasma exchange (TPE), which allows the replacement of coagulation factors while avoiding fluid overload. The highest evidence stems from a registry of children with thrombocytopenia-associated multiple organ failure (TAMOF). TAMOF is usually defined by thrombocytopenia, microangiopathic haemolysis, hemodynamic failure and ischaemic organ failure [57]. TAMOF is believed to be part of a spectrum of syndromes with disseminated microvascular thromboses that include DIC, TTP and haemolytic-uraemic syndrome (HUS). Patients with TAMOF have clinical DIC in addition to thrombotic microangiopathy. Fortenberry et al. published a study of 81 critically ill children with TAMOF, of which 74% received TPE. Adjusting for multiple confounders, they showed that the use of TPE was independently associated with a twofold decrease in mortality [57]. Multicentre randomized clinical trials are necessary to determine a causal relationship. Due to the lack of solid evidence, the paediatric surviving sepsis cannot suggest for or against the use of TPE in children with sepsis-associated TAMOF [58]. However, they suggest against using TPE in children in the absence of TAMOF.

Take-Home Messages

- Sickle cell patients can present with several life-threatening conditions that require intensive management. Despite their varied presentation, in most cases the single most lifesaving and morbidity-reducing intervention is to transfuse packed red blood cells in a timely manner. Patients with acute chest syndrome should be monitored for respiratory decline and treated with antibiotics and exchange transfusion if declining. Multi organ dysfunction syndrome (MODS) is a rapidly progressing disease, and prompt initiation of an exchange transfusion is critical.
- Patients with haemophilia can present with limb and life-threatening bleeding. It is important to treat with the appropriate factor product before initiating a full diagnostic workup.
- A child with thalassaemia is at increased risk for sepsis and needs supportive care and antibiotic coverage that takes into account that many of these children may not have a spleen.
- Catastrophic antiphospholipid syndrome is a potentially life-threatening condition associated with rapid onset of widespread thromboses and multi-organ failure. Triple therapy, with anticoagulation, steroids and plasma exchange or IVIG, is most successful at increasing survival.
- Critically ill children with immune thrombocytopenia (ITP) who present with moderate bleeding should be treated with a short course of corticosteroids, intravenous immunoglobulin (IVIG) or anti-D therapy for Rh(D)-positive children. In patients with ITP refractory to first-line treatments, a thrombopoietin receptor agonist (TPO-RA, either romiplostim or eltrombopag) should be used. Life-threatening bleeding should be managed with the concomitant administration of high-dose methylprednisone, IVIG and TPO-RA, as well as high-dose platelet transfusion doses to correct platelet counts as quickly as possible.
- Most patients with thrombotic thrombocytopenic purpura (TTP) will present with a triad of microangiopathic haemolytic anaemia, neurologic symptoms and thrombocytopenia. Autoantibodies against ADAMTS-13 will lead to ultra-large von Willebrand factor (UVWF) multimers that will trigger platelet adhesion to the

endothelium, leading to microthrombi and organ failure. Therapeutic plasma exchange has become a standard therapy for patients with TTP because it replaces ADAMTS-13 and removes both ULVWF and ADAMTS-13 inhibitors. Some experts will add steroids and will consider rituximab, an anti-CD20 monoclonal antibody, for refractory cases.

- Disseminated intravascular coagulation (DIC), a syndrome characterized by excessive activation of coagulation, resulting in both haemorrhage and thrombosis, can be triggered by a variety of clinical conditions, such as sepsis (the most frequent cause), trauma or malignancy. The International Society of Thrombosis and Haemostasis uses four tests to define DIC: platelet counts, elevated fibrin-related markers (such as d-dimers), prolonged prothrombin time and hypofibrinogenaemia. The only evidence-based treatment is heparin. In a subgroup of patients with DIC and thrombotic microangiopathy, known as thrombocytopenia-associated multiple organ failure (TAMOF), the use of TPE seems to be associated with improved outcomes although the current evidence is based on observational studies, not randomized trials.

? Questions

1. A 15-year-old male with sickle cell disease was admitted to the hospital for 3 days for an acute pain crisis. Despite management with IV opioids, he continues to report significantly worsening pain. Labs drawn today are significant for haemoglobin of 50 g/dL (baseline of 80 g/dL), platelet count of 40×10^9/L (baseline 190×10^9/L.), AST 345 U/L, ALT 235 U/L and creatinine 270 μmol/L, and his urine output has declined significantly. He is stable on room air but is complaining of significant chest pain and shortness of breath. What is the most important next step for this patient?
   A. Transfuse platelets
   B. Initiate dialysis
   C. Prepare for an exchange transfusion
   D. Increase his pain medication
   E. Obtain a CXR to evaluate chest pain

2. A 6-year-old male with haemophilia A presents to the emergency department after falling off the monkey bars at school and landing on his head. He had a brief loss of consciousness but is now awake and crying in pain. He has a factor at home, but it was not administered prior to arriving at the emergency department. What is the most important next step in the management of this patient?
   A. Order emergent head imaging to evaluate for a head bleed
   B. Check his factor VIII level
   C. Infuse factor VIII at 50 units/kg
   D. Provide analgesia for his head pain
   E. Observe for an hour and discharge home if his symptoms improve

3. A 12-year-old male with transfusion-dependent beta-thalassaemia presents with fever, headache, neck rigidity and altered mental status. His vitals on admission are significant for a temperature of 38.9 C, heart rate of 115 beats per minute and blood pressure of 70/30 mmHg. He is admitted to the PICU for management of meningitis and sepsis. Which one of these factors does not predispose this patient to sepsis?

A. History of transfusion dependence
B. A history of splenectomy
C. Non-compliance with prophylactic penicillin
D. History of iron overload with poor compliance with chelation therapy
E. Compliance with all childhood vaccines

4. A 4-year-old patient is admitted to the PICU for spontaneous subdural haemorrhage and severe thrombocytopenia (platelet count $4 \times 10^9/L$). A diagnosis of immune thrombocytopenia is suspected. Which of the following treatments should not be considered?
   A. Methylprednisone
   B. Intravenous immunoglobulin (IVIG)
   C. Rituximab
   D. Thrombopoietin receptor agonist (TPO-RA)
   E. Platelet transfusion

5. A 6-year-old patient is admitted to the PICU with altered mental status, anaemia (Hb 67 g/L) with schistocytes on the smear and thrombocytopenia (platelet count $27 \times 10^9/L$). Which of the following is the most appropriate first treatment?
   A. Platelet transfusion
   B. Therapeutic plasma exchange once ADAMTS-13 levels have been shown to be <10%
   C. Rituximab
   D. Intravenous immunoglobulin (IVIG)
   E. Emergent therapeutic plasma exchange

6. A 12-year-old patient is admitted to the PICU with septic shock, intubated and ventilated on an adrenalin perfusion. The nurse is concerned for significant oozing around the central line, bloody streaks in the endotracheal tube as well as the inability to draw blood because it clots immediately. Which of the following treatments is indicated?
   A. Thrombomodulin
   B. Activated protein C
   C. Recombinant tissue factor pathway inhibitor
   D. Heparin
   E. Therapeutic plasma exchange (TPE)

Answers

1. C. This patient is presenting with signs of multi-organ failure. While managing his organ failure with supportive care such as dialysis and optimizing pain management are important, the most important life-saving intervention is the prompt initiation of an exchange transfusion to decrease the amount of Hb S.
2. C. For potential life-threatening bleeding in a patient with haemophilia, treatment should be initiated first before any other intervention takes place. Delaying factor infusion to obtain imaging or check factor levels could potentially be deadly to this patient. Because of his underlying bleeding disorder and the possibility of a life-threatening bleed, observation only would likely increase the risk for significant morbidity and mortality.

3. E. Patients with thalassaemia are at an increased risk of sepsis due to chronic transfusion therapy, a history of splenectomy and a history of iron overload. Additionally, non-compliance with penicillin also increases the risk of infection with bacterial organisms. Receiving childhood vaccines is one way to prevent developing life-threatening sepsis.
4. C: In a patient with ITP, life-threatening bleeding should be managed with the concomitant administration of high-dose methylprednisone, IVIG and TPO-RA, as well as high-dose platelet transfusion doses to correct platelet counts as quickly as possible. Rituximab is considered for patients with refractory thrombotic thrombocytopenic purpura (TTP).
5. E: Therapeutic plasma exchange (TTP) has become a standard therapy for patients with TTP because it replaces ADAMTS-13 and removes both ULVWF and ADAMTS-13 inhibitors. TTP should be started as soon as the diagnosis of TTP is even suspected to avoid worsening cerebral dysfunction.
6. D: In patients with disseminated intravascular coagulation (DIC), which is characterized by excessive activation of coagulation, resulting in both haemorrhage and thrombosis, the only evidence-based treatment is heparin infusion. There is no benefit from thrombomodulin, activated protein C or recombinant tissue factor pathway inhibitor. Therapeutic plasma exchange (TPE) might be beneficial in patients with thrombocytopenia-associated multiple organ failure (TAMOF), a subset of DIC defined by thrombocytopenia, microangiopathic haemolysis, haemodynamic failure and ischaemic organ failure. However, since this patient did not have documented thrombocytopenia and microangiopathic haemolysis, TPE would not be the first-line treatment.

References

1. Sundd P, Gladwin MT, Novelli EM. Pathophysiology of sickle cell disease. Annu Rev Pathol. 2019;14:263–92.
2. White JG. Ultrastructural features of erythrocyte and hemoglobin sickling. Arch Intern Med. 1974;133(4):545–62.
3. Hassell KL, Eckman JR, Lane PA. Acute multiorgan failure syndrome: a potentially catastrophic complication of severe sickle cell pain episodes. Am J Med. 1994;96(2):155–62.
4. Hiran S. Multiorgan dysfunction syndrome in sickle cell disease. J Assoc Physicians India. 2005;53:19–22.
5. Desai PC, Ataga KI. The acute chest syndrome of sickle cell disease. Expert Opin Pharmacother. 2013;14(8):991–9.
6. Jain S, Bakshi N, Krishnamurti L. Acute chest syndrome in children with sickle cell disease. Pediatr Allergy Immunol Pulmonol. 2017;30(4):191–201.
7. Castro O, Brambilla DJ, Thorington B, Reindorf CA, Scott RB, Gillette P, et al. The acute chest syndrome in sickle cell disease: incidence and risk factors. The cooperative study of sickle cell disease. Blood. 1994;84(2):643–9.
8. Dean D, Neumayr L, Kelly DM, Ballas SK, Kleman K, Robertson S, et al. Chlamydia pneumoniae and acute chest syndrome in patients with sickle cell disease. J Pediatr Hematol Oncol. 2003;25(1):46–55.
9. Neumayr L, Lennette E, Kelly D, Earles A, Embury S, Groncy P, et al. Mycoplasma disease and acute chest syndrome in sickle cell disease. Pediatrics. 2003;112(1 Pt 1):87–95.
10. Melton CW, Haynes J. Sickle acute lung injury: role of prevention and early aggressive intervention strategies on outcome. Clin Chest Med. 2006;27(3):487–502. vii
11. Kassim AA, Galadanci NA, Pruthi S, DeBaun MR. How I treat and manage strokes in sickle cell disease. Blood. 2015;125(22):3401–10.

12. DeBaun MR, Jordan LC, King AA, Schatz J, Vichinsky E, Fox CK, et al. American Society of Hematology 2020 guidelines for sickle cell disease: prevention, diagnosis, and treatment of cerebrovascular disease in children and adults. Blood Adv. 2020;4(8):1554–88.
13. Steiner ME, Zantek ND, Stanworth SJ, Parker RI, Valentine SL, Lehmann LE, et al. Recommendations on RBC transfusion support in children with hematologic and oncologic diagnoses from the pediatric critical care transfusion and anemia expertise initiative. Pediatr Crit Care Med. 2018;19:S149–56.
14. Kuo KHM, Ward R, Kaya B, Howard J, Telfer P. A comparison of chronic manual and automated red blood cell exchange transfusion in sickle cell disease patients. Br J Haematol. 2015;170(3):425–8.
15. Rees DC, Robinson S, Howard J. How I manage red cell transfusions in patients with sickle cell disease. Br J Haematol. 2018;180(4):607–17.
16. Oldenburg J, Ananyeva NM, Saenko EL. Molecular basis of haemophilia A. Haemophilia. 2004;10(Suppl 4):133–9.
17. Goodeve AC. Hemophilia B: molecular pathogenesis and mutation analysis. J Thromb Haemost. 2015;13(7):1184–95.
18. Srivastava A, Brewer AK, Mauser-Bunschoten EP, Key NS, Kitchen S, Llinas A, et al. Guidelines for the management of hemophilia. Haemophilia. 2013;19(1):e1–47.
19. National Hemophilia Foundation Medical and Scientific Advisory Council. Guidelines for emergency department management of individuals with hemophilia and other bleeding disorders [Internet]. https://static1.squarespace.com/static/566b210340667a1cc1623840/t/5dcf0c338636542f1c352dbe/1573850163994/252+ER+Management.pdf
20. Holme PA, Tjønnfjord GE, Batorova A. Continuous infusion of coagulation factor concentrates during intensive treatment. Haemophilia. 2018;24(1):24–32.
21. Tebo C, Gibson C, Mazer-Amirshahi M. Hemophilia and von Willebrand disease: a review of emergency department management. J Emerg Med. 2020;58(5):756–66.
22. Marengo-Rowe AJ. The thalassemias and related disorders. Proc (Bayl Univ Med Cent). 2007;20(1):27–31.
23. Saliba AN, Atoui A, Labban M, Hamade H, Bou-Fakhredin R, Mufarrij A, et al. Thalassemia in the emergency department: special considerations for a rare disease. Ann Hematol. 2020;99(9):1967–77.
24. Borgna-Pignatti C, Rugolotto S, De Stefano P, Piga A, Di Gregorio F, Gamberini MR, et al. Survival and disease complications in thalassemia major. Ann N Y Acad Sci. 1998;850:227–31.
25. Rahav G, Volach V, Shapiro M, Rund D, Rachmilewitz EA, Goldfarb A. Severe infections in thalassaemic patients: prevalence and predisposing factors. Br J Haematol. 2006;133(6):667–74.
26. Wanachiwanawin W. Infections in E-beta thalassemia. J Pediatr Hematol Oncol. 2000;22(6):581–7.
27. Cervera R, Rodríguez-Pintó I, Espinosa G. The diagnosis and clinical management of the catastrophic antiphospholipid syndrome: a comprehensive review. J Autoimmun. 2018;92:1–11.
28. Cervera R, Piette JC, Font J, Khamashta MA, Shoenfeld Y, Camps MT, et al. Antiphospholipid syndrome: clinical and immunologic manifestations and patterns of disease expression in a cohort of 1,000 patients. Arthritis Rheum. 2002;46(4):1019–27.
29. Asherson RA, Cervera R, de Groot PG, Erkan D, Boffa MC, Piette JC, et al. Catastrophic antiphospholipid syndrome: international consensus statement on classification criteria and treatment guidelines. Lupus. 2003;12(7):530–4.
30. Erkan D, Espinosa G, Cervera R. Catastrophic antiphospholipid syndrome: updated diagnostic algorithms. Autoimmun Rev. 2010;10(2):74–9.
31. Rodríguez-Pintó I, Espinosa G, Erkan D, Shoenfeld Y, Cervera R, CAPS Registry Project Group. The effect of triple therapy on the mortality of catastrophic anti-phospholipid syndrome patients. Rheumatology (Oxford). 2018;57(7):1264–70.
32. Berman H, Rodríguez-Pintó I, Cervera R, Morel N, Costedoat-Chalumeau N, Erkan D, et al. Rituximab use in the catastrophic antiphospholipid syndrome: descriptive analysis of the CAPS registry patients receiving rituximab. Autoimmun Rev. 2013;12(11):1085–90.
33. Quintana-López G, Rodríguez-Pintó I, Maldonado-Cañón K, Espinosa G, Diaz-Rojas J, Cervera R. Cost-effectiveness analysis of treatments for the first episode of catastrophic antiphospholipid syndrome: a study based on the catastrophic antiphospholipid syndrome registry. Lupus. 2022;31(2):194–201.

34. Zufferey A, Kapur R, Semple J. Pathogenesis and therapeutic mechanisms in immune thrombocytopenia (ITP). JCM. 2017;6(2):16.
35. D'Orazio JA, Neely J, Farhoudi N. ITP in children: pathophysiology and current treatment approaches. J Pediatr Hematol Oncol. 2013;35(1):1–13.
36. Neunert C, Terrell DR, Arnold DM, Buchanan G, Cines DB, Cooper N, et al. American Society of Hematology 2019 guidelines for immune thrombocytopenia. Blood Adv. 2019;3(23):3829–66.
37. Provan D, Stasi R, Newland AC, Blanchette VS, Bolton-Maggs P, Bussel JB, et al. International consensus report on the investigation and management of primary immune thrombocytopenia. Blood. 2010,115(2):168–86.
38. Lowe EJ, Werner EJ. Thrombotic thrombocytopenic purpura and hemolytic uremic syndrome in children and adolescents. Semin Thromb Hemost. 2005;31(6):717–30.
39. Manea M, Karpman D. Molecular basis of ADAMTS13 dysfunction in thrombotic thrombocytopenic purpura. Pediatr Nephrol. 2009;24(3):447–58.
40. Rubinstein MA, Kagan BM, Macgillviray MH, Merliss R, Sacks H. Unusual remission in a case of thrombotic thrombocytopenic purpura syndrome following fresh blood exchange transfusions. Ann Intern Med. 1959;51:1409–19.
41. Levy GG, Nichols WC, Lian EC, Foroud T, McClintick JN, McGee BM, et al. Mutations in a member of the ADAMTS gene family cause thrombotic thrombocytopenic purpura. Nature. 2001;413(6855):488–94.
42. Rock GA, Shumak KH, Buskard NA, Blanchette VS, Kelton JG, Nair RC, et al. Comparison of plasma exchange with plasma infusion in the treatment of thrombotic thrombocytopenic purpura. N Engl J Med. 1991;325(6):393–7.
43. Bell WR, Braine HG, Ness PM, Kickler TS. Improved survival in thrombotic thrombocytopenic purpura–hemolytic uremic syndrome: clinical experience in 108 patients. N Engl J Med. 1991;325(6):398–403.
44. Joly BS, Coppo P, Veyradier A. Thrombotic thrombocytopenic purpura. Blood. 2017;129(21):2836–46.
45. Zwicker JI, Muia J, Dolatshahi L, Westfield LA, Nieters P, Rodrigues A, et al. Adjuvant low-dose rituximab and plasma exchange for acquired TTP. Blood. 2019;134(13):1106–9.
46. Swisher KK, Terrell DR, Vesely SK, Kremer Hovinga JA, Lämmle B, George JN. Clinical outcomes after platelet transfusions in patients with thrombotic thrombocytopenic purpura. Transfusion. 2009;49(5):873–87.
47. Levi M, ten Cate H. Disseminated intravascular coagulation. N Engl J Med. 1999;341(8):586–92.
48. Bakhtiari K, Meijers JCM, de Jonge E, Levi M. Prospective validation of the International Society of Thrombosis and Haemostasis scoring system for disseminated intravascular coagulation*. Crit Care Med. 2004;32(12):2416–21.
49. Gando S, Iba T, Eguchi Y, Ohtomo Y, Okamoto K, Koseki K, et al. A multicenter, prospective validation of disseminated intravascular coagulation diagnostic criteria for critically ill patients: comparing current criteria*. Crit Care Med. 2006;34(3):625–31.
50. Iba T, Di Nisio M, Thachil J, Wada H, Asakura H, Sato K, et al. Revision of the Japanese Association for Acute Medicine (JAAM) disseminated intravascular coagulation (DIC) diagnostic criteria using antithrombin activity. Crit Care. 2016;20(1):287.
51. Wang C, Chi C, Guo L, Wang X, Guo L, Sun J, et al. Heparin therapy reduces 28-day mortality in adult severe sepsis patients: a systematic review and meta-analysis. Crit Care. 2014;18(5):563.
52. Warren BL, Eid A, Singer P, Pillay SS, Carl P, Novak I, et al. High-dose antithrombin III in severe sepsis: a randomized controlled trial. JAMA. 2001;286(15):1869.
53. Bernard GR, Vincent JL, Laterre PF, LaRosa SP, Dhainaut JF, Lopez-Rodriguez A, et al. Efficacy and safety of recombinant human activated protein C for severe sepsis. N Engl J Med. 2001;344(10):699–709.
54. Dhainaut JF, Antonelli M, Wright P, Desachy A, Reignier J, Lavoue S, et al. Extended drotrecogin alfa (activated) treatment in patients with prolonged septic shock. Intensive Care Med. 2009;35(7):1187–95.
55. Abraham E, Reinhart K, Opal S, Demeyer I, Doig C, Rodriguez AL, et al. Efficacy and safety of tifacogin (recombinant tissue factor pathway inhibitor) in severe sepsis: a randomized controlled trial. JAMA. 2003;290(2):238.

56. Vincent JL, Francois B, Zabolotskikh I, Daga MK, Lascarrou JB, Kirov MY, et al. Effect of a recombinant human soluble thrombomodulin on mortality in patients with sepsis-associated coagulopathy: the SCARLET randomized clinical trial. JAMA. 2019;321(20):1993.
57. Fortenberry JD, Nguyen T, Grunwell JR, Aneja RK, Wheeler D, Hall M, et al. Therapeutic plasma exchange in children with thrombocytopenia-associated multiple organ failure: the thrombocytopenia-associated multiple organ failure network prospective experience. Crit Care Med. 2019;47(3):e173–81.
58. Weiss SL, Chair CV, Peters MJ, Chair CV, Alhazzani W, Flori HR, et al. Surviving sepsis campaign international guidelines for the management of septic shock and sepsis-associated organ dysfunction in children. Pediatr Crit Care Med. 2020;21(2):55.

Transfusion Medicine in the Pediatric Intensive Care Unit

Sonia Labarinas and Oliver Karam

Contents

J. Brierley et al. (eds.), *ESPNIC Children's Intensive Care Textbook*,
https://doi.org/10.1007/978-3-031-64762-8_40

Learning Objectives

- Recognize the current indications for different blood product transfusions and understand which are evidence-based and which are not
- Identify the different types of transfusion reactions or complications and describe their management

40.1 Introduction

Critically ill children are at high risk of receiving blood products during their stay in the pediatric intensive care unit (PICU). These transfusions are frequently beneficial but can be associated with notable risks. Therefore, it is of major importance to make the decision to transfuse based on the patient's individual characteristics, using the latest evidence, always accounting for the possible side effects as well as costs.

In this chapter, we will review the rationale for red blood cell (RBC), plasma, and platelet transfusions in the PICU.

40.2 Red Blood Cells

40.2.1 Anemia and O_2 Delivery

Critically ill children are at high risk of developing anemia [1]. As oxygen delivery (DO_2), the process of delivering O_2 to the cells, depends on cardiac output and arterial concentration of O_2 (CaO_2), anemia decreases O_2 delivery because of lower hemoglobin (Hb) content.

$$DO_2 = \text{cardiac output}\left(\text{stroke volume} \times \text{heart rate}\right) \times CaO_2$$

CaO_2 is defined by the formula:

$$CaO_2\left(\text{mL}\,O_2/100\,\text{mL}\right) = \left(\text{Hb} \times SaO_2 \times 1.34\right) + \left(0.003 \times PaO_2\right)$$

Systemic DO_2 is directly proportional to Hb concentration; therefore, the more effective way of increasing DO_2 in anemic patients is assumed to be transfusing red blood cells (RBC). The transfusion goal is ultimately to improve cellular energy production (adenosine triphosphate (ATP) production), which will translate into O_2 consumption (VO_2).

In normal physiologic conditions, DO_2 is 3–5 times greater than VO_2, allowing VO_2 to remain stable even if DO_2 decreases somewhat. However, if DO_2 drops below a "critical threshold," compensatory mechanisms will be overwhelmed, VO_2 will decrease proportionally, and tissue hypoxemia will occur.

It seems intuitive to think that RBC transfusion will increase DO_2 and VO_2 [2–4]. Nevertheless, host characteristics that may impair those mechanisms, like sepsis leading to mitochondrial dysfunction [5], have to be considered. Therefore, in those situations, the benefit of increasing tissue DO_2 will not be achieved and could even be detrimental [6]. A systematic review showed that, although RBC transfusion increases

Hb levels in all observational studies and DO_2 levels in most, it failed to increase VO_2 and improve lactate levels in most [7].

The blood products themselves, which are stored in blood banks, are not similar to the patient's own blood and might not be able to circulate as well and might induce an immune response [8].

There are also compensatory mechanisms to mitigate the effects of anemia. For example, a decrease in RBC causes a decrease in blood viscosity, which in turn decreases cardiac afterload, therefore increasing cardiac output and finally DO_2 [9].

Although multiple observational studies suggested that RBCs are stored for more than 14 days [8, 10], these findings were not confirmed in a recent randomized controlled trial [2].

40.2.2 When Should We Transfuse?

In 2018, a panel of 42 international experts, the Pediatric Critical Care Transfusion and Anemia Expertise Initiative (TAXI), published evidence-based and expert consensus-based recommendations on RBC transfusion in critically ill children [11].

Their recommendations for RBC transfusions are:

1. **Hemorrhagic Shock and Severe Bleeding**

   In a scenario of massive bleeding, RBC transfusion is indicated to improve DO_2 and maintain intra-vascular volume, with concomitant administration of plasma and platelets (ratio: 1/1/1 or 2/1/1) [7, 12]. The amount of transfusions should be based on blood loss estimation as well as hemodynamic status.
2. **Critically Ill Children Without Severe Bleeding**

   Many studies have evaluated the optimal Hb transfusion threshold in critically ill adults (TRICC trial) [13] and children [14]. The latter study, named TRIPICU, aimed to compare a restrictive transfusion strategy (transfusion if Hb < 7 g/dL) with a liberal strategy (transfusion if Hb < 9.5 g/dL) in stable or stabilized critically ill children (not hypotensive and no changes in hemodynamic support in the last 2 h). In this study, the authors showed that the outcomes (mortality and multiorgan dysfunction) were not significantly worse in the restrictive group and recommended not to administer RBC transfusion if stable hemodynamics and Hb > 7 g/dL.
3. **Cardiac Patients**

   In children with biventricular physiology and no remaining cyanotic heart defect as well as adequate postoperative hemodynamics, Cholette et al. support a restrictive transfusion therapy of Hb 7 g/dL [15]. In patients with persisting cyanotic heart disease, the current evidence suggests a postoperative level of 9 g/dL is sufficient [15].

40.3 Plasma

Plasma is a biological product that contains the noncellular portion of blood obtained from whole blood after centrifugation or plasmapheresis. Because of the ability of the coagulation proteins, especially factors V and VIII, plasma has to be stored at or below −18 °C. Plasma frozen within 8 h of collection is called fresh frozen plasma (FFP).

As plasma contains cytokines and various other bioactive substances, in addition to coagulation factors, it has been presumed that plasma transfusions could induce transfusion-associated immunomodulation (TRIM), which has been described in all blood product transfusions. Observational studies have shown that plasma transfusions were associated with worse clinical outcomes in critically ill children [16, 17] and adults [18, 19].

40.3.1 When Should We Transfuse?

As plasma contains coagulation factors, its most frequent indication is to correct abnormal coagulation tests. For the pediatric patient, the usual dose of FFP is 10–15 mL/kg.

1. **Massive Transfusions**

   Patients with massive bleeding suffer from dilutional coagulopathy and also from coagulation factor consumption. Those can be corrected with plasma administration, the current recommendations being a 1:1:1 strategy [7, 12].

2. **Non-massive Bleeding**

   Experts consensus guidelines advise transfusions in non-massively bleeding patients only if the international normalized ratio (INR) or the activated partial thromboplastin time (aPTT) is more than 1.5× normal. Nevertheless, the effect of FFP seems to be minimal when INR is <2.5 or aPTT <60 [20]. Therefore, it seems reasonable to use those higher thresholds in *non-massively bleeding* patients.

3. **Disseminated Intravascular Coagulation (DIC) in Conjunction with Active Bleeding**

   Similarly to patients with non-massive bleeding, there is no evidence that plasma transfusion should be given for an INR <2.5 or an aPTT <60 to patients with DIC and non-life-threatening bleeding.

4. **Non-bleeding Patients**

   Plasma should *not* be used as volume replacement, because there is no benefit over other colloids (purified albumin) or crystalloids [21] although there is growing animal evidence that plasma transfusions can improve the glycocalyx in various critical scenarios [22, 23].

   Plasma should *not* be used either to correct abnormal INR or aPTT in non-bleeding patients who have no planned surgery or invasive procedures because there is no correlation between coagulation tests and the risk of bleeding [24].

5. **Single Clotting Factor Deficiencies**

   Plasma should only be transfused if a specific concentration is not available.

6. **Reversal of Warfarin Effect**

   Warfarin causes a functional deficit of factors II, VII, IX, and X, as well as proteins C and S. Plasma should be administered if there is evidence of severe bleeding and if prothrombin complex (which contains concentrated factors I, VII, IX, and X) is unavailable.

7. **Hereditary Angioedema (Quincke Edema)**
   The purpose of treatment of acute episodes is to halt the progression of the edema as soon as possible. The standard and most efficient treatment should be C1 inhibitor concentrate. Plasma transfusions could be used instead if this treatment is not available.

40.4 Platelets

Thrombocytopenia affects up to a quarter of critically ill children during their ICU stay [25]. There are various causes of thrombocytopenia in the ICU, among which the main etiologies remain sepsis, DIC, thrombocytopenia-associated multiorgan failure, hemolytic uremic syndrome, drug-induced (heparin), massive transfusion, and hemolytic uremic syndrome.

In critically ill children, each mL/kg is independently associated with a 1% increase in mortality [26]. Even in children on ECMO, where the risk of bleeding is up to 70%, platelet transfusions are independently associated with an increased risk of bleeding the following day [27]. The only platelet transfusion randomized controlled trial published so far showed that, in preterm infants, a liberal platelet transfusion strategy (transfusing for a platelet count of 50×10^9 cells/L) causes an increased risk of bleeding and death, when compared to a restrictive platelet transfusion strategy (transfusing for a platelet count of 25×10^9 cells/L) [28].

40.4.1 When Should We Transfuse?

Although thrombocytopenia is associated with increased mortality in critically ill children as well as a longer PICU length of stay [25], so are platelet transfusions [26]. Therefore, the balance between benefits and harm must be carefully evaluated. For children, the platelet dose is usually 5–10 mL/kg [26].

General indications for platelet transfusions:

- In the absence of high-quality evidence, platelet transfusion should be considered in situations of actively bleeding patients and a platelet count $<50 \times 10^9$/L.
- There is a lack of evidence to support a defined platelet level for prophylactic platelet transfusion in critically ill children. However, as most evidence comes from oncology patients, the American Society of Clinical Oncology Clinical Practice Guidelines have recently published guidelines, recommending a prophylactic platelet transfusion of 10×10^9/L in most oncology situations [29].
- In non-bleeding patients with severe thrombocytopenia, most clinicians will transfuse platelets prior to surgical intervention (typically, if $<100 \times 10^9$/L) or lumbar puncture or insertion of central lines (typically, if $<50 \times 10^9$/L). However, there is little evidence to support these thresholds.
- Excessive bleeding while undergoing cardiopulmonary bypass or extracorporeal membrane oxygenation (ECMO). Children on ECMO are usually maintained with a platelet count greater than 80×10^9/L despite a lack of association between platelet count and bleeding on ECMO [26].

40.4.2 When Should We Not Transfuse?

- Children with idiopathic thrombocytopenic purpura (ITP) should not be transfused with platelets unless life-threatening hemorrhage.
- Similarly, children with thrombotic thrombocytopenic purpura (TTP) should not receive platelet transfusions as this may cause worsening thrombosis.
- Heparin-induced thrombocytopenia is also a contraindication to platelet transfusion if the patient is not bleeding significantly.

40.5 Blood Product Modifications

40.5.1 Leukoreduction

Leukoreduction consists of filtering red blood cell components shortly after their collection, allowing to removal of donor leukocytes prior to transfusion. Current filters have a pore size of 4 μm, which allows platelet and deformable RBC passage but holds leukocytes. Thanks to that process, red blood components contain $<1.0 \times 10^6$ leukocytes/unit [30]. Other benefits of this technique are the restriction of blood-borne infection transmission (such as Epstein-Barr virus, cytomegalovirus, and human T-cell lymphocytic virus), as these are intracellular pathogens, filtering pro-inflammatory mediators, and decreasing HLA antibody production [31]. One of the disadvantages of leukoreduction is the inadvertent removal of RBC (up to 10%). As of today, approximately 80% of all RBC transfused are leukoreduced, as this has been the standard in most European countries and Canada for many years.

40.5.2 Irradiated Blood Products

T-cell lymphocytes are present in blood products and tend to proliferate in the host after transfusion. This can lead to transfusion-associated graft-versus-host disease. 25–50 Gy of radiation applied to cellular blood components will prevent donor T lymphocytes from replicating. Plasma does not require irradiation as it does not contain significant white blood cells.

One of the disadvantages of irradiation is a shortened RBC half-life and increased potassium release, which decreases the storage duration from 42 days to less than 28 days. For this reason, irradiation is usually performed right before blood transfusion. The British Committee for Standards in Haematology blood transfusion task force published guidelines for the use of irradiated blood components in 2011 [32]. They recommend irradiation for: (1) all severe T-lymphocyte immunodeficiency syndromes; (2) all patients after autologous or allogeneic stem cell transplantation from the time of conditioning therapy until a patient is receiving graft-versus-host disease prophylaxis or if on any immunosuppressant therapy; (3) allogeneic blood transfused to stem cell donors should also be irradiated up to 7 days prior to harvesting all donations from first or second-degree relatives, even when immunocompetent patient; (4) all patients with Hodgkin lymphoma at any stage; (5) patients with aplastic anemia receiving immunosuppressant therapy; (6) all red cells for intrauterine transfusion; (7) red cells for neonatal exchange if prior intrauterine treatment; (8) for all other neonatal cases, if irradiation does not delay transfusion; (9) irradiation is not necessary for children with HIV; and (10) irradiation is also unnecessary for children undergoing cardiac surgery.

At some institutions, patients receiving solid organ transplants also receive irradiated blood products.

40.5.3 Pathogen Reduction

1. **Solvent/Detergent-Treated Plasma (SDP)**

   SDP is a pooled plasma product collected from more than 1000 donors. After routine donors screen for nonenveloped viruses (pre-donation), the pooled plasma product is filtered first time to remove cells and cell fragments and therefore intracellular pathogens. The product is then treated with tri-N-butyl-phosphate for pathogen and white blood cell inactivation. A second filtration removes bacteria and parasites. This plasma product is then packed and frozen. Compared with regular plasma, SDP is practically cell-free and contains significantly lower residual platelet concentrations and negligible amounts of microparticles due to its manufacturing and filtering process. There are no large multicentric and randomized trials comparing the efficacy or safety of regular plasma vs SDP products. However, observational studies have shown that SDP is independently associated with a lower risk of mortality in critically ill children [33].
2. **Amotosalen**

   Another technology involved amotosalen (INTERCEPT™ Blood System, Cerus Corp, Concord, CA), a molecule that irreversibly blocks the replication of DNA and RNA, preventing the proliferation of susceptible pathogens. Once inside a pathogen, amotosalen inserts itself in between the nucleic acid base pairs, and, upon illumination with ultraviolet light, forms an interstrand crosslink, which binds the DNA or RNA together and prevents replication. The reaction requires ultraviolet light and will not continue in its absence, making the product safe.

Treating plasma and platelets with amotosalen reduces the risk of transfusion-transmitted infections for patients, eliminates cytomegalovirus (CMV) from the products, and eliminates the need for irradiation to prevent transfusion-associated graft-vs-host disease.

40.6 Transfusion Reactions and Complications

Transfusions of blood products may cause different types of reactions which may be immediate (during or within 6 h of the transfusion) or delayed (days, weeks, or months later).

40.6.1 Early-Onset Reactions

1. **Transfusion-Related Acute Lung Injury (TRALI)**
   Acute onset of respiratory failure is associated with hypoxemia and bilateral infiltrates on X-ray with the absence of left atrial hypertension. Treatment is primarily supportive with adequate oxygenation and ventilation, sometimes requiring noninvasive or invasive mechanical ventilation and discontinuing blood product transfusion. Some authors even proposed to associate this definition with any ALI/ARDS recognized within 72 h of the transfusion [34].
2. **Transfusion-Associated Circulatory Overload (TACO)**
   Blood transfusions can lead to circulatory overload, by shifting the Frank-Starling curve to the right. Four of the five following criteria need to be observed within 6 h of transfusion, according to the British Haemovigilance Scheme (Serious Hazards of Transfusion (SHOT)) and the International Society of Blood Transfusion (ISBT) [35]: (1) acute respiratory distress, (2) tachycardia, (3) increased blood pressure, (4) acute or evolving pulmonary edema, and (5) documentation of positive fluid balance.
   The incidence of TACO is not well-known in children. Some authors have described an incidence change between 1.5% and 76% depending on the criteria used which suggests that different diagnostic criteria should be used [36].
3. **Hemolytic Reactions**
   They are caused by lysis of RBCs due to immunological incompatibility between donor and recipient blood. ABO mismatch is the most frequent and most severe of the blood group incompatibilities. In most instances, the cause is mistransfusion, when a patient received an RBC unit that was prepared for another patient. This is believed to be the most severe reaction, which results in hemolysis and death (in up to 10% of the cases).
4. **Febrile Non-hemolytic Reactions**
   These reactions are defined as an increase in the temperature of at least 1 °C during a transfusion in the absence of another cause. Other symptoms could present as chills, dyspnea, nausea, and vomiting. These reactions are cytokine-mediated and are usually prevented with leuko-reduction blood products. These reactions can often be successfully treated with antipyretics and antihistamines.
5. **Allergic/Anaphylactic Reactions**
   Most anaphylactic reactions are thought to be secondary to contact between donor allergens and recipient antibodies (IgE) inducing a type I hypersensitivity reaction. In a retrospective study conducted from 2002 to 2018, Yanagisawa et al. described an incidence of 3.6% (2742 children) of allergic/anaphylactic reactions [37]. Clinically, the reaction is similar to anaphylaxis from other causes and may present as urticaria solely due to digestive disorders, respiratory distress, and severe shock. When such a reaction is suspected, transfusion should be stopped, and supportive treatment must be adapted to the clinical presentation.
   In critically ill children, acute transfusion reactions may be underestimated as these symptoms could be attributed to the patient's underlying disease process.

40.6.2 Delayed Transfusion Reactions

1. **Transfusion Associated Graft-Versus-Host Disease (TA-GVHD)**
   TA-GVHD is a rare and fatal complication of blood transfusion where donor lymphocytes produce an immune-mediated destructive response against the recipient's tissues. Symptoms may include a constellation of fever, rash, gastrointestinal symptoms, liver failure, and pancytopenia. All of those may lead to hemorrhage and severe infections. Patients with immune deficiencies as well as premature babies are believed to be at higher risk for this complication. In 2015, Kopolovic et al. conducted a systematic review where they found not all patients with TA-GVHD had an underlying immunodeficiency or other known risk factors. Their findings are supported by the notion that TA-GVHD is principally attributable to viable donor lymphocytes present in the transfused component [38]. The best-proven intervention so far for TA-GVHD prevention is irradiation of blood products as well as leukoreduction for patients with impaired immunity [39]. Unfortunately, there is no effective treatment except for supportive care.
2. **Hemolytic Delayed Reactions**
   This complication is frequent among patients requiring chronic transfusions, such as sickle cell disease patients. It is probably resulting from the high incidence of alloimmunization in this population group. The culprit antibodies may not have been detected by cross-match or may have appeared after the transfusion. Prevention results in using best-matched RBCs, especially in the setting of chronic transfusions. Immunotherapy should also be considered in some instances [40].
3. **Post-transfusion Purpura (PTP)**
   PTP is an acute episode of severe thrombocytopenia occurring approximately 1 week after transfusion. It is believed to be associated with alloimmunization by platelet-specific antigens. This thrombocytopenia is refractory to platelet transfusion. Treatment includes steroids, plasmapheresis, and immunoglobulins. Prevention is also thought to be achieved thanks to leukoreduction and, when appropriate, irradiation [39].

40.6.3 Infectious Risks

The safety of blood products has improved over time thanks to notable improvements in donor screening and testing [41]. Blood is tested at least for the following infectious agents: hepatitis A, B, and C, human immunodeficiency virus (HIV), human T-cell lymphotropic virus (HTLV), West Nile virus (seasonal), and syphilis. ◘ Table 40.1 shows the incidences for HIV and hepatitis B and C, for various blood products.

Cytomegalovirus (CMV), EBV, and HTLV are transmitted by leukocytes, hence related to cellular blood product transfusions. Immunocompromised patients are highly susceptible to those related infections, which are a significant cause of mortality after stem cell transplantation. The transfusion of CMV-negative blood products is achieved by transfusing blood products from CMV-negative patients or the filtration of cellular blood products with third-generation leuko-reduction filters [42]. The transmission of EBV and HTLV has also decreased thanks to leukoreduction.

Table 40.1 Incidence of infectious disease transfusions risks based on Heiden et al. [44] and on Stramer [45]

	RBC	Plasma	SDP
HIV 1 + 2	1: 2.1 million	1: 10 million	No reported cases
Hepatitis C	1: 1.9 million	1: 50 million	No reported cases
Hepatitis B	1: 200,000–500,000	1: 1–2 million	No reported cases

RBC red blood cells, *HIV* human immunodeficiency virus, *SDP* solvent detergent treated plasma

Bacterial contamination is more frequent with platelets (1:1000–1:3000) than with RBC units (1:500000) or plasma because they are stored at room temperature for up to 5–7 days, which increases the risk of bacterial growth, even if they are inspected for bacterial contamination before being released [43]. The most common microorganisms identified are Gram-negative bacteria such as *Klebsiella pneumoniae*, *Serratia marcescens*, and *Pseudomonas species* and Gram-positive such as *Staphylococcus aureus*, *Staphylococcus epidermidis*, and *Bacillus cereus*. Those can be transmitted by an infection from the donor in the process of blood collection or during handling. When bacterial transmission is suspected, transfusion has to be stopped and broad-spectrum antibiotics started. In addition, the rest of the unit should be sent to the blood bank, for additional analyses.

Take-Home Messages

- Blood product transfusions can be a life-saving treatment and are frequently used in critically ill children. Years of experience and research have helped improve safety and establish evidence-based recommendations for their administration as severe complications are not uncommon after their use.
- As with any given treatment, the decision to transfuse RBC, plasma, and platelets should be based on the individual patient's characteristics and only administered if the benefits outweigh the potential risks. Further knowledge will lead to better transfusion strategies in critically ill children.

Questions

1. A 3-year-old patient is treated for *Streptococcus pneumoniae* sepsis in the PICU, on epinephrine and norepinephrine that you are still titrating up. His blood pressure is 70/30, heart rate is 170 beats per minute, and saturation is 98%. His labs show: white blood cell count of 4000×10^6 cells/L, hemoglobin of 6 g/dL, platelets of 100×10^9 cells/L, and lactate of 5 mmol/L. Which of the following interventions is the most appropriate?
   A. Order RBC to transfuse the patient
   B. Order platelets to transfuse the patient
   C. Administer 20 mL/kg bolus of normosaline to improve hemodynamics
   D. Order plasma to improve hemodynamics
   E. Increase pressors

2. A 2-year-old patient diagnosed in utero with hypoplastic left heart syndrome underwent a Norwood procedure shortly after birth. He finally was able to be discharged home but came back 2 weeks after for fever, rhinorrhea, cough, and upper respiratory distress. His physical exam shows mild retractions and nasal flaring. His saturation is 60% on room air, heart rate is 150 beats per minute, and blood pressure is 75/40 mmHg. His capillary refill is delayed to 4 s. His lab results show hemoglobin of 8.5 g/dL, platelets of 200 × 10^9cells/L, white blood cell count of 17,000 × 10^6 cells/L, and lactate of 0.8 mmol/L. What is the best next intervention for this patient?
   A. Immediately intubate the patient, give a fluid bolus, and order RBC
   B. Give a bolus of 20 mL/kg of normal saline (NaCl 0.9%)
   C. Consider antibiotics and order RBC
   D. Start noninvasive positive pressure ventilation and give a bolus of 20 cc/kg of normal saline
   E. Order antibiotics and give a fluid bolus of normal saline

3. An 8-year-old 25 kg male with chronic liver disease is admitted to the PICU for suspected sepsis. He is started on broad-spectrum antibiotics. The nurse calls you after the patient has an episode of hematemesis that she quantified as 600 mL of bright red blood. The patient looks distressed. His saturation is 95%, heart rate is 150 beats per minute, and blood pressure is 80/60 mmHg. His labs show hemoglobin of 8.5 g/dL (the previous one 2 h earlier 10.5 g/dL), platelets of 90 x10^9cells/L, and his prothrombin time is 25 s, partial thromboplastin time (PTT) is 50 s, INR is 4, and fibrinogen is 150 mg/dL. What would be your best therapeutic management next?
   A. Intubate the patient, perform an endoscopy, and order RBC STAT
   B. Order RBC while waiting for the liver team
   C. Transfuse with RBC slowly over 4 h and observe the patient carefully
   D. Order RBC, platelets, and plasma and transfuse with a 1:1:1 strategy
   E. Transfuse with 10 mL/kg of plasma as the major issue is coagulopathy secondary to liver disease

4. A 3-year-old patient is admitted to the PICU with a diagnosis of suspected immune thrombocytopenia with a platelet count of 9 x10^9cells/L for observation, as the floor is not comfortable with such thrombocytopenia. He is otherwise asymptomatic and has some bruises and petechia in the lower extremities. His mother reported upper respiratory symptoms 2 weeks prior to his visit to the emergency department and was worried when he started having more frequent bruises. His vitals show saturation—100%, heart rate—90 beats per minute, and blood pressure—95/45 mmHg. His labs show hemoglobin of 10.5 g/dL, platelets of 9 × 10^9cells/L, and his prothrombin time is 10 s, PTT is 25 s, and INR is 1.2. What is your next best intervention?
   A. Order platelets (10 mL/kg) and transfuse over 1 h
   B. Monitor the patient in the ICU for bleeding and take preventing measures (avoiding risks of falls and nonsteroidal anti-inflammatory drugs) but refrain from transfusing platelets
   C. Order plasma, RBC, and platelets and transfuse 1:1:1
   D. Order broad-spectrum antibiotics and perform a head CT
   E. Order and transfuse RBC and platelets

5. A 15-year-old female has a diagnosis of acute lymphocytic leukemia. As it is the second time she relapses, she is considered for bone marrow transplantation. She is at a high risk of receiving multiple blood products and has already required multiple transfusions in the course of her disease. In addition to avoiding blood products, if clinically appropriate, which of the following products or procedures will help prevent HLA alloimmunization from blood product therapy?
   A. Washed RBCs
   B. Fresh (<5 days old) RBCs
   C. Leukodepletion RBCs
   D. Corticosteroid therapy prior to transfusions
   E. Gamma-irradiated RBC

Answers

1. A: This patient is not hemodynamically stable and has a deficit in oxygen as reflected by the high lactates. Therefore, a RBC transfusion is appropriate. Considering there is no bleeding, plasma or platelet transfusions are not required. Further fluid boluses will only cause more hemodilution and worsen anemia.
2. C: This patient with cyanotic heart disease has a hemoglobin level below 9.5. Transfusing RBC should be strongly considered. In addition, considering the postoperative period, the respiratory distress, and the leukocytosis, a bacterial infection should be suspected and antibiotics should be considered.
3. D: This patient is believed to have lost about 600 mL of blood, out of a blood volume of about 25 kg × 60 mL/kg = 1500 mL. He is hypotensive and in shock. In massive bleeding, the transfusion strategy should provide RBC, plasma, and platelets, correct the anemia, and restore hemostasis.
4. B: A patient with immune thrombocytopenia should not receive platelet transfusion in the absence of life-threatening bleeding as this will only increase the risks of poor outcomes. However, it is reasonable to avoid intracranial bleeding by refraining from nonsteroidal anti-inflammatory drugs and decreasing risks of falls as well as monitoring the patient in the PICU, which will allow for prompt recognition of intracranial bleeding.
5. E: The best way to avoid HLA alloimmunization is gamma irradiation of RBC units as this will prevent donor T lymphocytes from replicating. Leukoreduction through filtering also decreases the number of donor lymphocytes but not to the same extent as irradiation.

References

1. Bateman ST, Lacroix J, Boven K, Forbes P, Barton R, Thomas NJ, et al. Anemia, blood loss, and blood transfusions in north American children in the intensive care unit. Am J Respir Crit Care Med. 2008;178(1):26–33.
2. Tucci M, Lacroix J, Fergusson D, Doctor A, Hebert P, Berg RA, et al. The age of blood in pediatric intensive care units (ABC PICU): study protocol for a randomized controlled trial. Trials. 2018;19(1):404.
3. Walsh TS, McArdle F, McLellan SA, Maciver C, Maginnis M, Prescott RJ, et al. Does the storage time of transfused red blood cells influence regional or global indexes of tissue oxygenation in anemic critically ill patients? Crit Care Med. 2004;32(2):364–71.

4. Doctor A, Cholette JM, Remy KE, Argent A, Carson JL, Valentine SL, et al. Recommendations on RBC transfusion in general critically ill children based on hemoglobin and/or physiologic thresholds from the pediatric critical care transfusion and anemia expertise initiative. Pediatr Crit Care Med. 2018;19(9S Suppl 1):S98–S113.
5. Vanhorebeek I, De Vos R, Mesotten D, Wouters PJ, De Wolf-Peeters C, Van den Berghe G. Protection of hepatocyte mitochondrial ultrastructure and function by strict blood glucose control with insulin in critically ill patients. Lancet. 2005;365(9453):53–9.
6. Doctor A, Stamler JS. Nitric oxide transport in blood: a third gas in the respiratory cycle. Compr Physiol. 2011;1(1):541–68.
7. Napolitano LM, Kurek S, Luchette FA, Corwin HL, Barie PS, Tisherman SA, et al. Clinical practice guideline: red blood cell transfusion in adult trauma and critical care. Crit Care Med. 2009;37(12):3124–57.
8. Karam O, Tucci M, Toledano BJ, Robitaille N, Cousineau J, Thibault L, et al. Length of storage and in vitro immunomodulation induced by prestorage leukoreduced red blood cells. Transfusion. 2009;49(11):2326–34.
9. Weiskopf RB, Viele MK, Feiner J, Kelley S, Lieberman J, Noorani M, et al. Human cardiovascular and metabolic response to acute, severe isovolemic anemia. JAMA. 1998;279(3):217–21.
10. Gauvin F, Spinella PC, Lacroix J, Choker G, Ducruet T, Karam O, et al. Association between length of storage of transfused red blood cells and multiple organ dysfunction syndrome in pediatric intensive care patients. Transfusion. 2010;50(9):1902–13.
11. Valentine SL, Bembea MM, Muszynski JA, Cholette JM, Doctor A, Spinella PC, et al. Consensus recommendations for RBC transfusion practice in critically ill children from the pediatric critical care transfusion and anemia expertise initiative. Pediatr Crit Care Med. 2018;19(9):884–98.
12. Holcomb JB, Zarzabal LA, Michalek JE, Kozar RA, Spinella PC, Perkins JG, et al. Increased platelet: RBC ratios are associated with improved survival after massive transfusion. J Trauma. 2011;71(2 Suppl 3):S318–28.
13. Hebert PC. Transfusion requirements in critical care (TRICC): a multicentre, randomized, controlled clinical study. Transfusion requirements in critical care investigators and the Canadian critical care trials group. Br J Anaesth. 1998;81(Suppl 1):25–33.
14. Lacroix J, Hebert PC, Hutchison JS, Hume HA, Tucci M, Ducruet T, et al. Transfusion strategies for patients in pediatric intensive care units. N Engl J Med. 2007;356(16):1609–19.
15. Cholette JM, Willems A, Valentine SL, Bateman ST, Schwartz SM, Pediatric Critical Care Transfusion and Anemia Expertise Initiative (TAXI), et al. Recommendations on RBC transfusion in infants and children with acquired and congenital heart disease from the pediatric critical care transfusion and anemia expertise initiative. Pediatr Crit Care Med. 2018;19(9S Suppl 1):S137–48.
16. Church GD, Matthay MA, Liu K, Milet M, Flori HR. Blood product transfusions and clinical outcomes in pediatric patients with acute lung injury. Pediatr Crit Care Med. 2009;10(3):297–302.
17. Karam O, Tucci M, Bateman ST, Ducruet T, Spinella PC, Randolph AG, et al. Association between length of storage of red blood cell units and outcome of critically ill children: a prospective observational study. Crit Care. 2010;14(2):R57.
18. Khan H, Belsher J, Yilmaz M, Afessa B, Winters JL, Moore SB, et al. Fresh-frozen plasma and platelet transfusions are associated with development of acute lung injury in critically ill medical patients. Chest. 2007;131(5):1308–14.
19. Sarani B, Dunkman WJ, Dean L, Sonnad S, Rohrbach JI, Gracias VH. Transfusion of fresh frozen plasma in critically ill surgical patients is associated with an increased risk of infection. Crit Care Med. 2008;36(4):1114–8.
20. Karam O, Demaret P, Shefler A, Leteurtre S, Spinella PC, Stanworth SJ, et al. Indications and effects of plasma transfusions in critically ill children. Am J Respir Crit Care Med. 2015;191(12):1395–402.
21. Finfer S, Bellomo R, Boyce N, French J, Myburgh J, Norton R, et al. A comparison of albumin and saline for fluid resuscitation in the intensive care unit. N Engl J Med. 2004;350(22):2247–56.
22. Vigiola Cruz M, Carney BC, Luker JN, Monger KW, Vazquez JS, Moffatt LT, et al. Plasma ameliorates endothelial dysfunction in burn injury. J Surg Res. 2019;233:459–66.
23. Diebel ME, Diebel LN, Liberati DM. Protective effects of plasma products on the endothelial-glycocalyx barrier following trauma-hemorrhagic shock: is sphingosine-1 phosphate responsible? J Trauma Acute Care Surg. 2019;87(5):1061–9.

24. Segal JB, Dzik WH, Transfusion Medicine/Hemostasis Clinical Trials Network. Paucity of studies to support that abnormal coagulation test results predict bleeding in the setting of invasive procedures: an evidence-based review. Transfusion. 2005;45(9):1413–25.
25. Krishnan J, Morrison W, Simone S, Ackerman A. Implications of thrombocytopenia and platelet course on pediatric intensive care unit outcomes. Pediatr Crit Care Med. 2008;9(5):502–5.
26. Nellis ME, Karam O, Mauer E, Cushing MM, Davis PJ, Steiner ME, et al. Platelet transfusion practices in critically ill children. Crit Care Med. 2018;46(8):1309–17.
27. Cashen K, Dalton H, Reeder RW, Saini A, Zuppa AF, Shanley TP, et al. Platelet transfusion practice and related outcomes in pediatric extracorporeal membrane oxygenation. Pediatr Crit Care Med. 2020;21(2):178–85.
28. Curley A, Stanworth SJ, Willoughby K, Fustolo-Gunnink SF, Venkatesh V, Hudson C, et al. Randomized trial of platelet-transfusion thresholds in neonates. N Engl J Med. 2019;380(3):242–51.
29. Schiffer CA, Bohlke K, Anderson KC. Platelet transfusion for patients with cancer: American society of clinical oncology clinical practice guideline update summary. J Oncol Pract. 2018;14(2):129–33.
30. Kim Y, Xia BT, Chang AL, Pritts TA. Role of leukoreduction of packed red blood cell units in trauma patients: a review. Int J Hematol Res. 2016;2(2):124–9.
31. Jackman RP, Deng X, Bolgiano D, Utter GH, Schechterly C, Lebedeva M, et al. Leukoreduction and ultraviolet treatment reduce both the magnitude and the duration of the HLA antibody response. Transfusion. 2014;54(3):672–80.
32. Treleaven J, Gennery A, Marsh J, Norfolk D, Page L, Parker A, et al. Guidelines on the use of irradiated blood components prepared by the British Committee for Standards in Haematology blood transfusion task force. Br J Haematol. 2011;152(1):35–51.
33. Camazine MN, Karam O, Colvin R, Leteurtre S, Demaret P, Tucci M, et al. Outcomes related to the use of frozen plasma or pooled solvent/detergent-treated plasma in critically ill children. Pediatr Crit Care Med. 2017;18(5):e215–23.
34. Marik PE, Corwin HL. Acute lung injury following blood transfusion: expanding the definition. Crit Care Med. 2008;36(11):3080–4.
35. Goldman M, Land K, Robillard P, Wiersum-Osselton J. Development of standard definitions for surveillance of complications related to blood donation. Vox Sang. 2016;110(2):185–8.
36. De Cloedt L, Emeriaud G, Lefebvre É, Kleiber N, Robitaille N, Jarlot C, et al. Transfusion-associated circulatory overload in a pediatric intensive care unit: different incidences with different diagnostic criteria. Transfusion. 2018;58(4):1037–44.
37. Yanagisawa R, Tatsuzawa Y, Ono T, Kobayashi J, Tokutake Y, Hidaka E, et al. Analysis of clinical presentations of allergic transfusion reactions and febrile non-haemolytic transfusion reactions in paediatric patients. Vox Sang. 2019;114(8):826–34.
38. Kopolovic I, Ostro J, Tsubota H, Lin Y, Cserti-Gazdewich CM, Messner HA, et al. A systematic review of transfusion-associated graft-versus-host disease. Blood. 2015;126(3):406–14.
39. Williamson LM, Stainsby D, Jones H, Love E, Chapman CE, Navarrete C, et al. The impact of universal leukodepletion of the blood supply on hemovigilance reports of posttransfusion purpura and transfusion-associated graft-versus-host disease. Transfusion. 2007;47(8):1455–67.
40. Pirenne F. Prevention of delayed hemolytic transfusion reaction. Transfus Clin Biol. 2019;26(2):99–101.
41. Bolton-Maggs PH, Cohen H. Serious hazards of transfusion (SHOT) haemovigilance and progress is improving transfusion safety. Br J Haematol. 2013;163(3):303–14.
42. Mainou M, Alahdab F, Tobian AA, Asi N, Mohammed K, Murad MH, et al. Reducing the risk of transfusion-transmitted cytomegalovirus infection: a systematic review and meta-analysis. Transfusion. 2016;56(6 Pt 2):1569–80.
43. Levy JH, Neal MD, Herman JH. Bacterial contamination of platelets for transfusion: strategies for prevention. Crit Care. 2018;22(1):271.
44. Heiden M, Seitz R. Quality of therapeutic plasma-requirements for marketing authorization. Thromb Res. 2002;107(Suppl 1):S47–51.
45. Stramer SL. Current risks of transfusion-transmitted agents: a review. Arch Pathol Lab Med. 2007;131(5):702–7.

Specific Situations

Contents

Sepsis and Septic Shock

Niha Peshimam, Isadora Rodriguez, and Simon Nadel

Contents

J. Brierley et al. (eds.), *ESPNIC Children's Intensive Care Textbook*,
https://doi.org/10.1007/978-3-031-64762-8_41

1. **Learning Objectives**
   - This is an introduction to definitions, pathophysiology, aetiology, management, and outcome of sepsis and septic shock in children. The student is introduced to major references and summaries of current thinking to give them a background in this important subject in critical care.

41.1 Introduction

Sepsis is a common, complex syndrome caused by the host's dysregulated response to infection [1]. Sepsis continues to be a major burden on health care services in both developed and developing countries, despite implementation of good hygiene practices and effective, universal immunisation programmes [2]. If not treated in a timely manner, sepsis can rapidly progress to septic shock, with associated multiple organ dysfunction and eventually death from multiple organ failure. Early recognition and timely diagnosis of sepsis, together with appropriate management consisting of prompt use of empiric antimicrobials, aggressive fluid resuscitation, and early escalation of care have been shown to reduce mortality.

41.2 Evolving Definitions of Sepsis

The International Pediatric Sepsis Conference (IPSC) in 2005 published definitions and criteria for diagnosing sepsis, severe sepsis, and septic shock in children [3]. This was based on the then existing definitions for adult sepsis with modifications based on age and differences in physiology in children (see ◘ Table 41.1 for definitions).

In 2016, the 'adult' definition of sepsis and septic shock was revised, and new criteria were published (Sepsis 3). 'Sepsis' was defined as life-threatening organ dys-

◘ Table 41.1 Definitions of systemic inflammatory response syndrome (SIRS), infection, sepsis, severe sepsis, and septic shock in children

SIRS (systemic inflammatory response syndrome)
The presence of at least two of the following four criteria, one of which must be abnormal temperature or leukocyte count: • Core temperature of >38.5 C or <36 C • Tachycardia is defined as a mean heart rate >2 SD above the normal for their age in the absence of external stimulus, chronic drugs, or painful stimuli; or otherwise unexplained persistent elevation over a 0.5- to 4-h time period or for children <1 year old, bradycardia is defined as a mean heart rate <10th percentile for age in the absence of external vagal stimulus, beta-blocker drugs, or congenital heart disease; or otherwise unexplained persistent depression over a 0.5-h time period • Mean respiratory rate >2 SD above normal for age or mechanical ventilation for an acute process not related to underlying neuromuscular disease or the receipt of general anaesthesia • Leukocyte count elevated or depressed for age (not secondary to chemotherapy-induced leukopenia) or >10% immature neutrophils
Infection

(continued)

Table 41.1 (continued)

A suspected or proven (by positive culture, tissue stain, or polymerase chain reaction test) infection caused by any pathogen or a clinical syndrome associated with a high probability of infection. Evidence of infection includes positive findings on clinical exam, imaging, or laboratory tests (e.g., white blood cells in a normally sterile body fluid, perforated viscus, chest radiograph consistent with pneumonia, petechial or purpuric rash, or purpura fulminans)
Sepsis
SIRS in the presence of or as a result of suspected or proven infection
Severe sepsis
Sepsis plus one of the following: Cardiovascular organ dysfunction or acute respiratory distress syndrome OR two or more other organ dysfunctions Septic shock Sepsis and cardiovascular organ dysfunction

SD standard deviation, *SIRS* systemic inflammatory response syndrome
Published by the International Pediatric Sepsis Conference in 2005) [1]

function caused by a dysregulated host response to infection, and 'septic shock' was defined as the subset of sepsis with circulatory and cellular/metabolic dysfunction associated with a higher risk of mortality (see Table 41.2 for 'adult' definitions of sepsis) [4]. However, it is unclear to what extent the adult definitions can be used for paediatric patients.

In 2020, the Surviving Sepsis Campaign published guidelines for the management of septic shock and sepsis-associated organ dysfunction in children. Sepsis definition was accepted if either the 2005 or 2016 adaptation was used. Septic shock was defined as severe infection leading to cardiovascular dysfunction (including hypotension, need for vasoactive medications or impaired perfusion) and 'Sepsis-associated organ dysfunction' as severe infection leading to cardiovascular and/or non-cardiovascular dysfunction [1].

More recently in 2023, the new International Consensus for Pediatric Sepsis and Septic Shock published the Phoenix Sepsis Score [5]. This system was developed using the best-performing subscores used in other organ dysfunction scoring systems, and it should be used for patients who are less than 18 years old but are not newborns or neonates with corrected gestational age younger than 37 weeks [6]. The current recommendation is not to use the definitions from 2005 as well as not using the term 'severe sepsis,' simply because the term 'sepsis' should already indicate life-threatening organ dysfunction and consequently, severe disease.

This change comes about mostly due to limitations of the criteria for SIRS including its poor predictive properties, as sepsis can manifest in a diverse range of symptoms, and use of the term *severe sepsis*, which is now deemed redundant. Survey data also found that most paediatric clinicians used the term *sepsis* to refer to infection with life-threatening organ dysfunction, which differs from the IPSC paediatric sepsis criteria [5].

Table 41.2 Definitions for sepsis and septic shock in adults

Sepsis is defined as life-threatening organ dysfunction caused by a dysregulated host response to infection
Organ dysfunction can be identified as an acute change in total SOFA score ⩾2 points consequent to the infection • The baseline SOFA score can be assumed to be zero in patients not known to have pre-existing organ dysfunction • A SOFA score ⩾2 reflects an overall mortality risk of approximately 10% in a general hospital population with suspected infection. Even patients presenting with modest dysfunction can deteriorate further, emphasising the seriousness of this condition and the need for prompt and appropriate intervention, if not already being instituted
In lay terms, **sepsis is a life-threatening condition that arises when the body's response to an infection injures its own tissues and organs**
Patients with suspected infection who are likely to have a prolonged ICU stay or to die in the hospital can be promptly identified at the bedside with **qSOFA**, that is, alteration in mental status, systolic blood pressure ≤100 mm Hg, or respiratory rate ⩾22 min
Septic shock is a subset of sepsis in which underlying circulatory and cellular/metabolic abnormalities are profound enough to substantially increase mortality
Patients with septic shock can be identified with a clinical construct of sepsis with persisting hypotension requiring vasopressors to maintain MAP ⩾65 mm hg and having a serum lactate level >2 mmol/L (18 mg/dL) despite adequate volume resuscitation. With these criteria, hospital mortality is in excess of 40%

ICU intensive care unit, *MAP* mean arterial pressure, *qSOFA* quick SOFA, *SOFA* sequential (sepsis-related) organ failure assessment

Published by the Third International Consensus Definitions for Sepsis and Septic Shock

Furthermore, the Phoenix Sepsis Score was validated using a diverse population from higher and lower income countries and designed to be feasible in low resource settings. The data however comes from patients deriving from the community and does not encompass hospital acquired infections. It also does not include objective scoring for other potentially important microcirculation biomarkers such as urine output and renal and liver function, even though they are usually readily accessible [6].

It is important to note that the Phoenix Sepsis Score is indicated for diagnosis of sepsis (i.e. infection with life-threatening organ dysfunction) and not as a screening tool for possible sepsis before organ dysfunction is overt. It is highly recommended that local screening tools to look for early signs of sepsis should continue to be used. Phoenix criteria are not designed to replace other screening tools [5].

A patient is then considered with sepsis if they score more than 2 points in the Phoenix Sepsis Score (see Table 41.3), which indicates a potentially life-threatening organ dysfunction (respiratory, cardiovascular, coagulation, and/or neurological systems) with the suspicion or confirmation of infection. In addition, septic shock is defined by children with sepsis who score at least 1 point in the cardiovascular component [5].

The new iteration of Surviving Sepsis Campaign Guidelines is under preparation to update the existing evidence.

41.3 Aetiology

Evolution of sepsis is not merely dependent on the causative organism but includes several host factors such as age of the patient, likely source of infection, underlying host factors, immunocompromised state, presence of indwelling devices, chronic co-morbidities, and time to or delay in recognition.

The common causative organisms implicated in the aetiology of sepsis in children vary based on age and underlying condition, as well as geographical location. While the most frequently identified pathogens are bacteria and viruses; fungi and parasites can also cause the clinical syndrome of sepsis. A significant proportion of children with sepsis will have no pathogen identified.

Group B streptococci (GBS), *Escherichia coli* (E. coli), and Listeria monocytogenes are commonly found to be responsible for sepsis presenting in the neonatal period [7]. Increased vigilance and the use of peripartum antibiotics given to the mother have reduced the incidence of GBS sepsis.

Perinatally acquired Herpes simplex virus (HSV) infection can cause fulminant sepsis in neonates, leading to rapid deterioration and death. Enterovirus and Parechoviruses may also cause a similar sepsis syndrome in neonates and young infants.

H. influenzae type b (Hib), *Neisseria meningitidis*, and *Streptococcus pneumoniae* are common causes of sepsis in children under 5 years of age. Improved availability of effective vaccines has significantly reduced incidence of sepsis caused by these organisms [7]. Toxic shock syndrome caused by toxin-producing strains of *Staphylococcus aureus* and *Streptococcus pyogenes* (Group A streptococci, GAS) continue to remain important additional causes of sepsis in children.

Children with frequent hospital admissions or receiving repeated courses of antibiotics may be prone to infections with methicillin-resistant Staphylococcus aureus (MRSA), Carbapenem-resistant Enterobacteriaceae, and vancomycin-resistant enterococci.

Immunocompromised children and those with chronic co-morbidities are at increased risk for sepsis caused by gram-negative organisms, particularly *Pseudomonas aeruginosa*, as well as alpha-haemolytic streptococci and fungi [1, 7].

Coagulase-negative Staphylococcus should be suspected in children with indwelling vascular catheters and other indwelling devices [1, 7].

Children with splenic dysfunction or congenital or acquired asplenia are prone to pneumococcal and Salmonella infection.

Viral-induced sepsis is not uncommon and while respiratory syncytial virus (RSV) and influenza virus are well-known causes for hospitalisation of infants, human metapneumovirus, rhinovirus, and adenovirus are being increasingly identified.

Covid-19-related illness in children may present with a hyper-inflammatory syndrome, often affecting the myocardium and causing shock, mimicking septic shock and should be evaluated in children as part of the differential diagnosis of sepsis [8].

It is important to be aware that sepsis can also be caused by malaria, dengue fever, rickettsial, and other endemic or epidemic infections, so inquiry for travel or other epidemiological clues should be sought [7].

Table 41.3 Phoenix sepsis score[a]

Variables	0 Points	1 Points	2 Points	3 Points
Respiratory (0–3 points)	$PaO_2:FiO_2$ ≥400 or $SpO_2:FiO_2$ ≥292[b]	$PaO_2:FiO_2$ <400 on any respiratory support or $SpO_2:FiO_2$ <292 on any respiratory support[b,c]	$PaO_2:FiO_2$ 100-200 and IMV or $SpO_2:FiO_2$ 148–220 and IMV[b]	$PaO_2:FiO_2$ <100 and IMV or $SpO_2:FiO_2$ <148 and IMV[b]
Cardiovascular (0–6 points)	No vasoactive medications[d] Lactate <5 mmol/L[e]	1 point each (up to 3) 1 vasoactive medication[d] Lactate 5-10.9 mmol/L	2 points each (up to 6) ≥2 vasoactive medications[d] Lactate ≥11 mmol/L[e]	
Mean arterial pressure, mmHg[g] Age based[f]				
<1 months 1–11 months 1–<2 years 2–<5 years 5–<12 years 12–17 years	>30 >38 >43 >44 >48 >51	17–30 25–38 31–43 32–44 36–48 38–51	<17 <25 <31 <32 <36 <38	
Coagulation (0–2 points)h	Platelets ≥100 × 10^3/μL International normalised ratio ≤1.3 D-dimer ≤2 mg/L FEU Fibrinogen ≥100 mg/dL	1 point each (maximum 2 points) Platelets <100 × 10^3/μL International normalised ratio >1.3 D-dimer >2 mg/L FEU Fibrinogen <100 mg/dL		
Neurological (0–2 points)I	Glasgow coma scale score >10; pupils reactive[j]	Glasgow coma scale ≤10[j]	Fixed pupils bilaterally	
Phoenix sepsis criteria				
Sepsis Suspected infection and Phoenix sepsis score ≥2 points				
Septic shock Sepsis with ≥1 cardiovascular point(s)				

(continued)

Table 41.3 (continued)

FEU fibrinogen equivalent units, *IMV* invasive mechanical ventilation, *INR* international normalised ratio of prothrombin time, *MAP* mean arterial pressure, *PaO2:FiO2* arterial partial pressure of oxygen to fraction of inspired oxygen ratio, *SpO2* oxygen saturation measured by pulse oximetry (only SpO_2 of 97%). SI conversion factor: To convert lactate from mmol/L tomg/dL, divide by 0.111

[a] The score may be calculated in the absence of some variables (e.g. even if lactate level is not measured and vasoactive medications are not used, a cardiovascular score can still be ascertained using blood pressure). It is expected that laboratory tests and other measurements will be obtained at the discretion of the medical team based on clinical judgement. Unmeasured variables contribute no points to the score. Ages are not adjusted for prematurity, and the criteria do not apply to birth hospitalisations, neonates whose postconceptional age is younger than 37 weeks, or those 18 years of age or older

[b] SpO_2:FiO_2 ratio is only calculated if SpO_2 is 97% or less

[c] The respiratory dysfunction of 1 point can be assessed in any patient receiving oxygen, high-flow, non-invasive positive pressure, or IMV respiratory support and includes a PaO_2:FiO_2 ratio of less than 200 and a SpO_2:FiO_2 ratio of less than 220 in children who are not receiving IMV. For children receiving IMV with a PaO_2:FiO_2 less than 200 and SpO_2:FiO_2 less than 220, see criteria for 2 and 3 points

[d] Vasoactive medications include any dose of epinephrine, norepinephrine, dopamine, dobutamine, milrinone, and/or vasopressin (for shock)

[e] Lactate reference range is 0.5–2.2 mmol/L. Lactate can be arterial or venous

[f] Age is not adjusted for prematurity, and the criteria do not apply to birth hospitalisations, children whose postconceptional age is younger than 37 weeks, or those 18 years or older

[g] Use measured MAP preferentially (invasive arterial if available or non-invasive oscillometric), and if measured MAP is not available, a calculated MAP (1/3 × systolic + 2/3 × diastolic) may be used as an alternative

[h] Coagulation variable reference ranges: Platelets, 150–450 × 10^9/L; D-dimer, <0.5 mg/L FEU; fibrinogen, 180–410 mg/dL. The INR reference range is based on the local reference prothrombin time

[i] The neurological dysfunction subscore was pragmatically validated in both sedated and nonsedated patients and those receiving or not receiving IMV support

[j] The Glasgow coma scale score measures level of consciousness based on verbal, eye, and motor response (range, 3–15, with a higher score indicating better neurological function)

41.4 Identifying the Child with Sepsis

Not all children with sepsis will present with fever, and many may have non-specific symptoms. Thus, clinicians should have a high index of suspicion when reviewing a child who presents with non-specific features, as this may be the early presentation of sepsis. A large number of health care systems now use Paediatric Early Warning Scores (PEWS) in both the emergency department and for patients admitted to the ward, which may help to improve early identification of the deteriorating child [9, 10].

Clinicians should take a thorough history to ascertain whether the patient has risk factors for sepsis, followed by a detailed physical examination.

Signs and symptoms that should raise suspicion of sepsis are listed in Table 41.4 [11].

Table 41.4 Signs and symptoms that should prompt clinical concern for sepsis

Fever >38 C	Hypothermia
Tachypnoea	Apnoea
Difficulty in breathing/respiratory distress	Cyanotic/mottled skin/ashen appearance
Tachycardia	Bradycardia
Abnormal capillary refill time (>3 s)	Reduced urine output
Weak pulses	Non-blanching rash
Altered mental status (irritability, Inappropriate crying, confused)	Inappropriate drowsiness (difficult to arouse, lethargic, or obtunded)

Emergency departments should have a screening tool and sepsis bundle of care to help with early identification of the septic child, timely management, and appropriate escalation. Multiple quality improvement projects have demonstrated that the use of a sepsis bundle is associated with improved outcome [1, 12].

Diagnostic tests to identify patient with sepsis are limited to non-specific biomarkers indicating an acute inflammatory response such as white blood cell count and differential, C-reactive protein (CRP), and procalcitonin (PCT). However, none of these tests are sensitive or specific enough for accurate diagnosis [13]. The healthcare costs of performing a PCT test are significantly higher when compared with CRP or white cell count. In addition, there are situations in which a markedly elevated procalcitonin is not predictive, for example, in the setting of moderate to severe acute kidney injury. Based on studies performed in adults, PCT is a useful prognostic marker that can be used for monitoring therapeutic response and can help guide safe antibiotic de-escalation/rationalisation [14].

Newer molecular tests (e.g. polymerase chain reaction, 16S ribosomal nucleic acid (RNA)) to identify both bacterial and viral infections maybe useful for rapid diagnosis or if standard microbiological techniques fail to identify the infecting pathogen, but these are expensive and are not widely available.

Blood lactate measurement provides a rapid and indirect estimation of cardiac output and is available as a point of care test to assist in the evaluation of the child with signs of shock. In adults and children, a blood lactate measurement of >2 mmol/L is an indication of poor perfusion and/or cellular/metabolic dysfunction, associated with septic shock [15]. While not helpful in the determination of the aetiology of shock, lactate level may aid in decisions regarding adequacy of shock resuscitation [16]. While tissue hypoperfusion is usually the most common cause for elevated blood lactate level, persistently elevated lactate level non-response to appropriate therapy, together with the absence of signs of hypoperfusion should prompt the clinician to consider alternate causes of lactic acidosis such as liver dysfunction, state of nutritional deficiency (e.g. thiamine deficiency), ingested drugs or toxins affecting cellular metabolism, or malignancy.

41.5 Pathophysiology

The pathophysiology of sepsis is complex. The host's immune system is activated by bacterial cell wall components (e.g. endotoxin, peptidoglycan, lipoteichoic acid) or bacterial exotoxins (e.g. Staphylococcal enterotoxin B, toxic shock syndrome toxin-1, Pseudomonas exotoxin A, M protein of haemolytic group A streptococci), or cellular and other components of fungi, viruses, or parasites.
Activation of host inflammatory cells including neutrophils, macrophages, lymphocytes, and.

endothelial cells leads to the production of proinflammatory cytokines such as tumour necrosis factor alpha (TNFa) and interleukin-1 (IL-1) [17]. This amplifies host cell activation and production of downstream mediators such as prostaglandins, leukotrienes, platelet-activating factor, and phospholipase A2. When these proinflammatory mediators are released in an uncontrolled and dysregulated manner, dysfunction of the endothelium, capillary leakage, a prothrombotic state, and myocardial dysfunction occurs. These changes. ultimately result in multiple organ dysfunction [18].

Hypotension in sepsis is thought to be a consequence of vasodilation due to impaired endothelial function, upregulation of nitric oxide secretion, and redistribution of intravascular fluid.

Myocardial dysfunction results from reduced venous return, decreased nitric oxide release, cytokine dysregulation, and release of myocardial depressant factors.

Hypoperfusion secondary to vasodilation results in acute tubular necrosis, which is one of the presumed mechanisms leading to acute kidney injury in sepsis [19]. Endothelial dysfunction contributes to the development of disseminated microvascular coagulation leading to impaired cellular and tissue perfusion and contributes to the multiple organ dysfunction and organ failure.

41.6 Antimicrobial Therapy

Evidence suggests that early and prompt administration of antibiotics is crucial to optimise outcome in patients with sepsis and septic shock [20].

Guidelines recommend that broad-spectrum antibiotics should be given within 1 h of presentation [1]. Empiric broad-spectrum antimicrobials should be selected, depending on known epidemiology and local antimicrobial resistance patterns, travel history, and factoring in the likely source of infection, presence of any indwelling devices, immunocompromised state if present, recent hospital admissions, and known colonisation with specific pathogens [11]. Clinicians should be guided by their local antimicrobial policy but can also refer to the recommendations from national guidelines and the Surviving Sepsis Campaign Guidelines.

All efforts should be made to collect relevant microbiological specimens, including blood, urine, sputum, and CSF (if necessary and safe to do so) prior to starting antibiotics. However, diagnostic tests should not delay antibiotic administration. Lumbar puncture may be deferred due to haemodynamic instability, concerns of raised intracranial pressure, abnormal coagulation, or infection at the lumbar puncture site.

As soon as clinically feasible, interventions to achieve source control should be implemented [1]. This may include removal of suspected infected indwelling devices, abscess drainage, debridement of necrotic soft tissue, and drainage of a septic joint or empyema.

Antimicrobial stewardship should be employed, which includes de-escalation of antibiotics when appropriate to reduce potential drug toxicity as well as avoidance of prolonged use. Appropriate antimicrobial stewardship involves cessation of antimicrobials if an alternative non-infectious aetiology for the clinical presentation is determined; and switching to a narrower spectrum antimicrobial as soon as possible based on microbiological data [21]. This decision should be made based on clinical improvement, site of infection, and whether source control has been achieved, together with identification of infecting pathogen with accompanying antimicrobial sensitivities. Close consultation with infectious disease specialists in complex cases is advised.

41.7 Vascular Access and Fluid Therapy

Hypovolaemia in the child with sepsis is a consequence of capillary leak, vasodilation, and fluid loss, which can be corrected with appropriate fluid resuscitation. Vascular access must be obtained rapidly when sepsis or septic shock is suspected. Ideally, the child should have two wide-bore peripheral venous cannulae inserted. If the child has septic shock and venous access has not been established within 5 min, interosseous access should be obtained. A blood gas should be obtained for lactate, glucose, and acid-base status.

Other investigations including full blood count, clotting screen, and renal and liver function tests should be obtained. In children who have no evidence of cardiovascular compromise as demonstrated by tachycardia, abnormal perfusion, or hypotension, fluid bolus therapy should not be given; they should be commenced on maintenance fluid therapy instead [22]. Children who are shocked should receive fluid boluses of 10–20 mL/kg aliquots with strict monitoring of heart rate, capillary refill time, blood pressure, and urine output and lactate levels. To assess response and need for further fluid administration after each bolus, it is necessary to repeat clinical examination to check for evidence of fluid overload by evaluating for new or worsening hepatomegaly, new or increasing oxygen requirement, basal crepitations, or radiographic evidence of pulmonary oedema. Fluid boluses up to 60 mL/kg can be given within the first hour in settings with access to advanced intensive care [22, 23]. In lower resource settings that do not have provision for advanced intensive care, fluid blouses in the first hour should not exceed 40 mL/kg and should only be given in the presence of hypotension [22, 23]. The child should be re-assessed regularly following each fluid bolus to evaluate response and to check for signs of fluid overload.

Early consultation and consideration of escalation to the Paediatric Intensive Care Unit is essential.

While there is limited data in the paediatric population, randomised control trials (RCTs) in adults have shown that the use of crystalloid fluids containing high concentrations of chloride for resuscitation is associated with an increased risk of hyperchloremic acidosis, acute kidney injury, coagulopathy, and mortality when compared with balanced or buffered crystalloid solutions such as Ringer's lactate or Plasma-Lyte [24, 25]. The routine use of colloid solutions such as 5% Human Albumin Solution or Gelofusine for resuscitation is now not recommended as they have been shown to exhibit no advantage over crystalloids, are more expensive, less easily available, and carry an increased risk of infection or coagulopathy [1, 22].

41.8 Vasoactive Agents

In children who have received 40–60 mL/kg of fluid resuscitation within an hour and who remain shocked, commencement of vasoactive medications is strongly recommended [1]. These children may continue to receive fluid boluses if appropriate together with vasoactive agents to try to reverse shock, but if shock persists, these children will require tracheal intubation and invasive ventilation. Some children may be managed with non-invasive positive pressure ventilation, but this depends on the clinical situation, patient response, and resources.

Previously dopamine was commonly used as the first-line vasoactive drug in the management of children with septic shock. Based on randomised control trials which have concluded that there are increased adverse effects with the use of dopamine in comparison to epinephrine and norepinephrine, current practice has moved towards the use of either epinephrine and norepinephrine as first-line vasoactive agents, both of which have vasopressor and inotropic effects [1, 26, 27].

If there is a delay or difficulty in obtaining central access, vasoactive agents can be administered through peripheral or intraosseous access [1, 28]. Both epinephrine and norepinephrine can be administered in dilute concentrations peripherally if necessary due to lack of central venous access. Excessive tachycardia may preclude the use of epinephrine. The published data on the safety of administering vasoactive medications peripherally in children is limited, and the clinicians should attempt to obtain central venous access as soon as feasible.

As there is no good evidence comparing the use of epinephrine and norepinephrine in children with fluid refractory shock, the choice of agent depends on the treating clinician's preference, local policy, and an assessment of physiology. Epinephrine is often used to manage shock associated with a low cardiac output state while norepinephrine is often used to manage shock where vasodilatation and decreased systemic vascular resistance are present.

The previously used classification of shock into 'warm shock' and 'cold shock' is now outdated as there was poor correlation between clinical assessment, cardiac index, and systemic vascular resistance when measured using advanced monitoring techniques [1].

Vasoactive agents should be titrated to a mean arterial pressure (MAP) between the fifth and 50th percentile for the age, adequate urine output, and adequate peripheral perfusion.

Vasopressin-receptor agonists (e.g. vasopressin or terlipressin) may be used in catecholamine-resistant shock, and inodilators (e.g. milrinone or dobutamine) can be considered if the child remains in shock with evidence of low cardiac output. These therapies are typically initiated in the intensive care unit setting where advanced haemodynamic monitoring is available. For more information, please see ◘ Table 41.5 [29].

Table 41.5 Most commonly used vasoactive drugs

	Consider if	Receptor	Effect	Side effects
Adrenaline	Signs of low cardiac output (cold peripheries, prolonged CRT, poor peripheral pulses, etc.)	Beta (lower doses) Alpha (higher doses)	Increased heart rate and contractility	Tachycardia Increased myocardial oxygen consumption Splanchnic constriction
Noradrenaline	Vasodilatation (hypotension, bounding pulses, etc.)	Alpha predominantly	Increased blood vessel constriction	Tachycardia Increased myocardial oxygen consumption Hepatic and mesenteric ischaemia
Vasopressin	Second line if not responsive to noradrenaline and adrenaline	V1 and V2	Increased blood vessel constriction	Hypertension Angina Tremor Vertigo Water intoxication Peripheral ischaemia
Milrinone	If persistent clinical evidence of hyporperfusion and cardiac dysfunction despite other vasoactive agents	Nonreceptor mediated inhibitor of cAMP phosphodiesterase III isoenzyme	Improve cardiac contractility Peripheral vasodilatation	Arrhythmias Hypotension Liver and GI dysfunction Thrombocytopaenia

41.9 Corticosteroids

Children who are at high risk for adrenal insufficiency, such as those with chronic or recent treatment with steroids or congenital or acquired adrenal insufficiency, should receive stress dose hydrocortisone early. Low dose hydrocortisone can also be used in children who remain in refractory shock after the use of fluid and vasoactive agents; however, there is not good evidence of their benefit [30, 31].

41.10 Respiratory Support

All children with sepsis should be given additional oxygen by facemask early, unless they are able to maintain their transcutaneous oxygen saturation >95% while breathing in room air. Children who need additional respiratory support but who do not have a clear indication for tracheal intubation and mechanical ventilation can be trialled on non-invasive respiratory support. This may reduce the work of breathing and improve oxygenation, thereby avoiding the need for intubation [32].

Definitive indications for mechanical ventilation include acute or incipient respiratory failure, non-response to non-invasive respiratory support, persistent shock despite acute fluid resuscitation of 40–60 mL/kg in 1 h, persistent hypoxemia, or inability to safely maintain the airway.

Rapid sequence induction of anaesthesia followed by tracheal intubation by the most experienced clinician is advised. Administration of general anaesthetic drugs and muscle relaxants along with the transition to positive pressure ventilation can reduce venous return and precipitate cardiac arrest. Induction agents such as propofol or benzodiazepines that may cause cardiac depression or vasodilatation should be avoided. Use of reduced doses of induction agents in the child with shock is also recommended [1].

Mechanical ventilation should be lung protective with minimal tolerated tidal volumes and peak pressures, high positive end expiratory pressure, together with efforts to minimise the amount of inspired oxygen while ensuring adequate oxygenation [33–35]. Based on the possibility of pulmonary oedema due to capillary leak, and the development of sepsis-induced paediatric acute respiratory distress syndrome (PARDS), a higher positive end expiratory pressure (PEEP) may be required for recruitment of alveoli, to prevent alveolar collapse and improve oxygenation [33–35].

Nitric oxide therapy is not routinely used in the management of children with sepsis-induced PARDS. However, children who have pulmonary hypertension or severe right ventricular dysfunction confirmed by echocardiography should be commenced on nitric oxide if refractory hypoxaemia remains a challenge despite optimisation of oxygenation strategies [36].

41.11 Monitoring the Child with Septic Shock

All children with sepsis should have basic monitoring which includes continuous monitoring of transcutaneous oxygen saturation, electrocardiography (ECG), and non-invasive blood pressure measurement.

In children who are in shock and receiving resuscitation fluid therapy and vasoactive agents, an indwelling arterial catheter for continuous invasive blood pressure measurement should be placed.

High blood lactate level may be an indication of incomplete resuscitation or should prompt the clinician to think of an alternative diagnosis.

Previously central venous pressure (CVP) measurements were used to guide the on-going resuscitation of patients with septic shock. This practice is no longer recommended as CVP monitoring has poor predictive value for assessing fluid responsiveness and is affected by several physiological factors [1]. However, placement of a central venous line may aid rapid fluid administration and the use of high-dose vasoactive agents.

There are a variety of advanced tools to monitor on-going resuscitation in children with septic shock. Several devices exist which are used for the non-invasive measurement of cardiac output and peripheral vascular resistance. These newer tools may not only give us more accurate information about fluid responsiveness and volume status but can also provide values for cardiac output and tissue perfusion. The detailed description of these methods is beyond the scope of this review.

41.12 Electrolytes and Metabolites

Electrolyte disturbances are commonly found in children with sepsis and septic shock, specifically hypoglycaemia, hypocalcaemia, hypokalaemia, and hypomagnesaemia. Plasma electrolytes should be monitored regularly and optimised when necessary.
If present, hypoglycaemia should be corrected by rapid infusion of IV dextrose. The routine use of insulin to maintain glucose within a tight normal range is not recommended [1, 37]. Adjunctive insulin treatment should only be considered if hyperglycaemia is associated with clinical compromise despite control of glucose administration [37]. Calcium plays an important role in myocardial contractility; ionised blood calcium levels should be maintained above 1 mmol/L.

Hypomagnesemia may exacerbate cardiac dysrhythmias but should be treated cautiously as magnesium sulphate can worsen hypotension.

41.13 Blood and Blood Product Transfusion

Blood haemoglobin level determines the oxygen carrying capacity of blood, thus affecting tissue oxygen delivery. Children who remain in shock despite fluid resuscitation and initiation of vasoactive agents may benefit from packed red blood cell transfusion if haemoglobin is <7 g/dL [38].

Disseminated intravascular coagulopathy is common in children with septic shock and may require transfusion with platelets, fresh frozen plasma, and/or cryoprecipitate to manage significant bleeding. There is no evidence to recommend prophylactic transfusion of red blood cells, platelets, or plasma in children with septic shock, even with coagulopathy. Children with very low platelet counts (<20,000/ mm^3) are at a significantly higher risk for bleeding and should be given platelet transfusion [1].

41.14 Refractory Septic Shock

The European Society of Paediatric and Neonatal Intensive Care has defined refractory septic shock in children as the association of high blood lactate with high vasoactive agent/inotrope doses associated with myocardial dysfunction [39]. Possible reversible causes should be evaluated and treated if found.

The presence of refractory shock is associated with a significantly higher mortality, and these patients should be considered for adjunctive therapies or extracorporeal support.

41.15 Renal Replacement Therapy

Fluid overload is associated with increased morbidity and possibly mortality in critically ill children [40]. There is no evidence that routine use of renal replacement therapy (RRT) is associated with improved outcomes [41]. Common indications for initiation of RRT in children with septic shock include fluid overload unresponsive to fluid restriction and diuretic therapy, acute kidney injury, and persistent lactic acidosis. The use of RRT requires both clinician and nursing expertise and the insertion of large vascular catheters for haemofiltration or dialysis in patients with coagulopathy and is not available in all centres.

There is no guidance on the optimal time to initiate RRT, and it should be commenced at the discretion of the treating team after the benefits have been weighed against possible risks.

41.16 Therapeutic Plasma Exchange/Plasmapheresis

While the role of therapeutic plasma exchange in the management of children with septic shock is not clearly established, small anecdotal studies have shown some benefit for patients with thrombocytopaenia-associated multiple organ failure (TAMOF) [42].

TAMOF is an inflammatory phenotype of sepsis-induced multiple organ dysfunction in children. It is identified by new-onset thrombocytopenia and evolving multiple organ dysfunction. If suspected, management should be discussed with a paediatric haematologist.

41.17 Immunoglobulin Therapy

A meta-analysis has demonstrated the benefits of intravenous immunoglobulin (IVIG) in the management of children with toxic shock syndrome, and it is used as an adjunct to antibiotics and source control [43]. However, there is no evidence that supports routine use of IVIG in the management of children with septic shock apart from those with toxic shock syndrome [44].

41.18 Extracorporeal Membrane Oxygenation (ECMO)

Extracorporeal Membrane Oxygenation (ECMO) has been suggested as a treatment for children with refractory septic shock, where anecdotal reports of its use have demonstrated up to 50% survival [45].

41.19 Conclusion

Paediatric sepsis and septic shock continue to be associated with significant morbidity and mortality worldwide. All children with septic shock should receive early empiric antimicrobial therapy and aggressive fluid therapy. All emergency departments should have guidelines and protocols in place for the management of sepsis. Sepsis bundles, protocols, and guidelines ensure standardised care and have been shown to improve outcome.

Take-Home Messages

- Early diagnosis and rapid initiation of appropriate therapy, including antimicrobial treatment, fluid resuscitation, introduction of vasoactive agents, escalation to critical care, and involvement of senior decision-makers are all essential to try to improve the outcome of sepsis and septic shock in children.
- Excellent evidence-based guidelines are in place for the management of sepsis and septic shock in the developed and developing world, and following these guidelines has led to improvements in outcome.
- Further research is required in many aspects of sepsis therapy in children in an attempt to further improve outcomes.
- Prevention by vaccination has led to major reductions in community-acquired bacterial sepsis in children, but further preventative measures are required if we are to further reduce sepsis-related mortality worldwide.

References

1. Weiss SL, Peters MJ, Alhazzani W, et al. Surviving sepsis campaign international guidelines for the management of septic shock and sepsis-associated organ dysfunction in children. Pediatr Crit Care Med. 2020;21:e52–e106.
2. Fleischmann-Struzek C, Goldfarb DM, Schlattmann P, et al. The global burden of paediatric and neonatal sepsis: a systematic review. Lancet Respir Med. 2018;6:223–30.
3. Goldstein B, Giroir B, Randolph A, et al. International pediatric sepsis consensus conference: definitions for sepsis and organ dysfunction in pediatrics. Pediatr Crit Care Med. 2005;6:2–8.
4. Singer M, Deutschman CS, Seymour CW, et al. The third international consensus definitions for sepsis and septic shock (sepsis-3). JAMA. 2016;315:801–10.
5. Schlapbach LJ, Watson RS, Sorce LR, et al. International consensus criteria for pediatric sepsis and septic shock. JAMA. 2024;331(8):665–74. https://doi.org/10.1001/jama.2024.0179.
6. Sanchez-Pinto LN, Bennett TD, DeWitt PE, et al. Development and validation of the phoenix criteria for pediatric sepsis and septic shock. JAMA. 2024;331(8):675–86. https://doi.org/10.1001/jama.2024.0196.
7. Randolph AG, McCulloh RJ. Pediatric sepsis: important considerations for diagnosing and managing severe infections in infants, children, and adolescents. Virulence. 2014;5:179–89.
8. Whittaker E, Bamford A, Kenny J, et al. Clinical characteristics of 58 children with a pediatric inflammatory multisystem syndrome temporally associated with SARS-CoV-2. JAMA. 2020;324:259–69.
9. Lambert V, Matthews A, MacDonell R, et al. Paediatric early warning systems for detecting and responding to clinical deterioration in children: a systematic review. BMJ Open. 2017;7:e014497.
10. Parshuram CS, Duncan HP, Joffe AR, et al. Multicentre validation of the bedside paediatric early warning system score: a severity of illness score to detect evolving critical illness in hospitalised children. Crit Care. 2011;15:R184.
11. Overview| Sepsis: recognition, diagnosis and early management| Guidance| NICE. https://www.nice.org.uk/guidance/ng51. Accessed 18 July 2021.
12. Evans IVR, Phillips GS, Alpern ER, et al. Association between the New York sepsis care mandate and in-hospital mortality for pediatric sepsis. JAMA. 2018;320:358–67.
13. Downes KJ, Fitzgerald JC, Weiss SL. Utility of procalcitonin as a biomarker for sepsis in children. J Clin Microbiol. 2020;58:e01851–19.
14. Lanziotti VS, Póvoa P, Soares M, et al. Use of biomarkers in pediatric sepsis: literature review. Rev Bras Ter Intensiva. 2016;28:472–82.

15. Rhodes A, Evans LE, Alhazzani W, et al. Surviving sepsis campaign: international guidelines for management of sepsis and septic shock: 2016. Crit Care Med. 2017;45:486–552.
16. Schlapbach LJ, MacLaren G, Festa M, et al. Prediction of pediatric sepsis mortality within 1 h of intensive care admission. Intensive Care Med. 2017;43:1085–96.
17. Gotts JE, Matthay MA. Sepsis: pathophysiology and clinical management. BMJ. 2016;353:i1585.
18. Kenet G, Strauss T, Kaplinsky C, et al. Hemostasis and thrombosis in critically ill children. Semin Thromb Hemost. 2008;34:451–8.
19. Shum H-P, Yan W-W, Chan TM. Recent knowledge on the pathophysiology of septic acute kidney injury: a narrative review. J Crit Care. 2016;31:82–9.
20. Schlapbach LJ, Weiss SL, Wolf J. Reducing collateral damage from mandates for time to antibiotics in pediatric sepsis-primum non nocere. JAMA Pediatr. 2019;173:409–10.
21. Godbout EJ, Pakyz AL, Markley JD, et al. Pediatric antimicrobial stewardship: state of the art. Curr Infect Dis Rep. 2018;20:39.
22. Maitland K, Kiguli S, Opoka RO, et al. Mortality after fluid bolus in African children with severe infection. N Engl J Med. 2011;364:2483–95.
23. Inwald DP, Canter R, Woolfall K, et al. Restricted fluid bolus volume in early septic shock: results of the fluids in shock pilot trial. Arch Dis Child. 2019;104:426–31.
24. Emrath ET, Fortenberry JD, Travers C, et al. Resuscitation with balanced fluids is associated with improved survival in pediatric severe sepsis. Crit Care Med. 2017;45:1177–83.
25. Semler MW, Self WH, Wanderer JP, et al. Balanced crystalloids versus saline in critically ill adults. N Engl J Med. 2018;378:829–39.
26. Ventura AMC, Shieh HH, Bousso A, et al. Double-blind prospective randomized controlled trial of dopamine versus epinephrine as first-line vasoactive drugs in pediatric septic shock. Crit Care Med. 2015;43:2292–302.
27. Ramaswamy KN, Singhi S, Jayashree M, et al. Double-blind randomized clinical trial comparing dopamine and epinephrine in pediatric fluid-refractory hypotensive septic shock. Pediatr Crit Care Med. 2016;17:e502–12.
28. Lampin ME, Rousseaux J, Botte A, et al. Noradrenaline use for septic shock in children: doses, routes of administration and complications. Acta Paediatr. 2012;101:e426–30.
29. Nichols, DG, Donald H, and Mark C. Rogers. Rogers' textbook of pediatric intensive care. (2016.
30. Rygard SL, Butler E, Granholm A, et al. Low-dose corticosteroids for adult patients with septic shock: a systematic review with meta-analysis and trial sequential analysis. Intensive Care Med. 2018;44:1003–16.
31. Venkatesh B, Finfer S, Cohen J, et al. Adjunctive glucocorticoid therapy in patients with septic shock. N Engl J Med. 2018;378:797–808.
32. Abadesso C, Nunes P, Silvestre C, et al. Non-invasive ventilation in acute respiratory failure in children. Pediatr Rep. 2012;4:e16.
33. Khemani RG, Smith L, Lopez-Fernandez YM, et al. Paediatric acute respiratory distress syndrome incidence and epidemiology (PARDIE): an international, observational study. Lancet Respir Med. 2019;7:115–28.
34. Kneyber MCJ, de Luca D, Calderini E, et al. Recommendations for mechanical ventilation of critically ill children from the paediatric mechanical ventilation consensus conference (PEMVECC). Intensive Care Med. 2017;43:1764–80.
35. The Pediatric Acute Lung Injury Consensus Conference Group. Pediatric acute respiratory distress syndrome: consensus recommendations from the pediatric acute lung injury consensus conference. Pediatr Crit Care Med. 2015;16:428–39.
36. Macrae DJ, Field D, Mercier J-C, et al. Inhaled nitric oxide therapy in neonates and children: reaching a European consensus. Intensive Care Med. 2004;30:372–80.
37. Chen L, Li T, Fang F, et al. Tight glycemic control in critically ill pediatric patients: a systematic review and meta-analysis. Crit Care. 2018;22:57.
38. Muszynski JA, Guzzetta NA, Hall MW, et al. Recommendations on RBC transfusions for critically ill children with non-hemorrhagic shock from the pediatric critical care transfusion and anemia expertise initiative. Pediatr Crit Care Med. 2018;19(9S, Suppl. 1):S121–6.
39. Morin L, Ray S, Wilson C, et al. Refractory septic shock in children: a European Society of Paediatric and Neonatal Intensive Care definition. Intensive Care Med. 2016;42:1948–57.

40. Sinitsky L, Walls D, Nadel S, et al. Fluid overload at 48 hours is associated with respiratory morbidity but not mortality in a general PICU: retrospective cohort study. Pediatr Crit Care Med. 2015;16:205–9.
41. Miao H, Wang F, Xiong X, et al. Clinical benefits of high-volume hemofiltration in critically ill pediatric patients with severe sepsis: a retrospective cohort study. Blood Purif. 2018;45:18–27.
42. Fortenberry JD, Nguyen T, Grunwell JR, et al. Therapeutic plasma exchange in children with thrombocytopenia-associated multiple organ failure: the thrombocytopenia-associated multiple organ failure network prospective experience. Crit Care Med. 2019;47:e173–81.
43. Parks T, Wilson C, Curtis N, et al. Polyspecific intravenous immunoglobulin in clindamycin-treated patients with streptococcal toxic shock syndrome: a systematic review and meta-analysis. Clin Infect Dis. 2018;67:1434–6.
44. Alejandria MM, Lansang MAD, Dans LF, et al. Intravenous immunoglobulin for treating sepsis, severe sepsis and septic shock. Cochrane Database Syst Rev. 2013;9:CD001090.
45. Oberender F, Ganeshalingham A, Fortenberry JD, et al. Venoarterial extracorporeal membrane oxygenation versus conventional therapy in severe pediatric septic shock. Pediatr Crit Care Med. 2018;19:965–72.

Hemorrhagic Shock in Children

Gilles Orliaguet, Caroline Durracher, and Estelle Vergnaud

Contents

J. Brierley et al. (eds.), *ESPNIC Children's Intensive Care Textbook*,
https://doi.org/10.1007/978-3-031-64762-8_42

Learning Objectives

- To present the pattern and specificities of hemorrhagic shock in children and describe the aims of management, which mainly relies upon the concept of damage control resuscitation, including damage control hemostasis and damage control surgery.

42.1 Introduction

Hemorrhagic shock is a failure of the circulatory system to provide sufficient oxygen to the cells due to sudden and severe blood loss. Hemorrhagic shock is a situation at high risk of morbidity and mortality [1–3]. It can occur in medical (e.g. digestive hemorrhage in a child with esophageal varices), surgical (e.g. bleeding post-tonsillectomy) or traumatic circumstances (ruptured spleen, complex trauma to the pelvis, penetrating wound, etc.) [3]. However, trauma remains the primary cause of hemorrhagic shock in children [4]. In addition, hemorrhagic shock is the main cause of death in trauma and remains a major cause of perioperative cardiac arrest [1, 5] and therefore requires rapid intervention, which is a critical prognosis factor [4, 6]. Diagnosis mainly relies upon physical examination and is usually easy in case of external bleeding. However, diagnosis may be difficult in children because of some pathophysiological particularities, especially in case of internal hemorrhage. The outcome widely depends upon an early and effective treatment. The management relies upon the concept of damage control resuscitation (DCR) which combines control of the hemorrhagic lesion (mostly damage control surgery (DCS); more rarely interventional radiology or endoscopy), hemodynamic resuscitation to maintain adequate tissue perfusion and oxygenation, as well as hematologic resuscitation (damage control hemostasis (DCH)) to reverse coagulation disorders [7–9]. Therefore, this chapter will present the specificities of hemorrhagic shock in children, including the diagnostic elements, and will focus on the management of hemorrhagic shock, including the particularities arising from applying DCR in children.

42.2 Diagnosis of Hemorrhagic Shock

Hemorrhagic shock is suspected when clinical signs and symptoms of tissue hypoperfusion are associated with evident (external hemorrhage) or possible (internal hemorrhage) active bleeding [6]. The diagnosis is confirmed when hemorrhage is shown to be the cause of shock. Internal hemorrhage is more difficult to recognize than external bleeding, especially in children. For example, the abdominal cavity of a child may contain a large volume of blood without being obviously distended. Similarly, in children under 18–24 months of age, a large intracranial hematoma (e.g. epidural hematoma) can lead to hemorrhagic shock [10, 11] while there is no obvious external bleeding.

Clinical signs and symptoms depend upon the volume of blood loss, the speed of bleeding, the age and the patient's condition (possible associated comorbidities). Usual signs of shock include tachycardia, tachypnea, increased capillary refill time (>3 s) and progressive consciousness disorders. However, in infants and young children, blood pressure is maintained longer than in adults and adolescents [2] despite severe bleeding, predominantly due to a very intense sympathetic vasoconstriction in response to hypovolemia. Thus, in young children, systemic hypotension occurs only following a reduction of more than 30–40% in the circulating blood volume [3, 12]. Systemic hypotension related to hemorrhagic shock in children shortly precedes cardiovascular collapse or even cardiac arrest. Different definitions of systemic hypotension have been proposed for children [13–15]. In order to simplify, the following definition of hypotension may be considered in children between 1 and 10 years of age [14]:

- Systolic blood pressure (SBP) $< (70 + [2 \times \text{age in years}])$ mmHg or
- Mean arterial pressure (MAP) $< (40 + [1.5 \times \text{age in years}])$

The shock index (heart rate/systolic blood pressure) pediatric age-adjusted (SIPA) is a recently proposed index that may help identify critically injured children [16, 17]. Threshold values included SIPA >1.22 (ages 4–6), >1.0 [7–12] and >0.9 (13–16 years). An increased SIPA is superior to age-adjusted hypotension to identify injured children likely to require an emergency operation, endotracheal intubation or early blood transfusion. Therefore, SIPA could be useful in helping to early identify children suffering from severe hemorrhage.

Clinical examination may sometimes be sufficient to diagnose hemorrhagic shock. However, some complementary examinations are helpful. In addition to anemia and coagulation disorders, hyperglycemia, metabolic acidosis and hyperlactatemia may be observed, indicating cellular hypoperfusion. In the case of internal bleeding, further investigations are often necessary to confirm the bleeding and its origin, such as a chest X-ray to look for hemothorax, abdominal ultrasound to diagnose a hemoperitoneum, cerebral CT scan to identify an epidural hematoma, etc.

42.3 Management of Hemorrhagic Shock in Children

42.3.1 Context of Damage Control Resuscitation in Children

The majority of the recent literature regarding the management of hemorrhagic shock has been published in the setting of adult trauma patients and has shown a dramatic reduction in mortality after major trauma hemorrhage [18]. In recent years, hemorrhagic shock resuscitation practice has changed from targeting a restoration of normal blood pressure to DCR [8]. DCR is a management strategy, used in military conflicts with reported success, which prioritizes early correction of coagulation disorders [19]. DCR has been incorporated into management in many civilian trauma centers, including pediatric trauma centers [9]. The concept of DCR prioritizes short-term physiological recovery and is based mostly on resuscitative maneuvers targeting the lethal triad (coagulopathy—acidosis—hypothermia) in association with DCS (▣ Fig. 42.1). The damage control strategy starts on the scene (i.e. at the scene of an accident or home) and continues during transport and admission to the hospital. In the context of DCR, the well-established ABC sequence is replaced by the <C> ABC sequence, indicating that the priority is to minimize blood loss and maximize tissue oxygenation in order to optimize outcome [19].

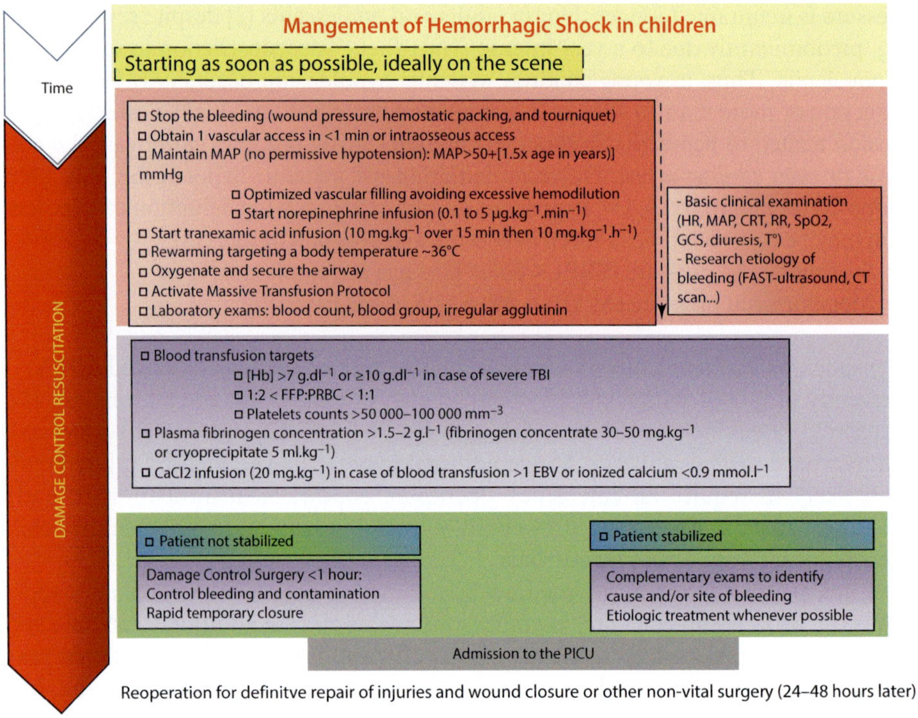

Fig. 42.1 Damage control resuscitation in children with hemorrhagic shock. *MAP* mean arterial pressure, *HR* heart rate, *CRT* capillary refill time, *RR* respiratory rate, SpO_2 pulsed oximetry, *GCS* Glasgow Comas Scale score, *T°* body temperature, *[Hb]* hemoglobin concentration, *FFP* fresh frozen plasma, *PRBC* packed red blood cells, $CaCl_2$ calcium chloride, *EBV* estimated blood volume, *PICU* pediatric intensive care unit

The different components of the DCR strategy in adults include: (1) stop the bleed, (2) rewarm rapidly, (3) limit crystalloid/colloid infusion, (4) permissive hypotension, (5) early ratio-based blood component therapy, (6) correct coagulation disorders and (7) damage control surgery [20]. While the concept of DCR was described first in adults, it may also be applied to children with severe bleeding but with some adaptations considering the impact that physiological particularities of children could have on management.

42.3.2 Stop the Bleed

Pelvic binders, direct compression and tourniquet use are essential (prehospital) interventions that save lives. Prehospital hemorrhage control has been so successful in the USA that the Department of Homeland Security and the American College of Surgeons launched the campaign 'STOP the Bleed' in 2015 (Department of Homeland Security. STOP the bleed [Internet]. 2016. Available from: ▶ https://www.dhs.gov/stopthebleed). The goal of this campaign is to train bystanders to help in case of a bleeding emergency, with an application of direct pressure and tourniquet use. Recent studies have confirmed the usefulness of tourniquets for reducing the volume of intravenous (IV) fluids and blood transfusion, finally improving survival in children suffering from war casualties [21, 22].

42.3.3 Rapid Rewarming

A proportionally larger skin surface area and reduced physiological warming capacities expose children to an increased risk of hypothermia [23], substantially aggravating the coagulopathy of hemorrhagic shock [8, 9]. As in adults, there is a direct relationship between the severity of hypothermia on hospital admission and the risk of death [24]. Prevention, or at least treatment, of hypothermia, is therefore fundamental from the very first stages of management [7]. It is mandatory to monitor body temperature and to prevent/treat hypothermia with all available means (survival blanket, temperature control in the ambulance and resuscitation room, use of active skin and fluid warming systems).

42.3.4 Permissive Hypotension in Children

Permissive hypotension is a strategy based on studies showing that trauma patients with uncontrolled hemorrhagic shock worsen following a large volume of IV fluid and increased intravascular hydrostatic pressure [8, 20, 25]. However, permissive hypotension is not recommended in patients with associated head injuries [25, 26], and there is currently no evidence supporting the use of permissive hypotension in pediatrics [9]. In addition, there is a major concern for the use of this strategy based on the physiologic response of pediatric patients to hypovolemia. In fact, the tremendous efficiency of the sympathetic nervous system in children to maintain blood pressure means that systemic hypotension is a late sign of hemorrhagic shock and represents a critical and uncompensated state, which may be closely followed by cardiac arrest [7–9]. Permissive hypotension in children is therefore not recommended due to lack of evidence, physiologic considerations and high rates of concomitant head injury.

42.3.5 Fluids and Drugs Administration

In case of circulatory failure caused by hemorrhage, volume administration is required [27]. Isotonic crystalloids are recommended as the initial resuscitation fluid for infants and children. If there are signs of systemic hypoperfusion (i.e. increased capillary refill time), an IV bolus of 10–20 $mL.kg^{-1}$ of an isotonic crystalloid must be administered, even if the systemic blood pressure is still normal. There is a growing body of evidence that balanced crystalloids should be preferred to normal saline as they induce less hyperchloraemic acidosis [28–30]. On the other hand, glucose-containing solutions must be avoided unless there is hypoglycemia.

Some authors advocate for early vasopressor support (norepinephrine) to restore blood pressure and perfusion (cerebral perfusion pressure), especially in brain-damaged patients. Moreover, owing to consciousness disorders and/or progressive respiratory failure, some patients will need tracheal intubation and mechanical ventilation.

42.4 Damage Control Hemostatic

Coagulation disorders may occur early in the setting of hemorrhagic shock [31]. In fact, coagulopathy in hemorrhagic shock may evolve because of hemodilution from IV fluids and blood products administration, consumptive coagulopathy and exacerbation from hypothermia and acidosis frequently present during resuscitation [8]. In life-threatening hemorrhagic shock, limiting the use of crystalloids in favor of a regimen of massive blood transfusion (MBT) may be required to minimize hemodilution. Therefore, hemostatic resuscitation is a transfusion strategy that targets coagulopathy with early blood product administration. There are different possibilities for combining packed red blood cells (PRBC), fresh frozen plasma (FFP), platelet concentrates (PC) and other blood products in delivering MBT so that the regimen used should be in accordance with local protocols. An MBT should be activated in the case of persistent bleeding in a child who has required volume expansion of half a blood mass or more or immediately if there are clinico-biological signs of coagulopathy (e.g. bruising, mucocutaneous bleeding, prolongation of activated clotting time and prothrombin time and/or INR, thrombocytopenia and hypofibrinogenemia). Unfortunately, there is currently no validated MBT in pediatrics explaining the wide variations in clinical practice from one center to another [3, 32]. However, this clinical situation must be anticipated in each hospital, in conjunction with the local blood transfusion center, in order to be able to deliver packs of blood products rapidly. These packs (composed, for example, of 1 PRBC, 1 FFP and 2 PC) will be administered according to the child's body weight (e.g. <10 kg = 1 pack, 10–30 kg = 2 packs and >30 kg = 3 packs). This is consistent with recent recommendations for therapeutic plasma transfusion, which recommend transfusing plasma in combination with red blood cell concentrates with an FFP:PRBC ratio of 1:2–1:1 in the event of massive hemorrhage and the implementation of MBT in centers that typically manage patients with massive hemorrhage [33, 34]. These recommendations also call for the implementation of early PC transfusion, usually at the time of the second transfusion prescription [35]. Fibrinogen administration is also required for massive transfusion or in case of fibrinogen concentration <1.5–2 $g.L^{-1}$ (fibrinogen concentrate 30–50 $mg.kg^{-1}$ or cryoprecipitate 5 $mL.kg^{-1}$) [35]. Finally, the administration of calcium (CaCl2 20 $mg.kg^{-1}$) is decided in case of transfusion of more than one blood volume or in case of ionized calcium <0.9 $mmol.L^{-1}$ [35]. On the other hand, the indications to transfuse a patient who is no longer bleeding and has been stabilized are not consensual. A low hemoglobin level is certainly an important indication, but the threshold for blood transfusion varies among physicians but may probably be set around 7 $g.dL^{-1}$ in stable children [36, 37]. In fact, multiple factors are usually considered in addition to hemoglobin level before starting a blood transfusion, mainly including severity and risk of persistent bleeding [38, 39], the prospect of surgery, prevention of cellular dysoxia and improvement of oxygen transport [36, 37]. Thus, the transfusion starter should probably be set to 9–10 $g.dL^{-1}$ if the patient is actively bleeding, unstable or has a brain (e.g. severe head injury) or heart condition.

Some biological tests must be collected immediately, such as blood group, irregular agglutinin, blood counts and coagulation exams. It is always required to order a complete blood phenotype, even when the patient's condition is so severe that the results cannot be expected before starting a transfusion. Other specimens may also be useful to guide further resuscitation, such as ionograms (kalemia, ionized calcium, renal function and liver enzymes), lactatemia and repeated bedside hemoglobin concentration determinations to guide PRBC transfusion. Blood gases help optimize ventilator settings, while lactatemia determination helps monitor the progression of shock [40, 41]. Functional coagulation assessment such as viscoelastic assays (e.g. thromboelastometry or thromboelastography), providing a dynamic, rapid and global approach to hemostasis including fibrinolysis, could optimize blood products transfusion and fibrinogen supply [42]. However, further studies are required before recommending its routine use in children.

Tranexamic acid (TXA) is an antifibrinolytic agent that reversibly binds to plasminogen at the lysine-binding site, preventing the binding of plasminogen to fibrin and the subsequent degradation of fibrin, thereby decreasing fibrinolysis. It effectively reduces bleeding and blood product transfusion in a large number of adult and pediatric perioperative and trauma settings [43–45]. TXA administration has been shown to be independently associated with decreased morbidity and mortality in pediatric trauma patients in a war setting [46]. Based on TXA pharmacokinetics, some authors recommend a dosing regimen of 10–30 $mg.kg^{-1}$ as loading dose (2 g maximum) followed by 5–10 $mg.kg^{-1}.h^{-1}$ maintenance infusion rate for pediatric trauma and surgery [43]. In the trauma setting, the reduction in mortality is greater when TXA is given within 3 h of the injury [47].

42.5 Damage Control Surgery (DCS)

DCS is a concept of shortened laparotomy to prioritize short-term physiological recovery over anatomical reconstruction in seriously injured trauma patients [7]. Appropriate selection of patients for DCS is crucial. Indeed, attempts at primary definitive repair of injuries in patients with severe physiological impairment may lead to poor outcomes or unplanned abbreviated procedures. Conversely, inappropriate use of DCS may deny patients with adequate physiological conditions the benefit of effective early management, with the subsequent risk of unnecessary additional procedures and increased morbidity and mortality [19]. The first step of DCS is hemorrhage control. Sometimes, interventional radiology procedures are necessary to achieve hemostasis. The second priority is the limitation of contamination by controlling the spillage of intestinal contents or urine from hollow viscus injuries. Abdominal closure is the final step of DCS; however, fascial closure is typically not recommended, because of the postoperative risk of intra-abdominal hypertension (IAH) with abdominal compartment syndrome (ACS). Once the physiologic status has normalized, definitive repair of all injuries and abdominal closure can be considered, generally 24–48 h later [19]. DCS is associated with dramatically increased survival of the most seriously injured patients [48]. DCS should not be undertaken separately from DCR; in fact, the two procedures represent different steps of the same strategy and are integral parts of each other, with DCS being the endpoint of DCR.

42.6 Assessment of the Effectiveness of Treatment

The effectiveness of treatment is assessed first on usual hemodynamic parameters, including MAP. It is clinically more relevant to monitor MAP than systolic and diastolic arterial pressures because MAP is directly measured by the oscillometric method of noninvasive blood pressure (NIBP) monitoring devices and is the driving perfusion pressure for organs. Nevertheless, clinical signs may be insufficient to assess precisely hemodynamic status, while NIBP measurements may be inaccurate [49, 50]. Therefore, it is often necessary to invasively monitor blood pressure, as soon as possible, especially in the most severe cases. Invasive blood pressure monitoring allows continuous and reliable monitoring of MAP and regular blood sampling. Unlike in adults, in children, the respiratory variation of the pulsed pressure (ΔPP) does not reliably predict the response to volume expansion [51]. In pediatric resuscitation, monitoring is based on various noninvasive and/or invasive hemodynamic monitoring tools [52, 53], among which cardiac ultrasound plays a major role [54]. Hemodynamic management may also benefit from cardiac output (CO) and/or stroke volume (SV) monitoring [54], combined with assessment of organ perfusion/oxygenation (lactate, $ScVO_2$ and regional O_2 oxygenation via NIRS) [55].

Clinical monitoring should follow regularly the evolution of clinical signs of shock, including notably hourly diuresis to identify the onset of acute renal failure (ARF). The definition of ARF is based on the modified RIFLE classification for pediatrics (pRIFLE): estimated creatinine clearance decreased by at least 25% or urine output <0.5 mL.kg^{-1}.h^{-1} for 8 h [56]. The remaining biological tests should help detect and/or monitor possible organ dysfunctions related to hemorrhagic shock (liver function, blood ionogram, blood glucose, acid-base balance and $ScVO_2$) (◘ Table 42.1) [4].

◘ **Table 42.1** Indication and frequency of complementary investigations for the follow-up of the bleeding child

Complementary exams	Indication	Frequency
Bedside hemoglobin concentration	Assessment of the effectiveness of blood transfusion and indirect assessment of ongoing bleeding	On admission and 15–30 min following blood transfusion
Blood count	Anemia management and optimization of RBC transfusion	On admission and every 4–6 h until bleeding has stopped
Platelets count	Search for thrombocytopenia and optimization of platelet transfusion	On admission and every 4–6 h until bleeding has stopped

(continued)

Table 42.1 (continued)

Complementary exams	Indication	Frequency
Coagulation screening tests with clotting factors and fibrinogen	Optimization of FFP transfusion and fibrinogen administration	On admission and every 6–24 h until bleeding has stopped
Arterial blood gas	Assessment of acid-base balance, lactatemia and optimization of ventilator settings	On admission and every 2 h until patient is stabilized
Blood ionogram	Assessment of kalemia, ionized calcium level, renal and liver function	On admission and every 6–8 h until patient is stabilized
Search for red blood cells or hemoglobin in the urine	Search for hematuria, hemoglobinemia and hemoglobinuria	On admission and every 6–8 h according to urine color
Chest X-ray	Assessment of ARDS or TRALI	According to the evolution
Abdominal ultrasound	Assessment of a hemoperitoneum	Every 24–48 h

RBC red blood cells, *FFP* fresh frozen plasma, *ARDS* acute respiratory distress syndrome, *TRALI* transfusion-related acute lung injury

Take-Home Messages

- Hemorrhagic shock is an emergency at high risk of morbidity and mortality in children.
- Clinical diagnosis is based on physical examination and is usually easy in case of external bleeding but sometimes difficult in case of internal hemorrhage.
- Outcome depends on early and aggressive treatment, starting on the scene.
- Management principle of hemorrhagic shock is based on damage control resuscitation, which prioritizes short-term physiological recovery.
- Damage control resuscitation mainly relies on resuscitative maneuvers targeting the lethal triad (coagulopathy—acidosis—hypothermia) in association with damage control surgery.
- The main steps of the strategy include stopping the bleeding, rewarming actively, limiting the administration of crystalloids and colloids, infusing tranexamic acid and vasopressor and activating the massive transfusion protocol.
- Permissive hypotension is contraindicated in children because hypotension is a late sign of shock and represents a critical and decompensated situation.
- Damage control surgery aims at quickly controlling bleeding and contamination with rapid temporary closure.
- Definitive surgical repair of injuries may be performed, hours or days, later on a stabilized patient.

References

1. Bhananker SM, Ramamoorthy C, Geiduschek JM, Posner KL, Domino KB, Haberkern CM, et al. Anesthesia-related cardiac arrest in children: update from the pediatric perioperative cardiac arrest registry. Anesth Analg. 2007;105(2):344–50.
2. Fisher JD, Nelson DG, Beyersdorf H, Satkowiak LJ. Clinical spectrum of shock in the pediatric emergency department. Pediatr Emerg Care. 2010;26(9):622–5.
3. McKiernan CA, Lieberman SA. Circulatory shock in children: an overview. Pediatr Rev. 2005;26(12):451–60.
4. Orliaguet G. Choc hémorragique et stratégie transfusionnelle. In: Paut O, Orliaguet G, editors. Réanimation pédiatrique. Paris: Springer Verlag; 2013. p. 27–50.
5. Bouglé A, Harrois A, Duranteau J. Prise en charge du choc hémorragique en réanimation pédiatrique. Réanimation. 2008;17:153–61.
6. Stylianos S. Outcomes from pediatric solid organ injury: role of standardized care guidelines. Curr Opin Pediatr. 2005;17(3):402–6.
7. Tran A, Campbell BT. The art and science of pediatric damage control. Semin Pediatr Surg. 2017;26(1):21–6.
8. Hughes NT, Burd RS, Teach SJ. Damage control resuscitation: permissive hypotension and massive transfusion protocols. Pediatr Emerg Care. 2014;30(9):651–6; quiz 7–8
9. Gilley M, Beno S. Damage control resuscitation in pediatric trauma. Curr Opin Pediatr. 2018;30(3):338–43.
10. Ciurea AV, Kapsalaki EZ, Coman TC, Roberts JL, Robinson JS 3rd, Tascu A, et al. Supratentorial epidural hematoma of traumatic etiology in infants. Childs Nerv Syst. 2007;23(3):335–41.
11. Ciurea AV, Gorgan MR, Tascu A, Sandu AM, Rizea RE. Traumatic brain injury in infants and toddlers, 0–3 years old. J Med Life. 2011;4(3):234–43.
12. Schwaitzberg SD, Bergman KS, Harris BH. A pediatric trauma model of continuous hemorrhage. J Pediatr Surg. 1988;23(7):605–9.
13. Dellinger RP, Levy MM, Rhodes A, Annane D, Gerlach H, Opal SM, et al. Surviving sepsis campaign: international guidelines for management of severe sepsis and septic shock, 2012. Intensive Care Med. 2013;39(2):165–228.
14. Haque IU, Zaritsky AL. Analysis of the evidence for the lower limit of systolic and mean arterial pressure in children. Pediatr Crit Care Med. 2007;8(2):138–44.
15. Nafiu OO, Voepel-Lewis T, Morris M, Chimbira WT, Malviya S, Reynolds PI, et al. How do pediatric anesthesiologists define intraoperative hypotension? Paediatr Anaesth. 2009;19(11):1048–53.
16. Acker SN, Bredbeck B, Partrick DA, Kulungowski AM, Barnett CC, Bensard DD. Shock index, pediatric age-adjusted (SIPA) is more accurate than age-adjusted hypotension for trauma team activation. Surgery. 2017;161(3):803–7.
17. Arbuthnot M, Armstrong LB, Mooney DP. Can we safely decrease intensive care unit admissions for children with high grade isolated solid organ injuries? Using the shock index, pediatric age-adjusted and hematocrit to modify APSA admission guidelines. J Pediatr Surg. 2017;52(6):989–92.
18. Cole E, Weaver A, Gall L, West A, Nevin D, Tallach R, et al. A decade of damage control resuscitation: new transfusion practice, new survivors, new directions. Ann Surg. 2019;273(6):1215–20.
19. Lamb CM, MacGoey P, Navarro AP, Brooks AJ. Damage control surgery in the era of damage control resuscitation. Br J Anaesth. 2014;113(2):242–9.
20. Simmons JW, Powell MF. Acute traumatic coagulopathy: pathophysiology and resuscitation. Br J Anaesth. 2016;117(suppl 3):iii31–43.
21. Kragh JF Jr, Cooper A, Aden JK, Dubick MA, Baer DG, Wade CE, et al. Survey of trauma registry data on tourniquet use in pediatric war casualties. Pediatr Emerg Care. 2012;28(12):1361–5.
22. Sokol KK, Black GE, Azarow KS, Long W, Martin MJ, Eckert MJ. Prehospital interventions in severely injured pediatric patients: rethinking the ABCs. J Trauma Acute Care Surg. 2015;79(6):983–9; discussion 9–90
23. Hamele M, Poss WB, Sweney J. Disaster preparedness, pediatric considerations in primary blast injury, chemical, and biological terrorism. World J Crit Care Med. 2014;3(1):15–23.
24. Waibel BH, Durham CA, Newell MA, Schlitzkus LL, Sagraves SG, Rotondo MF. Impact of hypothermia in the rural, pediatric trauma patient. Pediatr Crit Care Med. 2010;11(2):199–204.

25. Giannoudi M, Harwood P. Damage control resuscitation: lessons learned. Eur J Trauma Emerg Surg. 2016;42(3):273–82.
26. Kochanek PM, Tasker RC, Carney N, Totten AM, Adelson PD, Selden NR, Davis-O'Reilly C, Hart EL, Bell MJ, Bratton SL, Grant GA, Kissoon N, Reuter-Rice KE, Vavilala MS, Wainwright MS. Guidelines for the Management of Pediatric Severe Traumatic Brain Injury, Third Edition: Update of the Brain Trauma Foundation Guidelines, Executive Summary. Pediatr Crit Care Med. 2019;20:280–89.
27. Van de Voorde P, Turner NM , Djakow J, de Lucas N, Martinez-Mejias A, Biarent D, Bingham R, Brissaud O, Hoffmann F, Johannes GB, Lauritsen T, Maconochie I. European Resuscitation Council Guidelines 2021: Paediatric Life Support. Resuscitation 2021;161:327–87.
28. Fuhrman DY, Kellum JA. Hyperchloremic IV solutions: have we seen enough?...or "Still good medicine?". Pediatr Crit Care Med. 2018;19(2):171–2.
29. Stenson EK, Cvijanovich NZ, Anas N, Allen GL, Thomas NJ, Bigham MT, et al. Hyperchloremia is associated with complicated course and mortality in pediatric patients with septic shock. Pediatr Crit Care Med. 2018;19(2):155–60.
30. Emrath ET, Fortenberry JD, Travers C, McCracken CE, Hebbar KB. Resuscitation with balanced fluids is associated with improved survival in pediatric severe sepsis. Crit Care Med. 2017;45(7):1177–83.
31. Choi PM, Vogel AM. Acute coagulopathy in pediatric trauma. Curr Opin Pediatr. 2014;26(3):343–9.
32. Dehmer JJ, Adamson WT. Massive transfusion and blood product use in the pediatric trauma patient. Semin Pediatr Surg. 2010;19(4):286–91.
33. Cunningham ME, Rosenfeld EH, Zhu H, Naik-Mathuria BJ, Russell RT, Vogel AM. A high ratio of plasma: RBC improves survival in massively transfused injured children. J Surg Res. 2019;233:213–20.
34. Noland DK, Apelt N, Greenwell C, Tweed J, Notrica DM, Garcia NM, et al. Massive transfusion in pediatric trauma: an ATOMAC perspective. J Pediatr Surg. 2019;54(2):345–9.
35. Kietaibl S, Ahmed A, Afshari A, Albaladejo P, Aldecoa C, Barauskas G, De Robertis E, Faraoni D, Filipescu DC, Fries D, Godier A, Haas T, Jacob M, Lancé MD, Llau JV, Meier J, Molnar Z, Mora L, Rahe-Meyer N, Samama CM, Scarlatescu E, Schlimp C, Wikkelsø AJ, Zacharowski K. Management of severe peri-operative bleeding: Guidelines from the European Society of Anaesthesiology and Intensive Care: Second update 2022. Eur J Anaesthesiol. 2023;40:226–304.
36. Doctor A, Cholette JM, Remy KE, Argent A, Carson JL, Valentine SL, et al. Recommendations on RBC transfusion in general critically ill children based on hemoglobin and/or physiologic thresholds from the pediatric critical care transfusion and anemia expertise initiative. Pediatr Crit Care Med. 2018;19(9S Suppl 1):S98–S113.
37. Lacroix J, Tucci M, Du Pont-Thibodeau G. Red blood cell transfusion decision making in critically ill children. Curr Opin Pediatr. 2015;27(3):286–91.
38. Nellis ME, Tucci M, Lacroix J, Spinella PC, Haque KD, Stock A, et al. Bleeding assessment scale in critically ill children (BASIC): physician-driven diagnostic criteria for bleeding severity. Crit Care Med. 2019;47(12):1766–72.
39. Nellis ME, Levasseur J, Stribling J, Faustino EVS, Zantek ND, Sheth S, et al. Bleeding scales applicable to critically ill children: a systematic review. Pediatr Crit Care Med. 2019;20(7):603–7.
40. Morin L, Ray S, Wilson C, Remy S, Benissa MR, Jansen NJG, et al. Refractory septic shock in children: a European society of paediatric and neonatal intensive care definition. Intensive Care Med. 2016;42(12):1948–57.
41. Hatherill M, Waggie Z, Purves L, Reynolds L, Argent A. Mortality and the nature of metabolic acidosis in children with shock. Intensive Care Med. 2003;29(2):286–91.
42. Drucker NA, Wang SK, Newton C. Pediatric trauma-related coagulopathy: balanced resuscitation, goal-directed therapy and viscoelastic assays. Semin Pediatr Surg. 2019;28(1):61–6.
43. Goobie SM, Faraoni D. Tranexamic acid and perioperative bleeding in children: what do we still need to know? Curr Opin Anaesthesiol. 2019;32(3):343–52.
44. Goobie SM, Zurakowski D, Glotzbecker MP, McCann ME, Hedequist D, Brustowicz RM, et al. Tranexamic acid is efficacious at decreasing the rate of blood loss in adolescent scoliosis surgery: a randomized placebo-controlled trial. J Bone Joint Surg Am. 2018;100(23):2024–32.
45. collaborators C-t. Effects of tranexamic acid on death, disability, vascular occlusive events and other morbidities in patients with acute traumatic brain injury (CRASH-3): a randomised, placebo-controlled trial. Lancet. 2019;394(10210):1713–23.

46. Eckert MJ, Wertin TM, Tyner SD, Nelson DW, Izenberg S, Martin MJ. Tranexamic acid administration to pediatric trauma patients in a combat setting: the pediatric trauma and tranexamic acid study (PED-TRAX). J Trauma Acute Care Surg. 2014;77(6):852–8.
47. Roberts I, Shakur H, Coats T, Hunt B, Balogun E, Barnetson L, et al. The CRASH-2 trial: a randomised controlled trial and economic evaluation of the effects of tranexamic acid on death, vascular occlusive events and transfusion requirement in bleeding trauma patients. Health Technol Assess. 2013;17(10):1–79.
48. Rotondo MF, Schwab CW, McGonigal MD, Phillips GR 3rd, Fruchterman TM, Kauder DR, et al. 'Damage control': an approach for improved survival in exsanguinating penetrating abdominal injury. J Trauma. 1993;35(3):375–82; discussion 82–3
49. Vallet B, Blanloeil Y, Cholley B, Orliaguet G, Pierre S, Tavernier B, et al. Guidelines for perioperative haemodynamic optimization. Société française d'anesthésie et de réanimation. Ann Fr Anesth Reanim. 2013;32(6):454–62.
50. Lobos AT, Lee S, Menon K. Capillary refill time and cardiac output in children undergoing cardiac catheterization. Pediatr Crit Care Med. 2012;13(2):136–40.
51. Gan H, Cannesson M, Chandler JR, Ansermino JM. Predicting fluid responsiveness in children: a systematic review. Anesth Analg. 2013;117(6):1380–92.
52. Marik PE. Noninvasive cardiac output monitors: a state-of the-art review. J Cardiothorac Vasc Anesth. 2013;27(1):121–34.
53. Suehiro K, Joosten A, Murphy LS, Desebbe O, Alexander B, Kim SH, et al. Accuracy and precision of minimally-invasive cardiac output monitoring in children: a systematic review and meta-analysis. J Clin Monit Comput. 2016;30(5):603–20.
54. Brissaud O, Guichoux J, Villega F, Orliaguet G. Quelle évaluation hémodynamique non invasive en réanimation pédiatrique en 2009 ? [What non invasive haemodynamic assessment in paediatric intensive care unit in 2009?]. Ann Fr Anesth Reanim. 2010;29(3):233–41.
55. Turner NM. Intraoperative hypotension in neonates: when and how should we intervene? Curr Opin Anaesthesiol. 2015;28(3):308–13.
56. Ichai C, Vinsonneau C, Souweine B, Armando F, Canet E, Clec'h C, et al. Acute kidney injury in the perioperative period and in intensive care units (excluding renal replacement therapies). Anaesth Crit Care Pain Med. 2016;35(2):151–65.

Abdominal Trauma

Lucas Rabaux and Géraldine Hery

Contents

J. Brierley et al. (eds.), *ESPNIC Children's Intensive Care Textbook*,
https://doi.org/10.1007/978-3-031-64762-8_43

43.1 Introduction

Trauma remains the leading cause of death in children over 1 year of age in industrial countries [1]. It is a frequent situation that any clinician dealing with surgery or emergencies should be aware of.

Children present certain physiological characteristics that have already been discussed in this book and that should guide the clinician in the assessment of a traumatized child.

The most frequently injured organs are by order: spleen, liver, kidney, pancreas, and intestine.

Several elements are now widely agreed: Ultrasound first in a monotraumatized, hemodynamically stable child, CT scan in case of lesions found during the first examinations and in a polytraumatized child. Non-operative treatment should always be considered and is effective in more than 90% of cases. Some other elements are still debate length of hospitalization, need, and management of the follow-up.

In this chapter, we will first discuss solid organ injury. They shared a common management, so we will detail the spleen management, and then focus on particularities for the liver, renal, and pancreas.

43.2 Spleen

43.2.1 Frequency

The spleen is the most frequently injured solid organ in pediatric abdominal trauma. Splenic trauma is found in 25–30% [2] of blunt pediatric abdominal trauma, although it is frequently associated with other organ injuries.

43.2.2 Trauma Mechanism

The mechanisms are not different from adults although there are some specificities when it comes to children. The leading cause is road car accidents whether the child is a pedestrian or a passenger [1]. The lesions are more severe than adults, due to the position of the seat belt, a less protective iliac crest, a more elastic rib cage, and a greater transmission of force [3]. Sports accidents (contact sports or speed sports such as horseback riding and cycling) represent the second cause of spleen injuries. Regarding children, abdominal traumas due to child abuse must not be missed.

43.2.3 Diagnosis

43.2.3.1 Clinical

Pain in the left hypochondrium and flank, or referred to the left shoulder, is the main symptom for spleen trauma, along with a history of direct trauma. The clinical examination is mandatory because, apart from the patient's complaint, an abrasion or ecchymosis of the left hypochondrium and, furthermore, painful palpation is very indicative of spleen trauma.

43.2.3.2 Imaging and Biology

In monotrauma patients, diagnosis is evocated by abdominal ultrasound. It will be supplemented by a CT scan in case of suspicion of spleen trauma [2]. In case of clinically stable patient with a hemoglobin and hematocrit in normal ranges, some studies propose not to perform a CT scan systematically to lower radiations [4–6].

In polytraumatized children, a CT scan should be performed immediately.

In addition to imaging, biological tests are performed to identify and evaluate potential bleeding, to look for associated lesions, and to anticipate further treatment. It includes hemoglobin, hemostasis, blood group, liver function test, and lipase serum level.

43.2.3.3 Grade Classification

Injury grades for spleen, liver, and kidney are mostly classified according to the recommendations of the AAST (◘ Table 43.1), based on CT findings. There are other classifications which include clinical evaluation and spleen anatomy [2].

◘ **Table 43.1** AAST spleen injury scale

AAST grade and type of injury	Description
I	
Hematoma	Subcapsular, <10% of surface area
Laceration	Capsular tear, <1 cm of parenchymal depth
II	
Hematoma	Subcapsular, 10–50% of surface area; intraparenchymal, <5 cm in diameter
Laceration	1–3 cm in parenchymal depth
III	
Hematoma	Subcapsular, >50% of surface area; ruptured subcapsular or parenchymal hematoma; intraparenchymal hematoma, >5 cm in diameter
Laceration	>3 cm parenchymal depth or involving trabecular vessels
IV	
Laceration	Laceration involves segmental or hilar vessels producing major devascularization (>25% of spleen)
V	
Laceration	Completely shattered spleen
Vascular	Hilar vascular injury that devascularized spleen

43.2.4 Treatment

It must be done in an expert center as the effectiveness of non-operative management (NOM) depends on the availability of a technical platform and trained physicians.

43.2.4.1 Non-operative Management

NOM is the gold standard for spleen trauma. It involves hospitalization with clinical, biological, and possibly radiological monitoring. It has a rate of success of 90–95% [7]. The failure of non-operative management classically occurs in the first 12 h after admission, with a peak in the first 4 h [8]. The question is therefore to determine when intervention is necessary.

43.2.4.2 Arterial Embolization

Arterial embolization can be used in patients with arterial blush on imaging and ongoing hemorrhage, requiring repeated transfusions, but responding to resuscitation [7]. Prophylactic embolization in hemodynamically stable patients, even if arterial blush is noted on imaging, is not indicated [9].

43.2.4.3 Surgery

Surgery is only indicated for hemodynamically unstable patients who are not responding to active resuscitation (more than 40 mL/kg or 4 units of PBRC) and who present with high-grade lesions on imaging [2]. Surgeons should try as much as possible to preserve a functional piece of spleen, especially as the child is young (<5 years) [10] to prevent the risk of overwhelming sepsis, using splenorraphy rather than splenectomy when possible.

43.2.5 Monitoring

The main concern is the duration of stay and the type of care unit. There is not a consensus between American and European surgeons. APSA published recommendations in 2000 [11] that have been widely applied and criticized [5] reviewed in 2019 [9]. What stands out about these recommendations is that they are safe and protective. They are based on the CT grade, to which it seems reasonable to associate the hemodynamic status of the patient [2, 5]. Our current management is resumed in our algorithm (◘ Fig. 43.1).

43.2.6 Follow-Up

43.2.6.1 Complications

The two main long-term injuries are pseudo-aneurysms and secondary splenic rupture with massive hemorrhage.

The incidence of pseudo-aneurysms is 0.4–17% [12]. They are more frequent in the high grades near the hilum [13].

The incidence of secondary splenic rupture is 0.2–0.3% [14].

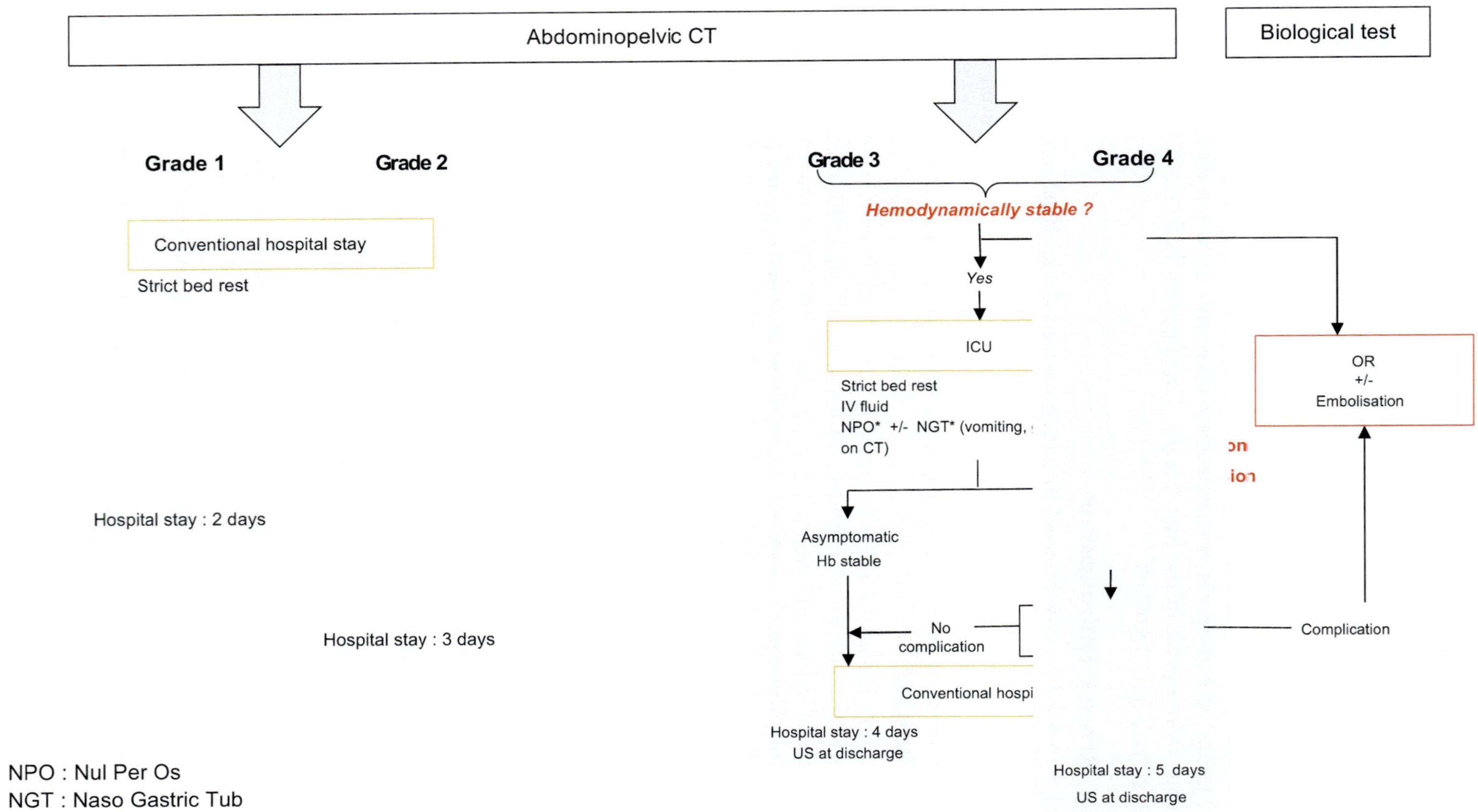

Fig. 43.1 Proposed algorithm for the management of abdominal solid organ injuries

43.2.6.2 Control Imaging

This is one of the most controversial topics in the management of spleen trauma.

For asymptomatic, uncomplicated, low-grade (grade I and II) lesions, routine follow-up imaging is not indicated [12].

For high-grade lesions, a follow-up by ultrasound seems reasonable. We suggest to perform US the last day of hospitalization and 1 month after the trauma.

43.2.6.3 Vaccination

We think that patients with high-grade splenic trauma > III should be considered hyposplenic and vaccination programs should be started at 14 days [2]. There is no consensus regarding the duration of prophylaxis antibiotic therapy; in our center, we give it for 6 months, and we stopped it after control of spleen accuracy test.

43.3 Liver

43.3.1 Frequency

Liver trauma represents 15% of abdominal trauma [15]. It is the leading cause of death with pediatric solid organ injury, mostly by hemorrhage.

43.3.2 Trauma Mechanism

They are the same as for the spleen. The leading cause is road car accidents, followed by sports accidents and child abuse.

The liver is the largest organ in the body in children. Two injury mechanisms explain its damage: A direct impact with a compressive force or a sudden deceleration with traction along livers' attachment points [15]. Bleeding comes from the portal vein, hepatic artery, and hepatic veins and is usually intense initially but tends to subside. Rupture of the bile ducts is likely when the fracture is nearby the hilum and leads to bile leakage that is diagnosed secondarily. The right lobe, particularly the segment VII, is the most frequently affected part of the liver.

43.3.3 Diagnosis

43.3.3.1 Clinical

Pain in the right hypochondrium and flank, along with a history of direct trauma or sudden deceleration. Sometimes, the referred pain in the right shoulder is the first complain of the child. The physician should then look for abrasion or ecchymosis of the right hypochondrium.

In addition, it is mandatory to search for hepatic lesions in case of right thoracic trauma.

Table 43.2 AAST liver injury scale

Grade[a]	Type	Injury description
I	Hematoma	Subcapsular, <10% surface area
	Laceration	Capsular tear, <1 cm parenchymal depth
II	Hematoma	Subcapsular, 10–50% surface area, intraparenchymal <10 cm in diameter
	Laceration	1–3 cm parenchymal depth, <10 cm in length
III	Hematoma	Subcapsular, >50% surface area or expanding; ruptured subcapsular or parenchymal hematoma, intraparenchymal hematoma ≥10 cm or expanding
	Laceration	>3 cm parenchymal depth
IV	Laceration	Parenchymal disruption involving 25–75% of hepatic lobe or 1–3 Couinaud's segments within the single lobe
V	Laceration	Parenchymal disruption involving >75% of hepatic lobe or >3 Couinaud's segments within the single lobe
	Vascular	Juxtavenous hepatic injuries, i.e., retrohepatic vena cava/central major hepatic veins
VI	Vascular	Hepatic avulsion

AAST American Association for the Surgery of Trauma
[a] Advance one grade for multiple injuries, up to grade III

43.3.3.2 Imaging and Biology

Regarding imaging and biology, liver's trauma management is the same as for the spleen.

Notice that cytolysis is frequent, very suggestive of liver trauma but not correlated with severity [16].

43.3.3.3 Grade Classification

The most common classification used is the AAST classification based on CT injury (Table 43.2).

43.3.4 Treatment

An expert center should be the first option even more than for spleen trauma due the late livers' specific complications that could occur.

43.3.4.1 Non-operative Management

NOM is the gold standard for liver trauma. It involves hospitalization, clinical, biological, and possibly radiological monitoring. It has a rate of success of 90–95% [15].

The question is therefore to determine when intervention is necessary.

43.3.4.2 Arterial Embolization

Arterial embolization can be used in patients with arterial blush on imaging AND ongoing hemorrhage, requiring repeated transfusions, but responding to resuscitation. Prophylactic embolization in hemodynamically stable patients, even if arterial blush is noted on imaging, is not indicated [9].

43.3.4.3 Surgery

Surgery is only indicated for hemodynamically unstable patients who are not responding to active resuscitation (more than 40 mL/kg or 4 units of PBRC) and who present with high-grade lesions on imaging [15].

The gold standard procedure for surgical management of liver trauma is perihepatic packing. Even if it is described as less successful in children than adults because of the flexibility of the ribs, and the major risk of abdominal compartment syndrome, it is a safest procedure, when you are not in a pediatric hepato-biliary center [15]. If the bleeding persists, transfer in an expert center should be proposed, as the next surgical steps are a pringles maneuver, and in third line of treatment total vascular exclusion of the liver.

43.3.5 Monitoring

There is no consensus on follow-up. However, it seems that one should be more cautious than for the spleen and the monitoring should be clinically as well as radiologically.

Studies seem to show a relatively low but significant complication rate, particularly in patients with symptoms [15]. It is therefore essential to know specific complications and there symptoms.

43.3.6 Complications

43.3.6.1 Vascular Complications

Pseudo-aneurysms can occur up to 5–10 days after the trauma [17]. They are in a large proportion of cases asymptomatic. They can rupture and cause secondary bleeding.

Hemobilia can occur and can be diagnosed with the triad : pain, icter and gastrohemorrahage. When diagnoed, pseudo anevrysms are mostly treated by embolization.

Bilhemia corresponds to a bilio-sus-hepatic fistula which leads to jaundice by the passage of bile into the blood. Biologically, there is a dissociation between the very high level of bilirubinemia and the low level of alkaline phosphatases. It is exceptional, usually it heals spontaneously; sometimes, a drainage in the bile duct is necessary.

43.3.6.2 Biliary Peritonitis

This is a diffuse biliary leak. It appears between the second and fifth day, but can appear later. The clinic is a peritonitis (pain, fever, generalized contracture). It is confirmed by ultrasound and puncture under ultrasound. It requires surgical exploration or abdominal drainage and secondary endoscopic treatments as biliary stent or naso-biliary drainage may be helpful

43.3.6.3 Bilioma

This is the most frequent complication [18] up to 4%. They occur within a week [19]. They can be asymptomatic or associated with symptoms such as fever, right hypochondrium pain, and feeding intolerance. Its treatment is an echoguided puncture-drainage. It can evolve to an abscess, which gives the same symptoms. Its treatment is also based on an echoguided puncture-drainage.

43.3.7 Follow-Up

43.3.7.1 Control Imaging

We recommend a US at discharge, and 1 month after the trauma with a clinical consultation to watch for any above-mentioned symptoms.

43.4 Kidney

43.4.1 Frequency

Renal trauma occurs in 10–20% of all pediatric blunt abdominal trauma cases [20, 21].

43.4.2 Trauma Mechanism

Pediatric renal injuries are usually caused by deceleration forces causing renal crushing against the ribs or the column or direct trauma to the flank due to falls, sports injuries, bicycle, or motor vehicle accidents [22, 23].

43.4.3 Diagnosis

43.4.3.1 Clinical

Renal injuries should be suspected in all cases with an adequate mechanism of injury and flank hematoma and pain or fractured lower ribs. Due to the underlying high-energy mechanisms causing blunt renal injuries, concomitant injuries of the liver, spleen, and bowel have to be look for.

Table 43.3 AAST renal injury scale

Grade	Type	Description
I	Contusion	Microscopic or gross hematuria. Urological studies normal
	Hematoma	Subcapsular, non-expanding without parenchymal laceration
II	Hematoma	Non-expanding perirenal hematoma confined to renal retroperitoneum
	Laceration	<1.0 cm parenchymal depth of renal cortex with no urinary extravasation
III	Laceration	>1.0 cm parenchymal depth of renal cortex w/out collecting system rupture or urinary extravasation
IV	Laceration	Parenchymal laceration extending through renal cortex, medulla, and collecting system
	Vascular	Main renal artery or vein injury with contained hemorrhage
V	Laceration	Completely shattered kidney
	Vascular	Avulsion at renal hilum that devascularizes kidney

43.4.3.2 Biology and Radiology

Urinalysis, hematocrit, and baseline creatinine levels have to be performed at first. The principal symptom of renal injury is hematuria. Microscopic hematuria (defined as four or more red blood cells per high-power field) is usually find in case of renal trauma, but major injuries as pedicle injuries or arterial thrombosis car occur without hematuria [24] (Table 43.3, 43.4).

Ultrasound examination can help to identify patients with need of further investigations and as a follow-up examination for parenchymal lesions, urinomas, or hematomas, but it cannot detect renal vascular injury.

Contrast-enhanced computed tomography (CECT) with a delayed urographic phase is considered the gold standard for grading renal injuries. Its negative predictive value of renal trauma is as high as 99.8% [25, 26]. Therefore, some studies [27] recommend performing CT as initial imaging modality in pediatric patients with abdominal trauma and visible or microscopic hematuria.

43.4.4 Treatment

43.4.4.1 Non-operative Management

Prolonged observation is now not necessary in patients with grade I and II injuries. Conservative treatment should also be performed in grade III injuries, and in case of hemodynamically stable patient, it should be considered at first in grades IV and V.

Generally, conservative treatment is associated with high success rates with renal salvage rates exceeding 90% [28].

Table 43.4 AAST pancreatic injury scale

Grade[a]	Injury type	Description of injury
I	Hematoma	Minor contusion without duct injury
	Laceration	Superficial laceration without duct injury
II	Hematoma	Major contusion without duct injury or tissue loss
	Laceration	Major laceration without duct injury or tissue loss
III	Laceration	Distal transection or parenchymal injury with duct injury
IV	Laceration	Proximal transection or parenchymal injury involving the ampulla or the bile duct
V	Laceration	Massive disruption of pancreatic head

[a] Advance one grade for multiple injuries up to grade III

Conservative treatment consists of bed rest, frequent vital sign evaluation, hemoglobin/hematocrit measurements, and pain therapy. The length of bed rest is not clearly defined, but generally the "grade bed rest" is also used in renal trauma. It seems that there is no need for systematic urinary catheter or antibiotic prophylaxis.

43.4.4.2 Surgical Treatment

In clinically unstable patients with no response to resuscitation, immediate surgical intervention has to be performed [29]. Discussed indications for surgical exploration are massive urinary extravasation, extensive (>20%) non-viable tissue, and arterial injury

The surgeon can try a renorrhaphy is it seems possible, a partial nephrectomy or nephrectomy in case of threatening bleeding not accessible to embolization [30].

43.4.5 Complications

The therapeutic consequences of the development of urinoma and extravasation of urine remain a matter of debate. Most urinomas are asymptomatic and will resolve in up to 90% of the patients without major intervention [31].

Most of patients with urinoma can be successfully treated with percutaneous drainage and/or ureteral stent placement [32].

Decrease in renal function at follow-up directly correlates with renal injury grade [33].

Follow-up should be performed on the long term in order to evaluate the renal function.

Hypertension after renal trauma is usually seen during the initial hospitalization, rather than during the long-term follow-up.

43.5 Pancreas

43.5.1 Frequency

The pancreas is the least injured solid organ occurring after a blunt abdominal trauma in children. Injury rates range from 1% to 12% of blunt injuries in children with a male gender more commonly affected [34, 35].

43.5.2 Trauma Mechanism

The majority of pancreatic injuries in children occurs after blunt trauma [36]. Bicycle accidents due to direct trauma by handlebar are the most common cause before injury to pedestrians by automobiles, child abuse, and injury to automobile occupants in motor vehicle accidents.

Whereas in adults pancreatic trauma is rarely isolated, in children the majority of pancreatic injuries are isolated.

43.5.3 Diagnosis

43.5.3.1 Clinical

The diagnosis of pancreatic injuries represents a challenge, as the clinical signs are highly non-specific, especially in the early post-traumatic period. Patients usually present with epigastric, right upper quadrant, or back pain associated with nausea and vomiting that can occur with a delay of hours or even days before the onset of abdominal symptoms. Presence of soft tissue ecchymosis in case of handlebar injuries in the right upper quadrant or in the epigastric region must lead to look for pancreatic and duodenal injury.

43.5.3.2 Radiological and Biological

Diagnosis can be suspected in case of high lipase blood serum level from 2 to 12 h after injury [37]. Some studies showed that high level of lipase serum ($\gg$1800 UI:L) is correlated with high-grade pancreatic injury.

Hepatic biology and usual HB level should be associated with the first blood sample [38].

Radiology is necessary to confirm the diagnosis of pancreatic trauma.

Ultrasound is often the first examination done in emergency care unit. It can show free peritoneal fluid and sometimes damage of other organs (spleen and liver).

CT scan is commonly used to detect pancreatic trauma but if it is realized just after the injury it might be repeated 24 h after if the suspicion of trauma persist.

MRCP and/or ERCP is usually used in days after the trauma in order to evaluate the pancreatic duct lesions (complete rupture or not) [39].

43.5.4 Treatment

43.5.4.1 Non-operative Management

Grade I and II blunt pancreatic injuries in children are treated non-operatively.

43

The non-operative approach in this case includes a monitoring of the child's clinical condition, repeated radiological investigations, and monitoring lipase serum levels.

In high-grade pancreatic injury, in case of non-operative management, some studies ask for fasting and parenteral nutrition [34], with a close follow-up in order to detect post-trauma complications such as pancreatic pseudocyst [40, 41].

In case of disrupt pancreatic duct, some studies recommend the insertion of a stent by ERCP in the pancreatic duct [42].

Complications such as pancreatic pseudocyst can be treated by endoscopic gastrocyst pigtail or percutaneous drainage.

43.5.4.2 Surgery

There is a lot of variability in the literature concerning the high-grade pancreatic injury treatment. No randomized studies are available.

Some advocate for operative surgical intervention arguing a lower risk of secondary complications and a lower length stay in hospital.

If the distal part of the pancreatic duct is damaged, spleen sparing distal pancreatectomy can be proposed, if it concerns the proximal pancreatic duct or pancreatic head, roux-en-Y pancreaticojejunostomy with preservation of pancreatic tail is performed.

However, head injuries are very complex to manage, and non-operative management is usually used in the first place to avoid complex surgery [35].

If both pancreatic head and duodenum are injured, radical pancreaticoduodenectomy can be proposed [43–45].

43.5.5 Follow-Up

As high lipase serum level is statistically related to pseudocyst formation, patients with high level should be monitored by lipase levels and ultrasound [38].

Pseudocyst can occur long time after the trauma and should be look for in case of recurrent abdominal pain after an abdominal trauma.

Long-term complications are rare in both management ways, and chronic endocrine and exocrine dysfunction are rarely seen even in patients with high-grade lesions [41, 46].

References

1. Mendelson KG, Fallat ME. Pediatric injuries: prevention to resolution. Surg Clin North Am. 2007;87(1):207–28, viii. https://doi.org/10.1016/j.suc.2006.09.016.
2. Coccolini F, Montori G, Catena F, Kluger Y, Biffl W, Moore EE, Reva V, Bing C, Bala M, Fugazzola P, Bahouth H, Marzi I, Velmahos G, Ivatury R, Soreide K, Horer T, Ten Broek R, Pereira BM, Fraga GP, Inaba K, Kashuk J, Parry N, Masiakos PT, Mylonas KS, Kirkpatrick A,

Abu-Zidan F, Gomes CA, Benatti SV, Naidoo N, Salvetti F, Maccatrozzo S, Agnoletti V, Gamberini E, Solaini L, Costanzo A, Celotti A, Tomasoni M, Khokha V, Arvieux C, Napolitano L, Handolin L, Pisano M, Magnone S, Spain DA, de Moya M, Davis KA, De Angelis N, Leppaniemi A, Ferrada P, Latifi R, Navarro DC, Otomo Y, Coimbra R, Maier RV, Moore F, Rizoli S, Sakakushev B, Galante JM, Chiara O, Cimbanassi S, Mefire AC, Weber D, Ceresoli M, Peitzman AB, Wehlie L, Sartelli M, Di Saverio S, Ansaloni L. Splenic trauma: WSES classification and guidelines for adult and pediatric patients. World J Emerg Surg. 2017;12:40. https://doi.org/10.1186/s13017-017-0151-4.

3. Santschi M, Echavé V, Laflamme S, McFadden N, Cyr C. Seat-belt injuries in children involved in motor vehicle crashes. Can J Surg. 2005;48(5):373–6.
4. Holmes JF, Sokolove PE, Brant WE, Palchak MJ, Vance CW, Owings JT, Kuppermann N. Identification of children with intra-abdominal injuries after blunt trauma. Ann Emerg Med. 2002;39(5):500–9. https://doi.org/10.1067/mem.2002.122900.
5. McVay MR, Kokoska ER, Jackson RJ, Smith SD. Throwing out the "grade" book: management of isolated spleen and liver injury based on hemodynamic status. J Pediatr Surg. 2008;43(6):1072–6. https://doi.org/10.1016/j.jpedsurg.2008.02.031.
6. Gaffley M, Neff LP, Sieren LM, Zeller KA, Pranikoff T, Rush T, Petty JK. Evaluation of an evidence-based guideline to reduce CT use in the assessment of blunt pediatric abdominal trauma. J Pediatr Surg. 2021;56(2):297–301. https://doi.org/10.1016/j.jpedsurg.2020.07.002. Epub 2020 Jul 23.
7. Dariel A, Soyer T, Dingemann J, Pini-Prato A, Martinez L, Faure A, Oumarou M, Hassid S, Dabadie A, De Coppi P, Gorter R, Doi T, Antunovic SS, Kakar M, Morini F, Hall NJ. European Pediatric Surgeons' Association survey on the use of splenic embolization in blunt splenic trauma in children. Eur J Pediatr Surg. 2022;32(6):497–503. https://doi.org/10.1055/s-0042-1749643. Epub 2022 Jul 26.
8. Holmes JH IV, Wiebe DJ, Tataria M, Mattix KD, Mooney DP, Scaife ER, Brown RL, Groner JI, Brundage SI, Tres Scherer LR III, Nance ML. The failure of nonoperative management in pediatric solid organ injury: a multi-institutional experience. J Trauma. 2005;59(6):1309–13. https://doi.org/10.1097/01.ta.0000197366.38404.79.
9. Gates RL, Price M, Cameron DB, Somme S, Ricca R, Oyetunji TA, Guner YS, Gosain A, Baird R, Lal DR, Jancelewicz T, Shelton J, Diefenbach KA, Grabowski J, Kawaguchi A, Dasgupta R, Downard C, Goldin A, Petty JK, Stylianos S, Williams R. Non-operative management of solid organ injuries in children: an American Pediatric Surgical Association Outcomes and Evidence Based Practice Committee systematic review. J Pediatr Surg. 2019;54(8):1519–26. https://doi.org/10.1016/j.jpedsurg.2019.01.012. Epub 2019 Jan 31.
10. Leone G, Pizzigallo E. Bacterial infections following splenectomy for malignant and nonmalignant hematologic diseases. Mediterr J Hematol Infect Dis. 2015;7(1):e2015057. https://doi.org/10.4084/MJHID.2015.057.
11. Stylianos S. Evidence-based guidelines for resource utilization in children with isolated spleen or liver injury. The APSA Trauma Committee. J Pediatr Surg. 2000;35(2):164–7; discussion 167–9. https://doi.org/10.1016/s0022-3468(00)90003-4.
12. Durkin N, Deganello A, Sellars ME, Sidhu PS, Davenport M, Makin E. Post-traumatic liver and splenic pseudoaneurysms in children: diagnosis, management, and follow-up screening using contrast enhanced ultrasound (CEUS). J Pediatr Surg. 2016;51(2):289–92. https://doi.org/10.1016/j.jpedsurg.2015.10.074. Epub 2015 Nov 10.
13. Notrica DM, Eubanks JW III, Tuggle DW, Maxson RT, Letton RW, Garcia NM, Alder AC, Lawson KA, St Peter SD, Megison S, Garcia-Filion P. Nonoperative management of blunt liver and spleen injury in children: evaluation of the ATOMAC guideline using GRADE. J Trauma Acute Care Surg. 2015;79(4):683–93. https://doi.org/10.1097/TA.0000000000000808.
14. Huebner S, Reed MH. Analysis of the value of imaging as part of the follow-up of splenic injury in children. Pediatr Radiol. 2001;31(12):852–5. https://doi.org/10.1007/s002470100004.
15. van As AB, Millar AJ. Management of paediatric liver trauma. Pediatr Surg Int. 2017;33(4):445–53. https://doi.org/10.1007/s00383-016-4046-3. Epub 2016 Dec 27.
16. Weber B, Lackner I, Braun CK, Kalbitz M, Huber-Lang M, Pressmar J. Laboratory markers in the management of pediatric polytrauma: current role and areas of future research. Front Pediatr. 2021;9:622753. https://doi.org/10.3389/fped.2021.622753.

17. Gow KW, Murphy JJ III, Blair GK, Stringer DA, Culham JA, Fraser GC. Splanchnic artery pseudo-aneurysms secondary to blunt abdominal trauma in children. J Pediatr Surg. 1996;31(6):812–5. https://doi.org/10.1016/s0022-3468(96)90140-2.
18. Giss SR, Dobrilovic N, Brown RL, Garcia VF. Complications of nonoperative management of pediatric blunt hepatic injury: diagnosis, management, and outcomes. J Trauma. 2006;61(2):334–9. https://doi.org/10.1097/01.ta.0000197605.27190.2c.
19. Tamura N, Ishihara S, Kuriyama A, Watanabe S, Suzuki K. Long-term follow-up after non-operative management of biloma due to blunt liver injury. World J Surg. 2015;39(1):179–83. https://doi.org/10.1007/s00268-014-2780-z.
20. Singer G, Arneitz C, Tschauner S, Castellani C, Till H. Trauma in pediatric urology. Semin Pediatr Surg. 2021;30(4):151085. https://doi.org/10.1016/j.sempedsurg.2021.151085. Epub 2021 Jul 14.
21. Petrone P, Perez-Calvo J, Brathwaite CEM, Islam S, Joseph DK. Traumatic kidney injuries: a systematic review and meta-analysis. Int J Surg. 2020;74:13–21. https://doi.org/10.1016/j.ijsu.2019.12.013. Epub 2019 Dec 21.
22. Ishida Y, Tyroch AH, Emami N, McLean SF. Characteristics and management of blunt renal injury in children. J Emerg Trauma Shock. 2017;10(3):140–5. https://doi.org/10.4103/JETS.JETS_93_16.
23. Gerstenbluth RE, Spirnak JP, Elder JS. Sports participation and high grade renal injuries in children. J Urol. 2002;168(6):2575–8. https://doi.org/10.1097/01.ju.0000037535.88844.cc.
24. Nguyen MM, Das S. Pediatric renal trauma. Urology. 2002;59(5):762–6; discussion 766–7. https://doi.org/10.1016/s0090-4295(02)01548-0.
25. Brown SL, Haas C, Dinchman KH, Elder JS, Spirnak JP. Radiologic evaluation of pediatric blunt renal trauma in patients with microscopic hematuria. World J Surg. 2001;25(12):1557–60. https://doi.org/10.1007/s00268-001-0149-6.
26. Chowdhary SK, Pimpalwar A, Narasimhan KL, Katariya S, Rao KL. Blunt injury of the abdomen: a plea for CT. Pediatr Radiol. 2000;30(11):798–800. https://doi.org/10.1007/s002470000330.
27. Dalton BGA, Dehmer JJ, Shah SR. Blunt renal trauma. J Pediatr Intensive Care. 2015;4(1):16–20. https://doi.org/10.1055/s-0035-1554984.
28. Redmond EJ, Kiddoo DA, Metcalfe PD. Contemporary management of pediatric high grade renal trauma: 10 year experience at a level 1 trauma centre. J Pediatr Urol. 2020;16(5):656.e1–5. https://doi.org/10.1016/j.jpurol.2020.06.033. Epub 2020 Jul 6.
29. Morey AF, Brandes S, Dugi DD III, Armstrong JH, Breyer BN, Broghammer JA, Erickson BA, Holzbeierlein J, Hudak SJ, Pruitt JH, Reston JT, Santucci RA, Smith TG III, Wessells H, American Urological Association. Urotrauma: AUA guideline. J Urol. 2014;192(2):327–35. https://doi.org/10.1016/j.juro.2014.05.004. Epub 2014 May 20.
30. Okur MH, Arslan S, Aydogdu B, Arslan MS, Goya C, Zeytun H, Basuguy E, Uygun I, Çigdem MK, Önen A, Otcu S. Management of high-grade renal injury in children. Eur J Trauma Emerg Surg. 2017;43(1):99–104. https://doi.org/10.1007/s00068-016-0636-y. Epub 2016 Feb 1.
31. Matthews LA, Smith EM, Spirnak JP. Nonoperative treatment of major blunt renal lacerations with urinary extravasation. J Urol. 1997;157(6):2056–8.
32. Umbreit EC, Routh JC, Husmann DA. Nonoperative management of nonvascular grade IV blunt renal trauma in children: meta-analysis and systematic review. Urology. 2009;74(3):579–82. https://doi.org/10.1016/j.urology.2009.04.049. Epub 2009 Jul 9.
33. Tasian GE, Aaronson DS, McAninch JW. Evaluation of renal function after major renal injury: correlation with the American Association for the Surgery of Trauma Injury Scale. J Urol. 2010;183(1):196–200. https://doi.org/10.1016/j.juro.2009.08.149.
34. Haugaard MV, Wettergren A, Hillingsø JG, Gluud C, Penninga L. Non-operative versus operative treatment for blunt pancreatic trauma in children. Cochrane Database Syst Rev. 2014;(2):CD009746. https://doi.org/10.1002/14651858.CD009746.pub2.
35. Englum BR, Gulack BC, Rice HE, Scarborough JE, Adibe OO. Management of blunt pancreatic trauma in children: review of the National Trauma Data Bank. J Pediatr Surg. 2016;51(9):1526–31. https://doi.org/10.1016/j.jpedsurg.2016.05.003. Epub 2016 May 31.
36. Takishima T, Sugimoto K, Asari Y, Kikuno T, Hirata M, Kakita A, Ohwada T, Maekawa K. Characteristics of pancreatic injury in children: a comparison with such injury in adults. J Pediatr Surg. 1996;31(7):896–900. https://doi.org/10.1016/s0022-3468(96)90405-4.
37. Nadler EP, Gardner M, Schall LC, Lynch JM, Ford HR. Management of blunt pancreatic injury in children. J Trauma. 1999;47(6):1098–103. https://doi.org/10.1097/00005373-199912000-00020.

38. Herman R, Guire KE, Burd RS, Mooney DP, Ehlrich PF. Utility of amylase and lipase as predictors of grade of injury or outcomes in pediatric patients with pancreatic trauma. J Pediatr Surg. 2011;46(5):923–6. https://doi.org/10.1016/j.jpedsurg.2011.02.033.
39. Bosboom D, Braam AW, Blickman JG, Wijnen RM. The role of imaging studies in pancreatic injury due to blunt abdominal trauma in children. Eur J Radiol. 2006;59(1):3–7. https://doi.org/10.1016/j.ejrad.2006.03.010. Epub 2006 Jun 15.
40. Mattix KD, Tataria M, Holmes J, Kristoffersen K, Brown R, Groner J, Scaife E, Mooney D, Nance M, Scherer L. Pediatric pancreatic trauma: predictors of nonoperative management failure and associated outcomes. J Pediatr Surg. 2007;42(2):340–4. https://doi.org/10.1016/j.jpedsurg.2006.10.006.
41. Wales PW, Shuckett B, Kim PC. Long-term outcome after nonoperative management of complete traumatic pancreatic transection in children. J Pediatr Surg. 2001;36(5):823–7. https://doi.org/10.1053/jpsu.2001.22970.
42. Canty TG Sr, Weinman D. Management of major pancreatic duct injuries in children. J Trauma. 2001;50(6):1001–7. https://doi.org/10.1097/00005373-200106000-00005.
43. Jurić I, Pogorelić Z, Biocić M, Todorić D, Furlan D, Susnjar T. Management of blunt pancreatic trauma in children. Surg Today. 2009;39(2):115–9. https://doi.org/10.1007/s00595-008-3823-6. Epub 2009 Feb 7.
44. Kolar I. One early and three delayed distal pancreatectomies without splenectomy and with preservation of the splenic vessels after traumatic transection of the distal pancreas in children. Eur J Pediatr Surg. 2005;15(2):132–6. https://doi.org/10.1055/s-2004-830345.
45. Meier DE, Coln CD, Hicks BA, Guzzetta PC. Early operation in children with pancreas transection. J Pediatr Surg. 2001;36(2):341–4. https://doi.org/10.1053/jpsu.2001.20711.
46. de Blaauw I, Winkelhorst JT, Rieu PN, van der Staak FH, Wijnen MH, Severijnen RS, van Vugt AB, Wijnen RM. Pancreatic injury in children: good outcome of nonoperative treatment. J Pediatr Surg. 2008;43(9):1640–3. https://doi.org/10.1016/j.jpedsurg.2008.03.061.

Immunosuppressed Patients

Jef Willems and Omer Aziz

Contents

J. Brierley et al. (eds.), *ESPNIC Children's Intensive Care Textbook*,
https://doi.org/10.1007/978-3-031-64762-8_44

44

Learning Objectives

After studying this chapter, you should be able to

- Recognize which patients on the PICU should be suspected of having a primary immune deficiency (PID) and to acquire knowledge in the approach of PID-related complications.
- Recognize which patient on the PICU should be suspected of having hemophagocytic lymphohistiocytosis (HLH) and to understand the approach of HLH-related complications.
- Understand organ dysfunction requiring pediatric critical care in the post-hematopoietic stem cell transplantation patient.

44.1 Introduction

Immunocompromised patients account for a disproportionate amount of the overall mortality and morbidity in the pediatric critical care. This is a reflection of the challenges of managing this relatively fragile although clinically heterogenous group of patients. The majority of these patients are immunocompromised as a results of treatment of their primary pathology, such as post-chemotherapy for oncological patients, immunosuppression post-organ transplant, and post-hematopoietic stem cell transplantation (HSCT). The post-HSCT patients are a specific cohort of patients, which will be discussed further later in this chapter. Management of the post-HSCT patient poses particular challenges not only from a clinical perspective, but also from an ethical perspective given the often guarded outcome of these patients on the pediatric intensive care. Patients with primary immunodeficiency disease (PID) may also present to the pediatric critical care; hence, a recognition of this condition is also important and briefly covered in this chapter.

44.2 Primary Immunodeficiency (PID)

Primary immunodeficiency disease (PID) refers to a vast heterogeneous group of more than 150 conditions in which there are inborn errors affecting immunity [1]. Overall prevalence of PID is reported to be between 1:2000 and 1:10,000 [2]. Clinical manifestations of PID include increased susceptibility to autoimmunity, malignancy, and infectious diseases [3]. An estimated 9% of pediatric patients with a diagnosis of PID will require critical care admission, and this rises to 29% of PID who have been treated with bone marrow transplantation [4].

When considering immunodeficiency in the critical care setting, it is important to differentiate between primary and secondary immunodeficiency. Although PID is due to an inherent error resulting in aberrant immunological function, secondary immunodeficiency results from conditions that are acquired or as a result of treatment, for example, immunosuppressive therapy, malnutrition, invasive catheters, and acquired viral or bacterial infections [3]. Secondary immunodeficiency is far more

Table 44.1 Types of PID

Classification	Subtypes and examples	Clinical features
Adaptive immunity: (T-cell and B-cells) Responsible for humoral and cell-mediated immunity. Most T-cell defects also lead to B-cell dysfunction hence resulting in combined immunodeficiency	*T-cell*: Autoimmune regulator gene mutation *B-cell*: X-linked gammaglobulinemia, specific antibody deficiency *Combined immunodeficiency*: Wiskott-Aldrich, ataxia telangiectasia, DiGeorge syndrome, severe combined immunodeficiency disease (SCID)	*T-cell immunodeficiency*: Lymphopenia *B-cell immunodeficiency*: Recurrent respiratory tract infections, severe sinus infections, failure to thrive, hearing impairment, diarrhea *Combined immunodeficiency*: SCID: Failure to thrive, severe infections usually within infancy
Innate immunity: (Phagocytes, dendritic cells, complement proteins) Responsible for initiation of the immune response to a potential pathogen	*Phagocyte*: Chronic granulomatous disease, hyper-IgE syndrome, leukocyte adhesion deficiency *Complement defects*	Recurrent and/or difficult to treat pyogenic infections affecting skin or other organs

Adopted from McCusker et al. (2011)

common compared to PID in the critical care setting. However, the critical care practitioner should be aware of clinical features which raise the possibility of PID in order to undertake the appropriate investigation and have early consultation with the immunology and infectious disease teams. This is particularly important as early diagnosis of PID is essential to reduce the morbidity and mortality that is associated with these disorders [1]. Furthermore, the critical care practitioner may be involved in caring for a patient with PID, who requires critical care for an associated condition, for example, congenital heart defect in a patient with DiGeorge syndrome.

PID has a vast array of clinical presentations; however, susceptibility to infection is a common feature for almost all of the PID conditions [1]. Often, recurrent and chronic infection leading to end organ damage, as well as invasive infection by opportunistic or atypical organisms, is the presenting feature of PID, rather than a severe infection by a virulent organism [3].

PID is classified into those that affect the innate immune system and those that affect the adaptive immune system (see Table 44.1).

The critical care management is aimed at good supportive care of any potential infection or any resulting organ dysfunction. Features which may lead to suspect PID include: recurrent infections, difficult to treat infections, infections with low virulence pathogen, as well as other constitutional symptoms such as failure to thrive. Hence, early discussion with infectious disease/immunology teams would be essential.

44.3 Hemophagocytic Lymphohistiocytosis (HLH)

Hemophagocytic lymphohistiocytosis (HLH) is a life-threatening condition associated with an almost universal mortality if not identified and treated aggressively. HLH is characterized by an unregulated immune response with resultant hyperinflammation and multi-organ failure. The incidence of HLH has been reported to be 1–2 per million in Europe and Japan [5]. A Swedish study indicated a prevalence of 1 in 50,000 live births [6]. The true incidence and prevalence of HLH is, however, not established given that it is a condition that may go unrecognized and the clinical features may be attributed to other conditions such as sepsis and multi-organ failure.

The term HLH is taken from the histological appearance of activated macrophages (histocytes) engulfing host blood cells and their progenitors, which may be evident in various different reticuloendothelial tissue biopsies such as from the bone marrow, lymph nodes, or the spleen [7]. The demonstration of hemophagocytosis is, however, not an essential criteria for the diagnosis of HLH, and may only be evident in between 20% and 50% of bone marrow aspirates for patients with HLH [8]. Furthermore, the histological appearance of hemophagocytosis is not specific to HLH [9]. The diagnosis of HLH is based upon clinical and laboratory criteria. However, a high clinical suspicion is needed in order to consider this relatively uncommon condition [5].

HLH is divided into familial (primary) and secondary forms (FHLH and sHLH, respectively). Both types of HLH culminate in the activated but ineffective innate system (including natural killer cells (NK cells), cytotoxic T lymphocytes (CTLs), and macrophages), which leads to a cytokine storm and thus the clinical features leading to organ damage and the resultant mortality and morbidity associated with HLH.

- FHLH is due to a genetic defect that usually results from a mutation encoding for a gene that is responsible for a protein involved in the immune pathway system. Being already clinically described in the 1950s, it was not until 1999 when the first genetic mutation associated with FHLH was identified [10].
- Most common triggers for sHLH are viral infections (29%) [11] (mainly Epstein-Barr virus (EBV) but also cytomegalovirus (CMV), parvovirus, herpes simplex virus, and human immunodeficiency virus [5]). Malignancy, predominantly hematological in nature but can also be solid tumors, is overall the second most common cause for sHLH (27%). Other infections, including bacterial, fungal, and parasitic infections, account for 20% of the sHLH triggers [11]. Autoimmune and rheumatological (in which case HLH is also referred to as macrophage activation syndrome—MAS) conditions are also associated in 7% of sHLH.

This distinction between FHLH and sHLH is not, however, complete as HLH may be triggered by, for example, an infection in someone who has a genetic defect consistent with FHLH. The clinical presentation of FHLH and sHLH is similar, although FHLH tends to present in infancy in up to 80% of cases [12], whereas the age of presentation for sHLH is more variable. Similarly, the initial treatment of FHLH and sHLH is also the same, namely immunosuppression as well as the treatment of any potential trigger. However, the only curative option for FHLH is bone marrow transplantation. Hence, identification of FHLH is integral to the initial work-up of any patient presenting with clinical features consistent with HLH.

There is also an increased incidence of HLH in several PID syndromes including but not limited to conditions associated with defective cellular granules such as Chediak-Higashi syndrome and Griscelli syndrome, which as well as with recurrent infections and albinism are associated with increased risk of HLH [5]. X-linked lymphoproliferative disease carries, in addition to an increased risk of lymphoma, also a predisposition to EBV infection, as well as an increased risk of EBV-associated HLH.

44.3.1 Clinical Diagnosis

Initial symptoms are very non-specific and may overlap with other clinical conditions in which there is inflammation; hence, a strong clinical suspicion is needed in order to diagnose HLH [9]. Fever, hepatosplenomegaly, and cytopenia are typical symptoms associated with HLH [13]. The typical laboratory findings of HLH include: elevated levels of ferritin, transaminases and triglycerides, and coagulopathy with low fibrinogen levels. The differential diagnosis of HLH includes disseminated infection, malignancies, and autoimmune conditions [13]. This is further complicated by the fact that all of these conditions may also precipitate HLH.

Given the complexities of diagnosing HLH as above, the Histiocyte Society developed the diagnostic criteria for HLH in 1991, which was updated in 2004 [13] (◘ Table 44.2).

Other features of HLH may also include skin rashes, jaundice, and edema [13]. Neurological signs and symptoms including focal neurological signs, seizures, and encephalopathy may be seen. CNS-HLH is associated with pleocytosis and elevated protein levels in the cerebral spinal fluid and with characteristic changes on MRI head including: periventricular white matter changes, meningeal enhancement, diffusion restriction, and possibly necrosis [9].

The pathological role of ferritin in inflammation is subject to debate; however, ferritin levels do correlate with the degree of inflammation [14]. Ferritin levels of greater than 10,000 μg/L are highly specific (96%) and sensitive (90%) for HLH, allowing HLH to be distinguished from other inflammatory conditions [15].

44.3.2 Treatment

The evolving pattern of organ dysfunction in the HLH patient may mean that critical care admission is required. Furthermore, given more than 40% of HLH may be diagnosed in the critical care setting [16], makes it essential that the intensivist is aware of not only of the clinical situations to consider HLH but also the potential evolution of organ failure. Reason for critical care admission in order of reducing frequency includes respiratory failure, neurological deterioration (seizures or encephalopathy), circulatory failure, renal failure, liver failure, and bleeding diatheses; often, patients having more than one organ system affected [16]. Hence, the critical care manage-

Table 44.2 2004 Histiocyte criteria for the diagnosis of HLH [13]

Diagnosis of HLH requires either criteria 1 OR 2 need to be fulfilled
Criteria 1: Molecular diagnosis consistent with HLH: Demonstration of the mutations consistent with FHLH
Criteria 2: Five out of the eight features below need to be met
Fever
Splenomegaly
Cytopenias, affecting more than 2 of the 3 cell lineages in the blood film: *Hemoglobin <90 g/L (in infants <4 weeks: Hemoglobin <100 g/L)* *Platelets <100 × 10^9/L* *Neutrophils <1.0 × 10^9/L*
Hypertriglyceridemia and/or hypofibrinogenemia *Fasting triglycerides ≥3.0 mmol/L (i.e., ≥265 mg/dL)* *Fibrinogen ≤1.5 g/L*
Hemophagocytosis in bone marrow or spleen or lymph nodes No evidence of malignancy
Low or absent NK-cell activity
Ferritin ≥500 μg/L
Soluble CD25 (i.e., soluble IL-2 receptor) ≥2400 U/mL

ment would involve appropriate organ support including ventilation, inotropic support, renal replacement therapy, as well as coagulation support in the form of blood products. Patients with HLH who require extracorporeal membrane oxygenation (ECMO) are reported to have a significantly lower survival to hospital discharge compared to non-HLH patients who require ECMO (30% versus 59% survival) [17]. Organ support is maintained while treatment for HLH is initiated. It is essential that any potential infection is identified and treated.

The management of HLH involves immunosuppressive treatment with etoposide and steroids in the induction phase followed by cyclosporin A for maintenance. Even in the absence of any active infection, the patient is on prophylactic antimicrobials. Patients with CNS-HLH will receive intrathecal methotrexate. Usually, patients with HLH would be expected to show a response with stabilization in clinical condition within 48 h of initiation of steroids. If, however, there is no response within 1 week then other immunosuppressive agents such as anakinra or antithymocyte, globulin may be considered [18].

HSCT is considered a curative treatment in FHLH once clinically stable.

44.4 Hematopoietic Stem Cell Transplantation (HSCT)

44.4.1 General Considerations

Patients undergoing HSCT may be limited in numbers but represent a unique population in PICU and may be considered some of the sickest patients on your unit. Up to 19–35% of HSCT patients will need PICU admission, with many of them requiring repeated admissions.

HSCT is widely performed as curative treatment for an increasing number of conditions which are otherwise fatal or incurable and associated with significant morbidity. It involves intravenous transfusion of hematopoietic stem cells. These have been harvested from HLA-matched related or unrelated donors (allogenic), or from the patient itself (autologous). Prior to the transplantation, the patient receives conditioning therapy in order to destroy residual malignancy and to attenuate immune response. After HSCT, the patient receives immune suppression to avoid graft rejection and prophylactic anti-infectious treatment. After the transplantation and a phase of aplasia, engraftment occurs, with an early and late phase (before and after100 days).

Box 44.1: Key Information Upon Admission of a HSCT Patient on PICU

Underlying disease—Malignant (high-risk solid tumors as neuroblastoma; hematologic as leukemia (*AML adverse outcome*) and myelodysplasia) or non-malignant (metabolic disorders with enzyme deficiency (*better outcome*), primary immunodeficiencies, autoimmune pathology, bone marrow failure syndromes)

HSCT modality—Autologous (*better outcome*) vs. allogenic (via leukapheresis or cord blood)

Conditioning regimen—Chemotherapy, immunotherapy, or total body irradiation (TBI); myeloablative versus reduced-intensity conditioning (RIC—*better outcome*)

Immune suppression—Steroids, calcineurin inhibitors

Prophylactic treatment—Steroids (GVHD), antiviral drugs (HSV or CMV infection (*CMV reactivation worse outcome*)), ursodeoxycholic acid (VOD)

Timeline of key events—Onset symptoms of organ dysfunction (*worse outcome in early phase*)

Essential for the effective management of the post-HSCT patient on the PICU is an understanding of the factors which have led the patient to the point of admission to the intensive care (Box ▶ 44.1) as well as an understanding of the trajectory of organ failure (Box ▶ 44.2 and ▶ 44.3). A multidisciplinary approach, coordinated by the pediatric intensivist, with close involvement of pediatric oncologists, HSCT specialists, immunologists, ID specialists, and other specialists (respiratory team, nephrologist, cardiologist, hepatologist), pediatric radiologists, microbiologists, pathologists, and pharmacists, is mandatory. Early warning systems may help identifying patients requiring PICU admission in a timely manner [19].

Historically, HSCT patients requiring PICU have been considered having a poor prognosis [20]; better understanding of pathophysiology, refining of HSCT techniques, and conditioning regimens, as well as earlier recognition and support of organ failure, have resulted in a better prognosis of these patients, with overall survival to PICU discharge now well above 75% [21]. This, however, remains a poorer outcome compared to the overall survival rates on the PICU.

44.4.2 Approach to the HSCT Patient with Organ Failure

44.4.2.1 Respiratory Failure

Acute respiratory failure (ARF) after pediatric HSCT is a major reason for PICU admission. Incidence is 10–25%, with higher numbers for allogenic HSCT. Pulmonary complications after HSCT usually present as cough, fever, dyspnea, and hypoxia. Distinction between early (<100 days) and late (>100 days) ARF is made. The etiology is diverse [22] (◘ Table 44.3):

An **aggressive diagnostic approach** is warranted, with extensive infectious testing, including rapid molecular diagnostics, broncho-alveolar lavage, and imaging including CT and echocardiography.

Awaiting the results, prompt initiation of broad-spectrum antibiotics, antivirals, and antifungals is advocated. In case of IPS, pulse dose corticoids can be given, but also treatment with etanercept, a TNF-α blocking agent, has been advocated [24].

Many children with ARF will require respiratory support, most of them invasive mechanical ventilation (IMV). A trial of non-invasive ventilation (NIV) may be warranted [25], though mucosal and skin lesions may complicate adequate attachment of an interface. Whether NIV improves outcome is subject to debate [26].

When IMV is indicated, patients usually meet ARDS criteria and a lung-protective ventilation strategy with high PEEP, low tidal volume, eventually prone ventilation, and with permissive hypercapnia and hypoxia, should be adapted. High-frequency oscillation (HFO) can be used without evidence about superiority to conventional IMV. Inhaled nitric oxide (iNO) may be of additional value in case of pulmonary hypertension. Fluid overload needs to be aggressively treated with diuretics and renal replacement therapy (RRT).

The need for IMV reflects high mortality, with survival to PICU discharge in 30–58% [21, 25, 27], with increasingly worse outcome when associated with an infection, IPS [28], combined with the need for CRRT, or with severe hypoxemia (mortality close to 100% when oxygenation index >25). Withdrawal of IMV may follow multidisciplinary ethical discussions, and prognostication by senior experts.

Though extracorporeal membrane oxygenation (ECMO) has been used in refractory ARF in pediatric HSCT recipients, most centers will not offer this modality since outcome is very poor.

44.4.2.2 Acute Kidney Injury (AKI)

Depending on which criteria used an AKI incidence of 20–50% has been reported in pediatric HSCT recipients, with need for RRT in 5–10% [29]. It is often associated with other organ dysfunction, notably ARF. As in AKI in other clinical settings, biomarkers may be poor indicators of severity. Multiple factors contribute to AKI

Table 44.3 Etiology of ARF post-HSCT

Infectious causes
Viral infections – Incidence up to 60% in HSCT recipients – Usually self-limiting but associated with later-on allo-immune activation [23] – Early: Common community-acquired viral infections – Late: Herpesviruses and adenovirus
Bacterial infections – Early: Hospital-acquired pneumonia (gram-positive and gram-negative) – Late: Infections with encapsulated micro-organisms
Fungal infections – Aspergillus and Candida infections are common
Non-infectious causes—Rule out fluid overload and cardiogenic pulmonary edema!
Transfusion-related acute lung injury (TRALI)
TA-TMA (Box ▶ 44.3): Especially if pulmonary hypertension present
Idiopathic pulmonary syndrome (IPS) – Early-presenting disease entity resulting from allo-immune pulmonary damage – Acute hypoxia, dyspnea, cough, and fever in the absence of infection and cardiac failure – Bilateral multi-lobar infiltrates on imaging – Strong association with aGVHD (Box ▶ 44.3) – Features of diffuse pulmonary hemorrhage (may be occult), acute respiratory distress syndrome (ARDS), and acute interstitial pneumonitis
Peri-engraftment syndrome – Inflammatory symptoms including fever, rash, and respiratory symptoms, occurring during neutrophile recovery – Usually a good response to (judicious) steroid therapy
Bronchiolitis obliterans syndrome (BOS) and bronchiolitis obliterans organizing pneumonia (BOOP) – Late-onset manifestations of allo-immune damage – Leading to irreversible lung damage with poor prognosis

occurring early after HSCT: nephrotoxic drugs including cytostatic drugs, pre-HSCT episodes of AKI (tumor lysis syndrome, sepsis, hemolysis, hemorrhagic cystitis), and especially fluid overload (FO), due to often vast amounts of IV fluids, drug solutions, and blood products which are administered during this phase of HSCT. Pulmonary and cardiac problems as well as infection may contribute to FO. There is a clear association between SOS (Box ▶ 44.3) and AKI, presumably with similar pathophysiology as hepato-renal syndrome [30].

Clinical signs of FO as weight gain and edema should be promptly recognized and aggressively treated with diuretics and meticulous fluid management, crucially also prior to PICU admission [31]. Early RRT may be indicated in those patients with FO refractory to this strategy (FO > 10% is considered a threshold for intervention [32]), as return to euvolemia is crucial for survival [33]. The need for RRT in HSCT recipients correlates with high mortality, with survival to PICU discharge of 33–45% to be expected [20, 21, 34].

44.4.2.3 Acute Encephalopathy

Severe central nervous system (CNS) complications are seen in 10–15% of HSCT recipients, frequently lead to PICU admission and are directly or indirectly associated with increased mortality [35]. Central nervous complications in the very early phase after HSCT are often related to aplasia, with besides CNS infections (Box ▶ 44.2) also rarely intracranial bleeding.

One of the most frequently seen complications is **posterior reversible encephalopathy syndrome (PRES)**, usually occurring in the earlier stages after HSCT. It is related to the use of CNIs, especially tacrolimus and cyclosporine (often regardless of levels), and characterized by acute encephalopathy, headache, vomiting, hypertension, cortical blindness, and seizures. Magnetic resonance imaging shows characteristic subcortical/cortical hyperintensity in T2-weighted sequences, preferentially but not only in the parieto-occipital regions. With prompt and aggressive treatment of hypertension and adaptation of immunosuppressive therapy, this condition is usually reversible [36], but life-threatening complications such as severe cerebral edema and intracranial hemorrhage are possible. Other important measures are seizure control and supportive care including correction of thrombocytopenia and coagulopathy.

Seizures frequently occur and may be due to drug toxicity (many drugs used during the HSCT process being neurotoxic, e.g., busulfan, cyclosporin, but also cryopreservatives used for stem cell infusion), or due to metabolic disturbances, cerebrovascular disorders, and CNS infections [37].

Box 44.2: Immune Reconstitution and Infections

Immune reconstitution is a complex process in which first (within weeks) innate immunity (neutrophils, monocytes, natural killer cells but also the mucosal barriers which contain innate immunity), then adaptive immunity (B and T lymphocytes) recover. Quantitative recovery does not imply normal functioning of the components of the immune system, which can take many years to succeed. Many post-transplant complications as infections or GVHD, but also relapse and secondary malignancies, are due to aspects of immune reconstitution and equally affect the success of this process. Increasing insights in these mechanisms lead to better strategies to reduce GVHD and infections [38].

Different types of infections occur at different phases of immune reconstitution.

Often, PICU admission for (septic) shock, ARF, or CNS involvement is required:

- Early (pre-engraftment): Profound aplasia, impairment of mucosal barriers, and presence of indwelling catheters result in a high risk for hospital-acquired bacterial meningitis and blood stream infections (BSIs). Prompt antibiotic treatment targeting gram-positive and gram-negative organisms is mandatory. Also, opportunistic infections may occur, with herpes simplex virus (HSV) causing viral encephalitis or BK polyomavirus causing hemorrhagic cystitis. Invasive aspergillosis (rarely causing CNS infection without a pulmonary focus) may occur already now, but more frequently presents in a later phase.

- Late (after engraftment): Reduced risk for BSI, except in GVHD. Predominantly viral infections occur. CMV infection can be devastating, viral load needs to be followed carefully, and pre-emptive therapy with ganciclovir started early. Also, adenovirus (both local and disseminated disease) and HHV-6 (encephalitis) can cause major morbidity.

Box 44.3: Early HSCT-Related Morbidity

Acute Graft-Versus-Host Disease (aGVHD)

What happens? Activation of the immune system, both innate and adaptive due to HSCT-related damage to the host tissue.

Who's at risk? Younger children, HSCT for malignancies, and especially HLA-mismatch between donor and recipient. Incidence of clinically important aGVHD ranges from 30% to 60% [39].

Presentation? Typically skin, gastrointestinal tract, and liver, but also eyes may be involved. Gut involvement itself can lead to severe fluid and electrolyte imbalances, requiring PICU admission. Surgical approach for major gastrointestinal complications may be required.

What can we do? The condition warrants increased intensity of immunosuppression (high-dose steroid therapy in first tier), after active infection is excluded, but this also predisposes the patient to further infections.

Outcome? Clinical gradation into stages I–IV is associated with increased morbidity and risk of mortality. There is a strong association with IPS and PRES. Two-year survival of children requiring high-dose steroids is 55%, in case of steroid-refractory aGVHD 32% [40].

Veno-Occlusive Disease (VOD)

What happens? Toxicity from the conditioning regimen may result in production of pro-inflammatory cytokines causing endothelial activation, damaging of sinusoidal cells, and post-sinusoidal portal hypertension. Subsequently, hepatocellular dysfunction and accumulation of metabolites further enhance this inflammation and can lead to liver failure and multi-organ dysfunction. Also referred to as sinusoidal obstruction syndrome (SOS).

Who's at risk? Children at younger age (<1 year), conditioning regimens containing busulfan, children with high-risk neuroblastoma, FHLH, and osteopetrosis [30].

Clinical picture? Weight gain, ascites, or hepatomegaly. A rise in bilirubin levels or transfusion refractory thrombopenia. Ultrasound findings as reversal of portal flow, renal and pulmonary failure occur at a later stage.

What can we do? Administration of defibrotide is the mainstay in the therapeutic approach [41].

Outcome? Mortality rate is high when multi-organ dysfunction occurs.

Transplant-Associated Thrombotic MicroAngiopathy (TA-TMA)

What happens? TA-TMA represents an intriguing and incompletely understood disease entity, in which vascular injury of multifactorial origin (conditioning regiment as well as infection) in genetically predisposed patients leads to microangiopathy with hemolysis and thrombocyte consumption. TA-TMA has many features in common with atypical hemolytic uremic syndrome, in which the alternative complement cascade is excessively activated [42].

Who's at risk? Incidence can be as high as 15% of HSCT recipients but is probably underreported.

Clinical picture? A high index of suspicion is required to diagnose TA-TMA, since multiple organs may be affected, with kidney disease (proteinuria and hypertension) and pulmonary vascular disease (hypoxic ARF and pulmonary hypertension), but also gastro-intestinal (ischemic bowel disease, frank gastrointestinal blood loss, and bowel strictures) and CNS involvement (seizures, stroke, or encephalopathy). Hemolysis and thrombocytopenia in the absence of coagulopathy lead to high transfusion requirement. Serositis with pleural and pericardial effusions and ascites. Echocardiography may show signs of right ventricular failure and pulmonary hypertension.

What can we do? Interruption of CNI therapy and plasmapheresis. Infections and GVHD have to be aggressively treated. Improved insights in the pathophysiology have resulted in more targeted (complement-blocking) therapies, with eculizumab being the most readily available drug.

Outcome? Mortality, especially in the presence of multi-organ failure, is high.

Take-Home Messages

- Immunosuppressed patients represent a small but challenging PICU population.
- A high index of suspicion is required to identify those patients without previously established diagnosis of PID or HLH.
- A thorough understanding of the HSCT process is crucial in approaching organ failure in its different stages.
- A multidisciplinary approach is key to a successful diagnostic and therapeutic approach of critically ill immunosuppressed children.
- A patient- and family-centered approach is crucial in conducting ethical decision-making when prognosis is poor.

References

1. McCusker C, Warrington R. Primary immunodeficiency. Allergy Asthma Clin Immunol. 2011;7:S11.
2. Boyle JM, Buckley RH. Population prevalence of diagnosed primary immunodeficiency diseases in the United States. J Clin Immunol. 2007;27(5):497–502.
3. Turvey SE, Bonilla FA, Junker AK. Primary immunodeficiency diseases: a practical guide for clinicians. Postgrad Med J. 2009;85:660–6.
4. Ödek Ç, Kendirli T, Doğu F, Yaman A, Vatansever G, Çipe F, et al. Patients with primary immunodeficiencies in pediatric intensive care unit: outcomes and mortality-related risk factors. J Clin Immunol. 2014;34(3):309–15.
5. Contino A, Trombatone G, Times F. Hemophagocytic lymphohistiocytosis in paediatric patients: a review. J Blood Disord Symptoms Treat. 2018;2(1):1–5.
6. Meeths M, Horne A, Sabel M, Bryceson YT, Henter JI. Incidence and clinical presentation of primary hemophagocytic lymphohistiocytosis in Sweden. Pediatr Blood Cancer. 2015;62(2):346–52.

7. Madkaikar M, Shabrish S, Desai M. Current updates on classification, diagnosis and treatment of hemophagocytic lymphohistiocytosis (HLH). Indian J Pediatr. 2016;83:434–43.
8. Gupta A, Weitzman S, Abdelhaleem M. The role of hemophagocytosis in bone marrow aspirates in the diagnosis of hemophagocytic lymphohistiocytosis. Pediatr Blood Cancer. 2008;50:192–4.
9. Jordan MB, Allen CE, Greenberg J, Henry M, Hermiston ML, Kumar A, et al. Challenges in the diagnosis of hemophagocytic lymphohistiocytosis: recommendations from the North American Consortium for Histiocytosis (NACHO). Pediatr Blood Cancer. 2019;66:e27929.
10. Stepp SE, Dufourcq-Lagelouse R, Le Deist F, Bhawan S, Certain S, Mathew PA, et al. Perforin gene defects in familial hemophagocytic lymphohistiocytosis. Science (80-). 1999;286(5446):1957–9.
11. George M. Hemophagocytic lymphohistiocytosis: review of etiologies and management. J Blood Med. 2014;5:69.
12. Janka GE. Familial and acquired hemophagocytic lymphohistiocytosis. Annu Rev Med. 2012;63:233–46.
13. Henter JI, Horne AC, Aricó M, Egeler RM, Filipovich AH, Imashuku S, et al. HLH-2004: diagnostic and therapeutic guidelines for hemophagocytic lymphohistiocytosis. Pediatr Blood Cancer. 2007;48:124–31.
14. Kernan KF, Carcillo JA. Hyperferritinemia and inflammation. Int Immunol. 2017;29(9):401–9.
15. Allen CE, Yu X, Kozinetz CA, McClain KL. Highly elevated ferritin levels and the diagnosis of hemophagocytic lymphohistiocytosis. Pediatr Blood Cancer. 2008;50(6):1227–35.
16. Buyse S, Teixeira L, Galicier L, Mariotte E, Lemiale V, Seguin A, et al. Critical care management of patients with hemophagocytic lymphohistiocytosis. Intensive Care Med. 2010;36(10):1695–702.
17. Cashen K, Chu RL, Klein J, Rycus PT, Costello JM. Extracorporeal membrane oxygenation outcomes in children with hemophagocytic lymphohistiocytosis. Perfus (United Kingdom). 2017;32(2):151–6.
18. Hines M. Diagnosis, treatment, and management of hemophagocytic lymphohistiocytosis in the critical care unit. In: Critical care of the pediatric immunocompromised hematology/oncology patient: an evidence-based guide. Springer; 2018. p. 159–82.
19. Cater DT, Tori AJ, Moser EAS, Rowan CM. Modification and assessment of the bedside pediatric early warning score in the pediatric allogeneic hematopoietic cell transplant population. Pediatr Crit Care Med. 2018;19(5):483–8.
20. Balit CR, Horan R, Dorofaeff T, Frndova H, Doyle J, Cox PN. Pediatric hematopoietic stem cell transplant and intensive care: have things changed? Pediatr Crit Care Med. 2016;17(3):e109–16.
21. Zinter MS, Dvorak CC, Spicer A, Cowan MJ, Sapru A. New insights into multicenter PICU mortality among pediatric hematopoietic stem cell transplant patients. Crit Care Med. 2015;43(9):1986–94.
22. Chima RS, Abulebda K, Jodele S. Advances in critical care of the pediatric hematopoietic stem cell transplant patient. Pediatr Clin N Am. 2013;60:689–707.
23. Versluys AB, Rossen JWA, van Ewijk B, Schuurman R, Bierings MB, Boelens JJ. Strong association between respiratory viral infection early after hematopoietic stem cell transplantation and the development of life-threatening acute and chronic alloimmune lung syndromes. Biol Blood Marrow Transplant. 2010;16(6):782–91.
24. Yanik GA, Horowitz MM, Weisdorf DJ, Logan BR, Ho VT, Soiffer RJ, et al. Randomized, double-blind, placebo-controlled trial of soluble tumor necrosis factor receptor: enbrel (etanercept) for the treatment of idiopathic pneumonia syndrome after allogeneic stem cell transplantation: blood and marrow transplant clinical trials network protocol. Biol Blood Marrow Transplant. 2014;20(6):858–64.
25. Van Gestel JPJ, Bierings MB, Dauger S, Dalle JH, Pavlíček P, Sedláček P, et al. Outcome of invasive mechanical ventilation after pediatric allogeneic hematopoietic SCT: results from a prospective, multicenter registry. Bone Marrow Transplant. 2014;49(10):1287–92.
26. Peters MJ, Agbeko R, Davis P, Klein N, Zenasni Z, Jones A, et al. Randomized study of early continuous positive airways pressure in acute respiratory failure in children with impaired immunity (SCARF) ISRCTN82853500. Pediatr Crit Care Med. 2018;19(10):939–48.
27. Rowan CM, Hege KM, Speicher RH, Goodman M, Perkins SM, Slaven JE, et al. Oxygenation index predicts mortality in pediatric stem cell transplant recipients requiring mechanical ventilation. Pediatr Transplant. 2012;16(6):645–50.

28. Sano H, Kobayashi R, Iguchi A, Suzuki D, Kishimoto K, Yasuda K, et al. Risk factor analysis of idiopathic pneumonia syndrome after allogeneic hematopoietic SCT in children. Bone Marrow Transplant. 2014;49(1):38–41.
29. Raina R, Herrera N, Krishnappa V, Sethi SK, Deep A, Kao WM, et al. Hematopoietic stem cell transplantation and acute kidney injury in children: a comprehensive review. Pediatr Transplant. 2017; https://doi.org/10.1111/petr.12935.
30. Cheuk DKL, Wang P, Lee TL, Chiang AKS, Ha SY, Lau YL, et al. Risk factors and mortality predictors of hepatic veno-occlusive disease after pediatric hematopoietic stem cell transplantation. Bone Marrow Transplant. 2007;40(10):935–44.
31. Benoit G, Phan V, Duval M, Champagne M, Litalien C, Merouani A. Fluid balance of pediatric hematopoietic stem cell transplant recipients and intensive care unit admission. Pediatr Nephrol. 2007;22(3):441–7.
32. Davis AL, Carcillo JA, Aneja RK, Deymann AJ, Lin JC, Nguyen TC, et al. American College of Critical Care Medicine clinical practice parameters for hemodynamic support of pediatric and neonatal septic shock. Crit Care Med. 2017;45(6):1061–93.
33. Michael M, Kuehnle I, Goldstein SL. Fluid overload and acute renal failure in pediatric stem cell transplant patients. Pediatr Nephrol. 2004;19(1):91–5.
34. Rajasekaran S, Jones DP, Avent Y, Shaffer ML, Elbahlawan L, Henderson N, et al. Outcomes of hematopoietic stem cell transplant patients who received continuous renal replacement therapy in a pediatric oncology intensive care unit. Pediatr Crit Care Med. 2010;11(6):699–706.
35. Cordelli DM, Masetti R, Zama D, Toni F, Castelli I, Ricci E, et al. Central nervous system complications in children receiving chemotherapy or hematopoietic stem cell transplantation. Front Pediatr. 2017;5:105.
36. Won SC, Kwon SY, Han JW, Choi SY, Lyu CJ. Posterior reversible encephalopathy syndrome in childhood with hematologic/oncologic diseases. J Pediatr Hematol Oncol. 2009;31(7):505–8.
37. Cordelli DM, Masetti R, Zama D, Gueraldi D, Rondelli R, Cottone C, et al. Etiology, characteristics and outcome of seizures after pediatric hematopoietic stem cell transplantation. Seizure. 2014;23(2):140–5.
38. Bosch M, Khan FM, Storek J. Immune reconstitution after hematopoietic cell transplantation. Curr Opin Hematol. 2012;19:324–55.
39. Faraci M, Caviglia I, Biral E, Morreale G, Giardino S, Garbarino L, et al. Acute graft-versus-host disease in pediatric allogeneic hematopoietic stem cell transplantation. Single-center experience during 10 yr. Pediatr Transplant. 2012;16(8):887–93.
40. MacMillan ML, Holtan SG, Rashidi A, DeFor TE, Blazar BR, Weisdorf DJ. Pediatric acute GVHD: clinical phenotype and response to upfront steroids. Bone Marrow Transplant. 2020;55(1):165–71.
41. Mahadeo KM, Bajwa R, Abdel-Azim H, Lehmann LE, Duncan C, Zantek N, et al. Diagnosis, grading, and treatment recommendations for children, adolescents, and young adults with sinusoidal obstructive syndrome: an international expert position statement. Lancet Haematol. 2020;7:e61–72.
42. Jodele S, Dandoy CE, Myers KC, El-Bietar J, Nelson A, Wallace G, et al. New approaches in the diagnosis, pathophysiology, and treatment of pediatric hematopoietic stem cell transplantation-associated thrombotic microangiopathy. Transfus Apher Sci. 2016;54:181–90.

Paediatric Onco-Critical Care

POKER (PICU Oncology Kids in Europe Research Group), a Section of ESPNIC

Roelie Wösten-van Asperen

Contents

J. Brierley et al. (eds.), *ESPNIC Children's Intensive Care Textbook*,
https://doi.org/10.1007/978-3-031-64762-8_45

Learning Objectives

After studying this chapter, you should be able to:

- Gain insight in conditions requiring PICU admission resulting from cancer and/or from complications related to therapy directed against the malignant disease.
- Recognise and effectively manage the most important emergencies in paediatric cancer patients.
- Recognise the different inflammatory conditions in critically ill cancer patients.

45.1 Introduction

With more than 3.7 million new cases and 1.9 million deaths each year among adults and children, cancer represents the second most important cause of death and morbidity in Europe among all age groups. New treatments—from precision medicine to immunotherapy—have translated into improved survival and cure rates: currently, 5-year all-cancer survival has increased to almost 80% in children [1]. Despite this progress, death rates from cancer remain substantial and challenging. About 40% of all cancer patients require admission to the paediatric ICU (PICU) at some point during the disease course [2]. PICU mortality rates of paediatric cancer patients are far higher when compared to current mortality rates of the general PICU population [3].

Accelerating progress against cancer may be associated with an increased number of patients who require life-sustaining therapies for disease or therapy-related events over the coming years. The standard of care for the management of paediatric cancer patients admitted to PICU is, in most cases, similar to those applied to other patients. However, the care for critically ill cancer patients is strongly influenced not only by the reason for the need for ICU treatment, but also by the unique features of the underlying disease and cancer treatment. An understanding of the underlying disease and the treatment-related complications is crucial in determining the best management of these patients.

The goal of this chapter is to provide an overview on the pathophysiology, diagnosis, and management of six key conditions requiring PICU admission resulting from the cancer itself and/or from complications related to therapy directed against the malignant disease.

45.2 Tumour Lysis Syndrome

Paediatric tumour lysis syndrome (pTLS) was first reported 1968 by Holland and Holland in five children with acute lymphoblastic leukaemia involving the treatment with allopurinol, hydration therapy, alkalinisation, mannitol, and haemodialysis to prevent renal failure [4]. While pTLS may occur spontaneously, it is usually observed after initiation of a specific tumour therapy. Obviously, there are risk factors for pTLS pertaining to cancer mass, cell lysis potential, renal function, and adequacy of supportive care. A gentle approach by specific tumour treatment protocols to avoid prompt massive cell lysis appears to be paramount for securing organ functions and well-being in children [5–7].

45.2.1 Pathophysiology

The pathophysiology of tumour lysis syndrome (TLS) has been reviewed elsewhere [8, 9]. When tumour cells lyse, potassium and phosphate as minerals, and a high load of nucleic acids are released which are further converted to hypoxanthine, xanthine, and finally uric acid, the end product in humans (◘ Fig. 45.1). Uric acid has a p*Ka* ~5.5 and is poorly soluble in water; at normal concentrations and physiological blood pH, 99% is in the ionised form [10]. The intracellular phosphorous content in malignant cell lines may be four times as high as the amount in normal cells [11]. In plasma homeostasis, one half of phosphate is ionised (present as $H_2PO_4^-$ and HPO_4^{2-}), 40% forms complexes with other ions such as calcium, sodium, and magnesium, and approximately 10% is bound to proteins [12]. In excess, calcium/phosphate formation

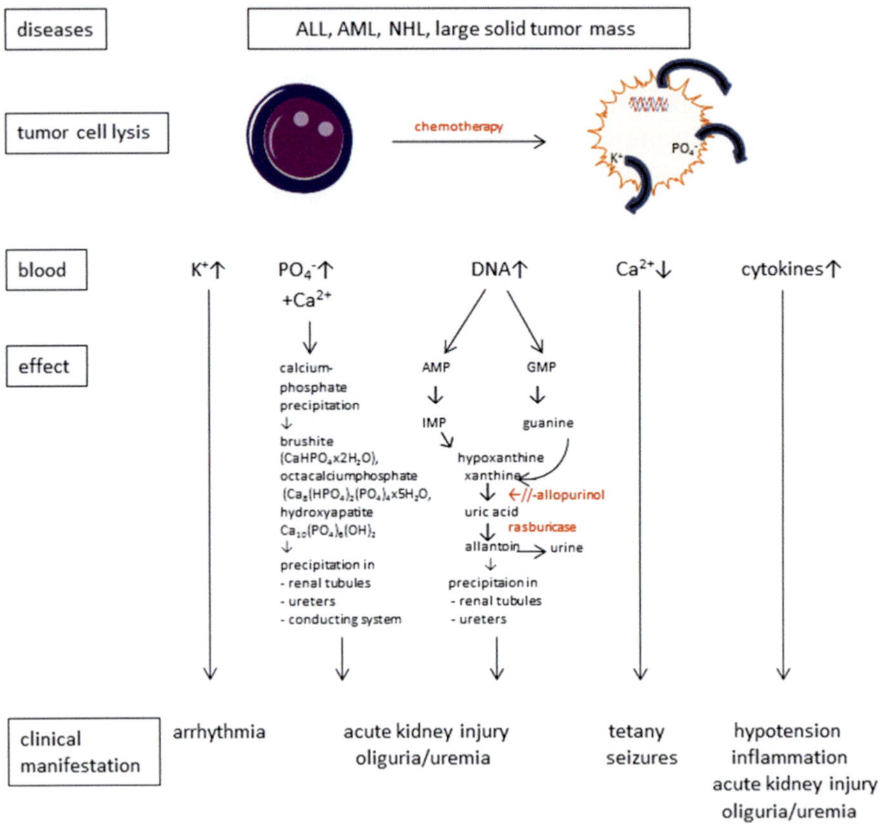

◘ **Fig. 45.1** Diagram illustrating the effects of tumor cell lysis in diseases like ALL, AML, NHL, and large solid tumor masses. Chemotherapy causes tumor cell lysis, releasing potassium (K+), phosphate ($PO4^{3-}$), and DNA into the blood. This leads to increased potassium and phosphate levels, calcium decrease, and elevated cytokines. Effects include calcium-phosphate precipitation, DNA breakdown into uric acid, and potential kidney injury. Clinical manifestations are arrhythmia, acute kidney injury, oliguria/uremia, tetany, seizures, hypotension, and inflammation. Allopurinol and rasburicase are noted for uric acid management. Abbreviations: ALL acute lymphatic leukemia, AML acute myeloid leukemia, NHL non-Hodgkin lymphoma, DNA deoxyribonucleic acid, AMP adenosine-monophosphate, GMP guanosine-monophosphate, IMP inosine-monophosphate involves especially brushite ($CaHPO_4·2H_2O$), octacalcium phosphate ($Ca_8(HPO_4)_2(PO_4)_4·5H_2O$), and hydroxyapatite ($Ca_{10}(PO_4)_6(OH)_2$) generation and transformation [13, 14]. The precipitation of calcium/phosphate compounds is difficult to foresee and may not be predictable by passing the so-called solubility product factor 6 mmol × mmol/L (60 mg × mg/dL) (which solely uses plasma calcium and phosphate concentrations), but depends on a myriad of factors such as magnesium, albumin, fetuin A, bicarbonate, and glomerular filtration rate [15]. Hyperphosphataemia may induce hypocalcaemia resulting in tetany, arrhythmia and seizures, and crystals consisting of calcium phosphate, uric acid, or xanthine may precipitate in the renal tubules causing acute kidney injury, vasoconstriction, impaired autoregulation, decreased blood flow, and inflammation by cytokine release. High levels of both uric acid and phosphate promote precipitation of crystals in tubules. Calcium phosphate may also precipitate outside the kidney, e.g. in the cardiac conducting system resulting in possibly fatal arrhythmias, or in soft tissue (a rare event in paediatrics).

45.2.2 Diagnosis

The tumour lysis syndrome can be classified as laboratory or clinical. Laboratory TLS is characterised by two or more of the following metabolic abnormalities, including hyperuricaemia (uric acid ≥475 μmol/L), hyperkalaemia (potassium ≥6 mmol/L), hyperphosphataemia (phosphate ≥1.63 mmol/L), hypocalcaemia (calcium ≤1.75 mmol/L), or a 25% change from baseline for any of these parameters. Clinical TLS involves arrhythmia, seizures, sudden death, and acute kidney injury represented by a serum creatinine ≥1.5 times the upper limit of normal [8]. In addition, posterior reversible encephalopathy syndrome may be more frequently incurred by children suffering from pTLS [16, 17].

45.2.3 Treatment

Tumour therapy should be delayed until prophylactic measures for pTLS can be initiated. Children at risk of pTLS should receive large amounts of intravenous fluids (0.45–0.9% saline at 3000 mL/m^2/day, 200 mL/kg/day if <10 kg) to improve renal perfusion and glomerular filtration and to avoid metabolic acidosis which promotes the precipitation of uric acid crystals [18]. Furosemide or mannitol may be indicated in case of low urine output (<2 mL/kg/h).

In haematological disorders, tumour cell mass can be easily reduced by leukapheresis or exchange transfusions which in general do not present with procedure-related adverse events [19]. To reduce uric acid levels in blood and organs, allopurinol (10 mg/kg/day oral in 3 doses, 200 mg/m^2/day iv) may be used; however, drawbacks of this kind of treatment are the effect delay by 1–2 days to achieve a significant reduction in uric acid levels, and the risk of xanthine nephropathy and urolithiasis [20]. As an alternative to allopurinol, rasburicase can be used.

Rasburicase is a recombinant form of the enzyme urate oxidase inherited by most mammals except humans converting uric acid into allantoin, a highly water-soluble compound which may be easily excreted by the urine. The recommended dosing schedule for children is 0.1–0.2 mg/kg once daily for up to 7 days including pre-treatment dosages for children with high-risk diseases such as mature B-cell non-Hodgkin lymphoma [21, 22]. Even in highest risk diseases such as B-ALL and Burkitt lymphoma stage III/IV with LDH ≥500 U/L, the introduction of rasburicase reduced the incidence of pTLS (from 16% to 12%) and the incidence of anuria from 9% to 6% in 348 children [23]. A single dose of rasburicase 0.2 mg/kg lowers increased uric acid concentrations in blood by 86% within 4 h compared to an only 12% reduction when giving allopurinol (300 mg/m^2 in three doses daily) [24]. Because of high costs (a 1.5 mg vial is ≈ €100), there have been attempts to establish less intensive/expensive dosing schedules aiming at sufficiently low uric acid concentrations in blood. A single dose of 1.5 mg prevented clinical TLS in 72% of 186 patients with laboratory TLS of which 56% were children [25]. These findings were confirmed in 48 children with successful normalisation of uric acid concentrations regardless of weight base dosage regimens vs. a fixed dose of 7.5 mg [26]. According to individual risk stratification highlighting very high white blood cell counts (>100 × 10^9/L), stage 3 and 4 lymphoma, and high tumour burden neuroblastoma, rasburicase may also be used prophylactically as single dosage administration followed by a second dose in case of initial uric acid concentrations >600 µmol/L [27]. Thus, glomerular filtration rate will be maintained within normal values or recover completely in those children with initial compromise. Rasburicase should not be used in patients with glucose-6-phosphate dehydrogenase deficiency as hydrogen peroxide, a breakdown product of uric acid, may cause methaemoglobinaemia and haemolysis. In a Cochrane Database Systematic Review on pTLS, allopurinol was not graded inferior to the newer recombinant urate oxidase preparation rasburicase despite a slower reduction of uric acid because of less adverse effects [28]. Currently, allopurinol is preferred in patients who are at low risk of pTLS (ALCL, T-cell-non-Hodgkin lymphoma, pre-B-ALL/AML with WBC <100 × 10^9/L) and rasburicase in patients who are at high risk of pTLS (B-cell non-Hodgkin lymphoma, ALL, ALL/AML with WBC >100 × 10^9/L, high-grade lymphoma (diffuse large B-cell lymphoma, T-NHL) with "bulky disease": LDH > 2 × upper limit of normal or large tumour mass on CT (e.g. >10 cm), and any haematological malignancy with acute kidney injury).

Alkalinisation is no longer recommended as high urine pH increases the solubility of uric acid but decreases the solubility of calcium phosphate products; if used at all alkalinisation should be stopped once hyperphosphataemia develops [29]. Of note, in a rat model of acute urate nephropathy treatment with acetazolamide and $NaHCO_3$ to achieve uric acid excretion by the urine, alkalinisation did not stop decline in renal plasma flow and glomerular filtration or increase in tubular pressure, compared to moderately induced diuresis by low-dose furosemide [30].

Children with hyperkalaemia at risk of arrhythmia can be treated with oral or rectal polystyrene sulphonate, glucose and insulin, β-mimetics, or calcium gluconate; hyperphosphataemia will be attenuated by oral sevelamer hydrochloride 50–200 mg/kg/day [31]. Symptomatic hypocalcaemia may be treated with the lowest dosage of calcium to relieve symptoms thus avoiding accelerated calcium phosphate precipitation.

Of course, renal replacement therapy, especially continuous hemodiafiltration, may restore all kinds of electrolyte disturbances in plasma immediately [32]. Interestingly, haemodialysis/hemofiltration dose and mode of continuous renal replacement therapy are no significant factors for survival/nonsurvival [33]. Usually, the need for renal replacement therapy can be prevented by restriction of potassium and phosphorous intake and by intravenous fluids, phosphate binders, and rasburicase.

45.3 Hyperleukocytosis

Hyperleukocytosis is defined as a peripheral white blood cell (WBC) count of >100,000/μL. It typically occurs in haematological malignancies, in children particularly in acute lymphoblastic leukaemia (ALL) and acute myeloid leukaemia (AML). Reported incidence of hyperleukocytosis at diagnosis ranges between 10% and 30% in ALL, 12% and 25% in AML, and ~19% in ambiguous lineage leukaemias [34–36]. Risk factors include infants <1 year, ALL with T-cell phenotype, 11q23 rearrangement or t(9;22), AML morphologic subtypes M4 and M5, acute promyelocytic leukaemia (M3), and inv(16) or FLT3-ITD rearrangements [35, 37]. Hyperleukocytosis itself is associated with severe complications and high morbidity. An increased risk of fatal bleeding and mortality is associated with WBC >500,000/μL in ALL and >100,000/μL in AML. Here, hyperleukocytosis is an independent risk factor for early death before day 15 in AML. Patients with WBC >200,000/μL of with FAB M4/M5 subtype are at even higher risk [38]. Thus, not alone cell number but cell type (lymphoblastic, myeloblastic, monocytic, etc.) as well determines the risk of fatal complications and poor outcome. Such complications mainly arise due to leukostasis (bleeding, infarction, obstruction of the terminal vessels, circulatory failure), disseminated intravascular coagulation (DIC), and tumour lysis. As hyperleukocytosis and its complications significantly contribute to early mortality of children with haematological cancers and are immediately life-threatening, monitoring and therapy must be started without delay.

45.3.1 Pathophysiology

The pathophysiology of hyperleukocytosis-induced leukostasis and bleeding is not completely understood. Two main theories are discussed [39]. The rheological theory highlights leukostasis due to increased blood viscosity. Hyperleukocytosis increases the cellular fraction and cytocrit (haematocrit plus leukocrit) and therefore viscosity, while a decreased deformability of leukaemic blasts occludes micro-vessels and impedes blood flow. The second theory relates to the blast-endothelial interface. Blast secreted cytokines such as TNF-α and IL-β and adhesion receptors such as VCAM-1 have been shown to mediate blast recruitment and adhesion to the endothelium with consecutive endothelial cell damage [37]. High metabolic activity of blasts may contribute to local hypoxaemia. As a consequence of likely both mechanisms, hyperleukocytosis may lead to tissue damage, haemorrhagic, and thromboembolic events. Furthermore, together both theories provide explanation, at least in part, why larger AML myeloblasts cause leukostasis more frequently and at lower blast counts compared to smaller ALL lymphoblasts; and why clinical symptoms and complications remain linked to leukaemic subtype rather than mere cell number. While an increased risk of fatal bleeding and leukostasis is attributed to hyperleukocytosis of >400,000/μL in ALL, such complications are seen at >150,000/μL in myeloblastic AML (FAB M1/M2) and with >100,000/μL in mono- or myelomonocytic AML subtypes (FAB M4/M5) [40, 41]. In promyelocytic AML (FAB M3), fatal disseminated coagulation and bleeding even are observed with no more than >10,000–20,000/μL, underlining that cell numbers provide no more arbitrary thresholds for risk assessment and emergency interventions [38].

45.3.2 Diagnosis

Hyperleukocytosis is diagnosed from a simple peripheral blood count. It requires an immediate differentiation of predominantly mature leukocytes as in infection (such as with pertussis or staphylococci) from leukoblasts in haematological malignancy. Hyperleukocytosis due to infection requires no specific treatment. Any hyperleukocytosis with suspicion of acute leukaemia, however, warrants time-critical management. Because the leukaemic subtype significantly affects morbidity and mortality as well as management of hyperleukocytosis, an emergency subtype allocation (microscopic examination of blood smears) is mandatory. Particular focus must be to diagnose high-risk hyperleukocytosis of FAB M3, M4, or M5. Where unavailable, an experienced paediatric haematologist-oncologist and/or the local study centre must be contacted. Children with critical leukaemic hyperleukocytosis need to be monitored in a PICU.

45.3.3 Treatment

Hyperleukocytosis with impending haemorrhage and leukostasis is a medical emergency. Principal management consists of intensive supportive care and cytoreduction (◘ Table 45.1).

Supportive care aims to prevent bleeding and tumour lysis syndrome. It comprises intensive monitoring of clinical and laboratory parameters. In adults, serum lactate has been suggested as an early indicator of impending leukostasis [42]. Careful hydration with monitoring of fluid balance and diuresis is required, and concurrent administration of allopurinol (with urine alkalinisation) or rasburicase is indicated. Because red blood cell transfusions contribute to increased cytocrit and blood viscosity as well as volume overload, they should be applied with caution. Decreased plasminogen levels <60% have been identified as additional risk factor for fatal bleeding [41]. However, the management or better prevention of bleeding remains challenging, due to disturbances in both coagulation and fibrinolytic cascades. "Physiologic" substitution of both pro- and anti-coagulatory factors with fresh-frozen plasma may contribute to volume overload, whereas specific factor preparations may aggravate disequilibrium. Similarly, platelet transfusion thresholds for thrombocytopenia must take into account individual risks of haemorrhage and thrombosis. Patients with leukostasis, bleeding, and active tumour lysis are at high risk for multi-organ failure. In addition to intensive monitoring, respiratory and renal replacement support should be available.

To prevent and treat hyperleukocytosis-induced bleeding and leukostasis, early cytoreduction is mandatory. As a critical problem, supporting a cytokine-triggered leukostasis theory, induction chemotherapy can initially aggravate leukostasis, DIC, and tumour lysis syndrome. Therefore, current strategies prefer an early low-dose chemotherapy pre-phase. Established paediatric oncology treatment protocols provide specific recommendations, such as cytarabine or hydroxyurea in myeloid leukaemias and steroids in ALL. For example, the German AML-BFM group recommends a starting dose of 40 mg/m^2 cytarabine and in case of insufficient cytoreduction within 12–24 h a 100 mg/m^2/day continuous infusion. If cytoreduction remains insuf-

Table 45.1 Hyperleukocytosis with risk of bleeding and leukostasis—treatment measures (*from AML-BFM 2012 protocol*)

Monitoring on paediatric intensive care unit
Careful hydration and fluid balancing (Potassium-free, ~3000 mL/m²/day; e.g. glucose 5% plus NaCl 10% 30 mL per each 1 L) (Consider furosemide with insufficient diuresis)
Rasburicase or allopurinol with urine alkalinisation (e.g. By adding sodium bicarbonate 8.4% 40 mL per each 1 L hydration fluid) (Aim for urine pH 7–8; in case of hyperphosphataemia stop alkalinisation, pH ~7)
No immediate anaemia replacement to avoid increase in cytocrit (Target haemoglobin 6–8 g/dL)
Coagulation status including fibrinogen, plasminogen, antithrombin III
Fresh-frozen plasma for plasmatic coagulopathy
Platelet transfusion at <20,000/μL (During ET or LA and initial cytoreduction aim >60,000/μL)
Delay diagnostic lumbar puncture until after cytoreduction
Cytarabine 40 mg/m² In case of insufficient response after 24 h 100 mg/m²/day continuous infusion In case of insufficient response after another 24 h initiation of anthracyclines
Consider exchange transfusion of leukapheresis For AML with hyperleukocytosis >200,000/μL or For AML with >100,000/μL and early signs of leukostasis, bleeding or coagulopathies or For AML FAB M4/M5 with >100,000/μL

ficient, early anthracyclines are recommended [41]. With blast reduction <50,000/μL or on day 5 at latest, intensive induction chemotherapy is begun.

While strategies such as emergency cranial or pulmonary irradiation for central nervous or pulmonary leukostasis provide little evidence to support their use, blast removal by exchange transfusion (ET) or leukapheresis (LA) has entered emergency protocols of some paediatric oncology groups while remaining controversial in others [39]. Opponents argue that fatal complications often occur before ET/LA can be initiated, that ET/LA may be inefficient at cost of additional intervention-associated complications and that ET/LA may delay chemotherapy. For example, a meta-analysis of AML treatment studies in children or adults from 1980s to 2012 did not reveal a reduction in early death rate with leukapheresis nor with low-dose chemotherapy induction [43]. In the Nordic Society of Paediatric Haematology and Oncology (NOPHO) AML registry, hyperleukocytosis of >200,000/μL was associated with an increased risk of early death. While ET or LA remained without impact on survival, 26% of patients never reached first protocol chemotherapy induction. The authors therefore conclude a lack of convincing evidence to recommend ET/LA in these patients and advocate rapid initiation of intensive chemotherapy [44]. In contrast, supporting the use of ET/LA, the AML-BFM group shows a trend towards decreased early death rate due to bleeding or leukostasis for ET or LA and strongly recommends ET/LA for children with AML and hyperleukocytosis >200,000/μL. With FAB M4/M5 subtypes or with clinical symptoms of bleeding, coagulopathy or leukostasis ET/LA is even recommended as of >100,000/μL [41].

Comparing LA and ET approach, a targeted apheresis of leukocytes/leukoblasts from the blood stream without additional disturbance of other components appears as intriguing strategy. However, in many clinical settings leukapheresis procedure will require longer set-up time compared to conventional exchange transfusion or be technically unavailable for small children and infants or at emergency hours. With both procedures, large-bore catheters with decreased mechanical destruction or traumatic activation of leukoblasts appear of advantage, whereas their insertion bears additional risk in thrombocytopenic or bleeding patients. While indispensable to generate sufficient flow for LA devices, smaller-calibre central lines suffice for ET. Furthermore, sodium citrate anticoagulation during LA may induce a critical decrease in circulating calcium and requires meticulous monitoring, particularly in small children. Calcium supplementation on the other hand can trigger calcium phosphate precipitation with impact on renal function in tumour lysis syndrome [43]. Therefore, ET may be of advantage in correcting metabolic disturbances and coagulation and providing correction of anaemia without volume overload or hyperviscosity. Yet, no studies have compared efficacy, complications, or benefit of both strategies.

Based on the pathophysiologic theory of blast-endothelial interaction via cytokines and cell adhesion molecules, the use of steroids such as dexamethasone (in non-ALL hyperleukocytosis) appears as intriguing molecularly targeted strategy to inhibit up-regulation of adhesion molecules, cytokine-mediated blast activation and endothelial damage [37], as well as cytokine-mediated systemic inflammatory response that may contribute to hyperviscosity due to capillary leak. However as yet, clinical evidence and risk/benefit analyses are lacking.

Emergency treatment of hyperleukocytosis, a life-threatening early complication in children with acute leukaemia, demands optimal and timely cytoreduction and supportive care provided by an interdisciplinary paediatric oncology and critical care team. With team experience contributing to improved patient outcome, treatment should be centralised at experienced centres [38]. Where diagnosed outside of such centres, immediate consultation should be sought and provided on initial measures and optimal timing of patient transfer.

45.4 Mediastinal Tumours

Both benign and malignant tumours occur in the mediastinum, including neurogenic tumours, lymphoma, germ cell tumours, thymoma, and lipoma. Normal thymus or thymic hyperplasia may be confused with a tumour especially in young children. Imaging plays a pivotal role in these cases by localising the lesions in a mediastinal compartment (anterior, middle, or posterior) and providing the diagnosis based on the specific imaging features. Large mediastinal tumours are more likely to cause airway compression in children than adults because of the combination of the relatively smaller size and greater compressibility of the paediatric airways. Hence, timely management of these lesions is critical to avoid respiratory compromise.

45.4.1 Symptoms

The mediastinum can be divided into three compartments: anterior (superior and inferior segments), middle, and posterior. Masses originating in one compartment may frequently cross over to another. In the paediatric population, most masses are found in the anterior mediastinum. Anterior mediastinal masses are characteristic of Hodgkin and non-Hodgkin lymphoma and less frequently neuroblastoma, germ cell tumours, or other sarcomas [45, 46].

These tumours may cause airway, major vessel, and cardiac compression [46]. Common symptoms of airway obstruction include shortness of breath, cough, stridor, and dyspnoea. Depending on the location of the mass and the degree of pressure on the heart and blood vessels, a mediastinal mass may produce circulatory symptoms, such as venous congestion (vena cava superior syndrome) and pulmonary oedema, or decreased cardiac output due to reduced filling pressures [47, 48]. The vena cava superior syndrome is characterised by oedema of the head, neck, and arms, often with cyanosis, plethora, and distended superficial vessels. As a consequence, thrombosis, cerebral oedema, and/or hemodynamic instability secondary to decreased venous return may develop [47].The severity of the symptoms can vary with posture, with the patient usually adopting a posture himself, where breathing is as easy as possible. Often, a upright position is preferred; in severe cases, the patient may also want to sleep upright.

Although respiratory or circulatory symptoms are often present at presentation, the most significant risk of serious collapse usually occurs after sedation or anaesthesia is given. Therefore, great caution should be exercised before giving sedation or anaesthesia to a patient with a mass in the mediastinum. Life-threatening complications from general anaesthesia are estimated to occur in 15% of cases [49–51]. This is primarily due to decreased lung volumes and compliance, bronchial and tracheal smooth muscle relaxation, and complete collapse of the trachea, bronchi or major vessels due to increased intrathoracic pressure positive by positive pressure ventilation. Masses located at or below the level of the carina may cause an inability to ventilate or oxygenate despite endotracheal intubation [46]. In addition, there is the potential for hemodynamic compromise due to decreased left-ventricular preload and cardiac output when the mass compresses the right cardiac chambers, superior vena cava (SVC), pulmonary arteries, or pulmonary veins [46, 50]. Recommendations for children with mediastinal masses who are undergoing general anaesthesia include maintaining spontaneous ventilation throughout the procedure, avoidance of muscle relaxants and positive pressure ventilation, immediate availability of airway manipulation tools (reinforced tracheal tubes, mainstem bronchus intubation, rigid bronchoscopy), and the availability of cardiopulmonary bypass [46, 52].

45.4.2 Treatment

Because some tumours are fast-growing, there is a preference to start therapy immediately. This means that there is a desire for quick diagnostics by performing a chest computed tomography (CT) and taking a biopsy, both interventions that often require sedation or anaesthesia. Given the risk of problems, a risk assessment and plan of approach is made in a multidisciplinary consultation with the oncologist, radiologist, surgeon, anaesthesiologist, and intensivist [49]. A high risk of perioperative cardiorespiratory collapse and anaesthesia is a contraindication for diagnostic procedures. Tissue that can be obtained relatively easily elsewhere in the body (neck, axilla, groin) for diagnostics without sedation or anaesthesia may be an alternative option [53]. If not, the patient should be treated empirically with intravenous corticosteroids and/or chemotherapy which usually results in the mass rapidly shrinking. If preoperative steroid treatment is given for a short period (usually 5 days), it is still possible to make a conclusive diagnosis [54].

Extracorporeal membrane oxygenation (ECMO) may be used to support a patient through diagnosis and treatment of a mediastinal mass [55]. Supportive care management includes tumour lysis syndrome precautions when steroid treatment is started, elevation of the head of the bed to decrease hydrostatic pressure, supplemental oxygen, and anticoagulation for any thrombosis-related SVC obstruction [56].

45.5 Posterior Reversible Encephalopathy Syndrome (PRES)

Posterior reversible encephalopathy syndrome (PRES) was first described by Hinchey in 1996 [57]. Its exact prevalence and pathogenesis are not well described and understood; nevertheless, PRES is one of the most frequent neurological complications in haematology-oncology paediatric patients leading to frequent admission in PICU. In children with acute lymphoblastic leukaemia, cumulative occurrence ranges from 1.7% at 1 month, to 3.7% at 1 year [58].

45.5.1 Pathophysiology

Subcortical vasogenic brain oedema occurs, but PRES precise pathogenesis remains unclear due to absence of an available animal model and difficulties to obtain biopsies. There are two theories on the pathophysiology of PRES. High blood pressure or high variations of blood pressure could outstrip cerebrovascular auto-regulatory mechanisms. This leads to cerebral hyper-perfusion, which could induce damage to the blood-brain barrier, with interstitial plasma macromolecules extravasation, responsible for significant endothelial dysfunction. Due to endothelial permeability, circulating cytokines could maintain and worsen vasogenic oedema [59, 60]. Another theory, based on direct endothelial dysfunction mechanisms, comes from the observation that PRES was also described in normotensive or hypotensive patients. Immune response trough activation of T lymphocytes could induce cytokine secretion like tumour-necrosis factor (TNF)-α and vascular endothelial growth factor (VEGF), which could directly injure the blood-brain barrier. According to the latter overall theory, hypertension is considered a symptomatic consequence of PRES rather than its primary cause [61]. Some risk factors of PRES occurrence have been identified based on simple univariate analysis: immunosuppressive treatments (e.g. cyclosporine), cytotoxic chemotherapies (e.g. L-Asparaginase, cytarabine, methotrexate), tumour lysis syndrome, graft-versus-host disease, infection, haematopoietic stem cell transplantation, thrombotic micro-angiopathy, and corticosteroids. Hypomagnesaemia and hypercalcaemia could also be contributing factors, maybe through their effect on cell membrane stability [62].

45.5.2 Diagnosis

No definition consensus exists so far, and the diagnosis of PRES will be based on series of compatible signs and the absence of any differential aetiology. It is based on both clinical symptoms and radiological findings:

- Acute or Sub-acute Neurological Symptoms: Encephalopathy and coma (from confusion to deep stupor), headache, visual disturbances, focal neurological deficit, seizure, and status epilepticus, with or without associated intracranial hypertension.
- Imaging: Brain MRI is the best exam to confirm PRES, and to help excluding differential diagnosis (such as infectious or autoimmune encephalitis, cerebral malignancy, progressive multifocal leukoencephalopathy). Nevertheless, there is currently no radiological consensus criteria of PRES, nor any pathognomonic signs. Vasogenic oedema is characterised by hyperintensity on FLAIR and T2-weighted sequences, more or less asymmetric, but always bilateral. Restricted diffusion can also be seen (15–30% of cases). PRES predominantly affects parieto-occipital areas, but may also impair frontal or temporal lobes, the cerebellum, or the posterior fossa. Subcortical white matter is always altered, with more or less associated cortex involvement.
- Cerebral spine fluid analysis remains normal (helps differentiating from infectious or inflammatory aetiologies).
- No electroencephalography alteration is specific of PRES, but published data are scarce [63].
- Outcome: Complete reversibility is frequent but some patients present with persistent neurological symptoms (mainly due to intracranial bleeding complications) and death may also occur in around 3% [64].

45.5.3 Treatment

No guidelines exist on how to manage PRES. Suspected causative agent should be withheld, when clearly identified. Blood pressure should be monitored and maintained in normal ranges with appropriate anti-hypertensive medications, but no randomised controlled trial is available to suggest the most appropriate strategy. In case of status epilepticus, valporic acid and clonazepam should be favoured to prevent the effects of phenytoin, carbamazepine, and phenobarbital on cytochrome P450 induction, and their endothelial direct toxicity [65]. Secondary seizure prophylaxis is recommended, levetiracetam being preferred, but there are no data about treatment duration. Besides, like in any patient with brain damage, secondary cerebral insults of systemic origin have to be prevented, monitored, and treated, especially dys-magnesaemia and dys-calcaemia in this setting. Specific immune treatment effects may be assessed in the near future like anti-TNF-α or anti-VEGF antibodies, based on PRES hypothesised pathogenesis [61].

45.6 Intracranial Hypertension

Intracranial hypertension in oncologic paediatric patients may be promoted by different conditions. Brain tumours are the most common solid neoplasms in paediatric age and may raise intracranial pressure potentially creating a life-threatening condition. Acute haemorrhages or venous thrombosis may cause acute neurologic symptoms or a progressive increase of intracranial pressure. Central nervous system infections may occur, promoting intracranial hypertension. That way, during an onset of oncological disease or during the course of patient's treatment, a child could be exposed to intracranial hypertension.

Personnel must be prepared to recognise the signs of this acute condition, assessing neurological status of the patient according to international resuscitation guidelines and applying multiparametric monitoring [66, 67].

45.6.1 Pathophysiology

Intracranial space is composed by three compartments located inside a rigid skull: brain, cerebrospinal fluid (CSF), and blood. When the mass of one compartment increases, the others try to compensate reducing their volume up to a threshold level beyond which a dramatic rise of intracranial pressure occurs.

Considering the first compartment (the brain), intracranial hypertension in oncologic patients is frequently due to the mass effect made by a brain neoplasm. Both supratentorial and infratentorial masses may produce a rise of intracranial pressure. This effect is amplified by the vasogenic oedema usually developing around the tumour. Typically, the brain component takes up more space, due to the presence of a neoplasm so CSF and blood (uncompressible elements) move to extracranial spaces (spinal subarachnoid space or bloodstream) to maintain an equilibrium [68].

Another mechanism of an increasing brain compartment is the obstruction of blood venous flow due to cerebral venous sinus thrombosis. Thrombosis in oncologic patients may be due to dysregulation of coagulation cascade usually promoted by toxic effect of therapy. Considering this adverse reaction, the most frequently involved drugs are L-asparaginase and steroids [69–71]. Intracranial hypertension is mainly due to the presence of venous infarcts with a following brain swelling.

A mass effect may be also created by cerebral abscesses, that are possible complications in these immunocompromised patients. Oncologic children treated with chemotherapy or following a bone marrow transplant are at higher risk for central nervous system infections. They are exposed to all community or nosocomial infective agents. *Aspergillus*, *Bacillus cereus*, and *Candida* are typical involved agents

[72–74]. However, during central nervous system infections brain oedema promoted by meningitis or encephalitis may occur too.

Considering the second compartment (CSF), it is important to underline that infratentorial neoplasms (mainly medulloblastomas, astrocytomas, ependymomas) may frequently block flow of CSF in the fourth ventricle [75]. They are very aggressive lesions because two mechanisms of intracranial hypertension (mass and obstruction of CSF) work together.

Finally, considering the third compartment (blood), it may increase if haemorrhage occurs. Oncologic patients are at risk of bleeding because of the low number of platelets (following therapies or due to the oncologic disease itself) or abnormal coagulation (due to hepatic insufficiency or presence of sepsis and disseminated intravascular coagulation) [76].

Intracranial hypertension may affect cerebral perfusion and develop a potential compression of falx cerebri, falx cerebelli, and tentorium cerebelli with a life-threating risk of cerebral herniation. However, the variable time course may promote different effect on intracranial pressure rise curve and symptoms may develop with a slow or acute clinical onset.

45.6.2 Symptoms and Clinical Signs of Intracranial Hypertension

Symptoms might differ depending on the duration of the underlying pathology. If solid brain tumours cause intracranial hypertension, the onset of symptoms becomes discrete and worsens over a longer time period, lasting up to several months. Children then suffer from progressive headaches, nausea and sober vomiting, and ataxia if the tumour is located in the fossa posterior. Reduced vigilance, which is the main symptom of acute elevation of intracranial pressure in the acute setting, appears rather rarely before the diagnosis is established.

Somnolence or coma as a sign of acute intracranial hypertension can be assessed by the Glasgow Coma Scale (GCS), assessing the patients' verbal, oculomotoric, and motoric responses to different stimuli. A maximum score of 15 in the GCS represents a fully alert and oriented patient; the minimum score of 3 represents a deeply comatose patient with no reactions to any stimuli. Additionally, focal or generalised seizures represent typical signs of acute intracranial processes as well as hemiparesis. In the infant, a full and bulging fontanelle might occur.

Uni- or bilateral dilated and fixed pupils as well as the so-called Cushing triad (irregular breathing patterns, bradycardia, and arterial hypertension) are urgent signs of cerebral or cerebellar herniation which should lead to prompt diagnostics and treatment [77].

45.6.3 Diagnostics

The mainstay of diagnostics in intracranial hypertension is cerebral imaging by cranial computed tomography (cCT) or cranial magnetic resonance imaging (cMRI). As cCT, in general, is easier accessible and performed faster, it is the imaging modality of choice in case of an emergency. Cerebral haemorrhage, oedema, and tumour can be diagnosed with high sensitivity. Vascular processes like ischaemic stroke and sinusoidal vein thrombosis as well as acute infectious diseases like abscesses often require a cCT with contrast enhancement. Soft tissue processes will be better diagnosed with MRI, e.g. leukaemic meningitis, PRES, or early general hypoxic encephalopathy. MRI investigations do not use radiation, so cMRI will be preferred if no immediate consequences of the imaging are suggested.

If the patient is in a stable clinical condition and intracranial hypertension should be ruled out as one different possible diagnosis, less elaborate diagnostic procedures can be performed. Inspection of the eyes' retina with evaluation of the papilla can rule out or confirm the presence of papilledema. When interpreting this symptom one has to keep in mind that in the acute setting, it might be too early for developing papilledema, and, on the other hand, resolution of this finding might also take several days or even weeks after successful treatment of intracranial hypertension [78, 79].

45

Oedema of the optic nerve can also be evaluated by ultrasound. The use of the optic nerve sheath density might be helpful as shown in some case series performed in patients with traumatic brain injury. Another ultrasound technique for detection of intracranial hypertension could be transcranial Doppler. Decreased (diastolic) velocity, increased resistance index, or either decreased or increased pulsatility indexes of the middle cerebral artery might indicate intracranial hypertension. This technique requires experience, so that inter-individual differences are not deniable. And, infratentorial processes might be overseen by this method [80–82].

45.6.4 Therapy

Many therapeutic options are not well-validated, and in addition, they are mostly investigated in traumatic brain injury. The transmission to intracranial hypertension due to various causes in paediatric cancer patients is questionable but describes clinical routine in many departments.

45.6.4.1 Conservative Treatment Strategies

1. Ensuring Vital Signs

   The first important step in treatment of intracranial hypertension is ensuring vital signs by enabling normoxia (oxygen saturation >96%, arterial oxygen tension 80–200 mmHg), normotension (see also below in topic cerebral perfusion pressure), normocapnia ($PaCO_2$ 35–45 mmHg), and normothermia. Hyperventilation with subsequent hypocapnia leads to cerebral vasoconstriction and should only be considered "last resort" option for short-term reduction in otherwise uncontrolled elevated intracranial pressure [83–85].

   Mechanical ventilation in the acute setting might become necessary if deeply reduced vigilance occurs with a GCS score <9. Sedation and analgesia then help to reduce pain and discomfort, and thus might lead to additional decrease in intracranial pressure.

2. Corticosteroids

   Corticosteroids are widely used to reduce perifocal oedema or other inflammatory processes due to infection in paediatric cancer patients. Already in the 1980s, serial CT studies have shown the reduction of perifocal oedema in brain tumours [86]. However, a recent review on the effect of dexamethasone on oedema reduction in adults with gliomas found conflicting results [87]. No clear positive or negative effects were shown for the use of adjunctive therapy in brain abscesses or acute subarachnoid haemorrhages [88, 89]. The only clear recommendation against steroid therapy derives from a large randomised trial in traumatic brain injury where it led to a worse outcome [90]. Dexamethasone therapy in children with acute or chronic intracranial hypertension will therefore be an individualised decision based on the underlying disease and pathophysiologic mechanisms.

3. Hyperosmolar Therapies:

   Hyperosmolar therapies like mannitol or hypertonic saline increase serum osmolarity and consequently reduce intracellular oedema. Case series demonstrated that both treatment options lead to a short-term decrease of intracranial pressure, whereas the newest results were published with hypertonic saline solutions. Due to the older age of studies concerning mannitol, the actual Brain Trauma Foundation guideline for TBI in children only recommends hypertonic saline. An effective dose could be 3 mL/kg body weight of NaCl 3% as bolus i.v. in 15 minutes. Serum sodium levels should not exceed 155 mmol/L [91, 92].

45.6.4.2 Surgical Treatment Strategies

Surgical therapy can sometimes be an option in intracranial hypertension in paediatric cancer patients. This procedure might be a relative contraindication due to severe thrombocytopenia or coagulopathy. The possible benefits always have to be outweighed against the enhanced risk of bleeding.

1. Monitoring Intracranial Pressure

   A value of 20 mmHg is considered the upper threshold of normal for intracranial pressure measured indirectly via lumbar puncture. In certain clinical situations (e.g. general cerebral oedema due to chemotoxicity with GCS of 8), one might want to measure intracranial pressure ICP continuously or repetitively. The derived values can then be used for guidance of therapy.

   In general, there are two possibilities for ICP monitoring used in children, either an external ventricular drainage EVD or an intraparenchymal catheter. The EVD is probably more invasive with higher risks like bleeding but has two advantages: (a) cerebrospinal fluid CSF drainage to lower the ICP and (b) access to CSF for investigation (e.g. in case of suggested infection).

   Once an ICP monitoring device is installed, the cerebral perfusion pressure can be calculated by subtraction of the ICP from the mean arterial pressure MAP (CPP = MAP – ICP). Of note, in this case the blood pressure transducer should be placed at the height of the external acoustic meatus. Recommendations for target CPP exist for TBI but could be adapted to cancer patients with ICH. Target CPP range from a minimum of 40 mmHg in infants and rise to 60 mmHg in adolescents. The upper threshold not to exceed should be 70 mmHg [93, 94].

2. Surgery of Space-consuming Processes

   If space-consuming processes are surgically accessible and the reason for intracranial hypertension, the treatment of choice should be the surgical intervention for removing or reducing the process. Indications could be a solid tumour, metastases, brain abscess, haemorrhages or hematomas, etc.

3. Decompressive Craniotomy

   If ICH cannot be controlled by conservative and surgical procedures, decompressive craniotomy could become a last option for lowering intracranial pressure. Two RCTs in TBI in adults have been published so far [95, 96]. The results are not completely convincing, so that recommendations for children with severe TBI leave it to an individualised decision-making.

45.7 Sepsis and Non-infectious Inflammatory Conditions

Children with cancer have an increased risk of febrile neutropenia and sepsis due to high-intensity cytotoxic protocols. Chemotherapy-induced leuko- and neutropenia along with broken physiological barriers and indwelling central venous accesses warrants that these children should be considered extremely susceptible to life-threatening infections. This is especially evident during intensified chemotherapy phases (remission induction and re-induction) where patients are particularly susceptible for febrile neutropenia and infections [97]. Cumulative incidence of PICU admission for severe sepsis in all paediatric oncology patients may be as high as 8% with death and/or multiple organ failure in 33% [98]. Sepsis is the leading cause for PICU admission in children with leukaemia and the third most frequent cause in haematopoietic stem cell transplant (HSCT) patients [99, 100]. Furthermore, it is important to acknowledge that not only are these children susceptible to common pathogens but they are also at risk of opportunistic bacteria along with viral and fungal infections and should be treated accordingly.

45.7.1 Sepsis Definition

Accurate and uniform use of sepsis definitions is crucial in conducting future research and in identifying these patients with increased risk. As SIRS criteria lack specificity in detection of those patients with higher risk of mortality, the Third International Consensus Definitions for Sepsis and Septic shock were published by the Adult Sepsis Definition taskforce in 2016 [101]. In January 2024, the Society of Critical Care Medicine Pediatric Sepsis Definition Task Force updated the criteria for sepsis and septic shock in children [102]. The task force developed a data-driven sepsis-related organ dysfunction score, the Phoenix Sepsis Score (PSS), which focused on dysfunction of the respiratory, cardiovascular, coagulation, and/or neurological systems [103]. A Phoenix Sepsis Score of 2 or more identified sepsis among critically ill children with suspected or confirmed infection.

Since children with neutropenia are unable to present a sufficient inflammatory response to infections, traditional signs such as heat, redness, pain, swelling, or even fever does not always appear. This is particularly true to children exposed to steroid therapy in whom localised pain or discrete symptoms can be the only sign of an upcoming infection. Therefore, a thorough history and physical examination should be performed with special attention to potential sites of infection and if in doubt of sepsis or infection the children should be treated as such.

Early IV or port access with blood cultures for bacteria and fungi from all lumens of central venous access devices, urine-, stools-, tracheal-, wound-, or spinal fluid cultures should be performed. Furthermore, blood samples containing at least CBC, CRP, electrolytes, and BUN/creatinine should also be acquired. Multiple biomarkers have been evaluated as possible markers of sepsis. However, despite promising results, no single biomarker has prevailed. This is probably is due to the complexity of the sepsis syndrome in a heterogeneous patent population [104, 105].

45.7.2 Micro-organisms and Antibiotics

To guide antimicrobial therapy, obtaining repetitive blood cultures is crucial. Nevertheless, blood cultures in the neutropenic patient are of low diagnostic yield with positive cultures in 10–40%. Especially when initial cultures are negative, the probability to obtain positive cultures in the following days is even lower [106]. In this view and as antimicrobial drugs are lifesaving in invasive bacterial infections, the empiric use of broad-spectrum antibiotics, often in combination regimens, is mandatory. Classically, especially gram-negatives are targeted (*P. aeruginosa* and *E. coli* being the most prevalent). However, with increased use of indwelling IV catheters, the importance of blood stream infections with gram positives is increasing (especially *S. aureus*).

Good knowledge of local bacterial resistance patterns is essential when choosing correct antibiotics. Antibiotic resistance arising from genetic selection under antibiotic pressure is a well-known phenomenon; however, most gram-negatives are susceptible to piperacillin-tazobactam and carbapenems. Extended-spectrum β-lactamase producing Enterobacteriaceae (ESBL-Ent) and even carbapenem-resistant Enterobacteriaceae (CRE) are increasingly present in chronically ill children and may cause life-threatening infections [107, 108]. As such, third- and fourth-generation cephalosporins are no longer considered adequate empiric treatment. Good surveillance to document individual colonisation patterns before sepsis occurs, thus avoiding inadequate antibiotic regimens, is crucial.

Resistance rates may be very different between age groups and countries, and even between different units within a hospital. Faster initiation improves outcome and adequate antibiotic therapy should be initiated within 30–60 min [109]. Right dosage is extremely important as well, and as many paediatric oncologic patients suffer a certain degree of renal insufficiency, potential nephrotoxicity needs to be taken into account. Therapeutic drug monitoring (TDM) is widely used in certain drugs (vancomycin/amikacin/voriconazole), and PK/PD research in view of optimising dosing schedules for many other antimicrobials is ongoing and may change our practice significantly [110].

As there is a sharp decline in development of new antimicrobials, we have to keep the known drugs as effective as possible. The term antibiotic stewardship (ABS) includes all initiatives to promote responsible antibiotic usage. The goal is to preserve the effectiveness but also to protect patients from unintended effects, such as toxicity and increasing bacterial resistance. Antibiotic stewardship interventions may be restrictive (e.g. formulary restriction, antimicrobial cycling) or persuasive (e.g. audit and feedback, education, guidelines) in nature. Multidisciplinary ABS teams including a paediatric infectious diseases specialist, a microbiologist, a clinical pharmacist, an infection control specialist, and of course the bedside clinicians (paediatric intensivist and oncologist) are suggested for optimal management of these patients [111].

Besides the bacterial infections seen in neutropenic patients, fungal infections may also be devastating. In *Candida* bloodstream infections, mortality rates in paediatric oncology patients are very high [112]. Especially *non-albicans* strains, with significant resistance to fluconazole, are notorious. Diagnosis can be challenging and PCR and candida mannan/aspergillus galactomannan can assist in differentiation between colonisation and invasive infections. In respiratory illness, more invasive approach including broncho-alveolar lavage or biopsies may be needed. Adequate antifungal treatment based on antimycogram and removal of indwelling catheters are cornerstones of the approach.

Viral infections are very common in patients with febrile neutropenia. Depending on the diagnostic tools used (with multiplex PCR for respiratory viruses widely available), respiratory viruses can be detected in up to 57% of these patients. The majority of these cases can be considered single viral infections, about one-fifths as a viral co-infection in children with also bacterial infections. Most commonly detected viruses are respiratory syncytial virus (RSV), human rhinovirus (HRV), parainfluenza virus (PIV), and influenza virus. PICU admission (mainly due to respiratory failure) and mortality are both relatively low in single viral infections. In a patient with diagnosis of a single viral infection, a positive clinical development, and negative bacterial tests, IV antibiotics may be halted early. As such, extensive viral testing may facilitate an antibiotic stewardship intervention [113]. Cytomegalovirus infections are quite common in paediatric oncology patients as well, with incidence of up to 10% in patients with prolonged febrile neutropenia. Usually reactivation occurs in a non-intense phase where also lymphopenia is prominent. PICU admission and organ failure are rare [114].

45.7.3 Septic Shock Management and Organ Support

The American College of Critical Care Medicine Clinical Practice Parameters for Hemodynamic Support of Pediatric and Neonatal Septic Shock offers a useful framework for the approach of paediatric oncology patients in septic shock [115]. The cornerstones are early recognition and early fluid resuscitation and antibiotics. Recognition bundles and early warning systems have been developed, usually assigning high risk to patients with malignancies or stem cell transplantation. Aggressive fluid resuscitation with crystalloids in aliquots of 20 mL/kg and circulatory support with catecholamines improves outcome. Where in the paediatric oncology group the clinical picture of "warm shock" is predominant, norepinephrine is by many preferred, while epinephrine is first-line drug in cold shock patients. However, if dopamine is easily available and well-known in the local settings, dopamine can be used as first-line support. Awaiting insertion of central venous access, these drugs can be administered via peripheral intravenous access.

As many of the paediatric oncology patients have previously been on corticoid therapy, administration of glucocorticoids should be considered in catecholamine-resistant shock.

Extracorporeal techniques may improve outcome. CRRT may be beneficial in fluid overloaded patients, and as many oncology or HSCT patients have pre-existent kidney failure, they are at increased risk for this [116]. Extracorporeal membrane oxygenation (ECMO) may be considered a last therapeutic resort. Considerable morbidity is associated with ECMO and due to survival rates <50% in children without comorbidity and much lower mortality in oncology patients careful oncologic prognostication needs to be taken into account before ECMO therapy is initiated [117, 118]. Though more data are required to further predict which patients are eligible for ECMO, increasingly reports of good outcome in well-selected patients are available, and, this modality needs to be considered in paediatric oncology patients with septic shock as well [119, 120].

45.7.4 Special Circumstances

There are a few situations that deserve special attention. Besides sepsis, other inflammatory conditions may be considered when a paediatric cancer patient with fever is admitted to PICU. New immunomodulating therapies as CAR-T-cell therapy can induce a cytokine release syndrome (CRS) [121]. CRS can be quite difficult to differentiate from sepsis since the syndrome is characterised by fever and multiple organ dysfunction. CRS should be suspected in patients having received immune therapy, such as CAR-T-cell therapy, bispecific T-cell-engaging therapy, or haploidentical HCT. Treatment regimes in light cases of CRS include fluids, antipyretics, and antihistamine treatment, while the severe cases are treated with anti-inflammatory drugs including tocilizumab (IL-6 receptor antagonist) and/or steroids [121]. However, before initiating steroid therapy a specialist in haematology should be consulted as steroid therapy could deplete or eradicate CAR-T cells.

Another inflammatory condition which can occur in paediatric cancer patients is secondary haemophagocytic lymphohistiocytosis (HLH). HLH is a life-threatening condition caused by uncontrolled immune activation and results in early death if not adequately treated. HLH shares features of sepsis or systemic inflammatory response syndrome (SIRS) and in case of a life-threatening emergency, the severity of disease and not the classification should guide initial treatment. Proper treatment includes suppression of hyperinflammation, maximal supportive care, appropriate antibiotic therapy, and elimination of triggers [122]. HLH is triggered by various stimuli, such as infections or the malignancy itself, and can result in uncontrolled immune activation of ineffective NK cells or CTLs [122, 123]. This dysfunction is followed by excessive macrophage activity with elevated levels of circulating cytokines (e.g. INF-γ, TNFα, and IL-6), which leads to the characteristic symptoms (e.g. fever) and laboratory findings (e.g. elevation of pro-inflammatory cytokines, hyperferritinaemia) [122, 123]. Diagnosing HLH is the first critical step towards a successful therapy. It is important to note that there is no single specific feature for HLH, including haemophagocytosis, and characteristic findings are only observed at late stages of disease, but the combination of prolonged fever, enlargement of liver or spleen, and cytopenia are suspicious for a diagnosis of HLH [122, 123]. In paediatrics, the HLH Study Group of the Histiocyte Society has proposed a set of criteria (◘ Table 45.2) to aid routine diagnostic workup and to establish a common basis for clinical trials [124]. In patients with a clinical picture of sepsis, the search for a causative trigger is mandatory and disease-specific treatment is self-evident. This includes appropriate broad-spectrum antibiotic treatment (until culture results) and antiviral therapy in patients

45

Table 45.2 Diagnosis of secondary HLH requires at least five of eight criteria listed below

Fever ≥38.5 °C
Splenomegaly
Cytopenias (affecting ≥2 lineages) Haemoglobin <9 g/dL Platelets $<100 \times 10^9$/L Neutrophils $<1.0 \times 10^9$/L
Hypertriglyceridaemia and/or hypofibrinogenaemia Triglycerides ≥265 mg/dL Fibrinogen ≤150 mg/dL
Haemophagocytosis in bone marrow or spleen or lymph nodes
Low or absent NK cell activity
Ferritin ≥500 μg/L
Soluble IL-2 receptor ≥2400 U/mL

with ongoing viral infections. Prophylactic antifungal therapy may be beneficial for patients with profound neutropenia. In patients with incipient organ failure, intravenous immunoglobulin treatment may be considered. Suppression of hyperinflammation should not be postponed and may include the use of dexamethasone, etoposide, and/or anakinra. It is important to note that immunosuppressive therapy may interfere with the patient's immune system, which is compromised in patients with HLH, but is also important to contain the infectious agent. Therefore, concomitant use of immunosuppressive therapy in patients with infections is critical and careful use of available therapies is mandatory.

HSCT patients also warrant special attention. These patients have often received higher amounts of toxic treatment and suffer neutropenia for longer periods of time. In order to host the new bone marrow, these patients are also often treated with immunosuppressive medication, which often have nephrotoxic side effects. This renders the HSCT patients not only more susceptible to the classical infections but also at increased risk of opportunistic, viral, and fungal infections. Nephrotoxicity can also play an important role when choosing appropriate antibiotic strategy. Close clinical monitoring and prompt empiric treatment with broad-spectrum antibiotics in patients with suspected infection are imperative. Donor granulocyte infusions can on special occasions be considered.

Central line-associated bloodstream infections (CLABSI) are both deadly and costly [125]. Generally, the central line can be exchanged, removed, or attempted salvage with lock therapy. Due to greater difficulties with vascular access in children compared to adults, more providers favour treatment of CLABSI instead of catheter removal. Choosing the correct antimicrobial therapy includes covering classical opportunistic pathogens until microbial resistance has been examined and targeted therapy can be initiated.

Acknowledgements Angela Amigoni, Pediatric Intensive Care Unit, Department of Woman's and Child's Health, Padua University Hospital, Padua, Italy; Roman Crazzolara, Department of Paediatrics, Paediatric Intensive Care Unit, Medical University of Innsbruck, Innsbruck, Austria; Jenny Potratz, Department of General Pediatrics-Intensive Care Medicine, University Children's Hospital Münster, Münster, Germany; Jeppe Sylvest Angaard Nielsen, Department of Neonatology and Paediatric Intensive Care, Rigshospitalet, Copenhagen, Denmark; Eva Tschiedel and Christian Dohna-Schwake, Kinderklinik I, University Medicine Essen, Essen, Germany; Solene Remy and Frederic Valla, Pediatric Intensive Care Unit, Hôpital Universitaire Femme Mère Enfant, Hospices Civils de Lyon, Lyon-Bron, France; Martin Krause, Department of Pediatrics, Universitätsklinikum Schleswig-Holstein, Kiel, Germany; Jef Willems, Department of Pediatric Intensive Care, Ghent University Hospital, Ghent, Belgium; Roelie Wösten-van Asperen, Department of Paediatric Intensive Care, University Medical Centre Utrecht/Wilhelmina Children's Hospital, Utrecht, the Netherlands; on behalf of the POKER (PICU Oncology Kids in Europe Research group) research consortium.

References

1. Gatta G, Botta L, Rossi S, Aareleid T, Bielska-Lasota M, Clavel J, Dimitrova N, Jakab Z, Kaatsch P, Lacour B, Mallone S, Marcos-Gragera R, Minicozzi P, Sánchez-Pérez MJ, Sant M, Santaquilani M, Stiller C, Tavilla A, Trama A, Visser O, Peris-Bonet R, EUROCARE Working Group. Childhood cancer survival in Europe 1999–2007: results of EUROCARE-5—a population-based study. Lancet Oncol. 2014;15(1):35–47.
2. Dalton HJ, Slonim AD, Pollack MM. Multicenter outcome of pediatric oncology patients requiring intensive care. Pediatr Hematol Oncol. 2003;20(8):643–9.
3. Wösten-van Asperen RM, van Gestel JPJ, van Grotel M, Tschiedel E, Dohna-Schwake C, Valla FV, Willems J, Angaard Nielsen JS, Krause MF, Potratz J, van den Heuvel-Eibrink MM, Brierley J, POKER (PICU Oncology Kids in Europe Research group) Research Consortium. PICU mortality of children with cancer admitted to pediatric intensive care unit: a systematic review and meta-analysis. Crit Rev Oncol Hematol. 2019;142:153–63.
4. Holland P, Holland NH. Prevention and management of acute hyperuricemia in childhood leukemia. J Pediatr. 1968;72(3):358–66.
5. Ozdemir MA, Karakukcu M, Patrioglu T, Torun YA, Kose M. Management of hyperleukocytosis and prevention of tumor lysis syndrome with low-dose prednisone continuous infusion in children with acute lymphoblastic leukemia. Acta Haematol. 2009;121(1):56–62.
6. Samochatova EV, Maschan AA, Shelikhova LN, Myakova NV, Beloqurova MB, Khlebnikova OP, et al. Therapy of advanced-stage mature B-cell lymphoma and leukemia in children and adolescents with rituximab and reduced intensity induction chemotherapy (B-NHL 2004M protocol): The results of a multicenter study. J Pediatr Hematol Oncol. 2014;36(5):395–401.
7. Sondhi V, Sharma A, Taneja M, Arora B, Banavali SD. L-Asparginase administration reduces white blood cell count and prevents tumor lysis syndrome in children with hyperleukocytic acute lymphoblastic leukemia. Acta Haematol. 2015;133(1):6–9.
8. Cairo MS, Bishop M. Tumour lysis syndrome: new therapeutic strategies and classification. Br J Haematol. 2004;127(1):3–11.
9. Howard SC, Jones DP, Pui CH. The tumor lysis syndrome. N Engl J Med. 2011;364(19):1844–54.
10. Klinenberg JR, Goldfinger SE, Seegmiller JE. The effectiveness of the xanthine oxidase inhibitor allopurinol in the treatment of gout. Ann Intern Med. 1965;62:639–47.
11. Frei E III, Bentzel CJ, Rieselbach R, Block JB. Renal complications of neoplastic disease. J Chronic Dis. 1963;16:757–76.
12. Granjon D, Bonny O, Edwards A. Coupling between phosphate and calcium homeostasis: a mathematical model. Am J Physiol Renal Physiol. 2017;313(6):F1181–99.

13. Eidelman N, Chow LC, Brown WE. Calcium phosphate saturation levels in ultrafiltered serum. Calcif Tissue Int. 1987;40(2):71–8.
14. Carino A, Ludwig C, Cervellino A, Müller E, Testino A. Formation and transformation of calcium phosphate phases under biologically relevant conditions: experiments and modelling. Acta Biomater. 2018;74:478–88.
15. Bielesz B, Reiter T, Marculsescu R, Gleiss A, Bojic M, Kieweg H, et al. Calcification propensity of serum is independent of excretory renal function. Sci Rep. 2017;7(1):17941.
16. Malbora B, Avci Z, Dönmez F, Alioglu B, Baskin E, Alehan F, et al. Posterior reversible leukoencephalopathy syndrome in children with hematologic disorders. Turk J Haematol. 2010;27(3):168–76.
17. Suzuki D, Kobayashi R, Iquchi A, Sano H, Kishimoto K, Yasuda K, et al. Tumor lysis syndrome as a risk factor for posterior reversible encephalopathy syndrome in children with hematological malignancies. Int J Hematol. 2014;100(5):485–9.
18. Cairo MS, Coiffier B, Reiter A, Younes A, TLS Expert Panel. Recommendations for the evaluation of risk and prophylaxis of tumour lysis syndrome (TLS) in adults and children with malignant disease: an expert TLS panel consensus. Br J Haematol. 2010;149(4):578–86.
19. Haase R, Merkel N, Diwan O, Elsner K, Kramm CM. Leukapheresis and exchange transfusion in children with leukemia and hyperleukocytosis. A single center experience. Klin Pädiatr. 2009;221(6):374–8.
20. LaRosa C, McMullen L, Bakdash S, Ellis D, Krishnamurti L, Wu HY, et al. Acute renal failure from xanthine nephropathy during management of acute leukemia. Pediatr Nephrol. 2007;22(1):132–5.
21. Shin HY, Kang HJ, Park ES, Choi HS, Ahn HS, Kim HK, et al. Recombinant urate oxidase (rasburicase) for the treatment of hyperuricemia in pediatric patients with hematologic malignancies: results of a compassionate prospective multicenter study in Korea. Pediatr Blood Cancer. 2006;46(4):439–45.
22. Galardy PJ, Hochberg J, Perkins SL, Harrison L, Goldman S, Cairo MS. Rasburicase in the prevention of laboratory/clinical tumour lysis syndrome in children with advanced mature B-NHL: a Children's Oncology Group report. Br J Haematol. 2013;163(3):365–72.
23. Wössmann W, Schrappe M, Meyer U, Zimmermann M, Reiter A. Incidence of tumor lysis syndrome in children with advanced stage Burkitt's lymphoma/leukemia before and after introduction of prophylactic use of urate oxidase. Ann Hematol. 2003;82(3):160–5.
24. Goldman SC, Holcenberg JS, Finklestein JZ, Hutchinson R, Kreissman S, Johnson FL, et al. A randomized comparison between rasburicase and allopurinol in children with lymphoma or leukemia at high risk for tumor lysis. Blood. 2001;97(10):2998–3003.
25. Philips A, Radhakrishnan V, Ganesan P, Ramamurthy J, Dhanushkodi M, Sagar TG. Efficacy of single dose rasburicase (1.5 mg) for prophylaxis and management of laboratory tumor lysis syndrome. Indian J Hematol Blood Transfus. 2018;34(4):618–22.
26. Savva DA, Herrera N, Rohatqi R. Comparison of fixed versus traditional weight-based dosing of rasburicase in a paediatric population. Pediatr Blood Cancer. 2018;65(10):e27236.
27. Syrimi E, Gunasekera S, Norton A, Velangi M, Motwani J, Hiwarkar P. Single dose rasburicase is a clinically effective pharmacoeconomic approach for preventing tumour lysis syndrome in children with high tumour burden. Br J Haematol. 2018;181(5):696–8.
28. Cheuk DK, Chiang AK, Chan GC, Ha SY. Urate oxidase for the prevention and treatment of tumor lysis syndrome in children with cancer. Cochrane Database Syst Rev. 2017;3(3):CD006945.
29. Jones GL, Will A, Jackson GH, Webb NJ, Rule S, The British Committee for Standards in Haematology. Guidelines for the management of tumour lysis syndrome in adults and children with haematologic malignancies on behalf of the British Committee for Standards in Haematology. Br J Haematol. 2015;169(5):661–71.
30. Conger JD, Falk SA. Intrarenal dynamics in the pathogenesis and prevention of acute urate nephropathy. J Clin Invest. 1977;59(5):786–93.
31. Kahlon DK, Dinand V, Yadav SP, Sachdeva A. Sevelamer is an effective drug in treating hyperphosphatemia due to tumor lysis syndrome in children: a developing world experience. Indian J Hematol Blood Transfus. 2016;32(1):78–82.
32. Tan HK, Bellomo R, M'Pis DA, Ronco C. Phosphatemic control during acute renal failure: intermittent hemodialysis versus continuous hemodiafiltration. Int J Artif Organs. 2001;24(4):186–91.

33. Fleming GM, Walters S, Goldstein SL, Alexander SR, Baum MA, Blowey DL, et al. Nonrenal indications for continuous renal replacement therapy: a report from the Prospective Pediatric Continuous Renal Replacement Therapy Registry group. Pediatr Crit Care Med. 2012;13(5):e299–304.
34. Ruggiero A, Rizzo D, Amato M, Riccardi R. Management of hyperleucocytosis. Curr Treat Opt in Oncol. 2016;17(2):7.
35. Sung L, Aplenc R, Alonzo TA, Gerbing RB, Gamis AS. Predictors and short-term outcomes of hyperleucocytosis in children with acute myeloid leukemia: a report from the Children's Oncology Group. Haematologica. 2012;97(11):1770–2.
36. Gerr H, Zimmermann M, Schrappe M, Dworzak M, Ludwig W-D, Bradtke J, Moericke A, Schabath R, Creutzig U, Reinhardt D. Acute leukaemias of ambigous lineage in children: characterization, prognosis and therapy recommendations. Br J Haematol. 2019;149(1):84–92.
37. Porcu P, Cripe LD, Ng EW, Bhatia S, Danielson CM, Orazi A, McCarthy LJ. Hyperleukocytic leukemias and leukostasis: a review of pathophysiology, clinical presentation and management. Leuk Lymphoma. 2000;39(1–2):1–18.
38. Creutzig U, Zimmermann M, Reinhardt D, Dworzak M, Stary J, Lehrnbecher T. Early deaths and treatment-related mortality in children undergoing therapy for acute myeloid leukemia: analysis of the multicenter clinical trials AML-BFM 93 and AML-BFM 98. J Clin Oncol. 2004;22(21):4384–93.
39. Ganzel C, Becker J, Mintz PD, Lazarus HM, Rowe JM. Hyperleukocytosis, leukostasis and leukapheresis: practice management. Blood Rev. 2012;26(3):117–22.
40. Lowe EJ, Pui CH, Hancock ML, Geiger TL, Khan RB, Sandlund JT. Early complications in children with acute lymphoblastic leukemia presenting with hyperleukocytosis. Pediatr Blood Cancer. 2005;45(1):10–5.
41. Creutzig U, Rössig C, Dworzak M, Stary J, von Stackelberg A, Wössmann W, Zimmermann M, Reinhardt D. Exchange transfusion and leukapheresis in pediatric patients with AML with high risk of early death by bleeding and leukostasis. Pediatr Blood Cancer. 2016;63(4):640–5.
42. Stemmler J, Wittmann GW, Hacker U, Heinemann V. Leukapheresis in chronic myelomonocytic leukemia with leukostasis syndrome: elevated serum lactate levels as an early sign of microcirculation failure. Leuk Lymphoma. 2002;43(7):1427–30.
43. Oberoi S, Lehrnbecher T, Phillips B, Hitzler J, Ethier MC, Beyene J, Sung L. Leukapheresis and low-dose chemotherapy do not reduce early mortality in acute myeloid leukemia hyperleukocytosis: a systematic review and meta-analysis. Leuk Res. 2014;38(4):460–8.
44. Zeller B, Glosli H, Forestier E, Ha SY, Jahnukainen K, Jónsson ÓG, Lausen B, Palle J, Hasle H, Abrahamsson J, NOPHO AML working group. Hyperleucocytosis in paediatric acute myeloid leukaemia—the challenge of white blood cell counts above 200 × 10^9/l. The NOPHO experience 1984–2014. Br J Haematol. 2017;178(3):448–56.
45. Ward E, DeSantis C, Robbins A, Kohler B, Jemal A. Childhood and adolescent cancer statistics, 2014. CA Cancer J Clin. 2014;64(2):83–103.
46. Pearson JK, Tan GM. Pediatric anterior mediastinal mass: a review article. Semin Cardiothorac Vasc Anesth. 2015;19(3):248–54.
47. Wilson LD, Detterbeck FC, Yahalom J. Clinical practice. Superior vena cava syndrome with malignant causes. N Engl J Med. 2007;356(18):1862–9.
48. Blank RS, de Souza DG. Anesthetic management of patients with an anterior mediastinal mass: continuing professional development. Can J Anaesth. 2011;58:853–59, 860–7.
49. Acker SN, Linton J, Tan GM, Garrington TP, Bruny J, Hilden JM, Hoffman LM, Partrick DA. A multidisciplinary approach to the management of anterior mediastinal masses in children. J Pediatr Surg. 2015;50(5):875–8.
50. Garey CL, Laituri CA, Valusek PA, St Peter SD, Snyder CL. Management of anterior mediastinal masses in children. Eur J Pediatr Surg. 2011;21(5):310–3.
51. Ng A, Bennett J, Bromley P, Davies P, Morland B. Anaesthetic outcome and predictive risk factors in children with mediastinal tumours. Pediatr Blood Cancer. 2007;48(2):160–4.
52. Anghelescu DL, Burgoyne LL, Liu T, Li CS, Pui CH, Hudson MM, Furman WL, Sandlund JT. Clinical and diagnostic imaging findings predict anesthetic complications in children presenting with malignant mediastinal masses. Paediatr Anaesth. 2007;17(11):1090–8.

53. Malik R, Mullassery D, Kleine-Brueggeney M, Atra A, Gour A, Sunderland R, Okoye B. Anterior mediastinal masses—a multidisciplinary pathway for safe diagnostic procedures. J Pediatr Surg. 2019;54(2):251–4.
54. Hack HA, Wright NB, Wynn RF. The anaesthetic management of children with anterior mediastinal masses. Anaesthesia. 2008;63(8):837–46.
55. Frey TK, Chopra A, Lin RJ, Levy RJ, Gruber P, Rheingold SR, Hoehn KS. A child with anterior mediastinal mass supported with veno-arterial extracorporeal membrane oxygenation. Pediatr Crit Care Med. 2006;7(5):479–81.
56. McCurdy MT, Shanholtz CB. Oncologic emergencies. Crit Care Med. 2012;40(7):2212–22.
57. Hinchey J, Chaves C, Appignani B, Breen J, Pao L, Wang A, et al. A reversible posterior leukoencephalopathy syndrome. N Engl J Med. 1996;334(8):494–500.
58. Anastasopoulou S, Eriksson MA, Heyman M, Wang C, Niinimäki R, Mikkel S, et al. Posterior reversible encephalopathy syndrome in children with acute lymphoblastic leukemia: clinical characteristics, risk factors, course, and outcome of disease. Pediatr Blood Cancer. 2019;66(5):e27594.
59. Fugate JE, Rabinstein AA. Posterior reversible encephalopathy syndrome: clinical and radiological manifestations, pathophysiology, and outstanding questions. Lancet Neurol. 2015;14(9):914–25.
60. Gasparini S, Ferlazzo E, Sueri C, Cianci V, Ascoli M, Cavalli SM, et al. Hypertension, seizures, and epilepsy: a review on pathophysiology and management. Neurol Sci. 2019;40(9):1775–83.
61. Marra A, Vargas M, Striano P, Del Guercio L, Buonanno P, Servillo G. Posterior reversible encephalopathy syndrome: the endothelial hypotheses. Med Hypotheses. 2014;82(5):619–22.
62. Ghali MGZ, Davanzo J, Leo M, Rizk E. Posterior reversible encephalopathy syndrome in pediatric patients: pathophysiology, diagnosis, and management. Leuk Lymphoma. 2019;60(10):2365–72.
63. Murray K, Amin U, Maciver S, Benbadis SR. EEG Findings in posterior reversible encephalopathy syndrome. Clin EEG Neurosci. 2019;50(5):366–9.
64. Zama D, Gasperini P, Berger M, Petris M, De Pasquale MD, Cesaro S, et al. A survey on hematology-oncology pediatric AIEOP centres: the challenge of posterior reversible encephalopathy syndrome. Eur J Haematol. 2018;100(1):75–82.
65. Bechstein WO. Neurotoxicity of calcineurin inhibitors: impact and clinical management. Transpl Int. 2000;13(5):313–26.
66. Kelly KM, Lange B. Oncologic emergencies. Pediatr Clin North Am. 1997;44(4):809–30.
67. Prusakowski MK, Cannone D. Pediatric oncologic emergencies. Hematol Oncol Clin North Am. 2017;31(6):959–80.
68. Shaffner DH, Nichols DG, editors. Rogers textbook of pediatric intensive care. 5th ed. Lippincott Williams & Wilkins; 2015.
69. Ghanem KM, Dhayni RM, Al-Aridi C, Tarek N, Tamim H, Chan AKC, Saab R, Abboud MR, El-Solh H, Muwakkit SA. Cerebral sinus venous thrombosis during childhood acute lymphoblastic leukemia therapy: risk factors and management. Pediatr Blood Cancer. 2017;64(12).
70. Millan NC, Pastrana A, Guitter MR, Zubizarreta PA, Monges MS, Felice MS. Acute and subacute neurological toxicity in children treated for acute lymphoblastic leukemia. Leuk Res. 2018;65:86–93.
71. Ranta S, Tuckuviene R, Mäkipernaa A, Albertsen BK, Frisk T, Tedgård U, Jónsson ÓG, Pruunsild K, Gretenkort Andersson N, Winther Gunnes M, Saulyte Trakymiene S, Frandsen T, Heyman M, Ruud E, Helgestad J. Cerebral sinus venous thromboses in children with acute lymphoblastic leukaemia—a multicentre study from the Nordic Society of Paediatric Haematology and Oncology. Br J Haematol. 2015;168(4):547–52.
72. Sadarangani M, Harvey M, McDonald A, Speert DP, Dix D. Brain abscesses due to Aspergillus nidulans infection during induction chemotherapy for acute lymphoblastic leukemia. J Pediatr Hematol Oncol. 2015;37(6):e384–6.
73. Dotis J, Iosifidis E, Roilides E. Central nervous system aspergillosis in children: a systematic review of reported cases. Int J Infect Dis. 2007;11(5):381–93.
74. Dabscheck G, Silverman L, Ullrich NJ. Bacillus cereus cerebral abscess during induction chemotherapy for childhood acute leukemia. J Pediatr Hematol Oncol. 2015;37(7):568–9.
75. Wong TT, Liang ML, Chen HH, Chang FC. Hydrocephalus with brain tumors in children. Childs Nerv Syst. 2011;27(10):1723–34.

76. Noje C, Cohen K, Jordan LC. Hemorrhagic and ischemic stroke in children with cancer. Pediatr Neurol. 2013;49(4):237–42.
77. Tasker RC, Czosnyka M. Intracranial hypertension and brain monitoring. In: Peditric critical care. 3rd ed. Mosby Elsevier.
78. Fernández-García MÁ, Cantarín-Extremera V, Andión-Catalán M, Duat-Rodríguez A, Jiménez-Echevarría S, Bermejo-Arnedo I, Hortigüela-Saeta M, Rekarte-García S, Babín-López L, Ruano Domínguez D. Secondary intracranial hypertension in pediatric patients with leukemia. Pediatr Neurol. 2017;77:48–53.
79. Rigi M, Almarzouqi SJ, Morgan ML, Lee AG. Papilledema: epidemiology, etiology, and clinical management. Eye Brain. 2015;7:47–57.
80. Robba C, Santori G, Czosnyka M, Corradi F, Bragazzi N, Padayachy L, Taccone FS, Citerio G. Optic nerve sheath diameter measured sonographically as non-invasive estimator of intracranial pressure: a systematic review and meta-analysis. Intensive Care Med. 2018;44(8):1284–94.
81. Rasulo FA, Bertuetti R, Robba C, Lusenti F, Cantoni A, Bernini M, Girardini A, Calza S, Piva S, Fagoni N, Latronico N. The accuracy of transcranial Doppler in excluding intracranial hypertension following acute brain injury: a multicenter prospective pilot study. Crit Care. 2017;21(1):44.
82. Robba C, Bacigaluppi S, Cardim D, Donnelly J, Bertuccio A, Czosnyka M. Non-invasive assessment of intracranial pressure. Acta Neurol Scand. 2016;134(1):4–21.
83. Oddo M, Bösel J. Participants in the International Multidisciplinary Consensus Conference on Multimodality Monitoring. Monitoring of brain and systemic oxygenation in neurocritical care patients. Neurocrit Care. 2014;21:103–20.
84. Bohman L-E, Levine JM. Fever and therapeutic normothermia in severe brain injury: an update. Curr Opin Crit Care. 2014;20(2):182–8.
85. Smith CM, Adelson PD, Chang Y-F, Brown SD, Kochanek PM, Clark RSB, Bayir H, Hinchberger J, Bell MJ. Brain-systemic temperature gradient is temperature-dependent in children with severe traumatic brain injury. Pediatr Crit Care Med. 2011;12(4):449–54.
86. Müller W, Kretzschmar K, Schicketanz KH. CT-analyses of cerebral tumors under steroid therapy. Neuroradiology. 1984;26(4):293–8.
87. Jessurun CAC, Hulsbergen AFC, Cho LD, Aglio LS, Nandoe Tewarie RD, Broekman MLD. Evidence-based dexamethasone dosing in malignant brain tumors: what do we really know? J Neurooncol. 2019;144(2):249–64.
88. Mohney N, Williamson CA, Rothman E, Ball R, Sheehan KM, Pandey AS, Fletcher JJ, Jacobs TL, Thompson BG, Rajajee V. A propensity score analysis of the impact of dexamethasone use on delayed cerebral ischemia and poor functional outcomes after subarachnoid hemorrhage. World Neurosurg. 2018;109:e655–61.
89. Simjian T, Muskens IS, Lamba N, Yunusa I, Wong K, Veronneau R, Kronenburg A, Brouwers HB, Smith TR, Mekary RA, Broekman MLD. Dexamethasone administration and mortality in patients with brain abscess: a systematic review and meta-analysis. World Neurosurg. 2018;115:257–63.
90. Edwards P, Arango M, Balica L, Cottingham R, El-Sayed H, Farrell B, Fernandes J, Gogichaisvili T, Golden N, Hartzenberg B, et al. Final results of MRC CRASH, a randomised placebo-controlled trial of intravenous corticosteroid in adults with head injury-outcomes at 6 months. Lancet. 2005;365(9475):1957–9.
91. Shein SL, Ferguson NM, Kochanek PM, Bayir H, Clark RS, Fink EL, Tyler-Kabara EC, Wisniewski SR, Tian Y, Balasubramani GK, Bell MJ. Effectiveness of pharmacological therapies for intracranial hypertension in children with severe traumatic brain injury—results from an automated data collection system time-synched to drug administration. Pediatr Crit Care Med. 2016;17(3):236–45.
92. Kochanek PM, Tasker RC, Carney N, Totten AM, Adelson PD, Selden NR, Davis-O'Reilly C, Hart EL, Bell MJ, Bratton SL, Grant GA, Kissoon N, Reuter-Rice KE, Vavilala MS, Wainwright MS. Guidelines for the management of pediatric severe traumatic brain injury, third edition: update of the Brain Trauma Foundation Guidelines, executive summary. Neurosurgery. 2019;84(6):1169–78.
93. Chambers IR, Jones PA, Lo TYM, Forsyth RJ, Fulton B, Andrews PJD, Mendelow AD, Minns RA. Critical thresholds of intracranial pressure and cerebral perfusion pressure related to age in paediatric head injury. J Neurol Neurosurg Psychiatry. 2006;77(2):234–40.

94. Kochanek PM, Carney N, Adelson PD, Ashwal S, Bell MJ, Bratton S, Carson S, Chesnut RM, Ghajar J, Goldstein B, Grant GA, Kissoon N, Peterson K, Selden NR, Tasker RC, Tong KA, Vavilala MS, Wainwright MS, Warden CR, American Academy of Pediatrics-Section on Neurological Surgery; American Association of Neurological Surgeons/Congress of Neurological Surgeons; Child Neurology Society; European Society of Pediatric and Neonatal Intensive Care; Neurocritical Care Society; Pediatric Neurocritical Care Research Group; Society of Critical Care Medicine; Paediatric Intensive Care Society UK; Society for Neuroscience in Anesthesiology and Critical Care; World Federation of Pediatric Intensive and Critical Care Societies. Guidelines for the acute medical management of severe traumatic brain injury in infants, children, and adolescents—second edition. Pediatr Crit Care Med. 2012;13(Suppl 1):S1–82.
95. Cooper DJ, Rosenfeld JV, Murray L, Arabi YM, Davies AR, D'Urso P, Kossmann T, Ponsford J, Seppelt I, Reilly P, Wolfe R, DECRA Trial Investigators; Australian and New Zealand Intensive Care Society Clinical Trials Group. Decompressive craniectomy in diffuse traumatic brain injury. N Engl J Med. 2011;364(16):1493–502.
96. Hutchinson PJ, Kolias AG, Timofeev IS, Corteen EA, Czosnyka M, Timothy J, Anderson I, Bulters DO, Belli A, Eynon CA, Wadley J, Mendelow AD, Mitchell PM, Wilson MH, Critchley G, Sahuquillo J, Unterberg A, Servadei F, Teasdale GM, Pickard JD, Menon DK, Murray GD, Kirkpatrick PJ, RESCUEicp Trial Collaborators. Trial of decompressive craniectomy for traumatic intracranial hypertension. N Engl J Med. 2016;375(12):1119–30.
97. Inaba H, Pei D, Wolf J, Howard SC, Hayden RT, Go M, Varechtchouk O, Hahn T, Buaboonnam J, Metzger ML, Rubnitz JE, Ribeiro RC, Sandlund JT, Jeha S, Cheng C, Evans WE, Relling MV, Pui CH. Infection-related complications during treatment for childhood acute lymphoblastic leukemia. Ann Oncol. 2017;28(2):386–92.
98. Aljabari S, Balch A, Larsen GY, Fluchel M, Workman JK. Severe sepsis-associated morbidity and mortality among critically ill children with cancer. J Pediatr Intensive Care. 2019;8(3):122–9.
99. Singer K, Subbaiah P, Hutchinson R, Odetola F, Shanley TP. Clinical course of sepsis in children with acute leukemia admitted to the pediatric intensive care unit. Pediatr Crit Care Med. 2011;12(6):649–54.
100. Pillon M, Amigoni A, Contin A, Cattelan M, Carraro E, Campagnano E, Tumino M, Calore E, Marzollo A, Mainardi C, Boaro MP, Nizzero M, Pettenazzo A, Basso G, Messina C. Risk factors and outcomes related to pediatric intensive care unit admission after hematopoietic stem cell transplantation: a single-center experience. Biol Blood Marrow Transplant. 2017;23(8):1335–41.
101. Singer M, Deutschman CS, Seymour CW, Shankar-Hari M, Annane D, Bauer M, Bellomo R, Bernard GR, Chiche JD, Coopersmith CM, Hotchkiss RS, Levy MM, Marshall JC, Martin GS, Opal SM, Rubenfeld GD, van der Poll T, Vincent JL, Angus DC. The third international consensus definitions for sepsis and septic shock (sepsis-3). JAMA. 2016;315(8):801–10.
102. Schlapbach LJ, Watson RS, Sorce LR, et al: International consensus criteria for pediatric sepsis and septic shock. JAMA. 2024;331(8):665–74.
103. Sanchez-Pinto LN, Bennett TD, DeWitt PE, et al: Development and validation of the phoenix criteria for pediatric sepsis and septic shock. JAMA. 2024;331(8):675–86.
104. Schuetz P, Christ-Crain M, Müller B. Procalcitonin and other biomarkers for the assessment of disease severity and guidance of treatment in bacterial infections. Adv Sepsis. 2008;6(3):82–9.
105. Lanziotti VS, Póvoa P, Soares M, Silva JR, Barbosa AP, Salluh JI. Use of biomarkers in pediatric sepsis: literature review. Rev Bras Ter Intensiva. 2016;28(4):472–82.
106. Neemann K, Yonts AB, Qiu F, Simonsen K, Lowas S, Freifeld A. Blood cultures for persistent fever in neutropenic pediatric patients are of low diagnostic yield. J Pediatr Inf Dis Soc. 2016;5(2):218–21.
107. Benner KW, Prabhakaran P, Lowros AS. Epidemiology of infections due to extended-spectrum Beta-lactamase-producing bacteria in a pediatric intensive care unit. J Pediatr Pharmacol Ther. 2014;19(2):83–90.
108. Logan LK. Carbapenem-resistant enterobacteriaceae: an emerging problem in children. Clin Infect Dis. 2012;55(6):852–9.
109. Fletcher M, Hodgkiss H, Zhang S, Browning R, Hadden C, Hoffman T, Winick N, McCavit TL. Prompt administration of antibiotics is associated with improved outcomes in febrile neutropenia in children with cancer. Pediatr Blood Cancer. 2013;60(8):1299–306.

110. De Cock PAJG, van Dijkman SC, de Jaeger A, Willems J, Carlier M, Verstraete AG, Delanghe JR, Robays H, Vande Walle J, Della Pasqua OE, De Paepe P. Dose optimization of piperacillin/tazobactam in critically ill children. J Antimicrob Chemother. 2017;72(7):2002–11.
111. Dellit TH, Owens RC, McGowan JE Jr, Gerding DN, Weinstein RA, Burke JP, Huskins WC, Paterson DL, Fishman NO, Carpenter CF, Brennan PJ, Billeter M, Hooton TM, Infectious Diseases Society of America; Society for Healthcare Epidemiology of America. Infectious Diseases Society of America and the Society for Healthcare Epidemiology of America guidelines for developing an institutional program to enhance antimicrobial stewardship. Clin Infect Dis. 2007;44(2):159–77.
112. Vogiatzi L, Ilia S, Sideri G, Vagelakoudi E, Vassilopoulou M, Sdougka M, Briassoulis G, Papadatos I, Kalabalikis P, Sianidou L, Roilides E. Invasive candidiasis in pediatric intensive care in Greece: a nationwide study. Intensive Care Med. 2013;39(12):2188–95.
113. Torres JP, De la Maza V, Kors L, Villarroel M, Piemonte P, Izquierdo G, Salgado C, Tordecilla J, Contardo V, Farfán MJ, Mejías A, Ramilo O, Santolaya ME. Respiratory viral infections and coinfections in children with cancer, fever and neutropenia: clinical outcome of infections caused by different respiratory viruses. Pediatr Infect Dis J. 2016;35(9):949–54.
114. Jain R, Trehan A, Mishra B, Singh R, Saud B, Bansal D. Cytomegalovirus disease in children with acute lymphoblastic leukemia. Pediatr Hematol Oncol. 2016;33(4):239–47.
115. Davis AL, Carcillo JA, Aneja RK, Deymann AJ, Lin JC, Nguyen TC, Okhuysen-Cawley RS, Relvas MS, Rozenfeld RA, Skippen PW, Stojadinovic BJ, Williams EA, Yeh TS, Balamuth F, Brierley J, de Caen AR, Cheifetz IM, Choong K, Conway E Jr, Cornell T, Doctor A, Dugas MA, Feldman JD, Fitzgerald JC, Flori HR, Fortenberry JD, Graciano AL, Greenwald BM, Hall MW, Han YY, Hernan LJ, Irazuzta JE, Iselin E, van der Jagt EW, Jeffries HE, Kache S, Katyal C, Kissoon N, Kon AA, Kutko MC, MacLaren G, Maul T, Mehta R, Odetola F, Parbuoni K, Paul R, Peters MJ, Ranjit S, Reuter-Rice KE, Schnitzler EJ, Scott HF, Torres A Jr, Weingarten-Arams J, Weiss SL, Zimmerman JJ, Zuckerberg AL. American College of Critical Care Medicine clinical practice parameters for hemodynamic support of pediatric and neonatal septic shock. Crit Care Med. 2017;45(6):1061–93.
116. Benoit G, Phan V, Duval M, Champagne M, Litalien C, Merouani A. Fluid balance of pediatric hematopoietic stem cell transplant recipients and intensive care unit admission. Pediatr Nephrol. 2007;22(3):441–7.
117. Gow KW, Heiss KF, Wulkan ML, Katzenstein HM, Rosenberg ES, Heard ML, Rycus PT, Fortenberry JD. Extracorporeal life support for support of children with malignancy and respiratory or cardiac failure: the extracorporeal life support experience. Crit Care Med. 2009;37(4):1308–16.
118. Chang TH, Wu ET, Lu CY, Huang SC, Yang TI, Wang CC, Chen JM, Lee PI, Huang LM, Chang LY. Pathogens and outcomes in pediatric septic shock patients supported by extracorporeal membrane oxygenation. J Microbiol Immunol Infect. 2018;51(3):385–91.
119. Smith S, Butt W, Best D, MacLaren G. Long-term survival after extracorporeal life support in children with neutropenic sepsis. Intensive Care Med. 2016;42(5):942–3.
120. Gorjup V, Fister M, Noc M, Rajic V, Ribaric SF. Treatment of sepsis and ARDS with extracorporeal membrane oxygenation and interventional lung assist membrane ventilator in a patient with acute lymphoblastic leukemia. Respir Care. 2012;57(7):1178–81.
121. Frey NV, Porter DL. Cytokine release syndrome with novel therapeutics for acute lymphoblastic leukemia. Hematol Am Soc Hematol Educ Program. 2016;2016(1):567–72.
122. Jordan MB, Allen CE, Weitzman S, Filipovich AH, McClain KL. How I treat hemophagocytic lymphohistiocytosis. Blood. 2011;118(15):4041–52.
123. Janka GE, Lehmberg K. Hemophagocytic lymphohistiocytosis: pathogenesis and treatment. Hematology Am Soc Hematol Educ Program. 2013;2013:605–11.
124. Henter JI, Horne A, Aricó M, Egeler RM, Filipovich AH, Imashuku S, Ladisch S, McClain K, Webb D, Winiarski J, Janka G. HLH-2004: diagnostic and therapeutic guidelines for hemophagocytic lymphohistiocytosis. Pediatr Blood Cancer. 2007;48(2):124–31.
125. National Healthcare Safety Network. Bloodstream infection event (central line-associated bloodstream infection and non-central line-associated bloodstream Infection). http://www.cdc.gov/nhsn/PDFs/pscManual/4PSC_CLABScurrent.pdf. Accessed 16 Nov 2015.

End-of-Life Nursing for Children and Families in ICU

Ashleigh E. Butler and Joseph C. Manning

Contents

J. Brierley et al. (eds.), *ESPNIC Children's Intensive Care Textbook*,
https://doi.org/10.1007/978-3-031-64762-8_46

Learning Objectives

After completing this chapter, the learner will be able to:

- Understand experiences and care needs of families with a child in the PICU.
- Identify strategies to enhance family-centered care within the PICU setting.
- Identify and discuss important elements of the end-of-life care experience for families in an ICU environment.
- Describe practical aspects of nursing care to support a family in the ICU when their child is dying.
- Identify and discuss important elements of the post-death and bereavement care experience for families after a child's death in an ICU environment.
- Describe practical aspects of nursing care to support a bereaved family in an ICU environment and after they have returned home.

46.1 Introduction

Families (that may include parents, siblings, and other extended family members and friends) of children that are critically ill or injured and admitted to the PICU have unique but interconnected experiences, needs, and outcomes [1–3]. It is important for all professionals working within the PICU setting to understand, support, and work in partnership with families during the child's care pathway in order to optimize their experiences and outcomes [4]. This chapter begins with an overview of the experiences, needs, and care considerations for families in the PICU, and proposes strategies to enhance family-centered care practices and address unmet needs. The chapter then focuses specifically on the care needs of families when their child is at end of life and when they have died. Practical approaches that can be used by PICU professionals to support families during these times are outlined.

46.2 Experiences and Care Needs of Families in the PICU

Having a critically ill or injured child that is being cared for within the PICU setting is often an adverse experience for families, specifically parents, provoking negative emotions that can include anxiety, stress, sadness, and fear [2, 3]. The acuity of their child's condition, prognostic uncertainty, the environment, and changes to parental role are all recognized as stressors [2]. Furthermore, parents of children with long-term conditions/medical complexity identify that lack of continuity and coordination of care exacerbate negative experiences [5]. Congruent with the variation in parental responses to the PICU, the needs of parents can also vary. However, commonly reported needs include: (a) being physically close to their child; (b) being recognized as a team member through all professional interactions; (c) participation in decision-making for their child; (d) opportunities to ask questions, be present, be involved, and have choice [6]; and (e) have available, detailed, well-timed and honest information that is delivered sensitively [2, 7]. PICU professionals are

Table 46.1 Principles of family-centered care

Information sharing	– Open, objective, and unbiased information – Accessible and involves a two-way process between professionals and families
Respect and honoring differences	– Respecting diversity that may include cultural and linguistic traditions and care preferences
Partnership and collaboration	– Decisions that best fit the needs, strengths, values, and abilities of all involved – Decisions made in partnership with families at the level they choose
Negotiation	– Proposed outcomes of medical care plans are flexible
Care in Context of family and community	– All care and decision-making reflects the child within the context of his/her family – Comprehension of wider ecosystem in which the child and family exists (e.g. home, school, daily activities, and their community) should also be considered

Adapted from Kuo et al. [8]

pivotal to ensuring that these parental needs are met through mobilizing a Family-Centered Care delivery model as part of their unit standard practice. As outlined in Table 46.1, this can be achieved through partnership, working with families in ways which values their expertise and insights, as well as open communication that is built on honesty and respect [8].

Whilst the experiences and needs of PICU siblings remains largely under researched, it is evident that they can also be negatively affected by having a brother or sister that is critically ill/injured. Fears, sadness, anxieties, and relative neglect of their own needs are evident in qualitative accounts of siblings. This is attributable to a range of factors that include: (a) changes in parental presence and parental behavior; (b) social disruptions due to substitute caregivers; (c) undertaking age-inappropriate adult responsibilities (e.g. care of other siblings or domestic duties); (d) repetitive exposure to distressing content in the PICU (e.g. strange environment, the technology, other patients, observing negative emotions of other relatives), and (e) fear and anxiety for their sibling's wellbeing [9]. Many siblings have intermittent access to the PICU, their parents, and information. As such, many siblings have uncertainties regarding the history of the critical illness for their brother/sister and the care pathway [10]. In order to support the needs of siblings, PICU professionals need to consider these and discuss with parents. Furthermore, when siblings are present in the PICU, professionals need to ensure that they have opportunity to seek timely and reliable information that is age/developmentally appropriate, and have a safe and open space to discuss their thoughts and how they are feeling. The "SIBS" framework (Table 46.2) is useful approach to supporting siblings whilst they have a brother or sister that is critically ill/injured on the PICU [11].

Table 46.2 "SIBS" framework for supporting siblings

*S*upport	Includes preparing the siblings for hospital visitation
*I*nformation	Ensuring that professionals are available to support the delivery of developmentally appropriate information
*B*alance	Supporting parents to have access and time with the siblings and distraction from the immediate crisis/experience
*S*ensitivity to time and resources	Professionals offer choice and sustainable solutions

46.3 When a Child Dies in the PICU

46.3.1 Family Experiences of End-of-Life Care in the PICU

The death of a child is one of the most difficult and traumatic things a family can experience. This is particularly true in an ICU setting, where a child's death is commonly the result of a sudden and unexpected illness or injury. Traditionally, the critical care environment is designed for the provision of high-quality, high-technology, life-saving care. As a result, the physical and social environments of the ICU are often inadequately prepared for the provision of end-of-life care for a dying child and their family [12, 13]. However, developing an understanding of the family experience of a child's death in an ICU setting can enable nurses to provide high-quality end of life care to children and their families, despite the challenges that the environment may pose.

There are many important aspects of end-of-life care for children and their families in an ICU setting that can significantly impact the overall experience. Families often report a more positive end-of-life experience when their parental role is supported and maintained [12, 14–18], when they can touch and hold their child [12, 13, 17–19], when their child is treated as an individual [16, 17, 20, 21], when they receive sensitive but open and honest communication [12, 15–18, 21–23], when they receive both practical and emotional support from staff [12, 15, 21–24], when there are sufficient practical resources available [12, 20, 23, 24], when they are afforded privacy and time to say goodbye to their child [12, 16, 17, 23, 25], and when they are supported to engage in memory-making activities with their child [19, 24]. Conversely, when parents are not supported to hold and care for their child or when they perceive that staff are not being open and honest with them, they report feeling disempowered, unsupported, and alone when their child was dying [12, 18, 20, 22, 23], with these feelings and memories persisting for years after their child's death [16, 20].

46.3.2 Supporting Families When Their Child Is Dying: Some Practical Suggestions

When a child is dying in an ICU, *facilitating the parental role* wherever possible is vital. Parents often want to be close to their child, whether that means holding them in a recliner chair or offering a full-sized hospital bed to cuddle in [12, 13, 16–19, 22, 25, 26].

They frequently want to help care for their child and should be supported to provide eye and mouth care, pressure area care, hygiene care, or assistance with feeding (if provided) to the extent they desire [14–16, 22]. In addition, many parents appreciate the removal of unnecessary tubes, lines, and equipment, so that they can hold their child more easily [13]. This is particularly true for any tubing that obscures the child's face.

Many families also want and need support to *engage in memory-making activities* with their child [19, 23]. There are many activities and mementos that can be created in conjunction with parents and families, such as memory books, hand and footprints, photographs (both professional and personal), locks of hair, or obtaining printouts of their child's ECG trace [14, 17, 21–23, 26]. In addition, *modifying the environment* to provide the family with privacy and dignity allows them to say goodbye to their child in their own time and in their own way. Offering to move the child and family to a private room or a quiet, out of the way space is appreciated by families, so that their dying child is not "on display" [12, 16, 17, 21–23]. Additionally, many families appreciate having *practical resources,* such a separate space where they can take a break, sleep, shower, or meet with other family members, as well as regularly being offered something to eat and drink [12, 15, 17, 20, 23]. Finally, *offering staff support* is an important aspect of caring for the families of dying children. Parents appreciate staff who genuinely care about them and their child and who offer comfort, emotional support, and guidance through the physical, emotional, and practical processes of dying [12, 17, 18, 20, 22].

46.4 After a Child Has Died in the ICU

46.4.1 Family Experiences of Post-death and Bereavement Care in the ICU

For families, the death of a child in the ICU marks the beginning of a very difficult, confusing, and lonely journey. Most families have never experienced the death of a loved one in a hospital setting, much less an ICU, so they are unfamiliar with the processes and procedures which surround death in this environment. Often, families are unsure of how to say goodbye to their child [14, 19]. They do not know how long they can stay with their child's body in the ICU, whether they can visit their child in the mortuary, or whether there are other practical or legal requirements which must take place [14]. Once they leave the hospital, many families are also unsure of how to manage their grief and how to identify and obtain any supports they might need [14, 19].

Receiving support and care from their child's nurse is highly valued by families, both in the immediate post-death phase and after they have left the hospital and returned home. Families rely on the nursing staff to guide and support them through the process of saying goodbye, leaving their child's body in the hospital, and returning home [13, 14, 17, 19, 24]. It is particularly meaningful to families if the supporting nurse is someone that they already have a relationship with, and someone who knew and cared for their child [14, 21]. When this support is provided, parents report feeling "cushioned from the starkness of life" after their child's death, and better able to undertake activities such as washing and dressing their child's body or packing up their belongings [14, 19]. Without this support, parents often feel isolated and abandoned in the ICU [19]. This is particularly important during the immediate hours after death. Whilst offering a private space for families to be with their child's body is important, it is equally important to ensure that families know the bedside nurse is still present to care for them and their child's body, even if they are not present in the room. Otherwise, families can feel as though staff have simply moved on to other tasks or other patients [14]. Ongoing support and contact from staff is also important to families after they have gone home; without it families feel as though they and their child have been forgotten [14, 19, 22, 27].

46.4.2 Supporting Families After a Child's Death: Some Practical Suggestions

One of the most important elements of supporting families after a child's death is simply *being present*. Families want and need nurses to be emotionally and physically present with them in the ICU to answer questions, support their emotional and psychological needs, and offer practical supports, such as something to eat or drink [17, 19, 23, 28]. In addition, *providing guidance and information* on the usual procedures surrounding death is usually very appreciated by families [14]. Key pieces of information may include how long they can remain in the ICU, how to help care for their child's body, how to visit their child in the mortuary, or what happens if their child's death needs to be investigated by a Coroner [14, 17, 21, 23]. This also extends to the provision of information about normal grief processes, local support groups and counselling services, or funeral providers who offer services for children [14, 19, 22, 23].

Finally, *offering follow-up contact* is highly valued by bereaved families. Follow-up contact can take many forms; from sending a bereavement card on behalf of the PICU or making a phone call, through to offering a formalized bereavement follow-up program [14, 17, 19, 21, 22, 24, 26–28]. Parent's value seeing familiar staff at their child's funeral, and when key dates such as birthdays or anniversaries are acknowledged. The provision of an annual ICU memorial or remembrance day is also valued by bereaved families as a way to remember their child and reconnect to the hospital [27]. ◘ Figure 46.1 also outlines several practical suggestions that were specifically identified by bereaved parents as helpful when they were in the ICU with their dying child and during their bereavement. Many of these can be easily implemented into care without significant cost or the need for specialized training and can have a significant impact on the family's end-of-life care experience in the ICU.

During Hospitalization	During the Dying Phase	During Bereavement
Information and communication Ensure open and honest communication Clear, early discussions of the likelihood of or potential for death Offer Tacit "permission" to withdraw life support Provide verbal and written/visual information, including picture and diagrams Maintain a photo board introducing the staff working on each shift	**The hours before death** A private room in an unobtrusive, quiet area of the PICU De-medicalize the environment as much as possible Provide space for extended family/friends Allocate a familiar nurse and doctor Offer professional photographs of the child	**The delivery of follow-up care** Ongoing contact with staff familiar to the family Staff presence at funeral Ensure whole family is followed up Timing of follow-up: 1 wk, 2–3 mo, ongoing for 12 mo Specific attention to anniversaries or special dates (eg, birthdays, mother's/father's day)
The provision of resources Provide a parent room with bathrooms, kitchens, a laundry, snacks, toiletries, phone chargers, internet access, and comfortable seating Organize/assist with ordered meals for parents/siblings Provide parent accommodation within the hospital, close to the PICU Improve parking facilities, with reduced cost for families of critically ill children	**The hours after death** Provide ongoing parent support from staff in the hours after death Provide information on how to visit the child in the morgue Improve the visitation room within the morgue Walk parents out of PICU and to their car Assist with transport home for parents Waive parking fees for bereaved parents	**The provision of information** Give a list of local funeral directors, counselors, and grief groups, who specialize in children's deaths Provide a "What happens next?" guideline, both for the post mortem examination process and for organizing funerals/going home Be cautious with how much information is given Clearly label all maill correspondence with sender and contents
The environment Orientate parents to hospital and local community services (supermarkets, restaurants) Improve environment: natural lighting, bigger rooms, more color Make PICU entrance processes simpler and easier Place a window in PICU entrance Doors Give explanations when asking parents to wait outside		**Connecting to other bereaved parents** Organize a parent support group for bereaved PICU parents from the hospital Develop a "buddy system" for parents in hospital before their child dies
Support Refer/connect parents to External support services as early as possible Provide a support worker for siblings Offer assistance explaining the situation to siblings		

Fig. 46.1 Practical suggestions for nursing care of the family when a child is dying in the ICU. (Reproduced with permission from Butler et al. [23])

Take-Home Messages

- PICU professionals need to be skilled in working with and supporting families during their time on the PICU, irrespective of the child's pathway or outcome.
- Facilitating the parental role for parents during and after the death of their child is crucial to providing high-quality end-of-life care.
- The provision of a quiet, private space for the child and family at the end of life is important.
- Families need physical, emotional, and practical support and guidance from staff as they move through the dying process with their child.
- Being physically and emotionally present with families after a child's death is highly valued.
- Many families need information about the procedures surrounding death, such as how to visit their child in the mortuary.
- Offering and engaging in follow-up contact or bereavement support is important to ensure families do not feel forgotten or abandoned by the hospital or the staff.

References

1. Manning JC, Pinto NP, Rennick JE, Colville G, Curley MA. Conceptualizing post intensive care syndrome in children—the PICS-p framework. Pediatr Crit Care Med. 2018;19(4):298–300.
2. Abela KM, Wardell D, Rozmus C, LoBiondo-Wood G. Impact of pediatric critical illness and injury on families: an updated systematic review. J Pediatr Nurs. 2020;51:21–31.
3. Shudy M, De Almeida ML, Ly S, Landon C, Groft S, Jenkins TL, et al. Impact of pediatric critical illness and injury on families: a systematic literature review. Pediatrics. 2006;118(Suppl 3):S203–S18.
4. Phiri PG, Chan CW, Wong C. The scope of family-centred care practices, and the facilitators and barriers to implementation of family-centred care for hospitalised children and their families in developing countries: an integrative review. J Pediatr Nurs. 2020;55:10–28.
5. Henderson CM, Williams EP, Shapiro MC, Hahn E, Wright-Sexton L, Hutton N, et al. "Stuck in the ICU": caring for children with chronic critical illness. Pediatr Crit Care Med. 2017;18(11):e561–e8.
6. Meert KL, Clark J, Eggly S. Family-centered care in the pediatric intensive care unit. Pediatr Clin N Am. 2013;60(3):761–72. https://doi.org/10.1016/j.pcl.2013.02.011.
7. Greenway TL, Rosenthal MS, Murtha TD, Kandil SB, Talento DL, Couloures KG. Barriers to communication in a PICU: a qualitative investigation of family and provider perceptions*. Pediatr Crit Care Med. 2019;20(9):e415.
8. Kuo DZ, Houtrow AJ, Arango P, Kuhlthau KA, Simmons JM, Neff JM. Family-centered care: current applications and future directions in pediatric health care. Matern Child Health J. 2012;16(2):297–305.
9. Shudy M, de Almeida ML, Ly S, Landon C, Groft S, Jenkins TL, et al. Impact of pediatric critical illness and injury on families: a systematic literature review. Pediatrics. 2006;118(Suppl 3):S203–18. https://doi.org/10.1542/peds.2006-0951B.
10. Manning JC. Stories of survival: exploring long-term psychosocial well-being in childhood survivors of acute life threatening critical illness: a multiple-case study. PhD Thesis, University of Nottingham. 2015.
11. Fleitas J. When Jack fell down… Jill came tumbling after: siblings in the web of illness and disability. MCN Am J Matern Child Nurs. 2000;25(5):267–73.
12. Butler AE, Hall H, Willetts G, Copnell B. Family experience and PICU death: a meta-synthesis. Pediatrics. 2015;136(4):e961–e73.
13. Falkenburg JL, Tibboel D, Ganzevoort RR, Gischler S, Hagoort J, van Dijk M. Parental physical proximity in end-of-life care in the PICU. Pediatr Crit Care Med. 2016;17(5):e212–e7.

14. Butler AE, Hall H, Copnell B. Becoming a team: the nature of the parent-healthcare provider relationship when a child is dying in the pediatric intensive care unit. J Pediatr Nurs. 2018;40:e26–32.
15. Currie ER, Christian BJ, Hinds PS, Perna SJ, Robinson C, Day S, et al. Parent perspectives of neonatal intensive care at the end-of-life. J Pediatr Nurs. 2016;31(5):478–89.
16. McGraw SA, Truog RD, Solomon MZ, Cohen-Bearak A, Sellers DE, Meyer EC. "I was able to still be her mom" parenting at end of life in the PICU. Pediatr Crit Care Med. 2012;13(6):e350.
17. Meert KL, Briller SH, Myers Schim S, Thurston C, Kabel A. Examining the needs of bereaved parents in the pediatric intensive care unit: a qualitative study. Death Stud. 2009;33(8):712–40.
18. Mitchell S, Spry JL, Hill E, Coad J, Dale J, Plunkett A. Parental experiences of end of life care decision-making for children with life-limiting conditions in the paediatric intensive care unit: a qualitative interview study. BMJ Open. 2019;9(5):e028548.
19. Butler AE, Hall H, Copnell B. The changing nature of relationships between parents and healthcare providers when a child dies in the paediatric intensive care unit. J Adv Nurs. 2018;74(1):89–99.
20. Falkenburg JL, Tibboel D, Ganzevoort RR, Gischler SJ, van Dijk M. The importance of parental connectedness and relationships with healthcare professionals in end-of-life care in the PICU. Pediatr Crit Care Med. 2018;19(3):e157–e63.
21. October T, Dryden-Palmer K, Copnell B, Meert KL. Caring for parents after the death of a child. Pediatr Crit Care Med. 2018;19(8):S61.
22. Baughcum AE, Fortney CA, Winning AM, Shultz EL, Keim MC, Humphrey LM, et al. Perspectives from bereaved parents on improving end of life care in the NICU. Clin Pract Pediatr Psychol. 2017;5(4):392.
23. Butler AE, Copnell B, Hall H. When a child dies in the PICU: practice recommendations from a qualitative study of bereaved parents. Pediatr Crit Care Med. 2019;20(9):e447–e51.
24. Butler AE, Copnell B, Hall H. The impact of the social and physical environments on parent–healthcare provider relationships when a child dies in PICU: findings from a grounded theory study. Intensive Crit Care Nurs. 2019;50:28–35.
25. Brooten D, Youngblut JM, Caicedo C, Dankanich J. Parents: wish I had done, wish I had not done, and coping after child NICU/PICU death. J Am Assoc Nurse Pract. 2019;31(3):175–83.
26. Levick J, Fannon J, Bodemann J, Munch S, Ahern K. NICU bereavement care and follow-up support for families and staff. Adv Neonatal Care. 2017;17(6):451–60.
27. Macdonald ME, Liben S, Carnevale FA, Rennick JE, Wolf SL, Meloche D, et al. Parental perspectives on hospital staff members' acts of kindness and commemoration after a child's death. Pediatrics. 2005;116(4):884–90.
28. Brooten D, Youngblut JM, Seagrave L, Caicedo C, Hawthorne D, Hidalgo I, et al. Parent's perceptions of health care providers actions around child ICU death: what helped, what did not. Am J Hospice Palliat Med. 2013;30(1):40–9.

Further Reading

Baughcum AE, Fortney CA, Winning AM, et al. Perspectives from bereaved parents on improving end of life care in the NICU. Clinical Pract Pediatr Psychol. 2017;5:392–403. https://doi.org/10.1037/cpp0000221.

Butler A, Copnell B, Hall H. When a child dies in the PICU: practice recommendations from a qualitative study of bereaved parents*. Pediatr Crit Care Med. 2019;20:e447–51. https://doi.org/10.1097/PCC.0000000000002040.

Fleitas J. When Jack fell down… Jill came tumbling after: siblings in the web of illness and disability. MCN Am J Matern Child Nurs. 2000;25(5):267–73.

Kuo DZ, Houtrow AJ, Arango P, Kuhlthau KA, Simmons JM, Neff JM. Family-centered care: current applications and future directions in pediatric health care. Matern Child Health J. 2012;16(2):297–305.

Levick J, Fannon J, Bodemann J, Munch S, Ahern K. NICU bereavement care and follow-up support for families and staff. Adv Neonatal Care. 2017;17(6):451–60.

Manning JC, Pinto NP, Rennick JE, Colville G, Curley MA. Conceptualizing post intensive care syndrome in children—the PICS-p framework. Pediatr Crit Care Med. 2018;19(4):298–300.

October T, Dryden-Palmer K, Copnell B, Meert KL. Caring for parents after the death of a child. Pediatr Crit Care Med. 2018;19(8S Suppl 2):S61–8. https://doi.org/10.1097/PCC.0000000000001466.

Paediatric Organ Donation

Yemi Jegede

Contents

J. Brierley et al. (eds.), *ESPNIC Children's Intensive Care Textbook*,
https://doi.org/10.1007/978-3-031-64762-8_47

Learning Objectives

By the end of this chapter, you will be able to:

- Explain why every potential paediatric donor matters.
- Describe ethical principles of organ donation.
- Understand how to maintain ethics in paediatric organ donation.
- Define how to diagnose death using circulatory criteria and neurological criteria.
- List the pre-conditions for brain-stem testing.
- Describe the components of the brain-stem test in children vs. neonates.
- Outline the process of DCD and recognise potential ethical issues associated with DCD.
- Understand how to potentially maximise DCD donation outcomes.
- Recognise the importance of DBD relative to DCD.
- Describe the physiological changes that accompany brain-stem ischaemia and the effect they have on potential organ transplant viability.
- Outline the process of DBD and the place of donor optimisation.
- Explain how to identify potential donors.
- Specify when and how to approach potential donor families.
- Understand why working collaboratively with specialist organ donation teams is advantageous.
- Recognise and explain what makes a successful deceased donor program.

47.1 Introduction

47.1.1 Importance of Deceased Organ Donation

Organ donation is defined as the act of giving one or more organs (or parts thereof), without compensation, for transplantation into someone else. Organ donation is a very personal yet complex decision, intertwined with medical, legal, religious, cultural, and ethical issues [1].

Since the successful first kidney transplants in the 1950s, organ transplant has become an established practice worldwide and is often the only treatment for end organ liver and heart failure. In renal and intestinal failure, organ donation considerably enhances the quality of life for the recipients as it takes away their reliance on dialysis and parental nutrition, respectively; these therapies save lives but have life limiting side effects. Additionally, they place an ongoing economic burden on society which is considerably reduced following transplantation.

One deceased donor can potentially save nine lives [2, 3].

Despite this, the societal and individual benefits of organ donation continue to be limited because the ongoing demand for organs is greater than the number of available organs.

In 2018, over 150,000 patients in Europe were registered on organ transplant waiting lists, in the same year there were only 34,221 transplants performed [4].

Deceased donation does not meet the need for transplantable organs in all countries, it is non-existent in many. Because of this, many countries rely on living donation as a source of kidney and liver transplants. Many unethical and unacceptable practises can stem from this such as organ trafficking as well as morbidity and even mortality in the donor. There is therefore a need for all countries to work towards establishing effective deceased donor programs.

Consequently, understanding the deceased donation process and the issues that may interrupt and prevent donation is paramount in ensuring that this scarce resource is used effectively in line with the wishes of potential donors for the benefit of potential recipients.

Accordingly, the consideration of organ donation should be an integral part of good quality end-of-life care.

47.2 Paediatric Perspective

Learning Objective

- Understand and explain why every potential paediatric donor matters.

Death in childhood is a rare event in high-income countries; therefore, the number of potential deceased organ donors will always be small.

In infancy, prematurity and congenital malformations are the most common causes of death later in early childhood metabolic disease and malignancy become additional causes. Trauma secondary to accidents becomes increasingly more common in later childhood.

Improvements in illness and accident prevention such as immunisation and road safety measures mean that death in childhood is becoming less and less common.

Increased accessibility and improvements in the delivery of paediatric and neonatal critical care have also decreased the death rate in children.

Proportionally more children die in the critical care setting in comparison to adults.

However, there are significantly lower numbers of deceased donors for any given child compared with an adult.

Within paediatric ICU, most deaths result from withholding or withdrawal of life-sustaining treatment. This is often after prolonged periods of attempted organ support.

Many of these children die with significant organ impairment or have underlying malignant, genetic, or metabolic diseases which make them unsuitable donors.

The incidence of traumatic brain injury has fortunately been steadily declining thanks to public health measures such as decreasing speed limits on roads and the wearing of cycle helmets. The survival from traumatic brain injury has also increased due to improvements in paediatric neuro intensive care. This means that the pool of potential paediatric donors following neurological determination of death has not increased in the last 10 years and seems to be declining.

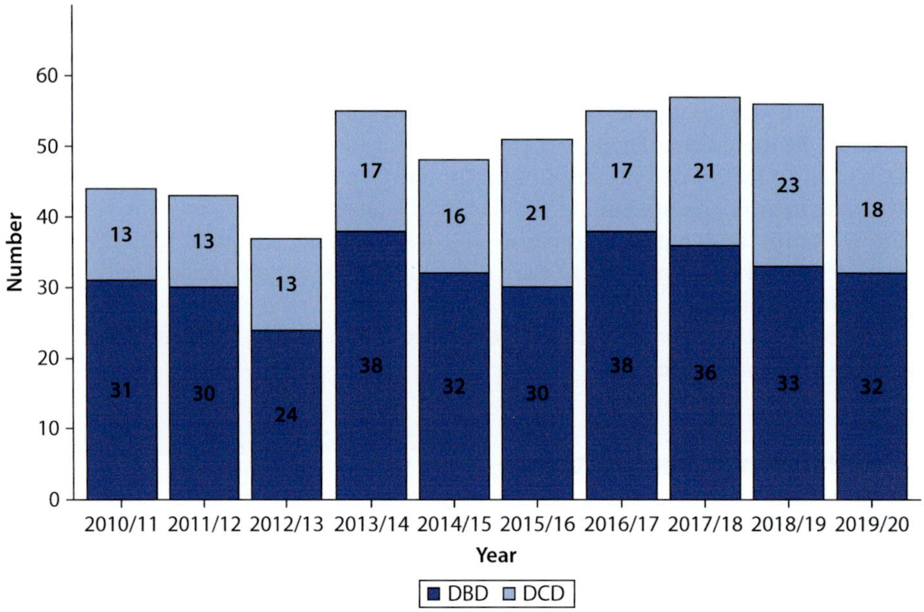

Donors aged less than 18 by donor type, 1 April 2010–31 March 2020 NHSBT [20]

In the UK, as with adults, the proportion of DCD donors has increased in paediatrics and now form a significant proportion of the paediatric donor pool. In the USA, according to organ procurement and transplantation data as of May 20, 2018, rates increased from under 2% of all deceased paediatric donations prior to 2000 to 15% of all paediatric deceased donations from 2013 to 2018.

Since the NHSBT donation task force of 2008, there has been an overall increase in donation of 50% in the UK population. However, paediatric donation rates did not increase until 2013 and have been static since.

This is because the donor pool in paediatrics is very small compared to adults.

However, the need for paediatric organs is increasing due to the increasing numbers of children surviving either acute or chronic organ failure.

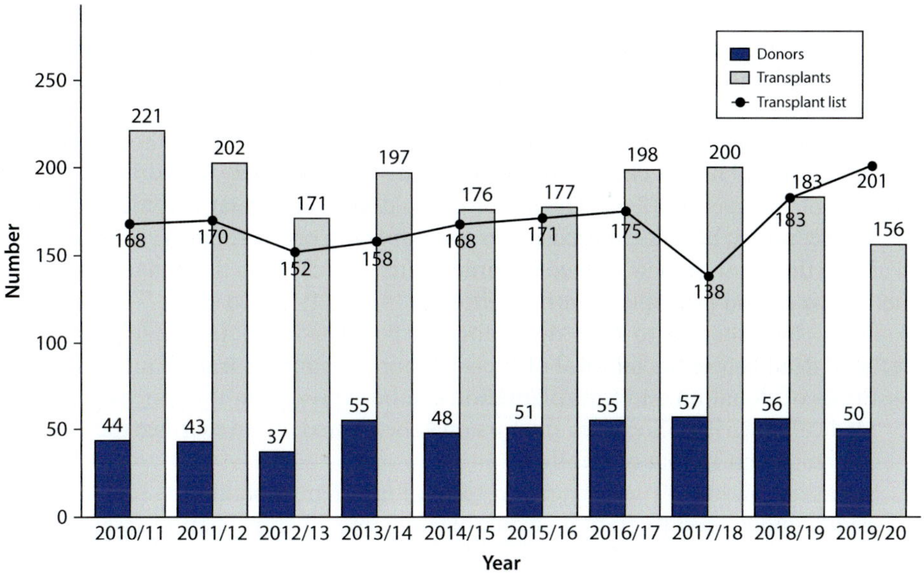

Number of deceased paediatric (less than 18 years) donors, transplants, and active transplant list in the UK, 1 April 2010–31 March 2020 [20]

In the UK, children form approx. 2% of the active transplant waiting list. There have been between 150 and 200 children every year on the active transplant list for the last 10 years. These numbers do not tell the whole story as there are also children who are taken off the active list because of intercurrent illness or because they have become too ill to be considered for a transplant.

Because of size discrepancy, it is not always possible to use adult organs in small children.

Increasing the donor pool by using living related donation or splitting adult organs such as in liver transplantation is not likely to fully address the shortfall in paediatric organs, which results in children waiting on average 2.5 times longer for an organ than an adult [5].

47.3 Ethics of Deceased Donation

Learning Objectives

- Understand and be able to explain the ethical principles of organ donation.
- Understand how to maintain ethics in paediatric organ donation.

47.3.1 What Makes Deceased Donation Ethical

From the point of view of the donor, deceased donation is essentially an act of altruism where the moral value of an individual's action is focused on the beneficial impact to another individual, without the possibility of getting anything in return [6]. Because most people would accept an organ for themselves or a member of their family if it was needed to save their life, deceased donation can also be viewed through the lens of human solidarity. Especially considering that an individual is far more likely to need a transplant than they are likely to become a donor over the course of their lifetime.

Deceased donation confers a wider benefit to society because those dying of organ failure will have a chance to live and contribute to society, one donor can save the lives of nine people [2, 3]. The use of organ donation to treat chronic organ failure has economic benefits as it costs less than ongoing organ support.

From the point of view of medical practitioners involved in the donation process, there is the ethical principle of nonmaleficence—the duty not to harm. This principle is upheld by adhering to the "dead donor rule" which requires that patients be declared dead before the removal of life-sustaining organs for transplantation [7].

Ethics of donation and transplantation can be expressed in three areas [8]:

1. Medical integrity—Societies' doctors must be trusted not to sacrifice the interests of one patient to that of another.
2. Scientific validity—The science and technology of transplantation must be sufficiently understood to grant a favourable outcome for transplant recipients.
3. Consent—This must be freely given without coercion, based on accurate information, adequately presented and properly understood.

It is not difficult to see how a clinician's ethical commitment to a dying patient can be displaced by a commitment to those waiting for organ transplant.

However, good medical practice as stipulated by the General medical Council UK (GMC) guidance describes what it means to be a good doctor. It states that a good doctor will make the care of their patient their first concern, they will maintain trust between themselves and their patients by being open, honest and by acting with integrity. This means a good doctor will not sacrifice the interests of one patient to that of another.

The ethics of donation is underpinned by having a transparent and robust consent process which protects the autonomy of the individual. Such a robust process will lead to increased societal trust in the donation process which in turn will maximise the number of consented donors.

An ethically valid informed consent process should consist of a transparent discussion which presents a family with all available end-of-life care options. The discussion should allow the family to reach a choice that is best for them. This should include information regarding the urgent need for organs and counselling regarding the consolation that many families may feel following donation knowing that their loved one has done something to help others.

There are differing ways a society may choose to gain consent for organ donation from its citizens:

47.3.1.1 Implicit or Presumed Consent

World Health Organization (WHO) defines presumed consent as a system that permits material to be removed from the body of a deceased person for transplantation and, in some countries, for anatomical study or research, unless the person had expressed his or her opposition before death by filing an objection with an identified office or an informed party which reports that the deceased definitely voiced an objection to donation [9]; this is consent without specific action denoting consent and inaction is taken as a sign of consent [10]. This form of consent is not applicable to children as consent for organ donation will be sort from those who have parental responsibility for the child.

47.3.1.2 Explicit Consent

This requires individuals to "opt-in" by proactively stating their wishes to be a donor by, for example, signing a donor registrar or agreeing that their parents sign one on their behalf.

Those with parental responsibility may know the wishes of their child with regards to donation, they may imagine what their child would have wished if asked or if they were old enough to understand the concept of donation. Or they may decide purely on their own intrinsic altruistic values as parents to give consent to donation.

Whatever the case clinicians have a responsibility to make sure that those who want to donate their organs can do so and that the consent process is informed and voluntary.

Equally families who do not want to donate their child's organs should not feel pressured into doing so.

47.3.2 Ethical Framework

Drawing up an ethical framework for decision-making when considering paediatric organ donation will help to establish a consistent ethical approach across all regions. Ensuring that all patients and families wishes are respected regardless of where they live.

▶ Example

For example, UK donation ethics committee paediatric recommendations 2015

- Recommendation 1

  Provided decisions are not against their child's interests, parents' values and beliefs should be allowed to determine whether they wish their child to be an organ donor, and if so whether to consent to interventions aimed at increasing the chances of a successful donation. Where a family is willing to consent to the removal of organs that are viable for transplantation, then the hospital has a responsibility to make this happen if it is possible. A decision made by a child with capacity that they would not want to donate organs after their death should always be respected.
- Recommendation 2

  Where a family is willing to consent to the removal of organs that are viable for transplantation, then the hospital has a responsibility to make this happen if it is possible.
- Recommendation 3

  A decision made by a child with capacity that they would not want to donate organs after their death should always be respected.
- Recommendation 4

  Where a child has indicated willingness to donate (for example by registering on the ODR), has not expressed a view either way or lacks the capacity to make such a decision, then clinicians should work with the child's family to reach a decision that takes account of any information about the child's views but also works for the family as a whole.

- Recommendation 5
  It would be ethically acceptable for organ donation from anencephalic infants to proceed with the consent of the parents after death has been confirmed by circulatory criteria.
- Recommendation 6
  Consistent with our earlier recommendation, the parents' values and beliefs should be allowed to determine whether their anencephalic child is intubated and ventilated, provided this is not against the child's interests. Precautionary sedation and analgesia would be needed to ensure this condition is met.
- Recommendation 7
  Health Departments and those responsible for coronial services in England, Wales and Northern Ireland might consider how the formal agreement on organ and tissue donation between the Procurator Fiscal Service and the Scottish Transplant Group could be adapted to work in the rest of the UK.
- Recommendation 8
  Consideration should be given to reviewing the Royal College of Pathologists and Royal College of Paediatrics and Child Health protocol for post mortems to identify the cause of sudden unexpected death in infancy in the context of organ donation.
- Recommendation 9
  When parents would like to donate their child's organs for transplantation but this is not clinically possible, clinicians should attempt wherever possible to accept such organs for research, if this is an acceptable alternative to the parents. ◀

47.4 Understanding the Diagnosis of Death Using Circulatory and Neurological Criteria

Learning Objectives

- Define how to diagnose death using circulatory criteria and neurological criteria.
- Be able to state the pre-conditions for brain-stem testing.
- To be able to describe the components of the brain-stem test in children vs. neonates.

Death is the irreversible loss of the capacity for consciousness, combined with irreversible loss of the capacity to breathe [10].

Consciousness is the state of wakefulness (arousal) and awareness of self and environment.

Death is the result of the irreversible loss of these functions in the brain either from intracranial causes such as trauma or haemorrhage or from cardiopulmonary arrest where impaired cerebral perfusion results in irreversible damage to the brain. The capacity to breathe and the capacity for consciousness are both functions of the brain and unlike any other organ the brain is both essential and irreplaceable [10, 11].

47.4.1 All Human Death Is Death of the Brain

Confirmation of death may seem simple at first glance but over time it has become more challenging. Due to the growing sophistication of medical science, we are now in a position where a person can have a heartbeat and appear to demonstrate breathing at the same time as having an irreversible loss of the capacity for consciousness because they are receiving mechanical ventilation.

The diagnosis of death and confirmation of death are done using the most appropriate criteria for the circumstances.

47.4.1.1 Somatic Criteria

- Decomposition or rigor mortis when death has occurred sometime ago.
- Examination for signs of life or evidence of internal organ failure are not required as death is obvious.

47.4.1.2 Circulatory Criteria

- Heart stops beating there is a cessation of the circulation.
- Within 15 s of absent cerebral circulation consciousness is lost, the EEG becomes isoelectric [12, 13]. Breathing stops.
- The brain suffers anoxic damage when the cerebral circulation is stopped.

Across all cultures, somatic and circulatory criteria are naturally recognised as a way to diagnosis death both in and out of the medical setting.

When resuscitation can be attempted, it is only successful if the circulation can be restored and cerebral circulation maintained.

47.4.1.3 Neurological Criteria

Previously called brain-stem death, we have now moved away from an anatomically based definition of death to one that is based on the permanent loss of function.

Diagnosis of death using neurological criteria or neurological determination of death.

- Requires that the patient meets certain pre-conditions that ensure that the clinical state of coma (loss of brain-stem function) is not treatable or reversible.
- If the pre-conditions are satisfied, then a series of clinical tests can be done to confirm the absence of brain-stem function.

These tests are necessary when it is not possible to determine death using somatic or circulatory criteria.

Specifically, in mechanically ventilated patients where the circulation and the appearance of breathing can be maintained even when there is an irreversible loss of the capacity for consciousness, combined with irreversible loss of the capacity to breathe, i.e., death.

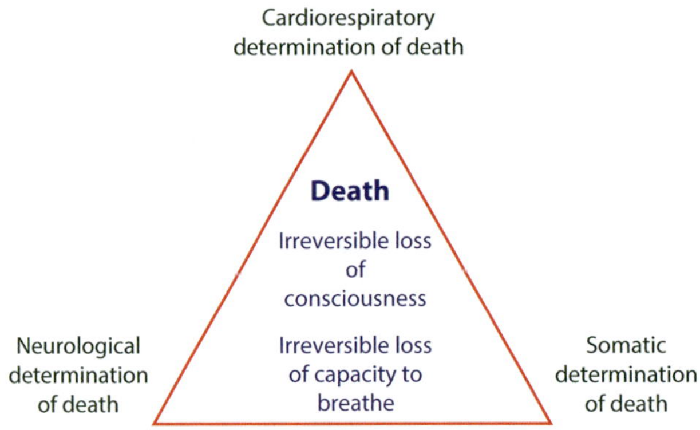

The relationship between the various criteria for the diagnosis and confirmation of death [10].

47.5 How to Diagnose Death Using Circulatory Criteria

In circumstances where there are no clear (somatic) signs that death has occurred, the point of cardiac arrest at which death occurs is identified by the following conditions:

The simultaneous and irreversible onset of apnoea and unconsciousness in the absence of the circulation.

Full and extensive attempts at reversal of any contributing cause to the cardiorespiratory arrest have been made the following potential contributing factors have been considered:

Body temperature, endocrine, metabolic, and biochemical abnormalities

One of the following is fulfilled:

- The individual meets the criteria for not attempting cardiopulmonary resuscitation
- Attempts at cardiopulmonary resuscitation have failed
- Treatment aimed at sustaining life has been withdrawn because it has been decided to be of no further benefit to the patient and not in his/her best interest to continue and/or is in respect of the patient's wishes via an advance decision to refuse treatment

The individual should be observed by the person responsible for confirming death for a minimum of 5 min to establish that irreversible cardiorespiratory arrest has occurred.

The absence of mechanical cardiac function is normally confirmed using a combination of the following:

- Absence of a central pulse on palpation
- Absence of heart sounds on auscultation. These criteria will normally suffice in the primary care setting.

However, their use can be supplemented in the hospital setting by one or more of the following:

- Absence of pulsatile flow using direct intra-arterial pressure monitoring
- Absence of contractile activity using echocardiography

Any spontaneous return of cardiac or respiratory activity during this period of observation should prompt a further 5 min observation from the next point of cardiorespiratory arrest.

After 5 min of continued cardiorespiratory arrest, the absence of the following should be confirmed:
- Pupillary responses to light
- Corneal reflexes
- Any motor response to supra-orbital pressure

The time of death is recorded as the time at which these criteria are fulfilled.

It is obviously inappropriate to initiate any intervention that has the potential to restore cerebral perfusion after death has been confirmed.

47.6 How to Diagnose Death Using Neurological Criteria [13]

Neurologically determination of death will almost always take place in a critical care setting where the patient is ventilated.

To diagnose death using neurological criteria, certain **preconditions** must be met:
- The patient must be in a deep coma with no intrinsic ability to breathe. This must result from an irreversible and untreatable injury of known cause.
- Prior to testing, the patient must be in a stable physiological condition.
- Other potential causes of apnoea and coma must be excluded. If these potential causes are correctable, these must be corrected before testing can be performed.
- Core temperature must be more than or equal to 36 °C as profound hypothermia is associated with loss of brain-stem reflexes.
- Peripheral nerve stimulator or another recognised method should be used to confirm that adequate neuromuscular function is present [13].
- The clinical team must be confident that there are no sedative or neuromuscular agents contributing to the coma or apnoea. Absence of neuro blocking agents can be confirmed by using a peripheral nerve stimulator, if necessary.

Particular care needs to be taken in the following RED FLAG circumstances as they cause the absence of brain-stem reflexes, or may lead to ***reversible*** coma or apnoea.
- In renal and hepatic impairment, excluding the residual effect of sedatives can be a challenge if there are doubts measuring serum concentrations can be useful, e.g., Midazolam <5 mcg/L Thiopental <10 mg/L.
- In prolonged infusions of fentanyl as total body clearance of fentanyl is highly variable and context sensitive [14].
- In conditions where intracranial compliance may be increased such as therapeutic decompressive craniectomy [13].
- If steroids have been given for space-occupying lesions or if the aetiology is primarily located in the brain-stem or posterior fossa [13].

Recommended that clinical testing is undertaken:
- More than 6 h after the loss of brain-stem reflexes and discontinuation of sedative drugs.

- More than 24 h after the loss of brain-stem reflexes where the primary cause is hypoxic brain injury.
- More than 24 h after the restoration of normothermia after therapeutic hypothermia.

47.7 UK Procedure for Neurological Determination of Death [13]

» The diagnosis of death by neurological criteria should be made by at least two medical practitioners. Both medical practitioners should have been registered with the General Medical Council (or equivalent Professional Body) for more than five years and be competent in the assessment of a patient who may be deceased following the irreversible cessation of brain-stem function and competent in the conduct and interpretation of the brain-stem examination. Both doctors should be competent in the diagnosis of death by neurological criteria, both should be paediatricians or paediatric intensivists and one should be a consultant.

» Testing should be undertaken by the nominated doctors acting together and must always be performed on two occasions. A complete set of tests should be performed on each occasion, i.e., a total of two sets of tests will be performed. Doctor One may perform the tests while Doctor Two observes; this would constitute the first set. Roles may be reversed for the second set. The tests, in particular the apnoea test, are therefore performed only twice in total. [A code of practice for the diagnosis and confirmation of death—Academy of Royal Medical Colleges 2008 updated January 2025.

Temperature, respiratory, circulatory, metabolic, or endocrine parameters for testing If prior to testing any cardiovascular or respiratory instability is present, exclude possibility that this is the cause of observed coma and apnoea For infants/children with congenital cyanotic heart disease oxygen levels should be kept in their normal range If there is any clinical reason to expect endocrine disturbances, then it is obligatory to ensure appropriate hormonal assays are undertaken	
Respiratory	Normal if possible—**$PaCO_2$ < 6.0 kPa, PaO_2 > 10 kPa** and **pH 7.35–7.45**
Cardiovascular	Mean arterial pressure should be consistently maintained at age-appropriate levels
Core temp aim	Greater or equal to 36 degrees C
Na	**125–160 mmol/L** Levels below 125 or above 160 mmol/L are associated with unresponsiveness
K	**>2 mmol/L** Serum potassium of less than 2 mmol/L may be associated severe neuromuscular weakness

(continued)

Mg	**0.5–3.0 mmol/L** Serum levels less than 0.5 mmol/L or greater than 3.0 mmol/L may be associated severe neuromuscular weakness
PO_4	**<3 mmol/L** Serum phosphate of more than 3 mmol/L may be associated severe neuromuscular weakness
Blood glucose	**3.0–20 mmol/L** before each brain-stem test
The reflexes for brain stem function include: – Pupillary response to light – Corneal reflex – Vestibulo-ocular reflex (caloric test) – Motor response to pain in the distribution of cranial nerve V (i.e., facial grimace or other motor response to supra-orbital pressure) – Gag and cough reflex in response to oropharyngeal stimulation and suction through an endotracheal tube or tracheostomy – Respiratory response to rise in arterial blood partial pressure of carbon dioxide ($PaCO_2$)	
Brain-stem reflexes	
Pupils (pupillary response to light)	Fixed in diameter and unresponsive to light
Corneal (blink) reflex	Absent when fine piece of gauze wiped across cornea
Eye movement Vestibular-ocular reflex (caloric test)	Absent with head flexed 30° when each ear is instilled with 20–50 mL of Ice-cold water (Each ear drum should be clearly visualised before the test)
Motor response	No motor response within the cranial nerve or somatic distribution in response to supraorbital pressure (Reflex limb and trunk movements (spinal reflexes) may still be present)
Gag	No gag reflex following stimulation to the posterior pharynx
Cough	No cough reflex following suction catheter placed down the trachea to the carina

Apnoea test	
End tidal carbon dioxide can be used to guide the starting of each apnoea test but should not replace the pre and post arterial $PaCO_2$ Oxygenation and cardiovascular stability should be maintained through each apnoea test	
PCO_2	**Starting arterial Co2 of at least 5.3 Kpa with an increase of at least 2.7 kpa**
pH	**Arterial ph less than 7.3 at the end of the test**

(continued)

Cease ventilation	
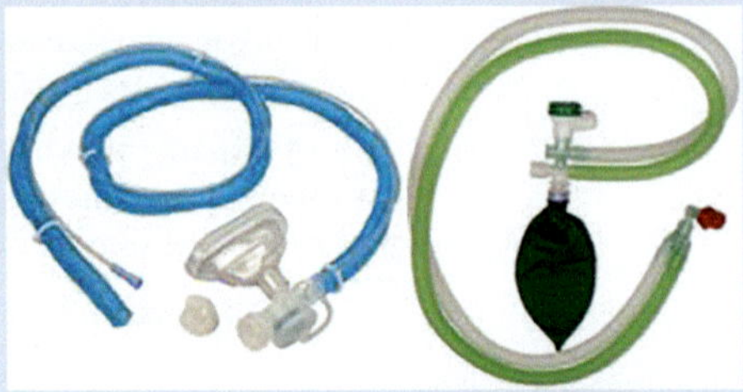	
Either use a CPAP circuit (e.g., Mapleson C or Ayres T piece) or disconnect the patient from the ventilator and administer oxygen via a catheter in the trachea through the endotracheal tube at a rate of 2–6 L/min There should be no spontaneous respiration within a minimum of 5 min following disconnection from the ventilator [UK donation practice favours the use of the Mapleson C as it allows visualisation of breathing (if it is present) as well as allowing a lung recruitment manoeuvre afterwards	
After 5 min	Confirm that the $PaCO_2$ has increased from the starting level by 2.7 kpa or more resulting in an arterial CO2 of at least 8 kpa
Recruitment manoeuvres	At the conclusion of the apnoea test, manual recruitment manoeuvres should be carried out before resuming mechanical ventilation and ventilation parameters normalised
Time of death	When both sets of tests have been completed

47.7.1 Neurological Determination of Death in the Neonate

Until 2015, it was not possible to determine death using neurological criteria in infants less than 2 months of age in the UK. In 2008, "A Code of Practice for the Diagnosis and Confirmation of Death" was published and it concluded that, "it is rarely possible confidently to diagnose brainstem death at this age."

In 2015, the Royal college of Paediatric and Child health UK (RCPCH) published Guidance for the Determination of death using neurological criteria in infants from 37 weeks corrected gestation to 2 months post term. The updated 2025 guidance reinforces this guidance and goes further stating that determination of death using neurological criteria can be reliably performed in infants from 37 weeks corrected gestation usuing the same criteria as adults [13].

Recently, organ donation from infants less than 6 months old has increased. Primarily because of the use of en bloc kidneys from small donors in renal transplantation and the development of hepatocyte transplants. Hepatocytes can be retrieved from very small infants.

- Essentially the diagnosis of death using neurological criteria is the same as for older children
- Absent brain-stem reflexes
- Absent motor responses
- No respiratory response to hypercarbia

The 2025 updated guidance states that as in the previous guidance:

There must be a clear rise in the partial pressure of carbon dioxide ($PaCO_2$) greater than 2.7 kPa above baseline of at least 5.3 kPa to >8.0 kPa with no response at that level. However, the interval between a complete set of tests must be at least 24 hours in children less than 2 years old or less than 2 years corrected in premature neonates. In children greater than 2 years old no delay is required between tests as long as the patients baseline parameters return to appropriate pre-test levels [13].

Similarity within the UK Code of Practice (2008) for the diagnosis of death after cardiorespiratory arrest and in a patient in a coma.

Diagnosing and confirming death after cardiorespiratory arrest (circulatory criteria)	Diagnosis and confirmation of death in a patient in a coma (neurological criteria)
Demonstration of loss of the capacity for consciousness	
Absence of the pupillary response to light	Absence of the pupillary response to light
Absence of the corneal reflex	Absence of the corneal reflex
Absence of any motor response to supra-orbital pressure	Absence of any motor response to supra-orbital pressure
Demonstration of loss of the capacity to breathe	
Five minutes observation of maintained cardiorespiratory arrest	Five minutes apnoea test to demonstrate no spontaneous respiratory effort
Academy of Medical Royal Colleges: A Code of Practice for the Diagnosis and Confirmation of Death, Academy of Medical Royal Colleges, London (2008)	

47.8 Donation Processes

Organ donation practises vary across the world. In many countries there is no option for deceased donation, in others deceased donation is limited to DBD only.

The process by which potential donors are identified, families approached, and consent obtained will also vary from country to country.

These variations may reflect the differing medical, legal, religious, cultural, ethical issues, and resources that every nation is subject to.

47.8.1 UK Example

▶ Example

Deceased organ donation in the UK is a nationally structured process which at its centre has the idea that the consideration of organ donation should be an integral part of good quality end-of-life care.

Every patient who meets the referral criteria should be identified and referred to the organ donation service. In the UK, there is both DCD and DBD donation [15]. ◀

47.8.2 Donation After Circulatory (Cardiac) Death DCD

Learning Objectives

- Be able to outline process of DCD and recognise potential ethical issues associated with DCD.
- Understand how to potentially maximise DCD donation outcomes.

DCD is the retrieval of organs for the purposes of transplantation when death has been confirmed using circulatory criteria.

The focus of DCD is to provide a donation option for patients who will never meet the neurological criteria for the diagnosis of death.

DCD also meets the needs of a small number of families who are uncertain/uncomfortable regarding the use of neurological criteria to diagnose death (brain death), but nevertheless wish to consent to donation. As it meets their need to witness the ending of life when the heart stops beating.

Therefore, there are benefits for both transplant patients as well as deceased patients and their families who wish to donate organs after death.

DCD occurs after there has been a withdrawal of life-sustaining treatment in the best interests of the patient. As continuation of therapy is futile and of no benefit to the patient; potentially resulting in the prolongation of suffering to the patient and to the family without hope of recovery.

The prospect of DCD can raise ethical concerns.

There may be a perceived conflict of interest for clinicians who are involved in the decision to withdrawal life-sustaining treatment and the process of gaining consent for donation.

To prevent this:

The decision to withdrawal life-sustaining treatment (WLST) should always be independent of the consideration of the patient as an organ donor.

However:

The UK Donation Ethics Committee in their 2011 guidance Ethical framework for controlled donation after circulatory death considered that:

> *There is no ethical dilemma if the treating clinician wishes to make contact with the SNOD (specialist nurse for organ donation) at an early stage, while the patient is seriously ill and death is likely, but before a formal decision has been made to withdraw life-sustaining treatment.*

End-of-life care conversations should be held with the family and it is only when the family fully understand and accept the decision to WLST that an approach can made to them to discuss potential organ donation. It is advisable to separate these discussions in time.

No members of the transplant or donor coordination teams should be involved in the decision to withdrawal life-sustaining treatments.

Other concerns may centre around the acceptability of interventions that are done before or after death to facilitate donation:

Pre-mortem interventions to facilitate controlled DCD that may be considered acceptable and unacceptable [10].

Acceptable interventions	Unacceptable interventions
Discussing a potential donor with the donor transplant coordinator before the patient's death and checking the organ donor register	Anything that causes or places the person at risk of serious harm or distress
Approaching the relatives about donation before the patient's death	Donor transplant coordinator caring for the potential donor while they are still alive
Seeking details of the patient's medical history relevant to donation	Systemic heparinisation in circumstances where this might accelerate death (e.g., recent intracranial bleed)
Taking blood and testing blood or serum samples	Femoral cannulation
Maintenance of life-sustaining treatment	CPR
Delaying the withdrawal of treatment	Involvement of the retrieval team and the recipient's clinical team in the care of the potential donor
Changing a patient's location for treatment withdrawal	

Or

Over the uncertainties concerning the time at which death can be confirmed after the mechanical cessation of the circulation. These include the possibility of the return of spontaneous circulation after asystole and possible return of cerebral blood flow (auto-resuscitation).

The dead donor rule needs to be maintained—the requirement that organ retrieval must not cause the death of the patient put another way the patient must be dead before organs are retrieved.

It is essential that when using circulatory criteria for the diagnosis of death for organ donation that there should be agreement not to attempt further resuscitation, there should be a minimum period of observation and there should be no activities that might restore cerebral circulation.

There is irreversible and therefore permanent cessation of function because it will neither return spontaneously nor will it return as a result of medical action because this will not be attempted.

If death is the irreversible loss of the capacity for consciousness, combined with irreversible loss of the capacity to breathe. Then how long should we wait after the cessation of circulation before we are sure of irreversibility?

Organ donation after circulatory determination makes it necessary to develop detailed guidelines on how doctors should employ circulatory respiratory tests for death in patients who are potential organ donors [16].

After 65 s of asystole studies show that patients do not undergo "auto-resuscitation" [16, 17]. The interval between cessation of mechanical circulation and the declaration of death must be long enough to exclude the possibility of auto-resuscitation. Because the database for cases of auto-resuscitation is so small and contains no infants or young children, it makes sense to include a longer interval than 65 s.

After a review of auto-resuscitation data, the Ethics Committee of the society of critical care medicine suggested a minimum of 2 min and a maximum of 5 min for the observation period. Transient resumption of cardiac activity was reported in a study of 1999 patients 14% of the time after retrospective analysis of ECG and blood pressure waveforms. All of the events occurred within 4 min and 20 s after a period of pulselessness [18].

This is clear evidence that a 5-min interval between the cessation of mechanical circulation and the declaration of death is sufficient [19].

Low output states can occur when the pulse is impalpable and therefore there is a risk that palpation of the pulse under these circumstances may not be reliable enough to recognise the cessation of circulation [16].

Therefore, the use of intra-arterial pressure monitoring or echo cardiography to determine mechanical asystole is recommended, where possible.

Mechanical asystole is enough and additional electrical asystole is not necessary because the standard for declaring death requires the absence of circulation, not the absence of cardiac electrical function.

47.8.2.1 Warm Ischaemic Injury in DCD

Organs from DCD donors are exposed to longer warm ischaemia than organs from comparable DBD donors.

Functional warm ischaemia time is considered to begin when the patients systolic arterial pressure decreases below 50 mmHg, the arterial oxygen saturation decreases below 70%, or both.

Ischaemic injury increases the risks of primary graft failure. Therefore, organ retrieval may not occur if the time interval from withdrawal of treatment (or onset of functional warm ischaemia) is prolonged.

UK functional warm ischaemia criteria for DCD organ retrieval [20].

Organ	Minimum functional warm ischaemia time (min)	Comments
Kidney	120	Plus a further 120 min in selected donors. DCD kidneys have a higher incidence of delayed graft function, but have similar long-term function to DBD grafts
Liver	30	May be limited to 20 min in sub-optimal donors. Outcomes from DCD liver transplantation are acceptable, but there is greater postoperative morbidity and a higher incidence of graft failure and biliary complications compared with DBD grafts

(continued)

Organ	Minimum functional warm ischaemia time (min)	Comments
Lung	60	Time to re-inflation of the lungs rather than cold perfusion. DCD may represent an important source of additional lung grafts, particularly when combined with ex vivo perfusion techniques
Pancreas	30	

To facilitate the best donation outcome in accordance with the donor family wishes:

- Withdrawal of treatment should be delayed until retrieval teams are in place to retrieve the organs.
- Delays in organ allocation and retrieval should be minimised as prolonging this process will cause increased stress and suffering for the donor family and can result in withdrawal of consent for donation.
- WLST should be done as close as possible to the operating room where organ retrieval is to take place. As organs should be removed as quickly as possible after death has been declared. This must be done without comprising the patients' right to comfort or their access to close friends and family. In many UK paediatric centres, this place will be the anaesthetic room adjacent to the operating room.
- WLST that leads to organ donation should follow the same local guidelines or practises of any other WLST done on the PICU. So, the PICU team are not perceived to have a conflict of interest in treatment-withdrawal decisions. Operational policies should be in place to underpin this.

47.8.3 Donation After Neurological Determination of Death DBD

Learning Objectives
- Recognise the importance of DBD relative to DCD.
- Be able to describe the physiological changes that accompany brain-stem ischaemia and the effect they have on potential organ transplant viability.
- Outline the process of DBD and the place of donor optimisation.

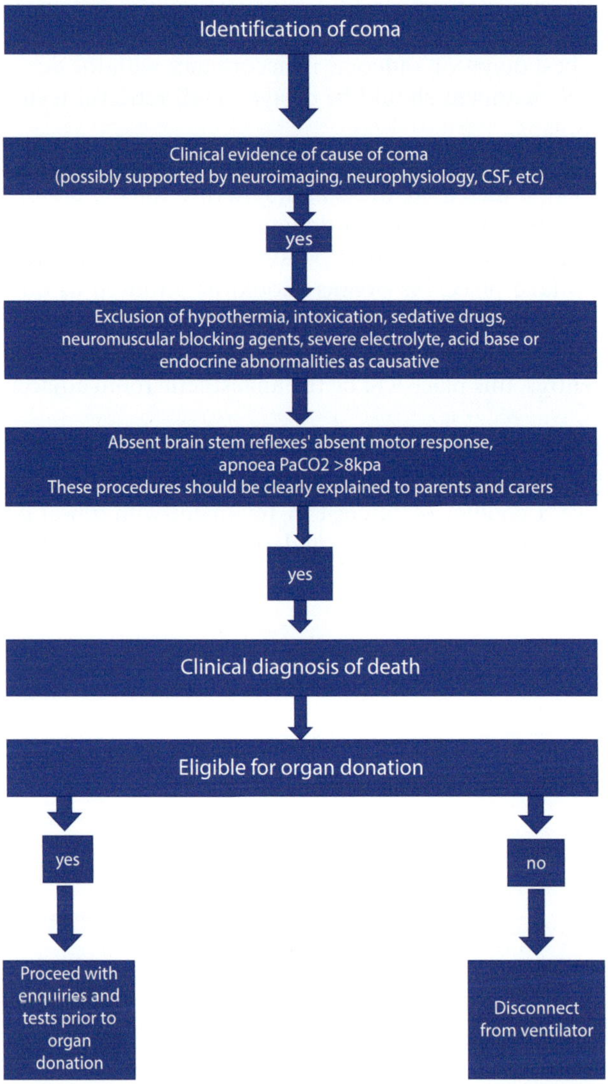

Donation after neurological determination of death brain death means that donor surgery can be carried out with the physiological circulation more or less intact ensuring better graft perfusion in comparison to DCD.

In the UK, on average 3.6 organs are transplanted per DBD donor compared to 2.1 per DCD donor [20].

There has been a decrease in the incidence of death diagnosed by neurological criteria both in adults and children in recent years [21, 22]. Probably because of improvements in road safety and in the delivery of neurocritical care management for traumatic brain injury and intracranial haemorrhage [23–25].

It is therefore essential that all those who fulfil the criteria for the diagnosis of death using neurological criteria should have brain-stem testing performed. As this also allows clinicians to give a definitive diagnosis of death rather than relying on circulatory criteria which can only be fulfilled in mechanically ventilated patients when life-sustaining therapy is withdrawn in the patients' best interests.

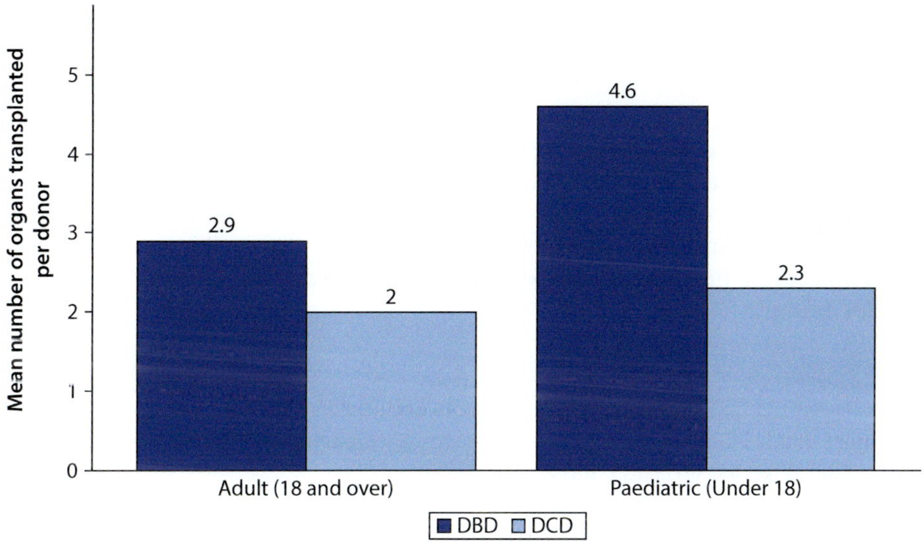

Mean number of organs transplanted per donor by age group and donor type, 1 April 2019–31 March 2020 [20]

After the determination of death using neurological criteria has been done, there are several things that will endanger the viability of potential organs for donation which come about as a result of the physiological changes that take place when brain-stem ischaemia occurs.

Death is the result of cerebral herniation through the foramen magnum due to raised intracranial pressure leading to brainstem ischaemia:

- At the top of the brain-stem pontine, ischaemia results increased parasympathetic and sympathetic activity leading to bradycardia, hypertension, and irregular breathing—Cushing's triad.
- As ischaemia spreads down the brainstem, there is damage to the parasympathetic innervated structures in the medulla leading to unopposed sympathetic drive, this is called a "catecholamine surge" or "autonomic storm." Increased levels of dopamine, adrenalin, and noradrenaline cause vasoconstriction, hypertension, tachycardia, and increased myocardial oxygen demand. Overtime these hormones are depleted, resulting in hypotension.

- Loss of vasomotor tone and hypotension occur with inferior brainstem ischaemia involving the spinal cord.

As perfusion stops in the hypothalamus and pituitary, the resultant neuro endocrine failure causes:
- Hypothermia—Resulting in possible arrhythmias, insulin resistance, and coagulopathy [26].
- Decreased circulating levels of adrenocorticotrophic hormone (ACTH)—This may impair the stress response of the donor [26, 27].
- Decreased thyroid stimulating hormone—Can cause functional hypothyroidism which may affect the donor heart as decreased T3 diminishes cardiac contractility [26].
- Decreased antidiuretic hormone—Loss of ADH causes Diabetes Insipidus leading to free water loss, hypovolaemia, and hypernatremia [26].

The catecholamine surge, metabolic derangement, and ischaemic injury precipitate a pro inflammatory response which provokes disseminated intravascular coagulation and platelet dysfunction which may lead to donor graft damage.

Use of a donor optimisation bundle will ensure that there is optimal maintenance of the haemodynamic and metabolic state in the donor. This will increase graft viability and ensure that the patient's and family's wish to donate is honoured.

For example

▶ Example

A 7-year-old child involved in a road traffic accident has suffered a catastrophic brain injury and is admitted to the paediatric intensive care unit. The patient is intubated and ventilated but has no central intravenous access.

Death is suspected using neurological criteria and the preconditions for brain-stem testing are met.

Brain-stem testing is performed and death is confirmed.

The parents give consent for organ donation.

Haemodynamic instability develops, a central line is inserted, pressors are started, and donation goes ahead in accordance with the wishes of the parents. ◀

▶ Example

"Paediatric donor optimisation care bundle"

Donor Optimisation Care Bundle – Paediatric (37 wks CGA - 15 yrs)

Patient Name__________________ Date of Birth__________________

Unit Number__________________ Date __________________

Cardiovascular — Y N/A

1. Monitor cardiovascular state aim for normal parameters[1] ☐ ■
2. Measure CVP (4 – 10 mmHg) (if suitable access available) ☐ ☐
3. Review intravascular fluid status and correct hypovolaemia with isotonic Fluid boluses (10mls/kg aliquot) ☐ ■
4. Measure central venous oxygen saturation (maintain >70%) ☐ ■
5. Measure cardiac output if appropriate (non-invasive monitoring is appropriate if available) ☐ ☐
6. Commence vasopressin where vasopressor required, wean or stop catecholamine pressors as able ☐ ☐
7. Commence dopamine / noradrenaline to maintain MAP as required ☐ ☐
8. Introduce adrenaline / dobutamine if echo indicates poor cardiac function ☐ ☐
9. Consider esmolol / labetalol in cases of persistent hypertension in the absence of vasopressors. ☐ ☐

Respiratory

(>1 month old - pH > 7.25 PaO_2 ≥ 10 kPa)
(37wk CGA - <1 month old pH >7.2 PaO2 >8kPa)

1. Perform lung recruitment manoeuvres (following apnoea tests, disconnections, suctions, de-saturations). ☐ ■
2. Review ventilation, ensure lung protective strategy (Tidal volumes 6- 8ml/kg (< 1month old 4-6mls/kg) and optimum PEEP (5 – 10 cm H_2O), PIP <30cmH_2O) ☐ ■
3. Maintain regular chest physio incl. suctioning as per unit protocol ☐ ■
4. Maintain 30 – 45 degrees head of bed elevation ☐ ■
5. If appropriate use a cuffed endotracheal tube and ensure it is adequately inflated (consider changing to cuffed tube if indicated) ☐ ☐
6. Patient positioning (side, back, side) as per unit protocol ☐ ■
7. Where available, and in the context of lung donation, perform bronchoscopy, bronchial lavage and - toilet for therapeutic purposes ☐ ☐

Fluids and metabolic management — Y N/A

1. Review fluid administration. IV crystalloid maintenance fluid (or NG water where appropriate) to maintain Na^+ < 150 mmol/l ☐ ■
2. Maintain urine output between 1.0 – 2.0ml/kg/hr (If > 4ml/kg/hr, consider Diabetes insipidus and treat promptly with vasopressin and/or DDAVP.) ☐ ■
3. Administer methylprednisolone ☐ ■
4. Start insulin infusion if necessary to maintain blood sugar (4 –12 mmol/l) ☐ ■
5. Continue NG feeding as appropriate, ensure prescribed gastric protection as unit policy ☐ ☐
6. Correct electrolyte abnormalities (maintain Na, K, Ca, Phos, and Mg within normal ranges) ☐ ■

Thrombo-embolic prevention

1. Ensure prevention measures in place as per unit policy ☐ ☐

Lines, Monitoring and Investigations (if not already completed)

1. Insert arterial line ☐ ■
2. Continue hourly observations as per critical care policy ☐ ■
3. Perform CXR (post recruitment procedure where possible) ☐ ■
4. Perform a 12-lead ECG ☐ ■
5. Send Troponin level in all cardiac arrest cases (and follow-up sample where patient in PICU > 24 hours) ☐ ☐
6. Where available, perform an echocardiogram ☐ ☐

Other

1. Maintain normothermia using active warming /cooling where required ☐ ■
2. Review and stop all unnecessary medications ☐ ■
3. Consideration for blood sampling volumes[2] ☐ ■
4. Family considerations and support throughout ☐ ■

Paediatric Donor Optimisation Care Bundle 2016

Drug	Standard infusion	Diluent	Rate of infusion	Dose
Dopamine	15mg/kg in 50mls (max 800mg in 50ml)	NaCl 0.9% OR Glucose 5%	1ml /hr = 5 micrograms/kg/min	<10 micrograms/kg/min
Noradrenaline	0.3mg / kg in 50mls (max concentration 8mg in 5ml)	Glucose 5%/ Na Cl 0.9%	1ml/hr = 0.1 micrograms/kg/min (of standard infusion)	0-0.5 micrograms/kg/min (maximum rate = 5mls/hr of standard infusion)
Vasopressin/ Argipressin	20 units in 50ml diluent	NaCl 0.9% / Glucose 5%	0.0003 units/kg/min = 0.045ml/kg/hr	0.0003-0.001units/kg/min (Max dose 6 u/hr)[3]
Vasopressin - treatment for Diabetes Insipidus[4]	2-5 units / litre diluent	NaCl 0.9% / Glucose 5%	ml for ml replacement of urine output	N/A
Adrenaline	0.3mg /kg in 50ml	Glucose 5%	1 ml /hr = 0.1micrograms/kg/min (of standard infusion)	0-0.5micrograms/kg/min
Dobutamine	30mg/kg in 50mls	Glucose 5%, 10% / Nacl 0.9%	1ml/hr = 10micrograms/kg/min	5-20 micrograms/kg/min

Esmolol	10mg/ml (pre-diluted)	50-300 micrograms/kg/min (max 500 micrograms/kg/min)	IV continuous infusion – titrated to response
Labetalol	5mg/ml (neat)	0.5 – 3 milligrams/kg/hr (max 5 milligrams/kg/hr)	IV continuous infusion – titrate to response

Drug	Dose	Administration
Methylprednisolone	15milligrams/kg (max 1g)	IV infusion over 1 hour
DDAVP (desmopressin)	1 month – 12 years 400 nanograms 12-18 years 1-4 micrograms	IV bolus
Insulin (50 units in 50ml)	0.1units/kg/hr	IV continuous infusion – titrated to response

Bibliography / References

1. European Paediatric Advanced Life Support 4th ed (2016). European Resuscitation Council. Lippincott Williams & Wilkins

2. SOP 5058 – Neonatal and Infant Organ Donation

3. Rozenfeld V, Cheng JW. The role of vasopressin in the treatment of vasodilation in shock states. Ann Pharmacother. 2000; 34:250-4

4. Ralston.C & Butt. W Continuous vasopressin replacement in diabetes incipidus. Arch Dis. Child. 1990 65; 896-897 doi 10.1136/adc.65.8.896

5. Mallory GB Jr, Schecter MG, Elidemir O, Management of the Paediatric Organ donor to optimise lung donation. Paediatric Pulmonol. 2009 Jun; 44(6):536-46

5. Paediatric Formulary Committee. *BNF for Children* (2015 -2016) London: BMJ Group, Pharmaceutical Press, and RCPCH Publications; (2015)

6. Optimisation care bundle http://www.odt.nhs.uk/pdf/dbd_care_bundle.pdf

7. Shemie. S Organ donation management in Canada; recommendations of the forum on medical management to optimise donor organ potential. 2006. Mar 14; 174(6):s13-s30

Systolic BP - Age specific ranges (mmHg) – EPALS guidance[1]	
0-1 month	50-60 mmHg
1-12 months	70-80 mmHg
1-10 years	70+(2 x age(yrs)) to 90+(2 x age(yrs))
> 10 yrs	90-120 mmHg

Paediatric Donor Optimisation Care Bundle 2016

Donor Optimisation Care Bundle – Paediatric (37 wks CGA - 15 yrs)

Patient Name______________ Date of Birth______________

Unit Number______________ Date ______________

Physiological Parameters / Goals **Tick ✓ = achieved, x = not achieved**

	O/A	+1hr	+2hrs	+4hrs	+6hrs	+8hrs	+10hrs	+12hrs	+14hrs	+16hrs	+18hrs
Target Systolic BP (primary goal) .... /mmHg	☐	☐	☐	☐	☐	☐	☐	☐	☐	☐	☐
CVP 4 – 10 mmHg (secondary goal)	☐	☐	☐	☐	☐	☐	☐	☐	☐	☐	☐
$PaO_2 \geq 10.0$ kPa (>1month) (37wk CGA - < 1month old PaO2 >8 kPa and pH> 7.2) $FiO_2 < 0.4$ as able	☐	☐	☐	☐	☐	☐	☐	☐	☐	☐	☐
$PaCO_2$ 5 – 6.5 kPa (or higher as long as pH > 7.25)	☐	☐	☐	☐	☐	☐	☐	☐	☐	☐	☐
$ScvO_2 > 70\%$	☐	☐	☐	☐	☐	☐	☐	☐	☐	☐	☐
Cardiac index > 2.5 - 6 l/min/m²	☐	☐	☐	☐	☐	☐	☐	☐	☐	☐	☐
SVRI 400– 1200 dynes*sec/cm⁵/m²	☐	☐	☐	☐	☐	☐	☐	☐	☐	☐	☐
Temperature 36 – 37°C	☐	☐	☐	☐	☐	☐	☐	☐	☐	☐	☐
Blood glucose 4.0 – 12 mmol/l	☐	☐	☐	☐	☐	☐	☐	☐	☐	☐	☐
Maintain Na < 150mmol/l	☐	☐	☐	☐	☐	☐	☐	☐	☐	☐	☐
Urine output 1- 2 ml/kg/hour	☐	☐	☐	☐	☐	☐	☐	☐	☐	☐	☐
Signature / Print Name											
Date / Time											

Paediatric Donor Optimisation Care Bundle 2016

◀

47.8.4 Donor Identification and Referral

Learning Objectives

- Explain how to identify potential donors.
- To be able to specify when and how to approach potential donor families.
- Understand why working collaboratively with specialist organ donation teams is advantageous.

Consideration of donation should be a routine part of high-quality end-of-life care. All potential donors should be identified in a timely fashion.

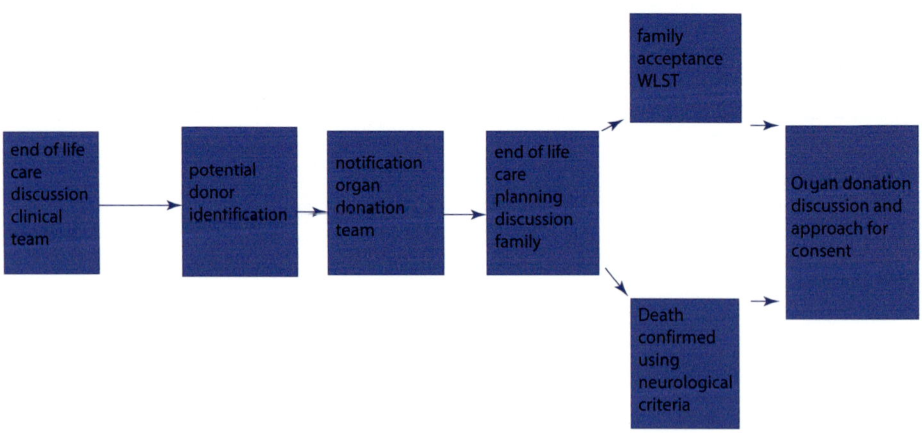

In the UK, Specialist nurses for organ donation support potential donor families and the operational processes of organ donation.

They support donor families through the end-of-life care process and are able to provide specific information which can be tailored to the needs of the family.

NICE guidelines recommend that patients should be referred to the SNODs as soon as there is an

- Intention to withdrawal life-sustaining treatment or
- Perform brain-stem testing.

These two instances are absolute triggers for SNOD referral/notification and should happen regardless of whether the treating team think that there is or is no potential for donation.

Other absolute triggers in UK paediatric practise are:

- Death is likely to happen in the next 48 h.
- The family have raised the question of donation.

Additionally, to make sure no potential donors are missed. The UK National organ donation committee—subgroup in paediatrics has conducted research into the use of paediatric extended notification triggers such as:

- Re-orientation of care discussions including palliative care.
- Early end-of-life care planning.

It is envisaged that at notification the SNOD and clinical team will plan the timing and nature of discussions going forward leading up to the mobilisation of the SNOD, if required.

Early involvement of the Specialist Nurse—Organ donation leads to prompt and pre-emptive advice regarding:

- Identification and the resolution of potential Coronial/Procurator fiscal (legal) issues.
- Rapid screening and assessment of donor eligibility.
- Early tissue typing and virology screening.
- Access to advice on neurological determination of death testing especially useful for those who rarely perform such tests in paediatrics.
- Advice regarding the use of the donor care bundle to support physiological optimisation in potential DBD donors.

Most importan tly early involvement of the SNOD teams promotes and facilitates a collaborative approach in planning and conducting the approach to the family to ask for consent to donation.

Research has shown that SNOD involvement increases consent rates:

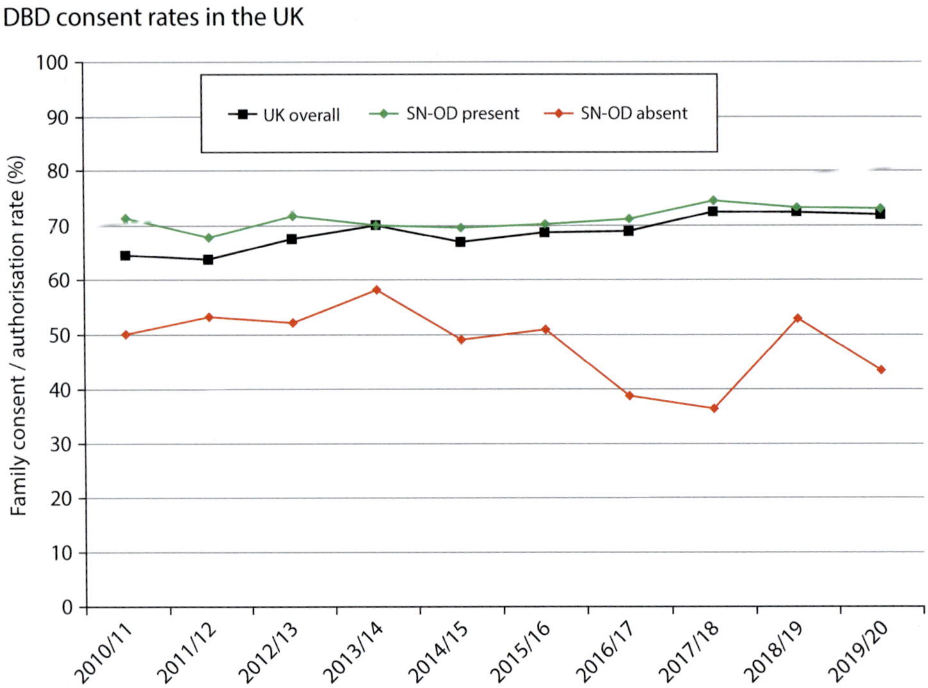

Three key stages in the approach of families

- Planning
- Confirming understanding of the acceptance of loss
- Discussing donation

Approaching families to gain consent for organ donation is more successful when the full expertise of the specialist team is utilised.

Paediatric teams generally pride themselves on their family-centred practise, their communication skills, and on their sensitivity when delivering bad news.

We are naturally very protective of our patients and their families and work hard to gain and preserve trust in challenging end-of-life care situations over many conversations with them.

Therefore, it can be difficult having an outside team become involved at the end of what often has been a protracted and distressing time for the treating teams.

Paediatric donation is a rare occurrence; therefore, most PICU consultants may only be directly involved with a handful of these cases in a career.

SNODs receive extensive training in communication and family support which is particularly focused on guiding families through end-of-life care journey. The SNODs are approaching families on a regular basis. Almost exclusively this will be with adult patients. However, there is a considerable amount of overlap in the process and dynamic of these conversations.

It is important that the PICU team accepts that SNOD involvement is the standard of care as per current professional guidance in the UK.

NICE guidelines recommend that a patient should be referred as a potential donor as soon as the intention to either withdraw life-sustaining treatments or perform brain-stem death tests has been reached.

Once the SNOD has been notified, bilateral planning discussions can be held regarding the timing of tests and conversations with the family.

Decisions can be made about who will be present in the conversations and how they will be introduced to the family. The team can discuss how the discussion will be structured and who will say what. This will allow the SNOD and clinical team to consider carefully when the possibility of organ donation is best raised with the family.

Donation must not be raised until the family fully understand that their child has died as will be the case following the diagnosis of death using neurological criteria

Or

When the intention to withdrawal life-sustaining treatment has been discussed, understood, and agreed to by the family.

Potential donation should never influence the decision to WLST. The decision to stop treatment should be based on what is in the child's best interests. The donation conversation is only relevant as part of the overall discussion of end-life-care when the family fully understand and accept that their child will die. This conversation should be separate in time to the initial WLST and diagnosis of death using neurological criteria discussion.

In most cases the discussion to confirm the acceptance of loss will be led by a senior clinician before making the transition to the specialist nurse to lead the discussion about donation.

The discussion around donation should be presented positively and never in an apologetic way.

47.8.5 Organ Retrieval

The organ retrieval team is responsible for retrieving those organs for which consent has been given and for which a suitable recipient has been identified or when appropriate organs where consent has been obtained for them to be used in clinical research.

There is a variation in the number of organs that are retrieved from each donor. The organ retrieval rate is higher in paediatrics than it is in adults 4.6 vs. 2.9 per DBD donor [20].

Not all organs retrieved are transplantable, this can be because of perceived poor function in the organ or rarely because of no suitable recipient.

The retrieval process incorporates assessment of organ suitability at several stages:

- By retrieval surgeons while organs are still in the donor to exclude the presence of potential contraindications to donation that could risk potential recipients.
- When organs are removed, they are reassessed individually and the quality is relayed to the transplanting team.
- On arrival at transplant centre, organs are checked again by the surgeon to check quality before proceeding to transplant.

There are various international and national guidelines regarding organ retrieval but these are not always consistent. However, the final decision as to whether a retrieved organ is transplanted rests with the transplant surgeon.

In the UK, a National Organ Retrieval Service (NORS) was commissioned in 2010. This ensures that there are fully staffed retrieval teams available 24 h a day, 7 days a week to retrieve donated organs from any hospital in the UK.

47.9 International Perspectives

Learning Objective

- Recognise and explain what makes a successful deceased donor program.

Rates of deceased donation vary markedly across the world. Organ donation rates have traditionally been expressed as donors per million population (pmp), this accurately measures the activity but not the effectiveness of donor programs. A number of factors can influence the number of potential donors [28].

- Incidence of life-threatening trauma and intracranial haemorrhage
- Availability of intensive care facilities
- Consent rates
- Legal constraints in a number of countries

A more meaningful measure would be the proportion of potential donors who become actual donors (conversion rate) in the UK, the Potential Donor Audit can provide this figure and is used to identify areas where practise can be improved in order to increase the conversion rate.

This national database is updated by the specialist nurses for organ donation and aims to capture details on all deaths on intensive care to see whether potential donors were referred in line with national guidance.

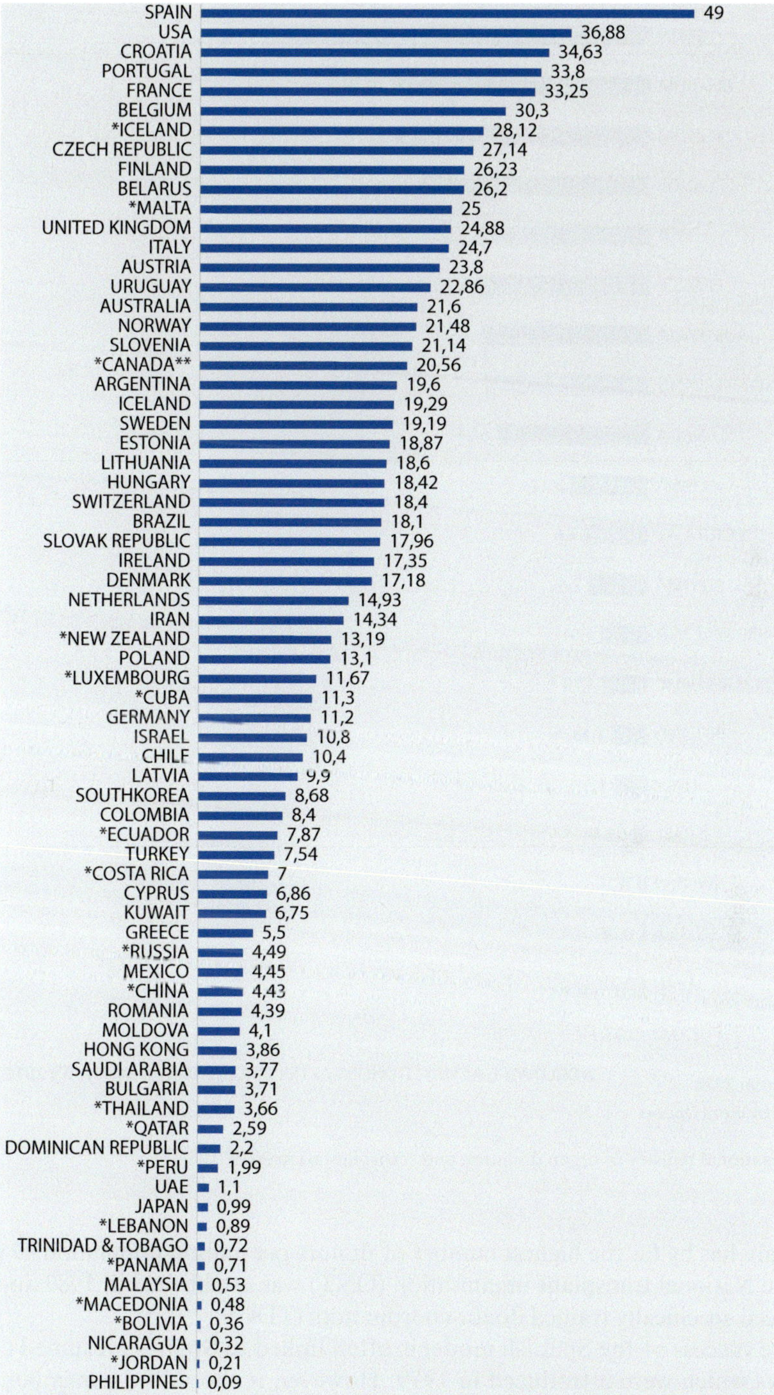

WORLDWIDE ACTUAL DECEASED ORGAN DONORS RATE 2019 (pmp)

*** Data from 2018**
**** Total Utilized donors**

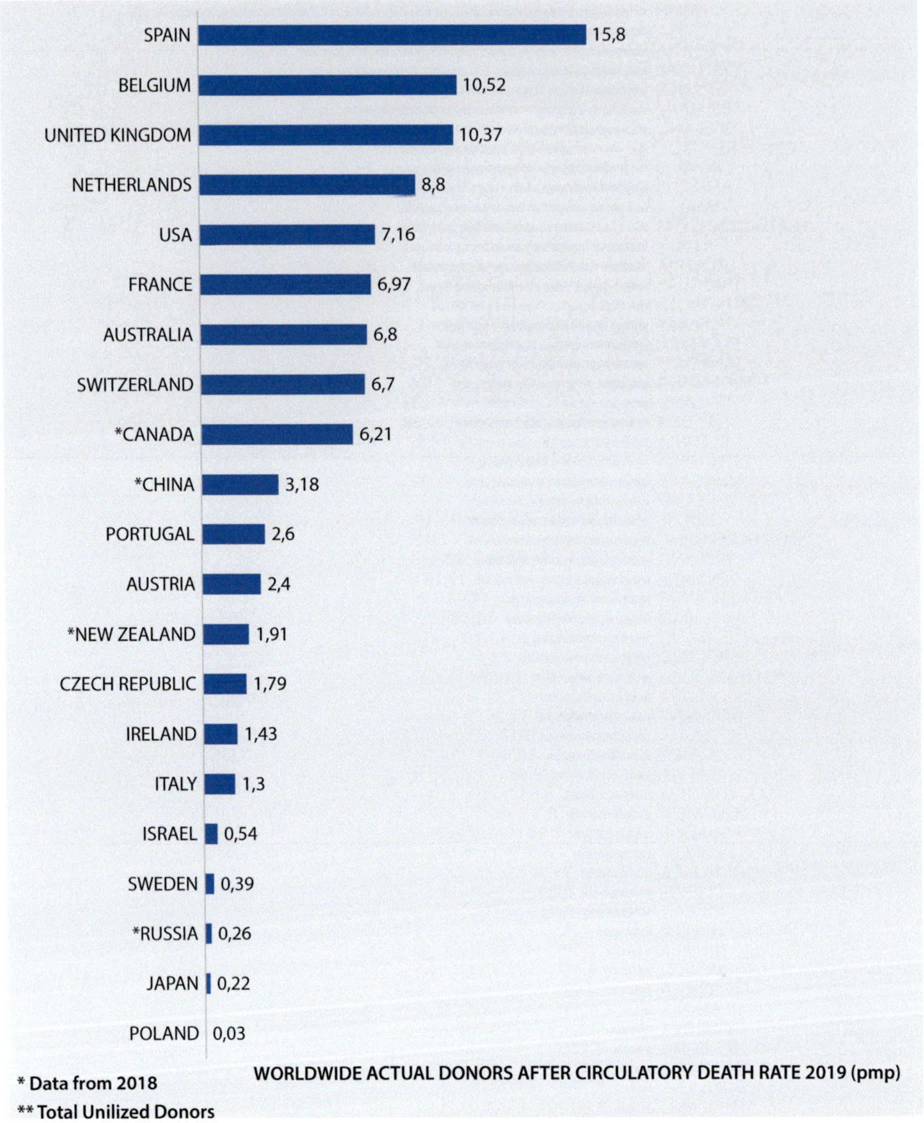

International registry in organ donation and transplantation 2019

Spain

- Spain has by far the highest number of donors per million population 49 pmp.
- The National transplant organisation (ONT) was established in 1989 and introduced specifically trained donor coordinators (TDC).
- The success of the Spanish model is often linked to Spain's presumed consent laws which were introduced in 1979. However, it should be remembered that relatives still have the final say when it comes to consent. Donation rates only began to rise with the establishment of ONT and the introduction of TDCs in 1989.

- The Spanish model also has a Quality Assurance Programme as a tool to define and monitor the potential of deceased donation and evaluate areas where improvement is possible.
- TCDs directly report to the medical director of the hospital and are independent of the transplant team.

USA
- 36.8 pmp.
- In the USA, the National Organ transplant act (NOTA) of 1984 established an organ procurement and transplantation network (OPTN). Since 1986, the United Network for Organ Sharing (UNOS) has held the federal contract as the OPTN, acting through 11 regions.
- The Center for Medicare and Medicaid services (CMS) requires hospitals to identify and refer all potential donors to the local organ procurement organisation (OPO).
- Hospitals use objective clinical criteria for contacting the OPO, for example, ventilator-dependent patients with a Glasgow coma scale of 5 or less.
- Specially trained personnel speak to families about the option of donation.

	California, USA	Spain	South Africa	New Zealand	Sweden	Germany	UK
Deceased organ donor rate per million population (pmp) 2019	36.88 (whole USA)	49	No published data	13.19	19.19	11.2	24.88
Length of DCD program	At least 20 years	DCD programs have existed since 1980s with controlled DCD starting in 2009 19 paediatric cases from 2012 to 2020	Since 2016 Only 1 paediatric case	Since 2008 mainly adults		No DCD	
DCD pmp	7.16	15.8	No published data	1.91	0.39	N/A	10.37
Share DCD/DBD Per year (2020)	DCD 90 (24%) DBD 288 (76%) in 2020	1777 deceased donors DCD 621 (35%) DBD 1156 (65%) in 2020 incl 37 paediatric (5DCD 32 DBD) 268 living donors	60% DBD 40% living related	DCD 10–15% DBD 85–90% Only 1–2 paediatric donors per year	DCD in some hospitals but no paediatric DCD 2016–2020 25 paediatric DBD donors	Total 826 donors 774 DBD 52 living related in 2020	1577 deceased donors DCD 631 (40%) DBD 946 (60%) In April 2019/March 2020 50 paediatric 18 DCD 36% 32 DBD 64%

National Centralised Donation agency	UNOS is the private, non-profit organisation that manages the nation's organ transplant system under contract with the federal government	Nationwide organisation called Organización Nacional de Trasplantes (ONT) which is part of the National Health System	Donation services are run provincially	Nationwide centralised agency—Organ Donation New Zealand (ODNZ)	Regional system	Centralised national donation agency	NHS blood and transplant (NHSBT)
Specialist approach team	Family services team, coordinators who are specifically trained to provide grief/bereavement support and speak with families about the option of donation	Donor coordinator teams lead by physicians, mostly intensivists, part time dedicated to donation and transplantation activities. Teams consist in nurses and physicians that are in hospital, mostly in the ICU/PICU, who are specifically trained as donor coordinators	No specialist team—nurse-led approach	No specialist team—local intensive care specialist does approach	Specialist nurses in some regions Approaches mainly physician led	A local coordinator usually a physician or the treating physician	Specifically trained Specialist nurses for organ donation (SNOD) Employed by NHSBT make the family approach in collaboration with local intensive care team

(continued)

	California, USA	Spain	South Africa	New Zealand	Sweden	Germany	UK
National guidance for paediatric donation	No national policies regarding paediatric organ donation outside of allocation policies. UNOS sets paediatric allocation policies	National guidance	Local guidance	National guideline which follows the Australia and New Zealand Intensive Care Society Statement on Death and Organ Donation 2019	National guidelines with local policies	Local hospital guidance	National guidance from: NHSBT, Royal College of Paediatrics and Child Health (RCPCH), National Institute for Clinical Excellence (NICE)

Countries with the highest deceased donation numbers have some or all these things in common:
- Systematic donor programs integrated into the health care system run by specially trained staff who can manage the donation process.
- Clear guidelines for notification of the specialist team regarding potential donors.
- Specialist organ donation team independent of the transplant team.
- A quality improvement tool to define and monitor the potential of deceased donation and evaluate areas where improvement is possible.

Take-Home Messages
- Consideration of potential organ donation is an integral part of high-quality end-of-life care.
- Demand for paediatric transplant organs exceeds supply.
- The ethics of organ donation is maintained through medical integrity, the scientific validity of transplantation and a robust consent process.
- Drawing up an ethical framework for decision-making when considering paediatric organ donation will help to establish a consistent ethical approach across all regions. Ensuring that all patients and families wishes are respected regardless of where they live.
- Death is the irreversible loss of the capacity for consciousness, combined with irreversible loss of the capacity to breathe. Death can be determined using cardiorespiratory or neurological criteria.
- DCD donation after circulatory determination death following withdrawal of life-sustaining therapy (WLST).
- DBD donation after neurological determination of death following brain-stem testing.
- Patients should be referred as a potential donor as soon as the intention to either withdraw life-sustaining treatments or perform brain-stem testing has been reached.
- Potential donation should never influence the decision to WLST. The decision to stop treatment should be based on what is in the child's best interests.
- Use of specialist teams in collaboration with treating teams to approach and support donor families increases the donor consent rate.

Acknowledgements Dr. Andre Vercueil Adult Instensivist, Intensive Care Medicine, King's College Hospital London, London, UK.

Lucy Dames London Organ Donation Service, National Blood and Transplant UK, London, UK.

Dr. Fredrik Hugosson and Dr. Manne Karlsson, Pediatric national clinical lead for organ donation in Sweden.

Dr. Saraswati Kache, MD Clinical Professor Division of Critical Care, Department of Pediatrics Lucile Packard Children's Hospital Stanford, USA.

Sandy Andrada, Regional Director Donor Network West, USA.

Dr. Med. Carl-Ludwig Fischer-Fröhlich coordinator Region Baden-Württemberg Organisationszentrale, Germany.

Dr. Beatriz Dominguez-Gil Director General Organización Nacional de Trasplantes, Spain.

Prof Mignon McCulloch Head of Clinical Unit: Renal and Organ Transplant, Red Cross War Memorial Children's Hospital, South Africa.

Dr. J Ritchie National Clinical Lead, Organ Donation, New Zealand.

References

1. Gruessner R. Organ donation. Encyclopedia Britannica. https://www.britannica.com/topic/organ-donation.
2. Munshi L, Murugan R. Intensive care of the deceased multiorgan donor: one donor, nine lives. In: Subramaniam K, Sakai T, editors. Anesthesia and perioperative care for organ transplantation. New York: Springer; 2017.
3. Subramaniam K, Sakai T, editors. Anesthesia and perioperative care for organ transplantation. New York: Springer; 2017.
4. European directorate for the quality of medicines and health care—EDQM, vol. 24; 2019.
5. NHS Blood and Transplant figures from the active heart transplant waiting list—19 September 2019.
6. Dalal AR. Philosophy of organ donation: review of ethical facets. World J Transplant. 2015;5(2):44–51.
7. Truog R, Robinson W. Role of brain death and the dead-donor rule in the ethics of organ transplantation. Crit Care Med. 2003;31(9):2391–6.
8. Dunstan GR. The ethics of organ donation. Br Med Bull. 1997;53(4):921–39.
9. Saunders B. Normative consent and opt-out organ donation. J Med Ethics. 2010;36(2):84–7.
10. Gardiner D, Shemie S, Manara A, Opdam H. International perspective on the diagnosis of death. Br J Anaesth. 2012;108(Suppl_1):i14–28.
11. Moss J, Rockoff M. EEG monitoring during cardiac arrest and resuscitation. JAMA J Am Med Assoc. 1980;244:2750.
12. Losasso TJ, Muzzi DA, Meyer FB, Sharbrough FW. Electroencephalographic monitoring of cerebral function during asystole and successful cardiopulmonary resuscitation. Anesth Analg. 1992;75:1021–4.
13. Academy of Royal Medical Colleges. A code of practice for the diagnosis and confirmation of death. Academy of Royal Medical Colleges; 2008.
14. Katz R, Kelly HW. Pharmacokinetics of continuous infusions of fentanyl in critically ill children. Crit Care Med. 1993;21(7):995–1000.
15. NICE CnG135[1] and NHS Blood and Transplant (NHSBT) Best Practice Guidance on timely identification and referral of potential donors.
16. DeVita MA, Snyder JV, Arnold RM, Siminoff LA. Observations of withdrawal of life-sustaining treatment from patients who became non-heart-beating organ donors. Crit Care Med. 2000;28(6):1709–12.
17. Ethics Committee, American College of Critical Care Medicine; Society of Critical Care Medicine. Recommendations for non-heart beating organ donation. Society of Critical Care Medicine. Crit Care Med. 2001;29(9):1826–31.
18. Dhanani S, Hornby L, van Beinum A, Scales NB, et al., Canadian Critical Care Trials Group; Canadian Donation and Transplantation Research Program. Resumption of cardiac activity after withdrawal of life-sustaining measures. N Engl J Med. 2021;384(4):345–52.
19. Department of Health Organ Donation after Circulatory Death. 2010. Report of a consensus meeting. Intensive Care Society, NHS Blood and Transplant, and British Transplantation Society.
20. Organ donation and transplant. Paediatric Care. https://www.odt.nhs.uk/deceased-donation/best-practice-guidance/paediatric-care/.
21. Watson CJE, Dark JH. Organ transplantation: historical perspective and current practice. Br J Anaesth. 2012;108(Suppl 1):i29.
22. World Health Organization. European Health for all database. http://www.euro.who.int/hfadb.
23. Clayton TJ, Nelson RJ, Manara AR. Reduction in mortality from severe heads injury following introduction of a protocol for intensive care management. Br J Anaesth. 2004;93:761–88.

24. Patel HC, Menon DK, Tebbs S, et al. Specialist neurocritical care and outcome from head injury. Intensive Care Med. 2002;28:547–5389.
25. Diringer MN, Edwards DF. Admission to a neurologic/neurosurgical intensive care unit is associated with reduced mortality rate after intracerebral haemorrhage. Crit Care Med. 2001;29(3):635–40.
26. Ranasinghe AM, Bonser RS. Endocrine changes in brain death and transplantation. Best Pract Res Clin Endocrinol Metab. 2011;25(5):799–812.
27. Dimopoulou I, Tsagarakis S, Anthi A, et al. High prevalence of decreased cortisol reserve in brain-dead potential organ donors. Crit Care Med. 2003;31(4):1113–7.
28. Rudge C, Matesanz R, Delmonico FL, Chapman J. International practices of organ donation. Br J Anaesth. 2012;108(Suppl_1):i48–55.

Toxicology in Pediatric ICU

Dhiren Gupta and Sandeep Dhingra

Contents

J. Brierley et al. (eds.), *ESPNIC Children's Intensive Care Textbook*,
https://doi.org/10.1007/978-3-031-64762-8_48

Learning Objectives

- Familiarity with epidemiology and demographics of childhood intoxications.
- Knowledge about signs and symptoms of common poisonings, and identification of toxidromes.
- Basic approach to managing a poisoned child.
- Indications of admitting a child with intoxication to pediatric intensive care unit.
- Knowledge of advanced elimination techniques including extracorporeal methods.

48.1 Introduction

Poisoning in children is one of the most frequently encountered medical emergency worldwide and represents a substantial number of avoidable admissions to the pediatric intensive care unit (PICU). Children form over 50% of human toxin exposures with a majority (76.6%) being unintentional. Intentional exposures are mostly seen in the adolescent age group with female preponderance and constitute roughly 10% of total exposures [1]. Patients with toxin exposure present a challenge both to diagnose and manage due to a variety of routes and plethora of available toxins. Children younger than 5 years are most susceptible to accidental poisoning due to their inquisitive nature and mouthing instincts.

Poisoning constitutes about 0.5–7.5% of the emergency department (ED) visits [2, 3], and shows a bimodal peak with a majority of children being in ≤5 years and ≥13 years age group. The 2020 National Poison Data System (NPDS) annual report [3], an annual report by American Association of Poison Control Centres (AAPCC) reporting poisoning data in the United States, notified nearly 2.2 million human exposures in the year 2019. Children up to 5 years of age constituted 42.8% of human exposures while those in the ≥13 years age group accounted for 8.24% of total exposures. The five leading toxin exposures in children were personal care products and cosmetics (11.4%), household cleaning substances (10.5%), analgesics (8.97%), toys and foreign bodies (7.17%), dietary supplements, herbals, and homeopathic medications (5.06%). Pharmaceutical agents are the most common intentional toxins ingested, while pesticides are common non-pharmaceutical toxins, encountered in suicidal attempts. Amongst the unintentional toxins in both age groups, carbon monoxide (CO) is an important inhaled toxin while venom injected by snake bites and insect stings are usual biological toxins needing PICU care.

Toxic substances can lead to poisoning when ingested, inhaled, injected, or absorbed through contact with skin or mucous membranes. Monitoring and treatment of such children is best done in a critical care setting as the evolution of a poisoned child is unpredictable. Constant vigil for early identification of complications, and appropriate rapid intervention, is the key to prevent deterioration in such patients. The percentage of children who will need PICU care varies from 8% to 11.5% [4, 5].

The emergency department (ED) physician should be acquainted with the management of common poisonings based on recent available information of the area. Readily accessible substances are encountered more frequently as compared to the highly toxic ones. Knowledge about them can help in early institution of therapy. The main objective in management of any poisoned patient is support of vital functions and self or assisted elimination of the toxin. Identification of poisoning with the intent of self-harm is essential, as this could suggest mental health issues in the child. The average mortality rate due to poisoning is around 1% in developed countries with a range of 3–5% in developing countries [6, 7].

48.2 Clinical Presentation

Children with toxin exposure can present in diverse ways and complaints are usually non-specific. Neurological and gastrointestinal symptoms are common as they mimic the frequency of poisonings from ingesting pharmaceuticals. A detailed history noting the type and quantity of exposure is essential whenever toxic exposure is suspected. Details concerning time of exposure, time to presentation, history of coughing, choking or vomiting, alteration in sensorium and interventions done prior to presentation helps immensely in counselling and planning the management. Additionally, information regarding last meal, chronic illness and medication thereof in the child and family members, should be sought.

Vital questions in history

- What is the agent
- Form and route of exposure
- When and how much
- Symptoms and temporal sequence
- Interventions prior to reporting
- Any chronic illness and medication intake

Essential examination findings

- Confirm route of exposure
- Vital parameters including SpO_2
- Examine mucosa and signs of drug abuse
- Eye signs including pupils
- Abnormal odors
- Consciousness

Every child should be examined thoroughly after undressing for signs of toxin exposure from all possible routes including intravenous. This practice can prevent missing out cases of envenomation and child abuse. Clinical examination should focus on changes in skin, mucosa, eye findings, abnormalities of central and autonomic nervous system, and the presence of any unusual odors. Characteristic combination of symptoms and signs may give clue to the identification of a toxidrome.

Toxidrome is a constellation of signs and symptoms which when present together suggest a particular type of poison. Combination of symptoms at presentation, mental status changes, vital parameters, clinical findings, and investigation results help to identify the class of toxin which can aid in initiation of appropriate treatment [8, 9]. Common toxidromes encountered in pediatric poisoning (◘ Table 48.1) are cholinergic and anticholinergic, sympathomimetic, sedative/hypnotic, and opioid.

Table 48.1 Common toxidromes and their features

Common toxidromes				
Type	**Mental status**	**Pupils**	**Symptoms**	**Causative agents**
Sympathomimetic (stimulant)	Hyperalert, agitation, restlessness, paranoia hallucination	Mydriasis	Insomnia, hyperthermia, tachycardia, tremor, excessive motor activity	Amphetamines, ADHD medications, phencyclidine, cathinones, cocaine, other stimulants
Sedative/hypnotic	Confusion, sedation, stupor, delirium, hallucination	Variable	Blurred vision, diplopia, nystagmus, paresthesia, slurred speech, ataxia	Benzodiazepines, barbiturates
Opioids	CNS depression, coma	Miosis	Hypothermia, unresponsiveness, bradycardia, bradypnea, shallow respiration, hypotension, decreased bowel sounds	Narcotic agents, heroin, clonidine
Anticholinergic[a]	Agitation, hallucination, delirium, coma	Mydriasis	Fever, tachycardia, flushing, dry skin, urinary retention, blurred vision, ileus, seizures, myoclonus, hallucinations, psychosis, coma	Antihistamines, antidepressants, scopolamine, sleep preparations, certain mushrooms
Cholinergic[b]	Confusion, coma	Miosis	Bradycardia, salivation, lacrimation, urination, defecation, gastrointestinal distress (diarrhea), emesis	Organophosphates, carbamates, insecticides, black widow spider bites, certain mushrooms

[a] Mnemonic: Hot as a hare, dry as a bone, red as a beet, mad as a hatter
[b] Mnemonic: SLUDGE

48

Majority of children remain asymptomatic even after exposure, suggesting that the substance was non-toxic or the amount was insignificant. This contrasts with intentional poisoning in adolescents who deteriorate rapidly and need intensive care. Poisoning with oral hypoglycemics, iron, clonidine, alcohols and opioids, barbiturates, antidepressants and anti-psychotics, cocaine, and caustic substances though infrequent, can be potentially fatal in small children even if ingested in small quantities [10].

48.3 Initial Management

A poisoned child represents an emergency with wide-ranging multi-organ pathophysiology. Resuscitation, decontamination, and supportive care are the three pillars of effective initial management. On suspicion of a toxic exposure, preliminary management should be directed towards stabilization of the patient's condition utilizing the fundamentals of resuscitation, the ABCs (airway, breathing, and circulation), and obtaining a reliable intravenous access. The letters D, E, and F can be used to elaborate the initial stabilization mnemonic to denote **d**econtamination, assessment of **d**isability, **d**rugs, **e**limination, **E**CG, and **f**ever [11].

Airway management takes precedence over all other steps as compromise to airway-protective reflexes and concern for aspiration dictates the need to secure the airway. Rapid sequence intubation (RSI) with pre-oxygenation and paralysis is the best approach to securing the airway [12]. Oro-tracheal intubation is preferred over naso-tracheal intubation as the latter is technically more difficult, associated with increased chance of sinusitis, trauma, sinus otitis, and is technically more difficult [13, 14]. Airway adjuncts and facilities to establish a surgical airway (cricothyrotomy) should be immediately available lest tracheal intubation fails. Criteria for endotracheal intubation and assisted ventilation are enumerated in ◘ Table 48.2. Breathing should be monitored to assess the adequacy of respiration. In case ventilation is initiated, settings on the ventilator should be titrated to the underlying lung physiology.

Circulation and cardiovascular abnormalities in the form of arrhythmias, hypertension, hypotension, and conduction abnormalities may be seen in a wide variety of drug ingestions. Specific management of cardiovascular derangements can be initiated in the ED and needs to be continued in the ICU under adequate monitoring. Fluid resuscitation can be individualized and is based on administration of crystalloids. Inotropes and vasopressors should be added early in the course of management of shock.

◘ **Table 48.2** Indications for intubation and ventilatory support

Airway	Upper airway obstruction unresponsive to airway adjuncts/positioning
Consciousness	Apnea/bradypnea/hypoventilation Absent gag and cough reflexes
Respiratory failure	Hypoxia ($PaO_2 < 60$ mmHg or $SpO_2 < 90\%$ on $FiO_2 > 0.6$) Hypercarbia ($PaO_2 > 50$ mmHg and pH < 7.30)
Cardiovascular instability	Fluid refractory shock unresponsive to first-line inotropes Metabolic acidosis
Secretion	Excessive oral/bronchial secretions
CNS	Raised ICP requiring hyperventilation/GCS < 9
Pulmonary	Pulmonary hypertension Pulmonary hemorrhage

The disability assessment involves a concise neurological examination, and includes consciousness level, pupillary shape, size, and reactivity to assess cerebral and brainstem function.

Drugs used in the initial management are limited to dextrose for hypoglycemia, oxygen in cases of hypoxemia and naloxone for reversal of respiratory depression in patients suspected with opioid poisoning.

Decontamination methods are urgently employed for the prevention of further absorption of toxin and are mainly useful in dermal and ocular exposures. Once a mainstay of poisoning through gastrointestinal (GI) route, they are no longer recommended unless patients who present very early (<1 h after ingestion) or for patients who have ingested large doses of poisonous substances for which antidotes do not exist [15]. If contemplated, GI decontamination should be started as early as possible in the ED. Starting GI decontamination later in the PICU does not improve the outcome as measured by mortality and length of stay [16].

Activated charcoal is a common decontaminating agent which works by adsorbing the toxins within the GI lumen, thereby limiting their absorption. A dose of 1 g/kg mixed with water in a concentration of 8 mL/g is used. It is ineffective in poisonings by alcohol, corrosives, and metals.

In a majority of children, the clinical condition rather than the specific substance ingested directs the management. Supportive care includes observation of vitals, temperature control, airway protection, hydration, nutrition, respiratory, hemodynamic and electrocardiac monitoring, maintaining oxygenation and ventilation, correction of electrolyte and acid–base disturbances, glycemic control, correction of perfusion abnormalities including hypertension, seizures, and keeping a note of ongoing medical problems and chronic medications.

Initial management
– Resuscitation—ABCs
– Vitals, SpO_2 and ECG
– Disability assessment
– Drugs—dextrose, oxygen, and naloxone
– Decontamination
– Charcoal
– Supportive care

48.4 Investigations

Investigations in cases of pediatric poisoning help in early identification of effects of toxins on the bodily functions, metabolic derangements, and progression of organ dysfunction if any. Routine hematological investigations including coagulation profile, biochemistries, blood gas including co-oximetry, serum lactate, and osmolarity, if available, should be undertaken [17]. When ingestion of a toxin is witnessed or with a confirmed history of exposure, toxicological screening tests are of limited value.

Table 48.3 Drug concentrations measured commonly

Acetaminophen	Methanol
Carbamazepine	Methemoglobin
Carboxyhemoglobin	Organophosphates
Digoxin	Phenobarbital
Ethanol	Phenytoin
Ethylene glycol	Salicylic acid
Iron	Theophylline
Lithium	Valproate

Screening tests for toxins are useful to confirm diagnosis in patients with unconfirmed exposures, which in turn can help in institution of specific therapy including administration of antidotes. It also helps in patients with mixed exposures and for monitoring response to therapy wherein both serum and urine screens can be sent [18]. The common drugs and toxins for which serum concentration levels can be measured are given in Table 48.3.

Electrocardiogram (ECG) is an essential investigation in all cases of systemic poisoning as toxins are known to produce cardiac dysrhythmias which may go undiagnosed clinically. ECG changes are commonly seen in drugs ingested inadvertently such as anti-arrhythmics, calcium channel blockers, and tricyclic antidepressants.

Routine investigations
– Hemogram
– Liver function tests
– BUN, serum creatinine
– Serum electrolytes (Na, K, Ca, Cl)
– Serum lactate
– Urine routine
– ECG

48.5 Criteria for PICU Admission

Validation attempts for admission to PICU based on severity scores (PRISM II/III, PIM II, APACHE II/III, SAPS II, etc.) have been unsuccessful for children with poisoning, thereby underscoring the importance of clinical judgement and experience in decision-making. The principle of "treating the patient and not the poison" underlies this approach [7], while at the same time one should remember that initially asymptomatic children may worsen later. Some well-established indications for admission to PICU [15] are enumerated in Table 48.4.

Table 48.4 Indications of admission to PICU

Acute respiratory failure	Need for respiratory support or airway adjuncts
	Respiratory distress as indicated by tachypnea for age, desaturation, marked distress
	Hypercarbia, hypoxemia, acidosis
	Airway obstruction, apnea, anaphylaxis
Hemodynamic instability or shock	Delayed capillary refill time of >3 s
	Non-palpable peripheral pulses
	Hypotension as described for age
	Need for inotropes
	Need for invasive hemodynamic monitoring
	Metabolic acidosis
	Arrythmias, ischemic changes on ECG
	Congestive heart failure
	Hypovolemia requiring fluid bolus
	Bleeding/hemorrhage
	Thrombocytopenia/severe anemia/coagulopathy
Neurological instability	Glasgow coma scale of <10
	Irritability, hallucinations, and delirium
	Features of raised intracranial pressure, seizures
	Intracranial hemorrhage
Metabolic disturbances	Serum sodium <125 mEq/L or >160 mEq/L
	Serum potassium <3 mEq/L or >6.5 mEq/L
	Blood glucose <30 mg/dL or >400 mg/dL
	Hypocalcemia (ionized calcium <0.8 mEq/L)
	Base deficit >–10
Patients exposed to intentional poisoning/suicidal cases	
Patients at risk of multi-organ dysfunction based on initial investigations	

48

48.6 Specific Management

The use of focused management strategies, including enhanced elimination techniques and antidotes, is limited to a small subset of cases. In all such patients, one must weigh the defined benefit against the risk of the intervention. When the substance to which the patient is exposed is unknown and the exposure unwitnessed, supportive therapy is instituted. A close watch for the development of complications or of a cluster of symptoms indicating a toxidrome is kept. In the event of incomplete or uncertain history, the findings on clinical examination, laboratory tests, and toxicological screening results can help in management.

Antidotes though used rarely can help in cases of specific toxin exposures. The local poison information center can provide information and help in selection of antidotes in such cases. Neutralizing the life-threatening potential of an ingested substance should be achieved early in the course of therapy. Efforts to decrease and delay absorption and to facilitate elimination of the systemically absorbed toxin must carry on simultaneously to minimize the harmful potential of the substance consumed. Advanced treatment modalities include whole bowel irrigation (WBI), multi-dose activated charcoal (MDAC), urine alkalinization, extracorporeal elimination, and use of antidotes.

48.6.1 Whole Bowel Irrigation

Whole bowel irrigation is a GI decontamination technique which increases the flow of toxin through the gut. Large amounts of osmotically balanced polyethylene glycol solution (PEG) is administered by placing a nasogastric/orogastric tube until the patient passes 2–3 clear liquid stools. It can be started safely in the ED and continued in PICU. Patients who have ingested contraband drugs for transportation (body packers) are traditionally managed using this technique. Ileus, intestinal obstruction, corrosive ingestion, and hypokalemia are some of the contraindications of WBI [15].

48.6.2 Multi-dose Activated Charcoal

Enhanced elimination can also be achieved by using multi-dose activated charcoal in patients who have ingested substances which have delayed absorption (slow-release preparations) and toxins which undergo entero-hepatic or entero-enteric circulation. Repeat doses of 0.5 g/kg of activated charcoal dissolved in water (8 mL/g) are used following an initial dose of 1 g/kg in MDAC.

48.6.3 Urine Alkalinization

Alkalinization of urine is a method of enhanced elimination which is used for weakly acidic toxins and drugs (salicylates, phenobarbital, methotrexate, chlorophenoxy herbicides, etc.). Acidic drugs get ionized in alkaline urine, preventing their resorption back into the tubules. Contraindications to urine alkalinization are renal impairment, fluid overload, and hypokalemia. Urine alkalinization is achieved by administering 2–3 mEq/kg of IV sodium bicarbonate solution prepared by adding 75–100 mEq of 8.4% $NaHCO_3$ to 425 mL of 5% dextrose (D5W), with 20–40 mEq/L of potassium chloride. D5W is the preferred fluid for dilution of $NaHCO_3$ as it restricts the risk of administering hypertonic fluid and probable hypernatremia. The recommended infusion rate is 1 mEq/kg/h with frequent testing of urine every 15–30 min for a target pH range of 7.5–8.5 [19]. Following achievement of the target urine pH, the infusion rate is continued at half the initial rate while urinary pH is tested every hourly. To aid in frequent urine testing, placement of a Foley's catheter becomes essential. Other laboratory parameters which must be closely monitored during alkalinization therapy include electrolyte measurements (to keep serum ionized calcium >1 mmol/L and serum potassium >4.0 mEq/L), and acid–base status (to keep arterial pH <7.50).

48.6.4 Extracorporeal Removal

Hemodialysis, hemofiltration, and continuous renal replacement therapy are extracorporeal treatments (ECTRs) sometimes used for removal of systemic toxins. Chemical and pharmacological properties of the toxin which makes it amenable to such therapy include a low volume of distribution (VD < 1 L/kg), low protein-binding capacity, low endogenous clearance, and low molecular weight [20]. Based on the type of ECTR used, various mechanisms which come into play are diffusion (hemodialysis, peritoneal dialysis), convection (hemofiltration), adsorption (hemoperfusion), and centrifugation/separation (therapeutic plasma exchange). Only a small minority of patients (0.1%) need ECTRs, as supportive measures are sufficient in a majority of toxic exposures [3].

Knowledge of the physical properties of the toxin is essential to select the appropriate ECTR technique for successful removal of toxin. ◘ Figure 48.1 depicts the stepwise approach for selection of ECTR technique [20]. In majority of the poison-

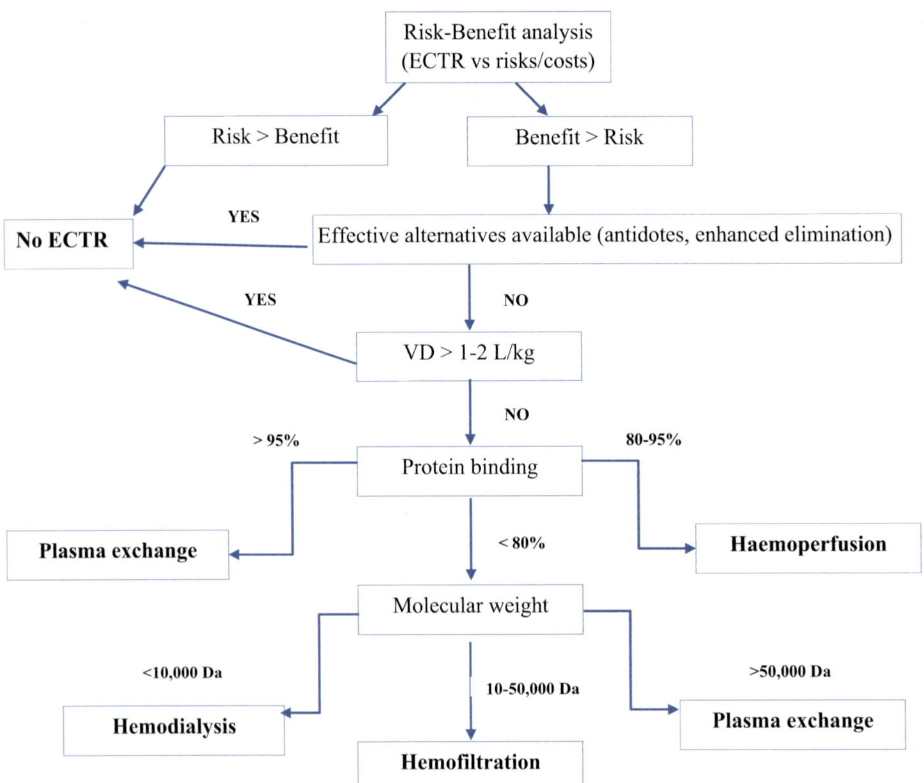

◘ **Fig. 48.1** Decision process for using ECTR technique

ings, intermittent hemodialysis is the preferred method as it leads to rapid poison removal. Concurrently it also addresses complications associated with severe intoxication which may include electrolyte disturbances, acid–base abnormalities, acute kidney injury (AKI), and volume overload.

Indications for extracorporeal therapy[a]
– Poisoning exposure must be severe
– Presence of life-threatening clinical signs (arrhythmias, respiratory failure, etc.)
– Absence of other life-saving alternatives (antidotes)
– ECTR must be capable of removing the poison from the blood compartment
– ECTR should significantly contribute to total body clearance
[a] Adapted from Extracorporeal Treatment in Poisoning workgroup (EXTRIP) guidelines [21]

48.6.5 Antidote Therapy

Antidotes though rarely indicated in commonly encountered poisonings play an important role in the management of severe specific toxin exposures. Once the toxin is identified by toxicological screen or accurate history, local poison centers can be contacted for guidance regarding use of antidotes. A list of common poisons and their antidotes is enumerated in ◘ Table 48.5.

Ask the following before antidote therapy
– Is the exposure to a specific substance confirmed
– Is the substance potentially toxic
– Is toxicity potentially lethal
– Can we stop absorption
– Can we enhance elimination
– Is there any specific antidote
– Is the intervention hazardous

Recommended emergency antidotes in PICU
– Activated charcoal
– Amyl nitrate
– Antivenin
– Calcium chloride
– Deferoxamine mesylate
– Digoxin immune Fab
– Ethanol
– Folic acid
– Fomepizole
– Glucagon
– Methylene blue 1%
– *N*-Acetylcysteine
– Naloxone
– Polyethylene glycol electrolyte solution
– Pralidoxime hydrochloride
– Pyridoxime
– Sodium bicarbonate
– Sodium nitrite 3%
– Thiamine hydrochloride
– Vitamin K_1

48.6.6 Lipid Emulsion Therapy

Lipid emulsion therapy (LET) has emerged as one of the newest advances in the management of critically ill patients with poisoning. LET which was initially investigated for treatment of anesthetic toxicity has now been increasingly used for lipid soluble toxin exposures. Though unproven, LET is thought to act as a "lipid sink" wherein it binds to lipophilic xenobiotics (e.g. tricyclic antidepressants, calcium channel blockers, cocaine, quetiapine, etc.) [22]. In the absence of any standard guidelines to its use in children, the proposed dose by American College of Medical Toxicology (ACMT) is 1.5 mL/kg bolus of 20% lipid emulsion followed by 0.25 mL/kg/min [23].

Table 48.5 Common poisons and their antidotes

Group	Poisons	Antidote
Agricultural pesticides	Organophosphates Malathion Acephate Fenitrothion Dichlorvos	Atropine sulfate
	Carbamates Propoxur Carbaryl Carbofuran	Pralidoxime
	Organochlorines Endosulfan Gamma benzene hexachloride chlordane	Cholestyramine
	Rodenticide Cholestyramine	Vitamin K
Industrial chemicals	Lead Mercury Arsenic	Calcium disodium edetate Dimercaprol D-Penicillamine Dimercaptosuccinic acid
	Methyl alcohol Ethylene glycol	Ethanol Folic acid/folinic acid Pyridoxine hydrochloride Folic acid Thiamine
	Cyanide	Amyl nitrite, sodium nitrite Sodium thiosulfate
	Methemoglobinemia-producing agents (nitrites, nitrates, dapsone, copper, aniline, naphthalene)	Methylene blue
Drugs	Acetaminophen Iron Benzodiazepines Opioids Isoniazid Digoxin Hypoglycemics	*N*-Acetylcysteine Desferoxamine Flumazenil Naloxone Pyridoxine Digoxin specific antibodies Dextrose, glucagon
Environmental toxins	Datura Snake bite Botulism	Physostigmine Anti-snake venom Botulinum antitoxin

48.7 Ancillary Support and Prevention

All patients with severe intoxications are at risk of ICU-related morbidities as with any other critically ill child. Risk of gastrointestinal hemorrhage is significantly increased in such patients with approximately 3/4th developing endoscopic evidence of gastric mucosal injury by 18 h of admission, with overt bleeding in 5% [24]. Proton-pump inhibitors or H_2-receptor antagonists should be used in all patients for prophylaxis against GI bleeding. Venous thromboembolism, ventilator-associated complications, hospital-acquired infections, and nutritional support are other areas of concern which must be addressed in all.

Majority of childhood poisonings are accidental in nature and are amenable to prevention. Three principal reasons which puts children at risk of poisoning are: improper storage of potentially toxic agents, lapse in caregiver attention, and children left unattended in other people's home [25]. Other significant risk factors include household stress, single parent, accessibility to toxic agents, unsupervised children, multiple siblings, and caretaking by grandparents [26–28].

Child-resistant packaging and safe storage decreases the incidence of childhood poisoning. Smaller volume prescribing, education about safe storage of medications, child-resistant lids, storage in lockable cupboards, and childproofing of households are other safety measures.

Take-Home Messages

- Poisoning and toxin exposures in children are mainly accidental.
- Exposures in adolescents are usually intentional and may involve multiple agents.
- Adolescent exposures are frequently associated with delay in seeking medical attention.
- Identification of toxidromes leads to early specific interventions.
- State poison control center should be contacted for reporting and guidance in all cases.
- Thorough clinical examination and lookout for risk factors helps in early institution of definitive therapy.
- Supportive management should be started early in the emergency department.
- In majority of the cases, clinical condition rather than the specifics of the substance guides the management.
- Intensive care maybe required in a small subset of patients for life-saving interventions.
- Childhood poisoning is amenable to preventive interventions.
- Intentional exposures are associated with worse outcome.

Summary

Childhood poisoning poses a challenge to the treating specialist since children are exposed to a wide variety of chemical, plant, and biological toxins in their daily life. There are limited studies to document the adverse effects of all the available drugs and chemicals, due to their ever changing nature, names, and ingredients. Role of local poison control centers has come to the forefront in guidance and data collection.

Many adolescents are also experimenting usage of synthetic drugs with a belief that they are legal substitutes for popular street drugs and are therefore safe. Alcohol exposure routes have also evolved with social media videos on how to take the "challenge" or revealing new ways to consume drugs and alcohol. This has led to a sharp rise in complexity of cases, especially in adults in whom exposure to multiple agents has become a norm. Energy drinks, typically containing caffeine, ingested alone or in combination with alcohol, leads to multiplication of the risks.

A symptom-based approach concentrating on the basics of resuscitation and supportive care, with a close watch on the development of complications helps in effective management of any child with toxin exposure. Mixed exposures, specific drugs, and toxins identified using toxicological screens are sometimes amenable to specific antidotes and advanced elimination methods.

Case Study

Presenting Complaints and History

A 4-year-old girl presented to the emergency with altered sensorium and vomiting within 30 min of accidental ingestion of a particular clearless fluid. It had been stored in an empty disposable water bottle, which was kept in the bottle holder of the car. On feeling thirsty while traveling, the girl took a sip of the substance thinking it to be water. She immediately started feeling dizzy and was brought to ED in an unconscious state with bluish discolouration of skin and mucosa.

▪ Questions

1. What are the common toxins which can lead to severe hypoxia on exposure?
2. What is the mechanism of action of the substance identified?
3. What are the systemic manifestations of the substance?
4. What are potential antidotes and management of this poisoning?

Physical Examination

On arrival, her airway was maintainable, breathing was deep and sighing, and GCS was 11. Pupils were equal, round, and reactive. She was cyanosed, peripheries were warm, and pulses were palpable.

Heart rate	Respiratory rate	Blood pressure	Temperature	SpO_2
138/min	26/min	112/74 mmHg	98.8 °F	46% (room air)

General: Unresponsive, cyanosed
Cardiovascular: Heart sounds normal with sinus rhythm
Pulmonary: Normal vesicular sounds, no wheeze or crackles
Neurological: Normal tone, normal deep tendon jerks, intact occulocephalic reflex, GCS-11

Initial Treatment

The patient was administered oxygen using a non-rebreathing mask. Routine lab investigations and blood gas analysis was conducted. The patient was intubated, as she remained hypoxic with GCS falling further. IV access was gained and maintenance fluids were started. She was shifted to PICU where further management was continued.

Details of Substance Ingested and Past Medical History

On further questioning, it was found that the father used to work in a printing press. The ingested substance was a chemical which is used as a "Fixer," and is added to various dyes and paints. The patient did not have any past medical illness and was not on any medication. There were no emotional or psychological stressors.

Diagnostic Testing

Hb	WBC/platelets	Electrolytes	AST/ALT	BUN/Creat
12.8 g/dL	11.4/3.2 × 10^3/cmm	Na—137 mEq/L K—3.8 mEq/L	48/41 IU/L	18/0.7 mg/dL

Arterial blood gas (FiO_2: 1.0): pH 7.48; PCO_2: 29 mmHg; PO_2: 248 mmHg
Carboxy Hb: 2.6%; MetHb: 34%, Colour of arterial blood - brown (Fig. 48.2)
Toxicology screen was negative for salicylates and ethanol

Hospital Course

The child was continued on invasive mechanical ventilation in the PICU. She required minimal pressure settings but remained hypoxic in spite of 100% oxygen. In view of severe methemoglobinemia (34%), she was administered 1 mg/kg of methylene blue which was followed by another dose as her metHb levels remained high with $SpO_2 < 80\%$. Repeat doses of methylene blue changed to colour of urine to greenish blue (Fig 48.3) and kept her metHb levels under 5% and oxygen saturation above 92%. She also developed anemia (Hb—6.5 g/dL) which was managed by transfusing packed cells. Vitamin C and *N*-acetyl cysteine were used as adjuvants utilizing their antioxidant property. The patient was extubated on day 2, and recovered completely by day 5 of admission.

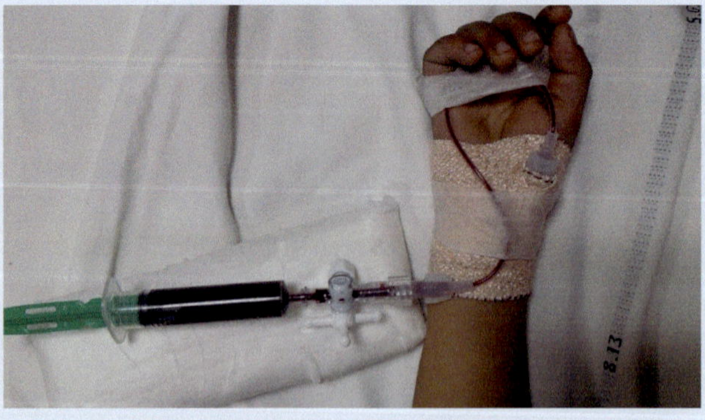

Fig. 48.2 Chocolate brown colored arterial blood due to methemoglobinemia

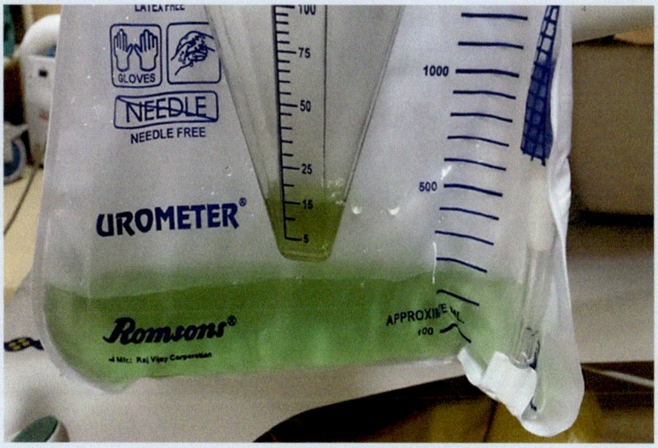

Fig. 48.3 Greenish blue urine on administration of methylene blue

Ancillary Tests

G-6-PD test—normal enzyme level (Fig. 48.3).

Answers

1. Hypoxia can be encountered in a vast variety of toxin exposures. Toxins usually cause anemic (carbon monoxide, methemoglobinemia, etc.) or histotoxic (cyanide, hydrogen sulphide, etc.) hypoxia. A wide range of drugs and chemicals when ingested, inhaled, or absorbed can lead to methemoglobinemia. Important chemicals include aniline and its derivatives, nitrites, and other oxidizing agents (benzocaine, naphthalene, etc.). Common drugs such as dapsone, antimalarials, and local anesthetics are also associated with methemoglobinemia.
2. The chemical implicated in the current case was most likely an aniline derivative which is a component of dyes, print, and photographic chemicals. On exposure to aniline, ferrous (Fe^{2+}) iron in hemoglobin oxidizes to ferric form (Fe^{3+}), resulting in the formation of methemoglobin, which is incapable of oxygen transport. Methemoglobinemia impairs the delivery of oxygen to tissues and results in signs and symptoms of hypoxemia whenever its concentration is >15%. Aniline and its derivatives may also cause hemolysis as was seen in this case. Aniline being an aromatic amine can lead to intoxication following ingestion, inhalation, or dermal absorption.
3. Aniline causes methemoglobinemia and hemolysis. Methemoglobin levels of 15–30%, lead to bluish discoloration of patient's skin, which is due to the dark color of methemoglobin. Levels above 30% lead to systemic hypoxia, cyanosis, and severe systemic effects.

Methemoglobin level (%)	Signs and symptoms
30–50	Headache, exhaustion, giddiness, tachycardia, breathing difficulty
50–70	Stupor, bradycardia, bradypnea, rhythm abnormalities, acid–base disturbance
60–70	Cardiac arrest, alteration of sensorium, coma, death

4. Methylene blue in the standard intravenous dose of 1–2 mg/kg of body weight (0.1–0.2 mL/kg of a 1% solution) is administered over 5–10 min. Response is normally observed within 30–60 min of infusion by noting a fall in methemoglobin level below 25%. Repeat doses can be given hourly if needed. The total dose over a 24 h period should not exceed 7 mg/kg, as in the G-6-PD-deficient individuals, methylene blue can itself cause hemolysis. Hyperbaric oxygen therapy, exchange transfusion, and rarely ECMO may be considered in patients who are refractory to methylene blue therapy.

References

1. Lamireau T, Llanas B, Kennedy A, Fayon M, Penouil F, Favarell-Garrigues JC, et al. Epidemiology of poisoning in children: a 7-year survey in a paediatric emergency care unit. Eur J Emerg Med. 2002;9:9–14.
2. Mintegi S, Fernández A, Alustiza J, Canduela V, Mongil I, Caubet I, et al. Emergency visits for childhood poisoning: a 2-year prospective multicenter survey in Spain. Pediatr Emerg Care. 2006;22:334–8.
3. Gummin DD, Mowry JB, Beuhler MC, Spyker DA, Brooks DE, Dibert KW, Rivers LJ, Pham NPT, Ryan ML. 2019 Annual report of the American Association of Poison Control Centers' National Poison Data System (NPDS): 37th annual report. Clin Toxicol. 2020;58(12):1360–541. https://doi.org/10.1080/15563650.2020.1834219.
4. Ergul AB, Torun YA. Retrospective evaluation of poisonings in a pediatric intensive care unit: 4 years of experience. J Clin Anal Med. 2018;9(4):278–83. https://doi.org/10.4328/JCAM.5660.
5. Even KM, Armsby CC, Bateman ST. Poisonings requiring admission to the pediatric intensive care unit: a 5-year review. Clin Toxicol (Phila). 2014;52(5):519–24. https://doi.org/10.3109/15563650.2014.909601.
6. Kirk MA. Use of the intensive care unit. In: Nelson LS, Lewin NA, Howland MA, Hoffman RS, Goldfrank LR, Flomenbaum NE, editors. Goldfrank's toxicologic emergencies. New York: McGraw Hill Medical; 2011. p. 148–54.
7. Patel MM, Travers CD, Stockwell JA, Geller RJ, Kamat PP, Grunwell JR. Analysis of interventions required in 12,021 children with acute intoxications admitted to PICUs. Pediatr Crit Care Med. 2017;18(7):e281–9. https://doi.org/10.1097/PCC.0000000000001187.
8. Holstege CP, Borek HA. Toxidromes. Crit Care Clin. 2012;28(4):479–98.
9. Nelson LS, Lewin NA, Howland MA, Hoffman R, Goldfrank L, Flomenbaum N. Initial evaluation of the patient: vital signs and toxic syndromes. In: Nelson LS, Lewin NA, Howland MA, Hoffman R, Goldfrank L, Flomenbaum N, editors. Goldfrank's toxicologic emergencies. 9th ed. New York: McGraw-Hill; 2011. p. 33–6.
10. Sachdeva DK, Stadnyk JM. Are one or two dangerous? Opioid exposure in toddlers. J Emerg Med. 2005;29(1):77–84.
11. Madden MA. Pediatric toxicology: emerging trends. J Pediatr Intensive Care. 2015;4(2):103–10. https://doi.org/10.1055/s-0035-1556753.
12. Adnet F, Borron SW, Finot MA, Lapandry C, Baud FJ. Intubation difficulty in poisoned patients: association with initial Glasgow Coma Scale score. Acad Emerg Med. 1998;5(2):123–7. https://doi.org/10.1111/j.1553-2712.1998.tb02596.x.
13. Salord F, Gaussorgues P, Marti-Flich J, Sirodot M, Allimant C, Lyonnet D, et al. Nosocomial maxillary sinusitis during mechanical ventilation: a prospective comparison of orotracheal versus the nasotracheal route for intubation. Intensive Care Med. 1990;16(6):390–3. https://doi.org/10.1007/BF01735177.
14. O'Connor MFKM, Hall JB. Airway management. In: Hall JBSG, Wood LDH, editors. Principles of critical care. 2nd ed. New York: Mc-Graw Hill; 1998.
15. Brent J, Burkhart K, Dargan P, Hatten B, Megarbane B, Palmer R, White J, editors. Critical care toxicology. Diagnosis and management of the critically poisoned patient. 2nd ed. Springer International Publishing; 2017.

16. Benson BE, Hoppu K, Troutman WG, Bedry R, Erdman A, Hojer J, et al. Position paper update: gastric lavage for gastrointestinal decontamination. Clin Toxicol (Phila). 2013;51(3):140–6. https://doi.org/10.3109/15563650.2013.770154.
17. Chyka PA, Holley JE, Mandrell TD, Sugathan P. Correlation of drug pharmacokinetics and effectiveness of multiple-dose activated charcoal therapy. Ann Emerg Med. 1995;25(3):356–62. https://doi.org/10.1016/S0196-0644(95)70295-4.
18. Tomaszewski C, Runge J, Gibbs M, Colucciello S, Price M. Evaluation of a rapid bedside toxicology screen in patients with drug toxicity. J Emerg Med. 2005;28(4):389–94. https://doi.org/10.1016/j.jemermed.2004.11.021.
19. Proudfoot AT, Krenzelok EP, Vale JA. Position paper on urine alkalinization. Clin Toxicol. 2004;42:1–26.
20. Ghannoum M, Roberts DM, Hoffman RS, Ouellet G, Roy L, Decker BS, et al. A stepwise approach for the management of poisoning with extracorporeal treatments. Semin Dial. 2014;27(4):362–70. https://doi.org/10.1111/sdi.12228.
21. Lavergne V, Nolin TD, Hoffman RS, Robert D, Gosselin S, Goldfarb DS, et al. The EXTRIP (Extracorporeal treatments in poisoning) workgroup: guideline methodology. Clin Toxicol. 2012;50:403–13.
22. Blaber MS, Khan JN, Brebner JA, McColm R. "Lipid rescue" for tricyclic antidepressant cardiotoxicity. J Emerg Med. 2012;43(3):465–7.
23. American College of Medical Toxicology. ACMT position statement: interim guidance for the use of lipid resuscitation therapy. J Med Toxicol. 2011;7(1):81–2.
24. Cook D, Guyatt G, Marshall J, Leasa D, Fuller H, Hall R, et al. A comparison of sucralfate and ranitidine for the prevention of upper gastrointestinal bleeding in patients requiring mechanical ventilation. Canadian Critical Care Trials Group. N Engl J Med. 1998;338(12):791–7.
25. Bryant S, Singer J. Management of toxic exposure in children. Emerg Med Clin North Am. 2003;21(1):101–19.
26. Calello DP, Henretig FM. Pediatric toxicology: specialized approach to the poisoned child. Emerg Med Clin North Am. 2014;32(1):29–52.
27. McFee RB, Caraccio TR. "Hang Up Your Pocketbook"—an easy intervention for the granny syndrome: grandparents as a risk factor in unintentional pediatric exposures to pharmaceuticals. J Am Osteopath Assoc. 2006;106(7):405–11.
28. Russo M, Pecker L, Wood J, et al. Grandparent involvement in exploratory pediatric poisonings: a hospital-based study. Clin Toxicol. 2013;51(7):592.

Burns in Children

Harish Bangalore

Contents

J. Brierley et al. (eds.), *ESPNIC Children's Intensive Care Textbook*,
https://doi.org/10.1007/978-3-031-64762-8_49

Learning Objectives

- To learn about who gets burnt, how, and what is the outcome of children with burns in the current era.
- To learn about how stabilize, resuscitate, and refer a child with thermal injuries including airway control, fluid resuscitation, and management of inhalation injuries.
- Recognize and understand how children with thermal injuries are managed in burn centers including treatment of infections, pain management, nutrition, thrombo-prophylaxis, and the hypermetabolic response.

49.1 Introduction

A burn can be defined as coagulative destruction of the skin and its structures by thermal, chemical, mechanical, or electrical injury. Thermal injuries account for more than 300,000 deaths annually and for 10 million disability adjusted life years lost each year, more than 95% of such occur in low- and middle-income countries [1]. The incidence, severity, length of hospital stay, and mortality globally due to burns is decreasing in the more developed countries [2]. It is a disease which is more prevalent in low socio-economic regions [3]. Most injuries in children less than 5 years of age are due to scalds and contact burns while flame burns are more common in older children. About a quarter of all burns occur in younger children, especially toddlers, with nearly three-quarters of the injuries being sustained at home. Non-accidental is suspected to be the cause in about 1% of all burn injuries [4].

Though about two-thirds of the burns are small [<10% Total Burn Surface Area (TBSA)], the infrequent occurrence, particularly of large burns (>30% TBSA) in comparison to other diseases and injuries, causes anxiety due to unfamiliarity with management [4, 5]. A structured approach is useful in the resuscitation, stabilization, and management. It is vital to recognize that burn management is essentially a surgical disease in which the input of a multi-disciplinary team in a specialized burns service is vital for larger or more complex injuries. The management of burns has generally improved over the last few decades and most children even with severe injuries are expected to survive with specialized burn care. The mortality in children with 90–100% burns is 55% but about 3% in the 30–39% group [6, 7]. The management of a severe burn injury is usually prolonged and is a continuum starting with the initial resuscitation, stabilization, and transfer, followed by definitive surgical management with excision and skin grafting when needed, nutritional management, treatment of infections and rehabilitation, both physically and psychologically.

49.2 Resuscitation and Stabilization

Case Scenario *A 8-year-old child was referred to you after her dress caught fire at a birthday party. She sustained a burn to most of her trunk, back, buttocks, upper limbs, and part of the lower limbs. How do you go about assessing, stabilizing, and resuscitating this child?*

The initial resuscitation of a child with thermal injuries should follow the ABCDE trauma principle with the assessment of airway, breathing, circulation, spine assessment, primary and secondary survey in line with guidelines. First aid is important—

cooling the burn with cool or tepid running tap water for 20 min within 3 h of the injury is useful. Ice should not be used for this purpose. In addition, "Stop, Drop and Roll" in flame injuries, isolating electrical power sources, and avoiding chemical cross contamination are important measures. All burning clothing should be removed including nappies and jewelry if any. It is prudent to keep the patient warm and avoid hypothermia while instituting first aid measures [8].

49.2.1 Airway and Lower Respiratory Tract

The airway and lower respiratory tract can be involved due to direct upper respiratory thermal injury, inhalation injury of the lower respiratory tract, and systemic toxicity due to inhalation of toxic material and gases.

The mucosa and airways above the glottis can be injured from exposure to intense heat largely confined to the supra-glottic region due to reflex closure of the glottis. This leads to edema and ulceration due to epithelial injury during the initial 24 h following injury. Burns in the oral cavity or blistering of the mucous membranes may provide suggestions of upper airway involvement. Occasionally, injuries to the front of the neck and aspiration of hot liquids may lead to upper airway edema and distortion of the anatomy. It is vital to understand that airway support may be extremely difficult when it is delayed. An experienced practitioner should intubate the child and a well-fitting cuffed endotracheal tube is preferred. A naso-gastric tube should be placed prior to intubation to counter gastric distention. Similarly, unplanned extubations can have serious consequences due to difficulty in obtaining an airway particularly after the initiation of fluid resuscitation. This can be avoided by being meticulous with securing the endo tracheal tube and ensuring adequate analgesia and sedation. In addition, cutting the endotracheal tube too short should be avoided due to risks of migration with facial edema. Nursing in the semi-upright position with moderate elevation of the head and trunk help reduce airway edema [9]. Supportive management is necessary while the inflammation, edema, and the injury to the supra-glottic area decreases over a few days.

The lower respiratory tract below the vocal cords can be involved by high humidity heat, superheated steam, and blast injuries, in addition to the smoke and particulate damage (<10 μm) and toxic injury due to inhaled chemical components. This leads to mucosal damage and inflammation and decreased mucosal clearance [10]. This clinically manifests as bronchoconstriction, bronchial edema, and casts. Lung parenchymal damage usually occurs after 24 h due to immune system activation and the resulting inflammation causing alveolar collapse, decreased particulate clearance and ventilation perfusion mismatch, and pulmonary vascular clots. This can manifest as pulmonary collapse and consolidation, edema, and pulmonary hypertension [11]. Inhalation injury causes pulmonary edema 2–3 days and pneumonia 7–14 days after injury. The circumstances of injury should be taken into consideration—scalds and open-air flame injuries are unlikely and burns in confined spaces are more likely to have inhalational injury. The suspicion of an inhalation and smoke injury is based on circumstantial and clinical features—smoke exposure, flame injuries in confined places, soot at the mouth and singing of the nasal hair, diminished consciousness and facial burns suggest inhalation injuries. The clinical signs of inhalation injury such as cough, wheezing, hoarseness, and dyspnea are delayed and are late manifestations.

Carbonaceous secretion is indicative but may be absent if it is cleared rapidly. In addition, early chest X rays are also unreliable for the diagnosis of inhalation injuries. Fiberoptic examination of the upper and lower respiratory tracts are the most reliable modality for diagnosis. Mucosal edema, erosions, and carbonaceous secretions are suggestive of inhalation injury [12].

The management of inhalation injury is largely supportive in addition to concomitant identification and treatment of toxic inhalational agents and fluid resuscitation. In intubated patients, supportive treatment based on established principles, acute respiratory distress syndrome management including open-lung strategy, limiting tidal volumes to <6 mL/kg and plateau pressures less than 30 cm of H_2O are useful. In addition, pulmonary toilet with regular inhalation of bronchodilators, *N*-acetyl cysteine and heparin, may help in the management of inhalational injuries [13–15]. At times, circumferential burns to the chest may need prompt escharotomies to aid in respiratory support to address decreased chest wall compliance. In severe inhalational injuries with hypoxemia refractory to standard management, prone positioning and inhaled nitric therapy could be beneficial. There is no role for prophylactic antibiotics or steroids in the treatment of inhalation injuries [16].

The identification and management of systemic toxicity due to carbon monoxide, cyanide and other toxic products of combustion are important considerations in the management of inhalation injuries.

Carbon monoxide is produced by incomplete combustion of hydrocarbon fuels. It causes hypoxemia by displacing oxygen from hemoglobin, due to the high affinity of carbon monoxide for hemoglobin, producing carboxyhemoglobin, which has 200 times more affinity for oxygen. In addition, it also binds to cytochromes causing decreased cellular oxygen utilization. A diminished consciousness in the setting of a flame injury in a confined space should suggest toxicity due to carbon monoxide. A routine pulse oximeter or partial pressure of oxygen measurements (pO_2) on a blood gas analysis are inadequate to diagnose carbon monoxide toxicity. Diagnosis is by co-oximetry measurement of carboxyhemoglobin levels in blood. Levels of carboxyhemoglobin of 15–20% cause headache and confusion and levels above 60% are fatal. The half-life of carbon monoxide is 5 h in air and is reduced to 60 min by administration of 100% oxygen. All children should be commenced on 100% humidified oxygen aiming for a saturation of >95% till co-oximetry is obtained to rule out carbon monoxide poisoning. This is continued till the carbon monoxide level is less than 10%. Hyperbaric oxygen is not currently recommended for management of its toxicity [17, 18]. It is important to note that there is not a good correlation with the carbon monoxide levels and morbidity. In addition, it is important to consider the time after the initial injury the level was taken as the levels decrease over time.

Cyanide gas exposure is thought to be frequent in smoke inhalation particularly with combustion of fabrics containing wool, nylon, silk, and plastics containing melamine and polyurethanes. Cyanide produces hypoxia at the cellular level by binding of the ferric ions in cytochrome-C oxidase blocking cellular aerobic metabolism. Clinical manifestations of cyanide toxicity include neurologic deficits, persistent and unexplained acidosis, and serum lactate greater than 8 mmol/L. As it is not possible to measure cyanide in the emergency care setting, supplementary cyanide intoxication should be suspected in the presence of alerted sensorium, seizures, metabolic acidosis, high lactate, and a low oxygen extraction. The treatment includes 100% oxygen, mechanical ventilation, blood pressure support, and administration of antidote. Hydroxocobalamin (70 mg/kg to a maximum of 5 g) acts as an antidote by combining with cyanide to form cyanocobalamin (Vitamin B12) which is excreted in the urine. It should be administered as soon as possible when cyanide intoxication is suspected. Side-effects are red coloring of skin and urine, urticarial eczema, and seldom anaphylactic shock. In addition, hydroxocobalamin interferes with the measurement of methemoglobin, oxyhemoglobin, and carboxyhemoglobin in the blood. Sodium thiosulfate and dicobalt EDTA are other antidotes [19].

Inhalation injuries are recognized to have an increased requirement for fluid resuscitation and are associated with a high mortality and morbidity [7]. Hence, early initiation of therapy and judicious fluid management are also important in the management of inhalation injuries [20, 21].

The key aspects of management of inhalation injuries is as shown in ◘ Fig. 49.1 of the Appendix.

The child had first aid measures instituted, was covered in a clean blanket, and transferred to the emergency department. The child was assessed in a systematic way, and it was noted that the child was conscious, had no stridor, or soot with normal saturations, tachycardia, normal blood pressure in one limb which was burn free but was in pain and distress and the extent of the flame injury was determined to be large at about 60% with the injury predominantly on the chest, back, buttocks, and lower limbs. Two large bore intravenous access were secured, and a decision made to intubate and transfer the child to a burn service for further treatment. The intubation was uneventful with no signs of inhalational injury noted and it was easy to ventilate and oxygenate. The burns area was covered with clean longitudinal strips of cling film.

49.2.2 Fluid Resuscitation After Thermal Injuries

Thermal injuries cause pathophysiological changes which induce a response in almost every organ of the body. The initial phase occurs in the first 24–72 h and consists of large fluid shifts with increased vascular permeability and intravascular fluid depletion due to a combination of direct tissue injury, imbalance between the capillary hydrostatic and osmotic gradient at the capillary level, changes in the endothelial glycocalyx, and release of inflammatory mediators [22, 23]. Fluid resuscitation is key during this phase and the goal is to replenish the intra-vascular fluid losses for this period. It is recognized that up to half of plasma water can be lost within 2–3 h in a burn injury of 40% TBSA [22, 24]. The period of intravascular fluid loss is maximum in the first 8–12 h over the burn injury and reduces subsequently. The rate and composition of fluid replacement should aim to mirror this pattern. Colloids are not usually beneficial during the first few hours due to a leak of the colloid into the interstitial space [25, 26].

Fluid resuscitation in thermal injuries has been attributed to improvements in outcomes since the 1940s by Oliver and Copeland. Over the years, several formulae have been utilized based on body weight, the burn surface area, and the composition of the fluid [27–31] (◘ Table 49.1). Most of these regimens advocate a higher rate of resuscitation within the first 8–12 h followed by a slower rate over the next 16 h. The composition of the fluid used is isotonic crystalloid (Ringer lactate) in regimens such as the Parklands and modified Brookes or a combination of crystalloid and colloid-based solutions in other regimens. The amount of fluid given should be directly pro-

Table 49.1 Fluid resuscitation formulae in children

Regimen name	Resuscitation regimen
Modified Parkland's	2–4 mL/kg/% burn + Maintenance per Holiday and Seagar < 30 kg of Ringer lactate over 24 h ½ over the first 8 h and ½ over the next 16 h
Shriners	4 mL/kg/% burn + 1500 mL/m^2 body of fluid in total divided over 24 h in three parts Ringer lactate with 50 mEq/L of Sodium bicarbonate over the first 8 h Ringer lactate only over the next 8 h Ringer lactate with 12.5 g/L of 25% Albumin over the last 8 h
Galveston	5000 mL/m^2 burn + 1500 mL/m^2 body of Ringer lactate over 24 h ½ over the first 8 h and ½ over the next 16 h

portional to the extent of the burn injury. A child's palm including fingers are roughly equal to 1% of the child's body surface area which can be used to roughly assist burn size estimates. The %TBSA should be calculated with the help of charts such as the Lund–Browder chart [32] (Fig. 49.2). Newer technology such as mobile applications can be used to estimate the percentage burns surface area. Erythema of the skin should not be counted in estimation of the burns surface area.

49

Children have important differences which need to be considered. The body surface area in children based on weight is higher than in adults and hence may lead to problems with under or over resuscitation when using the traditional weight-based formulae. It is generally thought that children have higher fluid resuscitation needs in burns than adults [33, 34]. The threshold at which additional resuscitation fluids is started in children is 10%. In children with circulatory shock, a crystalloid bolus of 20 mL/kg should be given. The fluid deficit is calculated per the Parkland formula (2–4 mL/kg/%TBSA) with the addition of maintenance fluid to children lesser than 30 kg. Smaller children have lower glycogen reserves, a larger surface area, and need the addition of 5% dextrose with Ringer lactate in younger children as a maintenance. Half of the total fluid calculated (2–4 mL/kg/%TBSA + maintenance fluid in a child <30 kg) is given over the first 8 h and the remainder over the next 16 h. Smaller children with a lower %TBSA are likely to have a higher contribution from maintenance fluids [35].

Regardless of the regimen used, it is important to balance adequate fluid resuscitation and avoidance of overzealous fluid resuscitation with regular titration based on end-goals of resuscitation [24, 36]. Urine output is the most common end point used to judge adequate resuscitation in children [37]. A combination of endpoints which help in titration of resuscitation fluids include urine output, hemodynamic stability with age-appropriate heart rate and blood pressure, resolution of metabolic and lactic acidosis. Advanced hemodynamic monitoring may also be useful in large burns [38, 39]. While it is recognized that fluid requirements may be higher in children, fluid resuscitation needs twice the predicted amounts per Parklands and oliguria should warrant a consideration of complications such as abdominal compartment syndrome or a low cardiac output state.

Practical challenges in children needing resuscitation for thermal injuries such difficult venous access should be considered. Two large-bore cannula should ideally be sited in non-burnt areas and resuscitation started as soon as possible after the injury. The use of intra-osseous access or central venous access with three-point securing should be considered through burnt skin if no other suitable site is available.

The child needed fluid resuscitation with 20 mL/kg boluses of Ringer lactate due to tachycardia and hypotension following induction for intubation. Resuscitation fluids with maintenance were commenced per the Parkland's formulae.

49.2.3 Transport to a Burn Service

Safe, controlled transfer of children to a burns service is paramount. After initial stabilization, a child should be discussed preferably in a conference call with the local team, transport team, and the specialist burn service. All burn networks must have well-circulated referral criteria to referring hospitals. The usual indications for a referral to a specialist burn center include burns >5% TBSA, any burns involving the face, feet, hands or perinium or over a joint, circumferential burns, burns with inhalation injuries, electrical and chemical burns. A succinct, brief history should include the mechanism of injury, previous relevant history, allergies, tetanus toxoid status, and treatment instituted to date. Details such as the estimated TBSA, size of endotracheal tube, evidence of airway injury, suspicion of inhalation injury and toxicity, the size and extent of injury, intravenous access, intravenous fluid resuscitation initiated and end points of perfusion—hemodynamics, lactate, urine output are essential.

The local surgical team should be involved in the initial discussions and the need for an escharotomy in circumferential limb and chest burns should be considered prior to transfer.

It cannot be stated enough that the endotracheal tubes need to be well secured—ties may be needed in case of facial burns. The tube should not be cut short as there is a risk of migration of the tube into the mouth with increasing facial edema with resuscitation. Signs of toxicity with carbon monoxide and cyanide should be considered and treatment initiated promptly before transport.

Two large bore well-functioning cannula are essential. It may be necessary to secure a central venous line if it is difficult to secure peripheral access when most of the skin surface area is burnt. The central venous access should be secured at three points. The fluids given to date, current fluids ongoing and the end points of resuscitation should recorded. The fluid resuscitation should continue through the transport journey. The peripheral pulses must be monitored in circumferential limb injuries. A naso-gastric tube and urine catheter should be placed before moving the child.

Children with burns loose heat quicker than adults and can develop hypothermia rapidly. The child should be covered with warm blankets and thermal blankets/warmers if necessary. The burn wounds should be covered with clean longitudinal strips of cling film. The temperature should be monitored through the journey and measures instituted to prevent hypothermia. The use of warm intravenous fluids may be necessary in large burns. A rectal temperature of 38 °C should be targeted. Ensure the child has adequate analgesia.

On arrival to the burns center, a formal and systematic handover in the presence of the transport team, anesthetist, intensive care, and burn surgical team should be done in a systematic manner with formal identification of all individuals and their roles in the team.

49.2.4 Ongoing Management: Surgical

At admission to the burns intensive care unit, an initial assessment of the burn injury is performed by an experienced burn surgeon and anesthetic team. The burn wound is thoroughly cleaned or debrided as part of the assessment and life or limb-saving interventions, such as escharotomies and fasciotomies, are performed if necessary.

Burn injuries are classified according to the depth of the burn involved [40] (Table 49.2). Burn injuries involving more superficial layers of the skin (superficial partial thickness) will heal with simple debridement, dressings, and supportive management. Burn involving deeper layers of the skin (deep dermal and full thickness) heal with secondary intention after a prolonged period if surgical excision and treatment is not initiated.

49

Burn injury is primarily a surgical disease. The basic principle of management of a burn injury is promoting the healing of skin which is likely to recover (superficial partial thickness) with debridement of dead tissue and autografting of deeper injuries (deep dermal and full thickness) to fasten healing and wound closure. Autografts are used for definitive wound cover. This is taken from unburnt areas of the body such as the scalp, back, abdomen, and back. Early total burn wound excision and skin grafting to achieve wound closure is the corner stone of surgical burn care management. This has been shown to reduce infection rates, reduce the length of hospital stay, and improve survival in burn patients, especially in children [41–43].

Table 49.2 Burn wound depth

Type	Level involved	Clinical features	Implication
Superficial	Epidermis only	Red, painful, no blisters,	Do not include erythema in TBSA Heals in 3–7 days
Superficial partial thickness	Epidermis and upper dermis without skin appendages	Red or pale pink, painful, blisters, brisk capillary refill	Heals in 1–2 weeks with non-adherent dressings
Deep dermal	Epidermis and dermis with skin appendages	Dark pink, red or white, mottled skin with capillary stains, delayed or absent capillary refill with dull/ variable sensation	Surgical intervention likely required
Full thickness	All skin layers or deeper with fat/ fascia	White, black, yellow, or brown, leathery appearance, no sensation, no capillary refill	Surgical intervention

After initial assessment and stabilization, surgical treatment is undertaken usually within the first 72 h. The burnt areas which are likely to heal are covered with dressings to keep them protected, promote healing, and prevent occurrence of infection. In large burns, there may be limited donor sites. Surgical expansion techniques such as mesh grafting and Meek grafts increase the surface area available for re-epithelization of wounds.

Some areas may need temporary coverage with allografts to protect autografts, which is known as sandwich grafting, or to promote healing of mixed depth areas or excised wounds that cannot be covered with autografts. Donor areas heal relatively quickly and can be harvested again once healed. Sometimes, dermal substitutes and dermal matrix templates are used to improve the quality of healing, particularly for functionally important or cosmetically sensitive areas.

A child with a large burn may need multiple surgical procedures not only during their acute admission but also to release scar contractures or to improve functional recovery as they grow up. Some areas may need to be re-grafted due to loss of previous autografts caused by mechanical trauma during routine nursing care and rehabilitation or, more commonly, secondary infections.

49.2.5 Ongoing Management: Medical

Ongoing management is necessary not only to aid in the healing process and facilitating adequate wound cover and skin growth but also to support the intense pathophysiological changes which occur following large thermal injuries after 24–72 h following the injury [22, 23].

The ongoing medical management supplements the surgical management of a burn injury and is as highlighted below.

49.2.5.1 Cardiovascular

The initial phase of a large burn causes a right and left ventricular myocardial depression, increased systemic and pulmonary vascular resistance. This is called as the "ebb phase" and is contributory to burn shock. This phase is followed by an intense "flow phase" with a hypermetabolic response which causes "cardiac stress," an increase in heart rate, blood pressure, increased myocardial oxygen consumption, and increased cardiac output following the initial 24–72 h and may persist up to 2 years [44].

Treatment during the ebb phase is largely supportive intensive care management of burn shock with judicious fluid management, and inotropic support. In the later period, the initiation of beta blockers to modulate the hypermetabolic response following adequate resuscitation and stability after the initial burn injury has been shown to decrease left ventricular work without affecting oxygen delivery or other cardiovascular parameters [45]. During the treatment of a child with a large thermal injury, there may be re-occurrence of shock due to infections necessitating temporary cessation of beta blockade.

49.2.5.2 Hypermetabolic Response

Large burns are characterized by an intense hypermetabolic response characterized by an increase in the resting energy expenditure (REE) and changes in almost every organ leading to multi-organ dysfunction. This causes changes in carbohydrate, protein, and lipid metabolism. Hyperglycemia, insulin resistance, associated with increased infections and poor wound healing; and increased lipolysis with increase in free fatty acids leading to fatty infiltration of all organs including the liver; and increased protein catabolism and breakdown leading to muscle wasting and decreased lean body mass are some of the effects of the hypermetabolic state. The cause of this response is not clear but is thought to be due to increased expression of catecholamines and glucocorticoids in addition to an inflammatory response. If not adequately recognized and treated, it leads to a severe catabolic state leading to wasting [45].

Several treatments are used to treat the hypermetabolic response. Early total burn wound excision and wound closure reduces the REE requirements and helps manage the hypermetabolic response. Nutritional support to meet the increased caloric requirements with a high caloric, high protein, low fat feed help in meeting the increased energy expenditure and aid wound healing. The core body temperature is increased in large burns by about 2 °C because of this phenomenon. Increasing the ambient temperature of the room from 25 to 33 °C in patients exceeding 60% TBSA decreased the REE from 2.0 to 1.4 times the REE [46]. Exercises and physical therapy can help build body muscle mass and children with large burn injuries [47].

Oxandrolone is a testosterone analogue with little virilizing potential and is used in children with large thermal injuries to help attenuate the hypermetabolic effects on lean muscle and body mass. In burn patients, oxandrolone has been shown to not only achieve an increase in muscle protein synthesis but also reduce weight loss, increase donor site healing, and has been shown to decrease the length of hospitalization [48–50].

Propranolol is used to attenuate the increased catecholamine response following the burn injury in the "flow" phase after a large burn injury after resuscitation from the "ebb phase." It has been shown to be safe and attenuates the catabolic effects of the hypermetabolic state with an improvement in lean body mass, decrease bone loss and REE in children [51].

49.2.5.3 Nutritional Support and Gastro-Intestinal Support

Early and adequate nutritional support is one of the key features of modern burn care which has resulted in improved outcomes for the last few decades. Nutritional needs in burns are increased due to a combination of factors such as needs for wound repair and healing, the catecholamine and inflammatory surge resulting in a hypermetabolic state and an impaired thermoregulation [52, 53].

The total energy expenditure in patients with >40% TBSA burns is 1.3–1.5 times the REE. In convalescent burns patients, optimal nutrition support has been shown to be 1.2 times the calculated REE [54]. The REE can be calculated by indirect calorimetry. Caloric requirement can also be calculated by using formulae derived from retrospective dietary analysis of children with burns needed to maintain body weight [55]. Curreri and Galveston formulae are examples of equations which help estimating the REE in children with burns. A diet which is high in carbohydrate and protein was shown to decrease muscle catabolism and improve lean body mass when compared to a formula with a high fat content [56]. A protein requirement of 1.5–3.0 g/kg/day is adequate [57]. Enteral nutrition is known to be superior to a combination of enteral and parenteral nutrition. This should be commenced as soon as possible (within 6–12 h) and has been shown to decrease the hypermetabolic response [58, 59]. The small intestine is more resistant to post burn ileus than the stomach and the colon. Hence, children with large burn wounds may benefit from naso-jejunal feeds.

A supplementation of zinc, copper, and selenium as well as Vitamin B1, C, D, and E is recommended in large burns [60]. Constipation is a common occurrence in children with burns and should be anticipated and appropriately treated.

The monitoring of nutritional adequacy in children with burn injuries is challenging and as weight may not reflect adequate nutrition due to the changes in body composition with a tendency to fat deposition and muscle wasting. Some techniques such as DEXA scan, CT scan, and ultrasound of the quadriceps may be helpful but of limited utility and challenging in acute settings [61].

49.2.5.4 Infection and Sepsis

Children with large burns may have episodes of infection due to a loss of the skin barrier, burn-induced immunosuppression, and complications of treatment such as vascular devices and catheters. Infections can cause significant morbidity and mortality due to multi-organ failure, particularly in the later phase of large burn injuries [62, 63]. A robust anti-microbial stewardship, regular surveillance for infections, and judicious use of antibiotics is important. A burn injury without any clinical signs of infection either local or systemic does not need antibiotics to prevent the occurrence of infection. Signs of infection such as fever, increased white cell count, and inflammatory response (C-reactive protein/Calcitonin) along with a good clinical examination helps in the diagnosis and appropriate management [64–67]. There maybe challenges in differentiating an acute inflammatory response following a large burn with a secondary infection. A hypermetabolic response may also produce signs like an infection. Regular screening swabs are necessary to tailor antimicrobial therapy appropriately. In addition, local measures such as debridement and showering are also helpful in controlling infections. Antimicrobials should be given for short periods of time and stopped as soon as possible as there is a risk of increase in resistant organism with prolonged courses of antimicrobials. It is prudent to note that the metabolism of antibiotics such as aminoglycosides maybe altered in large burns and dosing needs to be adjusted appropriately. Reactivation of viral and fungal infections also need to be considered when there is no response to antibiotics.

49.2.5.5 Lines and Thromboprophylaxis

Burn injuries produce a hypercoagulable state and are associated with an increased risk of line-related thrombosis [68]. Prophylactic anticoagulation is frequently used in some institutions in children with large burns with central venous access. The metabolism of low-molecular-weight heparin is increased, and the levels need to be monitored particularly if targeting therapeutic anti-coagulation [69–71].

It is important to be vigilant for central line-associated infections which can be caused due to gut translocation and bacterial seeding due to wound manipulation in addition to vicinity to open wounds. As both thrombosis and line-associated infections are not uncommon, some institutions routinely change central venous catheters every 7–10 days. In children with large burn injuries, central venous access may be challenging due to these issues.

49.2.5.6 Sedation and Pain Management

Pain management is an important aspect of management of burn injuries. This consists of both the acute management—immediate, with dressing change and with movement in raw areas. In addition, management of background pain is also important. Opioids are the main agent types of these medications are used for management of pain in burn injuries and in addition to agents such as Acetaminophen, non-steroidal anti-inflammatory agents, and Ketamine in some patients [72]. Pain management protocols should address both aspects of acute and background pain management in addition to escalation in case of poor control. Donor sites such as the scalp can also be very painful and regional blocks are sometimes used in pain management in donor areas. Measurement scales such as the visual analogue scales and the FLACC score in younger children are useful tools [73]. Pain management should involve a multi-disciplinary team which includes the anesthetists, intensivists, surgeons, nurses, and psychologists. This is important not only for rehabilitation and management but also for preventing long-term phycological issues such as post-traumatic stress syndrome.

Management of pain should consider tachyphylaxis, cycling of opioid analgesics in addition to non-pharmacological aspects such as play therapy and the input of psychologists in addition to creating a positive and motivational environment.

Sedation is frequently required for procedures such as dressing changes and must incorporate a protocol which is suitable for the local needs and capabilities.

Itching and neuropathic pain are aspects of burn management which need a similar approach with a guideline of escalation and a scoring system [74, 75]. Gabapentin in addition to antihistamines are an important agent which helps in this management [76].

The child admitted with the flame injury did well initially following the management of the acute resuscitative phase of burns. Her wound recovery was complicated by graft loss with Pseudomonas infection. Systemic and local anti-microbials directed at the sensitivities of the organism isolated was successful in treating the infection. Three more split skin grafts were required during her care. She was transferred from the intensive care to the ward after the initial resuscitation, debridement, and grafting but needed another brief period of admission to intensive care for the management of Pseudomonas sepsis. She was commenced on Propranolol and Oxandrolone after the initial resuscitation phase. Her nutritional recovery was good, and she was able to tolerate feeds well through her admission. She needed ongoing input of the psychologists, physiotherapists, and play therapist to help motivate her and manage her pain and anxiety. She made a good recovery and was discharged from the burns center 2 months after her admission with ongoing follow-up for nutritional follow-up, physiotherapy, and prevention of scar tissue and contractures.

49.3 Conclusion

The management of large burn injuries needs a multi-disciplinary team with the knowledge and experience to deal with the pathophysiology that occurs in both the acute phase and during the ongoing recovery and rehabilitation phase. With modern burn care, almost every burned child would be expected to survive with good recovery of form and function in even the largest of burn injuries. Psychological support for the child and their family as well as long term follow-up are also important considerations.

Appendix

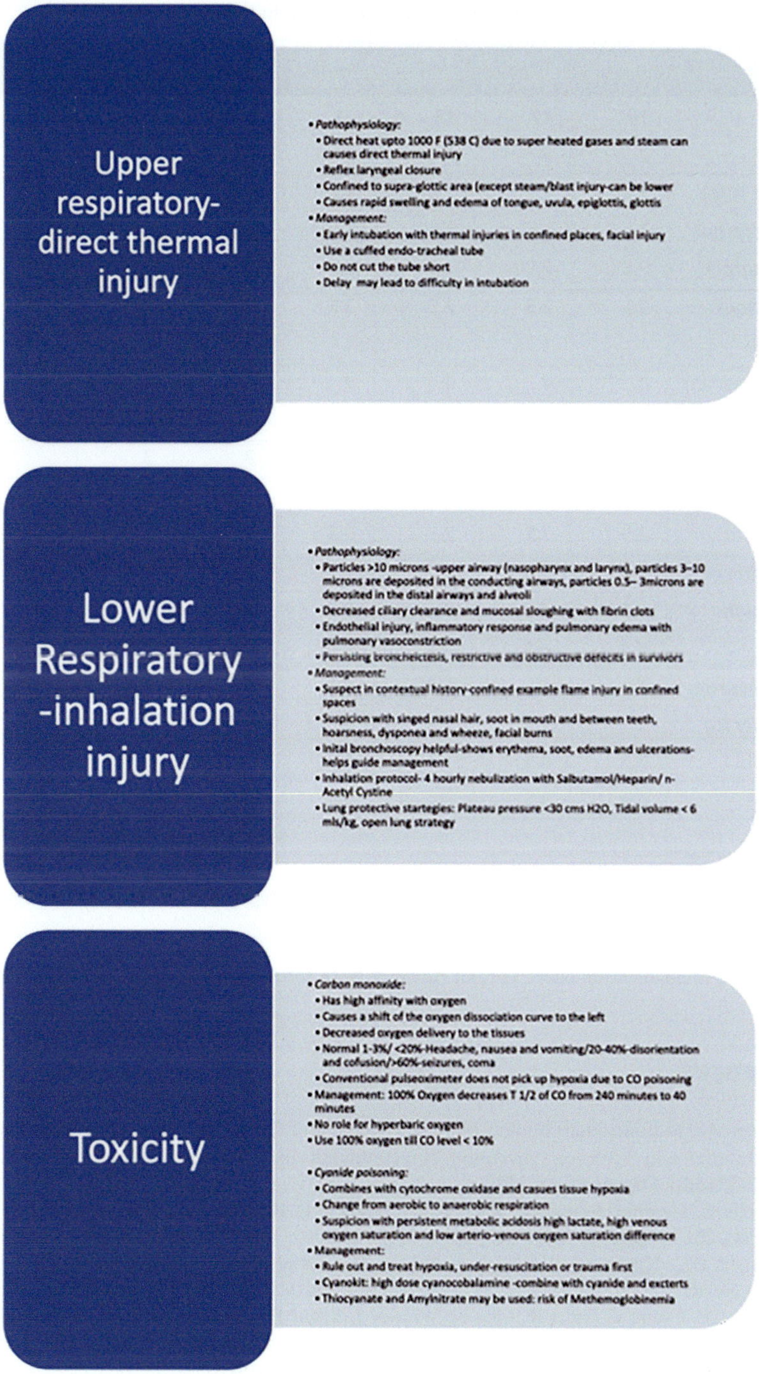

Fig. 49.1 Inhalation injury in burns

LUND AND BROWDER CHART

Commonly used in burn centers

Estimate of % Total Body Surface Area (TBSA) Burn by sum of individual areas

Area	Birth-1	1–4 Years	5–9 Years	10–14 Years	10–14 Years	Adult	Total
Head	***19***	***17***	***13***	***11***	***9***	***7***	
Neck	2	2	2	2	2	2	
Anterior trunk	13	13	13	13	13	13	
Posterior trunk	13	13	13	13	13	13	
Right buttock	2.5	2.5	2.5	2.5	2.5	2.5	
Left buttock	2.5	2.5	2.5	2.5	2.5	2.5	
Genitalia	1	1	1	1	1	1	
Right upper arm	4	4	4	4	4	4	
Left upper arm	4	4	4	4	4	4	
Right lower arm	3	3	3	3	3	3	
Left lower arm	3	3	3	3	3	3	
Right hand	2.5	2.5	2.5	2.5	2.5	2.5	
Left hand	2.5	2.5	2.5	2.5	2.5	2.5	
Right thigh	***5.5***	***6.5***	***8***	***8.5***	***9***	***9.5***	
Left thigh	***5.5***	***6.5***	***8***	***8.5***	***9***	***9.5***	
Right lower leg	***5***	***5***	***5.5***	***5.5***	***6.5***	***7***	
Left lower leg	***5***	***5***	***5.5***	***6***	***6.5***	***7***	
Right foot	3.5	3.5	3.5	3.5	3.5	3.5	
Left foot	3.5	3.5	3.5	3.5	3.5	3.5	
Total							

Rows in ***bold italics*** indicate areas of difference between adult and pediatric patients. All other areas are the same for adults and children.

Fig. 49.2 Lund-Browder chart. (From: Advance Burn Life Support Course 2017 [32])

References

1. Peden M. The injury chart book: a graphical overview of the global burden of injuries. Department of Injuries and Violence Prevention Noncommunicable Diseases and Mental Health Cluster, World Health Organization; 2002.
2. Smolle C, Cambiaso-daniel J, Forbes AA, Wurzer P, Branski LK, Huss F, et al. HHS Public Access. 2018;43(2):249–57.
3. Herbert HK, Hyder AA, Butchart A, Norton R. Global health: injuries and violence. Infect Dis Clin North Am. 2011;25(3):653–68, x. https://doi.org/10.1016/j.idc.2011.06.004.
4. Battle CE, Evans V, James K, Guy K, Whitley J, Evans PA. Epidemiology of burns and scalds in children presenting to the emergency department of a regional burns unit: a 7-year retrospective study. Burns Trauma. 2016;4(1):19. https://doi.org/10.1186/s41038-016-0047-7.
5. James SL, Abate D, Abate KH, Abay SM, Abbafati C, Abbasi N. Global, regional, and national incidence, prevalence, and years lived with disability for 354 diseases and injuries for 195 countries

and territories, 1990–2017: a systematic analysis for the global burden of disease study 2017. Lancet. 2017;392:1789–858.
6. Kraft R, Herndon DN, Al-Mousawi AM, Williams FN, Finnerty CC, Jeschke MG. Burn size and survival probability in paediatric patients in modern burn care: a prospective observational cohort study. Lancet. 2012;379(9820):1013–21. https://doi.org/10.1016/s0140-6736(11)61345-7.
7. Barrow RE, Spies M, Barrow LN, Herndon DN. Influence of demographics and inhalation injury on burn mortality in children. Burns. 2004;30(1):72–7. https://doi.org/10.1016/j.burns.2003.07.003.
8. Org.uk. [cited 2022 Jun 13]. http://www.cbtrust.org.uk/wp-content/uploads/2019/01/BBA-First-Aid-Guideline.
9. ISBI Practice Guidelines Committee, Ahuja RB, Gibran N, Greenhalgh D, Jeng J, Mackie D, et al. ISBI practice guidelines for burn care. Burns. 2016;42(5):953–1021. https://doi.org/10.1016/j.burns.2016.05.013.
10. Demling RH. Smoke inhalation lung injury: an update. Eplasty. 2008;8:e27.
11. Albright JM, Davis CS, Bird MD, Ramirez L, Kim H, Burnham EL, et al. The acute pulmonary inflammatory response to the graded severity of smoke inhalation injury. Crit Care Med. 2012;40(4):1113–21. https://doi.org/10.1097/CCM.0b013e3182374a67.
12. Pruitt BA Jr, Cioffi WG. Diagnosis and treatment of smoke inhalation. J Intensive Care Med. 1995;10(3):117–27. https://doi.org/10.1177/088506669501000303.
13. Miller AC, Rivero A, Ziad S, Smith DJ, Elamin EM. Influence of nebulized unfractionated heparin and N-acetylcysteine in acute lung injury after smoke inhalation injury. J Burn Care Res. 2009;30(2):249–56. https://doi.org/10.1097/BCR.0b013e318198a268.
14. Desai MH, Mlcak R, Richardson J, Nichols R, Herndon DN. Reduction in mortality in pediatric patients with inhalation injury with aerosolized heparin/acetylcystine therapy. J Burn Care Rehabil. 1998;19(3):210–2. https://doi.org/10.1097/00004630-199805000-00004.
15. The Pediatric Acute Lung Injury Consensus Conference Group. Pediatric acute respiratory distress syndrome: consensus recommendations from the pediatric acute lung injury consensus conference. Pediatr Crit Care Med. 2015;16(5):428–39. https://doi.org/10.1097/pcc.0000000000000350.
16. Thamm OC, Perbix W, Zinser MJ, Koenen P, Wafaisade A, Maegele M, et al. Early single-shot intravenous steroids do not affect pulmonary complications and mortality in burned or scalded patients. Burns. 2013;39(5):935–41. https://doi.org/10.1016/j.burns.2012.10.007.
17. Piantadosi CA. Diagnosis and treatment of carbon monoxide poisoning. Respir Care Clin N Am. 1999;5(2):183–202.
18. Buckley NA, Juurlink DN, Isbister G, Bennett MH, Lavonas EJ. Hyperbaric oxygen for carbon monoxide poisoning. Cochrane Libr. 2011; https://doi.org/10.1002/14651858.cd002041.pub3.
19. Mintegi S, Clerigue N, Tipo V, Ponticiello E, Lonati D, Burillo-Putze G, et al. Pediatric cyanide poisoning by fire smoke inhalation: a European expert consensus. Pediatr Emerg Care. 2013;29(11):1234–40. https://doi.org/10.1097/pec.0b013e3182aa4ee1.
20. Endorf FW, Gamelli RL. Inhalation injury, pulmonary perturbations, and fluid resuscitation. J Burn Care Res. 2007;28(1):80–3. https://doi.org/10.1097/bcr.0b013e31802c889f.
21. Navar PD, Saffle JR, Warden GD. Effect of inhalation injury on fluid resuscitation requirements after thermal injury. Am J Surg. 1985;150(6):716–20. https://doi.org/10.1016/0002-9610(85)90415-5.
22. Vaughn L, Beckel N. Severe burn injury, burn shock, and smoke inhalation injury in small animals. Part 1: Burn classification and pathophysiology: severe burn injury and smoke inhalation injury. J Vet Emerg Crit Care. 2012;22(2):179–86. https://doi.org/10.1111/j.1476-4431.2012.00727.x.
23. Nielson CB, Duethman NC, Howard JM, Moncure M, Wood JG. Burns: pathophysiology of systemic complications and current management. J Burn Care Res. 2017;38(1):e469–81. https://doi.org/10.1097/bcr.0000000000000355.
24. Barrow RE, Jeschke MG, Herndon DN. Early fluid resuscitation improves outcomes in severely burned children. Theatr Res Int. 2000;45(2):91–6. https://doi.org/10.1016/s0300-9572(00)00175-1.
25. Kramer GC, Gunther RA, Nerlich ML, Zweifach SS, Demling RH. Effect of dextran-70 on increased microvascular fluid and protein flux after thermal injury. Circ Shock. 1982;9(5):529–41.
26. Demling RH. Fluid replacement in burned patients. Surg Clin N Am. 1987;67(1):15–30. https://doi.org/10.1016/s0039-6109(16)44130-7.
27. Romanowski KS, Palmieri TL. Pediatric burn resuscitation: past, present, and future. Burns Trauma. 2017;5(1):26. https://doi.org/10.1186/s41038-017-0091-y.

28. Pruitt BA Jr, Mason AD Jr, Moncrief JA. Hemodynamic changes in the early postburn patient the influence of fluid administration and of a vasodilator (hydralazine). J Trauma. 1971;11(1):36–46. https://doi.org/10.1097/00005373-197101000-00003.
29. Baxter CR, Shires T. Physiological response to crystalloid resuscitation of severe burns. Ann N Y Acad Sci. 1968;150(3):874–94. https://doi.org/10.1111/j.1749-6632.1968.tb14738.x.
30. Fakhry SM, Alexander J, Smith D, Meyer AA, Peterson HD. Regional and institutional variation in burn care. J Burn Care Rehabil. 1995;16(1):85–90. https://doi.org/10.1097/00004630-199501000-00017.
31. Carvajal HF. Fluid resuscitation of pediatric burn victims: a critical appraisal. Pediatr Nephrol. 1994;8(3):357–66. https://doi.org/10.1007/bf00866366.
32. Pham TN, Bettencourt AP, Bozinko GM, Chang PH, Chung KK, Craig CK, et al. Advanced burn life support course. Ameriburn.org. 2017 [cited 2022 Jun 14]. http://ameriburn.org/wp-content/uploads/2019/08/2018-abls-providermanual.pdf.
33. Graves TA, Cioffi WG, McManus WF, Mason AD Jr, Pruitt BA Jr. Fluid resuscitation of infants and children with massive thermal injury. J Trauma. 1988;28(12):1656–9. https://doi.org/10.1097/00005373-198812000-00007.
34. Merrell SW, Saffle JR, Sullivan JJ, Navar PD, Kravitz M, Warden GD. Fluid resuscitation in thermally injured children. Am J Surg. 1986;152(6):664–9. https://doi.org/10.1016/0002-9610(86)90445-9.
35. Bangalore H, Ray S, Martin N. Intravenous maintenance fluids in resuscitation for thermal injuries in children. Burns. 2018;44(8):2102–4. https://doi.org/10.1016/j.burns.2018.05.019.
36. Pruitt BA Jr. Protection from excessive resuscitation: "pushing the pendulum back". J Trauma. 2000;49(3):567–8. https://doi.org/10.1097/00005373-200009000-00030.
37. Greenhalgh DG. Burn resuscitation: the results of the ISBI/ABA survey. Burns. 2010;36(2):176–82. https://doi.org/10.1016/j.burns.2009.09.004.

38. Stutchfield C, Davies A, Young A. Fluid resuscitation in paediatric burns: how do we get it right? A systematic review of the evidence. Arch Dis Child. 2019;104(3):280–5. https://doi.org/10.1136/archdischild-2017-314504.
39. Kraft R, Herndon DN, Branski LK, Finnerty CC, Leonard KR, Jeschke MG. Optimized fluid management improves outcomes of pediatric burn patients. J Surg Res. 2013;181(1):121–8. https://doi.org/10.1016/j.jss.2012.05.058.
40. Sebn L. Nhs.uk. [cited 2022 Jun 14]. https://www.lsebn.nhs.uk/website/X13911/files/LSEBN%20Burns%20Depth%20Assessment.pdf.
41. Bull JP, Fisher AJ. A study of mortality in a burns unit: a revised estimate. Ann Surg. 1954;139(3):269–74. https://doi.org/10.1097/00000658-195403000-00002.
42. Janzekovic Z. A new concept in the early excision and immediate grafting of burns. J Trauma. 1970;10(12):1103–8. https://doi.org/10.1097/00005373-197012000-00001.
43. Muller MJ, Herndon DN. The challenge of burns. Lancet. 1994;343(8891):216–20. https://doi.org/10.1016/s0140-6736(94)90995-4.
44. Williams FN, Herndon DN, Suman OE, Lee JO, Norbury WB, Branski LK, et al. Changes in cardiac physiology after severe burn injury. J Burn Care Res. 2011;32(2):269–74. https://doi.org/10.1097/BCR.0b013e31820aafcf.
45. Herndon DN, Barrow RE, Rutan TC, Minifee P, Jahoor F, Wolfe RR. Effect of propranolol administration on hemodynamic and metabolic responses of burned pediatric patients. Ann Surg. 1988;208(4):484–92. https://doi.org/10.1097/00000658-198810000-00010.
46. Wilmore DW, Mason AD Jr, Johnson DW, Pruitt BA Jr. Effect of ambient temperature on heat production and heat loss in burn patients. J Appl Physiol. 1975;38(4):593–7. https://doi.org/10.1152/jappl.1975.38.4.593.
47. Suman OE, Spies RJ, Celis MM, Mlcak RP, Herndon DN. Effects of a 12-wk resistance exercise program on skeletal muscle strength in children with burn injuries. J Appl Physiol. 2001;91(3):1168–75. https://doi.org/10.1152/jappl.2001.91.3.1168.
48. Hart DW, Wolf SE, Ramzy PI, Chinkes DL, Beauford RB, Ferrando AA, et al. Anabolic effects of oxandrolone after severe burn. Ann Surg. 2001;233(4):556–64. https://doi.org/10.1097/00000658-200104000-00012.
49. Wolf SE, Edelman LS, Kemalyan N, Donison L, Cross J, Underwood M, et al. Effects of oxandrolone on outcome measures in the severely burned: a multicenter prospective randomized double-blind trial. J Burn Care Res. 2006;27(2):131–9. https://doi.org/10.1097/01.bcr.0000202620.55751.4f.

50. Przkora R, Herndon DN, Suman OE. The effects of oxandrolone and exercise on muscle mass and function in children with severe burns. Pediatrics. 2007;119(1):e109–16. https://doi.org/10.1542/peds.2006-1548.
51. Finnerty CC, Herndon DN. Is propranolol of benefit in pediatric burn patients? Adv Surg. 2013;47:177–97. https://doi.org/10.1016/j.yasu.2013.02.001.
52. Wilmore DW, Aulick LH. Metabolic changes in burned patients. Surg Clin North Am. 1978;58(6):1173–87. https://doi.org/10.1016/s0039-6109(16)41685-3.
53. Lee JO, Benjamin D, Herndon DN. Nutrition support strategies for severely burned patients. Nutr Clin Pract. 2005;20(3):325–30. https://doi.org/10.1177/0115426505020003325.
54. Hart DW, Wolf SE, Herndon DN, Chinkes DL, Lal SO, Obeng MK, et al. Energy expenditure and caloric balance after burn: increased feeding leads to fat rather than lean mass accretion. Ann Surg. 2002;235(1):152–61. https://doi.org/10.1097/00000658-200201000-00020.
55. Hildreth MA, Herndon DN, Desai MH, Broemeling LD. Current treatment reduces calories required to maintain weight in pediatric patients with burns. J Burn Care Rehabil. 1990;11(5):405–9. https://doi.org/10.1097/00004630-199009000-00006.
56. Hart DW, Wolf SE, Zhang X-J, Chinkes DL, Buffalo MC, Matin SI, et al. Efficacy of a high-carbohydrate diet in catabolic illness. Crit Care Med. 2001;29(7):1318–24. https://doi.org/10.1097/00003246-200107000-00004.
57. Patterson BW, Nguyen T, Pierre E, Herndon DN, Wolfe RR. Urea and protein metabolism in burned children: effect of dietary protein intake. Metabolism. 1997;46(5):573–8. https://doi.org/10.1016/s0026-0495(97)90196-7.
58. Herndon D, Stein MD, Rutan TC, Abston S, Linares H. Failure of TPN supplementation to improve liver function, immunity, and mortality in thermally injured patients. J Trauma. 1987;27(2):195–204. https://doi.org/10.1097/00005373-198702000-00018.
59. Herndon DN, Barrow RE, Stein M, Linares H, Rutan TC, Rutan R, et al. Increased mortality with intravenous supplemental feeding in severely burned patients. J Burn Care Rehabil. 1989;10(4):309–13. https://doi.org/10.1097/00004630-198907000-00004.
60. Rousseau A-F, Losser M-R, Ichai C, Berger MM. ESPEN endorsed recommendations: nutritional therapy in major burns. Clin Nutr. 2013;32(4):497–502. https://doi.org/10.1016/j.clnu.2013.02.012.
61. Van Eyck A, Eerens S, Trouet D, Lauwers E, Wouters K, De Winter BY, et al. Body composition monitoring in children and adolescents: reproducibility and reference values. Eur J Pediatr. 2021;180(6):1721–32. https://doi.org/10.1007/s00431-021-03936-0.
62. Weber JM, Sheridan RL, Pasternack MS, Tompkins RG. Nosocomial infections in pediatric patients with burns. Am J Infect Control. 1997;25(3):195–201. https://doi.org/10.1016/s0196-6553(97)90004-3.
63. Sheridan RL, Ryan CM, Yin LM, Hurley J, Tompkins RG. Death in the burn unit: sterile multiple organ failure. Burns. 1998;24(4):307–11. https://doi.org/10.1016/s0305-4179(97)00062-4.
64. Neely AN, Smith WL, Warden GD. Efficacy of a rise in C-reactive protein serum levels as an early indicator of sepsis in burned children. J Burn Care Rehabil. 1998;19(2):102–5. https://doi.org/10.1097/00004630-199803000-00003.
65. Jeschke MG, Finnerty CC, Kulp GA, Kraft R, Herndon DN. Can we use C-reactive protein levels to predict severe infection or sepsis in severely burned patients? Int J Burns Trauma. 2013;3(3):137–43.
66. Lavrentieva A, Kontakiotis T, Lazaridis L, Tsotsolis N, Koumis J, Kyriazis G, et al. Inflammatory markers in patients with severe burn injury. Burns. 2007;33(2):189–94. https://doi.org/10.1016/j.burns.2006.07.001.
67. Sheridan RL. Sepsis in pediatric burn patients. Pediatr Crit Care Med. 2005;6(Suppl):S112–9. 10.1097/01.pcc.0000161577.27849.be
68. Harrington DT, Mozingo DW, Cancio L, Bird P, Jordan B, Goodwin CW. Thermally injured patients are at significant risk for thromboembolic complications. J Trauma. 2001;50(3):495–9. https://doi.org/10.1097/00005373-200103000-00014.
69. Vermaak PV, D'Asta F, Provins J, Farr M, Wilson YT. Thromboprophylaxis in adult and paediatric burn patients: a survey of practice in the United Kingdom. Burns. 2019;45(6):1379–85. https://doi.org/10.1016/j.burns.2019.04.003.
70. Nielsen DPD, Bangalore H, Borrows E. Comments upon "Thromboprophylaxis in adult and paediatric burn patients: a survey of practice in the United Kingdom". Burns. 2021;47(2):479–80. https://doi.org/10.1016/j.burns.2019.11.026.

71. Lin H, Faraklas I, Saffle J, Cochran A. Enoxaparin dose adjustment is associated with low incidence of venous thromboembolic events in acute burn patients. J Trauma. 2011;71(6):1557–61. https://doi.org/10.1097/TA.0b013e31823070f9.
72. Merkel SI, Voepel-Lewis T, Shayevitz JR, Malviya S. The FLACC: a behavioral scale for scoring postoperative pain in young children. Pediatr Nurs. 1997;23(3):293–7.
73. Summer GJ, Puntillo KA, Miaskowski C, Green PG, Levine JD. Burn injury pain: the continuing challenge. J Pain. 2007;8(7):533–48. https://doi.org/10.1016/j.jpain.2007.02.426.
74. Morris V, Murphy LM, Rosenberg M, Rosenberg L, Holzer CE III, Meyer WJ III. Itch assessment scale for the pediatric burn survivor. J Burn Care Res. 2012;33(3):419–24. https://doi.org/10.1097/bcr.0b013e3182372bfa.
75. Cuignet O, Pirson J, Soudon O, Zizi M. Effects of gabapentin on morphine consumption and pain in severely burned patients. Burns. 2007;33(1):81–6. https://doi.org/10.1016/j.burns.2006.04.020.
76. Schneider JC, Nadler DL, Herndon DN, Kowalske K, Matthews K, Wiechman SA, et al. Pruritus in pediatric burn survivors: defining the clinical course. J Burn Care Res. 2015;36(1):151–8. https://doi.org/10.1097/BCR.0000000000000145.

Surgical Neonates in PICU

Maria Chalia and Simon Hannam

Contents

J. Brierley et al. (eds.), *ESPNIC Children's Intensive Care Textbook*,
https://doi.org/10.1007/978-3-031-64762-8_50

Learning Objectives

- Be able to recognise surgical conditions and apply an initial management plan prior to surgical evaluation.
- Recognise the principles of pre- and post-operative care.
- Understand the differences in acute versus elective surgery.
- Be familiar with pain management and sedation options for surgical neonates.

50.1 Introduction

The care of surgical neonates can differ based on the underlying surgical conditions and comorbidities. However, there are key principles that apply to all neonates based on the physiology in the first month of life and key points in the assessment and management in both the preoperative and postoperative period. This chapter focuses on the initial assessment, preoperative preparation, common surgical conditions, and postoperative management.

50.2 Preoperative Care of Surgical Neonates

The initial assessment of a surgical neonate should include history taking and physical examination. A neonatal history should focus on maternal health during pregnancy, antenatal investigations, particularly scans, family history, risk factors for congenital infection, condition at birth, requirement for resuscitation, and the neonatal course leading up to surgery. The physical examination should identify any dysmorphic features and/or co-existing congenital anomalies that may lead to a unifying diagnosis and aid the perioperative management.

In the preoperative phase, the neonate is stabilised prior to surgery with key focus on airway, ventilation, and circulatory management. Also, ensure careful fluid management, infection risk, any renal or liver problems, any neurological concerns, and anticipation of the level of postoperative care required. There may be a need for multiple specialist input prior to surgery.

In an intubated and ventilated neonate, there needs to be clear documentation and communication with the anaesthetist about the method of intubation (nasal or oral), the size and position of the endotracheal tube (ETT) [1], and any previous airway difficulties. A recent chest X-ray should give accurate assessment of the ETT tip position. The corrected gestational age and weight, and/or the presence of facial dysmorphism, such as micrognathia may predict airway difficulties. Surgery for tracheo-oesophageal fistula and oesophageal atresia (TOF-OA) will need ear nose throat (ENT) specialist input.

Ventilation should be optimised prior to surgery with recent arterial or capillary gases. Neonates requiring inhaled nitric oxide (iNO) for ongoing management of pulmonary hypertension, might not be suitable for surgery. There are surgical cases where ventilation can only be optimised following surgical intervention for decompression. This would include severe necrotising enterocolitis or large lung lesions.

A preoperative cardiac assessment can be needed as some surgical conditions have a high association with cardiac anomalies. In such cases, an echocardiogram

(Echo) should be carried out. The presence of a heart defect or evidence of pulmonary hypertension may determine timing for surgery and may result in transfer to a surgical centre with cardiac expertise.

Prescribing intravenous fluids in neonates and especially preterm infants needs to be adjusted according to gestational age (◘ Table 50.1). Ensure regular glucose monitoring as neonatal hypoglycaemia has been associated with poor neurodevelopmental outcomes [4], and all fluids prescribed should be have a 10% dextrose concentration [5]. Peripheral perfusion and blood pressure need to be assessed. As a rule of thumb, the mean blood pressure should be around the same as the corrected gestational age in preterm infants. In hypovolaemia, 0.9% sodium chloride boluses (10–20 mL/kg) may be administered. Blood transfusions and other blood products (fresh frozen plasma or cryoprecipitate) may be required if the haemoglobin is low or coagulation is deranged. Human albumin solution (HAS) 4.5% can be administered in boluses of 10 mL/kg but should be used with caution as it may worsen tissue oedema. Consider and address the potential causes of hypovolaemia and hypotension. Inotropic support may be needed if there is evidence of cardiac impairment.

There should be an adequate period of nil by mouth (NBM) prior to surgery. If fully fed, a 4-h period of NBM is required for breast-fed and a 6-h period for formula-fed neonates [6]. Neonates that are fed via a naso-jejunal tube or a gastrostomy are at a lower risk of aspiration.

Secure intravenous access should be ensured. This can be using an umbilical venous catheter (UVC), a neonatal long line or peripheral venous access. A UVC can be kept in for a maximum of 7 days. Neonatal long lines can be 1 French (for small neonates <1 kg) or 2 French (single or double lumen) and can be kept in for a much longer period. It is important to bear in mind that the neonatal haemostatic system is in a prothrombotic state [7] and critically ill neonates are at a higher risk of thromboembolic phenomena, most likely due to the increased number of indwelling catheters [8]. Therefore, the minimum required central lines should be inserted, monitored, reviewed regularly, and removed as soon as possible. Invasive blood pressure monitoring via an umbilical arterial catheter or peripheral arterial line can be very useful in a critically ill neonate.

A complete set of laboratory investigations, including full blood count (FBC), urea and electrolytes, renal and liver function tests, C-reactive protein (CRP), coagulation screen, and blood grouping should be sent. Thrombocytopenia should be cor-

◘ Table 50.1 Daily maintenance fluid requirement in combination with insensible water losses

Birth weight (g)	Insensible losses (mL/kg/day)	Daily fluid requirement (mL/kg/day)		
		Day 1–2	Day 3–7	Day 8–30
<750	100+	100–200	120–200	120–180
750–1000	60–70	80–150	100–150	120–180
1001–1500	30–65	60–100	100–150	120–180
>1500	15–30	60–100	100–150	120–180

Adapted from Refs. [2, 3]

rected if the count is less than 100 × 10^9/L and further platelets should be available during the operation. Similarly, coagulation should be appropriately corrected with vitamin K, fresh frozen plasma, or cryoprecipitate. Potential abnormal renal and/or liver function may limit the pharmaceutical options for sedation and/or antibiotic cover, and the drug doses ought to be adjusted to renal and/or liver doses. DNA for storage should be considered where chromosomal analysis has not been carried out. Previous radiological films or other studies (i.e., contrast studies, computed tomography scans) should be reviewed.

Another important consideration prior to surgery is gastric decompression. A nasogastric tube should be in situ, and regularly aspirated. In certain cases, such as intestinal obstruction or necrotising enterocolitis, it should be on free drainage with an attached bag.

The neurological state of the neonate needs to be assessed, although this may be not fully achievable in those who are sedated and/or muscle relaxed. A cranial ultrasound scan prior to surgery is required, followed by a repeat one in the immediate postoperative period, for both preterm and term neonates. Bear in mind that there is a high association between neonatal seizures and critical illness or need for surgery [9–11]. Additionally, hypoxia or ischaemia events perioperatively can lead to morbidity and mortality. Continuous skin surface oxygen saturation monitoring is employed routinely as an index of skin and vital organ oxygenation; however, this does not necessarily reflect on end-organ perfusion. Some centres have, therefore, employed the use of near infrared spectroscopy (NIRS) with some evidence to support that the cerebral, renal and/or mesenteric perfusion as an adjunct tool in monitoring organ perfusion may aid clinical management [12–15].

50.3 Common Surgical Conditions

50.3.1 Tracheo-Oesophageal Fistula and Oesophageal Atresia

Oesophageal atresia (OA) with or without a tracheo-oesophageal fistula (TOF-OA) is a congenital anomaly with incidence of 1 in 3500 live births [16] that may have been suspected antenatally due to polyhydramnios and/or absence of a stomach bubble (◘ Fig. 50.1). It results in the neonate being unable to manage its secretions with a high risk of aspiration and breathing difficulties. Neonates present with excessive secretions, feeding difficulties, and/or respiratory distress in the first hours to days of life (◘ Fig. 50.2). A Replogle tube needs to be placed in the oesophageal pouch. This is a tube with multiple holes on either side which continuously aspirates secretions. Frequent flushing of its spare lumen with 0.9% sodium chloride (1–3 mL) is required every 15 min. Intubation is avoided preoperatively due to the potential risk of stomach and bowel distension.

The surgical priority is to assess the airway, identify the fistula and ligate it. This is followed by either a primary oesophageal anastomosis or a delayed closure. The latter is considered in cases of a long gap between the two oesophageal pouches, defined as >3 cm or >2 vertebral bodies [17, 18]. Oesophageal atresia or TOF-OA may be an isolated anomaly or part of a syndrome, such as Trisomy 18, 21, VACTERL

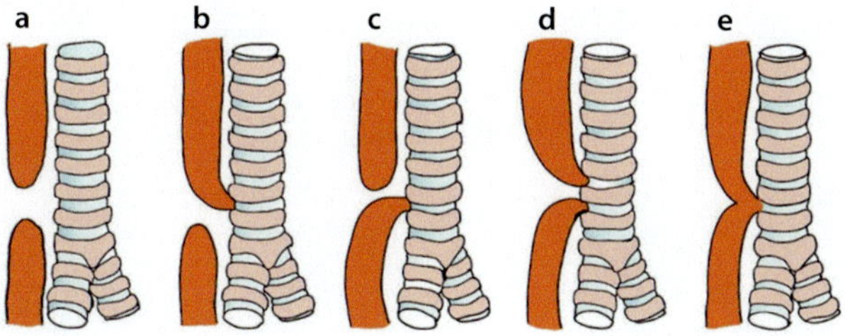

■ **Fig. 50.1** Types of oesophageal atresia with or without trachea-oesophageal fistula [17]. The commonest type is type C with 86% prevalence and the least common is type D

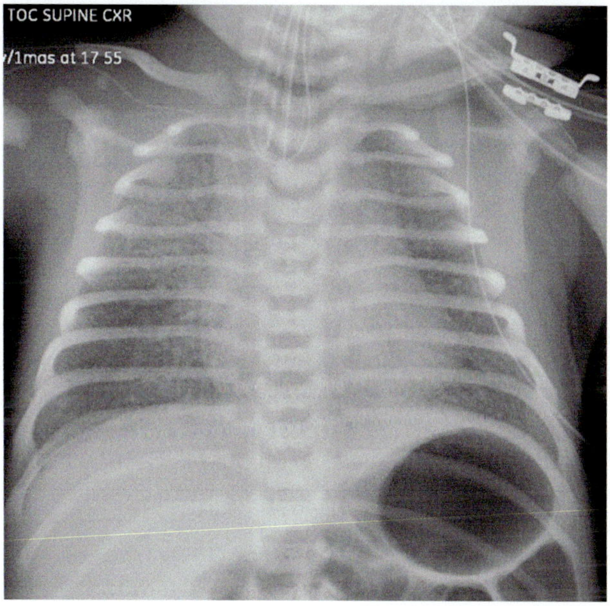

■ **Fig. 50.2** The nasogastric tube is coiled in the oesophagus in-keeping with oesophageal atresia. There is a large stomach bubble which suggests the presence of a trachea-oesophageal fistula. A Replogle tube is in situ

association (vertebral defects, anal atresia, cardiac defects, tracheo-oesophageal fistula, renal anomalies, and limb abnormalities). An Echo in the preoperative phase is essential for excluding any co-existing heart defects.

50.3.2 Congenital Diaphragmatic Hernia

The incidence of congenital diaphragmatic hernia (CDH) is 1 in 2500–3000 live births with left-sided CDH being more common. Intestinal contents and intrabdominal organs, such as the stomach, liver, and spleen herniate inside the pleural cavity, compressing the ipsilateral lung, the mediastinal structures, and the contralateral lung (■ Fig. 50.3). CDH can be associated with cardiac anomalies in 20% of cases [19] or other congenital or chromosomal anomalies in up to 25% of cases [20].

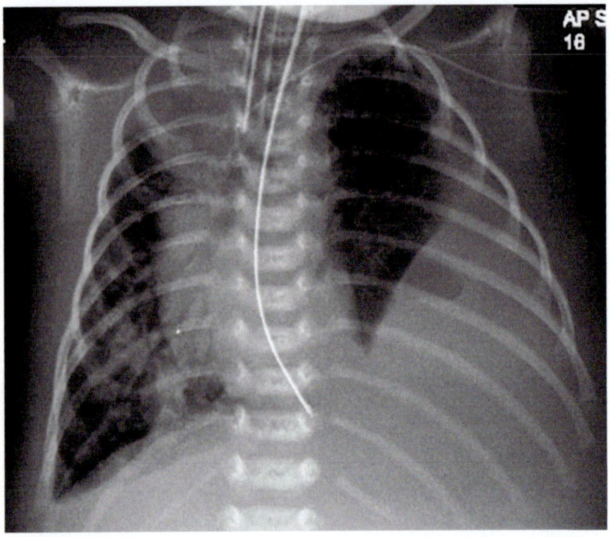

Fig. 50.3 Left-sided congenital diaphragmatic hernia with the stomach, spleen, part of the liver and bowel loops in the thorax

50

The degree of pulmonary hypoplasia can be evaluated using antenatal measurements based on ultrasound measurements of the lung size compared to the head circumference and the presence of the liver in the pleural cavity. The observed to expected lung area to head circumference ratio (O/E LHR) is corrected for gestational age and expressed as a percentage. A severe CDH has an O/E LHR of 15–25% and is associated with a 25% survival; a moderate CDH has a O/E LHR of 25–35% or 35–45% with liver herniation and is associated with 67% survival. Those with a mild CDH had a survival rate of 87% [21–23].

A fetoscopic endoluminal tracheal occlusion (FETO) is being offered in several maternity centres across Europe. A balloon is inflated in the foetal trachea and traps lung fluid which accumulates in the lung and promotes lung growth. The procedure has been shown to improve survival in those with severe CDH [24]. Such cases ought to be delivered in foetal medicine centres with trained staff to deflate the balloon prior to delivery.

On delivery, the neonate is intubated, intravenous access is obtained, and often paralysis is commenced. Different modes of ventilation can be used although high-frequency oscillation has recently been demonstrated to be inferior to conventional ventilation [25]. Also, the role of iNO is controversial. ECMO can be considered if there is no response to conventional therapy. Surgery is only carried out once the pulmonary hypertension has improved [26].

50.3.3 Abdominal Wall Defects

50.3.3.1 Exomphalos

In exomphalos, the abdominal contents herniate at the base of the umbilical cord with a protective sac around them. Elements of the cord can be seen over the sac at its apex, forming a normal looking umbilical cord. The incidence ranges from 1 in

4000 to 1 in 7000 live births with reports of concomitant anomalies from 29% to 88% [27–29]. The presence of liver in the sac, co-existing cardiac anomalies, or pulmonary hypoplasia increase the morbidity and mortality rate. One-year survival ranges from 92% with an isolated exomphalos to 81% in cases with multiple anomalies and 27% with chromosomal anomalies

Surgical approaches include staged tucks of the defect until final closure or allowing time for the muscle and skin to grow around the defect until it closes. Postoperatively, it takes time to establish feeds and central access for TPN administration is paramount.

50.3.3.2 Gastroschisis

Gastroschisis is another centrally located abdominal wall defect with two distinct differences from exomphalos: the intestine is not covered in a protective sac and the umbilicus is a separate anatomical structure, located to the left of the defect. It is also rarely associated with chromosomal abnormalities. In utero, the intestine is directly exposed to amniotic fluid and, becomes oedematous, indurated, and foreshortened. There is delayed peristalsis and ineffective absorption which may take weeks to improve.

Immediately after birth, the defect needs to be covered in cling film to minimise insensible losses and risk of injury. Attention needs to be paid to temperature stability as the large exposed intestinal surface increases the risk of hypothermia. A nasogastric tube should be inserted to aspirate the gastric contents and then placed on free drainage as there can be considerable amounts of bilious aspirates and the neonate can be born fluid depleted. Depending on perfusion, gases, and haemodynamic stability, fluid boluses are required in the form of 0.9% sodium chloride boluses or human albumin solution (HAS). At least 20 mL/kg should always be given as soon as possible. Due to the nature of the defect, umbilical lines are contraindicated and should not be attempted. Surgery may entail primary closure or a staged approach with serial silo tucks and can take many weeks to close. Establishing full enteral feeds can also be slow and central access for TPN administration is needed.

50.3.4 Intestinal Obstruction

Intestinal obstruction (◘ Table 50.2) can present antenatally with maternal polyhydramnios, and dilated, or hyperechogenic bowel. Presentation can also be postnatal. Symptoms and signs depend on the level of obstruction but include abdominal distension (◘ Fig. 50.4), bilious aspirates, vomiting, or failure to pass meconium in the first 24–48 h of life [30]. Bilious vomiting is a surgical emergency and needs to be urgently assessed within 4 h of presentation as there may be a malrotation with volvulus requiring surgery.

50.3.5 Necrotising Enterocolitis

Necrotising enterocolitis (NEC) is the most frequently seen surgical emergency in the preterm neonatal population with a mortality rate of 20–30% [31]. It is associated morbidity, including adverse neurodevelopmental outcomes. The incidence of NEC

Table 50.2 Types of anatomical or functional intestinal obstruction

Type	Presentation	Diagnosis	Treatment	Associations
Duodenal atresia	Immediately post birth	Double-bubble appearance	Duodeno-duodenostomy	Trisomy 21 (30%) VACTERL association Jejunal/ileal/anal atresia Annular pancreas
Duodenal web	Within the first few days of life with feed intolerance, abdominal distension, and vomiting	Double-bubble appearance if severely or completed obstructed	Duodenal web reduction	Trisomy 21 Malrotation Annular pancreas
Malrotation with volvulus	In the first week of life with bilious vomits and rapid deterioration in the instance of volvulus	Upper GI contrast study	Ladd's procedure for malrotation, correction of volvulus	Duodenal atresia/stenosis/web Gastroschisis/exomphalos Biliary system malformations Hypoplasia or agenesis of the dorsal pancreas Congenital diaphragmatic hernia, Heterotaxy, Choanal atresia Hypospadias
Jejuno-ileal atresia	Within the first 2 days of life with abdominal distension; bilious vomits	Triple bubble appearance in proximal atresia; multiple dilated loops proximal to the atresia	Resection and anastomosis or stoma formation	Other atresias
Imperforate anus	Within the first 2 days of life	Distended bowel loops with lack of air in the rectum	Low type—anoplasty, high type—colostomy	Oesophageal atresia VACTERL association Sacral agenesis and lower limb hypoplasia Anorectal malformations

(continued)

Table 50.2 (continued)

Type	Presentation	Diagnosis	Treatment	Associations
Meconium ileus	Immediately post birth; abdominal distension; bilious vomiting; failure to pass meconium within 24–48 h	Dilated bowel loops, air-fluid levels, 'groundglass' sign on X-ray Microcolon appearance on upper GI contrast study	Contrast enema; formation of stoma	Cystic fibrosis
Hirschprung's disease	Abdominal distension, failed to pass meconium, enterocolitis	Dilated bowel loops, absence of gas in rectum	Rectal biopsy at term equivalent age; formation ion of stoma	Trisomy 21

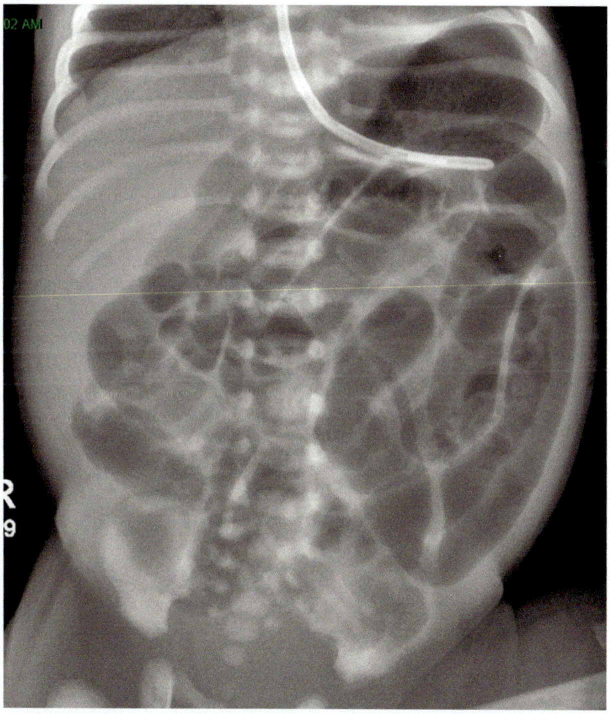

Fig. 50.4 Bowel loop dilatation with absent air in the rectum. Hirschsprung's disease or a more distal obstruction are possible causes

is inversely related to gestational age. NEC may present with feed intolerance, bilious aspirates, vomits, abdominal distension, and/or passing blood per rectum It can also present as sepsis with temperature instability, tachycardia, hypotension, desaturations, apnoea, and recurrent bradycardias. If not ventilated, the neonate might need intubation and adequate analgesia with morphine or an equivalent. Investigations may demonstrate metabolic acidosis, raised lactate, thrombocytopenia, deranged coagulation, raised CRP, and hyperglycaemia. Blood cultures may show the presence of a bacteriaemia.

Necrotising enterocolitis has typical appearances on abdominal X-ray with an abnormal gas pattern of the bowel, dilated loops, thickened bowel walls, pneumatosis coli and in severe cases, portal venous gas (◘ Fig. 50.5). If NEC is suspected, enteral feeds should be stopped with a nasogastric tube on free drainage. Triple antibiotics should be commenced to cover gram-positive and gram-negative bacteria. First-line treatment is benzyl penicillin, amikacin (or gentamicin), and metronidazole. A septic neonate with NEC may need volume replacement as well as inotropic support. Anaemia, thrombocytopenia, and any coagulopathy require addressing urgently with blood products. Investigations, including a FBC, biochemistry profile, CRP, and coagulation screen should be repeated regularly following the presentation of NEC.

The progress of NEC can be unpredictable and radiological findings are not always consistent with clinical severity. Not all neonates will require surgery in the acute or latent phase [32]. Failure of medical management, inability to ventilate, or intestinal perforation are absolute indications for surgery.

Intestinal perforation is a complication of NEC. It can also be seen in preterm neonates, without the usual findings of NEC on histopathology, and is referred to as

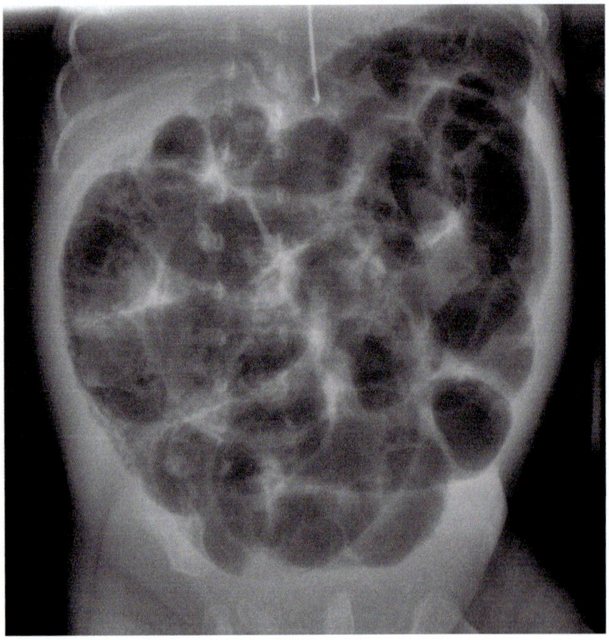

◘ **Fig. 50.5** Diffuse soap-bubble appearance within the bowel wall, bowel distension and bowel wall thickening, all findings consistent with necrotising enterocolitis

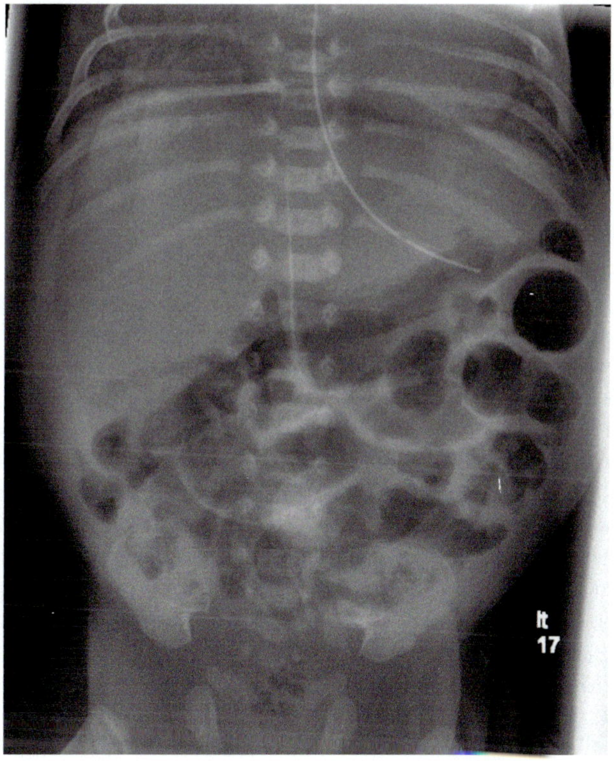

Fig. 50.6 Intestinal perforation following NEC with a pneumoperitoneum, free air under the diaphragm, Silver's sign (air around the falciform ligament) and Rigler's sign evident medially and in the left lower quadrant

spontaneous ileal perforation (SIP). Air below the diaphragm on an abdominal X-ray signifies intestinal perforation (Fig. 50.6). Other radiological signs of intestinal perforation include Rigler's sign, where air outlines both sides of the bowel wall, the football sign, where the abdominal cavity is outlined by gas, as seen with a massive pneumoperitoneum and the triangle sign, where a triangular air pocket is noted between three loops of bowel; urachus sign, secondary to the outline of the middle umbilical ligament [33, 34].

50.4 Postoperative Care of Surgical Neonates

Postoperative care commences with a focused handover between the surgical, anaesthetic, and intensive care teams. Information must be shared on the type of surgery and findings, airway and ventilation management, intravenous and arterial access, anaesthetic drugs used, and the amount of fluid and/or blood product supplementation required. Also, any other significant events that occurred during the operation or transportation of the neonate, such as any peri-arrest or cardio-respiratory arrest situations must be conveyed along with a clear surgical plan including the need for continuation of muscle relaxation, antibiotic cover, and a feeding plan.

A chest X-ray and blood gas must be obtained immediately to ensure correct positioning of the ETT and whether ventilator settings need adjusting. Ensure adequate analgesia and sedation. Neonates are more likely to have apnoeas or periods of shallow, periodic breathing postoperatively, which should be considered when weaning ventilation and planning for extubation.

In cases of an underlying cardiac anomaly and/or evidence of pulmonary hypertension, there may be a need for a repeat echo. A period of close invasive blood pressure monitoring may be required postoperatively, especially if there is ongoing inotropic support.

If a large volume of fluids has been administered during the operation, it is particularly important to monitor the blood pressure, peripheral perfusion, urine output, the presence of a metabolic acidosis, lactate, and serum sodium. A full set of bloods including a FBC, a coagulation screen, urea, and electrolytes, renal and liver function should be obtained. Na elevation of the CRP may be observed postoperatively. Fluid restriction may be warranted, especially in the presence of increased oedema. In the neonate, a standard fluid regime in the immediate postoperative period ranges from 100 to 120 mL/kg/day of 10% Dextrose with additives of sodium chloride and potassium chloride, given there is sufficient urine output and low or normal levels of potassium. If there is evidence of fluid overload, a period of fluid restriction to 60–80 mL/kg/day may be required. As muscle paralysis may contribute to generalised oedema, continuing with this therapy needs to be carefully considered. Ongoing fluid losses need to be monitored and replaced with 0.9% sodium chloride (with added 10 mmol potassium chloride in a 500 mL bag), stoma losses with the same solution if greater than 20 mL/kg/day, silo losses with 4.5% human albumin solution, and similarly chest drain losses.

If a prolonged period of NBM is anticipated, central access, if not already present, must be obtained for parenteral nutrition. Parenteral nutrition should address the calorie, protein, electrolyte, lipid, vitamin, and element requirements of the neonate. Electrolytes need to be monitored to ensure adequate supplementation. Enteral feeds should only be commenced following discussion with the surgical team and once there are minimal and clear gastric losses, bowel sounds present or bowel movements happening. In the presence of a newly sited stoma, feeds should be considered once it starts functioning with the presence of gas and/or output. High doses of opiate infusions may lead to gut dysmotility and ileus, which may hinder initiation of enteral feeds, so weaning should take place as soon as possible.

It is vital to closely monitor of pain symptoms with an appropriate neonatal tool, such as the Neonatal Pain, Agitation and Sedation Scale (N-PASS) [35]. A morphine infusion from 20 to 40 μg/kg/h or fentanyl infusion from 1 to 3 μg/kg/h are routinely used in neonates. Other agents such as clonidine or dexmedetomidine may be considered to help manage withdrawal symptoms. Although there is limited evidence on the use and safety of either, in preterm neonates [36, 37]. Urine catheterisation should be considered when using high doses of opiates or muscle relaxant agents. The latter should only be used after careful consideration such as where there is concern about an oesophageal atresia repair that is under tension or respiratory compromise due to abdominal distension.

As mentioned before, request a cranial ultrasound scan after surgery. In any case of cardiorespiratory arrest, prolonged muscle paralysis, or clinical evidence of seizures request an electroencephalogram. Further imaging such as computed tomography (CT) or magnetic resonance imaging (MRI) to exclude brain injury may be required.

During transportation to and from theatre and during surgery itself, neonates are at high risk of hypothermia. Hypothermia can lead to respiratory or cardio-respiratory compromise, inducing a catabolic state with resultant hypoglycaemia and electrolyte imbalance. It has been associated with an increase in morbidity and mortality when compared to neonates with normothermia and, therefore, efforts should be maximised to prevent it [38, 39]. Extra measures should be taken to ensure normothermia, such as warming the operating theatre room, use of a 'Bair Hugger' (a system comprising a reusable warming unit and single-use disposable warming blankets), minimising skin exposure, and warming up fluids prior to intravascular administration. In the postoperative period, similar action should be taken by minimising exposure and handling, increasing the incubator temperature for preterm neonates, or using an over-head heater for term neonates.

Throughout the perioperative phase, it is vital to ensure a close collaboration and communication with the surgical team in managing and planning future progress. An essential part of the postoperative phase should be to plan any possible surgical procedures required in the future and to establish appropriate follow-up and support in the community.

Take-Home Messages

- Obtain a thorough perinatal history.
- If there is one congenital anomaly, it is likely there is another.
- Ensure relevant investigations have been completed prior to surgery.
- Always consider DNA storage preoperatively.
- Avoid intubation preoperatively in infants with trachea-oesophageal fistula and oesophageal atresia.
- Volume replacement is essential in gastroschisis.
- Bilious vomiting in neonates is a time critical emergency.
- Intestinal perforation in NEC requires urgent surgical intervention.
- Analgesia is of paramount importance in the postoperative period.

References

1. Kempley ST, Moreiras JW, Petrone FL. Endotracheal tube length for neonatal intubation. Resuscitation. 2008;77(3):369–73.
2. Fanaroff AA, Martin RJ. Neonatal and perinatal medicine: diseases of the fetus and newborn. 10th ed. St. Louis: Mosby; 1997.
3. Dell KM. Fluid, electrolytes, and acid-base homeostasis. Philadelphia, PA: Elsevier/Saunders; 2015.
4. McKinlay CJD, Alsweiler JM, Anstice NS, Burakevych N, Chakraborty A, Chase JG, et al. Association of neonatal glycemia with neurodevelopmental outcomes at 4.5 years. JAMA Pediatr. 2017;171(10):972–83.
5. Basu SK, Kaiser JR, Guffey D, Minard CG, Guillet R, Gunn AJ, et al. Hypoglycaemia and hyperglycaemia are associated with unfavourable outcome in infants with hypoxic ischaemic encephalopathy: a post hoc analysis of the CoolCap Study. Arch Dis Child Fetal Neonatal Ed. 2016;101(2):F149–55.
6. American Society of Anesthesiologists Committee. Practice guidelines for preoperative fasting and the use of pharmacologic agents to reduce the risk of pulmonary aspiration: application to

healthy patients undergoing elective procedures: an updated report by the American Society of Anesthesiologists Committee on Standards and Practice Parameters. Anesthesiology. 2017;114(3):495–511.
7. Chalmers EA. Epidemiology of venous thromboembolism in neonates and children. Thromb Res. 2006;118(1):3–12.
8. Saxonhouse MA, Burchfield DJ. The evaluation and management of postnatal thromboses. J Perinatol. 2009;29(7):467–78.
9. Abend NS, Dlugos DJ, Clancy RR. A review of long-term EEG monitoring in critically ill children with hypoxic-ischemic encephalopathy, congenital heart disease, ECMO, and stroke. J Clin Neurophysiol. 2013;30(2):134–42.
10. Abend NS, Arndt DH, Carpenter JL, Chapman KE, Cornett KM, Gallentine WB, et al. Electrographic seizures in pediatric ICU patients: cohort study of risk factors and mortality. Neurology. 2013;81(4):383–91.
11. Naim MY, Gaynor JW, Chen J, Nicolson SC, Fuller S, Spray TL, et al. Subclinical seizures identified by postoperative electroencephalographic monitoring are common after neonatal cardiac surgery. J Thorac Cardiovasc Surg. 2015;150(1):169–78; discussion 78–80.
12. McNeill S, Gatenby JC, McElroy S, Engelhardt B. Normal cerebral, renal and abdominal regional oxygen saturations using near-infrared spectroscopy in preterm infants. J Perinatol. 2011;31(1):51–7.
13. Koch HW, Hansen TG. Perioperative use of cerebral and renal near-infrared spectroscopy in neonates: a 24-h observational study. Paediatr Anaesth. 2016;26(2):190–8.
14. Alderliesten T, Dix L, Baerts W, Caicedo A, van Huffel S, Naulaers G, et al. Reference values of regional cerebral oxygen saturation during the first 3 days of life in preterm neonates. Pediatr Res. 2016;79(1–1):55–64.
15. Metcalfe KHM, Stienstra R, McHoney M. NIRS as a biomarker of bowel ischaemia & surgical pathology: a meta-analysis of studies in newborns. Early Hum Dev. 2021;161:105437.
16. Shaw-Smith C. Oesophageal atresia, tracheo-oesophageal fistula, and the VACTERL association: review of genetics and epidemiology. J Med Genet. 2006;43(7):545–54.
17. Gross RE. The surgery of infancy and childhood. Philadelphia: WB Saunders; 1953.
18. Spitz L. Oesophageal atresia. Orphanet J Rare Dis. 2007;2:24.
19. Harting MT, Lally KP. The Congenital Diaphragmatic Hernia Study Group registry update. Semin Fetal Neonatal Med. 2014;19(6):370–5.
20. Beaumier CK, Beres AL, Puligandla PS, Skarsgard ED, Canadian Pediatric Surgery Network. Clinical characteristics and outcomes of patients with right congenital diaphragmatic hernia: a population-based study. J Pediatr Surg. 2015;50(5):731–3.
21. Done E, Gucciardo L, Van Mieghem T, Jani J, Cannie M, Van Schoubroeck D, et al. Prenatal diagnosis, prediction of outcome and in utero therapy of isolated congenital diaphragmatic hernia. Prenat Diagn. 2008;28(7):581–91.
22. Gucciardo L, Deprest J, Done E, Van Mieghem T, Van de Velde M, Gratacos E, et al. Prediction of outcome in isolated congenital diaphragmatic hernia and its consequences for fetal therapy. Best Pract Res Clin Obstet Gynaecol. 2008;22(1):123–38.
23. Snoek KG, Peters NCJ, van Rosmalen J, van Heijst AFJ, Eggink AJ, Sikkel E, et al. The validity of the observed-to-expected lung-to-head ratio in congenital diaphragmatic hernia in an era of standardized neonatal treatment; a multicenter study. Prenat Diagn. 2017;37(7):658–65.
24. Deprest JA, Nicolaides KH, Benachi A, Gratacos E, Ryan G, Persico N, et al. Randomized trial of fetal surgery for severe left diaphragmatic hernia. N Engl J Med. 2021;385(2):107–18.
25. van den Hout L, Tibboel D, Vijfhuize S, te Beest H, Hop W, Reiss I, et al. The VICI-trial: high frequency oscillation versus conventional mechanical ventilation in newborns with congenital diaphragmatic hernia: an international multicentre randomized controlled trial. BMC Pediatr. 2011;11:98.
26. Snoek KG, Reiss IK, Greenough A, Capolupo I, Urlesberger B, Wessel L, et al. Standardized postnatal management of infants with congenital diaphragmatic hernia in Europe: the CDH EURO Consortium Consensus—2015 update. Neonatology. 2016;110(1):66–74.
27. Gilbert WM, Nicolaides KH. Fetal omphalocele: associated malformations and chromosomal defects. Obstet Gynecol. 1987;70(4):633–5.
28. Rijhwani A, Davenport M, Dawrant M, Dimitriou G, Patel S, Greenough A, et al. Definitive surgical management of antenatally diagnosed exomphalos. J Pediatr Surg. 2005;40(3):516–22.

29. Tassin M, Descriaud C, Elie C, Houfflin Debarge V, Dumez Y, Perrotin F, et al. Omphalocele in the first trimester: prediction of perinatal outcome. Prenat Diagn. 2013;33(5):497–501.
30. Juang D, Snyder CL. Neonatal bowel obstruction. Surg Clin North Am. 2012;92(3):685–711, ix–x.
31. Fitzgibbons SC, Ching Y, Yu D, Carpenter J, Kenny M, Weldon C, et al. Mortality of necrotizing enterocolitis expressed by birth weight categories. J Pediatr Surg. 2009;44(6):1072–5; discussion 5–6.
32. Neu J. Necrotizing enterocolitis: the search for a unifying pathogenic theory leading to prevention. Pediatr Clin N Am. 1996;43(2):409–32.
33. Soni R, Katana A, Curry JI, Humphries PD, Huertas-Ceballos A. How to use abdominal X-rays in preterm infants suspected of developing necrotising enterocolitis. Arch Dis Child Educ Pract Ed. 2020;105(1):50–7.
34. Sureka B, Bansal K, Arora A. Pneumoperitoneum: what to look for in a radiograph? J Family Med Prim Care. 2015;4(3):477–8.
35. Hillman BA, Tabrizi MN, Gauda EB, Carson KA, Aucott SW. The Neonatal Pain, Agitation and Sedation Scale and the bedside nurse's assessment of neonates. J Perinatol. 2015;35(2):128–31.
36. Zankl A, Martin J, Davey JG, Osborn DA. Opioid treatment for opioid withdrawal in newborn infants. Cochrane Database Syst Rev. 2021;7:CD002059.
37. McDonald D, Palsgraf H, Shah P. Dexmedetomidine—an emerging option for sedation in neonatal patients. J Perinatol. 2022;42(7):845–55.
38. de Almeida MF, Guinsburg R, Sancho GA, Rosa IR, Lamy ZC, Martinez FE, et al. Hypothermia and early neonatal mortality in preterm infants. J Pediatr. 2014;164(2):271–5.e1.
39. Morehouse D, Williams L, Lloyd C, McCoy DS, Miller Walters E, Guzzetta CE, et al. Perioperative hypothermia in NICU infants: its occurrence and impact on infant outcomes. Adv Neonatal Care. 2014;14(3):154–64.

Transport of the Critically Ill Child

Timothy Wait and Padmanabhan Ramnarayan

Contents

J. Brierley et al. (eds.), *ESPNIC Children's Intensive Care Textbook*,
https://doi.org/10.1007/978-3-031-64762-8_51

Learning Objectives

- Understand the process of retrieval from the point of referral to the point of handover at the receiving centre.
- Learn a safe and organised approach to stabilisation and transport of the critically ill child.
- Recognise those situations requiring time-critical transport and outline an approach to these situations.
- Recognise the central importance of patient and staff safety to the transport process.

51.1 Introduction

Following centralisation of paediatric intensive care units (PICUs) in many parts of the world, critically ill children presenting to general hospitals usually need transfer to a hospital with a PICU. In the United Kingdom and Ireland, approximately half of unplanned admissions to PICUs are for transported children [1]. The majority of these transfers are performed by specialised paediatric critical care transport teams (PCCTs). Studies show that the use of a specialised team for transfer is associated with improved survival [2].

The transport environment represents a time of significant vulnerability for the critically ill child—therefore, a safe and organised approach to these scenarios is essential. In this chapter, we will cover the basic principles of referral triage, patient stabilisation prior to transport, the transport process including for time-critical transfers, and how to ensure patient and staff safety during the transport.

51.2 Referral to a PCCT

Referral to the regional PCCT should be made by the local hospital team at the earliest opportunity once the need for transfer is identified. In many settings, PCCTs also provide critical care advice even if transfer is not required—such advice may avoid the need for transfer if key interventions are initiated at an early stage. In general, the referral should be made by the most senior available clinician; however, some flexibility is required in high-acuity situations when it may be necessary for senior staff to remain at the bedside and a more junior member of staff to make the initial referral call.

A suggested structure for the initial referral call is shown in Box ► 51.1. Transport services typically make use of a referral proforma with the aim of promoting a standardised structure for referral and handover across the network—this improves efficiency of communication and reduces the risk that important details are missed. It is particularly important to establish at the outset of the call whether there is a need for a time-critical transfer, i.e. one where an urgent surgical procedure (e.g. evacuation of an extradural haematoma) is required.

Caring for a critically ill child can be stressful even for experienced clinicians. A polite and collegial approach to taking the initial referral is invaluable in this context, and the style of communication adopted should take this into account. Interruptions to the referring clinician can be quite disruptive, and should be avoided as far as possible. An exception to this general rule is use of the "read-back" method to confirm key details, a technique which promotes shared understanding and may even improve the flow of the conversation.

On conclusion of the initial referral call, the usual priorities are to discuss the case with the duty transport consultant and relay any further clinical advice to the local hospital team, to identify and secure an appropriate PICU bed, and to mobilise a retrieval team. In the UK, the target time from acceptance for transport to mobilisation of a retrieval team is within 30 min. The local hospital team should be contacted when the team mobilises to confirm an estimated time of arrival and to obtain a further clinical update.

Although the vast majority of referrals are telephone-based, telemedicine with real-time audiovisual communication is an alternative that has been shown in preliminary studies to improve the quality of referral and improve assessment of the patient's condition [3, 4].

Box 51.1: Suggested Structure for the Initial Referral Call

Referral details

- Name and contact number for referring clinician
- Patient's current location
- Patient's age and weight
- Need for time-critical transfer

Clinical details

- History up to the point of presentation
- Subsequent management and clinical progress
- Current physiologic status (suggest "ABCDE" structure)
- Results of investigations (blood gas analysis, imaging, laboratory investigations)

Summary/close

- Retrieval clinician summarises clinical scenario and offers management advice
- Next contact agreed

51.3 The Transport Process

51.3.1 Staffing and Equipment

A PCCT is usually made up as a minimum of three individuals—doctor, nurse, and ambulance technician—and supported by a transport consultant, although team composition may vary across healthcare settings. An advanced nurse practitioner (ANP) may take on the role of the retrieval doctor. The team members must be suitably trained, experienced, and equipped to provide ongoing critical care during the retrieval, and to undertake all necessary critical care procedures.

An extensive range of equipment is required in order to be self-sufficient in providing ongoing critical care, and must be stowed in a standardised fashion so that any item can be readily accessed when required. Use of a dedicated retrieval trolley allows for oxygen cylinders, suction unit, ventilator, syringe pumps, and monitoring equipment to be mounted on the trolley itself (◘ Fig. 51.1). Smaller items such as airway

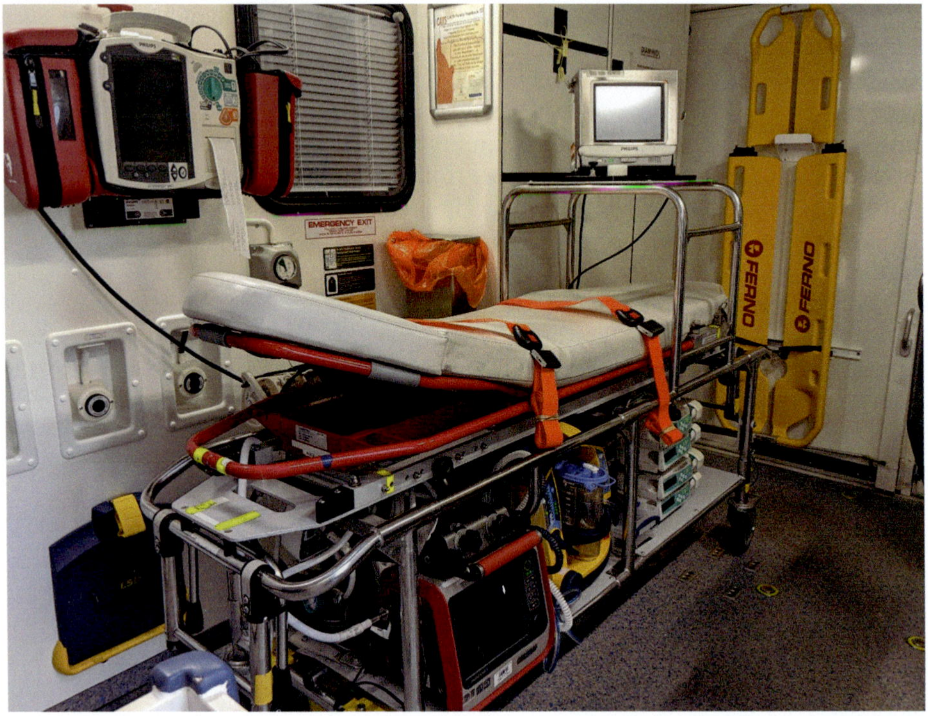

Fig. 51.1 Retrieval trolley installed in ambulance. Ventilator, suction unit, and syringe pumps are mounted on the near side of the trolley; oxygen cylinders and nitric oxide module are mounted on the far side of the trolley; and a transport monitor is mounted on a removable bridge. All equipment is secure in the event of a collision

equipment, vascular access equipment, chest drains, and drug pack are then stored in a set of equipment packs which may be carried to the patient's bedside. Finally, spares and infrequently used items may be kept in the ambulance.

Vehicle and equipment checks should be conducted by the team at the start of each shift using a written checklist, and a pre-departure checklist is then completed when the team mobilises (see Fig. 51.2 for an example checklist). Equipment packs must be re-stocked following each retrieval. The service must additionally maintain a schedule for replacement of stock at expiry, equipment servicing, vehicle maintenance, and vehicle deep cleaning.

51.3.2 Handover at Referring Centre

On arrival at the patient's bedside, the retrieval team should introduce themselves and establish whether there are any immediate concerns which would need to be addressed prior to full handover. Handover is then conducted in a structured fashion, covering history up to the point of presentation, subsequent management and clinical progress, current physiologic status, and results of investigations. It is helpful to review imaging (chest radiograph, CT scans) at close of handover, with particular attention to endotracheal tube position on the chest radiograph.

Retrieval Checklist

Before leaving base

Admin aware of destination	
Receiving centre has patient details	
Bed confirmed with nurse in charge	
Referring hospital contacted with ETA	
Image link and discharge summary requested	
Inverter on / ventilator and monitor charging	

Before leaving referring hospital

Transfer plan agreed with consultant	
Blood gas reviewed	
Chest X ray reviewed	
Infection control issues addressed	
Patient ID bracelet, allergies documented	

Adequate sedation / analgesia / paralysis	
Adequate monitoring including ETCO2	
Patient /lines / tubing secure	
Temperature management appropriate	
Medical gases O2 / NO sufficient for transfer	
Monitor / ventilator / syringe pumps charged	
Infusion drug volumes sufficient for transfer	
Airway bag / BVM / T piece	
Drug bag / plan for hypotension	

Clinical documentation (notes, radiology)	
EBM, blood spot (neonates only)	
Parent information given	
Admin advised re who is on board the ambulance	
Receiving unit updated	
Research bloods / paperwork	

Equipment checklist

	Base	RH	PICU
Retrieval form, clipboard and folder			
Mobile phones			
Equipment packs x3			
Airway bag			
Fridge drugs /controlled drugs /drug pouch			
ACR or BabyPOD			
iSTAT and cartridges			
Ventilator and tubing / mains plugged in			
Inhaled NO module			
Monitor and cables / mains plugged in			
Defib/spare battery			
Suction unit			
Syringe drivers			
Transwarmers – winter			
Thermos bag for EBM			
CPAP / HFNC kit			
Equipment cleaned	x	x	
Used equipment disposed	x	x	

Additional equipment for flight transfers

Sharps bin			
Aerosled clipdeck			
Nitric flight kit			

Fig. 51.2 Example retrieval checklist. (Adapted from Children's Acute Transport Service retrieval checklist)

51.3.3 Patient Stabilisation

Emergency equipment and drugs should be accessible prior to approaching the patient (Box ► 51.2). The stabilisation phase may be approached using an "Airway, Breathing, Circulation, Disability, Exposure" framework.

Box 51.2: Suggested Emergency Equipment and Drugs for Transport

- Mapleson C or F circuit with anaesthetic facemask, checked for leaks and patency, connected to oxygen cylinder at head end of trolley
- Self-inflating bag-valve-mask (as back-up device)
- Suction unit and Yankauer suction catheter
- Patient-specific airway bag:
  - Oropharyngeal airway
  - Laryngoscopes ×2

  - Endotracheal tubes ×3—anticipated size plus one size above and one below
  - Endotracheal tube stylet
  - Lubricating jelly
  - Syringe
  - Tape
  - Scissors
  - Magill forceps
  - Flexible suction catheters
  - Laryngeal mask airway
- Bougies (most easily stored in a tube fixed to the retrieval trolley)
- Emergency drug bag:
  - Drugs for rapid sequence induction
  - Pre-filled adrenaline syringe
  - Flushes and fluid boluses
  - Syringes, needles, and drug labels
  - Additional drugs selected on case-by-case basis
- Thoracostomy equipment (consider)
- Intraosseous access equipment (consider)

51.3.3.1 Airway

From a safety perspective, there should be a low threshold for endotracheal intubation prior to transport. When the intubation has been performed prior to arrival of the retrieval team, details of the procedure including drugs used, grade of laryngoscopy, and any difficulties encountered should be sought at handover. Use of personal protective equipment during airway management should be guided by local policy; however, airborne precautions should be considered when managing the airway of any child with undiagnosed respiratory tract infection, including suspected covid-19.

The endotracheal tube size should be confirmed as appropriate, and on occasion it may be necessary to exchange the tube over a bougie prior to transport. Cuffed endotracheal tubes are generally preferable in the transport environment, particularly when lung compliance is anticipated to deteriorate. Available evidence suggests that modern high-volume, low-pressure cuffed endotracheal tubes are not associated with an increased incidence of post-extubation stridor or subglottic stenosis [5–9]. The cuff should be inflated just enough to obliterate leak, and cuff pressure limited to ≤20 cmH_2O under normal circumstances.

The endotracheal tube position should be confirmed on chest radiograph and adjusted if necessary. In general, the tip of the endotracheal tube should be projected at the level of the T3 vertebral body. Due to the short length of the trachea, tube ties are insufficient to mitigate the risk of endotracheal tube displacement in small children. It is our practice to use the Melbourne strapping technique to secure the tube prior to transport (◘ Fig. 51.3).

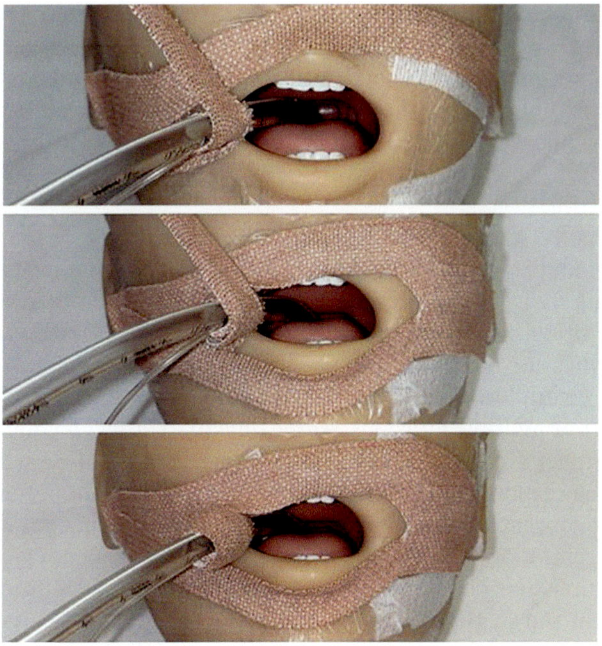

Fig. 51.3 Melbourne strapping technique. The upper limb of the first tape is secured across the maxilla and the lower limb wraps the tube from below at the ipsilateral corner of the mouth. The lower limb of the second tape is secured across the mandible and the upper limb wraps the tube from above at the contralateral corner of the mouth

51.3.3.2 Breathing

Intubated children should be established on a transport ventilator. Waveform capnography and pulse oximetry should be continuously monitored, and a sample should be obtained for blood gas analysis prior to departure. The pCO_2 from blood gas analysis may be correlated with the end-tidal CO_2 to allow adjustments to be made to minute ventilation during transport. It is helpful to carry a portable blood gas analyser such as the i-STAT system.

When selecting ventilator settings, the same principles may be applied as for any mechanically ventilated child. Of particular note, all ventilated children should receive at least 5 cmH_2O positive end expiratory pressure (PEEP) and a lung-protective ventilation strategy targeting 5–7 mL/kg tidal volume. Some degree of permissive hypercapnia is often appropriate, particularly for children with expiratory airflow obstruction in whom a low respiratory rate is essential. Patients with neurologic injury are an important exception to this rule, and should be ventilated to normocapnia as part of a neuroprotective strategy.

Transport of children requiring non-invasive respiratory support presents a less-controlled situation than transport of the intubated child. Equipment and drugs for intubation should be kept available in case of unanticipated deterioration *en route*. Attention should be paid to preventing patient distress during the journey. If safe to do so, a parent should accompany the child, and distractions such as books or videos may be helpful. Transport of children on high-flow humidified nasal cannula oxygen is feasible if appropriate equipment is available (for example, a Hamilton T1 transport ventilator and humidifier), but the effect of high flow rates on oxygen consumption needs to be taken into consideration.

51.3.3.3 Circulation

The haemodynamic status should be stabilised as far as possible prior to transport. Blood pressure and 3-lead electrocardiogram should be monitored. Movement and vibration during transport reduces the accuracy of oscillometric non-invasive blood pressure monitoring, and there should be a low threshold for continuous invasive arterial blood pressure monitoring.

In general, central venous access should be obtained for patients requiring inopressor support or multiple infusions. Adrenaline (0.01–1 mcg/kg/min) may be commenced by peripheral intravenous infusion or intraosseous infusion as a short-term measure, with close monitoring of the access site for extravasation. It may be prudent to avoid higher concentration adrenaline solutions in this setting, for example using a maximum concentration of 4 mg adrenaline in 50 mL 0.9% saline (the standard "single strength" adrenaline concentration for adult intensive care units in the UK [10]).

For neonatal shock, the possibility of duct-dependent congenital heart disease should be borne in mind and an intravenous infusion of dinoprostone (prostaglandin E2, 5–50 ng/kg/min) commenced if required. Intubation prior to transfer should be considered for patients established on dinoprostone dose greater than 15 ng/kg/min, due to the risk of apnoeas.

Enteral fluid and nutrition should be discontinued for transfer and consideration given to maintenance intravenous fluids. 0.9% saline with 5% dextrose at two-thirds predicted maintenance rate is a reasonable default fluid selection for the majority of situations [11–13].

51.3.3.4 Disability

Pre-intubation neurologic status should be documented for all children, and pupillary size and reactivity checked intermittently during the transfer. For children requiring neuroprotective measures, care should be taken that these are maintained during transport. 3% saline boluses (3 mL/kg) should be added to the emergency drug bag for children with clinical suspicion of raised intracranial pressure.

Analgosedation and muscle relaxation should be maintained in the intubated child using continuous infusions. The choice of agents is dependent on the clinical scenario; however, intravenous infusions of morphine (10–40 mcg/kg/h), midazolam (1–2 mcg/kg/min), and vecuronium (1–2 mcg/kg/min) are a reasonable default selection for the majority of situations. It should be noted that all of these infusions are relatively slow to reach steady state, and therefore intravenous bolus loading doses should be considered (for example, morphine 50–100 mcg/kg, midazolam 50–100 mcg/kg, and vecuronium 100 mcg/kg). There remains some controversy as to whether an intermittent bolus approach to muscle relaxation is acceptable.

Glucose should be checked intermittently. The possibility of metabolic disease should be borne in mind for children presenting with unexplained hypoglycaemia, and consideration given to empiric dextrose infusion (8 mg/kg/min IV) and specialist consultation.

51.3.3.5 Exposure

A nasogastric or orogastric tube should be placed for all intubated patients, the stomach contents aspirated, and the tube left on free drainage or intermittently aspirated during the transport phase. Placement of a urinary catheter should be considered, especially in cases of suspected raised intracranial pressure.

A head-to-toe examination should be documented prior to transport. Any child protection concerns must be clearly documented and handed over at the receiving centre. The safety of other siblings must also be considered.

Patient temperature should be continuously monitored. An oesophageal temperature probe is appropriate for intubated patients, and a skin or rectal temperature probe for non-intubated patients. Any infection control concerns must be communicated to the receiving centre prior to transport.

51.3.4 Packaging for Transport

Three key areas must be addressed when packaging for transport:

- Patient, lines, and equipment secure for transport and temperature management appropriate.
- Adequate supplies of medical gases, electrical power, and infusion drugs available to cover the duration of the transport phase.
- Emergency equipment and drugs accessible for the transport phase.

The patient must be secured during transport using appropriately rated equipment, for example, a BabyPOD™ for children ≤5 kg, an Ambulance Child Restraint (ACR®) for children 5–45 kg, and standard ambulance trolley straps for children >45 kg. If vehicle or trolley changes are required, such as during air transfers, a vacuum mattress or Aerosled® system may be used. Careful attention should be paid to padding of pressure areas and to temperature control. A warming device such as a TransWarmer® mattress should be considered for children <5 kg, and use of blankets and ambulance heating as required for older children.

All lines and tubes should be secured. Ventilator tubing should be secured to the patient and to the retrieval trolley or pod using medical tape, in order to minimise the risk of inadvertent traction on the endotracheal tube. The capnography line should run over the top of other lines and monitoring cables. Labelled infusion lines and monitoring cables should run in parallel towards the foot end of the trolley. An extension set with a three-way tap connected to its distal end should be run from a reliable additional point of intravenous access to allow administration of emergency drugs if required during transport.

Oxygen requirement for transport of a ventilated patient may be estimated based on gas flow to the ventilator and duration of transport from the point of disconnection from wall oxygen supply at the referring centre to the point of connection to wall oxygen supply at the receiving centre. For safety, an FiO_2 of 1.0 is assumed, the estimated volume is doubled, and use of the ambulance oxygen supply is not taken into consideration. The calculation is as follows:

$$\text{Oxygen availability for transport}\,(\text{L}) = 2 \times \text{gas flow}\,(\text{L/min}) \times \text{duration of transport phase}\,(\text{min})$$

For mechanically ventilated patients, the gas flow usually approximates the minute volume. An important exception is the Smiths Medical babyPAC™ ventilator, which consumes a minimum of 11 L/min gas flow when used with the "active-PEEP" mode. Oxygen consumption by non-invasive devices may be substantially greater than by mechanical ventilators. Of particular importance, high-flow humidified nasal cannula systems may deliver close to 100% oxygen at up to 60 L/min.

Oxygen cylinder capacities for commonly used cylinder types are shown in Box ▶ 51.3. For redundancy, at least two cylinders should be accessible during transport.

Anticipated volumes required for infusion drugs may be estimated as maximum anticipated infusion rate (mL/h) × duration of journey (h). Additional syringes should be prepared prior to departure if required. Adequate charge should be confirmed for all battery-powered equipment. The ambulance or aircraft oxygen supply and power supply should be used during the transport phase.

Emergency equipment and drugs (Box ▶ 51.1) must be kept accessible during the transport phase, and may conveniently be stowed on the retrieval trolley itself.

Prior to departure from the bed space, the retrieval consultant is updated by telephone and the receiving centre contacted with an update on the patient's condition and an estimated time of arrival. A pre-departure checklist should be completed (◘ Fig. 51.2).

Box 51.3: Oxygen Cylinder Capacities for Commonly Used Cylinder Types [14]

D—340 L
CD—460 L
ZD—605 L
E—680 L
F—1360 L
ZX—3040 L

51.3.5 The Transport Phase

The patient should be stabilised as far as possible prior to transport in order that interventions during the transport phase itself are kept to a minimum. If an emergency arises or interventions are required during road transport, it is usually safest for the ambulance to pull over to the side of the road. It may on rare occasions be necessary to divert to the nearest Emergency Department if it is not felt safe to continue to the destination unit. In these cases, every effort should be made to provide a pre-alert to the receiving department.

A parent should be allowed to accompany the child during transport where feasible, provided that this does not impede the delivery of clinical care by the transport team. Many parents find that this reduces their stress level during what can be a very distressing time [15]. The possibility of deterioration *en route*, and how this would be managed, must be clearly explained prior to departure.

51.3.6 Handover at Receiving Centre

On arrival to the bed space at the receiving centre, the transport team should introduce themselves and identify any immediate concerns which would need to be addressed prior to full handover. Handover should usually be conducted prior to transferring the patient off the transport trolley, in order that the receiving centre team are familiar with the clinical details prior to becoming involved in patient care.

51.4 Time-Critical Transfers

Time-critical transfer is most commonly required for neurosurgical emergencies, general surgical emergencies, and for secondary transfer of the major trauma patient to a major trauma centre. These transfers should usually be undertaken by the referring hospital team, as the harm caused by delay waiting for the arrival of a retrieval team typically outweighs the risks of non specialist transfer [16–18]. A suitably trained and experienced team should accompany the patient, usually a senior anaesthetist or intensivist and a senior intensive care nurse. A simplified checklist to support time-critical transfer is shown in ◘ Fig. 51.4.

The retrieval service may provide clinical advice and may assist with referral to the receiving centre. When the receiving centre is confirmed, the exact destination should be clarified (usually the Emergency Department or Operating Theatres) and contact details taken. The receiving department must be contacted directly with an estimated time of arrival and clinical status update.

Written policies for acceptance of time-critical transfers must be in place. With such policies in place, multiple telephone conversations between different clinicians can be avoided. ICU bed capacity should never be a barrier to time-critical transfer, and if necessary a secondary transfer may be performed once the time-critical intervention has been undertaken. These issues were highlighted in a Regulation 28 report issued in February 2017 regarding the death of an adult patient following delay in organising transfer for emergent hemicraniectomy [19].

Time critical transfer checklist

Communication:

- Local ambulance service aware – blue light transfer ☐
- Receiving department contacted with ETA ☐
- Images linked and notes copied ☐
- Receiving department contact number: ____________________

Ventilation:

- Sedated and paralysed ☐
- ET tube secure, depth confirmed ☐
- Adequate oxygen supply ☐
- Ventilator battery charged ☐

Monitoring:

- ETCO2 ☐
- SpO2 ☐
- BP – invasive or NIBP set to cycle ☐
- ECG ☐
- Monitor battery charged ☐

IV access and infusions:

- Minimum 2 points IV access ☐
- All lines secure ☐
- Adequate volumes of infusion drugs ☐
- Syringe pump batteries charged ☐

Emergency equipment:

- Map C/F circuit ☐
- BVM ☐
- Suction unit ☐
- Guedel airway ☐
- Laryngoscopes x2 ☐
- ET tubes x2, syringe, lubricant, tape, scissors ☐
- Bougie ☐
- LMA/iGel ☐
- Thoracostomy equipment (scalpel, spencer wells) ☐
- Vascular access equipment (consider IO) ☐

Emergency drugs:

- RSI drugs if not intubated ☐
- Adrenaline ☐
- Fluid boluses ☐
- Hypertonic saline boluses if required ☐
- Blood products if required ☐
- Plan for hypotension discussed ☐

Fig. 51.4 Example checklist for time-critical transfer

51.5 Air Transport

Air transport presents additional risk, complexity and cost in comparison to land transport, and anticipated benefits should be balanced against these potential harms. Helicopter transport is appropriate for journeys of intermediate duration or with difficult road access, while fixed wing transport is usually the only practicable option for journeys beyond the range of helicopter transport.

Many of the challenges of land transport are exaggerated in the air transport environment. Access to the patient may be limited, communication may be difficult, and noise, vibration, and turbulence may interfere with patient assessment and monitoring. The same principles apply to stabilisation and packaging as for any critical care transport. Particular attention should be paid to ensuring adequate supplies of oxygen, electrical power and infusion drugs, and emergency equipment and drugs should be readily accessible.

Reduction in atmospheric pressure at altitude results in a reduction in inspired partial pressure of oxygen (PiO_2) for a given inspired oxygen fraction (FiO_2). Fixed wing aircraft typically operate at a cabin pressure of 7000–8000 ft. Helicopter cabins are typically non-pressurised but these aircraft operate at altitudes below 10,000 ft. At 7000 ft, barometric pressure is approximately 78 kPa (vs. 101 kPa at sea level) resulting in a PiO_2 of 16 kPa at an FiO_2 of 0.21, and a PiO_2 of 78 kPa at an FiO_2 of 1.0.

Reduction in atmospheric pressure at altitude additionally results in the expansion of gas-filled cavities and in the tendency for dissolved gases to come out of solution. Air transport should be avoided for patients with undrained pneumothorax or other closed space gas collections, and should be avoided within approximately 24 h of deep-sea diving due to the risk of precipitating decompression sickness. Endotracheal tube cuff pressure should be re-adjusted on ascent and descent (◘ Fig. 51.5).

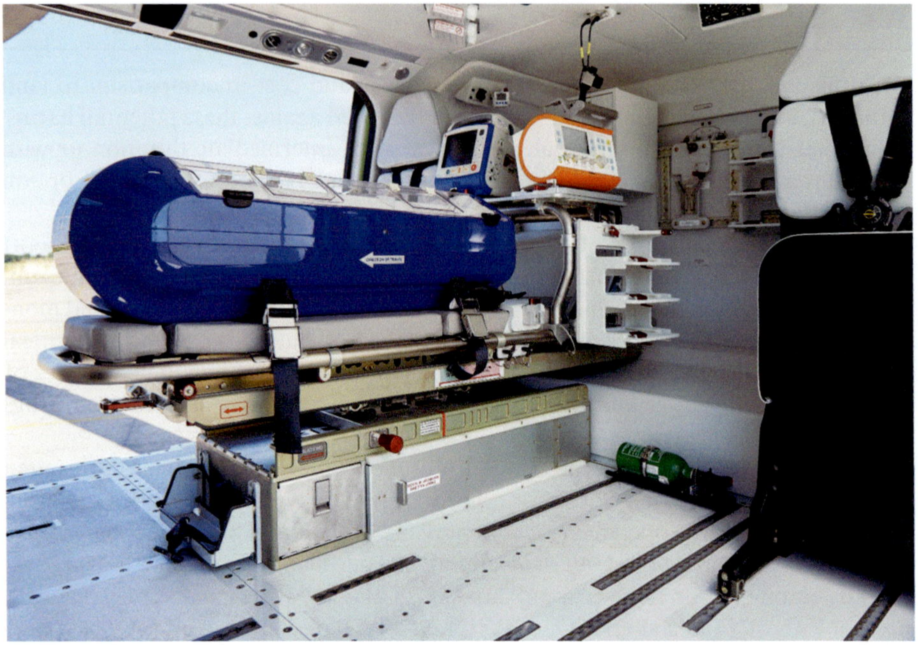

Fig. 51.5 Cabin interior of a specialised paediatric critical care transport helicopter. (Photograph courtesy of The Children's Air Ambulance, UK. Stretcher with BabyPOD™ mounted centrally in the cabin)

51.6 Safety and Clinical Governance

Patient safety during critical care transport is dependent on the ability of the team to function effectively in an unfamiliar environment at the referring and receiving hospitals, and in the remote environment of the transport phase itself. An organised approach and clear communication are essential to maintaining safety in such environments, and enable the team to respond effectively to unexpected developments. Simulation training may be very helpful to enable staff to familiarise themselves with standard operating procedures.

Attention must be paid to physical safety during the transport phase. Clinical staff should follow the direction of the ambulance technician or aircrew at all times, and in particular should not approach an aircraft until invited to do so by the crew. Use of lights and sirens is generally appropriate during road transport of the critically ill child in order to minimise delays due to heavy traffic, but provided the patient is stable a "time-critical" approach to the journey is not required. A small number of fatalities occur each year in the UK due to collisions involving ambulances [20], and based on data from prehospital care services in the USA, the ambulance collision rate is more than doubled when lights and sirens are used [21].

Clinical governance arrangements need to cover not only the transport service but also issues identified at the local hospital, at the receiving centre, and at a network level. Governance issues identified during the transport process but external to the transport service itself may be best reviewed at a regional level, with representation from local hospitals and PICUs.

Take-Home Messages

- Interhospital transport of the critically ill child should be carried out by a specialised paediatric critical care transport team wherever feasible.
- Stabilisation for transport may be approached using an "Airway, Breathing, Circulation, Disability, Exposure" structure.
- Three key considerations are addressed during packaging for transport:
  - Patient and equipment secure, temperature management appropriate.
  - Sufficient oxygen, electrical power and infusion drugs available.
  - Emergency equipment and drugs accessible.
- Written policies governing acceptance and transport for time-critical conditions must be in place to prevent unnecessary delay in organising transfer. Time-critical transfer should usually be performed by the referring hospital team.
- Clear communication and an organised approach are essential for patient safety in the transport environment.

References

1. PICANet 2019 annual report. https://www.picanet.org.uk/annual-reporting-and-publications/. Accessed 10 Feb 2020.
2. Ramnarayan P, et al. Effect of specialist retrieval teams on outcomes in children admitted to paediatric intensive care units in England and Wales: a retrospective cohort study. Lancet. 2010;376:698–704.
3. Ellenby MS, Marcin JP. The role of telemedicine in pediatric critical care. Crit Care Clin. 2015;31:275–90.
4. Harvey J, et al. The impact of telemedicine on pediatric critical care triage. Pediatr Crit Care Med. 2017;18:e555–60.
5. Newth CJ, et al. The use of cuffed versus uncuffed endotracheal tubes in pediatric intensive care. J Pediatr. 2004;144:333–7.
6. Weiss M, et al. Prospective randomized controlled multi-centre trial of cuffed or uncuffed endotracheal tubes in small children. Br J Anaesth. 2009;103:867–73.
7. Greaney D, et al. A retrospective observational study of acquired subglottic stenosis using low-pressure, high-volume cuffed endotracheal tubes. Paediatr Anaesth. 2018;28:1136–41.
8. de Wit M, et al. The incidence of postoperative respiratory complications: a retrospective analysis of cuffed vs uncuffed tracheal tubes in children 0–7 years of age. Paediatr Anaesth. 2018;28.210–7.
9. Chambers NA, et al. Cuffed vs. uncuffed tracheal tubes in children: a randomised controlled trial comparing leak, tidal volume and complications. Anaesthesia. 2018;73:160–8.
10. FICM guideline for medication concentrations in adult critical care areas. https://www.ficm.ac.uk/sites/default/files/ics-standard-medication-concentrations-2016.pdf.
11. McNab S, et al. Isotonic versus hypotonic solutions for maintenance intravenous fluid administration in children. Cochrane Database Syst Rev. 2014;(12):CD009457.
12. McNab S, et al. 140 mmol/L of sodium versus 77 mmol/L of sodium in maintenance intravenous fluid therapy for children in hospital (PIMS): a randomised controlled double-blind trial. Lancet. 2015;385:1190–7.
13. Torres SF, et al. Hypotonic and isotonic intravenous maintenance fluids in hospitalised paediatric patients: a randomised controlled trial. BMJ Paediatr Open. 2019;3:e000385.
14. BOC medical oxygen safety and technical data sheet. https://www.bochealthcare.co.uk/en/quality-and-safety/safety-and-technical-data/safety-data-sheets/safety-data-sheets.html. Accessed 10 Feb 2020.
15. Davies J, et al. Should parents accompany critically ill children during inter-hospital transport? Arch Dis Child. 2005;90:1270–3.

16. Rollin AM. Working together for the sick or injured child: the Tanner Report. Anaesthesia. 2006;61:1135–7.
17. Joint Statement from the Society of British Neurological Surgeons (SBNS) and the Royal College of Anaesthetists (RCoA) regarding the provision of emergency paediatric neurosurgical services. 2010. https://www.sbns.org.uk/index.php/policies-and-publications/protocol-and-guidelines-2/. Accessed 10 Feb 2020.
18. Royal College of Anaesthetists. Guidelines for the provision of paediatric anaesthesia services. 2020. https://www.rcoa.ac.uk/gpas/chapter-10. Accessed 10 Feb 2020.
19. Regulation 28: Report to prevent future deaths. 2017. https://www.judiciary.uk/wp-content/uploads/2017/02/Dennett-2017-0026.pdf.
20. Lutman D, et al. Ambulance and aeromedical accident rates during emergency retrieval in Great Britain. Emerg Med J. 2008;25:301–2.
21. Watanabe BL, et al. Is use of warning lights and sirens associated with increased risk of ambulance crashes? A contemporary analysis using National EMS Information System (NEMSIS) data. Ann Emerg Med. 2019;74:101–9.

Analgosedation in the Pediatric Intensive Care Unit

Pavla Pokorná, John van den Anker, Jonas Berner, and Dick Tibboel

Contents

J. Brierley et al. (eds.), *ESPNIC Children's Intensive Care Textbook*,
https://doi.org/10.1007/978-3-031-64762-8_52

Learning Objectives

This chapter will provide the readers with information about analgesia and sedation in the pediatric intensive care unit (PICU). The first part of the chapter summarizes the current knowledge about pain and distress in neonates, infants, and children. The second part focuses on various assessment scales and treatment interventions of pain and distress including preventive and therapeutic measures. Both non-pharmacological and pharmacological therapeutic procedures will be discussed. The final part (and Supplementary Data) guides the readers through the current level of knowledge of commonly used analgesic and sedative drugs. Because this chapter focuses mainly on analgesia and sedation in neonates, infants, and children admitted to PICUs, chronic or palliative, neuropathic and oncological pain, and its treatments are not included. These topics are considered beyond the scope of this chapter. *Read the summary of each section carefully to answer the questions correctly at the end.*

52.1 Introduction

Adequate analgesia and sedation are essential for neonates, infants, and children admitted to pediatric intensive care units (PICUs) [1–3]. Nowadays, guidelines and local practice protocols for analgesia and sedation are increasingly available [4–6]. In 2016, within this context, a multidisciplinary position paper was published guiding professionals in the assessment of pain, distress, withdrawal syndrome, and delirium in PICUs [7]. Unfortunately, sparse data are available on treatment algorithms based on efficacy and safety parameters for analgesics and sedatives under these conditions [8]. In addition, no benefits of protocolized analgosedation were found as compared to standard PICU care in children [9], and currently more than 50% of patients admitted to the PICU will perceive discomfort [10].

Consumption of analgesics and sedatives in critically ill newborns, infants, and children has increased over the last decade [11–15]. Recent published pharmacoepidemiological data on drug prescriptions based on more than 66,000 patients and extracted from the national database in the United States, showed that analgesic, sedative, and neuromuscular blocking drugs were used in 63.3% of all patients admitted to a total number of 161 PICUs (of which analgesics were administered in 58.4%, sedatives in 39.8%, and neuromuscular blocking agents in 17.3% of all patients) [16]. Fentanyl, morphine, and midazolam were the most commonly used drugs. In addition, a combination of analgesic and sedative drugs (>5 days opioids with benzodiazepines) has been shown to be a significant risk factor for the development of drug tolerance or withdrawal [16].

The goal of adequate analgosedation is to achieve maximum efficacy and safety. For this reason, the primary (efficacy) and secondary (safety) endpoints of analgosedation guide the conduct and design of clinical trials in a more systematic way [17], and are successfully implemented in daily clinical practice [18].

52.2 Two Basic Concepts: Pain and Distress

52.2.1 Definition of Pain

In 1979, the World Health Organization (WHO) adopted a general definition of pain [19] issued by the International Association for the Study of Pain (IASP, established in 1973 and available from: www.who. int): "Pain is an unpleasant sensory and emotional experience associated with actual or potential tissue damage and described in terms of such damage" [20–22]. In the meanwhile, the definitions of pain have been regularly revised and focused on children, and myths about effects of pain on the immature organism were convincingly denied [23]: "Pain is subjectively perceived and described experience while the pediatric population differs from adults in the manifestations of pain, and in the response to pain and treatment interventions" [24, 25]. *Nowadays, pain is considered worldwide as a biopsychosocial phenomenon* [26].

52.2.2 Developmental Aspects of Pain

Children experience pain different form adults primarily due to neurobiological changes during development and perceptions may vary from child to child [23, 27, 28]. Children feel pain like adults or likely more than adults due to the immature physiological mechanisms of the pain profile. The current concept of children's pain states that the child has a higher sensitivity to pain, a lower pain threshold, which decreases with the accumulation of painful procedures, a more pronounced reflex response to touch and normal manipulation as a painful procedure [29]. Developmental changes are, for example, the role of nociceptors for peripheral sensitization or hyperalgesia, as well as the role of the spinal cord for pain modulation which may change with age [4]. In general, the nociceptive pathways start functioning already at the 20th week of gestation [30] while the development of the relevant pathways, both ascending and descending, goes on beyond the neonatal period, and consequently inadequate stimuli may have a negative impact on the developing brain [28, 31–33].

52.2.3 The Conceptual Model of Pain

Pain is a multimodal phenomenon that includes four basic levels (perception, experience, suffering, and behavior) based on two "historical models", the biopsychosocial Engel's model of the disease (1977) and Loeser's conceptual model of pain (1983):

- Nociception—perception of pain during a painful stimulus (neurophysiological-somatic)
- Pain—unpleasant sensory and emotional experience (psychological-sensory)

- Distress—milder aspect of pain and suffering (theological and philosophical-affective)
- Behavior—altered by pain (medical and social-behavioral)

52.2.4 Incidence of Pain

In 2016, painful and stressful procedures were studied in neonates admitted to NICUs, the mean number (SD; range) of heel sticks was 16.0 (14.4; 1–86) per neonate while a non-systematic analgesic approach was used during the 7.5 (4.4) day study period [34]. In 2019, a comparable study showed that the mean number (interquartile range) of these procedures had decreased to 11 (5–23) per patient per day in the PICU [35]. This study showed also that ventilated patients were twice as much exposed to painful procedures as compared to non-ventilated patients, and endotracheal suctioning was the most frequent procedure in the PICU [35]. Epidemiological studies have evaluated pain treatment in different countries and recently in Europe [36–38]. Finally, pain can be classified according to its causes, the intensity and duration of painful stimuli, and the so-called "typological distribution of pain" or a synonym used as a pain profile [39–42] (◘ Table S1).

◘ **Table S1** General definitions of pain and distress

Acute pain	Extensive, nociceptive, and behavioral cascade triggered by tissue injury and generally subsides *within weeks*
Postoperative pain	Acute pain experienced post-surgery
Prolonged (or persistent) pain	Disease or treatment-related pain lasting for 1 month with the expectation of healing the damaged tissue
Chronic pain	More than 1 month (and 3 months, respectively) and no recovery of tissue damage is expected (while the following terms such as persistent and prolonged vs chronic pain are interchanged by authors)
Distress	Organism's response to aversive internal and external stimuli including discomfort, anxiety, etc.
Iatrogenic withdrawal syndrome	A clinical syndrome after stopping or reversing a drug after prolonged exposure to that drug [7]
Tolerance	A decrease in a drug's effect or the need to increase the dose to achieve the same effect [15]

(continued)

Table S1 (continued)

Physiological dependence	Requirement for continued administration of a sedative or analgesic to prevent signs of neonatal abstinence or withdrawal syndrome using NAS, and SOS, WAT-1, respectively
Delirium	Neurocognitive disorder due to a somatic illness or its treatment using DSM-5 criteria by American Psychiatric Association diagnostic and statistical manual of mental disorders, fifth edition (DSM-5) Washington, DC: American Psychiatric Association; published in 2013, and reviewed

52.3 Pain Assessment

Pain assessment scores were developed to assess the child's body's responses to various painful and stressful stimuli [7, 43]. Traditionally, symptoms of pain and suffering include, but are not limited, to facial expressions, crying, and body movements, muscle tension, and the nature of sleep. However, the ability to perceive pain is highly variable and may be influenced by various factors related to patients, care-givers, and/or environment (e.g., pain threshold, life period, ethnic or cultural group, current mental state, anticipation of impending pain, previous experience with pain, current disease, age). Moreover a distinction must be made between pain and anxiety because every pain results in distress but distress does not always relate to or causes pain to the child's body [7, 28] (Table S2). *Assessments of the child's body's responses to various painful and stressful stimuli are listed below:*

STEP 1. Observations depending on how children respond to stimuli

- *Non-verbal scales*: evaluations in the preverbal population (age <3 years) or unconscious children [44] who cannot describe harmful stimuli by self-report.
- *Verbal scales*: self-reports in children (age >3 years) who express noxious stimuli themselves [45, 46].

STEP 2. Observations depending on how the manifestations are evaluated

- *Physiologic variables:* age-appropriate parameters, e.g., respiratory rate (RR/min), heart rate (HR/min), saturation (SpO_2/% requires oxygen to stay at >95%), blood pressure (BP/mmHg).
- *Behavior variables:* e.g., facial expressions, crying, breathing patterns, arm and leg movements, excitement, calm, facial tension, alertness, muscle tone, or using standardized tools (e.g., poker chips, tables).

STEP 3. Observations obtained according to age, pain or sedation profile, cognitive function

- Recently, behavioral or multidimensional (physiologic and behavioral) instruments are adjusted according to age (e.g., preterm and term neonates, infants, toddlers, children), pain distribution (e.g., pre-procedural pain, acute/procedural, postoperative, prolonged, chronic) and level of cognitive impairment.

Table S2 Pain and sedation profile adjusted for PICU settings (adapted from Harris et al. [7] and Giordano [41]

Pain distribution	Duration	Procedures/validated scales
Pre-procedural/procedural (acute) pain	Acute pain mainly procedural pain lasting <72 h	e.g., heel lancing, venipuncture, insertion and removal of drains, intubation, arterial puncture, lumbar puncture, peripheral IV cannula insertion, central vein catheter insertion, nasogastric and rectal tube insertion, circumcision: (e.g., COMFORT, COMFORT-B, FLACC, NFCS, NIPS, NPASS, PIPP-r)
Postoperative pain	Pain lasting 24–48 h after surgery	e.g., small or large surgical procedures and cardiac surgeries: (e.g., CHEOPS, FLACC, MAPS, NFCS, CRIES Scale)
Prolonged pain	Pain lasting >72 h under specific conditions	e.g., mechanical ventilation in critically ill patients (related to treatment procedures, e.g., extracorporeal membrane oxygenation (ECMO) or therapeutic hypothermia (HT) or disease, e.g., peritonitis, necrotizing enterocolitis (NEC) (e.g., COMFORT, COMFORT-B, COMFORT-neo, NFCS, N-PASS, PAT)
Chronic pain	Pain lasting 1–6 months while most often the pain lasts 3–6 months	e.g., pain that may lead to permanent tissue damage (e.g., PedsQL)
Palliative care	Pain lasting part of the active overall care for child's body, mind and spirit and family support as well	e.g., it begins when illness is diagnosed, and continues regardless of whether or not a child receives treatment of specific disease (e.g., PaPaS scale)
Sedation	*Discomfort lasting over periods while "optimal sedation" is* a state in which the patient is somnolent, responsive to the environment but untroubled by it, and with no excessive movements	Preventing and reducing anxiety, discomfort and improving amnesia and sleep (e.g., COMFORT, COMFORT-B, COMFORT-neo) [7, 55]

In daily clinical practice, different scores are used in the PICU:

The use of care bundles is highly advocated [47].

For example

Scales used in the preverbal population (age < 3 years) are, e.g., neonatal facial coding system (NFCS), premature infant pain profile revised version (PIPP-r) or Swedish ALP-Neo scale for neonates, COMFORT scales under the age of three

52

[11, 44, 46, 48] or the Face, Legs, Activity, Cry, and Consolability (FLACC) scale in children aged 6–42 months undergoing a procedure [48].

Scales used in the verbal population (age > 3–12 years and 8–17 years, respectively) are, e.g., the verbal numeric scale (VNS) also called as the ▶ numeric rating scale (NRS), the visual analogue scale (VAS) [49] or the Cardiac Analgesic Assessment Tool (CAAT), COMFORT scales or Eastern Ontario Children's Hospital Pain Scale (CHEOPS). A recent ▶ systematic review of faces scales demonstrated that only a few have appropriately investigated ▶ psychometric properties and can be considered well established and validated such as: the Pieces of Hurt Tool, the ▶ Faces Pain Scale, the Faces Pain Scale-Revised, the Wong-Baker FACES Pain Scale [50].

In 2019, a total number of 65 scales is available for the preverbal population of which 65% are behavioral (e.g., neonatal infant pain score, NIPS), 35% multidimensional (e.g., COMFORT scales) while only 43% were validated for implementation in daily clinical practice [44], e.g., PIPP-r for preterm neonates, COMFORT for acute, procedural, prolonged pain, sedation under the age of three, FLACC or COMFORT-B (Behavior Scale) for disabled children and Down syndrome [51, 52]. The validation process included the evaluation of the criteria for validity, consistency, and reliability of scores feasible in daily clinical practice based on consensus standards for selection of health measurement tools (COSMIN) [53, 54].

Key step The COMFORT-B score is a reliable score assessing procedural or prolonged pain and sedation in children under 3 years of age [55]:

Summary

What score is appropriate for the patient?

- *The first criterion* is the ability to verbalize responses to stimuli (e.g., non-verbal vs verbal).
- *The second criterion* is if the appropriate variables are used for observation in the individual patient (e.g., physiology variables vs behavioral variables).
- *The third criterion* depends on age (preterm, term neonates and toddlers age <3 years vs. children >3–17 years), pain and sedation profile, cognitive functions and specific conditions (behavioral scale vs. multidimensional scale).
- The best score is the score recommended and validated for age, pain distribution or sedative profile and cognitive function and individualized for the patient.

52.4 Treatment Interventions

In 2018, the Working Group the Analgesic, Anesthetic, and Addiction Clinical Trial Translations, Innovations, Opportunities, and Networks (ACTTION; ▶ www.acttion.org) of the Pediatric Pain Research Consortium (PPRC) concluded that neonates and infants under 6 months of age are the most vulnerable population in terms of pain, its treatment, and long-term consequences [56]. As stated in line with objectives of adequate analgesia and sedation to achieve maximum efficacy and safety, that applies to children of all ages admitted to the PICU [7, 44].

STEP 1. Efficacy of analgesia and sedation

- This approach addresses medical and ethical issues such as untreated pain or distress as inadequate analgesia can have short-term consequences or even increased mortality [23, 27]. Moreover, uncontrolled pain and anxiety release stress hormones, delay the child's recovery process and prolong hospitalization due to various health complications [57, 58]. In addition, inadequate analgesia and sedation can have long-term consequences, e.g., induced hypersensitivity to pain and anxiety in later life or altered development of the nervous system [58–61].

STEP 2. Safety of analgesia and sedation

- This approach focuses primarily on immediate adverse or side effects of drugs (during or after treatment) measured by physiological variables or measures of behavior (e.g., hemodynamic profile, respiratory depression, constipation, urinary retention, chest rigidity, iatrogenic withdrawal syndrome, e.g., SOS or WAT-1, delirium, e.g., DMS-5), or short-term parameters (e.g., EEG, NIRS, BIS) or long-term "neurotoxicity" of the drug such as e.g., neurodevelopmental outcome measured by cognitive, behavioral, and observational functions [61–63]. These findings are compiled based on experimental data [28, 64, 65] and a few clinical studies [36, 66, 67].

STEP 3. PICU standardized indicators of quality of care

- The primary outcomes (i.e., reports related to the PICU) are, e.g., standardized mortality rate, length of stay (LOS) adjusted according to disease severity, secondary outcomes (i.e., reports related to use of analgesic and sedative drugs) are, e.g., duration of mechanical ventilation, incidence of withdrawal or delirium, drug consumption, and cumulative doses of analgosedative drugs [68].

52.4.1 Non-pharmacological Interventions

Non-pharmacological interventions are used as a first step alone or in combination with pharmacological interventions to prevent or reduce harmful stimuli [69]. Some techniques appear to be successful in neonates [70–72] as well in children [73, 74]. However, current evidence for a positive effect is low and more research is needed on various non-pharmacological interventions. In neonates, the most frequently used techniques are—e.g., facilitated tucking or non-nutritive sucking [72], massage [75], skin to skin techniques [76] or administration of sucrose 24% [77], glucose 30% and mother's milk. In addition, in children of all ages, the highest evidence is present for facilitated tucking or non-nutritive sucking and rocking/holding [73]. In children and adolescents also psychological interventions may be helpful to reduce procedural pain in particular [78]. *The general principles of non-pharmacological interventions also relevant for the PICU population are:*

- ensuring peace, comfort, and convenience
- suitable environment for peaceful sleep and rest and containment of circadian rhythm
- protection against unpleasant environmental influences
- involvement/presence of the parents
- distraction from pain such as music, movies; artificial intelligence
- soothing and soothing techniques

- synchronization and individualization of nursing interventions according to the patient's needs
- relaxation techniques, e.g., audio techniques or skin-to-skin techniques, e.g., Kangaroo care [79].

52.4.2 Pharmacological Interventions

Recently, recommendations published by the World Health Organization (WHO) in 2012 (available from: ▶ www.who.int) were originally used for treatment of chronic pain in children by the three-step ladder that has changed to the two-step ladder (mild, moderate to severe pain) and principles adopted for patients admitted to the PICU [7]. *Several guidelines have been published:*

- Guidelines for regional pediatric anesthesia and pain therapy provided by The European Society of Regional Anesthesia and Pain Therapy and the American Society of Regional Anesthesia and Pain Medicine [80].
- Guidelines, local practice protocols, and updated recommendations for analgesia and sedation used in PICUs [6].
- the National Cancer Institute, the American Pain Society, the British Pain Society, and The European Association for Palliative Care recommend that several opioids should be available for clinicians to ensure an optimal and individualized treatment approach [81, 82].
- The 2022 Society of Critical Care Medicine Clinical Practice Guideline [83].

According to the WHO recommendations, paracetamol and ibuprofen (nonsteroidal anti-inflammatory drugs, NSAIDs) are recommended for the treatment of mild pain, weak opioids (codeine and tramadol) for moderate or severely moderate pain while strong opioids for severe pain (hydromorphone, fentanyl, methadone morphine, oxycodone). Paracetamol, morphine, and fentanyl (or its derivates) are the most commonly used analgesics in the PICU. For postoperative pain in children less than 1 year of age, paracetamol was shown to be equipotent to morphine both during a clinical trial and subsequent daily clinical practice [84, 85]. However, paracetamol while used alone failed for procedural pain in neonates and young infants. In general, opioids are widely used for moderate and severe pain in the PICU and in case of so-called opiate-induced sedation. The most commonly used sedative drugs are benzodiazepines (midazolam, lorazepam) while α-adrenergic receptor agonists (clonidine, dexmedetomidine) are increasingly used as an alternative to midazolam due to their presumed favorable efficacy (sedation and add-on analgesia profile) and safety (hemodynamic profile).

For Example

Acute/procedural pain/sedation, the drugs of first choice are ultra-rapid-acting (alfentanil, remifentanil) or rapid-acting opioids (fentanyl and its derivatives), sedatives (midazolam, dexmedetomidine), or other drugs (ketamine, propofol).

Postoperative pain/sedation, first-line drugs are strong opioids (morphine, fentanyl and its derivates) with paracetamol or sedatives (midazolam, dexmedetomidine). In addition, paracetamol as well dexmedetomidine may have morphine-sparing effect (or opioid-sparing effect).

Prolonged and chronic pain/sedation weak opioids (tramadol) or strong opioids (morphine, fentanyl and its derivatives) with sedatives (midazolam, clonidine) and with the correct dose, duration of treatment, and combination therapy <5 days are used and titrated according to the desired effect and also to avoid withdrawal or delirium.

*Sedation (*mild to moderate), midazolam is a widely used drug for acute/procedural, postoperative and prolonged sedation that is increasingly replaced by clonidine and dexmedetomidine.

Withdrawal syndrome and delirium, α-adrenergic receptor agonists (clonidine, dexmedetomidine), benzodiazepines (diazepam, lorazepam, midazolam, oxazepam), the N-methyl-D-aspartate receptor (NMDA receptor or NMDAR) antagonists (ketamine) and barbiturates (phenobarbital) or dopamine, mainly D2, receptor antagonists and antipsychotic drugs (haloperidol) are used.

Key step the COMFORT-B score is a reliable tool for re-evaluation of acute and prolonged pain and sedation in children under 3 years of age who have been given analgesics or sedatives i.v [7] [55].

Summary

What treatment intervention is appropriate for the patient?

- *The first criterion* is the decision whether non-pharmacological intervention can be used as a first step alone or in combination with pharmacological interventions.
- *The second criterion*, if pharmacological intervention is required, is the choice of drug for analgesia—the choice of drug depends on the pain and sedation profile—analgesic drugs (non-opioids, opioids) alone or in combination with other drugs, e.g., paracetamol or ibuprofen for mild to moderate pain alone or in combination with weak opioids (tramadol) or strong opioids (morphine, fentanyl) for the treatment of moderate or severe pain. Sedative drugs (midazolam, clonidine, dexmedetomidine) alone or in combination with opioids for mild and moderate sedation. However, it is strongly recommended to select the age-appropriate drug, formulation, and dosage.
- *The third criterion* is the correct dose of the drug, the duration of treatment and the combination of drugs depending on the clinical indication—treatment phase (e.g., starting dose, maintenance dose, weaning from analgesia) and pain or sedation profile (e.g., acute/procedural, postoperative, prolonged). The dosing regimen is adjusted according to age (maturational factors), while non-maturational factors should also be considered (e.g., effects of liver or kidney damage, treatment modality such as ECMO, CPB, HT or CRRT—or the magnitude of inflammation, e.g., SIRS, on CYP3A4 polymorphism).

Take-Home Messages

- **To Date**

- Newborns, infants, and children at PICU are often exposed to painful and stressful stimuli and large differences exist between centers in the use of assessment tools and treatment protocols.

(continued)

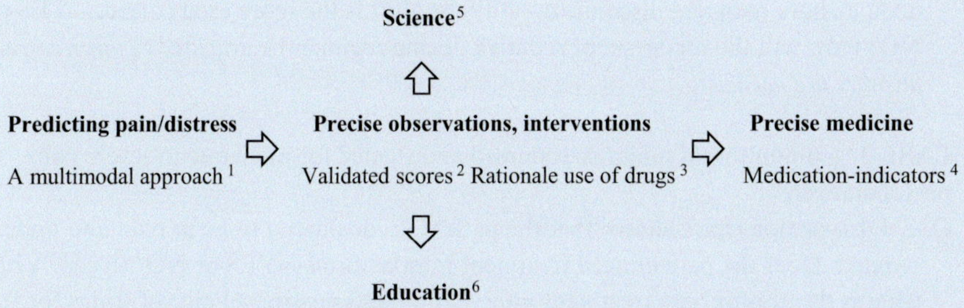

Fig. 52.1 Key steps to achieve adequate analgosedation in the PICU (adapted by ESPNIC). (1) A multimodal approach based on *the conceptual model of pain* (see the second part of this chapter). (2) Validated scores based on *the validation process* (see the third part of this chapter). (3) Rationale use of drugs based on *the multiple determinant concept* (see the chapter: Clinical Pharmacology in the Paediatric Intensive Care Unit and Supplementary Data). (4) Medication-indicators based on *the PICU standardized indicators of quality of care* related to analgesic and sedative drugs (see the fourth part of this chapter). (5) Science based on *scientific advice* on the primary (efficacy) and secondary (safety) endpoints of clinical trials on analgosedation [17]. (6) Education based on a systematic approach, for example on simulations based on the application of physiologically based pharmacokinetic/pharmacodynamic (PBPK/PD) modeling similarly to other drugs (see the chapter: Clinical Pharmacology in the Paediatric Intensive Care Unit)

- Preventive and treatment interventions are equally important because pain and stress as well inadequate treatment may have short- and long-term consequences.
- Dose adjustment of analgesic and sedative drugs is primarily based on pharmacodynamics; however, sparse evidence of the efficacy and safety of analgesics and sedatives drugs is available.
- Key steps to achieve the goals of adequate analgesia and sedation are maximum efficacy and safety based on the use of validated assessment scores, evidence-based non-pharmacological and pharmacological interventions, treatment indicators, and individualized approaches, see Fig. 52.1.

52.5 Conclusion

The multifactorial approach of adequate analgesia in the PICU reflects the multimodal phenomenon of pain and is based on validated re-evaluations and treatment interventions tailored to the individual patient. This population should be considered "pharmacologically" vulnerable, and inadequate analgosedation as well as the use of analgesic and sedative drugs may have negative effects on the developing brain.

Questions

CASE 1" a two-month-old patient is examined for acute/procedural pain"

Q1. FLACC = 10 by repeated measurements, does the patient have pain—YES or NO? Is the score used adequate for the age category—YES or NO? (*two correct answers are needed*)

CASE 2" a full-term neonate is examined and treated for prolonged pain and sedation"

Q2. The COMFORT-B scale = 24 by repeated measurements, does the full-term neonate have pain and discomfort—YES or NO? Is the score used correct—YES or NO? How will the analgesic or sedative dosing regimen be adjusted? *(three correct answers are needed)*

CASE 3 "a 6-month-old infant is examined and treated for moderate to severe pain postoperatively"

Q3. Observations have shown that the patient is considered to be in pain and undersedated. Does the patient need treatment interventions—YES or NO? In case YES, what is the appropriate treatment intervention and possible choice of drugs for the patient? (*three correct answers are needed*)

Answers

A1. The FLACC scale is correct (1), and YES (2) is correct (the patient is in acute pain)
Comments: The FLACC scale or Face, Legs, Activity, Cry, Consolability scale is a behavioral tool used to assess pain for children between the ages of 2 months and 7 years or disabled patients to measure procedural pain in preverbal population. The scale ranges from 0–10 with 0 representing no pain.

A2. The COMFORT-B scale is correct (1), and YES (2) is correct (the patient is in prolonged pain and discomfort). Therefore, a loading dose (mg/kg) of analgesic or sedative drugs must be given or a maintenance dose (mg/kg) must be increased (3).
Comments: The COMFORT-B score is the correct score used in the preverbal population suffering from prolonged pain and discomfort and measured by multimodal variables (movement, calmness, facial tension, alertness, respiration rate, muscle tone, etc.)

52

A3. YES, this is correct (1), and the patient is in moderate to severe postoperative pain and needs pharmacological intervention (2). For example, paracetamol in combination with opioids (morphine, fentanyl or its derivatives) and the right dose for age and pain profile are recommended (3).
Comments: Paracetamol in combination with opioids is a possible treatment for moderate to severe pain postoperatively in a 6-month-old infant. Appropriate variables (physiological and behavioral) should also be used to achieve the efficacy and safety of analgesia and sedation.

References

1. Poh YN, Poh PF, Buang SN, Lee JH. Sedation guidelines, protocols, and algorithms in PICUs: a systematic review. Pediatr Crit Care Med. 2014;15(9):885–92.
2. Mathews L. Pain in children: neglected, unaddressed and mismanaged. Indian J Palliat Care. 2011;17(Suppl):S70–3.
3. Tobias JD, Rasmussen GE. Pain management and sedation in the pediatric intensive care unit. Pediatr Clin North Am. 1994;41(6):1269–92.
4. Walker SM. Neonatal pain. Paediatr Anaesth. 2014;24(1):39–48.
5. Sperotto F, Mondardini MC, Dell'Oste C, Vitale F, Ferrario S, Lapi M, et al. Efficacy and safety of dexmedetomidine for prolonged sedation in the PICU: a prospective multicenter study (PROSDEX). Pediatr Crit Care Med. 2020;21(7):625–36.
6. Mondardini MC, Vasile B, Amigoni A, Baroncini S, Conio A, Mantovani A, et al. Update of recommendations for analgosedation in pediatric intensive care unit. Minerva Anestesiol. 2014;80(9):1018–29.

7. Harris J, Ramelet AS, van Dijk M, Pokorna P, Wielenga J, Tume L, et al. Clinical recommendations for pain, sedation, withdrawal and delirium assessment in critically ill infants and children: an ESPNIC position statement for healthcare professionals. Intensive Care Med. 2016;42(6):972–86.
8. Pokorna P, Tibboel D. Numbers, numbers: great, great…but?! Pediatr Crit Care Med. 2020;21(9):844–5.
9. Curley MA, Wypij D, Watson RS, Grant MJ, Asaro LA, Cheifetz IM, et al. Protocolized sedation vs usual care in pediatric patients mechanically ventilated for acute respiratory failure: a randomized clinical trial. JAMA. 2015;313(4):379–89.
10. Bosch-Alcaraz A, Jordan I, Benito-Aracil L, Saz-Roy M, Falco-Pegueroles A. Discomfort of the critically ill paediatric patient and correlated variables. Aust Crit Care. 2020;33:504.
11. Anand KJ, Sippell WG, Aynsley-Green A. Randomised trial of fentanyl anaesthesia in preterm babies undergoing surgery: effects on the stress response. Lancet. 1987;1(8524):62–6.
12. Carbajal R, Simon N. [Sedation and analgesia in children]. Arch Pediatr. 1995;2(11):1089–1096.
13. Carbajal R, Eriksson M, Courtois E, Anand KJ. [Sedation and analgesia for neonates in NICUs across Europe]. Arch Pediatr. 2015;22(5 Suppl 1):95–96.
14. Means LJ, Ferrari L, Mancuso TJ, Davidson P, Hackel A, Deshpande JK, et al. The pediatric sedation unit: a mechanism for safe pediatric sedation. Pediatrics. 1999;103(1):199–201.
15. Carbajal R, Eriksson M, Courtois E, Boyle E, Avila-Alvarez A, Andersen RD, et al. Sedation and analgesia practices in neonatal intensive care units (EUROPAIN): results from a prospective cohort study. Lancet Respir Med. 2015;3(10):796–812.
16. Patel AK, Trujillo-Rivera E, Faruqe F, Heneghan JH, Workman TE, Zeng-Treitler Q, et al. Sedation, analgesia, and neuromuscular blockade: an assessment of practices from 2009 to 2016 in a National Sample of 66,443 pediatric patients cared for in the ICU. Pediatr Crit Care Med. 2020;21:e599.
17. van Dijk M, Ceelie I, Tibboel D. Endpoints in pediatric pain studies. Eur J Clin Pharmacol. 2011;67(Suppl 1):61–6.
18. Neunhoeffer F, Kumpf M, Renk H, Hanelt M, Berneck N, Bosk A, et al. Nurse-driven pediatric analgesia and sedation protocol reduces withdrawal symptoms in critically ill medical pediatric patients. Paediatr Anaesth. 2015;25(8):786–94.
19. Devine R, Merskey H. The description of pain in psychiatric and general medical patients. J Psychosom Res. 1965;9(3):311–6.
20. Merskey H, Gillis A, Marszalek KS. A clinical investigation of reactions to pain. J Ment Sci. 1962;108:347–55.
21. Merskey H. Psychological aspects of pain. Postgrad Med J. 1968;44(510):297–306.
22. Merskey H. On the development of pain. Headache. 1970;10(3):116–23.
23. Anand KJ, Hickey PR. Pain and its effects in the human neonate and fetus. N Engl J Med. 1987;317(21):1321–9.
24. Treede RD. The International Association for the study of pain definition of pain: as valid in 2018 as in 1979, but in need of regularly updated footnotes. Pain Rep. 2018;3(2):e643.
25. Raja SN, Carr DB, Cohen M, Finnerup NB, Flor H, Gibson S, et al. The revised International Association for the study of pain definition of pain: concepts, challenges, and compromises. Pain. 2020;161:1976.
26. Darnall BD, Carr DB, Schatman ME. Pain psychology and the biopsychosocial model of pain treatment: ethical imperatives and social responsibility. Pain Med. 2017;18(8):1413–5.
27. Anand KJ, Sippell WG, Aynsley-Green A. Pain, anaesthesia, and babies. Lancet. 1987;2(8569):1210.
28. van den Hoogen NJ, de Kort AR, Allegaert KM, Joosten EA, Simons SHP, Tibboel D, et al. Developmental neurobiology as a guide for pharmacological management of pain in neonates. Semin Fetal Neonatal Med. 2019;24(4):101012.
29. Pancekauskaite G, Jankauskaite L. Paediatric pain medicine: pain differences, recognition and coping acute procedural pain in paediatric emergency room. Medicina (Kaunas). 2018;54(6):94.
30. Anand KJ. Pain assessment in preterm neonates. Pediatrics. 2007;119(3):605–7.
31. Beggs S, Torsney C, Drew LJ, Fitzgerald M. The postnatal reorganization of primary afferent input and dorsal horn cell receptive fields in the rat spinal cord is an activity-dependent process. Eur J Neurosci. 2002;16(7):1249–58.

32. Knaepen L, Patijn J, van Kleef M, Mulder M, Tibboel D, Joosten EA. Neonatal repetitive needle pricking: plasticity of the spinal nociceptive circuit and extended postoperative pain in later life. Dev Neurobiol. 2013;73(1):85–97.
33. den Hoogen NJV, Patijn J, Tibboel D, Joosten EA. Neonatal plasticity of the nociceptive system: mechanisms, effects, and treatment of repetitive painful procedures during NICU admittance. Curr Pharm Des. 2017;23(38):5902–10.
34. Courtois E, Droutman S, Magny JF, Merchaoui Z, Durrmeyer X, Roussel C, et al. Epidemiology and neonatal pain management of heelsticks in intensive care units: EPIPPAIN 2, a prospective observational study. Int J Nurs Stud. 2016;59:79–88.
35. Baarslag MA, Jhingoer S, Ista E, Allegaert K, Tibboel D, van Dijk M. How often do we perform painful and stressful procedures in the paediatric intensive care unit? A prospective observational study. Aust Crit Care. 2019;32(1):4–10.
36. Koizumi T, Kurosawa H. Survey of analgesia and sedation in pediatric intensive care units in Japan. Pediatr Int. 2020;62(5):535–41.
37. Tabacco B, Tacconi C, Amigoni A. Survey on monitoring analgesia and sedation in the Italian pediatric intensive care units. Minerva Anestesiol. 2017;83(10):1010–6.
38. Daverio M, et al. Pain and sedation management and monitoring in pediatric intensive care units across Europe: an ESPNIC survey. Crit Care. 2022;26(1):88.
39. Allegaert K, Tibboel D, van den Anker J. Pharmacological treatment of neonatal pain: in search of a new equipoise. Semin Fetal Neonatal Med. 2013;18(1):42–7.
40. Baarslag MA, Allegaert K, Van Den Anker JN, Knibbe CA, Van Dijk M, Simons SH, et al. Paracetamol and morphine for infant and neonatal pain; still a long way to go? Expert Rev Clin Pharmacol. 2017;10(1):111–26.
41. Durrmeyer X, Daoud P, Decobert F, Boileau P, Renolleau S, Zana-Taieb E, et al. Premedication for neonatal endotracheal intubation: results from the epidemiology of procedural pain in neonates study. Pediatr Crit Care Med. 2013;14(4):e169–75.
42. Short SR, Thienprayoon R. Pediatric palliative care in the intensive care unit and questions of quality: a review of the determinants and mechanisms of high-quality palliative care in the pediatric intensive care unit (PICU). Transl Pediatr. 2018;7(4):326–43.
43. van Dijk M, Tibboel D. Update on pain assessment in sick neonates and infants. Pediatr Clin North Am. 2012;59(5):1167–81.
44. Giordano V, Edobor J, Deindl P, Wildner B, Goeral K, Steinbauer P, et al. Pain and sedation scales for neonatal and pediatric patients in a preverbal stage of development: a systematic review. JAMA Pediatr. 2019;173:1186.
45. Valkenburg AJ, Tibboel D, van Dijk M. Pain sensitivity of children with Down syndrome and their siblings: quantitative sensory testing versus parental reports. Dev Med Child Neurol. 2015;57(11):1049–55.
46. Valkenburg AJ, de Leeuw TG, van Dijk M, Tibboel D. Pain in intellectually disabled children: towards evidence-based pharmacotherapy? Paediatr Drugs. 2015;17(5):339–48.
47. Ista E, Redivo J, Kananur P, Choong K, Colleti J, Needham D, Awojoodu R, Kudchadkar S. Assessing pain, both spontaneous wakening and breathing trials, choice of sedation, delirium monitoring/management, early exercise/mobility, and family engagement/empowerment bundle practices for critically ill children: an international survey of 161 PICUs in 18 countries. Crit Care Med. 2021;50(1):114–25.
48. Crellin DJ, Harrison D, Santamaria N, Huque H, Babl FE. The psychometric properties of the FLACC scale used to assess procedural pain. J Pain. 2018;19(8):862–72.
49. Bailey B, Daoust R, Doyon-Trottier E, Dauphin-Pierre S, Gravel J. Validation and properties of the verbal numeric scale in children with acute pain. Pain. 2010;149(2):216–21.
50. Tomlinson D, von Baeyer CL, Stinson JN, Sung L. A systematic review of faces scales for the self-report of pain intensity in children. Pediatrics. 2010;126(5):e1168–98.
51. Cascella M, Bimonte S, Saettini F, Muzio MR. The challenge of pain assessment in children with cognitive disabilities: features and clinical applicability of different observational tools. J Paediatr Child Health. 2019;55(2):129–35.
52. Terstegen C, Koot HM, de Boer JB, Tibboel D. Measuring pain in children with cognitive impairment: pain response to surgical procedures. Pain. 2003;103(1–2):187–98.
53. Playfor S, Jenkins I, Boyles C, Choonara I, Davies G, Haywood T, et al. Consensus guidelines on sedation and analgesia in critically ill children. Intensive Care Med. 2006;32(8):1125–36.

54. Kimberlin CL, Winterstein AG. Validity and reliability of measurement instruments used in research. Am J Health Syst Pharm. 2008;65(23):2276–84.
55. Ista E, van Dijk M, Tibboel D, de Hoog M. Assessment of sedation levels in pediatric intensive care patients can be improved by using the COMFORT "behavior" scale. Pediatr Crit Care Med. 2005;6(1):58–63.
56. Walco GA, Kopecky EA, Weisman SJ, Stinson J, Stevens B, Desjardins PJ, et al. Clinical trial designs and models for analgesic medications for acute pain in neonates, infants, toddlers, children, and adolescents: ACTTION recommendations. Pain. 2018;159(2):193–205.
57. Anand KJ, Sippell WG, Aynsley-Green A. Randomised trial of fentanyl anaesthesia in preterm babies undergoing surgery: effects on the stress response. Lancet. 1987;1(8527):243–8.
58. Weisman SJ, Bernstein B, Schechter NL. Consequences of inadequate analgesia during painful procedures in children. Arch Pediatr Adolesc Med. 1998;152(2):147–9.
59. Walker SM, Franck LS, Fitzgerald M, Myles J, Stocks J, Marlow N. Long-term impact of neonatal intensive care and surgery on somatosensory perception in children born extremely preterm. Pain. 2009;141(1–2):79–87.
60. Page GG. Are there long-term consequences of pain in newborn or very young infants? J Perinat Educ. 2004;13(3):10–7.
61. Walker SM. Long-term effects of neonatal pain. Semin Fetal Neonatal Med. 2019;24(4):101005.
62. de Graaf J, van Lingen RA, Simons SH, Anand KJ, Duivenvoorden HJ, Weisglas-Kuperus N, et al. Long-term effects of routine morphine infusion in mechanically ventilated neonates on children's functioning: five-year follow-up of a randomized controlled trial. Pain. 2011;152(6):1391–7.
63. de Graaf J, van Lingen RA, Valkenburg AJ, Weisglas-Kuperus N, Groot Jebbink L, Wijnberg-Williams B, et al. Does neonatal morphine use affect neuropsychological outcomes at 8 to 9 years of age? Pain. 2013;154(3):449–58.
64. Durrmeyer X, Vutskits L, Anand KJ, Rimensberger PC. Use of analgesic and sedative drugs in the NICU: integrating clinical trials and laboratory data. Pediatr Res. 2010;67(2):117–27.
65. van den Bosch GE, Dijk MV, Tibboel D, de Graaff JC. Long-term effects of early exposure to stress, pain, opioids and anaesthetics on pain sensitivity and neurocognition. Curr Pharm Des. 2017;23(38):5879–86.
66. Davidson AJ. Anesthesia and neurotoxicity to the developing brain: the clinical relevance. Paediatr Anaesth. 2011;21(7):716–21.
67. Schiller RM, Allegaert K, Hunfeld M, van den Bosch GE, van den Anker J, Tibboel D. Analgesics and sedatives in critically ill newborns and infants: the impact on long-term neurodevelopment. J Clin Pharmacol. 2018;58(Suppl 10):S140–S50.
68. Hughes RG, Blegen MA. Medication administration safety. In: Hughes RG, editor. Patient safety and quality: an evidence-based handbook for nurses. Advances in patient safety. Rockville; 2008.
69. Carbajal R, Greteau S, Arnaud C, Guedj R. [Pain in neonatology. Non-pharmacological treatment]. Arch Pediatr. 2015;22(2):217–221.
70. Stevens BJ, Yamada J, Estabrooks CA, Stinson J, Campbell F, Scott SD, et al. Pain in hospitalized children: effect of a multidimensional knowledge translation strategy on pain process and clinical outcomes. Pain. 2014;155(1):60–8.
71. Bueno M, Yamada J, Harrison D, Khan S, Ohlsson A, Adams-Webber T, et al. A systematic review and meta-analyses of nonsucrose sweet solutions for pain relief in neonates. Pain Res Manag. 2013;18(3):153–61.
72. Stevens B, Yamada J, Lee GY, Ohlsson A. Sucrose for analgesia in newborn infants undergoing painful procedures. Cochrane Database Syst Rev. 2013;(1):CD001069.
73. Pillai Riddell RR, Racine NM, Gennis HG, Turcotte K, Uman LS, Horton RE, et al. Non-pharmacological management of infant and young child procedural pain. Cochrane Database Syst Rev. 2015;2015(12):CD006275.
74. Pillai Riddell RR, Racine NM, Turcotte K, Uman LS, Horton RE, Din Osmun L, et al. Non-pharmacological management of infant and young child procedural pain. Cochrane Database Syst Rev. 2011;(10):CD006275.
75. Jain S, Kumar P, McMillan DD. Prior leg massage decreases pain responses to heel stick in preterm babies. J Paediatr Child Health. 2006;42(9):505–8.
76. Johnston C, Campbell-Yeo M, Disher T, Benoit B, Fernandes A, Streiner D, et al. Skin-to-skin care for procedural pain in neonates. Cochrane Database Syst Rev. 2017;2:CD008435.

77. Stevens B, Yamada J, Ohlsson A, Haliburton S, Shorkey A. Sucrose for analgesia in newborn infants undergoing painful procedures. Cochrane Database Syst Rev. 2016;7:CD001069.
78. Birnie KA, Noel M, Chambers CT, Uman LS, Parker JA. Psychological interventions for needle-related procedural pain and distress in children and adolescents. Cochrane Database Syst Rev. 2018;10:CD005179.
79. Jefferies AL, Canadian Paediatric Society, Fetus and Newborn Committee. Kangaroo care for the preterm infant and family. Paediatr Child Health. 2012;17(3):141–6.
80. Suresh S, Ecoffey C, Bosenberg A, Lonnqvist PA, de Oliveira GS Jr, de Leon Casasola O, et al. The European Society of Regional Anaesthesia and Pain Therapy/American Society of Regional Anesthesia and Pain Medicine recommendations on local anesthetics and adjuvants dosage in pediatric regional anesthesia. Reg Anesth Pain Med. 2018;43(2):211–6.
81. Chou R, Fanciullo GJ, Fine PG, Adler JA, Ballantyne JC, Davies P, et al. Clinical guidelines for the use of chronic opioid therapy in chronic noncancer pain. J Pain. 2009;10(2):113–30.
82. Caraceni A, Hanks G, Kaasa S, Bennett MI, Brunelli C, Cherny N, et al. Use of opioid analgesics in the treatment of cancer pain: evidence-based recommendations from the EAPC. Lancet Oncol. 2012;13(2):e58–68.
83. Smith HAB, Besunder JB, Betters KA, Johnson PN, Srinivasan V, Stormorken A, Farrington E, Golianu B, Godshall AJ, Acinelli L, Almgren C, Bailey CH, Boyd JM, Cisco MJ, Damian M, deAlmeida ML, Fehr J, Fenton KE, Gilliland F, Grant MJC, Howell J, Ruggles CA, Simone S, Su F, Sullivan JE, Tegtmeyer K, Traube C, Williams S, Berkenbosch JW. 2022 Society of Critical Care Medicine clinical practice guidelines on prevention and management of pain, agitation, neuromuscular blockade, and delirium in critically ill pediatric patients with consideration of the ICU environment and early mobility. Pediatr Crit Care Med. 2022;23(2):e74–e110.
84. Ceelie I, de Wildt SN, van Dijk M, van den Berg MM, van den Bosch GE, Duivenvoorden HJ, et al. Effect of intravenous paracetamol on postoperative morphine requirements in neonates and infants undergoing major noncardiac surgery: a randomized controlled trial. JAMA. 2013;309(2):149–54.
85. Baarslag MA, Ista E, de Leeuw T, van Rosmalen J, Tibboel D, van Dijk M, et al. Clinically effective implementation of intravenous paracetamol as primary analgesia after major surgery in neonates and young infants. Arch Dis Child. 2018;103(12):1168–9.
86. Vet NJ, Kleiber N, Ista E, de Hoog M, de Wildt SN. Sedation in critically ill children with respiratory failure. Front Pediatr. 2016;4:89.
87. Pacifici GM, Allegaert K. Clinical pharmacology of paracetamol in neonates: a review. Curr Ther Res Clin Exp. 2015;77:24–30.
88. Lundeberg S, Beck O, Olsson GL, Boreus LO. Rectal administration of morphine in children. Pharmacokinetic evaluation after a single-dose. Acta Anaesthesiol Scand. 1996;40(4):445–51.
89. O'Donnell FT, Rosen KR. Pediatric pain management: a review. Mo Med. 2014;111(3):231–7.
90. Goodarzi M. Comparison of epidural morphine, hydromorphone and fentanyl for postoperative pain control in children undergoing orthopaedic surgery. Paediatr Anaesth. 1999;9(5):419–22.
91. Hajimaghsoudi M, Bagherabadi M, Zarepur E, Ahmadi Hanzaei V. Intravenous versus subcutaneous midazolam using jet-injector in pediatric sedation; a randomized clinical trial. Emerg (Tehran). 2018;6(1):e53.
92. Vicencio-Rosas E, Perez-Guille MG, Flores-Perez C, Flores-Perez J, Trujillo-Jimenez F, Chavez-Pacheco JL. Buprenorphine and pain treatment in pediatric patients: an update. J Pain Res. 2018;11:549–59.
93. Soliman IE, Broadman LM, Hannallah RS, McGill WA. Comparison of the analgesic effects of EMLA (eutectic mixture of local anesthetics) to intradermal lidocaine infiltration prior to venous cannulation in unpremedicated children. Anesthesiology. 1988;68(5):804–6.
94. Bourdier S, Khelif N, Velasquez M, Usclade A, Rochette E, Pereira B, et al. Cold vibration (buzzy) versus anesthetic patch (EMLA) for pain prevention during cannulation in children: a randomized trial. Pediatr Emerg Care. 2019;37:86.
95. Lillieborg S, Otterbom I, Ahlen K. Topical anaesthesia in neonates, infants and children. Br J Anaesth. 2004;92(3):450; author reply -1.
96. Taddio A, Ohlsson A, Einarson TR, Stevens B, Koren G. A systematic review of lidocaine-prilocaine cream (EMLA) in the treatment of acute pain in neonates. Pediatrics. 1998;101(2):E1.

97. Ziesenitz VC, Vaughns JD, Koch G, Mikus G, van den Anker JN. Correction to: pharmacokinetics of fentanyl and its derivatives in children: a comprehensive review. Clin Pharmacokinet. 2018;57(3):393–417.
98. Chaves C, Remiao F, Cisternino S, Decleves X. Opioids and the blood-brain barrier: a dynamic interaction with consequences on drug disposition in brain. Curr Neuropharmacol. 2017;15(8):1156–73.
99. Packiasabapathy S, Sadhasivam S. Gender, genetics, and analgesia: understanding the differences in response to pain relief. J Pain Res. 2018;11:2729–39.
100. Smith HS. The metabolism of opioid agents and the clinical impact of their active metabolites. Clin J Pain. 2011;27(9):824–38.
101. Ghiasi N, Bhansali RK, Marwaha R. Lorazepam. Treasure Island: StatPearls; 2020.
102. Allegaert K, de Hoon J, Van Overmeire B, Devlieger H. Clinical pharmacology of non opioid analgesics in neonates. Verh K Acad Geneeskd Belg. 2005;67(5–6):289–315.
103. Allegaert K, Van den Anker JN, Verbesselt R, de Hoon J, Vanhole C, Tibboel D, et al. O-demethylation of tramadol in the first months of life. Eur J Clin Pharmacol. 2005;61(11):837–42.
104. Allegaert K, Rochette A, Veyckemans F. Developmental pharmacology of tramadol during infancy: ontogeny, pharmacogenetics and elimination clearance. Paediatr Anaesth. 2011;21(3):266–73.
105. Grond S, Sablotzki A. Clinical pharmacology of tramadol. Clin Pharmacokinet. 2004;43(13):879–923.
106. Dhawan BN, Cesselin F, Raghubir R, Reisine T, Bradley PB, Portoghese PS, et al.; International Union of Pharmacology. XII. Classification of opioid receptors. Pharmacol Rev. 1996;48(4):567–592.
107. James A, Williams J. Basic opioid pharmacology—an update. Br J Pain. 2020;14(2):115–21.
108. Pathan H, Williams J. Basic opioid pharmacology: an update. Br J Pain. 2012;6(1):11–6.
109. Stephenson RP. A modification of receptor theory. Br J Pharmacol Chemother. 1956;11(4):379–93.
110. Anand KJ, Aranda JV, Berde CB, Buckman S, Capparelli EV, Carlo WA, et al. Analgesia and anesthesia for neonates: study design and ethical issues. Clin Ther. 2005;27(6):814–43.
111. Anand KJ, Hall RW. Pharmacological therapy for analgesia and sedation in the newborn. Arch Dis Child Fetal Neonatal Ed. 2006;91(6):F448–53.
112. Anand KJ, Clark AE, Willson DF, Berger J, Meert KL, Zimmerman JJ, et al. Opioid analgesia in mechanically ventilated children: results from the multicenter measuring opioid tolerance induced by fentanyl study. Pediatr Crit Care Med. 2013;14(1):27–36.
113. Lemmens HJ, Burm AG, Bovill JG, Hennis PJ, Gladines MP. Pharmacodynamics of alfentanil. The role of plasma protein binding. Anesthesiology. 1992;76(1):65–70.
114. Goresky GV. Safety of alfentanil. Can J Anaesth. 1992;39(1):97.
115. Goresky GV, Koren G, Sabourin MA, Sale JP, Strunin L. The pharmacokinetics of alfentanil in children. Anesthesiology. 1987;67(5):654–9.
116. Ziesenitz VC, Vaughns JD, Koch G, Mikus G, van den Anker JN. Pharmacokinetics of fentanyl and its derivatives in children: a comprehensive review. Clin Pharmacokinet. 2018;57(2):125–49.
117. Saarenmaa E, Huttunen P, Leppaluoto J, Fellman V. Alfentanil as procedural pain relief in newborn infants. Arch Dis Child Fetal Neonatal Ed. 1996;75(2):F103–7.
118. Kwak HJ, Kim JY, Min SK, Kim JS, Kim JY. Optimal bolus dose of alfentanil for successful tracheal intubation during sevoflurane induction with and without nitrous oxide in children. Br J Anaesth. 2010;104(5):628–32.
119. Klees TM, Sheffels P, Dale O, Kharasch ED. Metabolism of alfentanil by cytochrome p4503a (cyp3a) enzymes. Drug Metab Dispos. 2005;33(3):303–11.
120. Meistelman C, Saint-Maurice C, Lepaul M, Levron JC, Loose JP, MacGee K. A comparison of alfentanil pharmacokinetics in children and adults. Anesthesiology. 1987;66(1):13–6.
121. Davis PJ, Cook DR. Clinical pharmacokinetics of the newer intravenous anaesthetic agents. Clin Pharmacokinet. 1986;11(1):18–35.
122. Davis PJ, Killian A, Stiller RL, Cook DR, Guthrie RD, Scierka AM. Pharmacokinetics of alfentanil in newborn premature infants and older children. Dev Pharmacol Ther. 1989;13(1):21–7.
123. Feierman DE, Lasker JM. Metabolism of fentanyl, a synthetic opioid analgesic, by human liver microsomes. Role of CYP3A4. Drug Metab Dispos. 1996;24(9):932–9.

124. Hagos FT, Horvat CM, Au AK, Conley YP, Li L, Poloyac SM, et al. Factors contributing to fentanyl pharmacokinetic variability among diagnostically diverse critically ill children. Clin Pharmacokinet. 2019;58(12):1567–76.
125. Favie LMA, Groenendaal F, van den Broek MPH, Rademaker CMA, de Haan TR, van Straaten HLM, et al. Pharmacokinetics of morphine in encephalopathic neonates treated with therapeutic hypothermia. PLoS One. 2019;14(2):e0211910.
126. Zeilmaker-Roest GA, van Rosmalen J, van Dijk M, Koomen E, Jansen NJG, Kneyber MCJ, et al. Intravenous morphine versus intravenous paracetamol after cardiac surgery in neonates and infants: a study protocol for a randomized controlled trial. Trials. 2018;19(1):318.
127. Knibbe CA, Krekels EH, van den Anker JN, DeJongh J, Santen GW, van Dijk M, et al. Morphine glucuronidation in preterm neonates, infants and children younger than 3 years. Clin Pharmacokinet. 2009;48(6):371–85.
128. Schnabel A, Reichl SU, Zahn PK, Pogatzki-Zahn E. Nalbuphine for postoperative pain treatment in children. Cochrane Database Syst Rev. 2014;2014(7):CD009583.
129. Sivak EL, Davis PJ. Review of the efficacy and safety of remifentanil for the prevention and treatment of pain during and after procedures and surgery. Local Reg Anesth. 2010;3:35–43.
130. Davis PJ, Wilson AS, Siewers RD, Pigula FA, Landsman IS. The effects of cardiopulmonary bypass on remifentanil kinetics in children undergoing atrial septal defect repair. Anesth Analg. 1999;89(4):904–8.
131. Lundeberg S, Roelofse JA. Aspects of pharmacokinetics and pharmacodynamics of sufentanil in pediatric practice. Paediatr Anaesth. 2011;21(3):274–9.
132. Wilde M, Pichini S, Pacifici R, Tagliabracci A, Busardo FP, Auwarter V, et al. Metabolic pathways and potencies of new fentanyl analogs. Front Pharmacol. 2019;10:238.
133. Wilson AS, Stiller RL, Davis PJ, Fedel G, Chakravorti S, Israel BA, et al. Fentanyl and alfentanil plasma protein binding in preterm and term neonates. Anesth Analg. 1997;84(2):315–8.
134. Moriarty C, Carroll W. Paracetamol: pharmacology, prescribing and controversies. Arch Dis Child Educ Pract Ed. 2016;101(6):331–4.
135. Allegaert K, Tibboel D, van den Anker J. Narcotic-sparing approaches and the shift toward paracetamol in neonatal intensive care. Handb Exp Pharmacol. 2020;261:491–506.
136. Mian P, Knibbe CAJ, Calvier EAM, Tibboel D, Allegaert K. Intravenous paracetamol dosing guidelines for pain management in (pre)term neonates using the paediatric study decision tree. Curr Pharm Des. 2017;23(38):5839–49.
137. Allegaert K. A critical review on the relevance of paracetamol for procedural pain management in neonates. Front Pediatr. 2020;8:89.
138. Kanabar DJ. A clinical and safety review of paracetamol and ibuprofen in children. Inflammopharmacology. 2017;25(1):1–9.
139. Ziesenitz VC, Zutter A, Erb TO, van den Anker JN. Efficacy and safety of ibuprofen in infants aged between 3 and 6 months. Paediatr Drugs. 2017;19(4):277–90.
140. van den Anker JN. Use of ibuprofen in paediatric populations. J R Soc Med. 2007;100(Suppl 48):18–22.
141. Van Overmeire B, Touw D, Schepens PJ, Kearns GL, van den Anker JN. Ibuprofen pharmacokinetics in preterm infants with patent ductus arteriosus. Clin Pharmacol Ther. 2001;70(4):336–43.
142. de Wildt SN, de Hoog M, Vinks AA, Joosten KF, van Dijk M, van den Anker JN. Pharmacodynamics of midazolam in pediatric intensive care patients. Ther Drug Monit. 2005;27(1):98–102.
143. Hammer GB. Sedation and analgesia in the pediatric intensive care unit following laryngotracheal reconstruction. Paediatr Anaesth. 2009;19(Suppl 1):166–79.
144. Wilson KC, Reardon C, Theodore AC, Farber HW. Propylene glycol toxicity: a severe iatrogenic illness in ICU patients receiving IV benzodiazepines: a case series and prospective, observational pilot study. Chest. 2005;128(3):1674–81.
145. Carney L, Kendrick J, Carr R. Safety and effectiveness of dexmedetomidine in the pediatric intensive care unit (SAD-PICU). Can J Hosp Pharm. 2013;66(1):21–7.
146. Perez-Guille MG, Toledo-Lopez A, Rivera-Espinosa L, Alemon-Medina R, Murata C, Lares-Asseff I, et al. Population pharmacokinetics and pharmacodynamics of dexmedetomidine in children undergoing ambulatory surgery. Anesth Analg. 2018;127(3):716–23.

147. Damian MA, Hammer GB, Elkomy MH, Frymoyer A, Drover DR, Su F. Pharmacokinetics of dexmedetomidine in infants and children after orthotopic liver transplantation. Anesth Analg. 2020;130(1):209–16.
148. Yasaei R, Saadabadi A. Clonidine. Treasure Island: StatPearls; 2020.
149. de Castro REV, Martins RSO, Prata-Barbosa A, de Magalhaes-Barbosa MC. Clonidine doses for sedation in the PICU. Pediatr Crit Care Med. 2020;21(1):110.
150. Pacifici GM. Clinical pharmacology of phenobarbital in neonates: effects, metabolism and pharmacokinetics. Curr Pediatr Rev. 2016;12(1):48–54.
151. Voller S, Flint RB, Stolk LM, Degraeuwe PLJ, Simons SHP, Pokorna P, et al. Model-based clinical dose optimization for phenobarbital in neonates: an illustration of the importance of data sharing and external validation. Eur J Pharm Sci. 2017;109S:S90–S7.
152. Michalickova D, Pokorna P, Tibboel D, Slanar O, Knibbe CAJ, Krekels EHJ. Rapid increase in clearance of phenobarbital in neonates on extracorporeal membrane oxygenation: a pilot retrospective population pharmacokinetic analysis. Pediatr Crit Care Med. 2020;21(9):e707–e15.
153. Pokorna P, Posch L, Sima M, Klement P, Slanar O, van den Anker J, et al. Severity of asphyxia is a covariate of phenobarbital clearance in newborns undergoing hypothermia. J Matern Fetal Neonatal Med. 2019;32(14):2302–9.
154. Favie LMA, Groenendaal F, van den Broek MPH, Rademaker CMA, de Haan TR, van Straaten HLM, et al. Phenobarbital, midazolam pharmacokinetics, effectiveness, and drug-drug interaction in asphyxiated neonates undergoing therapeutic hypothermia. Neonatology. 2019;116(2):154–62.
155. Folino TB, Muco E, Safadi AO, Parks LJ. Propofol. Treasure Island: StatPearls; 2020.
156. Secor T, Safadi AO, Gunderson S. Propofol toxicity. Treasure Island: StatPearls; 2020.
157. Preckel B, Bolten J. Pharmacology of modern volatile anaesthetics. Best Pract Res Clin Anaesthesiol. 2005;19(3):331–48.
158. Martin-Biggers J, Quick V, Spaccarotella K, Byrd-Bredbenner C. An exploratory study examining obesity risk in non-obese mothers of young children using a socioecological approach. Nutrients. 2018;10(6):781.
159. Palacios A, Mencia S, Llorente AM, Cruz J, Toledo B, Ordonez O, et al. Sevoflurane therapy for severe refractory bronchospasm in children. Pediatr Crit Care Med. 2016;17(8):e380–4.
160. Miller AL, Theodore D, Widrich J. Inhalational anesthetic. Treasure Island: StatPearls; 2020.
161. Sun L. Early childhood general anaesthesia exposure and neurocognitive development. Br J Anaesth. 2010;105(Suppl 1):i61–8.
162. Kumar M, Chawla R, Goyal M. Topical anesthesia. J Anaesthesiol Clin Pharmacol. 2015;31(4):450–6.
163. Foster JP, Taylor C, Spence K. Topical anaesthesia for needle-related pain in newborn infants. Cochrane Database Syst Rev. 2017;2:CD010331.
164. Brisman M, Ljung BML, Otterbom I, Larsson LE, Andreasson SE. Methaemoglobin formation after the use of EMLA cream in term neonates. Acta Paediatr. 1998;87(11):1191–4.

Further Reading

Allegaert K, van den Anker JN. Chapter xx. Sedation in the neonatal intensive care unit: international practice. In: Mason K, editor. Pediatric sedation outside the operating room, 3rd ed. Springer Verlag.
Yaffe SJ, Aranda CV. Neonatal and paediatric pharmacology: therapeutic principles in practice, 5th ed. 2020. isbn-13:978-0781795388.

Vital Support

Contents

Clinical Pharmacology in the Paediatric Intensive Care Unit

Pavla Pokorná, John van den Anker, and Dick Tibboel

Contents

J. Brierley et al. (eds.), *ESPNIC Children's Intensive Care Textbook*,
https://doi.org/10.1007/978-3-031-64762-8_53

Learning Objectives

This chapter will provide the readers with information how to use drugs in an effective and safe way in infants and children of all ages admitted to intensive care units.

The first part focuses on the basic principles of clinical pharmacology. In the second part, specific aspects are described to understand how development influences various pharmacokinetic processes. In the third part, other factors superimposed on these developmental changes will be analysed to understand variable responses to drugs under specific conditions. In the final part, evidence-based medicine for drug dosing in infants and children of all ages admitted to intensive care units will be highlighted.

Read the summary of each section carefully to answer the questions correctly at the end.

53.1 Introduction

In infants and children of all ages, many drugs are still prescribed in an off-label manner (i.e. drugs are used for an unapproved indication, dose or age group) despite major improvements in diagnostics, therapies and applied technology in intensive care medicine during recent years [1–3]. In neonatal intensive care units (NICUs), 34.0–95.6% of drugs are used off-label, whereas this percentage is 43.8–83.0% in paediatric intensive care units (PICUs) [4–8].

Many drugs administered in NICUs and PICUs are not approved for use in infants and children by the U.S. Food and Drug Administration (FDA) or European Medicines Agency (EMA) or have only limited approval [9]. This has resulted in the publication of a statement paper of the American Academy of Paediatrics (AAP) Committee on Drugs in 2014 [10], and very recently also a policy statement paper and recommendations for good clinical practice in Europe [11].

Preventable adverse drug reactions (ADRs) have been systematically reviewed by validated quality assessment criteria and ideally implemented in NICUs and PICUs. The dosing errors (e.g. frequency of administrations of antimicrobials) were found to be the most frequently documented errors in both intensive care settings [12]. However, large variations in assessment methods were identified varying from methods developed locally to those adapted based on existing definitions [13–17].

53.2 General Aspects of Clinical Pharmacology

Clinical pharmacology is the study of drugs in humans. To understand clinical pharmacology, the basic principles of pharmacology are shortly reviewed. Drug disposition is a general term that encompasses the four processes that determine drug and metabolite concentrations in plasma, in tissue and within cells. In general, drug disposition and action are determined by pharmacokinetics (PK), pharmacodynamics (PD) and pharmacogenetics (PG):

- *Pharmacokinetics* (PK): "what the body does to a drug" as described by the following processes: absorption, distribution, metabolism and excretion (ADME) and measured by PK parameters. Volume of distribution (Vd) and clearance (CL) are the primary PK parameters, and elimination half-life ($T_{1/2}$) is one of the secondary PK parameters calculated from the primary parameters and frequently used in daily clinical practice.

- *Pharmacodynamics* (PD): "what a drug does to the body." Drugs have different effects depending on the drug itself, the individual taking it and their environment. To simplify, drugs have wanted vs unwanted effects or desired vs undesired effects. For example, desired effects are relief in pain symptoms observed by various scores after administration of analgesic drugs or decrease in blood pressure after administration of antihypertensive drugs. Drugs are classified by its pharmacological effects (analgesic or antihypertensive) or its target (action on the central nervous system or cardiovascular system). Each drug may have short- or long-term desired and/or undesired effects.
- *Pharmacogenetics* (PG): "How people respond differently to drugs due to their genetic inheritance." The long-term goal of the use of pharmacogenetics is to help healthcare providers select the drugs and doses best suited for each person. It is part of the field of precision medicine which aims to treat each patient individually.

53.2.1 PK Processes: Its Language and Parameters

- *Absorption rate constant* (K_a): This is the fractional rate of drug absorption from the site of administration (e.g. gastrointestinal tract, skin, lungs) into the systemic circulation.
- *Bioavailability* (F): This is the ratio between the amount of drug that enters the systemic circulation and its dose. It ranges between 0 and 1.0 (0–100%). $F = 1.0$ (100%) applies to intravenous (IV) drug administration.
- *Volume of distribution* (Vd) is calculated as the ratio between the amount of drug in the body (dose) and Cpl of the drug = plasma concentration in blood at the defined time period: Vd = dose/Cpl. Unit: volume [L]; commonly reported as the ratio of Vd to body weight [L/kg].
- *Clearance* (CL) is calculated as the rate of elimination (metabolism and excretion) of a drug from the body and the Cpl of a drug per unit time: CL = elimination rate/Cpl. Unit: volume/time [L/h] and CL often refers to body weight or body surface area [L/h/kg or L/h/m^2]. For the basic terminology used in clinical pharmacology, see ◘ Table S1.

53.2.2 Dose and Dosing Interval

Dosage regimen (dose and dosing interval) is based on the primary PK parameters, and the following variables are used to calculate the loading dose (LD) and the maintenance dose (MD) rate. For drugs given IV, these doses are calculated as follows:

- **Dose rate** (mg/h) = dose (mg) divided by dosing interval (h)
- **Loading dose** (mg) = [Cpl (mg/L) × Vd (L)]/F
- **Maintenance dose rate** (mg/h) = [Cpl (mg/L) × CL (L/h)]/F

(Abbr.: *Cpl* represents the desired plasma concentration of a specific drug, *Vd* the volume of distribution, *CL* the clearance and *F* the bioavailability of the drug, $F = 1$ for IV administration and hours (h)).

For drugs not given IV, these doses need to be divided by the bioavailability (F):
- **Maintenance dose** = [CL (L/h) × C_{ss} (mg/L) × τ (h)]/F

(Abbr.: *τ* represents the dosing interval, *Css* represents the desired steady-state plasma concentration of a specific drug and *F* the bioavailability of the drug, *F* < 1 for oral administration and dosing interval (h))

53.2.3 Targeted Pharmacotherapy

Targeted pharmacotherapy is also called "tailored, individualized, personalized, customized, precise," and the synonyms are all meant to describe optimal pharmacotherapy—in other words to maximize drug efficacy and drug safety in an individual patient and for a certain condition [18–21]. Tailored medicine allows physicians to treat people using a personalized approach. It uses genetic information, lifestyle and environment to tailor a treatment plan for every individual patient. Tailored medicine can also help doctors create individual prevention strategies. There are different ways to reach targeted therapy:

The pharmacokinetic concept (ADME) is applied to reach tailored medicine including the right dose and dosing interval. This approach is so-called kinetically guided therapy and is also known as therapeutic drug monitoring (TDM) [22]. To illustrate how the pharmacokinetic concept (ADME) determines kinetically guided therapy, it is important to remember the basic principles for drug administration:

53

- STEP 1: in general, the initial loading dose (LD) of drugs is based on the volume of distribution (Vd) followed by a maintenance dose (MD) based on total body clearance (CL).
  Within this context, TDM is often needed for individualization of drug dosing as patients do not have the same dose-concentration-exposure relationship due to changes in ADME, see also below [22]:
- STEP 2: for aminoglycosides such as gentamicin, the initial loading dose (LD) is based on weight (body size) and the maintenance dose (MD) on weight and renal function and guided by mathematical equations for drugs administered IV.
  For example, gentamicin is a hydrophilic drug, distributed in the extracellular space ("large Vd drug") and predominantly excreted as parent drug via glomerular filtration ("renal CL drug"), while only about 5% is reabsorbed via the renal tubules. TDM may improve efficacy and safety by using surrogate endpoints such as peak concentrations being 8–12 times higher than the minimal inhibitory concentration (MIC) of the pathogen for which gentamicin has been prescribed to assure optimal efficacy. To prevent toxicity, a trough concentration of less than 1–2 mg/L will be aimed for [23, 24]. This results in:
- STEP 3: aim at a C_{min} = 1–2 mg/L to avoid toxicity [19].
- STEP 4: aim at a C_{max}/MIC ≥ 8 (8–12, resp.) to reach optimal efficacy, and that goal is clearly dependent on the MIC of the pathogen that needs to be treated, and these values vary per country and per hospital.

Key step to achieve the right dosage regimen (dose and dosing interval) for IV administered drugs in general:
- the loading dose (LD) [mg/kg] must be *increased* if volume of distribution increases

$Vd\uparrow \rightarrow C_{max}\downarrow$
- the loading dose (LD) [mg/kg] must be *decreased* if volume of distribution decreases
  $Vd\downarrow \rightarrow C_{max}\uparrow$ [based on TDM (C_{max})]
- the maintenance dose (MD) rate [mg/h/kg] must be *increased* if the drug elimination increases: $CL\uparrow \rightarrow C_{min}\downarrow$ and $T_{1/2}$ are shortened (drugs administered IV continuously) and the dosing frequency must be increased (drugs administered IV intermittently)
- the maintenance dose (MD) rate [mg/h/kg] must be *decreased* if drug elimination decreases $CL\downarrow \rightarrow C_{min}\uparrow$ and $T_{1/2}$ are prolonged (drugs administered IV continuously) and the dosing frequency must be decreased (drugs administered IV intermittently) [based on TDM (C_{min})]

(Abbr.: C_{max} *(mg/L)* represents the maximum concentration of a drug after drug administration, C_{min} *(mg/L)* the minimum concentration a drug reaches before the next dose is administered, $T_{1/2}$ *(h)* is the elimination half-life exploring the time required for the Cpl of the drug to reach half of its original Cpl, *MIC* the minimum inhibitory concentration).

53.2.4 Pharmacokinetic Models

Pharmacokinetic models of different complexity (one or more compartments) have been developed to describe the area under the concentration-time curve (AUC) as determined by measuring several blood (plasma) drug concentrations (Cpls) over a predetermined time period. For instance, a one-compartment PK model has been successfully used for phenobarbital therapy in neonates treated for asphyxia with therapeutic hypothermia [25].

A two-compartment model is used for example for clavulanic acid, while a three-compartment model has been used to describe the PK of amoxicillin in PICU patients [26].

Population pharmacokinetic models are models based on PK/PD (Pop-PK/PD) at the population level using usually sparse data analysis (e.g. demographics, Cpls, PK/PD parameters) by a non-linear mixed-effects modelling approach (NONMEM): *Non-linear effects* mean that the dependent variables (e.g. Cpls) are non-linearly related to the model and independent variable(s), *mixed effects* similarly as fixed effects explain that parameters do not vary, while *random effects* mean that parameters vary across individuals [27, 28].

Finally, physiology-based PK models (PBPK) are more complex models in which current knowledge on developmental physiology is used to simulate drug concentration-time profiles of children, infants and neonates but these new models are also developed and used for predicting transplacental transfer of frequently used drugs by pregnant women [29, 30].

Regulatory agencies are nowadays demanding population PK, population PK-PD and/or PBPK information during the different stages of new drug development in the paediatric age range.

53.2.5 General Factors

The major determinants of drug disposition are absorption, distribution, metabolism and excretion (ADME).

Drug absorption is affected by many factors including the physicochemical properties of a drug (most drugs are weak organic acids or bases existing in either unionized or ionized form).

In case of orally administered drugs, absorption depends among others on gastric emptying, gastroesophageal reflux, gastric acid production, intestinal transit time, composition of the intestinal microbiome and surface, intestinal permeability and the first-pass effect.

Drug distribution is also affected by several factors. There are differences in the sizes of body compartments (proportion of total body water, extracellular fluids, adipose tissue and muscle mass), protein-binding capacity—e.g. plasma, tissues, erythrocytes [31], myocardium [32]. For example, propofol binding to erythrocytes is clinically important as 48% is bound to albumin and 50% to erythrocytes, and due to hypoalbuminemia or anaemia, the free fraction of propofol increases significantly, potentially leading to toxicity. Drug distribution depends also on plasma protein concentrations (α-acid glycoprotein, albumin) or on penetration across the barriers—for example, the immature blood-brain barrier is more permeable for some anticonvulsive drugs [33]. Additionally, the physicochemical properties of a drug play a role ("large" Vd drugs—e.g. lipophilic drugs distribute more likely to other tissues compared to "low" Vd drugs—e.g. hydrophilic drugs). For the developmental changes in body water compartments and body fat, see ◘ Fig. 53.1.

Drug elimination reflects drug metabolism and excretion.

53

Drug metabolism is characterized by various phenotypic variants and is affected by multiple factors (e.g. genetic, environmental, constitutional) [34]. Drugs are subject to three phases of drug metabolism [35]: phase I—hydrolysis, oxidation and reduction via cytochrome P450 iso-enzymes (CYP450), phase II—glucuronidation and acetylation via uridine 5′-diphospho-glucuronosyltransferases (UGTs), the sulfotransferases (SULTs) and the glutathione S-transferase (GTS) pathways [36, 37]. The transporter-mediated uptake of drugs into the hepatocytes and efflux into the bile reflects the phase III hepatic pathway by the organic anion transporting polypeptides (OATPs), organic anion transporters (OATs) and organic cation transporters (OCTs) [38]. Data on drug metabolism are taken either from experimental studies (studies in vitro on phenotypic expression of mRNA and protein activity) or from clinical studies focusing on metabolic ratio after administration of a drug (midazolam) [39] or the prodrug (a biologically inactive compound which can be metabolized in the body to produce an active drug (acyclovir) [40, 41]. There are about 15–20% of 57 known active CY*P450* human genes reported relevant and involved in drug metabolism in various organs such as the liver, the kidney, the intestine, the skin, the brain and the lung [42]. As a consequence, to date some prescription recommendations are based on pharmacogenetics as developed by phenotypic definitions: total amount of active alleles to metabolize the drug is expressed as ultra-rapid metabolizer (UM), rapid metabolizer (RM), extensive metabolizer (EM), intermediate metabolizer (IM) and poor metabolizer (PM). In 2014, the Clinical Pharmacogenetics

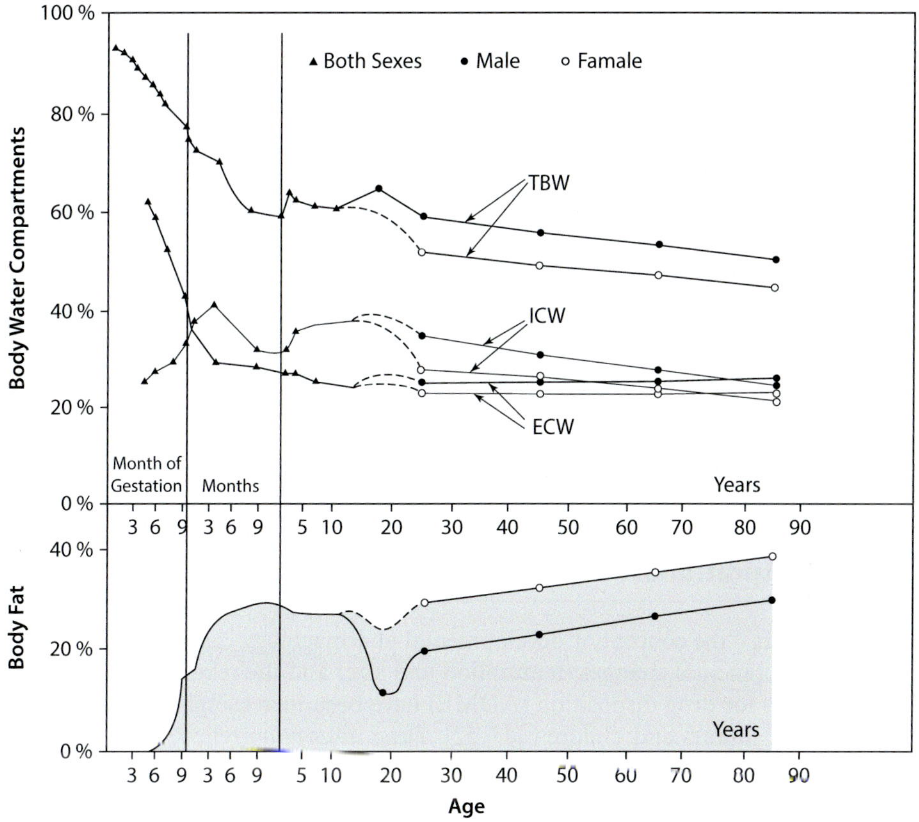

Fig. 53.1 A classical model of changes in body water compartments and body fat from early life to elderly [110]. *TBW* total body water, *ICW* intracellular water, *ECW* extracellular water and fat content of the body. (Adapted by Friis-Hansen B [110])

Implementation Consortium (CPIC) was established to translate genetic information about drug metabolism in daily clinical practice [43, 44]. For example, tramadol is metabolized to an active O-demethylated metabolite of tramadol acting as a potent μ-opioid agonist. However, in terms of PMs it is recommended to switch to another drug due to possible inadequate analgesic effect. The second example of drugs used in the PICU are proton pump inhibitors for those who are ultrarapid metabolizers (UMs) because effects may be insufficient due to an excessive high clearance and low plasma concentrations. In contrast to PMs of anticonvulsive drugs (phenytoin) in which the maintenance dose should be decreased up of 50% to avoid toxicity [45].

Drug excretion is the complex process involving the three major renal pathways: glomerular filtration rate (GFR) (free drugs and metabolites are filtered from plasma across the glomerular membrane into the urine), tubular reabsorption (drugs are reabsorbed from the tubule into the blood) and tubular excretion (the augmented passage of drugs from the plasma into the tubule by tubular transporters) [46]. Among other physiochemical drug properties, drug ionization is also important for the total amount of drug excreted from the body (urine pH determines the excretion of ionized acid or base drugs, while non-ionized drugs are reabsorbed from the tubule and excreted less).

Summary

- The primary PK parameters—Vd [L/kg] and CL [L/h/kg] are used to describe the main PK processes (distribution and elimination) for IV administered drugs.
- The primary PK parameters—Vd [L/kg] and CL [L/h/kg] are used to estimate the dosage adjustment: *the loading dose (LD) is guided by Vd* [L/kg] *and the maintenance dose (MD) rate by CL* [L/h/kg] *for IV administered drugs.*
- The major determinants of drug disposition (ADME) are responsible for pharmacological considerations: if the rate at which drugs are absorbed, distributed, metabolized or eliminated is changing, the dosage regimen needs to be adjusted.

53.3 Specific Aspects of Clinical Pharmacology

53.3.1 Maturational Factors

Over the years, "the concept of developmental pharmacology" as well as the impact of the developmental changes (maturation and size) and the relative roles of pharmacogenetics for drug disposition (ADME) have been increasingly applied to neonates, young infants and children [47–52]. *Drug absorption* reflects among others skin maturation processes, changes in body surface area (BSA) and changes in systemic bioavailability from the skin, the lung, the intestine and the rectum [53]. *Drug distribution* changes significantly during the first year primarily due to changes in relative percentage of total body water and fat to body weight, protein-binding capacity, membrane permeability and drug penetration across the barriers [33]. *Drug metabolism* develops uniquely over the years [34, 41]. The total CYP450 activity of foetal liver mostly expressed by SULT1A3/1A4 and CYP3A7 is about 30% and 60% of adult values. The activity of other CYP450 iso-enzymes is between 1 and 5% at birth and increases within weeks (CYP2C19—e.g. phenobarbital), months (CYP2E1—e.g. acetaminophen, CYP3A4—e.g. midazolam) and years (CYP1A2—e.g. caffeine, theophylline). Similarly, the UGT iso-enzymes (UGT1A9—e.g. acetaminophen) reaches adult activity by 10 years of age. Nevertheless, the high interindividual variability of expressed iso-enzymes is known due to genetic polymorphisms [54, 55]. *Drug excretion* is highly dependent on the processes of maturation of renal functions (increased renal perfusion). In a full-term neonate, the glomerular filtration rate (GFR) is about 10–20 mL/min/1.73 m^2 at birth, increases to 20–30 mL/min/1.73 m^2 during the first weeks of life and reaches adult values (70 mL/min/1.73 m^2) by 3–5 months and 6–12 months of age, respectively, while the tubular functions mature over the years [46].

Overall, the maturational factors ("almost predictable") may contribute to altered drug absorption—e.g. enhanced percutaneous absorption of corticoids [44] or povidone iodine occur in neonates [45], large drug distribution and low elimination—e.g. aminoglycosides [46] in the youngest population for review see [24]. The major maturational factors of drug disposition are summarized in (◘ Table S2).

For example, Vd (mg/L) of gentamicin is larger (due to age-related body compositions and enhanced the extracellular water), while CL (mg/L/kg) remains to be lower (due to immature and low renal excretion) in preterm neonates in comparison with full-term neonates or children or adults. So, these maturational changes determine in preterm neonates (GA ≤29 weeks, first week after birth) the once-daily dosage adjustment with higher LD (5 mg/kg) and lower MD rate (dosing interval of 48 h) of gentamicin the more immature the neonate is vs older children (2.5 mg/kg three times daily) [24].

53.3.2 Non-maturational Factors

Non-maturational factors of drug disposition (ADME) are superimposed on the developmental changes [56]. In the PICU, a multifactorial approach should be used and our knowledge of development, disease, treatment modality, comedication and genetics integrated in dose optimization [57]. The major non-maturational considerations during critical illness are related to the dynamic changes in physiological status (regional and systemic blood flow, body compartment proportions) and the physicochemical properties of a drug (drug solubility). These may lead to the variety of drug absorbing, distributing, metabolically transforming and eliminating multiple organ systems [58]. As a consequence, *drug absorption* may be altered or highly variable as it is known with orally administered sildenafil for the treatment of pulmonary hypertension (PH) in infants [59], *drug distribution* remains larger (hydrophilic drugs under sepsis)—e.g. ampicillin in neonates [60] or piperacillin/tazobactam in critically ill children [61, 62], while *drug elimination* reflects the state of the six primary eliminating organs for specific drugs (the lungs, skin, kidneys, liver, colon and lymph) and changes in drug metabolism during inflammation in the paediatric population [63, 64]. Finally, two major non-maturational factors were found to be relevant for drug elimination such as the decreased CYP 450 metabolic CL [65–67] and the increased (augmented) renal Cl [26, 68] under sepsis/systemic inflammatory response syndrome (SIRS) and are related to multiple organ failure syndrome. Within this concept, it is essential to identify biomarkers of acute renal failure (AKI) for drugs eliminated via the kidney and dose optimization under specific conditions [69, 70].

Hypothermia. The major pharmacological considerations [64] during therapeutic hypothermia (HT) [71] are related primarily to the physiological "adaptation" mechanisms lowering the body temperature (Tc) followed by rewarming. Changes in regional and systemic blood flow, enzymatic activity and compartment compositions, and also the impact of disease (post-cardiac arrest) [72] or the physicochemical properties of a drug are subject to several reviews [73]. Consequently, HT may contribute to decreased *drug distribution* (decreased peripheral compartment for lipophilic drugs) or reduced *drug elimination* (decreased metabolic capacity and organ perfusion for drugs eliminated via the liver or the kidneys) [74, 75]. This has been studied in a more systematic way by the Pharma Cool study group. This nationwide NICU-based study systematically evaluates the effects of HT on PK and PD of individual drugs [76]. HT does not affect PK of phenobarbital [77–79] apart from the influence of asphyxia severity [25], while CL has been found significantly reduced with amikacin excreted via kidney [80] or morphine metabolized in the liver [81].

ECMO. The major determinants of drug disposition (ADME) under extracorporeal membrane oxygenation (ECMO) [82] were reviewed for neonatal and paediatric ECMO populations (data *in vitro, in vivo* and *in silico*) [57, 83]. The pharmacological considerations are primarily related to drug-circuit interactions or priming volume and haemodilution. Vd increases due to drug sequestration by the ECMO circuit (e.g. lipophilic drugs are characterized by a higher octanol/water partition coefficient (log *P*) and tend to increase in drug loss in the circuit and larger Vd). ECMO-induced CL is variable and correlates more likely with many factors like ECMO-disease interactions. Recently, changes in drug disposition under ECMO have been found to be significant for analgesic and sedative drugs due to increased adsorption and Vd despite the new developed ECMO system [84, 85]. CL was highly influenced by renal replacement therapy (RRT) with clonidine [86] or strongly related to renal functions in case of vancomycin [87].

Renal replacement therapy (RRT) [88, 89]and *cardiopulmonary bypass* (CPB) [90] are the two treatment modalities with various impacts on drug disposition [81]. In summary, there are many factors they may influence PK of drugs such as continuous renal replacement therapy (CRRT) vs intermittent haemodialysis (IHD), the characteristics of the dialysis membrane(size), water solubility of drugs, protein-binding, the rate of blood flow and the duration of therapy with antimicrobials, for instance [89].

Overall, the non-maturational factors are responsible for changes in drug disposition (ADME) in neonates, infants and children under specific conditions and treatment modality compared to "control groups." These changes are highly variable and induced by many factors. For the major non-maturational factors of drug disposition, see (◘ Table S3).

53

For gentamicin, Vd (mg/L) in patients treated for severe sepsis remains to be much more variable or larger (due to changes in proportional body compositions and extremely enhanced extracellular water), while CL (mg/L/kg) of gentamicin remains either abnormal low (due to AKI or multiple organ failure or HT or PDA in neonates) or abnormal high (due to the augmented renal CL) compared with patient without severe sepsis. Therefore, the dosage regimen of gentamicin must be strongly individualized. So, the lower CL of gentamicin determines the extended once-daily dosage adjustment, while the higher LD (10 mg/kg) and prolonged dosing interval of gentamicin (dosing interval 48 h) of gentamicin are suggested to achieve efficacy (C_{max} of 15–20 mg/L) and to avoid toxicity (C_{min} <2 mg/L) of gentamicin (nephrotoxicity and ototoxicity) [91]. Compared to that previously reported dosage regimen using the LD (5 mg/kg) and the MD rate (dosing interval of 48 h) of gentamicin, (C_{max} <12 mg/L) and (C_{min} <2 mg/L) will be achieved in neonates [24] and 7 mg/kg in adults [92].

For amikacin, the first PD study evaluating outcome indicator sepsis in neonates was conducted by Sherwin [93], and the CL model proposed was based on weight and postmenstrual age. However, when this model was applied in the neonatal population including (weight 0.44–4.4 kg; PMA 24–41 weeks), CL ranges from 0.0155 to 0.428 L/h (which means 30-fold interindividual variability) and dose adjustment of amikacin did not reflect that high interindividual variability in CL, subsequently [94, 95].

Summary
- The major maturational factors of drug disposition are primarily responsible for differences in drug absorption, as well as a larger volume of distribution and a decreased total body clearance in neonates compared to infants, children and adults.
- The major non-maturational factors of drug disposition in addition to the developmental changes are responsible for additional changes in volume of distribution and total body clearance, necessitating further dosage adjustments.

53.4 Evidence-based Pharmacotherapy

53.4.1 Rational Use of Drugs

In 2019, the concept of the rational use of antimicrobials in neonates was introduced and the basic principles should be integrated in the PICU as the concept of overall rational use of specific drugs [96] see (◘ Fig. 53.2):
- Age-appropriate drug formulation
- Age-appropriate dose and dosing interval
- Accurate information of the drug
- Information of the drug indication
- Drug safety, efficacy, toxicity

53.4.2 Therapeutic Drug Monitoring

Therapeutic drug monitoring (TDM) is "the clinical practice of measuring specific drugs at designated intervals and use appropriate concentrations" [22]. TDM is relevant for neonates, infants and children [97, 98]. For example, Cpls of specific drugs (C_{min}, C_{max}) are used to avoid its toxicity (C_{min}—e.g. gentamicin), while (C_{max}) is used to achieve the maximum effect (C_{max}—e.g. gentamicin). The range of C_{min}–C_{max}) is

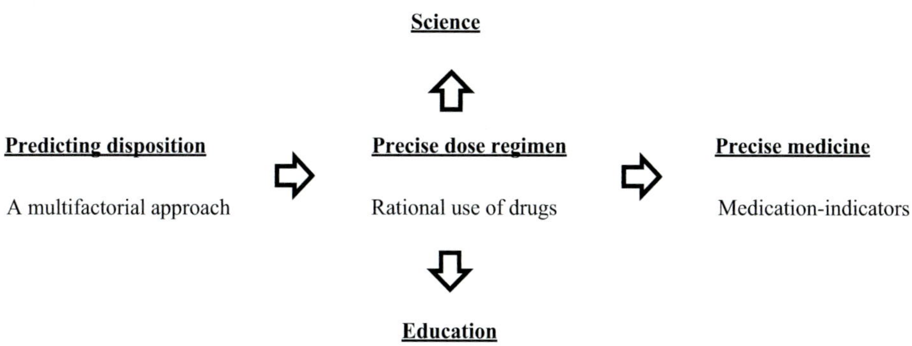

◘ **Fig. 53.2** Key steps to achieve goals of "precision medicine" in the paediatric intensive care unit (adapted by ESPNIC)

also called the therapeutic window. The most frequently monitored groups of drugs include aminoglycosides (gentamicin, amikacin, tobramycin), antipsychotics (quetiapine, risperidone), antidepressants (fluoxetine), glycopeptide (vancomycin), antiepileptics (valproate, lamotrigine and others), immunosuppressants (cyclosporine, methotrexate, mycophenolate mofetil), bronchodilators (theophylline, caffeine), cardiotonic drugs (digoxin), reverse transcriptase inhibitors (treatment of HIV infection), analgesics (paracetamol, acetylsalicylic acid)—used in toxicology, amiodarone, propranolol, etc. TDM is relevant to be used in the PICU for paediatric dosing [99] and pharmacology studies [100] (◘ Table S4) as the following considerations should be taken into account:

- *Patient-related*
  - preterm neonates, critically ill infants and children of all ages
- *Drug-related*
  - drugs with a narrow therapeutic window (aminoglycosides, vancomycin, digoxin)
  - insufficient drug response or adverse/toxic effects (phenobarbital, levetiracetam, valproate)
  - drug-drug interactions due to poor predictability of drug inducers/inhibitors (anticonvulsants)
- *Disease-related*
  - dynamically changing condition (sepsis, PDA, congenital heart diseases, seizures, multiple organ failure, AKI)
- *Treatment modality-related*
  - HT, ECMO, CBP, RRT
- *Miscellaneous*
  - poor predictability of PK/PD (congenital heart diseases)

53.4.3 Specific Drugs

This section will provide the readers with the systematic approach how the clinical pharmacology principles should be implemented in daily clinical practice in infants and children of all ages treated in the PICU.

In 2020, guidelines achieving therapeutic goals (the maximum efficacy and safety) are available for sepsis, septic shock [101, 102] and sepsis-associated organ dysfunction in neonates, infants and children [103]. For *antimicrobials,* the following guidelines to achieve the targeted therapy are: (1) prevention, (2) de-escalation and (3) antimicrobial dose optimization strategies (to improve efficacy/efficacy and prevent bacterial resistance) [104, 105]. Recently, the most used antimicrobials are β lactams, aminoglycosides and vancomycin in both NICU and PICU; however, evidence on dose optimization is for less than half of the papers [106]. TDM for antimicrobials [107], antifungals and antiviral drugs as well as the PBPK models using paediatric CL predictions [108] also for some "repurposed drugs"—e.g. chloroquine for SARS-CoV-2 in 2020 are recommended [109].

Take-Home Messages
To Date:
- Neonates, young infants and children are frequently exposed to off-label drugs, and large differences in treatment protocols exist between centres.
- Sparse evidence with large variations in assessment methods of medication errors and preventable ADRs are reported for both ICU settings.
- Lack of data published in international guidelines and recommendations still "prevent" a high level of evidence-based pharmacotherapy.
- Key steps towards achieving appropriate dose adjustments, drug efficacy and safety are based on successfully developed pharmacological concepts. These have been introduced, should be implemented and validated for ICU-dependent neonates, infants and children. "Take-Home Messages ends"

53.5 Conclusion

The multifactorial approach of drug prescriptions in the ICU is based on pharmacological concepts and increasingly applied to neonates, infants and children. This population should be considered as "pharmacologically" vulnerable, while the risk of known and unknown factors determining drug disposition is high. Prospectively conducted drug research supported by systematic knowledge and education remains a challenge.

Questions

Q1. *Which changes in drug disposition (ADME)* must be followed by the changes in dosage regimen (dose and dosing interval)—*four examples* must be listed at least (general recommendation)

Q2. How do *developmental factors* determine the right dosage regimen (dose and dosing interval)—*one example* must be listed for a neonate compared to an adult (age-appropriate recommendation)

Q3. How do *non-maturational* factors determine the right dose and dosing interval of a drug?—*one example* must be listed for a patient with or without condition (individualized recommendation)

Answers

A1. **Key step** towards achieving the right dosage regimen (dose and dosing interval) adjustment must be changed "precisely" in the following cases:
- the loading dose (LD) [mg/kg] must be *increased* if drug absorption decreases (K_a↓, T_{max}↑ and C_{max}↓, AUC↓) and/or if drug distribution increases (Vd↑, C_{max}↓)
- the loading dose (LD) [mg/kg] must be *decreased* if drug absorption increases (K_a↑, T_{max}↓ and C_{max}↑, AUC↑) and/or if drug distribution decreases (Vd↓, C_{max}↑)
- the maintenance dose (MD) [mg/kg] and the MD rate [mg/h/kg] must be *decreased* if drug elimination decreases (Cl↓, $T_{1/2}$↑, C_{min}↑) (drugs administered IV continuously) and the dosing frequency must be decreased (drugs administered IV intermittently)

- the maintenance dose (MD) [mg/kg] and the MD rate [mg/h/kg] must be *increased* if the drug elimination increases (Cl↑, $T_{1/2}$↓, C_{min}↓) (drugs administered IV continuously) and the dosing frequency must be increased (drugs administered IV intermittently)

A2. **Key step** towards achieving the right dosage regimen (dose and dosing interval) is based on *age-appropriate dose and dosing interval* adjusted for neonates, infants and children. For a neonate
- the loading dose (LD) [mg/kg] must be increased due to large Vd [L/kg]
- the maintenance dose (MD) [mg/kg] and a low MD rate [mg/h/kg] must be decreased due to low CL [L/h/kg]

A3. **Key step** towards achieving the right dosage regimen (dose and dosing interval) is based on *age-appropriate dosage regimen* adjusted for neonates, infants and children, however, should be *individualized* under specific condition correspondingly:
- the loading dose (LD) [mg/kg] must be increased/decreased due to large/decreased Vd [L/kg]
- the maintenance dose (MD) [mg/kg] and a low dose *maintenance* rate [mg/h/kg] must be increased/decreased due to increased = augmented/low CL [L/h/kg]

References

1. Lussky RC, Cifuentes RF, Siddappa AM. A history of neonatal medicine-past accomplishments, lessons learned, and future challenges. Part 1—the first century. J Pediatr Pharmacol Ther. 2005;10(2):76–89.
2. Lussky RC, Cifuentes RF, Siddappa AM. A history of neonatal medicine—Past accomplishments, lessons learned, and future challenges: part II—The 1990s, the new millennium, future challenges. J Pediatr Pharmacol Ther. 2005;10(3):143–58.
3. Carcillo JA. What's new in pediatric intensive care. Crit Care Med. 2006;34(9 Suppl):S183–90.
4. Czaja AS, Reiter PD, Schultz ML, Valuck RJ. Patterns of off-label prescribing in the pediatric intensive care unit and prioritizing future research. J Pediatr Pharmacol Ther. 2015;20(3):186–96.
5. Kouti L, Aletayeb M, Aletayeb SMH, Hardani AK, Eslami K. Pattern and extent of off-label and unlicensed drug use in neonatal intensive care units in Iran. BMC Pediatr. 2019;19(1):3.
6. Flint RB, van Beek F, Andriessen P, Zimmermann LJ, Liem KD, Reiss IKM, et al. Large differences in neonatal drug use between NICUs are common practice: time for consensus? Br J Clin Pharmacol. 2018;84(6):1313–23.
7. Costa H, Costa TX, Martins RR, Oliveira AG. Use of off-label and unlicensed medicines in neonatal intensive care. PLoS One. 2018;13(9):e0204427.
8. Nir-Neuman H, Abu-Kishk I, Toledano M, Heyman E, Ziv-Baran T, Berkovitch M. Unlicensed and off-label medication use in pediatric and neonatal intensive care units: no change over a decade. Adv Ther. 2018;35(7):1122–32.
9. Yang CP, Veltri MA, Anton B, Yaster M, Berkowitz ID. Food and Drug Administration approval for medications used in the pediatric intensive care unit: a continuing conundrum. Pediatr Crit Care Med. 2011;12(5):e195–9.
10. Frattarelli DA, Galinkin JL, Green TP, Johnson TD, Neville KA, Paul IM, et al. Off-label use of drugs in children. Pediatrics. 2014;133(3):563–7.
11. Schrier L, Hadjipanayis A, Stiris T, Ross-Russell RI, Valiulis A, Turner MA, et al. Off-label use of medicines in neonates, infants, children, and adolescents: a joint policy statement by the European Academy of Paediatrics and the European society for Developmental Perinatal and Pediatric Pharmacology. Eur J Pediatr. 2020;179(5):839–47.

12. Alghamdi AA, Keers RN, Sutherland A, Ashcroft DM. Prevalence and nature of medication errors and preventable adverse drug events in paediatric and neonatal intensive care settings: a systematic review. Drug Saf. 2019;42(12):1423–36.
13. Allan EL, Barker KN. Fundamentals of medication error research. Am J Hosp Pharm. 1990;47(3):555–71.
14. Billstein-Leber M, Carrillo CJD, Cassano AT, Moline K, Robertson JJ. ASHP guidelines on preventing medication errors in hospitals. Am J Health Syst Pharm. 2018;75(19):1493–517.
15. Allegaert K. Adverse drug events in pediatric intensive care are common, but improvement strategies exist and are effective. Rev Paul Pediatr. 2016;34(4):393–4.
16. Goldstein SL, Mottes T, Simpson K, Barclay C, Muething S, Haslam DB, et al. A sustained quality improvement program reduces nephrotoxic medication-associated acute kidney injury. Kidney Int. 2016;90(1):212–21.
17. Stoops C, Stone S, Evans E, Dill L, Henderson T, Griffin R, et al. Baby NINJA (nephrotoxic injury negated by just-in-time action): reduction of nephrotoxic medication-associated acute kidney injury in the neonatal intensive care unit. J Pediatr. 2019;215:223. 8.e6.
18. Scharplatz M, Puhan M, Steurer J, Bachmann LM. [Pharmacogenetics. Tailored therapy in medicine—opportunities and challenges]. Praxis (Bern 1994). 2004;93(10):359–65.
19. van den Anker J, Allegaert K. Clinical pharmacology in neonates and young infants: the benefit of a population-tailored approach. Expert Rev Clin Pharmacol. 2012;5(1):5–8.
20. Allegaert K. Neonates need tailored drug formulations. World J Clin Pediatr. 2013;2(1):1–5.
21. Leeder JS, Lantos J, Spielberg SP. Conference scene: pediatric pharmacogenomics and personalized medicine. Pharmacogenomics. 2010;11(12):1691–702.
22. Kang JS, Lee MH. Overview of therapeutic drug monitoring. Korean J Intern Med. 2009;24(1):1–10.
23. Kashuba AD, Bertino JS Jr, Nafziger AN. Dosing of aminoglycosides to rapidly attain pharmacodynamic goals and hasten therapeutic response by using individualized pharmacokinetic monitoring of patients with pneumonia caused by gram-negative organisms. Antimicrob Agents Chemother. 1998;42(7):1842–4.
24. Pacifici GM. Clinical pharmacokinetics of aminoglycosides in the neonate: a review. Eur J Clin Pharmacol. 2009;65(4):419–27.
25. Pokorna P, Posch L, Sima M, Klement P, Slanar O, van den Anker J, et al. Severity of asphyxia is a covariate of phenobarbital clearance in newborns undergoing hypothermia. J Matern Fetal Neonatal Med. 2019;32(14):2302–9.
26. De Cock PA, Standing JF, Barker CI, de Jaeger A, Dhont E, Carlier M, et al. Augmented renal clearance implies a need for increased amoxicillin-clavulanic acid dosing in critically ill children. Antimicrob Agents Chemother. 2015;59(11):7027–35.
27. Mould DR, Upton RN. Basic concepts in population modeling, simulation, and model-based drug development. CPT Pharmacometrics Syst Pharmacol. 2012;1:e6.
28. Mould DR, Upton RN. Basic concepts in population modeling, simulation, and model-based drug development—part 2: introduction to pharmacokinetic modeling methods. CPT Pharmacometrics Syst Pharmacol. 2013;2:e38.
29. Kuepfer L, Niederalt C, Wendl T, Schlender JF, Willmann S, Lippert J, et al. Applied concepts in PBPK modeling: how to build a PBPK/PD model. CPT Pharmacometrics Syst Pharmacol. 2016;5(10):516–31.
30. Hartmanshenn C, Scherholz M, Androulakis IP. Physiologically-based pharmacokinetic models: approaches for enabling personalized medicine. J Pharmacokinet Pharmacodyn. 2016;43(5):481–504.
31. Mazoit JX, Samii K. Binding of propofol to blood components: implications for pharmacokinetics and for pharmacodynamics. Br J Clin Pharmacol. 1999;47(1):35–42.
32. Robertson IM, Baryshnikova OK, Li MX, Sykes BD. Defining the binding site of levosimendan and its analogues in a regulatory cardiac troponin C-troponin I complex. Biochemistry. 2008;47(28):7485–95.
33. Cornford EM, Pardridge WM, Braun LD, Oldendorf WH. Increased blood–brain barrier transport of protein-bound anticonvulsant drugs in the newborn. J Cereb Blood Flow Metab. 1983;3(3):280–6.
34. Allegaert K, van den Anker JN, Naulaers G, de Hoon J. Determinants of drug metabolism in early neonatal life. Curr Clin Pharmacol. 2007;2(1):23–9.

35. Xu C, Li CY, Kong AN. Induction of phase I, II and III drug metabolism/transport by xenobiotics. Arch Pharm Res. 2005;28(3):249–68.
36. Hines RN, McCarver DG. The ontogeny of human drug-metabolizing enzymes: phase I oxidative enzymes. J Pharmacol Exp Ther. 2002;300(2):355–60.
37. McCarver DG, Hines RN. The ontogeny of human drug-metabolizing enzymes: phase II conjugation enzymes and regulatory mechanisms. J Pharmacol Exp Ther. 2002;300(2):361–6.
38. Roth M, Obaidat A, Hagenbuch B. OATPs, OATs and OCTs: the organic anion and cation transporters of the SLCO and SLC22A gene superfamilies. Br J Pharmacol. 2012;165(5):1260–87.
39. Klotz U. [Clinical pharmacology of midazolam]. Anaesthesiologie und Reanimation. 1989;14(6):347–354.
40. Wu KM. A new classification of prodrugs: regulatory perspectives. Pharmaceuticals (Basel). 2009;2(3):77–81.
41. Allegaert K, Verbesselt R, Rayyan M, Debeer A, de Hoon J. Urinary metabolites to assess in vivo ontogeny of hepatic drug metabolism in early neonatal life. Methods Find Exp Clin Pharmacol. 2007;29(4):251–6.
42. Ingelman-Sundberg M, Rodriguez-Antona C. Pharmacogenetics of drug-metabolizing enzymes: implications for a safer and more effective drug therapy. Philos Trans R Soc Lond B Biol Sci. 2005;360(1460):1563–70.
43. Caudle KE, Klein TE, Hoffman JM, Muller DJ, Whirl-Carrillo M, Gong L, et al. Incorporation of pharmacogenomics into routine clinical practice: the Clinical Pharmacogenetics Implementation Consortium (CPIC) guideline development process. Curr Drug Metab. 2014;15(2):209–17.
44. Zhou SQ, Skaar DJ, Jacobson PA, Huang RS. Pharmacogenomics of medications commonly used in the intensive care unit. Front Pharmacol. 2018;9:1436.
45. Klotz U. The role of pharmacogenetics in the metabolism of antiepileptic drugs: pharmacokinetic and therapeutic implications. Clin Pharmacokinet. 2007;46(4):271–9.
46. Lu H, Rosenbaum S. Developmental pharmacokinetics in pediatric populations. J Pediatr Pharmacol Ther. 2014;19(4):262–76.
47. Allegaert K, van de Velde M, van den Anker J. Neonatal clinical pharmacology. Paediatr Anaesth. 2014;24(1):30–8.
48. Kearns GL, Abdel-Rahman SM, Alander SW, Blowey DL, Leeder JS, Kauffman RE. Developmental pharmacology—drug disposition, action, and therapy in infants and children. N Engl J Med. 2003;349(12):1157–67.
49. Allegaert K. Developmental pharmacology—Special issues during childhood and adolescence. Drug Res (Stuttg). 2018;68(S1):S10–S1.
50. van den Anker J, Reed MD, Allegaert K, Kearns GL. Developmental changes in pharmacokinetics and pharmacodynamics. J Clin Pharmacol. 2018;58(Suppl 10):S10–25.
51. Lim SY, Pettit RS. Pharmacokinetic considerations in pediatric pharmacotherapy. Am J Health Syst Pharm. 2019;76(19):1472–80.
52. Leeder JS, Kearns GL, Spielberg SP, van den Anker J. Understanding the relative roles of pharmacogenetics and ontogeny in pediatric drug development and regulatory science. J Clin Pharmacol. 2010;50(12):1377–87.
53. Nicolas JM, Bouzom F, Hugues C, Ungell AL. Oral drug absorption in pediatrics: the intestinal wall, its developmental changes and current tools for predictions. Biopharm Drug Dispos. 2017;38(3):209–30.
54. Allegaert K, van Schaik RH, Vermeersch S, Verbesselt R, Cossey V, Vanhole C, et al. Postmenstrual age and CYP2D6 polymorphisms determine tramadol o-demethylation in critically ill neonates and infants. Pediatr Res. 2008;63(6):674–9.
55. Allegaert K, Vanhole C, Vermeersch S, Rayyan M, Verbesselt R, de Hoon J. Both postnatal and postmenstrual age contribute to the interindividual variability in tramadol glucuronidation in neonates. Early Hum Dev. 2008;84(5):325–30.
56. Allegaert K, Simons SHP, Tibboel D, Krekels EH, Knibbe CA, van den Anker JN. Non-maturational covariates for dynamic systems pharmacology models in neonates, infants, and children: filling the gaps beyond developmental pharmacology. Eur J Pharm Sci. 2017;109S:S27–31.
57. Raffaeli G, Pokorna P, Allegaert K, Mosca F, Cavallaro G, Wildschut ED, et al. Drug disposition and pharmacotherapy in neonatal ECMO: from fragmented data to integrated knowledge. Front Pediatr. 2019;7:360.

58. Boucher BA, Wood GC, Swanson JM. Pharmacokinetic changes in critical illness. Crit Care Clin. 2006;22(2):255–71. vi
59. Thakkar N, Gonzalez D, Cohen-Wolkowiez M, Massaro MM, Bernhardt J, Zane NR, et al. An opportunistic study evaluating pharmacokinetics of sildenafil for the treatment of pulmonary hypertension in infants. J Perinatol. 2016;36(9):744–7.
60. Kaplan JM, McCracken GH Jr, Horton LJ, Thomas ML, Davis N. Pharmacologic studies in neonates given large dosages of ampicillin. J Pediatr. 1974;84(4):571–7.
61. Cies JJ, Shankar V, Schlichting C, Kuti JL. Population pharmacokinetics of piperacillin/tazobactam in critically ill young children. Pediatr Infect Dis J. 2014;33(2):168–73.
62. Nichols K, Chung EK, Knoderer CA, Buenger LE, Healy DP, Dees J, et al. Population pharmacokinetics and pharmacodynamics of extended-infusion piperacillin and tazobactam in critically ill children. Antimicrob Agents Chemother. 2016;60(1):522–31.
63. Vet NJ, de Hoog M, Tibboel D, de Wildt SN. The effect of inflammation on drug metabolism: a focus on pediatrics. Drug Discov Today. 2011;16(9–10):435–42.
64. Carcillo JA, Doughty L, Kofos D, Frye RF, Kaplan SS, Sasser H, et al. Cytochrome P450 mediated-drug metabolism is reduced in children with sepsis-induced multiple organ failure. Intensive Care Med. 2003;29(6):980–4.
65. Brussee JM, Vet NJ, Krekels EHJ, Valkenburg AJ, Jacqz-Aigrain E, van Gerven JMA, et al. Predicting CYP3A-mediated midazolam metabolism in critically ill neonates, infants, children and adults with inflammation and organ failure. Br J Clin Pharmacol. 2018;84(2):358–68.
66. Vet NJ, de Hoog M, Tibboel D, de Wildt SN. The effect of critical illness and inflammation on midazolam therapy in children. Pediatr Crit Care Med. 2012;13(1):e48–50.
67. Vet NJ, Brussee JM, de Hoog M, Mooij MG, Verlaat CW, Jerchel IS, et al. Inflammation and organ failure severely affect midazolam clearance in critically ill children. Am J Respir Crit Care Med. 2016;194(1):58–66.
68. Dhont E, Van Der Heggen T, De Jaeger A, Vande Walle J, De Paepe P, De Cock PA. Augmented renal clearance in pediatric intensive care: are we undertreating our sickest patients? Pediatr Nephrol. 2020;35(1):25–39.
69. Zwiers AJ, de Wildt SN, Hop WC, Dorresteijn EM, Gischler SJ, Tibboel D, et al. Acute kidney injury is a frequent complication in critically ill neonates receiving extracorporeal membrane oxygenation: a 14-year cohort study. Crit Care. 2013,17(4):R151.
70. Buijs EA, Zwiers AJ, Ista E, Tibboel D, de Wildt SN. Biomarkers and clinical tools in critically ill children: are we heading toward tailored drug therapy? Biomark Med. 2012;6(3):239–57.
71. Jacobs SE, Berg M, Hunt R, Tarnow-Mordi WO, Inder TE, Davis PG. Cooling for newborns with hypoxic ischaemic encephalopathy. Cochrane Database Syst Rev. 2013;2013(1):CD003311.
72. Arpino PA, Greer DM. Practical pharmacologic aspects of therapeutic hypothermia after cardiac arrest. Pharmacotherapy. 2008;28(1):102–11.
73. Zanelli S, Buck M, Fairchild K. Physiologic and pharmacologic considerations for hypothermia therapy in neonates. J Perinatol. 2011;31(6):377–86.
74. Pokorna P, Wildschut ED, Vobruba V, van den Anker JN, Tibboel D. The impact of hypothermia on the pharmacokinetics of drugs used in neonates and young infants. Curr Pharm Des. 2015;21(39):5705–24.
75. van den Broek MP, Groenendaal F, Egberts AC, Rademaker CM. Effects of hypothermia on pharmacokinetics and pharmacodynamics: a systematic review of preclinical and clinical studies. Clin Pharmacokinet. 2010;49(5):277–94.
76. de Haan TR, Bijleveld YA, van der Lee JH, Groenendaal F, van den Broek MP, Rademaker CM, et al. Pharmacokinetics and pharmacodynamics of medication in asphyxiated newborns during controlled hypothermia. The PharmaCool multicenter study. BMC Pediatr. 2012;12:45.
77. Shellhaas RA, Ng CM, Dillon CH, Barks JD, Bhatt-Mehta V. Population pharmacokinetics of phenobarbital in infants with neonatal encephalopathy treated with therapeutic hypothermia. Pediatr Crit Care Med. 2013;14(2):194–202.
78. van den Broek MP, Groenendaal F, Toet MC, van Straaten HL, van Hasselt JG, Huitema AD, et al. Pharmacokinetics and clinical efficacy of phenobarbital in asphyxiated newborns treated with hypothermia: a thermopharmacological approach. Clin Pharmacokinet. 2012;51(10):671–9.
79. Sima M, Pokorna P, Hartinger J, Slanar O. Estimation of initial phenobarbital dosing in term neonates with moderate-to-severe hypoxic ischaemic encephalopathy following perinatal asphyxia. J Clin Pharm Ther. 2018;43(2):196–201.

80. Cristea S, Smits A, Kulo A, Knibbe CAJ, van Weissenbruch M, Krekels EHJ, et al. Amikacin pharmacokinetics to optimize dosing in neonates with perinatal asphyxia treated with hypothermia. Antimicrob Agents Chemother. 2017;61(12)
81. Favie LMA, Groenendaal F, van den Broek MPH, Rademaker CMA, de Haan TR, van Straaten HLM, et al. Pharmacokinetics of morphine in encephalopathic neonates treated with therapeutic hypothermia. PLoS One. 2019;14(2):e0211910.
82. Bartlett RH, Gazzaniga AB, Toomasian J, Coran AG, Roloff D, Rucker R. Extracorporeal membrane oxygenation (ECMO) in neonatal respiratory failure. 100 cases. Ann Surg. 1986;204(3):236–45.
83. Di Nardo M, Wildschut ED. Drugs pharmacokinetics during veno-venous extracorporeal membrane oxygenation in pediatrics. J Thorac Dis. 2018;10(Suppl 5):S642–S52.
84. Wildschut ED, Ahsman MJ, Allegaert K, Mathot RA, Tibboel D. Determinants of drug absorption in different ECMO circuits. Intensive Care Med. 2010;36(12):2109–16.
85. Zeilmaker GA, Pokorna P, Mian P, Wildschut ED, Knibbe CAJ, Krekels EHJ, et al. Pharmacokinetic considerations for pediatric patients receiving analgesia in the intensive care unit; targeting postoperative, ECMO and hypothermia patients. Expert Opin Drug Metab Toxicol. 2018;14(4):417–28.
86. Kleiber N, Mathot RAA, Ahsman MJ, Wildschut ED, Tibboel D, de Wildt SN. Population pharmacokinetics of intravenous clonidine for sedation during paediatric extracorporeal membrane oxygenation and continuous venovenous hemofiltration. Br J Clin Pharmacol. 2017;83(6):1227–39.
87. Lonabaugh KP, Lunsford KJ, Fang GY, Kaufman DA, Addison SD, Buck ML. Vancomycin dosing in pediatric extracorporeal membrane oxygenation: potential impacts of new technologies. J Pediatr Pharmacol Ther. 2017;22(5):358–63.
88. Bugge JF. Pharmacokinetics and drug dosing adjustments during continuous venovenous hemofiltration or hemodiafiltration in critically ill patients. Acta Anaesthesiol Scand. 2001;45(8):929–34.
89. Bugge JF. Influence of renal replacement therapy on pharmacokinetics in critically ill patients. Best Pract Res Clin Anaesthesiol. 2004;18(1):175–87.
90. van Saet A, de Wildt SN, Knibbe CA, Bogers AD, Stolker RJ, Tibboel D. The effect of adult and pediatric cardiopulmonary bypass on pharmacokinetic and pharmacodynamic parameters. Curr Clin Pharmacol. 2013;8(4):297–318.
91. Lanao JM, Calvo MV, Mesa JA, Martin-Suarez A, Carbajosa MT, Miguelez F, et al. Pharmacokinetic basis for the use of extended interval dosage regimens of gentamicin in neonates. J Antimicrob Chemother. 2004;54(1):193–8.
92. Cobussen M, Stassen PM, Posthouwer D, van Tiel FH, Savelkoul PHM, Havenith T, et al. Improving peak concentrations of a single dose regime of gentamicin in patients with sepsis in the emergency department. PLoS One. 2019;14(1):e0210012.
93. Sherwin CM, Svahn S, Van der Linden A, Broadbent RS, Medlicott NJ, Reith DM. Individualised dosing of amikacin in neonates: a pharmacokinetic/pharmacodynamic analysis. Eur J Clin Pharmacol. 2009;65(7):705–13.
94. van den Anker JN, Allegaert K. Individualized dosing of aminoglycosides in neonates: mission accomplished or work in progress? Eur J Clin Pharmacol. 2009;65(11):1159–60.
95. De Cock RF, Allegaert K, Sherwin CM, Nielsen EI, de Hoog M, van den Anker JN, et al. A neonatal amikacin covariate model can be used to predict ontogeny of other drugs eliminated through glomerular filtration in neonates. Pharm Res. 2014;31(3):754–67.
96. van den Anker J, Allegaert K. Rational use of antibiotics in neonates: still in search of tailored tools. Healthcare (Basel). 2019;7(1):28.
97. Pauwels S, Vermeersch P, Desmet K, Vanstapel F. Practice-oriented quality specifications for therapeutic drug monitoring. Clin Chem. 2014;60(3):559–60.
98. Koren G. Therapeutic drug monitoring principles in the neonate. National Academy of CLinical Biochemistry. Clin Chem. 1997;43(1):222–7.
99. Bartelink IH, Rademaker CM, Schobben AF, van den Anker JN. Guidelines on paediatric dosing on the basis of developmental physiology and pharmacokinetic considerations. Clin Pharmacokinet. 2006;45(11):1077–97.
100. Thakkar N, Salerno S, Hornik CP, Gonzalez D. Clinical pharmacology studies in critically ill children. Pharm Res. 2017;34(1):7–24.

101. Weiss SL, Peters MJ, Alhazzani W, Agus MSD, Flori HR, Inwald DP, et al. Surviving sepsis campaign international guidelines for the management of septic shock and sepsis-associated organ dysfunction in children. Intensive Care Med. 2020;46(Suppl 1):10–67.
102. Weiss SL, Peters MJ, Alhazzani W, Agus MSD, Flori HR, Inwald DP, et al. Executive summary: surviving sepsis campaign international guidelines for the management of septic shock and sepsis-associated organ dysfunction in children. Intensive Care Med. 2020;46(Suppl 1):1–9.
103. Fuchs A, Bielicki J, Mathur S, Sharland M, Van Den Anker JN. Reviewing the WHO guidelines for antibiotic use for sepsis in neonates and children. Paediatr Int Child Health. 2018;38(sup1):S3–S15.
104. Fontela PS, Quach C, Karim ME, Willson DF, Gilfoyle E, McNally JD, et al. Determinants of antibiotic tailoring in pediatric intensive care: a national survey. Pediatr Crit Care Med. 2017;18(9):e395–405.
105. van Donge T, Bielicki JA, van den Anker J, Pfister M. Key components for antibiotic dose optimization of sepsis in neonates and infants. Front Pediatr. 2018;6:325.
106. Hartman SJF, Bruggemann RJ, Orriens L, Dia N, Schreuder MF, de Wildt SN. Pharmacokinetics and target attainment of antibiotics in critically ill children: a systematic review of current literature. Clin Pharmacokinet. 2020;59(2):173–205.
107. Brinkmann A, Rohr AC, Koberer A, Fuchs T, Preisenberger J, Kruger WA, et al. [Therapeutic drug monitoring and individual dosing of antibiotics during sepsis: modern or just "trendy"?]. Med Klin Intensivmed Notfmed. 2018;113(2):82–93.
108. Calvier EAM, Nguyen TT, Johnson TN, Rostami-Hodjegan A, Tibboel D, Krekels EHJ, et al. Can population modelling principles be used to identify key PBPK parameters for paediatric clearance predictions? An innovative application of optimal design theory. Pharm Res. 2018;35(11):209.
109. Smit C, Peeters MYM, van den Anker JN, Knibbe CAJ. Chloroquine for SARS-CoV-2: implications of its unique pharmacokinetic and safety properties. Clin Pharmacokinet. 2020;59(6):659–69.
110. Friis-Hansen B. Body composition during growth. In vivo measurements and biochemical data correlated to differential anatomical growth. Pediatrics. 1971;47(1):Suppl 2:264+.

Further Reading

Yaffe SJ, Aranda CV. Neonatal and paediatric pharmacology: therapeutic principles in practice, 4th ed. isbn-13:978-0781795388

Continuous Kidney Replacement Therapy in Children

Mehak Bansal, Zaccaria Ricci, and Akash Deep

Contents

J. Brierley et al. (eds.), *ESPNIC Children's Intensive Care Textbook*,
https://doi.org/10.1007/978-3-031-64762-8_54

Learning Objectives

In this chapter, we will discuss the basic concepts of kidney replacement therapy in children with acute kidney injury. The indications of commencing kidney replacement therapy and the appropriate timing of initiation of kidney replacement therapy will be addressed in detail. The reader will also get an in-depth information of the various modalities, dose, and anticoagulation of kidney replacement therapy. Advantages and complications of each modality will also be discussed along with brief mention of challenges of delivering kidney replacement therapy in a pandemic state and in the neonatal period.

54.1 Introduction

Acute kidney injury (AKI) frequently occurs in children getting admitted to pediatric intensive care unit and requires initiation of kidney replacement therapy (KRT) of many patients. The decision to initiate KRT is quite complex and depends on both patient- and center-specific factors. Commencement of KRT warrants consideration on crucial issues like patient's hemodynamic stability, time to initiate KRT, which modality to choose, type of catheter, dose of KRT, and anticoagulation. Peritoneal dialysis continues to be the modality of choice for long-term KRT in cases of children with end-stage renal disease, but in cases of AKI, with the advancement in technology, there has been an increased emphasis on using continuous KRT (CKRT). In this chapter, we will be discussing various aspects of KRT in children.

54.2 Early Development

In 1977, Kramer et al demonstrated the efficacy of a unique system for ultrafiltration in patients with fluid overload [1]. The device consisted of a capillary hemofilter which utilized the patient's systemic arterial blood pressure to drive ultrafiltration. This novel technique, termed continuous arteriovenous hemofiltration (CAVH), was initially adopted as a technology independent alternative to hemodialysis. Over the last 25 years, the technology introduced by Peter Kramer has evolved and has been modified further to provide both convective and diffusive exchange of solutes for enhanced solute clearance. In order to achieve predictable and controlled ultrafiltration, pump-assisted systems were developed in early 1990s and replaced arterial blood pressure-driven systems. These pump-assisted techniques have collectively come to be known as continuous venovenous hemofiltration (CVVH). In the last decade, elaborate CVVH devices with added safety, ultrafiltration, and thermal control mechanisms have been introduced in clinical practice. These devices are a far cry from the simplistic design envisioned by Peter Kramer.

54.3 Mechanisms of Solute Removal in KRT

All the modalities of KRT—peritoneal dialysis (PD), intermittent hemodialysis (IHD), or continuous renal replacement therapy (CKRT)—are based on the transport of water and solutes across a semipermeable membrane in order to discard the waste products of the body and replace the excretory functions of the kidney. The four major transport mechanisms involved in KRT are ultrafiltration, diffusion, convection, and adsorption.

Ultrafiltration—It refers to the fluid removal driven by the hydrostatic pressure across a semipermeable membrane. The ultrafiltration rate depends upon the hydraulic permeability of the membrane, surface area of the membrane, and transmembrane pressure.

Diffusion—In diffusion, a dialysate fluid is administered on one side of the semipermeable membrane and the movement of the solutes occurs from high concentration to low concentration, resulting in equilibrium of the solute across the membrane via random Brownian motion. Usually, the dialysate is run counter-current to the blood flow to allow a sustained solute gradient and ensure more effective clearance. The amount of solute cleared depends on the concentration gradient and the size of the molecule. Diffusion is more effective in clearing low-molecular-weight solutes like urea and creatinine as opposed to high-molecular-weight solutes like cytokines and beta2 microglobulin.

Convection—It is the movement of the solutes across the semipermeable membrane by force of water, also termed as the solvent drag. The movement of the solute across the membrane depends upon the charge and size of the solute and the size of the pores of the semipermeable membrane. If a sterile solution is introduced pre- or post-membrane in the CKRT circuit (CVVH), a pressure gradient is generated, which promotes solvent drag across the membrane. The capability of the solute to cross the semipermeable membrane via convection is termed as sieving coefficient. It is the ratio of solute concentration in the effluent and the blood. The sieving coefficient can decline over a period of time as the large molecules can accumulate across the membrane surface, reducing the size of the pores. Convection facilitates the movement of moderate-sized molecules using solvent drag.

Adsorption—This mechanism removes the solutes from the blood as the solutes adhere to the membrane in the extracorporeal circuit. Adsorption can hence contribute to large size molecule removal, and the removal varies with size, charge, the structure of the molecule, and the characteristics of the semipermeable membrane. The removal of the solute via adsorption decreases with time as the membrane becomes saturated with the solutes.

54.4 Modalities of KRT

KRT can be intermittent or continuous, depending on the duration of treatment. Intermittent therapy lasts for less than 24 h; however, continuous therapy substitutes kidney functions for an extended period of time and continues for at least 24 h/day (◘ Fig. 54.1). The subcategories of CKRT are based on the primary methods of solute clearance. In slow continuous ultrafiltration (SCUF), the ultrafiltration removes the fluid from the blood and is applied to treat fluid overload. Solute removal is minimal in this technique due to slow rate of ultrafiltration (low rate of convection) and lack of dialysis. In continuous venovenous hemofiltration (CVVH), a replacement fluid is added pre- and/or post-filter and uses higher rates of convection for solute clearance. Continuous venovenous hemodialysis (CVVHD) uses dialysate

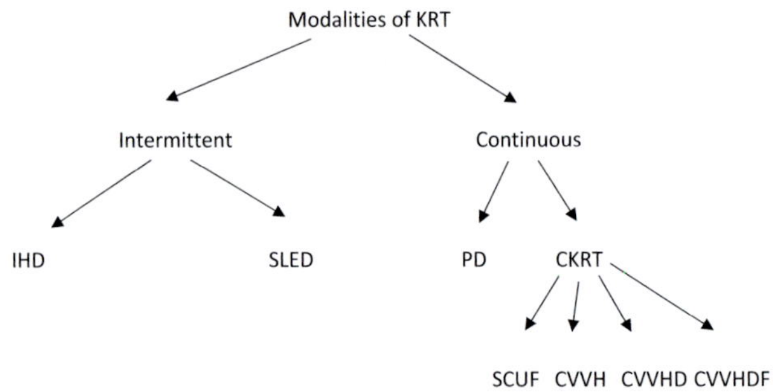

Fig. 54.1 Classification of modalities of renal replacement therapy (KRT) in children. *IHD* Intermittent—intermittent hemodialysis, *SLED* slow low efficiency dialysis, *PD* continuous—peritoneal dialysis, *SCUF* slow continuous ultrafiltration, *CKRT* continuous kidney replacement therapy, *CVVH* continuous venovenous hemofiltration, *CVVHD* continuous venovenous dialysis, *CVVHD* continuous venovenous hemodiafiltration

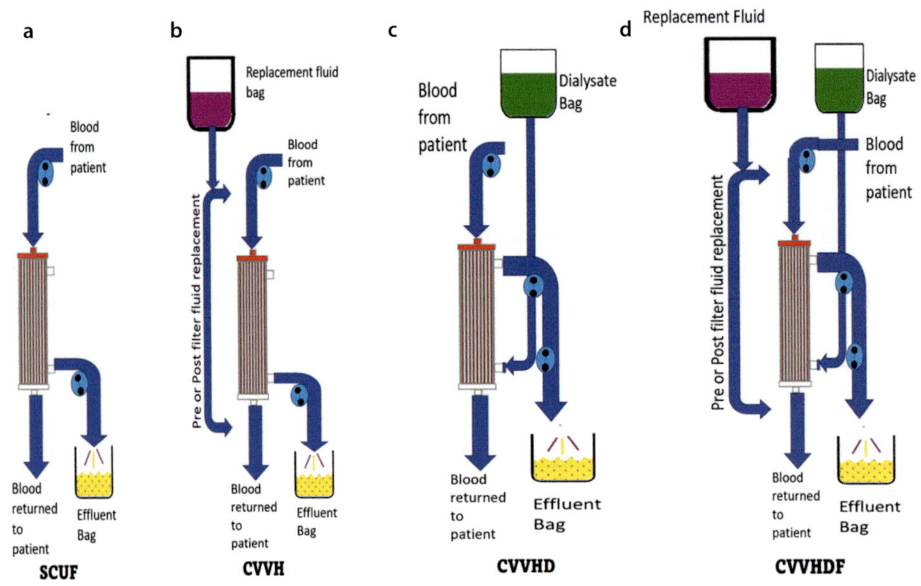

Fig. 54.2 Schematic diagram of various modalities of continuous kidney replacement therapy (CKRT). (**a**) Slow continuous ultrafiltration (SCUF) uses mechanism of ultrafiltration to remove the fluid from the blood. (**b**) Continuous venovenous hemofiltration (CVVH) uses convection for solute clearance and utilizes replacement fluid which is added pre- and post-filter. (**c**) Continuous venovenous hemodialysis (CVVHD) uses diffusive clearance and requires dialysate fluid. (**d**) Continuous venovenous hemodiafiltration (CVVHDF) uses **b** combined convection and diffusive clearance and requires both replacement and dialysate fluid

54

fluid to achieve diffusive clearance, and continuous venovenous hemodiafiltration (CVVHDF) uses both replacement and dialysate fluid for combined convection and diffusive clearance (Fig. 54.2).

The optimal modality for KRT is based on indication of the dialysis child's weight and size, overall clinical status, performance of the modality used, availability of the resources, and the expertise of the unit [2]. The decision to initiate intermittent or CKRT also depends upon the hemodynamic status of the child, with continuous modes being preferred in hemodynamically unstable patients. The availability of vascular access or the condition of the peritoneal membrane also determines the modality used. Two major studies done on children receiving KRT in pediatric intensive care units (PICU) of UK and United States demonstrated that CKRT was the preferred modality in children and was done in 57.9% and 46.5% of the total cases, respectively [3, 4]. PD was less commonly used but was the preferred modality in neonates and post-cardiac surgery infants. CKRT is nowadays preferred as it allows gradual fluid and solute clearance and is better tolerated in hemodynamically unstable patients as compared to IHD. When compared to PD, CKRT allows more accurate fluid removal, better control of ultrafiltration and the blood flow rates, along with the capability to adjust the composition of extracellular fluid. Among CKRT-based therapies, CVVH is believed to remove more of medium- and large-sized molecules because of convective-based clearance. Therefore, many nephrologists and intensivists prefer CVVH over diffusion-based clearance; however, we have insufficient data to prove it [5, 6].

54.5 Indications of KRT

The absolute indications of KRT are summarized in ◘ Table 54.1. The indications for KRT in sick children can be renal or nonrenal. A report from prospective pediatric continuous renal replacement therapy (ppCRRT) registry, which analyzed CKRT data from 13 centers in the United States, revealed that about 86% of the CKRTs were performed for renal indications (fluid overload and electrolyte disturbances), whereas the rest 15% of the CKRTs was done for nonrenal indications, such as drug intoxication, inborn errors of metabolism, and tumor lysis syndrome [1]. Nowadays, majority of the cases of AKI that receive KRT are associated with sepsis and multiorgan dysfunction and fluid overload [3].

◘ Table 54.1 Absolute indications of KRT

1. Fluid overload resistant to diuretics
2. Severe metabolic acidosis refractory to medical management
3. Hyperkalemia refractory to medical management
4. Uremic encephalopathy
Other indications for KRT
5. Poisoning with a dialyzable drug or toxin
6. Life-threatening electrolyte derangements not responding to medical management
7. Progressive azotemia or oliguria not responding to medical management

54.6 Timing of Initiation of KRT

In the absence of absolute indications of initiation of KRT, the decision to initiate KRT can be challenging. Theoretically, early initiation of KRT allows better control of metabolic disturbances, early removal of waste products, and excess fluid from the patient, which should improve outcomes in a patient with AKI. Furthermore, studies have demonstrated that 10–20% fluid overload at the time of initiation of CKRT was associated with increased mortality, laying emphasis on the early CKRT for fluid removal and providing room for adequate nutrition, medications, and blood products. A seminal publication from ppCRRT registry evaluated the impact of fluid overload in 297 patients and demonstrated 29.6% mortality in <10% fluid overload at the time of initiation of CKRT, 43.1% in cases with 10–20% fluid overload, and 65.6% mortality in cases with more than 20% fluid overload [7]. Zarbock et al. also showed survival benefit with early KRT initiation in patients with fluid overload and Neutrophil gelatinase-associated lipocalin (NGAL)-positive AKI further reiterating the early initiation of KRT in cases of fluid overload [8]. However, KRT can also expose the children to iatrogenic complications, such as bleeding, hypotension, infections, and hypothermia. A recent multinational randomized controlled trial—STAART AKI trial concluded that an accelerated renal replacement therapy was not associated with lower mortality at 90 days as compared to adult patients who received standard therapy [9]. Also, another study by Gaudry et al. reiterated that the timing of initiation has no survival benefit in patients with severe AKI in the absence of urgent indications to start KRT, further emphasizing that meticulous monitoring of patient with AKI can reduce the use of KRT and the complications associated with it [10]. It has currently not been established if timing of KRT in frail pediatric critically ill children may follow different indications and if in these patients an accelerated initiation of dialysis could be beneficial. Retrospective studies are only available so far and show that in children who started CKRT, those who received it closer to the admission day had a better outcome. These findings should be confirmed by a prospective pediatric trial.

Hence, given the possibility of risk factors involved in delaying the use of KRT in KDIGO stage 3 patient and considering the benefits of early KRT in patients with fluid accumulation, along with reduced risk of complications in delivering CKRT in today's practice, a personalized approach is warranted while starting KRT in critically sick children.

54.7 CKRT Devices–CKRT Devices

Several devices are now available commercially for use in CKRT modalities. The choice of CKRT device in children depends on the availability, cost, and local expertise. These devices are based on the principle that a high hydraulic permeability hemofilter connected to the patient's central venous access via a circuit is utilized to ultrafilter plasma in a slow but continuous manner. In most of the available CKRT machines, a peristaltic "arterial pump" helps to pump blood into the extracorporeal circuit and also to generate the hydrostatic pressure necessary for ultrafiltration in the hemofilter. Following ultrafiltration and convective solute exchange in the hemofilter, the blood is returned to the patient through the "venous" port of the vascular access. The dialysate used for diffusive solute clearance is pumped into and out of the hemofilter via its side-ports. The dialysate is separated from the blood by the hemofilter capillary membrane and flows in a counter-current path to the flow of the blood inside the capillary column. The flow of the dialysate into the hemofilter is controlled with one pump, while another pump administers the replacement filter into the extracorporeal circuit at the pre- or post-hemofilter location.

Pulsatile or piston action intravenous pumps (IV) were used in early versions of CKRT devices in order to control ultrafiltration rate during the procedure. These pumps can have error rate of up to 30%, are inaccurate for control of ultrafiltration, and have been largely abandoned. Ultrafiltration control error in the newer CKRT devices is only 1–2% of total ultrafiltration, resulting in improved control of therapy goals. Current generation of CKRT devices also provides for plug-in warming modules for the blood pathway, thus reducing the possibility of hypothermia.

Though a number of CKRT devices are available across the globe from different manufacturers, with distinctive features, the main issues of running CKRT in children are higher circuit extracorporeal volumes as compared to child's blood volume and relative higher blood flows, but most of the current devices designed for adults have been adapted for pediatric use with smaller lines and circuits. Currently, several pediatric specific devices are being created, which may revolutionize the pediatric CKRT practice.

Vascular Access—The success of the CKRT highly depends upon the quality of vascular access, which can be very challenging particularly in case of neonates and infants. The vascular access should ensure adequate blood flow to generate proper access and return pressures and to prevent related complications. By and large, as defined by the Poiseuille's law, the resistance in a tube is directly proportional to the length of the tube and inversely proportional to the fourth power of the radius. Therefore, the widest and the shortest vascular catheter will ensure adequate blood flow. The site of the vascular placement also determines the quality of the vascular access. The internal jugular vein (IJV) is preferred (right over left IJV) in view of its large caliber, direct entry to superior vena cava, and lower rates of recirculation. Femoral veins are easy to access, but not ideal and are considered the second choice, as they are associated with higher recirculation rates and flow interference secondary to movement of the children and increased intraabdominal pressure. In a child at risk for long-term KRT treatment, subclavian vein cannulation should be avoided due to high risk of stenosis at the puncture site, which may interfere with the future attempts of forming an arteriovenous graft or fistula in future, in case the patient develops chronic kidney disease. The ppCRRT registry evaluated the effect of size and location of the vascular access on the functional survival of CKRT circuit and found that circuit survival was significantly higher in larger-diameter catheters and when the vascular catheter was placed in IJV as compared to subclavian and femoral veins. In this study, the 48-h survival of 8 French catheters was higher (76%) as compared to 26% with 7 French catheters, and 5 French catheters were associated with poorest survival [11]. Neonates can accommodate a 7 French catheters in IJV in a relatively easy way, for running CKRT [12]. However, smaller catheters have been proposed by other authors to run neonatal dialysis and they provided acceptable results, in terms of filter life, down to 5 French.

Temporary uncuffed catheters are inserted at the bedside percutaneously. If the use of catheter is anticipated to last for more than few weeks, a tunneled, cuffed, double lumen catheter can be preferred [13]. The Kidney Disease: Improving Global Outcomes (KDIGO) guideline recommends the use of bedside ultrasound to obtain vascular access as it significantly reduces the risk of catheter placement failure and the complications, such as hematoma, arterial puncture, and thrombosis, associated with the catheter placement [14]. Also, the time taken for successful cannulation is also significantly reduced with use of real time ultrasound [15]. ◘ Table 54.2 shows recommended weight-based temporary catheter sizes in children. Daily assessment should be done regarding the need for the dialysis catheter, and it should be removed as soon as it is no longer required or replaced with more permanent access if long-term KRT treatment is predicted.

Hemofilter—There are various types of hemofilters available with various thickness, pore size, charge, and adsorptive features that determine the extent of solute removal. In general, hemofilter must be proportionate to patient's body surface area. Additional factor that needs to be considered while choosing the hemofilter is the priming volume of the hemofilter. AN-69 is a polyacrylonitrile membrane, which is preferred, as it has a higher sieving coefficient and a greater ability to remove the inflammatory mediators and the cytokines. However, it is associated with the release of bradykinin release syndrome especially when used with blood prime. It causes abrupt hypotension 5–10 min after the initiation of CKRT and can be prevented by buffering the blood to physiological pH while priming the circuit or by avoiding the use of AN-69 circuit. Other membrane available is polyarylethersulfone membranes (PAES), which is not associated with bradykinin release syndrome. The only available PAES membrane in pediatrics is HF 20 filter with a surface area of 0.2 m^2 and priming volume of 60 mL. Dedicated neonatal machines have filters with extremely low priming volumes.

Blood Priming—If the extracorporeal circuit volume of a hemofilter exceeds 10–15% of the patient's total blood volume, blood priming of the circuit is often required to prevent hemodilution and hypotension, especially in children weighing less than 10 kg. However, a packed red blood cell unit (PRBC) has a pH of 6.8, hematocrit 70% and high serum potassium levels and ionized calcium level of 0.3 mEq/dL and priming with blood can lead to hyperkalemia, hypocalcemia, delivery of acid load, and bradykinin release syndrome with AN-69 membrane. pH of the PRBCs can be corrected by mixing equal amount of bicarbonate and blood using Y-connector during priming process and to compensate for the low ionized calcium of the blood, intravenous calcium should be administered the return line or infused directly into the patient, in order to prevent hypocalcemia. Other maneuvers, such as, giving

54

◘ **Table 54.2** Suggested sizes of temporary catheters for continuous renal replacement therapy according to weight of the patient

Weight of the child	Vascular access catheter size
<10 kg	7 French
10–20 kg	8 French
>20 kg	11 French

packed cell transfusion directly to the patient and removing the blood into the circuit simultaneously (bypass system) and dialyzing the blood in the circuit to normalize the blood prime before connecting it to the patient (recirculation system) can be tried to prevent bradykinin release syndrome [16, 17].

CKRT Solutions—The main purpose of the CKRT solution is providing a safe and consistent metabolic control and adapt to the choice of therapy used—CVVH, CVVHD, or CVVHDF. The important characteristics of an ideal solution are physiological, reliable, easy to prepare, easy to store, inexpensive, easily available, and compatible. The CKRT solutions contain various concentrations of electrolytes, such as sodium, potassium, chloride, calcium, phosphorous, magnesium, and glucose. In general, the concentration of electrolytes should be equal in dialysate and replacement solutions. Historically, these solutions had lactate as the solution buffer; however, it resulted in the development of lactic acidosis, hypotension, and cardiac dysfunction [18]. Hence, modern, industry-made, and physiological solutions available are bicarbonate-based dialysate and replacement solutions and are the standard of care in children receiving CKRT. Many solutions may contain a small amount of lactate (3 mEq/L) along with bicarbonate (22–35 mEq/L) to provide stability and physiological pH to the solution. Concentration of calcium can be varied depending on the type of anticoagulation being used (citrate-based anticoagulation requires calcium-free solutions) [19].

54.8 CKRT Prescription (Table 54.3)

Blood Flow Rate (BFR)—In children, the recommended BFR is 3–10 mL/kg/min. In neonates and infants, relatively higher BFR of 10–12 mL/kg/min can be used, especially while using adult-sized CKRT machines, in order to generate sufficient access and return pressures and prevent clotting of the circuit. The ppCRRT regis-

Table 54.3 Continuous kidney replacement therapy prescription

Modality	CVVH, CVVHD, CVVHDF
Priming	Blood prime in case of children <10 kg or if the extracorporeal volume is >10% of patient's blood volume
Blood flow rate	3–10 mL/kg/min in children 10–12 mL/kg/min in infants and neonates
Dose or effluent volume	Depends on the indication –30–40 mL/kg/min or 2.5–3 L/1.73m^2/h
Ultrafiltration rate	0.5–2 mL/kg/h
Anticoagulation	Unfractionated heparin, regional citrate, prostacyclin, low-molecular-weight heparin, nafamostat mesylate

CVVH Continuous venovenous hemofiltration, *CVVHD* continuous venovenous dialysis, *CVVHD* continuous venovenous hemodiafiltration try reported a mean BFR of 97.9 mL/min (ranging from 10 to 350 mL/min), with mean BFR scaled to body weight of 5 mL/kg/min (0.6–53.6 mL/kg/min) [1]. The BFR generally depends on a number of factors, such as vascular access, CKRT machine, prescribed dose, and patient's hemodynamic stability. By placing a good-sized vascular access, BFR can be adjusted according to the size of the patient. Also, its preferable to start with low BFR and gradually increase it as per the patient's tolerance in order to prevent hemodynamic instability. However, higher BFR can prolong the life of the circuit by reducing the risk of filter clotting, but higher flows do not increase the small solute clearance, unlike intermittent hemodialysis.

Dose of CKRT—CKRT dose is equivalent to the total effluent volume, expressed in mL/kg/h. It estimates the clearance of small solutes from the blood, such as blood urea nitrogen. In 2000, Ronco et al. studied the impact of CKRT dose on the survival of the patients and found that intermediate and high groups had better outcome than the conventional dose group [20]. However, recent randomized control trials—Acute Renal Failure Network Study (ATN) and Randomized Evaluation of Normal vs Augmented Level (RENAL)—did not find any significant difference in the survival between less and more intensive CKRT groups [21, 22]. Therefore, based on these studies it is apparent that increasing the dose beyond 25 mL/kg/h offers no significant mortality benefit of adult patients. The delivered dose can be less than the prescribed dose and depends on a number of factors, like circuit clotting, vascular access issues, scheduled filter change, interruption in CKRT due to patient issues, and the dilutional effect due to prefilter replacement solution. KDIGO recommends an effluent dose of at least 25–30 mL/kg/h to achieve a dose delivery of 20–25 mL/kg/h [14]. By extrapolating the dose of 25–30 mL/kg/h on a 70 kg individual with body surface area (BSA) of 1.73 m^2, we can calculate the pediatric dose of approximately 2000 mL/1.73 m^2/h. Studies have shown that if more rapid clearance is required, such as hyperammonemia associated with acute liver failure, inborn errors of metabolism, and tumor lysis syndrome, higher CKRT dose of 8000 mL/1.73 m^2/h can be prescribed in order to target more rapid clearance of solute [23, 24]. While prescribing high dose keep a close watch on the electrolyte imbalance (sodium variations, hypokalemia, calcium and magnesium derangements, hypophosphatemia) and it is important to closely monitor them during CKRT sessions. In practice, the dose of CKRT is started at 2 L/1.73 m^2/h and titrated up based on the clearance of the solute.

Ultrafiltration—Ultrafiltration allows removal of excess fluid over a period of time, which makes room to administer nutrition, medications, and also provide solute clearance by convective mechanism. In patients where main aim is just solute removal, the aim should be to achieve an even fluid balance, which means that CKRT will remove all fluids received by the patient, minus the urine output. However, in patients with fluid overload, where we wish to remove fluids along with solute, CKRT machine can be set up to remove all the fluids received by the patient plus additional volume. The net ultrafiltration rate can be 0.5–2 mL/kg/h or 1–3% of the child's body volume per hour. The targeted ultrafiltration rate can be determined keeping in mind the percentage of fluid overload, hemodynamic stability of the patient, and his ability to tolerate fluid removal. Caution should be paid regarding excessively high rates (above 1.75 mL/kg/h) of netUF since it has been shown to be harmful in adult retrospective studies.

Anticoagulation—The significance of anticoagulation was highlighted by Brophy et al., who demonstrated that no anticoagulation reduces the life span of the CKRT circuit [25]. In children, the BFR is lower and the vascular access is of small caliber, both of these factors increase the risk of clotting. Various anticoagulants that can be used for CKRT circuit are heparin, prostacyclin, citrate, a combination of two anticoagulants, or no anticoagulant (◘ Table 54.4).

1. Unfractionated Heparin—It remains the most popular anticoagulant used. Heparin has its own set of advantages in terms of cost, ease of use, availability of activated clotting time (ACT) for dose titration, and possibility of reversal using protamine. However, it is associated with side effects associated with side effects such as heparin-2-induced thrombocytopenia (HIT), heparin resistance, and propensity to cause hemorrhage. Systemic anticoagulation is achieved by administering heparin bolus of 20 units per kilogram (kg) followed by infusion of 10–20 units/kg/h. Activated clotting time (ACT) is monitored while using heparin and is aimed at 180–220 s. If the ACT is low, then the dose of unfractionated heparin can be increased by 10–20%.
2. Citrate—Administration of citrate prefilter leads to chelation of the calcium in the extracorporeal circuit, which is an important co-factor in the clotting cascade. This makes the circuit hypocoagulable. A regular monitoring of the ionized calcium should be done in the CKRT circuit (<0.35 mmol/L) in order to maintain adequate anticoagulation. Citrate allows for regional anticoagulation of the circuit without any side effects of systemic anticoagulation. Citrate is administered into the circuit after removal from the patient but before entering the CKRT filter. Calcium is directly infused into the patient via central line to reverse the risk of anticoagulation and hypocalcemia. Various studies have demonstrated lesser hemorrhagic complications and better filter life with citrate as compared to heparin [26, 27].
3. Prostacyclin—Prostacyclin helps reduce filter clotting due to its anti-platelet and heparin sparing property. Deep et al have used prostacyclin-based anticoagulation in children with acute liver failure and demonstrated that prostacyclin is superior to other forms of anticoagulation in children with acute liver failure, with a mean circuit life of 2 days [28]. Therefore, prostacyclin is a good alternative to heparin and citrate, offering lesser side effects as compared to other anticoagulants. Also, a combination of heparin and prostacyclin can be used to minimize the heparin-induced side effects. Prostacyclin is administered at dose of 4 mg/kg/min.

◘ **Table 54.4** Commonly used anticoagulation regimens in CKRT

- Saline flushes
- Heparin (unfractionated heparin)
- Low-molecular-weight heparin
- Citrate regional anticoagulation
- Prostacyclin
- Nafamostat mesilate
- Danaparoid
- Hirudin/lepirudin
- Argatroban (thrombin inhibitor)

Nutrition during CKRT—The presence of AKI in a critically ill child enhances the hypercatabolic state and alters the carbohydrate, protein, and lipid metabolism. KRT further accelerates the catabolism and enhances nutritional losses which may further worsen the nutritional deficiencies. Furthermore, the fluid overload in AKI poses a huge challenge to the intensivist in providing nutrition. Hence, it is imperative to maximize the nutritional support to the child receiving KRT—2.5 g/kg/day of protein and 20–30% calories above the resting energy expenditure (REE).

Drug Dosing during CKRT—Certain drugs are removed significantly during CKRT, and dose adjustment of such drugs is required to prevent underdosing. Drug removal during KRT is influenced by the mode of renal replacement therapy, the frequency of KRT, and the flow rates used during KRT [29]. The pharmacokinetic properties of the drug also play a vital role, and the properties which cause increased clearance of the drug during CKRT are low molecular weight (<5000 Daltons), decreased plasma protein binding (<80%), low volume of distribution (<1 liter per kilogram of body weight), and less extrarenal clearance [30]. Therefore, appropriate drugs need to be selected on CKRT and drug dosages need to be optimized on CKRT keeping in mind the clearance of drugs on CKRT and altered hemodynamics in a sick child.

Complications of CKRT—Although CKRT is considered superior to intermittent hemodialysis in terms of hemodynamic stability and volume control, CKRT is associated with certain complications (◘ Table 54.5).

1. Hemodynamic Instability—One of the most important complications of CKRT is hypotension. Hypovolemia can be caused on CKRT due to characteristic difference between crystalloids used for priming the circuit and the child's blood. Aggressive fluid removal from the patient's blood can also contribute to hypovolemia. Higher blood flow rates used on commencing CKRT can also lead to rapid intravascular shifts, and hence, blood flow rates should be gradually increased. Myocardial dysfunction caused by negative inotropy and vasodilatory effects of acid-based dialysate solutions can also cause hypotension. Another contributing factor is cardiac arrythmias which can occur due to electrolyte imbalance caused by CKRT.
2. Acid Base Imbalance and Electrolyte Disturbances—Regional citrate anticoagulation use can cause acid base imbalance in two situations citrate accumulation and citrate overload. Impaired clearance of citrate in severe hepatic dysfunction results in citrate accumulation leading to increased anion gap metabolic acidosis and hypernatremia. In case of citrate overload, alkalemia can occur as each

◘ Table 54.5 Complications of CKRT

Technical complications	Clinical complications
• Vascular access failure • Circuit clotting • Occlusion of catheter • Inadequate blood flow for clearance • Tubing malfunction/separation • Air embolism • Loss of clearance over time	• Bleeding • Infection (catheter-related and bacteremia) • Hypothermia • Nutritional losses • Hypotension • Electrolyte disturbance

citrate ion is converted in liver to three bicarbonate ions. RCA also causes hypocalcemia and hypomagnesemia. Phosphate clearance is also high on CKRT due to large filter pore size and intercompartmental mass transfer. Also, phosphate and magnesium are not present in the commercially available solutions; therefore, they need to be replaced. Other electrolyte disturbances that can occur on CKRT are hypokalemia and hypocalcemia. Hence, strict monitoring of electrolytes should be done on CKRT. Stringent glucose monitoring should also be done on CKRT to achieve euglycemia. Dialysate solutions contain dextrose to provide nutrition and prevent hypoglycemia.

3. Catheter-Related Complications—Vascular catheter-related hemorrhagic complications can be reduced by inserting catheter under ultrasonographic guidance. Other issues with the catheter are catheter dysfunction, such as kinking, blocking that can lead to premature filter clotting. Catheter-related bloodstream infections can also occur, and strict hand hygiene and other preventing measures should be taken while accessing the vascular catheter.
4. Hypothermia—Extracorporeal radiant heat exchange leads to hypothermia in 5–50% of patients [31]. Thermal loss can increase the oxygen demand and increased daily energy requirements. Heat loss can also mask fevers and can cause delay in the recognition of infections.
5. Hematological Complications—Systemic anticoagulation like heparin, which is used to prevent filter clotting, can increase the risk of bleeding and its use is contraindicated in patients with severe coagulopathy. Those patients who receive heparin can also develop heparin-induced thrombocytopenia (HIT). RCA has got improved safety and less bleeding risk as compared to heparin. CKRT also decreases platelet concentration and impairs their aggregation due to clearance of proinflammatory platelet accumulating factors.
6. Loss of Vitamins and Minerals—Many water-soluble vitamins and essential minerals, such as vitamin D, vitamin C, vitamin E, selenium, manganese, zinc, and copper, are lost during CKRT and can become deficient in patients.

Peritoneal Dialysis—In resource-limited settings, PD is most commonly used modality, and is quite safe, effective, and useful. As opposed to other modalities of KRT, PD requires less technical expertise, resource allocation, and is more cost-effective. PD allows rapid commencement of therapy and provides slow continuous solute and water clearance via diffusion and ultrafiltration. Due to this property, acute PD is a good option in critically ill children with severe coagulopathy, difficult vascular access, and hemodynamic instability. Also, acute PD is extensively used in acute kidney following cardiac surgery in neonates, and has shown a significant decrease in the mortality [32]. Furthermore, PD is most widely used KRT modality in neonates, especially in preterm newborns less than 1 kg.

However, PD has certain drawbacks, and it is not effective in cases where we need urgent fluid removal, clearance of toxins, and rapid reversal of severe metabolic disturbances such as hyperkalemia and hyperammonemia. Also, PD catheter dysfunction, peri-catheter leaks, and poor dialysate flows can preclude successful KRT in critically ill children. PD is contraindicated in patients with recent abdominal surgery, diaphragmatic defects, intraabdominal sepsis, or intraabdominal malignancy. Relative contraindications are ventriculoperitoneal shunts, previous abdominal surgeries, and prune belly syndrome. In such cases, catheter placement can be very challenging as well as there is high chance of catheter dysfunction. Furthermore, in patients of severe acute respiratory distress syndrome with very high ventilatory settings, PD can be quite difficult, as respiratory status can worsen with PD fluid insertion.

PD Catheter Insertion—Earlier, rigid PD catheters were widely used as they are quite cheap and easy to insert. However, they can cause damage to the viscus. Also, rigid catheters have a greater chance of catheter dysfunction and peri-catheter leaks. Non-cuffed flexible percutaneous catheters is a viable option in unstable patients, as it can be placed at the bedside via Seldinger technique and can last up to 5–7 days. For longer use, soft and flexible Tenckhoff catheter with single or double dacron cuffs should be used. It has subcutaneous or tunnel placement, and the presence of dacron cuffs reduces the risk of leakage, infections, and catheter migration [33]. Tenckhoff catheter with a peel away sheath can be percutaneously placed in a sick child in a pediatric intensive care unit; however, surgical insertion of Tenckhoff catheter is routinely recommended for initiation of PD in children.

Cycling—Acute PD can be done manually or by using automated PD cycler. Manual PD is gravity-based, labor-intensive, and requires constant supervision to ensure accurate dwell volume and ultrafiltration volume. However, the automated cycler requires less manpower and machine is programmed to deliver the PD prescription. However, automated cyclers may not be feasible in newborns owing to dead space and non-availability of cyclers that can allow a very small fill volume.

Dialysate Composition—Commercially available PD solutions are conventional dextrose-based solutions and biocompatible PD solutions. Dextrose-containing solutions use dextrose as an osmotic agent to drive ultrafiltration and convection-based solute clearance and use lactate as a buffer. Dextrose also acts as an additional source of calories and nutrition. Biocompatible PD solutions have a neutral pH and lower amount of glucose degradation products. They use bicarbonate as a buffer and have lower lactate concentration. Hence, such solutions are advantageous in critically ill children with progressive lactic acidosis and multiorgan failure. In the absence of commercially available solutions, PD solutions can also be prepared in hospital pharmacies.

54

PD Prescription (◘ Table 54.6)—The recommended dose of PD in children is 10 mL/kg (300 mL/m^2 in children and 200 mL/m^2 in infants), but in case of high catabolic states, aggressive PD regimen (40–50 mL/kg or 800–1200 mLs/m^2) or longer dwell time should be followed to ensure adequate solute removal. Also, the dextrose concentration in the PD fluid can be increased from 2.5 to 4.25% after a few cycles to achieve more efficient ultrafiltration. Usual inflow time is 10–15 min, dwell time is 30–90 min, and outflow time can range from 20 to 30 min. In case of life-threatening hyperkalemia, frequent cycles with dwell time of 15–20 can be done until the potassium levels are lowered significantly. Reduction of the dwell time in hypercatabolic states increases the dialysate flow and the efficacy of the solute clearance [34]. A complete drainage of the effluent in every cycle must be ensured to prevent dialysate fluid accumulation in the peritoneal cavity, which can lead to abdominal distension and respiratory insufficiency. Heparin 250–1000 units per liter of dialysate fluid should be added to prevent clotting. There is no need of intraperitoneal antibiotics, if the patient is on systemic antibiotic cover. Electrolytes should be frequently monitored in a child on continuous PD, in particular potassium , which can later be added to the dialysate fluid in case of hypokalemia. A monitoring chart should be

Table 54.6 PD prescription

Manual or automated PD cycler
Catheter—Tenckhoff/Seldinger technique catheter
PD fluid: Dextrose 2.5–4.25%. In case of hypokalemia, add potassium chloride 3–4 mmol/L
Anticoagulation—add heparin—250–1000 units per liter of dialysate
PD dwell volume: Usual volume—10–20 mL/kg (300–600 mL/m²)
High volume—40–50 mL/kg or 1200 mLs/m² (depending upon the target solute clearance)
PD inflow time: 5–10 min (min)
PD dwell time: 30–60 min
PD outflow time: 20–25 min

kept at bedside that records exchange number, glucose concentration of the dialysate, volume of exchanges, amount of effluent and patient's weight, etc. Blood urea nitrogen, creatinine, electrolytes, and blood glucose should be monitored on a daily basis.

Complications of PD—Complications related to PD catheter are leakage around the PD catheter, kinking of the catheter, obstruction, and impaired drainage. Peritonitis is another major complication. Most common organisms responsible for causing peritonitis are Staphylococcus aureus and pseudomonas aeruginosa.

KRT during Unprecedented Pandemic State—CKRT remains the preferred mode of KRT among the critically sick children with AKI in a pandemic situation depending upon the availability of staff, equipment, and expertise. Even from logistics point of view, this holds true as not every pediatric ICU has got facilities such as reverse osmosis or RO system to deliver IHD. Also on CKRT one nurse can easily manage more than one patient, limiting the use of resources like personal protective equipment (PPE) in a COVID-19 pandemic state, which is not possible with IHD. Also, CKRT can be done bedside in isolation rooms or CKRT machines can be kept outside the intensive care units with extended tubings, which will limit the exposure to healthcare personnel [35].

However, in a pandemic situation, where hospitals are overwhelmed with patients , there is always a possibility of paucity of CKRT machines, trained staff, infusion pumps, and other consumables (hemofilter , circuit , replacement, and dialysate fluid) to run CKRT. In a situation where CKRT machines are limited, use of IHD is a feasible option in selected group of hemodynamically stable patients and peritoneal dialysis can be initiated in hemodynamically unstable patients. Also, prolonged intermittent KRT using conventional CKRT machines can also be done, which runs for 8–10 h with higher blood flow rates of 50–60 mL/kg/h instead of the usual recommended dose of 1.73 mL/m²/min or 35–45 mL/kg/h, which runs for 24 h [36]. Furthermore, in resource-limited setting machines can be alternated between 2 and 3 patients in 24 h or rotated once in 24 h among patients or whenever the circuit clots. If consumables are limited, then lower exchange rates of 20 mL/kg/h can be used in selected patients of AKI who are having fluid overload or are in hypercatabolic state. In-house replacement fluids can also be made by mixing saline and dextrose with desired electrolytes in case of deficiency of replacement fluids. Hence, delivering KRT in a pandemic situation can be extremely challenging and the intensivist must utilize the available resources in such situation with utmost efficacy and innovate new ideas to deliver KRT with available machines, resources, and consumables.

54.9 Future Directions

Dedicated Neonatal Machines. The biggest challenge in providing CKRT to newborns using standard machines is the priming volume required to prime the circuit and filter. In a 4 kg newborn, circulating blood volume is 320 mLs, and the minimal extracorporeal volume using the adult machine is 95 mLs, which essentially means that one-third of the blood is outside the patient's body. It can cause serious issues if they are not thought through; therefore, the circuit needs to be blood primed. So, the question for the clever person is "Can we have a smaller circuit with lesser priming volume required?"

Therefore, researchers around the globe started to work on getting this done—modification of the Aquadex machine which was used for ultrafiltration for adults to remove fluids in congestive heart failure, CARPEDIEM from Italy, NIDUS from Newcastle in the UK, and there is a Japanese circuit with priming volume of about 10 mLs.

Aquadex uses 33 mL circuit, was FDA approved in 2006 for ultrafiltration, and provides pre-filter CVVH. This cartoon shows the circuit—heparin-added prefilter, and so is replacement fluid, ACT-monitored post-filter.

In 2012, the Cardio-Renal, Pediatric Dialysis Emergency Machine (CARPEDIEM) launched the "fitted era" for pediatric CKRT. The project was born in the same place where 24 years earlier the first CAVH had been performed: in Vicenza, Italy. The aim was to develop a CKRT platform specifically dedicated to newborns and small infants in the weight range of 2.0–10 kg and with an approximate BSA of 0.15–0.5 m^2. Three circuits with surface areas of 0.075, 0.15, and 0.25 m^2 are available. The three small roller pumps move blood into a 27-mL (34 mL and 45 mL, respectively, with the bigger filters) total volume circuit. The solute clearance may reach 2 L/h/1.73 m^2 of BSA and/or 25–35 mL/kg/h in patients weighing less than 10 kg. To ensure a highly accurate fluid balance, the CARPEDIEM is equipped with gravimetric controls combined with an excellent scale sensitivity of 1 g for both infusion and effluent bags.

In 1995, the Newcastle group designed a novel HD circuit, which operated by different principles. It was driven by syringes and uncoupled the baby's blood flow capacity from the requirements of the dialysis filter. They have subsequently developed this device into the Newcastle infant dialysis and ultrafiltration system (Nidus). This syringe-driven machine repeatedly withdraws 5–12.5 mL aliquots of blood from a single-lumen central venous line, passes and returns it across a dialysis filter, and then back to the baby. At a blood flow rate of 20 mL/min, this processes 5 mL of blood each minute. The circuit has two operating syringes, a high-flux polysulfone 0.045, a heparin syringe, pumped dialysate, a pressure transducer and an air-detector, and self-primes with 4.3 mL of heparinized saline, giving a minimum operating volume of 9.3 mL. It records its precise operating status and syringe positions every one-tenth of a second, and has battery back-up. The circuits have been designed for up to 24 h of continuous use. This machine is now gone into clinical trial called IKID trial in the UK.

Though we have now dedicated neonatal CKRT machines, that does not end or solve a problem, it has to be ongoing education and training of the whole staff—medical, nursing with particular importance to access which needs to be the right catheter in the right location at the right time by the right person, and important consideration to drug removal during this therapy.

Precision CKRT—Recent guidelines have recommended a standard static prescribed dose of 20–25 mL/kg/h [14], as greater CKRT dose has not demonstrated any survival benefit or improvement in renal recovery in critically sick patients with AKI [21, 22]. However, all the studies studied fixed dose prescription which cannot determine whether fixed or dynamic CKRT dose is appropriate in critically sick patients with unpredictable clinical course and rapid changes in the clinical, physiological, and metabolic profile of the patients. Hence, the concept of precision CKRT has been proposed, emphasizing the CKRT dose should be dynamic and should be modified over time according to the clinical demands of the patient and if the standard dose is not able to achieve adequate fluid, metabolic, and electrolyte balance. For example, in a patient with hypercatabolic state, a greater dose of CKRT should be initiated to achieve adequate solute control. Later on, the dose can be reduced to the standard dose of 20–25 mL/kg/h if the clinical status of the patient improves and desired solute clearance is achieved. Quality indicators should be aimed while delivering CKRT in order to guide to optimal CKRT care.

54.10 Conclusions

Delivery of KRT in children with AKI remains a challenge, especially due to their small size. However, advancements in technology and new innovations in delivery of KRT have contributed to improved survival in patients with AKI. The clinician should always keep in mind the risks and the benefits of various modalities of CKRT and tailor the treatment according to the needs of the patient.

Take-Home Messages

- Acute kidney injury commonly occurs in children being admitted to pediatric intensive care units and many of them require commencement of renal replacement therapy.
- The choice of modality of renal replacement therapy is based on certain important patient and center-related factors, such as weight of the child, his clinical condition, hemodynamic stability, expertise of the staff, and availability of resources.
- Continuous renal replacement therapy has become the preferred modality to deliver renal replacement therapy as it allows accurate fluid removal, better solute clearance, and offers a better tolerance in hemodynamically unstable patients.
- Since early initiation of renal replacement therapy has not shown any mortality benefit, therefore, in the absence of absolute indications of commencement of renal replacement therapy, a personalized approach is warranted while initiating renal replacement therapy keeping in mind the risks involved in the delaying the initiation of renal replacement therapy.
- Continuous renal replacement therapy can be started with a dose of 20–25 mL/kg/h, but if rapid clearance is required especially in case of hypercatabolic states, then the dose of continuous renal replacement therapy can be increased in order to target better and rapid clearance of solutes.
- Heparin remains the most popular anticoagulant in renal replacement therapy owing to its low cost, ease of use, and possibility of reversal with protamine.

- Intermittent hemodialysis is very effective and allows faster removal of toxins and in situation of critical volume overload as compared to peritoneal dialysis and continuous renal replacement therapy in selected group of patients who are hemodynamically stable.
- Peritoneal dialysis remains the most commonly used modality in resource-limited settings and in neonates and preterm with acute kidney injury. It is quite safe and effective and requires less clinical expertise.

References

1. Symons JM, Chua AN, Somers MJ, et al. Demographic characteristics of pediatric continuous renal replacement therapy: a report of the prospective pediatric continuous renal replacement therapy registry. Clin J Am Soc Nephrol. 2007;2(4):732–8.
2. Pathak S, Pandey SS, Lazarus M, Mudey A, Nagrale A. Incidences and clinical outcomes of acute kidney injury in PICU: a prospective observational study. Int J Med Health Sci. 2017;6:101–5.
3. Westrope CA, Fleming S, Kapetanstrataki M, Parslow RC, Morris KP. Renal replacement therapy in the critically ill child. Pediatr Crit Care Med. 2018;19(3):210–7.
4. Beltramo F, DiCarlo J, Gruber JB, Taylor T, Totapally BR. Renal replacement therapy modalities in critically ill children. Pediatr Crit Care Med. 2019;20(1):e1–9.
5. Friedrich JO, Wald R, Bagshaw SM, Burns KE, Adhikari NK. Hemofiltration compared to hemodialysis for acute kidney injury: systematic review and meta-analysis. Crit Care. 2012;16(4):R146.
6. Ricci Z, Ronco C, Bachetoni A, et al. Solute removal during continuous renal replacement therapy in critically ill patients: convection versus diffusion. Crit Care. 2006;10(2):R67.
7. Sutherland SM, Zappitelli M, Alexander SR, et al. Fluid overload and mortality in children receiving continuous renal replacement therapy: the prospective pediatric continuous renal replacement therapy registry. Am J Kidney Dis. 2010;55(2):316–25.
8. Zarbock A, Kellum JA, Schmidt C, et al. Effect of early vs delayed initiation of renal replacement therapy on mortality in critically ill patients with acute kidney injury: the ELAIN randomized clinical trial. JAMA. 2016;315:2190–9.
9. STAKRT-AKI Investigators; Canadian Critical Care Trials Group; Australian and New Zealand Intensive Care Society Clinical Trials Group; United Kingdom Critical Care Research Group; Canadian Nephrology Trials Network; Irish Critical Care Trials Group, Bagshaw SM, Wald R, Adhikari NKJ, Bellomo R, da Costa BR, Dreyfuss D, Du B, Gallagher MP, Gaudry S, Hoste EA, Lamontagne F, Joannidis M, Landoni G, Liu KD, McAuley DF, McGuinness SP, Neyra JA, Nichol AD, Ostermann M, Palevsky PM, Pettilä V, Quenot JP, Qiu H, Rochwerg B, Schneider AG, Smith OM, Thomé F, Thorpe KE, Vaara S, Weir M, Wang AY, Young P, Zarbock A. Timing of initiation of renal-replacement therapy in acute kidney injury. N Engl J Med. 2020;383(3):240–51.
10. Gaudry S, Hajage D, Benichou N, et al. Delayed versus early initiation of renal replacement therapy for severe acute kidney injury: a systematic review and individual patient data meta-analysis of randomised clinical trials. Lancet. 2020;395(10235):1506–15.
11. Hackbarth R, Bunchman TE, Chua AN, et al. The effect of vascular access location and size on circuit survival in pediatric continuous renal replacement therapy: a report from the PPCKRT registry. Int J Artif Organs. 2007;30(12):1116–21.
12. Sutherland SM, Alexander SR. Continuous renal replacement therapy in children. Pediatr Nephrol. 2012;27(11):2007–16.
13. Macedo E, Mehta RL. Continuous dialysis therapies: core curriculum 2016. Am J Kidney Dis. 2016;68(4):645–57.
14. Kidney Disease: Improving Global Outcomes (KDIGO) Acute Kidney Injury Work Group. KDIGO clinical practical guideline for acute kidney injury. Kidney Int. 2012;2:1–138.
15. Rabindranath KS, Kumar E, Shail R, Vaux EC. Ultrasound use for the placement of haemodialysis catheters. Cochrane Database Syst Rev. 2011;(11):CD005279.
16. Brophy PD, Mottes TA, Kudelka TL, et al. AN-69 membrane reactions are pH-dependent and preventable. Am J Kidney Dis. 2001;38(1):173–8. https://doi.org/10.1053/ajkd.2001.25212.

17. Pasko DA, Mottes TA, Mueller BA. Pre dialysis of blood prime in continuous hemodialysis normalizes pH and electrolytes. Pediatr Nephrol. 2003;18(11):1177–83. https://doi.org/10.1007/s00467-003-1258-2.
18. Davenport A, Will EJ, Davison AM. Hyperlactataemia and metabolic acidosis during haemofiltration using lactate-buffered fluids. Nephron. 1991;59(3):461–5.
19. John JC, Taha S, Bunchman TE. Basics of continuous renal replacement therapy in pediatrics. Kidney Res Clin Pract. 2019;38(4):455–61.
20. VA/NIH Acute Renal Failure Trial Network, Palevsky PM, Zhang JH, et al. Intensity of renal support in critically ill patients with acute kidney injury [published correction appears in N Engl J Med. 2009 Dec 10;361(24):2391]. N Engl J Med. 2008;359(1):7–20. https://doi.org/10.1056/NEJMoa0802639.
21. Palevsky PM, O'Connor TZ, Chertow GM, Crowley ST, Zhang JH, Kellum JA, et al. Intensity of renal replacement therapy in acute kidney injury: perspective from within the Acute Renal Failure Trial Network Study. Crit Care. 2009;13:310.
22. RENAL Replacement Therapy Study Investigators, Bellomo R, Cass A, Cole L, Finfer S, Gallagher M, et al. Intensity of continuous renal-replacement therapy in critically ill patients. N Engl J Med. 2009;361:1627–38.
23. Spinale JM, Laskin BL, Sondheimer N, Swartz SJ, Goldstein SL. High-dose continuous renal replacement therapy for neonatal hyperammonemia. Pediatr Nephrol. 2013;28:983–6.
24. Fleming GM, Walters S, Goldstein SL, Alexander SR, Baum MA, Blowey DL, Bunchman TE, Chua AN, Fletcher SA, Flores FX, Fortenberry JD, Hackbarth R, McBryde K, Somers MJ, Symons JM, Brophy PD. Nonrenal indications for continuous renal replacement therapy: a report from the prospective pediatric continuous renal replacement therapy registry group. Pediatr Crit Care Med. 2012;13:e299–304.
25. Brophy PD, Somers MJ, Baum MA, Symons JM, McAfee N, Fortenberry JD, et al. Multi-centre evaluation of anticoagulation in patients receiving continuous renal replacement therapy (CKRT). Nephrol Dial Transpl. 2005;20:1416–21.
26. Fernández SN, Santiago MJ, López-Herce J, García M, Del Castillo J, Alcaraz AJ, et al. Citrate anticoagulation for CKRT in children: comparison with heparin. Biomed Res Int. 2014;2014:786301.
27. Sık G, Demirbuga A, Annayev A, Citak A. Regional citrate versus systemic heparin anticoagulation for continuous renal replacement therapy in critically ill children. Int J Artif Organs. 2020;43(4):234–41.
28. Deep A, Zoha M, Dutta KP. Prostacyclin as an anticoagulant for continuous renal replacement therapy in children. Blood Purif. 2017;43(4):279–89.
29. Jang SM, Infante S, Abdi PA. Drug dosing considerations in critically ill patients receiving continuous renal replacement therapy. Pharmacy (Basel). 2020;8(1):18.
30. Schetz M. Drug dosing in continuous renal replacement therapy: general rules. Curr Opin Crit Care. 2007;13(6):645–51.
31. Finkel KW, Podoll AS. Complications of continuous renal replacement therapy. Semin Dial. 2009;22(2):155–9. https://doi.org/10.1111/j.1525-139X.2008.00550.x. PMID: 19426420.
32. Bojan M, Gioanni S, Vouhé PR, Journois D, Pouard P. Early initiation of peritoneal dialysis in neonates and infants with acute kidney injury following cardiac surgery is associated with a significant decrease in mortality. Kidney Int. 2012;82(4):474–81.
33. Auron A, Warady BA, Simon S, Blowey DL, Srivastava T, Musharaf G, Alon US. Use of the multipurpose drainage catheter for the provision of acute peritoneal dialysis in infants and children. Am J Kidney Dis. 2007;49(5):650–5.
34. Vasudevan A, Phadke K, Yap HK. Peritoneal dialysis for the management of pediatric patients with acute kidney injury. Pediatr Nephrol. 2017;32(7):1145–56.
35. Deep A, Bansal M, Ricci Z. Acute kidney injury and special considerations during renal replacement therapy in children with coronavirus disease-19: perspective from the Critical Care Nephrology Section of the European Society of Paediatric and Neonatal Intensive Care. Blood Purif. 2021;50(2):150–60. https://doi.org/10.1159/000509677. Epub ahead of print. PMID: 32663827; PMCID: PMC7445370.
36. Palevsky PM, O'Connor TZ, Chertow GM, Crowley ST, Zhang JH, Kellum JA, et al. Intensity of renal replacement therapy in acute kidney injury: perspective from within the acute renal failure trial network study. Crit Care. 2009;13(4):310.

Role of Dietitian and Nutrition in Paediatric Critical Care

Luise V. Marino, Lynne Latten, and Corinne Jotterand Chaparro

Contents

J. Brierley et al. (eds.), *ESPNIC Children's Intensive Care Textbook*,
https://doi.org/10.1007/978-3-031-64762-8_55

Learning Objectives

Readers will learn how to consider to nutrition support of critically ill children, using a dietetic approach inclusive of the assessment of: Anthropometry (A), Biochemistry (B), Clinical considerations (C), Dietary (D) and Evaluation (E).

Learning objectives therefore for this chapter include;

1. To be able to define adequate growth in the context of critical illness.
2. To understand the purpose of completing routine nutrition bloods during critical illness and considerations for nutrition support.
3. To understand how the phases of critical illness affect energy and protein requirements.
4. To characterise the mode and type of nutrition support recommended in critically ill children.
5. To understand the implications of commonly used medications on gastrointestinal function.
6. To understand principles of developing a nutritional diagnosis and nutrition care plan.
7. To understand how often nutrition adequacy should be assessed and how often nutrition care plans should be reviewed.
8. To explore how the development and implementation of nutrition guidelines are associated with improve nutrition delivery and support in critically ill children.
9. To consider how audit and service evaluation of nutrition support contributes towards continuous quality improvement.
10. To understand principles of patient-centred care and goal setting with caregivers/parents, including strategies to reduce feeding difficulties and improve outcomes.

55.1 Introduction

This chapter will discuss and review the available data on considerations for nutrition support of critically ill children, using a dietetic approach inclusive of the assessment of: Anthropometry (A), Biochemistry (B), Clinical considerations (C), Dietary (D) and Evaluation (E) [1].

In high-income countries, the majority of admissions to PICU are children <12 months old (47%); length of stay (LOS) varies with 25% of children admitted for <24 h, 30% 1–3 days and 19% >7 days, with a mortality rate of 1.1–4% [2, 3]. In low- and middle-income countries, mortality rate among children is considerably higher ranging from 8.5 to 27.5% [4, 5].

55.2 Organising Nutrition Care

The role of the dietitian in PICU is to work within a multi-disciplinary team with an overarching goal of avoiding both under- and over-nutrition, positively impacting on short- and longer-term clinical outcomes. However, in order to develop a nutrition guideline inclusive of a nutrition care process, e.g. A, B, C, D and E, a guideline including how to complete nutrition assessment should be developed [6]. Implementation of guidelines may be enhanced where they are developed using a team approach of motivated volunteers including a physician, pharmacist, dietitian, nurse and nurse assistant, with the support from the local organisation management team, reporting to local nutrition steering groups or other organisational nutritional committees [7].

55.3 Anthropometry (A)

The European Society of Enteral and Parenteral Nutrition (ESPEN) and European Society for Paediatric Gastroenterology Hepatology and Nutrition (ESPGHAN) recommend using nutritional screening tools in hospitalised children to assess nutrition risk [8, 9]. However, to date none of these tools are sensitive or specific enough to accurately identify critically ill infants and children with increased nutrition risk [10–12]. All children admitted to a PICU should be considered to have nutrition risk, either due to inadequate intake, increased requirements or losses prior to PICU admission. This likely to be further exacerbated by fluid restriction and limited fluid allowance in which to provide nutrition support.

Valla et al. reported almost a quarter of children were malnourished on admission or experience a further decline in nutrition status during their PICU stay [13]. In addition, infants and children with congenital heart disease (CHD), who are underweight at the time of surgery, spend significantly longer in hospital [14]. Those with a low weight-for-age at the time of surgery are more likely to die at 12 months of age, irrespective of the severity of the cardiac defect [15], suggesting being underweight increases morbidity and mortality.

Dietitians are uniquely qualified to complete a thorough nutrition assessment on admission and throughout a PICU stay, which is essential particularly if there is a prolonged length of stay, as continued growth is important.

55.3.1 Quality Assurance Framework for the Measurement of Anthropometry

A nutrition assessment guideline should encompass a quality assurance framework to ensure anthropometric measurements are of the highest quality. Quality measures of anthropometry, especially of weight and body height, are important as they are used to determine; (1) drug dosing, (2) ventilator settings and (3) nutrition requirements, especially energy requirements. Therefore, inaccurate measures may negatively impact outcomes.

A quality assurance framework for anthropometrical measurements should be included in a nutrition guideline focusing on:

1. Principles that need to be embedded within a guideline to ensure measurements completed adhere to objectives and standards of a guideline.
2. Minimum knowledge and training standards with regard to nutrition basics and factors that may affect nutritional status.
3. These factors should feed into local entry and exit policies for nutrition support of critically ill children accounting for those who suffer from malnutrition or overweight/obesity.

4. Standard operating procedures for anthropometric measurements should be developed and implemented within the unit, ensuring that all healthcare professionals, including dietitians know how to make accurate measurements.
5. Competency frameworks should be developed, and all staff should be regularly assessed to ensure measures are being completed according to the unit standards.
6. For an individual, this framework can be used to establish an individual healthcare professional practice with regard to self-directed training, maintenance of training standards and entry and exit criteria for individual children's nutrition support [7, 16].
7. To ensure accurate and regular anthropometric measurements in critically ill children, the dietitians have various responsibilities (Table 55.1).

Table 55.1 Role of dietitians regarding anthropometry

1. Checking the availability of the equipment required
Weight – Bed/cots with weight balances incorporated – Digital class III medical scales able to weigh up to 10 kg – Patient transfer board with III digital scale and length measure for older children **Length** – Measuring rod with arms suitable for infants – Patient transfer board with III digital scale and length measure for older children **Circumferences and segment measures: head, mid-upper arm and ulna** – Disposable paper tape measure – Non-stretchable plastic covered tape measure (able to be cleaned between uses)
2. Classifying nutrition risk
At (or within 6 h) of admission
Ask the parent for their hand held record of the child's growth chart – Most parents of young children will have the child's growth chart available – Review recent growth trends, e.g. weight/length – Plot these measures in the patient electronic or paper hospital record **For infants born <37 weeks of gestational age at birth, measures of anthropometry should be corrected up to:** – 1 year of age in those born at a gestational age of 32–36 + 6 weeks – 2 years of age in those infants born at a gestational age of <32 weeks **All children should have anthropometry completed on admission** – Weight – Length, ulna length – Head circumference (<3 years of age) **These measures should then be plotted on the child's electronic or paper growth record and used to calculate z-scores for:** – weight for age <10 years of age – weight for height or body mass index – length for age – head circumference for age (<3 years of age) **Where there is no access to electronic growth records:** – Use the World Health Organization (WHO) Anthro Survey Analyser tool to calculate z-scores: ► https://worldhealthorg.shinyapps.io/anthro/

(continued)

55

Table 55.1 (continued)

Then, classify nutritional status using WHO criteria for acute and persistent malnutrition [17]	
Moderate acute malnutrition (MAM)	Children: weight-for-height or height-for-age < – 2 SD on WHO growth charts
Severe acute malnutrition 0–60 months (SAM)	All children: height-for-age and weight-for-height < –3 SD (stunting and wasting, respectively) on the WHO growth curve
Chronic/persistent malnutrition	Height-for-age < – 2 SD, i.e. stunted
Acute on chronic malnutrition	Acute weight loss in a stunted child
Malnutrition in older children (>5 years)	BMI < 5th centile SAM < –3 z-score
Overweight	BMI > +1 z-score
Obesity	BMI > +2 z-score
During the PICU stay	
All infants <12 months of age should have: – Weight repeated 1–2 per week – Length, ulna length repeated monthly – Head circumference (<3 years of age) repeated monthly **All children should have**: – Weight repeated 1 per week (infants/ children should be naked and weight of dressings/ equipment should be accounted for) – Mid-upper arm circumference measures may be used where children have organomegaly/ oedema – Length, ulna length repeated monthly – Head circumference (<3 years of age) repeated monthly – It may be easier to designate a measuring day on the unit	
At PICU discharge	
As part of a nutrition handover, a summary of anthropometry should be included providing an assessment of: – Recommendation for frequency of measures with regard to post-PICU rehabilitation – Growth, e.g. length/height-for-age z-scores – Weight gain, e.g. weight-for-height/ BMI or weight-for-age z-scores – Recommend strategies for ongoing nutrition support and exit criteria for when it may no longer be required, e.g. >–1 and <1 z-score	

Summary

- ALL children admitted to PICU will have nutrition risk and a nutrition review will be required, which is inclusive of anthropometry
- ALL staff should be trained in how to accurately complete, record and classify a child's growth
- ALL children should have their weight measured weekly, and length measured monthly

55.4 Biochemistry (B)

Dietitians are involved in the review of routinely collected biochemistry, in addition to the interpretation of pathophysiology for aberrant values (■ Table 55.2).

55.4.1 Refeeding Syndrome

Although refeeding syndrome in critically ill children has a low incidence of <9% [18], the consequences can be profound. As such, the role of the dietitian is to assess individual risk [19]. Before nutrition support is commenced, the following screening questions may be useful to consider;

- Does the child have acute persistent malnutrition <–2 weight-for-length z-scores or a history of poor intake for 7–10 days?
- Before nutrition support has been commenced, were serum electrolytes of sodium, potassium, magnesium or phosphorus on the lower end of the normal range?
- Is the child on multiple pharmacopeia including diuretics and inotropic support which may impact on electrolyte absorption or losses?
- In case, potassium, magnesium or phosphorus is decreased after the introduction of nutrition support, consider the other factor that may induce electrolyte abnormalities beside a possible refeeding syndrome

■ **Table 55.2** Role of dietitians regarding biochemistry

At (or within 6 h) of admission
Monitor: – Urea and electrolytes, liver function, calcium, phosphorus, magnesium, glucose, INR (blood clotting), lactate, full blood count, C-reactive protein
During the PICU stay
Monitor: – Urea and electrolytes, liver function, calcium, phosphorus, magnesium, glucose, INR (blood clotting), lactate, full blood count, C-reactive protein – If receiving parenteral nutrition (PN), review triglycerides 2–3 times per week – If CRP is <10 and there is concern regarding micronutrient deficiencies, complete nutrition-related bloods, e.g. serum zinc – If there is concern regarding vitamin D status, measure levels and provide therapeutic treatment where levels are <50 nmol for 4–8 weeks depending on local guidance
At PICU discharge
Monitor: – Urea and electrolytes, liver function, calcium, phosphorus, magnesium, glucose, INR (blood clotting), lactate, full blood count, C-reactive protein – If receiving PN, review triglycerides 2–3 times per week – If CRP is <10 and there is concern regarding micronutrient deficiencies, complete nutrition-related bloods, e.g. serum zinc – If there is concern regarding vitamin D status, measure levels and provide therapeutic treatment where levels are <50 nmol for 4–8 weeks depending on local guidance

Summary
- Dietitians are involved in the review of routinely collected biochemistry in addition to the interpretation of pathophysiology for aberrant value.
- Screening children with a history of poor intake or moderate acute/ persistent malnutrition may help reduce the risk of refeeding syndrome.
- Using a protocol to guide the management of electrolyte and micronutrient abnormalities may support appropriate supplementation.

55.5 Clinical (C)

In order to develop an appropriate nutrition, diagnosis and care plan dietitians are required to develop an understanding of metabolic changes and fuel utilisation during each phase of critical illness (Table 55.3). Critical illness is characterised by a cascade of endocrine and metabolic reactions, affecting all major organs (Fig. 55.1) [21, 22]. There are three notional phases of the stress response in critically ill children, suggested as follows:

- *Acute Phase*—characterised by increased vital organ function, which appears to have a much shorter duration in children than in adults. In the majority of children, there is an early resolution of the stress response with respect to counter regulatory hormones and glucose metabolism within 48 h.
- *Stable Phase*—stabilisation of weaning of vital organ support, incomplete resolution of stress response.
- *Recovery Phase*—clinical mobilisation with normalisation of neuroendocrine, immunological and metabolic alterations (may occur in a high dependency unit or ward setting) [21].

Table 55.3 Role of dietitians regarding clinical aspects

At (or within 6 h) of admission
– Assess impact of critical illness on ability to commence early enteral feeding – Set initial target intake of energy, based on resting energy expenditure (REE) calculated by Schofield [20] – Prescribe appropriate enteral nutrition formula
During the PICU stay
– Review clinical progress – Adjust energy targets as appropriate to changing clinical picture – Assess feed tolerance – Monitor nutrition intake and adjust feed plan to ensure consistent, appropriate intake – Adjust feeding targets in light of anthropometry measurements – Advocate for appropriate PN use if enteral nutrition is inadequate
At PICU discharge
– Devise appropriate feed/nutrition plan to aid ongoing nutritional rehabilitation – Ensure ongoing nutritional and anthropometry assessment within the ward environment

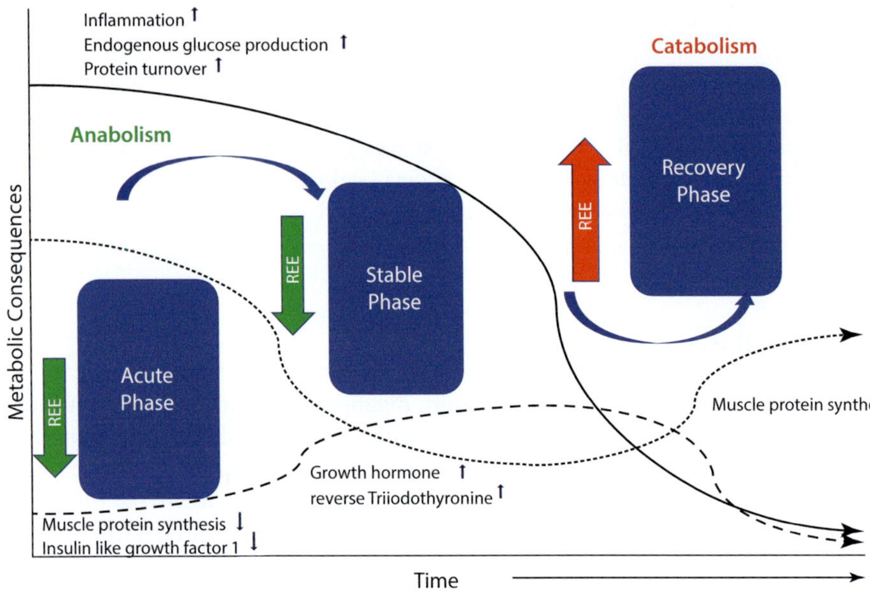

Fig. 55.1 Different phases of critical illness with corresponding neuro-endocrine, immunologic and metabolic changes (adapted from Joosten [21]). *REE* resting energy expenditure

55.6 Dietary (D)

Children admitted to PICU may have existing acute or persistent nutrition deficits, arising from sudden disease onset or due to chronic illness. The aim of nutritional support in critically ill children is not usually to reverse disease-related malnutrition, but to minimise a further decline in nutritional status through the provision of adequate amounts of macro- and micronutrients during an acute admission [23]. As such, the goal of nutrition support is to preserve life, maintain and improve cell function and support recovery into rehabilitation [24, 25].

Critically ill children are often unable to eat or drink, as a result of an endotracheal tube (ETT) in situ to facilitate mechanical ventilation or being too unwell to consume sufficient nutrition orally [25], as such it is common for enteral feeds to be commenced on admission. Early enteral feeds within 6–24 h of admission [26–30] may improve nutritional delivery particularly when used in conjunction with locally adapted feeding protocols [31–34]. Advancing nutrition support in a stepwise fashion has been shown to be an effective way to initiate and advance nutritional support until the goal volume for delivery is achieved [25, 31, 35, 36].

Where possible, nutrition support should be provided via the gastrointestinal tract (GIT), via a nasoenteric (NET) tube into the stomach or small bowel. The results of PepEPANIC trial showed that withholding PN for 1 week in the PICU was clinically superior to providing early PN; late PN resulted in fewer new infections, a shorter duration of dependency on intensive care and a shorter hospital stay [37–42].

Children with paediatric multisystem inflammatory syndrome temporally associated with COVID-19 (PIMS) or septic shock may have vasculitis changes in peripheral and visceral arteries including cerebrovascular, renal and gastrointestinal systems [43, 44]. In children with PIMS-TS, the GIT involvement has been reported in up to 35% of children with varying severity. In these instances, children may tolerate a peptide feed into the small bowel better. [44, 45]. The routine measurement of gastric residual volume is also not recommended [20]. During critical illness, micronutrient should be provided in sufficient amounts to meet reference nutrient intakes for age [46] (Table 55.4).

Table 55.4 Role of dietitians regarding dietary aspects [47, 48]

At (or within 6 h) of admission
On admission a dietitian should: – **Form a nutrition diagnosis by completing a nutrition assessment inclusive of** – Anthropometry—growth trends and current nutritional status – Biochemistry—routine biochemistry, assessing risk (if any) for refeeding syndrome – Clinical history—previous medical history and history at presentation – Diet history—previous dietary intake, presence of food allergies or intolerances – **Develop a nutrition care plan based on;** – Anthropometry—nutrition deficits – Biochemistry—aberrant values and the impact relative to the dietary prescription – Clinical history—as part of the current presentation, is the patient on any medication or life support that may impact on feeding tolerance? – Dietary intake—calculate estimated energy and protein requirements using Schofield equation, recommend the route of feeding, type of feed to be administered and goal rate/volume for feed with a plan to increase towards the goal rate in a stepwise fashion – Evaluation—the nutrition care plan should provide a date for a review and plan for follow-up. An important aspect of the evaluation and plan to review (1) prescribed versus actual intake, (2) review of fluid allowance for feed, (3) the use of nutrient energy dense feeds, (4) route and mode of feeding, (5) excess losses, e.g. vomiting or diarrhoea and provide recommendations for support with regard to commencing laxatives or reviewing the use of hyperosmolar medication. Carers should be kept informed as to the goals and plans with regard to nutrition support, along with expectation setting regarding oral intake post-extubation
During the PICU stay
– **The nutrition care plan should be reviewed on a daily basis for acutely ill children and should be inclusive of:** – Anthropometry—differences in weight/length – Biochemistry—aberrant values and the impact relative to the dietary prescription – Clinical history—is there any medication or life support that is impacting on feeding tolerance? – Dietary intake—re-calculate estimated energy and protein requirements using Schofield equation based on acute, stable or recovery phase, recommending the route of feeding, type of feed to be administered and goal rate/volume for feed with a plan to increase towards the goal rate in a stepwise fashion. – Evaluation—the nutrition care plan should provide a date for a review and plan for follow-up. An important aspect of the evaluation and plan to review (1) prescribed versus actual intake, (2) review of fluid allowance for feed, (3) the use of nutrient energy dense feeds, (4) route and mode of feeding, (5) excess losses, e.g. vomiting or diarrhoea and provide recommendations for support with regard to commencing laxatives or reviewing the use of hyperosmolar medication. Carers should be kept informed as to the goals and plans with regard to nutrition support, along with expectation setting regarding oral intake post-extubation

(continued)

Table 55.4 (continued)

At PICU discharge
– **A handover of nutrition care plan should be provided including plans for rehabilitation the plan should be inclusive of:** – Anthropometry—goals regarding nutritional rehabilitation (both over- and undernutrition) – Biochemistry—including the need for micronutrient supplementation to support recovery – Clinical history—ongoing issues that may impact on the ability to consume sufficient nutrition orally – Dietary intake—re-calculate estimated energy and protein requirements using Schofield equation based on the recovery phase, recommending the route of feeding, type of feed to be administered and goal rate/volume for feed or oral nutrition supplements. Carers should be kept informed as to the goals and plans with regard to nutrition support, along with expectation setting regarding oral intake post-extubation – Evaluation—the nutrition care plan should provide a date for a review along with an exit plan for nutrition support (as appropriate), a referral to speech and language therapists may be required for a swallowing assessment

55.7 Evaluation (E)

Evaluation and quality improvement is about providing safe, effective, patient-centred care, which is timely, and inclusive. Dietitians should be involved in regular service evaluation, audit and research. The purpose of which is to assess current practice on a PICU against a standard allows the creation of a "baseline," from which changes can be implemented to ensure the nutrition service is safe, effective, patient-centred, timely, efficient and equitable. The auditing process is cyclical, and after improvements have been made, re-auditing against the same standards will allow quantifiable demonstration of improvement (Table 55.5).

Summary

- Dietitians should be involved in evaluation, audit and research
- Dietitians are strongly involved in the evaluation of nutrition assessment and nutrition support throughout the PICU stay and at discharge. At PICU admission, dietitians have to evaluate whether all children have a nutrition risk assessment. During PICU stay, dietitians evaluate whether the feeding protocol is followed and determine the reasons for a discrepancy between the nutritional prescription and administration.
- Dietitians evaluate whether the PICU team including physicians and nurses has sufficient nutritional knowledge and competences, organise courses if needed in collaboration with the PICU team.

Table 55.5 Role of dietitians regarding evaluation

At (or within 6 h) of admission
– Review anthropometric measurements have been completed – Enteral feeding was commenced within target aim
During the PICU stay
– Weekly anthropometric measurements were completed – Review feed intake compared to feed prescribed – Was feeding protocol followed – Were energy targets adjusted to reflect changes in clinical condition
At PICU discharge
– Changes in anthropometric measurements from admission to discharge – Nutritional intake through admission – Ongoing growth measurements and related to outcomes

Take-Home Messages

- Dietetic support within a PICU is associated with improve nutritional status and outcomes in critically ill children.
- ***Anthropometry*** should be assessed on PICU admission, and regularly throughout the stay.
- ***Biochemistry*** should be regularly reviewed and micronutrient supplementation should be commenced in patients with deficient levels.
- ***Clinical outcomes*** may be improved with the timely commencement of nutrition support, and the use of nutrient energy dense feeds may aid in achieving nutrition targets.
- **Dietary considerations** should include the following:
  - Enteral feeding guidelines
  - Early enteral nutrition within 6–24 h of admission in haemodynamically stable children including those on vasoactive medication and extracorporeal life support
  - In the instance where whole protein feeds are poorly tolerated, the use of a peptide nutrient energy dense feed may improve tolerance
  - Continuous feeds may be better tolerated during the acute phase moving to intermittent bolus feeds during stable and recovery phases
- During the acute phase, energy requirements should not exceed basal metabolic rate; as children become stable, energy intake may be increased as estimated using Schofield equations.
- Withholding PN for 1 week in the PICU is recommended, as it was shown to be clinically superior to providing early PN.
- The use of pharmaconutrition such as glutamine and/ or micronutrients is not currently recommended as scientific data are missing.
- Parents should be kept informed as to the goals and plans with regard to nutrition support, along with expectation setting regarding oral intake post-extubation.
- **Evaluation** of nutritional practices should be performed regularly, mostly driven by dietitians and in collaboration with the PICU team.

References

1. Lacey K, Pritchett E. Nutrition care process and model: ADA adopts road map to quality care and outcomes management. J Am Diet Assoc. 2003;103(8):1061–72.
2. PICANET. PICANET annual report 2015. 2015.
3. Larsson Viksten J, et al. Children aged 0-16 admitted to Swedish intensive care units and paediatric intensive care units showed low mortality rates. Acta Paediatr. 2019;108(8):1460–6.
4. Ballot DE, et al. A comparison between raw and predicted mortality in a paediatric intensive care unit in South Africa. BMC Res Notes. 2018;11(1):829.
5. Haftu H, et al. Assessment of pattern and treatment outcome of patients admitted to pediatric intensive care unit, Ayder Referral Hospital, Tigray, Ethiopia, 2015. BMC Res Notes. 2018;11(1):339.
6. Tume LN, et al. Practical strategies to implement the ESPNIC nutrition clinical recommendations into PICU practice. Clin Nutr ESPEN. 2021;42:410–4.
7. Valla FV, et al. A training program for anthropometric measurements by a dedicated nutrition support team improves nutritional status assessment of the critically ill child. Pediatr Crit Care Med. 2015;16(3):e82–8.
8. Hartman C, et al. Malnutrition screening tools for hospitalized children. Curr Opin Clin Nutr Metab Care. 2012;15(3):303–9.
9. Chourdakis M, et al. Malnutrition risk in hospitalized children: use of 3 screening tools in a large European population. Am J Clin Nutr. 2016;103(5):1301–10.
10. Marino LV, Thomas PC, Beattie RM. Screening tools for paediatric malnutrition: are we there yet? Curr Opin Clin Nutr Metab Care. 2018;21(3):184–94.
11. Carter LE, et al. Screening for pediatric malnutrition at hospital admission: which screening tool is best? Nutr Clin Pract. 2020;35:951.
12. Huysentruyt K, et al. Accuracy of nutritional screening tools in assessing the risk of undernutrition in hospitalized children. J Pediatr Gastroenterol Nutr. 2015;61(2):159–66.
13. Valla FV, et al. Faltering growth in the critically ill child: prevalence, risk factors, and impaired outcome. Eur J Pediatr. 2018;177(3):345–53.
14. Marino LV, Magee A. A cross-sectional audit of the prevalence of stunting in children attending a regional paediatric cardiology service. Cardiol Young. 2016;26:787–9.
15. Mitting R, et al. Nutritional status and clinical outcome in postterm neonates undergoing surgery for congenital heart disease. Pediatr Crit Care Med. 2015;16:448.
16. Wootton S, Durkin K, Jackson A. Quality control issues related to assessment of body composition. Food Nutr Bull. 2014;35(2 Suppl):S79–85.
17. World Health Organization. Global database on child growth and malnutrition: child growth indicators and their interpretation. 2012. www.who.int/nutgrowhdb/about/introudction/en/index2.html.
18. Dunn RL, Stettler N, Mascarenhas MR. Refeeding syndrome in hospitalized pediatric patients. Nutr Clin Pract. 2003;18(4):327–32.
19. Byrnes MC, Stangenes J. Refeeding in the ICU: an adult and pediatric problem. Curr Opin Clin Nutr Metab Care. 2011;14(2):186–92.
20. Tume LN, et al. Nutritional support for children during critical illness: European Society of Pediatric and Neonatal Intensive Care (ESPNIC) metabolism, endocrine and nutrition section position statement and clinical recommendations. Intensive Care Med. 2020;46(3):411–25.
21. Joosten KF, Kerklaan D, Verbruggen SC. Nutritional support and the role of the stress response in critically ill children. Curr Opin Clin Nutr Metab Care. 2016;19(3):226–33.
22. Singer P, et al. ESPEN guideline on clinical nutrition in the intensive care unit. Clin Nutr. 2018;
23. Mehta NM, et al. Defining pediatric malnutrition: a paradigm shift toward etiology-related definitions. JPEN J Parenter Enteral Nutr. 2013;37(4):460–81.
24. Powell-Tuck J. Nutritional interventions in critical illness. Proc Nutr Soc. 2007;66(1):16–24.
25. Mehta NM, et al. Guidelines for the provision and assessment of nutrition support therapy in the pediatric critically ill patient: Society of Critical Care Medicine and American Society for Parenteral and Enteral Nutrition. Pediatr Crit Care Med. 2017;18(7):675–715.
26. D H. Congenital cardiac disease. In: Shaw V, Lawson M, editors. Clinical paediatric dietetics. Oxford: Blackwell Publishing; 2014.

27. Hulst JM, et al. Causes and consequences of inadequate substrate supply to pediatric ICU patients. Curr Opin Clin Nutr Metab Care. 2006;9(3):297–303.
28. Meyer R, et al. The impact of enteral feeding protocols on nutritional support in critically ill children. J Hum Nutr Diet. 2009;22(5):428–36.
29. Kerklaan D, et al. Worldwide survey of nutritional practices in PICUs. Pediatr Crit Care Med. 2016;17(1):10–8.
30. Briassoulis GC, Zavras NJ, Hatzis MT. Effectiveness and safety of a protocol for promotion of early intragastric feeding in critically ill children. Pediatr Crit Care Med. 2001;2(2):113–21.
31. Mehta NM, Compher C, A.S.P.E.N. Board of Directors. Clinical guidelines: nutrition support of the critically ill child. JPEN J Parenter Enteral Nutr. 2009;33(3):260–76.
32. Hamilton S, et al. A stepwise enteral nutrition algorithm for critically ill children helps achieve nutrient delivery goals*. Pediatr Crit Care Med. 2014;15(7):583–9.
33. Braudis NJ, et al. Enteral feeding algorithm for infants with hypoplastic left heart syndrome poststage I palliation. Pediatr Crit Care Med. 2009;10(4):460–6.
34. Zamberlan P, et al. Nutrition therapy in a pediatric intensive care unit: indications, monitoring, and complications. JPEN J Parenter Enteral Nutr. 2011;35:523.
35. Gentles E, et al. Delivery of enteral nutrition after the introduction of practice guidelines and participation of dietitians in pediatric critical care clinical teams. J Acad Nutr Diet. 2014;114(12):1974–80.e3.
36. Mara J, et al. An evaluation of enteral nutrition practices and nutritional provision in children during the entire length of stay in critical care. BMC Pediatr. 2014;14:186.
37. Koletzko B, et al. Use of parenteral nutrition in the pediatric ICU: should we panic because of PEPaNIC? Curr Opin Clin Nutr Metab Care. 2017;20(3):201–3.
38. Goulet O, Jochum F, Koletzko B. Early or late parenteral nutrition in critically ill children: practical implications of the PEPaNIC trial. Ann Nutr Metab. 2017;70(1):34–8.
39. Vanhorebeek I, et al. Effect of early supplemental parenteral nutrition in the paediatric ICU: a preplanned observational study of post-randomisation treatments in the PEPaNIC trial. Lancet Respir Med. 2017;5(6):475–83.
40. van Puffelen E, et al. Cost-effectiveness study of early versus late parenteral nutrition in critically ill children (PEPaNIC): preplanned secondary analysis of a multicentre randomised controlled trial. Crit Care. 2018;22(1):4.
41. Verstraete S, et al. Leukocyte telomere length in paediatric critical illness: effect of early parenteral nutrition. Crit Care. 2018;22(1):38.
42. Verstraete S, et al. Long-term developmental effects of withholding parenteral nutrition for 1 week in the paediatric intensive care unit: a 2-year follow-up of the PEPaNIC international, randomised, controlled trial. Lancet Respir Med. 2019;7(2):141–53.
43. The Royal College of Paediatrics and Child Health. Guidance: Paediatric multisystem inflammatory syndrome temporally associated with COVID-19. 2020.
44. Riphagen S, Gomez X, Gonzalez-Martinez C, Wilkinson N, Theocharis P. Hyperinflammatory shock in children during COVID-19 pandemic. Lancet. 2020;395:1607.
45. Fabi M, et al. Gastrointestinal presentation of Kawasaki disease: a red flag for severe disease? PLoS One. 2018;13(9):e0202658.
46. Marino LV, et al. Micronutrient status during paediatric critical illness: a scoping review. Clin Nutr. 2020;39(12):3571–93.
47. Eveleens RD, et al. Definitions, predictors and outcomes of feeding intolerance in critically ill children: a systematic review. Clin Nutr. 2020;39(3):685–93.
48. Marino LV, Johnson MJ, Beattie RM. Feeding intolerance in children with critical illness. Clin Nutr. 2020;39(3):609–11.

Psychology

Gillian Colville

Contents

J. Brierley et al. (eds.), *ESPNIC Children's Intensive Care Textbook*,
https://doi.org/10.1007/978-3-031-64762-8_56

Learning Objectives

In this chapter, the reader will learn about the main sources of psychological strain on children and families in PICU. For children, these are (a) potentially traumatising experiences, (b) difficulty recalling or understanding what is happening to them and (c) disturbing experiences which can occur in relation to delirium. It will also be explained that parents often suffer clinically significant rates of distress acutely and, in some cases, for many months after their child's admission to PICU. Illustrative examples of casework by a psychologist working in this setting will be provided, along with information about models of working with acute stress in medical settings, which may be helpful in guiding professional interactions in such a way that the risk of long-term psychological difficulties is minimised. Finally, an overview of the research on longer term psychological outcomes will be presented, providing the reader with an appreciation of how the majority of families naturally recover psychologically, but also drawing their attention to the fact that a minority will require further professional support in the longer term.

56.1 Introduction

As mortality rates have decreased in intensive care, there has been an increased focus on outcomes—emotional as well as physical—and a greater awareness of the potentially traumatising aspects of PICU admission for both the child and their family members. A new term, post-intensive care syndrome (PICS) [1], has been proposed to cover the constellation of difficulties adult ICU patients may experience as they recover from their critical illness. These include cognitive, social and psychological problems as well as fatigue and physical weakness. This conceptual framework has also recently been extended to embrace the experiences of family members, in relation to the critical care admission of a loved one (post-intensive care syndrome-family (PICS-F) [2] and specifically regarding the impact on patients and families in paediatric settings (post-intensive care syndrome-paediatric (PICS-p) [3]. The PICS-p framework emphasises the primacy of the family, including siblings, in the child's life and the importance of understanding how the child's illness and experiences on PICU interact with their developmental stage. In this chapter, the nature of the psychological strains relating to critical care treatment and its aftermath on patients and their parents are outlined, together with the latest evidence on how best to support them acutely and post-discharge.

56.2 Psychological Care of the Child

In the short term, the priorities in terms of psychologically informed support for children after PICU treatment are to encourage them to engage with the world again; to help them regain some kind of routine and to find appropriate forms of distraction for them, in the form of play activities.

The child's ability to adjust to what has happened will be delayed for some time, while their physical recovery is the main focus. They may require encouragement to eat and to mobilise in order to regain physical strength before they can begin to address recovery on a psychological level [4] and indeed may only report significant levels of distress many months later [5].

Apart from the general issues which arise whenever a child is admitted to hospital, which include separation from family, being in an unfamiliar place and the fear of pain, there are three aspects of the child's experience which are more specific to the fact that they are in critical care. These are (a) delirium, (b) contending with potentially traumatising experiences and (c) difficulties remembering or understanding what has happened.

(a) ***Paediatric Delirium*** In the past decade, there has been a growing appreciation of the prevalence of delirium in adult intensive care patients and its association with increased length of stay and mortality [6, 7] Recently, delirium assessment tools have been developed with PICU patients and their use incorporated into ESPNIC guidelines [8]. The true prevalence of delirium on PICU is unknown but as more units begin to assess it routinely, more data are becoming available, with one recent study estimating prevalence rates in patients admitted for 48 h or more, of 69% [9] using the Cornell Assessment of Pediatric Delirium (CAP-D) [10]. Furthermore, there is evidence that approximately one in three children experience strange hallucinatory or delusional experiences soon after weaning off the ventilator, and that memory for these experiences is an independent risk factor for the development of later post-traumatic stress symptoms [11].
As yet there is no consensus on pharmacological management, but it should be remembered that by definition delirium is a fluctuating condition which is self-limiting. There is a role for non-pharmacological interventions, such as strategies to increase the patient's orientation to their surroundings like providing favourite toys or blankets, or a daily activity plan on the wall. These have been found helpful with elderly patients, who often become delirious or confused when unwell, and have reduced their requirements for sedation [12]. Parental presence can be reassuring, although it is important to forewarn parents about the possibility of delirium, which can be quite distressing to witness. They can then they help gradually to orient and comfort their child (***See*** ▶ Case History 56.1).

(b) ***Potentially Traumatising Experiences***: As children begin to regain consciousness, they may start to remember the traumatic circumstances leading up to their admission, whether this was an accident or a period of rapid medical deterioration, and be troubled by this. They may also be distressed by what they witness on the unit such as the resuscitation of a neighbouring child [13]. Although a minority of children will go on to develop lasting symptoms of post-traumatic stress disorder (PTSD) (***See*** ▶ Box 56.1), the Pediatric Model of Traumatic Stress [14] suggests that it is possible to work preventatively with children in these situations by providing information in a timely way and helping to mobilise the child and family's natural coping resources.

(c) ***Memory and Understanding***: The 'Intensive care memory gap' [15] described by adult intensive care patients is also a feature of patients in paediatric settings. As a group, they also have more difficulty fully understanding what is happening, by virtue of their younger age. From the research data available, it seems that, apart from those associated with delirium as described above, most children's memories of PICU are neutral [16], with a significant minority of children remembering nothing at all about their admission. Some children will not be troubled by this lack of information, but others will require more details, once they are sufficiently recovered physically. Initially, and especially if they are in pain and debilitated by fatigue, they may only to be able to handle brief, age-appropriate

Box 56.1. Post-traumatic Stress Disorder (ICD-11 Code 6B40)

- Traumatic experience AND functional impairment
  - at least one symptom in each of the following three categories, lasting at least 1 month
- Re-experiencing (e.g. nightmares, flashbacks)
- Avoidance (e.g. avoiding talking about it, avoiding reminders)
- Feeling a continuous sense of threat (e.g. hypervigilance, exaggerated startle response)

  ▶ https://icd.who.int/en

explanations, which may need to be repeated several times. For younger children, or those with learning difficulties, the use of real-world toy figures may help to make explanations more tangible (***See*** ▶ Case History 56.2)

▪ Case History 56.1: Behavioural Management of Delirium

Teddy, 8-years-old, who was treated in PICU for a week for a respiratory infection, was very fearful in the days following extubation and finding it difficult to sleep. When he was referred to the unit psychologist, he confided that there were large 'creepy crawlies' on the ceiling above his bed. It was explained to his mother that this was likely to be delirium.

She found that she was unable to reassure her son initially, but that he became calmer when she stopped challenging him and agreed to sweep the 'creepy crawlies' away each morning when she came in. The symptoms gradually lessened and, in time, the child was able to understand that the creatures he had been scared of had not been real, and even to see the funny side of it.

▪ Case History 56.2: Psychological Support Post-injury

Susie, an 11-year-old child with mild learning difficulties, was involved in a road traffic collision while being driven to school by her mother and sustained a serious fracture to her femur. Her mother only sustained soft tissue injuries, but was briefly unconscious. Susie was extracted from the wreckage first and taken to hospital by ambulance on her own. Following surgery, she developed sepsis and required admission to PICU, where she was ventilated for 3 weeks. During her recovery on the general ward, Susie appeared withdrawn, angry and confused. She was referred to the unit psychologist in view of her distress. The psychologist obtained a detailed history of the main events of the accident and the PICU admission, in order to give a clear developmentally appropriate explanation to Susie, using real-world toy figures (***See*** ◘ Fig. 56.1) which were then photographed and made up into a story book, which she was given to keep. It emerged that the girl had not understood why her mother had not accompanied her to hospital.

Two months later, in a follow-up telephone call, Susie's parents reported that, after an initial period of being reluctant to return to school, her behaviour had largely returned to normal and that she had used the picture book to explain what had happened, to her classmates and her teacher

NB Personal details In the case histories have been changed to protect patient confidentiality

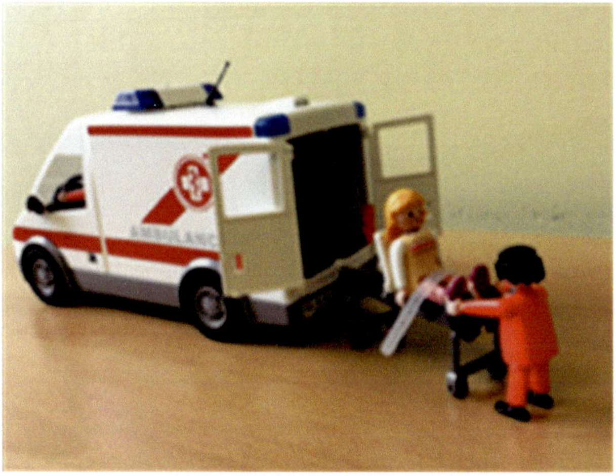

Fig. 56.1 Use of hospital play toys in explanations to children

56.3 Supporting Parents

In relation to supporting parents acutely on PICU, the emphasis is primarily preventative and should initially be focused on providing useful information—both about what is happening to their child and about normative psychological reactions in parents in this situation. The promotion of their normal coping strategies is also protective [14] against the development of PTSD. For example, if they usually cope with stress by making lists, it may be helpful to provide them with pen and paper and encourage them to identify what they most need to focus on in the short term and what can be left to deal with later. They can also be helped to think about who best to approach for emotional support. Sometimes other relatives such as grandparents are not able to provide as much support as parents need, because they are overwhelmed by their own anxieties about the child. In such a situation, a friend or colleague may be more practical help, or the parent may appreciate having an opportunity to talk over their worst fears with a professional such as, the unit psychologist, a social worker or a chaplain depending on preference and availability. At this early stage, it is important to acknowledge parents' long established needs for hope, proximity and clear information [17] and to be aware of the principles underpinning psychological first aid [18] (***See*** ▶ Box 56.2) which emphasises the value of creating a sense of safety, calm and connectedness, together with providing clear information and support. Increasingly, paediatric units are providing ICU diaries to parents in which to record their experiences and the child's progress [19] as there is evidence that these help to reduce PTSD symptoms in the relatives of adult ICU patients [20]. There are also a number of useful online resources about managing psychological adjustment in children and parents in medical settings (***See*** ▶ Box 56.3).

There is an assumption that the high-tech environment of PICU is particularly distressing for parents, but research has shown that the impact on their role as parents is a greater source of stress [21] and that their *subjective* fear that the child could die is much more predictive of later psychological distress that objective indices of risk [22].

Box 56.2. Psychological First Aid [18]

People do better over the long term if they are helped to:

- Feel safe
- Feel connected to others
- Feel calm
- Maintain hope
- Regain a sense of control by being able to help themselves
  ▶ https://www.who.int/mental_health/world-mental-health-day/ppt.pdf

Box 56.3. Useful Online Resources

- Information for professionals about PTSD in children ▶ https://www.nctsn.org/
- Downloadable information sheets for families about how to manage traumatic experiences ▶ https://www.healthcaretoolbox.org/
- Information for families about psychological recovery in the year following PICU dischargecite [23] ▶ https://www.georgespicu.org.uk/families/

In a series of qualitative interviews with children and their parents, Atkins et al. [23] describe the over-riding drive to return to 'normal' that characterises families' descriptions of the year following PICU discharge. For some, the definition of 'normal' has to take account of markedly changed circumstances, such as a new diagnosis or uncertainty about prognosis, and for older children, there is often a need to reassert their independence after a period of being unusually dependent on their parents. In time though most families were able to put together a family story about what happened and even to appreciate that has been some positive aspects to their experience, echoing another study which found evidence of significant post-traumatic growth in this population [24]. Another theme which emerged in these interviews was the need to prioritise supporting the child's *physical* recovery before addressing the psychological and social, leading the researchers to propose that a biopsychosocial model is useful to bear in mind in relation to advising or supporting families over this period [4]. A booklet based on the findings of this study is available online at ▶ https://www.georgespicu.org.uk/families/—(***See*** ◘ Fig. 56.2).

In the longer term, most parents feel their child is relatively unchanged by the experience of being treated in PICU [25] especially if like the majority, they are very young, although there is evidence that around one-third of older children report significant levels of PTSD symptoms [11]. However, parents are aware of a change in their relationship, in that they describe themselves as more fearful for their and children, acknowledging that this can lead to over-protectiveness [25] and a minority (5–28% of children and 10–21% of parents [26]) report significant PTSD symptoms

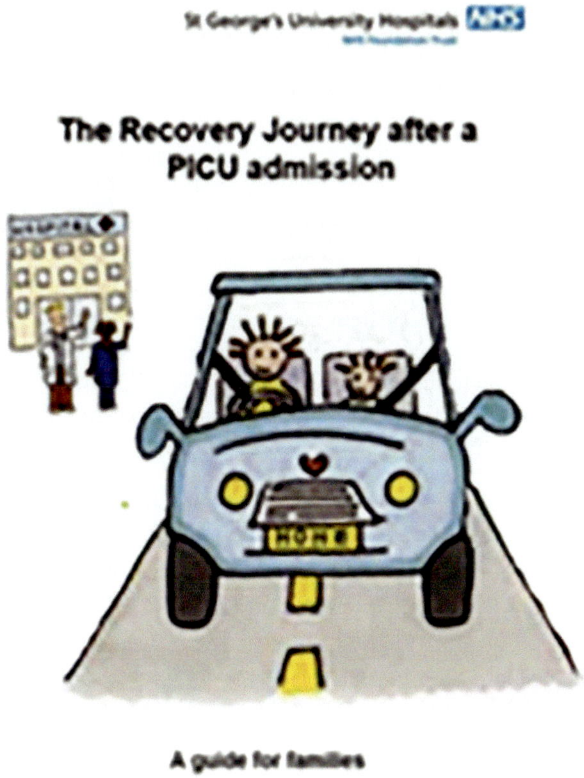

Fig. 56.2 Illustration from family information booklet [23]

even as much as a year later [5], which can have a significant impact on wider family functioning [27].

For children and parents with frank and persisting symptoms of post-traumatic stress, there are a number of evidence-based treatments available [28]. One example of a brief treatment which has been found to be effective in parents after PICU [29] is narrative exposure therapy [30]. Another is eye movement desensitisation reprocessing (EMDR) therapy [31]. Finally, the risk of complicated grief reactions has been found to be elevated in parents bereaved on PICU [32], who may consequently require additional support in the community after they leave the hospital.

Take-Home Messages

- The majority of families adjust well psychologically after PICU
- However, up to 28% of children and 21% parents report clinically significant levels of PTSD symptoms related to the child's PICU admission, within the year following discharge
- Delirium is a feature of children's experience of PICU and should be routinely assessed
- Psychological first aid is a useful framework to guide acute professional interactions with families
- Initially, families may only be able to focus on physical recovery—psychological issues may become more apparent later
- The child will be able to adjust better if they are provided with an explanation of what has happened to them, in developmentally appropriate language
- Complicated grief reactions are common in bereaved parents after PICU treatment

References

1. Needham DM, Davidson J, Cohen H, Hopkins RO, Weinert C, Wunsch H, et al. Improving long-term outcomes after discharge from intensive care unit: report from a stakeholders' conference. Crit Care Med. 2012;40:502–9.
2. Davidson JE, Jones C, Bienvenu OJ. Family response to critical illness: post intensive care syndrome- family. Crit Care Med. 2012;40(2):618–24.
3. Manning JC, Pinto NP, Rennick JE, Colville G, Curley MAQ. Conceptualizing post intensive care syndrome in children—the PICS-p framework. Pediatr Crit Care Med. 2018;19(4):298–300. https://doi.org/10.1097/PCC.0000000000001476.
4. Atkins E, Colville G, John M. A 'biopsychosocial' model for recovery: a grounded theory study of families' journeys after a paediatric intensive care admission. Intensive Crit Care Nurs. 2012;28(3):133–40.
5. Colville G, Pierce C. Patterns of post-traumatic stress symptoms in families after paediatric intensive care. Intensive Care Med. 2012;38:1523–31.
6. Ely EW, Shintani A, Truman B, Speroff T, Gordon SM, Harrell FE Jr, et al. Delirium as a predictor of mortality in mechanically ventilated patients in the intensive care unit. JAMA. 2004;291(14):1753–62.
7. Ely EW, Gautam S, Margolin R, Francis J, May L, Speroff T, et al. The impact of delirium in the intensive care unit on hospital length of stay. Intensive Care Med. 2001;27(12):1892–900.
8. Harris J, Ramelet AS, van Dijk M, Pokorna P, Wielenga J, Tume L, et al. Clinical recommendations for pain, sedation, withdrawal and delirium assessment in critically ill infants and children: an ESPNIC position statement for healthcare professionals. Intensive Care Med. 2016;42(6):972–86. https://doi.org/10.1007/s00134-016-4344-1.
9. Dervan LA, Di Gennaro JL, Farris RW, Watson RS. Delirium in a tertiary PICU: risk factors and outcomes. Pediatr Crit Care Med. 2020;21:21–32. https://doi.org/10.1097/PCC.0000000000002126.
10. Traube C, Silver G, Kearney J, Patel A, Atkinson TM, Yoon MJ, et al. Cornell assessment of pediatric delirium: a valid, rapid, observational tool for screening delirium in the PICU. Crit Care Med. 2014;42(3):656–63.
11. Colville G, Kerry S, Pierce C. Children's factual and delusional memories of intensive care. Am J Respir Crit Care Med. 2008;177:976–82.
12. Inouye SK, Westendorp RG, Saczynski JS. Delirium in elderly people. Lancet. 2014;383(9920):911–22.
13. Noyes J. 'Ventilator-dependent' children who spend prolonged periods of time in intensive care units when they no longer have a medical need or want to be there. J Clin Nurs. 2000;9:774–83.

14. Kazak AE, Kassam-Adams N, Schneider S, Zelikovsky N, Alderfer MA, Rourke M. An integrative model of pediatric medical traumatic stress. J Pediatr Psychol. 2006;31:343–55.
15. Griffiths RD, Jones C. Filling the intensive care memory gap? Intensive Care Med. 2001;27(2):344–6.
16. Playfor S, Thomas D, Choonara I. Recollection of children following intensive care. Arch Dis Child. 2000;83(5):445–8.
17. Molter NC. Needs of relatives of critically ill patients: a descriptive study. Heart Lung. 1979;8(2):332–9.
18. Hobfoll SE, Watson P, Bell CC, Bryant RA, Brymer MJ, Friedman MJ, et al. Five essential elements of immediate and mid-term mass trauma intervention: empirical evidence. Psychiatry. 2007;70:283–315.
19. Lynch F, Endacott R, Latour JM. Patient diaries: survey of paediatric intensive care units in the United Kingdom and Ireland. Nurs Crit Care. 2020;25(1):31–6. https://doi.org/10.1111/nicc.12472.
20. Jones C, Bäckman C, Capuzzo M, Egerod I, Flaatten H, Granja C, et al. Intensive care diaries reduce new onset post traumatic stress disorder following critical illness: a randomised, controlled trial. Crit Care. 2010;14(5):R168.
21. Curley MA, Wallace J. Effects of the nursing mutual participation model of care on parental stress in the pediatric intensive care unit—a replication. J Pediatr Nurs. 1992;7(6):377–85.
22. Balluffi A, Kassam-Adams N, Kazak A, Tucker M, Dominguez T, Helfaer M. Traumatic stress in parents admitted to the pediatric intensive care unit. Pediatr Crit Care Med. 2004;5:547–53.
23. Atkins E, John M, Colville G. Families' experiences of life in the year after a child's critical illness: navigating the road to a "new normal". J Pediatr Intensive Care. 2020;9:188–95. https://doi.org/10.1055/s-0040-1705132.
24. Colville G, Cream P. Post-traumatic growth in parents after a child's admission to intensive care: maybe Nietzsche was right? Intensive Care Med. 2009;35(5):919–23.
25. Colville G, Darkins J, Hesketh J, Bennett V, Alcock J, Noyes J. The impact on parents of a child's admission to intensive care: integration of qualitative findings from a cross-sectional study. Intensive Crit Care Nurs. 2009;25(2):72–9.
26. Nelson LP, Gold JI. Posttraumatic stress disorder in children and their parents following admission to the pediatric intensive care unit: a review. Pediatr Crit Care Med. 2012;13:338–47.
27. Riley AR, Williams CN, Moyer D, et al. Parental posttraumatic stress symptoms in the context of pediatric post intensive care syndrome: impact on the family and opportunities for intervention. Clin Pract Pediatr Psychol. 2021;9:156–66. https://doi.org/10.1037/cpp0000399.
28. National Institute for Health and Care Excellence (NICE). The management of PTSD in adults and children in primary and secondary care. NICE clinical guideline 116. Manchester: National Institute for Health and Care Excellence; 2018. www.nice.org.uk/guidance/NG116. Accessed 2 Mar 2020.
29. Colville GA. Narrative exposure therapy with parents who have been traumatized in pediatric settings: a case series. Clin Pract Pediatric Psychol 2017;5(2):161–169 https://doi.org/10.1037/cppp0000187.
30. Conijn T, De Roos C, Vreugdenhil HJI, Van Dijk-Lokkart EM, Wijburg FA, Haverman L. Effectiveness of time-limited eye movement desensitization reprocessing therapy for parents of children with a rare life-limiting illness: a randomized clinical trial. Orphanet J Rare Dis. 2022;17:328. https://doi.org/10.1186/s13023-022-02500-9.
31. Schauer M, Neuner F, Elbert T. Narrative exposure therapy: a short-term treatment for traumatic stress disorders. 2nd ed. Boston: Hogrefe Publishing; 2011.
32. Meert KL, Shear K, Newth CJ, Harrison R, Berger J, Zimmerman J, et al. Follow-up study of complicated grief among parents eighteen months after a child's death in the pediatric intensive care unit. J Palliat Med. 2011;14(2):207–14.

Ethics in Paediatric and Neonatal ICU

Hanaa Benjeddi and Joe Brierley

Contents

J. Brierley et al. (eds.), *ESPNIC Children's Intensive Care Textbook*,
https://doi.org/10.1007/978-3-031-64762-8_57

Learning Objectives

- To understand the basic moral theories used in contemporary bioethics.
- To understand the ethical and legal questions facing the children's intensive care team and the debates about different approaches to them.
- To understand the importance of ethical support to the modern ICU team.

57.1 Introduction

The term ethics has many meanings, but generally, for those working in paediatric and neonatal intensive care, it is most familiar from decision-making, often involving the limitation of life-sustaining treatments. However, several other relevant issues with a moral dimension affect daily ICU practice. How much should a country spend on health care, how much of this should be used for children and of this, how much for children's ICU beds? Related to this, what should the healthcare team be paid compared to other professions? Should ICU teams be allowed to strike for better pay and conditions or to persuade funders to spend more on health care, whether government or private providers.

Europe has an incredibly diverse population due to centuries of migration accelerated by recent issues such as globalisation and previous colonialism. This means that whereas in some countries, traditional state cultural norms, often predicated on religious traditions, have given way to a more secular approach, elsewhere, resistance to any such transition remains firm.

At its heart, ethics is about whether something is right or wrong. But who decides what is right or wrong? Where does our source of morality come from—is it personal or the state, or are there universal ethical norms to which even a God or the Gods must adhere? This is important to the ICU team because our team members, our patients and their families may have very different cultural norms.

This chapter will explore an elementary introduction to the moral theories most frequently used in health care and then consider a few important ethical areas in intensive care, including decisions to limit therapy, long-term technological support, consent in ICU, pandemics, research and innovative therapy, second opinions and international transfer for treatment.

57.2 Traditional Moral Theories

57

Whilst the sources of people's morality can vary, modern bioethical thinking is often traced, at least in Westernised countries, to the post-Second World War United States. It is often considered to have originated with the concepts of citizen's rights, equality and an overdue push against medical paternalism. Perhaps the most influential work, which still features in many an introduction to bioethics course, is Beauchamp and Childress's Principles of Biomedical Ethics, in which the authors develop a healthcare ethics approach using the *four principles* of autonomy, beneficence, non-maleficence and justice [1]. Whilst each principle was already well-established in moral philosophy, the new focus on health care was influential.

In short: Autonomy means allowing patients to make their own decision, beneficence the obligation to act for the benefit of the patient, non-maleficence to avoid harm and justice to ensure the fair distribution of healthcare resources.

Generically important, these foundation principles are arguably too limited to apply to children or the critically ill, and certainly to critically ill children. They often seem to be in conflict in any specific situation. Can using them help us know whether to provide a tracheostomy and long-term ventilation for a child with a progressive neurologically regressive disease? Whose autonomy are we discussing, is not this a harmful continuation of a prolonged dying process, but surely continuing existence is beneficial? Is this expensive undertaking just if other children live in extreme poverty in the same country?

Other models exist and need to be understood by the intensive care team. *Utilitarianism*, developed during the Enlightenment in the UK, suggests the correct action should be that which delivers the greatest good (with many definitions, e.g. pleasure or human flourishing) for the greatest number of people with the resources available. It is the outcome that determines the morality of any action. Attractive at the macro-level, utility classically meets challenge with individual claims to high-expense treatment such as ICU rather than more cost-effective preventative public health. It is often contrasted with *deontology*, associated with the German philosopher Immanuel Kant, in which it is the morality of the action itself that is most important rather than the outcome—so a universal generalisable moral law suggests that actions such as lying or stealing are always wrong, even if they lead to a better outcome.

Virtue ethics has been influential in health care and focuses on the role of character and virtue rather than the action or its outcome. It considers ethical issues in the broader sense of how we ought to live or perhaps even asks what sort of ICU teams we want to be. This is most readily found in the sets of values many institutions, or indeed ICUs, espouse in mission statements or similar core documents. However, whilst we might aspire to act as a virtuous individual might, it is not clear what this means in day-to-day PICU practice. Is there really an ideal nurse lead who others might copy? Should we run the ward round as the latest holder of the Nobel Peace Prize might?

Finally, and arguably the most useful to those working in PICU, is *feminist ethics* or the *ethics of care*, in which criticism of other ethical theories is advanced insofar as they have undervalued women's moral experience. The feminist approach focuses less on the transactional nature of moral decision-making but instead on people's relationships—the caring elements, with the child in PIC not an individual with rights, about whom decisions are made but a son, a cousin, a sister or a niece. It considers the vulnerabilities and needs of those involved far more than traditional moral theories, especially in our context the caring, loving relationships of the family.

57.3 Ethics in Modern PICU

What does ethics mean in the day-to-day PICU environment? Perhaps most frequently, the term is used when considering the moral issue involved in providing organ support for very sick children. 'I think this is unethical' is a phrase not infrequently muttered by teams caring for a child slowly dying with full ongoing ICU support. But what does this mean, is stopping and allowing the child to die if the parents want to carry on somehow more ethical? Who decides, and how? Decisions to limit life-sustaining treatments are some of the most challenging in paediatrics, especially as the child's death may follow.

57.4 Death

Given the increase in children living with life-limiting conditions, technological dependence and background complexity, one important area is the traditional concept that the time of human death should only be in the hands of a God. This model somewhat contradicts the modern medical paradigm in which most deaths have medical decisions made, ultimately determining the time of death. This might be as clear as the cessation of cardiopulmonary resuscitation, withdrawal of ECMO in a child with a catastrophic brain injury or a decision not to admit a dying child into the PICU. It is a valuable discussion to counter the meaningless, often unchallenged, statement that 'we want everything to be done'.

However, the nuanced approach to decision-making in this context with children and their parents requires the PIC team and referring specialists to develop thoughtful, compassionate communication methods.

The law, of course, varies hugely worldwide, even in Europe, a single continent. For example, some countries permit euthanasia in children, whereas others do not allow it in anyone. PIC teams must operate within the law of their state, yet might be fundamental in advocates for changing that law if they see a need, given the law is not static. Culture is another crucial variable—there are normative values in society, eventually represented in our statutes, occasionally supranational laws for some such as the European bodies, and for most countries, the application of Human Rights whether from bodies such as the UN, so the UN Convention of the Rights of the Child or the EU Human Rights Act.

However, there is more subtle cultural variability—whether between different areas of Europe, in which, for example, the likelihood of having a one-way wean of life-sustaining therapy on PIC at the end of life rather than dying during failed resuscitation varies by the region of Europe involved,) or in adult ICU the same dichotomy is related to the religious views of the treating clinician.

Organ donation and post-mortem examination both have many ethical components, though as so often with children, the child's best interest, parent decision-making.

57.5 Moral Injury

The question of how to resolve situations in which the PIC team and referring colleagues think carrying on life-sustaining therapy is in the child's best interests or, frankly, harmful to the child varies too. In some European countries, the PICU team are able to withdraw life-sustaining therapy irrespective of the parents' views; elsewhere, the PIC team can only do this with the approval of a court; in other countries, a child's parents can effectively determine what happens in this context.

Providing life-sustaining treatment for a child when the team think it is the wrong thing to do is an increasing part of modern PICU. The concept of moral distress was first highlighted in nursing students in the 1970s and involves healthcare workers being negatively affected by delivering treatment they disagree with. Initially, a nursing comment on the moral basis of some physician-determined treatments, often towards the end of life, it is now increasingly recognised as harm caused to those forced to deliver activities with which they ethically disagree, whether in military, healthcare or legal settings. The arguably pejorative term distress, with its association with fragility in those affected, is increasingly replaced with the term moral injury following criticism of the entire concept.

Nonetheless, we all have a responsibility to look after ourselves and our colleagues, as do the institutions which employ us.

Significant changes in the population admitted to PICU underpin some of the current ethical challenges. Survival rates have soared, though not entirely due to improvements in treatment but more due to changes in the decisions made about PICU provision. Admissions of children with chronic healthcare conditions now predominate in many units; complexity, severe neuro-disability, long-term technological dependence, and recurrent, prolonged admission are relatively new entrants to the PICU lexicon.

Parents now frequently understand complex PICU terminology and structures as they have either been there before or have children at home on mechanical support. This means open, transparent, compassionate partnership with families whilst maintaining child-centred care is now the standard for every PICU.

The role of gatekeeper to the high-expense resource of ICU is still the role of the intensivist, depending on whether the unit is closed or open.

57.6 Pandemics

During the COVID-19 pandemic, the ICU gatekeeper role became an international hot topic in adult medicine, but thankfully not with children. However, this role is the daily reality for many children's ICU teams in low-resource environments and requires clear objective frameworks to avoid any unconscious, as well as conscious, bias. Overwhelming demand is an occasional experience in annual RSV peaks but rare otherwise. Because of this, the children's ICU community is arguably less prepared for a future pandemic predominantly affecting children than their adult colleagues were before the COVID pandemic. The last serious work in most paediatric teams occurred around the H1N1 pandemic before the changes in the paediatric case mix described above. An update is required and was, somewhat ironically, called for just before the COVID-19 pandemic [2]. What is clear is that the standard, predominantly adult medicine-based, utilitarian paradigm of previous pandemic planning will need a recalibration for modern-day paediatrics.

57.7 Consent

Another challenging area is the consent for procedures that are or could be, in place in the ICU. Developed from the speciality of anaesthetics, adult ICU has assumed permission to treat patients because those treatments are urgent and life-saving treatment, usually in an unconscious, critically ill person, delivered by specialists who traditionally did not seek consent to provide anaesthesia. Paediatric ICU rather followed this lead, whereas, in the neonatal ICU, a strong infant's best interests standard meant that parents were not made offers they could not refuse.

However, is our patient the child, or more the family dyad with the parents who, for most children, we provide information to and seek consent from?

This is changing at different rates in different countries based on national legal and cultural norms. However, given that many children are admitted to ICU for prolonged periods, undergo recurrent admissions or are managed on life-sustaining technologies at home, the previous justifications seem inadequate. Which interventions should the ICU team seek specific consent for, what information standard is required, and what are the implications of refusing consent? Information from the UK suggests parents would like more chances to provide their consent, but they do not want this to get in the way of delivering treatments. (Brierley JME consent).

It is sensible for all ICUs to provide detailed information at admission about likely information, and depending on the local situation, suitable consent processes with the information the parents/child need to provide consent.

57.8 Research

Although the evidence base for much of what happens in the ICU is poor, this has improved in recent years. Part of this has been accepting that research must be a daily part of ICU practice. Randomised intervention trials are increasing, having been the exception around the turn of the century when observational reports predominated. With such a diverse population and low specific disease case numbers in most centres, collaborative national and international multi-centre studies are becoming the norm. Deferred consent is now standard, in which research can commence during the acute admission episode with consent for participation and retention of data obtained when there is more time for discussion.

Research aims to generate generalisable data without targeting benefit to the patient. Occasionally, when a child is very sick, and there are no evidence-based/standard treatment options, specialist teams may consider trying novel or compassionate treatments to treat the child. The ICU team may be asked to consider continuing life-sustaining therapy whilst such interventions are tried—whether operations or chemotherapy. The balance of the burdens and proposed benefits can be nuanced. The ICU team must advocate for the child whilst recognising the understandable desire of the family and treating clinicians to explore all options.

57.9 Second Opinions

Often, if a novel treatment is proposed, obtaining a second opinion from an independent specialist in the relevant specialities, including ICU, is ethically sensible. This can also be useful to reassure families if no such treatment is being considered, but the child's outcome seems poor.

Such opinions should be based on therapeutic disease-modifying treatments and be clear if different ethical norms between countries are relevant, such as discussing end-of-life treatments where euthanasia is legal in one country but not the other.

57.10 Ethics Support

There are little data about what ethical support should be available for the ICU team, but given that end-of-life and ethical issues feature highly on areas that ICU staff feel least prepared for and worry most about, support and training must be taken more seriously by the ICU management team, and institutions. They must be rapidly available and have suitable expertise.

References

1. Beauchamp TL, Childress JF. Principles of biomedical ethics. 8th ed. Oxford: Oxford University Press; 2019.
2. Brierley J, Playfor S, Ray S. Planning for next pandemic: call for new guidance. Lancet Respir Med. 2020;8(3):228–9.

Chaplains and Faith Support

Jim Linthicum and Joe Brierley

Contents

J. Brierley et al. (eds.), *ESPNIC Children's Intensive Care Textbook*,
https://doi.org/10.1007/978-3-031-64762-8_58

Learning Objectives

Understand the role of chaplaincy and faith support to children, families, and staff in pediatric and neonatal intensive care. Determine how spiritual support can help during periods of critical illness, and the rituals important for some during these episodes and in end-of-life care.

58.1 Introduction

> *Faith is irrational, but then so is the ICU.*
> PICU parent quote

Many would say the paediatric intensive care (PICU) has a rationality described by solid numbers and data, a claim Faith and religion do not make. However, the PICU is an environment where the rational medical world must coexist with religion and spirituality, not least in the most challenging cases. Both the families of critically ill children and many members of the PICU team seek support and meaning beyond the scientific. This chapter will explore the relationship by examining the ICU setting and the issues involving faith that can arise there, exploring them using a published Chaplaincy and Spiritual Care taxonomy to highlight not only those issues but also the interventions and, where possible, the outcomes, though not based so much on rationality but in reality, and perspective.

The children's or paediatric intensive care (PICU) environment represents a particularly challenging area where parents, usually the ultimate decision-makers for younger children, share serious decision-making in an unfamiliar, intimidating, and often scary environment. This is especially true when life-and-death critical-care decisions are made. These challenges can occur in various ways and touch different professional groups and vocations where creative interventions can be developed in the medical/psychosocial field, including Spiritual and Religious Care (SRC).

General taxonomies related to SRC have been created to enable analysis of the areas, though mostly in adult settings. However, in 2019, Zhong et al. published a predictive model for chaplain taxonomy patterns through latent class analysis in infants in a paediatric inpatient setting, [1] which Nash and colleagues extrapolated to the broader paediatric environment, including the PICU [2].

58.2 The Taxonomy

The taxonomy model used by both Zhong et al. and Nash is based on an item developed by Massey et al. known as the Advocate Chaplaincy Taxonomy [3]. The taxonomy consists of 100 items divided into three categories: Intended Effect, Methods, and Interventions [3]. 'The Intended Effects category purportedly refers to the outcome(s) a chaplain hopes to accomplish, whereas Methods describes how a chaplain hopes to achieve the desired outcome. Finally, Interventions refer to what a chaplain does to achieve the desired outcome' [1].

We will use this loose framework to explore and describe issues pertinent to providing SRC in a paediatric and neonatal ICU. In addition, as some of these issues will fit into the existing taxonomy, their context will be explored to see if distinctive features are present.

58.3 Setting

Before focusing on the specific location, there are certain assumptions regarding working in paediatrics. In her *Blogging Chaplains* entry, Kate Bradford defines them as:

1. Children have different spiritual needs to adults; children and adolescents are at different development stages: physically, cognitively, emotionally, and spiritually, depending on their age and life experience.
2. Children are more vulnerable and require significant safeguards around their care.
3. Paediatric chaplains often visit parents and relatives who have been traumatically impacted by serious illness or ongoing disability of their child. In this situation, chaplains might ask, "Who is the patient?"
4. Decisions are being made by parents, guardians, and medical staff on behalf of patients who cannot speak for themselves.
5. There is heightened intensity around childhood illness, triggering precipitation of anticipatory losses of hopes and dreams of the parents, family, and broader community.
6. Childhood illness, disability, and death alter family systems forever, indelibly changing siblings' lives.
7. When a young life does not reach its potential, there is a widespread belief that this is not fair, and there are related issues of injustice, blame, guilt, and shame.
8. Our culture perceives serious childhood illness, disability, and death as a reversal of natural order, and consequently does not cope well with these situations.
9. There is a responsibility on all practitioners to be aware of self and the way in which their actions affect the plasticity of the family system.

(*Blogging Chaplains Website*—**Distinctives of Paediatric Hospital Chaplaincy** Kate Bradford June 2015.)

The setting we use here as normative for our exploration will be a tertiary UK PICU where we have conducted some interviews with patients, families and staff earlier [4]. Examples of helpful Spiritual and Religious Care (SRC) practice will be reviewed in interventions, which provides data to make even the spiritual have some measurability.

Because responses to having a child in PICU, or being the child in PICU, and from staff caring for the child, are as unique as the critically ill child being discussed, generalisation is difficult, if not impossible, necessitating 'road brush' applications. Some of the catalysts regarding response include:

- Hope and a sense of future.
- Fear of that same future.
- Trust of the professionals dealing with the child and their decision-making, including staff's trust in themselves in challenging situations.
- Moral and ethical questions, particularly in times of disagreement.

- In terms of spiritual care, the 'bigger questions perhaps best described by Douglas Adams as "Life, the Universe and Everything"'.
- Ways to ensure that all parties feel heard and valued and have a shared understanding of the situation, possible consequences of treatment and an appreciation of why different interventions are being explored.

In Table 58.1 from Zhong et al., the frequencies of particular taxonomy items are shown by percentage in the three categories of Intended Effects, Methods and Outcomes [1] (Fig. 58.1).

As not all of the items were identified in the review a use greater than 10%, like the tables here, are selected to both be identified and then give descriptions for understanding use on the Paediatric ICU:

58.3.1 Intended Effect

Demonstrate caring and concern—interpretation of this can be subjective for both the giver and receiver. The term intended is essential here, and acknowledgement of the effectiveness of this can be based on it leading to a Method or Intervention.

Helping someone feel comforted—while more measurable than the previous item, the resulting Method or Intervention guides an understanding of the result.

Table 58.1 Frequencies (%) of taxonomy items used in more than 10% of chaplain visits

Category	Items	Initial visit ($n = 433$)	Follow-up visit ($n = 388$)	Total ($n = 821$)
Intended effect	Demonstrate caring and concern	326 (75%)	245 (63%)	571 (70%)
	Helping someone feel comforted	106 (24%)	123 (32%)	229 (28%)
	Faith affirmation	90 (21%)	102 (26%)	192 (23%)
	Build a relationship of care and support	101 (23%)	51 (13%)	152 (19%)
	Convey calm presence	62 (14%)	40 (10%)	122 (15%)
	Establish rapport and connectedness	33 (8%)	66 (17%)	99 (12%)
Method	Offer spiritual/religious support	419 (97%)	346 (89%)	765 (93%)
	Offer emotional support	35 (8%)	67 (17%)	102 (12%)
Intervention	Pray	383 (88%)	323 (83%)	706 (86%)
	Active listening	107 (25%)	111 (29%)	218 (27%)
	Compassionate touch	26 (6%)	55 (14%)	81 (10%)

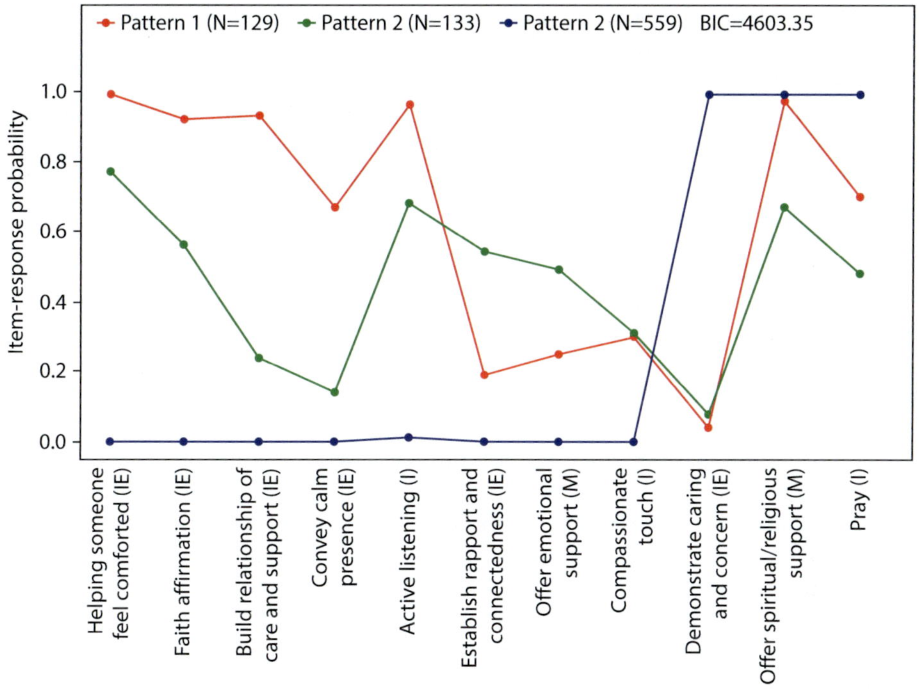

Fig. 58.1 Chaplain taxonomy patterns estimated using a 3-class LCA model analyzing the 11 most frequently delivered items to infants. *BIC* Bayesian information criterion, *I* intervention, *IE* intended effect, *M* method

Faith affirmation—Idiosyncratic and raises whether the SRC provider needs to be of that faith.

Build a relationship of care and support—While pertinent to the Paediatric ICU and includes all service users, it might sit more usefully in the Method section.

Convey calm presence—If considered part of SRC, this conveys an example of how all staff on the unit can provide this provision.

Establish rapport and connectedness—again, fits more appropriately into Methods.

58.3.2 Method

Offer spiritual/religious support—the critical intervention of any SRC, which needs to be unpacked for this chapter (see below).

Offer emotional support—often done in partnership with other psychosocial team members.

58.3.3 Intervention

Pray—while having expectations of Method can be interpreted in various ways that need, to an extent, to be made explicit for shared understanding between provider and receiver.

Active listening—again, an intervention is expected of all care providers. Therefore, if seen as a part of SRC, it demonstrates the involvement of a more general group.

Compassionate touch—In light of current controversies, this intervention needs, at best, to happen within very proscribed and mutually accepted boundaries. Often delivered by the medical and nursing teams, this again shows the mutuality of SRC work.

There is a sense of generality to all of these; however, they often lack both the specificity and humanity addressed in this chapter. Therefore, it is vital to start with descriptions that allow the models here to apply to PICUs internationally.

58.4 Who Carries Out This Work?

National and international RSC services differ greatly depending on perceived needs and resources available. Ideally, as religious and spiritual needs can often differ, practitioners must have a knowledge of the needs of specific faiths and the ability to widen their purview to the more general questions of spirituality. In recent years, the field of Chaplaincy has sometimes tried to embrace the latter with more enthusiasm than the former, although its remit can often seem more diffuse.

In our hospital, for example, spiritual can cover many of the issues mentioned above, including

- Hope for the present and future, sometimes requiring the hope to be reimagined and redrawn.
- Issues of meaning—why is this happening to me or my child?
- Existing belief structures and the comfort or challenges that they offer in a more specific situation setting.
- Relationships—not only externally, but also internally, particularly when difficult decisions have to be made (i.e. 'don't know if I can live with myself if I make that decision'—parent speaking to Jim Linthicum).
- Transcendence—not only in terms of relationship with a transcendent process or being but seeing the bigger picture.

This description helps define who carries out this work, for, while the RSC provider will often have some involvement in these situations, families, children, and staff often gravitate to those with whom they have already built a relationship of trust and with whom they feel a degree of comfort. This, as seen below, speaks to the need for all caregivers in the PICU to know how to provide RSC and when to refer to others.

58.5 How Does the Work Happen?

The first requirement for this provision is presence or simply being there. Seeing an RSC provider or someone who can provide such support creates availability and familiarity. It can often take time for a patient, family, or staff member to feel comfortable approaching or being approached by someone with whom they can discuss some of these issues. For that reason, RSC requires a practitioner known throughout the department. Nursing and medical staff often watch RSC interactions quietly from afar before deciding to trust the RSC provider, which forms a regular part of chaplaincy discussion.

Another requirement is the ability to journey with a patient, staff, or family member on their terms, not those of the RSC provider. This can be particularly difficult if there are disagreements about a child's best interests when the RSC provider can be perceived as advocating either for a particular medical procedure or against the suggestions of the experts. Families and clinicians can, if given enough time, usually reach an agreement about best interests, but part of the nature of PICU is that time is not always available, creating a challenge that, if not dealt with sensitively, can mean the RSC team potentially losing the trust of one or more of the participants involved.

The ability to signpost and build external relationships can feature in a relationship with a RSC provider. Sometimes, no matter how close a patient, family or staff member may be to the provider, the information is simply not within their gift. This can happen when dealing with people of other faiths or belief systems, as well as the provider's own. A knowledge of resources or, at the very least, how to access them is essential. End-of-life life care can be needed rapidly, so the RSC provider's knowledge or database needs to be up-to-date and readily accessible.

Signposting can also be a separate theme because some of the information or acts that are signposted already exist within the unit or hospital. Rituals can be both bespoke or existing and can be modified to the situation. Providing rituals can require a great deal of collaboration between the RSC and PICU team, and the RSC must be sensitive to the medical situation, after all, the primary reason for the child's situation.

One intervention sought on more than one occasion has been the marriage of those with a child in an end-of-life care situation, a process that has both legal and pastoral implications. As neither parent is dying, they cannot avail themselves of the State's willingness to provide for a deathbed wedding. In England, however, the State Church recognises the need for a wedding when the parent's child is severely ill or receiving end-of-life care. JL has participated in at least three of these situations, and other of the hospital's SRC practitioners have participated in others. This has not always meant that the child died, but meeting this pastoral need allowed the parents a degree of control in a situation where they otherwise felt out of control. (It must be noted that such an offering can differ from country to country.)

Most faiths have other rituals requested in the PICU, particularly if death seems imminent. These include baptism, the sacrament of the sick, prayers in the Christian tradition and many more when working across faiths. These fall well within the taxonomy of RSC, acknowledging the distinctiveness of this service.

Falkenburg et al., while showing the broadening dimension of this type of care from fundamental religion to complex spirituality, pointed out the serious 'existential issues that parents in particular deal with when facing speak[ing] of parent's connectedness with the deceased child and the hope of some kind of reuniting after one's own death' [5]. While this type of situation needs to be handled with care, particularly if the risk of familial self-destructiveness accompanies the end of the child's death, it again points to a distinctive offering of the RSC provider.

58.6 What Are the Processes?

Although much that is discussed here can seem to be vague, there are specific ways in which opportunities for engagement are possible.

Following up on the concept of presence, the need for an RSC provider to be seen and known is paramount, often occurring through regular ward visits and being **seen** as a part of the ward environment. With the importance of shielding and protecting patients, family and staff from infection during COVID-19, new and innovative ways were developed to make opportunities for interaction possible. Many chaplaincies around Britain developed methods of virtual communication. The most challenging part was establishing initial contact unless the service user had requested SRC. This process was helped by having at least one person on the ground when needed and maximising the use of the referral system.

Referrals to SCR providers have increased, not only due to COVID-19 but also in line with the growing move towards increased Data Protection and autonomy of the service user. There are still many paths open to such referrals, and they include the following:

- Staff referrals—The referrals are, with consent, made by a member of the ward staff, usually with a specific need described. Many SRC departments have developed or are developing electronic referral systems that work in line with the electronic recordkeeping systems of the Trust. These benefits are myriad, including a paper trail, greater accountability, recognition of the status of SRC as part of the treatment modality and the introduction of themes that can be addressed in the notes. This also allows SRC services, nationally and internationally, to share non-person-specific data and work together to build more uniform support. (For more, see how this affects taxonomy).
- Community referrals—These referrals are often based at the religious end of SRC and need to be handled carefully within the Confidentiality guidelines of the given health care system. Each SRC should have a way of assessing the actual desire of the patient, family, or staff in line with the request when used carefully, though it can offer opportunities to meet those in need who are not on the radar as well as offering the possibility of normalising the situation through connections with the local community.
- Self-referrals—Considering the situations in which the patients in the PICU find themselves, the term self here points primarily to the families and staff. Once again, the mechanisms for referral are essential. Information should be publicised and available for families and staff to access easily. Many SRC departments worldwide have a 24/7 on-call system pointing to both a practical and symbolic function, offering confidence that someone will be available in time of need. It is also important that what is promised can be delivered promptly; therefore, regular system audits offer a review of the systems in place. Staff must be aware of the parameters of the on-call system. One useful measure is to have Standard Operating Procedures with a minimum response time. For most SRCs, a 15-min phone response time is beneficial, ensuring staff know their needs are recognised and providing a timely discussion about arrival time and likely provision of support.
- Quality of referrals: Choi et al. found that many referrals to SRCs in adult ICUs are not made until end-of-life care is ongoing. Therefore, there is limited time for

relationship-building and care provision [6]. In the paediatric setting, referrals often come earlier, offering opportunities to bring depth to both the relationships and care provision. Data from our London tertiary paediatric care hospital measures initial visits and continuing care. Recognising the presence of confounding factors, each initial encounter was followed by at least 2.5 continuing care encounters, showing that earlier referral can make a difference to continuing care and demonstrating service users' desire for additional encounters. This finding showed a positive outcome in an area in which obtaining evidence is challenging.

Some other processes of service delivery in the ICU are determined by the condition of the child. Nash et al. showed the importance of Interpretive Spiritual Encounters, which can be addressed in various ways, including forms of activity [2]. Two factors influencing this are the patient or siblings' ability to respond to this form of interaction and the degree of working with the Play Team in an institution. The quality of the Play Department at this author's hospital is such that effective relationships are maintained in this area and can add the roles of SRC to the provision and exploration of processes.

This also highlights the importance of teamwork within the entire setting. Having RSC members as a part of the psychosocial team provides a truly holistic way of viewing patients, staff and families in which a wealth of expertise can be applied to needs. Our interviews suggested that families and patients see clear distinctions between Psychology and Chaplaincy [4]. In our centre, collaboration between psychology and chaplaincy, particularly supporting staff, clearly points to several positive ways of working together.

58.7 Distinctions

Notably, there are distinctions between the different ICU populations provided with RSC. The categories of the taxonomy, e.g., active listening or prayer, contain a generality that needs to be unpacked and nowhere is this as clear as in the provision for staff vs. patients and families. Two distinctive themes emerge for work with staff-staff support: moral injury and well-being.

Moral Injury: While relatively recently described, the concept of moral distress or now preferred injury is a longstanding concept. Issues of conscientious objection and challenge in having to perform procedures have, to an extent, been around since Hippocrates. Jameton named the modern iteration and described the process as: 'One or more negative self-directed emotions or attitudes that arise in response to one's perceived involvement in a situation that one perceives to be morally undesirable' [7]. Much of the increase in this can be attributed to factors like ever-developing processes that can improve parts of a patient's condition, prompting the question, just because we can, should we?

As meta-narratives inform much moral and ethical thinking of religion and spirituality, the role of RSC becomes a part of the conversation.

What then can RSC offer, particularly in situations where some staff believe that maintaining invasive treatment, and even sometimes life itself, is not in the child's best interests? As discussed previously, the first two requirements are being known to the staff and family as being trustworthy and being present. Listening holistically and non-judgmentally to the person and treating team is vital; this includes developing an explicit knowledge of the moral and ethical tenets of the family's faith, including the ability to assist in applying them in particular situations.

Both signposting and being an advocate also play a role. This requires a degree of familiarity with the setting regarding the available resources. It also requires a willingness to engage in the role of advocacy and being conscious of one's limitations as well as skills. Recognising these limitations, as well as developing a strong relationship with the institutional ethics body and staff support team, is imperative. In our experience, the ICU offers the greatest number of challenges that can lead to moral injury in modern children's hospitals, so it requires the development of specific competencies that go beyond those offered in Chaplaincy taxonomies.

Well-being: Looking after hospital staff well-being is a longstanding concept but recently become a more explicit concern, particularly during the COVID-19 pandemic. In the United Kingdom, the NHS Care Act defines well-being as a broad concept relating to the following areas in particular:

- personal dignity (including treatment of the individual with respect)
- physical and mental health and emotional well-being
- protection from abuse and neglect
- control by the individual over their day-to-day life (including over care and support provided and the way they are provided)
- participation in work, education, training or recreation
- social and economic well-being
- domestic, family and personal domains
- suitability of the individual's living accommodation
- the individual's contribution to society

While a comprehensive definition, its sheer size challenges the opportunity of providing it fully, particularly in a busy ICU. The breadth of the particular areas also demands that a variety of agencies, from hospital colleagues to administrative structures, be involved in the provision.

Narrowing it down, what specific role(s) can RSC providers play in maintaining well-being? Interestingly, while physical and mental health and emotional well-being are mentioned, there is nothing about the spiritual. Returning to our opening definition of spirituality, one would think that issues of hope, meaning, relationship and others should be considered. Therefore, RSC might usefully expand the categories, for example, adding spirituality to personal dignity, showing involvement in well-being, and considering many of the definitions of spirituality when helping deal with moral injury. The main message is that RSC can be crucial to the groups providing services to maintain healthcare staff well-being.

Other categories of staff support SRC are similar to those provided for patients and families. Staff will also seek involvement in rituals both as individuals and in groups. Calm presence, active listening, prayer, and various items from the taxonomy are also offered, showing that SRC staff support is both specific and general for those seeking it. Debriefs can play a significant part in the SRC work; however, much of this depends on methods already deployed in an institution and ensuring safe practice, as a poorly performed debrief can be harmful.

58.8 Themes

After looking at the who and how of SRC, reviewing any overarching themes that emerge within practice is important. Our interviews provided a list of themes arising from families and staff in the PICU at a London tertiary paediatric hospital [4]. Many parallels the themes encountered within the general work of SRC and constitute cause and effect with the taxonomy mentioned above. These themes are:

Staff

- Decision-making
- Control
- Rationalising the ICU
- Compartmentalising

Parent

- Perspective
- Hope
- Comfort
- Polarisation of religion

Shared

- SRC (Chaplaincy) as distinctive
- Miracles

These themes encompass a range of concerns held by many within the ICU, which cannot be addressed by medicine or science alone. They offer both challenges and possibilities that SRC can address directly and through work with other staff on the ward. The taxonomy can offer the methods, the themes, the content and the outcomes.

58.9 Outcomes

Measurement of outcomes within SRC can be difficult but not impossible. SRC departments worldwide continue to develop ways to measure, and to an extent even quantify their work. Often, outcomes are guided by Spiritual Care plans, making their success dependent on the adequacy of planning.

Two interesting examples come from the themes provided by our interviews:

Hope—The very nature of hope can be subjective. What part would SRC play in addressing this theme? Looking at one quote, certain parts of a Spiritual Care plan could immediately apply. '*So, there was a lot of hope involved… Really a time to pray and plead that things would get better.*' RC could address sources of hope, including metanarrative, describing what that hope looks like, is this the only hope available, what happens if what is hoped for does not happen and related questions. The outcomes would include the opportunity for the parent to articulate their hope and do some parallel planning by widening and reframing their hopes. At no point in this exercise should hope be taken away, but it can be reframed or expanded.

Miracles—Perhaps one of the most challenging themes, miracles, can offer one of the biggest challenges to all involved. *'Guess that one comes up a lot, around the conflicts that families face, around healing or believing that a miracle…'* (Staff member). *'Knowing… that against all odds, you know, God will sustain her, God will keep her.'* (Parent). Much like hope, miracles can represent a change in the understanding of the predicted future and seem unrealistic, which may make many staff feel uncomfortable. Again, the nature of what is sought can be explored with SRC, as the spectrum of miracles is so large and inclusive that even physical death for a deteriorating child can be deemed by some to be the miracle. What then would the outcome be? It would undoubtedly vary depending on whose need is being addressed and could be recorded, and assistance could be offered in looking after the patient, family, or staff member for whom an intervention is requested.

Increasingly, recognising some of the difficulties in quantifying the work of SRC, case studies have another way of measuring its outcomes. Even more than the ways of measuring outcomes suggested above, case studies allow a process approach that can be educative for other practitioners in similar situations. They can also help guide the language of record keeping, something progressively becoming an important part of SRC communication, and the importance of sharing helpful information shows what SRC brings as part of the wider team.

58.10 Resourcing and Training

The Paediatric ICU has an extensive range of professionals working within it, and, sometimes, the question arises of where SRC fits into the resourcing of a very costly department. In many countries, the law mandates minimum SRC cover to maintain equality and diversity, though this can have many forms, and there are rarely agreed standards of provision at a policy level, as opposed to perhaps at a less demanding guideline level.

The literature abounds on the positive effects of SRC and outcome figures can show both needs and interventions, the question remains concerning resourcing provision. While it is inappropriate in an international and cross-cultural chapter to look at figures and percentages, the data we present on SRC in Paediatric ICUs does suggest specific minimum provisions. These include a caregiver who is:

- A part of the ICU team. This means there will be a regular presence and appropriate knowledge of the team's procedures and cultures. Some hospitals have external SCR providers, which can mean that in challenging situations, additional time is needed to teach the process as well as the fact that when an SCR provider is only on-site during difficult times, they can be seen to represent only medical challenges.
- Available 24/7, generally as a part of the team well-known to the unit. Emergencies and challenges do not work to a 9–5 schedule, nor do calls to the PICU. Availability in times of crisis, while not a specific part of the taxonomy, is implied in many of its expectations.
- Can work across faiths and philosophies. Also, if providing cover for their own faith, having an intimate knowledge of it, including possible distortions.
- Trained to provide spiritual care.

While the last requirement appears self-evident, there is a need to both know about SCR provision and the ability and willingness to grow it. Perhaps one of the challenges in this field over the years is its failure to be perceived as having a distinct knowledge base. More recently, SCR training programmes have been developed to hone skills and offer experiential learning designed to improve practice, with many SCR providers now maintaining a learning portfolio that must be kept up to date to continue to practice.

58.11 Conclusion

While technology and methods can change, human nature remains consistent, which is why many issues highlighted here remain important, despite some being built on processes developed long ago. The taxonomy with which we started offers a framework and foundation, distinctive enough to define the subject but general enough for growth.

Our opening statement reminds us that the Paediatric ICU can be where 'irrationality meets irrationality'. However, that may lie in the rational and the necessary.

Take Home Messages

Chaplaincy and faith support are an important part of the ICU multidisciplinary team. It provides a unique basis for many families' world view and can be a crucial part of decision-making in ICU, including during end-of-life care. Religious rituals can be vital during critical illness for some people, and the ability of chaplains to provide pastoral support to both families and staff can be an important part of daily ICU.

References

1. Zhong X, Mazumdar M, Sharma V, Jandorf L, Welsh D, Marin DB. Predictive model for chaplain taxonomy patterns identified through latent class analysis among infants in a pediatric inpatient setting. J Health Care Chaplain. 2021;27(2):118–28. https://doi.org/10.1080/08854726.2019.1670537.
2. Nash P, Roberts E, Nash S, Darby K, Parwaz AA. Adapting the advocate health care taxonomy of chaplaincy for a pediatric hospital context: a pilot study. J Health Care Chaplain. 2019;25(2):61–75. https://doi.org/10.1080/08854726.2018.1473911.
3. Massey K, Barnes MJ, Villines D, Goldstein JD, Pierson ALH, Scherer C, Summerfelt WT. What do I do? Developing a taxonomy of chaplaincy activities and interventions for spiritual care in intensive care unit palliative care. BMC Palliat Care. 2015;14(1):10. https://doi.org/10.1186/s12904-015-0008-0.
4. Modan T, Linthicum J, Brierley J. 565: Exploring the role of religion and spirituality with parents and staff on a UK PICU. Crit Care Med. 2015;43(12):143. https://doi.org/10.1097/01.Ccm.0000474393.57783.3d.
5. Falkenburg JL, van Dijk M, Tibboel D, Ganzevoort RR. The fragile spirituality of parents whose children died in the pediatric intensive care unit. J Health Care Chaplain. 2020;26(3):117–30. https://doi.org/10.1080/08854726.2019.1670538.
6. Choi P, Chow V, Curlin F, Cox C. Intensive care clinicians' views on the role of chaplains. J Health Care Chaplain. 2019;25(3):89–98. https://doi.org/10.1080/08854726.2018.1538438.
7. Campbell SM, Ulrich CM, Grady C. A broader understanding of moral distress. Am J Bioeth. 2016;16(12):2–9. https://doi.org/10.1080/15265161.2016.1239782. PMID: 27901442.

Looking After People

Contents

Caring and Listening to Families in the ICU

Rufaro Ndokera and C. M. Pierce

Contents

J. Brierley et al. (eds.), *ESPNIC Children's Intensive Care Textbook*,
https://doi.org/10.1007/978-3-031-64762-8_59

59.1 Introduction

The care of children is fundamentally intertwined with the care of their families. In paediatric intensive care (PIC), where mortality is a rare outcome, there is an increased focus on morbidity. Children who experience intensive care are more likely to experience a range of physical, psychological and neurodevelopmental sequelae [1].

A PIC admission is a time of extreme stress for families, and it is important that we care and support them in a holistic way. Providing comprehensive care to the family reaches beyond the desire to deliver family-centred care it extends to trying to limit physical and psychological morbidity in the critically ill child. Focusing on the care of families has a cascade of implications. Limiting the acute stress for families facilitates their ability to engage in complex decision-making and advocacy, allowing them to support their convalescing child. This results in a reduction in the post-intensive care psychosocial morbidity for all members of the family.

Considering the care of families adds complexity to the acute care of the child. There are associations between our intervention to the patient and psychosocial outcomes in families. These negative outcomes may not become apparent during the time on PIC but can affect the family and the recovery of the child for months post-discharge. Poor communication episodes have been shown to contribute to the development of post-traumatic stress. Post-traumatic stress disorder (PTSD) in children can affect the psychological well-being of parents and vice versa. The consideration and care of the family is the responsibility of the whole team, not simply those allocated to specific roles and includes both practical and pastoral elements from the greater multidisciplinary team (MDT).

59.2 Family-Centred Care

Family-centred care is a key concept in the delivery of good paediatric care. This is defined as an 'approach to healthcare that is respectful and responsive to individual families' needs and values and in which partnership and collaboration are key concepts' [2, 3]. A family-centred approach ensures that the family unit remains part of the team caring for the child.

The definition of the family unit has changed over time. The traditional 'family' is defined as 'two or more people who are related by blood, marriage, and—occasionally—adoption' [4], but no longer describes the 'modern' family. Throughout this chapter, when referring to families, we encompass all close, biological, legal, and cultural relatives. Parent, again, is considered inclusively and 'refers to the child's primary caregivers and could include biological or adoptive parents, grandparents, and other guardians' [5].

59.2.1 The Parental Impact of Paediatric Intensive Care

Families will present to PIC in different ways, acutely, or as elective admissions. As such, they may appear to have vastly unique experiences. It is important for us to realise that the nature of a child's illness and their length of stay has not been shown to independently affect the parental stress response. A short stay may be just as traumatic to some as a much longer stay with an objectively sicker child [6, 7].

In the acute phase, parents report life coming to a 'halt', with up to half of parents experiencing acute stress symptoms and one-fifth meeting the full criteria for acute stress disorder [8, 9]. The interruption to daily life is significant. Less time is given to other family members, work, and self-care [10]. (See ◘ Table 59.1):

Many of these symptoms are seen in caregiver's post-discharge. Our understanding of the effects of a PIC admission on parents is gathering momentum. Surveys of parental psychological wellness show worse scores at later time points, possibly because parents feel the need to 'cope' and 'get through' the immediate insult. The focus is on the child's physical recovery before parental needs [12, 13]. Levels of anxiety and depression in caregivers of ICU graduates at 1 year post admission have been found to be close to double community rates [13]

The impact of stress disorders, post-traumatic stress (PTS), anxiety and depressive symptoms can be far reaching. Symptoms of psychological poor health impact on other family members, leading to family dysfunction and reduction in the quality of life for caregivers and the index child [6]. In addition, early distress in parents is associated with longer term psychological problems in their children [13]. A considerable number of parents have sleep problems which can lead to excessive fatigue, poor mood and difficulty performing effectively and efficiently. This is important because the parents are the key decision-makers and advocates for their child. Children are dependent on their caregivers for medical and emotional care and well-being. If symptoms of psychological difficulty cloud the caregiver's ability to engage, this can affect their ability to contribute to supporting and rehabilitating their child, both physically and emotionally [14]. A PIC admission does not equally affect all families. Some parents report positive post IC feelings, manifesting as enhanced relationships, changing life priorities, spiritual change and an increased appreciation of life [12, 15, 16].

◘ **Table 59.1** Symptoms experienced by parents with children on ICU

- Difficulty sleeping, feeling constantly exhausted
- Anxiety and worrying, panic attacks, phobias
- Depression
- Feeling very emotional (sad or irritable and angry)
- Feeling jittery, difficulty relaxing
- Going over what has happened repeatedly
- Nightmares, bad dreams
- Difficulty concentrating
- Overworking
- Stress and tension in relationships (particularly between parents)
- Difficulty coping with their child, or his or her siblings

Adapted from 'When your child is admitted to the intensive care unit' [11]

59.2.2 Paediatric Intensive Care and Its Effect on Siblings

Much of the literature about families in PIC is focused on the needs of the parents. Importantly, siblings may require support. It is often assumed that the parents will be providing the necessary support to siblings. However, parents have a significant burden during this period and may not be able to fully appreciate the needs of the well sibling nor be able to communicate and provide such support [17]. Changes in parental behaviour may be perceived more strongly by well siblings than by parents, making it challenging for parents to mitigate or address the siblings' changing needs. In addition to the stress from knowing your sibling is unwell, the changes in parenting behaviours, substitute caregivers, changes in routine, and uncertainty of the clinical situation can all impact the sibling. The implications of this and approaches to it will be dependent on the sibling's stage of growth and development [17].

After discharge from PICU, there can be changes in the relationships with parents reporting a deterioration in sibling relationships and in the relationship between the well sibling and their parents [18]. Members of the MDT can provide support to parents to understand and address the needs of well siblings [19].

59.3 PIC Survivorship: Morbidity

The PIC patients' medical needs are varied, complex and technical. The impact of our management decisions on the psychological well-being of these children needs to be carefully considered, especially those that may persist post-discharge. In this chapter, we consider the dynamic interaction outcomes can have on the wider family.

These issues have been conceptualised in the framework of post-intensive care syndrome–paediatric (PICS-p). This recognises the interdependency between the outcomes of the child and the family unit. Whilst recognising the heterogeny of the population with regards to baseline status, it highlights major areas that can be impacted by a PIC admission.

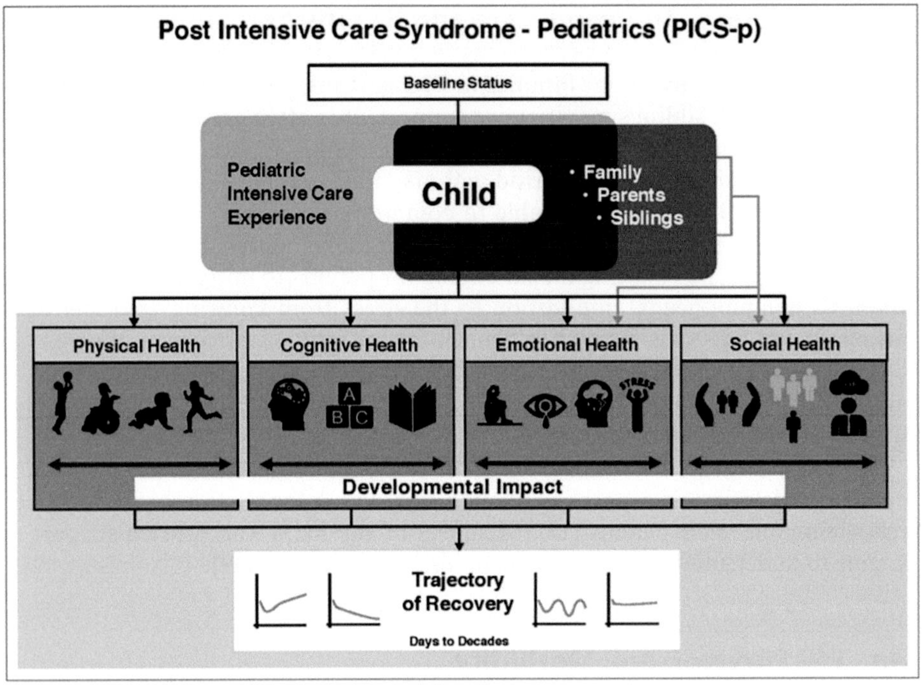

From 'Conceptualizing post intensive care syndrome in children—The PICS-p framework' [1]

Children who have spent time on PIC are more likely to have challenges, they are at higher risk of psychiatric, sleep and fatigue disorders than their healthy peers [20]. For those of school age, a reduction in IQ has been seen, although they remain within the normal range.

PIC graduates may experience post-traumatic symptoms. Importantly, this does not appear to directly correlate with memories of the period on ICU, but, in one study, around one-third of children reported a delusional, mostly negative, or scary memory. Those experiencing delusional memories were more at risk of post-traumatic stress symptoms. With these issues in mind, the prompt recognition and treatment of delirium in PIC is important [21].

59.4 Supporting the Parental Role

59.4.1 Visiting

Unrestricted visiting for parents is important. Separation of a parent from their child in the intensive care unit (ICU) can be a significant source of stress [15]. Conversely, the presence of familiar visitors has a positive psychological impact on patients in adult ICU, it is intuitive that this should extrapolate to the paediatric population [7, 22]. Family presence on the PICU, including wider family and siblings, helps orientate the child, provides socialisation and makes them feel safe and reassured. For siblings who may experience anxiety related to the unknowns of ICU, interacting with their ill sibling may dispel or reduce imagined concerns. The reality of care in the PICU may, in fact, be reassuring. This all contributes to reduced stress in the child, potentially reduced stress in parents and siblings, and, therefore, reduced psychological morbidity for the family [23–25]. Additionally, shared family experiences can help bring the family together. Ongoing interactions allow the unwell child to maintain and re-establish relationships during the admission and following discharge [17]. It may be necessary, for short periods, to limit the number of people at the bedside to avoid disrupting clinical care; however, the overall goal should be of minimal restriction [23].

Although parent's presence is encouraged, there may be unintended negative effects. Constant presence may lead to greater exposure to traumatic events and may cause significant distress for parents [15].

59.4.2 Delivering Care

Empowering parents in delivering care to their child with training and supervision whilst on IC contributes to increased family satisfaction [2, 3].

59.4.3 Ward Rounds, Decision-Making and Communication

Ward rounds are the point of clinical decision-making. Due to their complex nature, multiple attendees, need for confidentiality and opportunity for teaching, there have been questions about the appropriateness of parental presence. Bedside ward rounds with parental presence are the parental preference and improves parent satisfaction and may reduce their anxiety. Parents may not be directly engaged in the round, but their presence allows them to maintain their parental [7, 26–28].

59.4.4 Transitions

Transitional periods are acutely stressful to families [15]. The period between hospital admission and transfer to PIC can be a significant stressor, especially if this is prolonged. Discharge to the ward, local hospital or home can also be a challenging time. The reduction in nursing ratios, loss of 'community' in terms of the ICU family and the new ward environment can be difficult. It is important that we proactively prepare and support families for these transitions.

59.5 The Multidisciplinary Team

Most of the work doctors and nurses do in front-line intensive care services is about managing the quickly changing physiological status of their patients. These teams do not always have the time, capacity and experience to provide the necessary psychosocial support to their patients and families. Furthermore, patients are frequently under the care of multiple teams and how these teams coordinate their treatment strategies providing continuity of care has become an increasing challenge in modern medicine.

We know that both verbal and non-verbal communication is central to a families' experience of paediatric critical care. Poor communication can contribute to parental acute stress [15, 29] and in the bereaved, complicated grief response [30, 31].

The development of a robust psychosocial team alongside the medical team is important in providing families with continuity, guidance and support throughout their admission.

59.5.1 Family Liaison Service

Recognition of the challenges in delivering holistic, family-centred care on the ICU has led to the emergence of family liaison services (FLS) in PICU's. This service is ideally led by specialist family liaison nurses (FLN), working alongside the front-line team of doctors and nurses. The FLNs provide the essential, non-clinical support the family requires to move smoothly through the IC. They overcome issues related to lack of continuity, holistic support and practical guidance experienced by families during an ICU admission. FLNs traditionally have an ICU background with additional training in liaison, bereavement, ethics and psychological skills, making them uniquely placed to facilitate truly holistic care for the patient and family.

The FLNs aim to see every family in the first days of admission or make contact preadmission for those with a planned attendance. Their primary purpose is to meet the non-medical needs of families (psychological, social, family support), either directly, or through signposting to additional in-hospital or external resources [32]. FLNs also function as a conduit between the families and the medical team, improving communication by explaining medical progress in lay terms and providing the continuity of care that is so crucial for longer stay patients. The FLNs join the family during multidisciplinary meetings, providing support and advocacy. Given their significant training and IC background, they have the medical knowledge to understand the conditions and treatments which makes them uniquely placed to support families during an IC admission. The FLN team plays a vital role in screening families who may require support from the IC psychologist or social worker and encouraging families to make use of these services by de-stigmatising the process.

59.5.2 Psychology

Not all families will require input from psychology teams. However, we know that in a notable minority, there is significant psychological morbidity related to a child's PIC admission [16, 20]. Whereas children may have limited memories of their time on PIC [21], parents' memories may be more detailed and traumatic [7, 15]. It is known that the psychological adjustment of both children and parents following a PIC admission has a weak correlation with the severity of illness [6, 14, 19, 33–35]. The team psychologist aims to meet the psychological needs of families, as well as the children. They can be a useful intermediary, to establish which families may benefit from further psychological intervention. Sibling support by the IC psychologist can be invaluable, particularly around the time of death.

For some families, engagement in the acute phase may be limited as they may only be able to focus on 'coping' and 'holding themselves together'. Nonetheless, families should be made aware that they can have access to psychological support after an IC admission. Signposting the presence of the team highlights that we recognise the psychological burden of their situation and 'normalises' accessing it. In this period, the focus may be on normalising their response to their circumstances and directing them to the importance of self-care [36].

The PIC psychology team is also well-placed to provide education and written information for families. Written resources about the psychological burden of a child's PIC admission, how to understand and manage well siblings' responses during this time and how to support their unwell child's psychological rehabilitation are just a few of the valuable insights that the psychology team can provide. Written information allows parents to digest this in their own time and reference it throughout their journey.

For parents requiring intervention, the psychology team will judge what input may be beneficial and in what timeframe it might be delivered. If acute support is required, then the PIC team can address this. However, in certain circumstances, psychological intervention may be inappropriate until the child is well out of danger. In addition, in the post-discharge, rehabilitation phase, parental input may be more appropriately delivered by an adult psychology team, and potentially, closer to the child's base hospital if they have travelled a distance for IC care [19]. PIC psychologists remain an important part of the IC team, deeply considering, signposting and intervening in the psychological well-being of the whole family surrounding the child.

59.5.3 Religious and Spiritual Support

'Spirituality' and 'Religion' are distinct but related entities, 'Spirituality' relates to what it means to be human, 'Religion' is an organised set of beliefs and practices shared by a community or group [31]. Matters of faith, religion and spirituality may affect and influence a family's approach to illness, disability and end-of-life decision-making [37].

Religious and spiritual support in times of stress will be important to many families [31, 38]. Studies investigating the role of spiritual support highlight the importance of explicit spiritual or religious themes (prayer, faith, access to and care from clergy). Implicit themes were also identified, including insight and wisdom, reliance on values and virtues such as hope, trust and love [37].

Given the value of religious/spiritual support—providing access to these on the ICU allows receptive families an alternative and additional way to understand and navigate this challenging time. Access to major faith-based leaders and non-denominational practitioners should be possible. This can bring comfort to families and is especially important when religious matters are relevant to clinical decision-making. It is also beneficial to have such practitioners present during ethics meetings, to provide spiritual advocacy, giving the family confidence that spiritual matters important to them have been given due consideration [31].

59.5.4 Play Specialists

Play is an important way for children to explore and understand the world around them. Play specialists can become an integral part of the intensive care team, working alongside the medical and nursing staff, to improve a child's experience in the hospital. Importantly, play specialists also work with families and can support siblings through this time.

The role of a play specialist can be relevant pre-admission (for those with planned admission, e.g. post-op), during the acute phase, and in the rehabilitation phase for those who experience a mid- to long-term stay.

Play specialists facilitate play within the limits of a child's illness or injury; they provide fun and stimulation whilst trying to provide some normality in an otherwise stressful and scary environment. Their work can also help with reducing anxiety, preparing for treatment or providing distraction during a procedure. In the longer term patient, play specialists can help teams and families address issues such as challenging behaviour and communication problems. Providing structured and directed play activities in the rehabilitation phase of an acute illness helps empower parents to return to play and some normality, which can seem daunting after having seen your child so unwell [39].

59.6 Care of the Family at the End of Life

As a society, the death of a child is a rare occurrence and as such, the support received by families by their usual support network may be inadequate. Population-based studies demonstrate an increased risk of mortality in bereaved parents, more so in those whose children have died during childhood. In addition, there is an increased risk of both mental and physical health problems, marital breakdown and job loss among those bereaved [5].

For families where the end of their PIC journey is with the death of a child, the support and care provided by the PIC multidisciplinary team will hold lifelong impact and relevance.

59.7 When Death is Expected or Imminent

Most deaths on PIC occur following limitation or withdrawal of life sustaining therapies. This is important because it gives the whole team the opportunity to engage the family in the process, ask and anticipate their needs and support them through an incredibly painful and often frightening period. Maintaining open and honest communication with families when death is imminent is critical to the family's experience. There are many approaches to these conversations, but it is key to speak openly whilst considering the hopes and wishes of the family in a holistic way. It is important, even in anticipation of death, that the parental role as decision-maker and advocate is respected and honoured [40]. These conversations should include team members known to the family and the inclusion of nurse facilitators has a positive impact on the family's experience of the death of a child in an ICU [41].

59.8 Resuscitation

In circumstances where the end of life follows an attempt at cardiopulmonary resuscitation (CPR), families if they wish should be present during resuscitation. The benefits to the family are clear without a negative impact on the delivery of resuscitation [42]. Witnessing resuscitation attempts may also reduce markers of psychological distress in both the short- and longer term [43]. For families, observing the period of resuscitation helps them adjust to the loss of their child. Their presence allows them to see first-hand the medical efforts in resuscitation [44, 45]. Providing appropriately trained support for those family members during this period of resuscitation is essential.

59.9 After Death

The needs of parents immediately after the death of a child will be family-specific. We may have an opportunity to explore and accommodate these desires before death if it is anticipated. If not, we should be aware of the common themes that arise when speaking to bereaved parents about their experiences. Parents want to remain parents following the death of their child. Remaining in the parental role and allowing adjustment to the change in this relationship is crucial [31]. Being physically close to their child after death is important. For the recently bereaved, the concept of time may loosen and parents feel significant value in not feeling rushed or prematurely separated from their child. Being able to provide care and say goodbye in a respectful, quiet and private space is important to families after the death of a child [40]. Religious, spiritual and cultural differences in how families respond to the death of their child must be respected. Practically, there are various approaches to keeping the family together after death. Transfer to a hospice may allow access to a 'cold room' where a family could spend several days with their child after death. Some IC units have a similar room within the unit, allowing for families to gather and spend time with their child, in a non-medicalised environment [40, 46]. In the absence of such facilities, providing a quiet, private room creates a respectful, calm environment in which the family have space to grieve. Where possible, involving the parents in the washing and dressing of their child after death can help provide parents with a physical connection during this final experience [5]. Keepsakes, photographs and memory boxes should be offered to families to facilitate the transition away from hospital after the death of their child.

Parents are likely to be left with questions surrounding the death of their child. Although the medical team should be available and prepared to answer those questions contemporaneously, families may value the opportunity to come back to the team with questions once they have had time to gather their thoughts. It is also well-recognised that retaining information during times of stress and in the acute phase is limited [47]. In some units, the family liaison team will call the family regularly after the death of a child from the point the family leaves the hospital. This regular communication allows the FLT to check in with the family and provide any support or signposting they may require. Offering the family, a follow-up appointment after the death of a child to discuss and ask questions is deemed valuable [5, 48, 49]. The administrative tasks following the death of a child are unfamiliar and may seem overwhelming to families. Having a bereavement key worker can help the family navigate these processes. Ideally, this should be someone already known to the family. Families may need help and guidance with how to support the child's siblings. The siblings may also need ongoing support. Providing appropriate signposting, literature and resources to families to address such issues is important in the context of fully family-centred care [19, 50].

59.10 Bereavement Services

Bereavement support 'involves the care that acknowledges suffering and grief, provides guidance through the dying process and in the mourning period that follows' [31]. Establishing a robust bereavement program is essential to providing the support needed for our families. Bereavement support needs to be individual to the family's needs. Bereavement follow-up should be coordinated by the key worker, providing families with psychological and practical support.

59.11 Mediation, Feedback and Liaison

A liaison service has become an integral part of the Hospital team, improving communication and family satisfaction. In the United Kingdom, each trust has a Patient Advice and Liaison Service (PALS). PALS can prove highly successful in the de-escalation and resolution of conflicts and the subsequent reduction of complaints received [51]. Cases involving difficult decision-making and/or end-of-life care may, on occasion, cause significant conflict for staff and families. An approach based upon impartial mediation meets the needs of the family and staff. These needs may reach beyond the remit of in-house patient liaison services and external mediation services may need to be sought.

Feedback from users is an essential element in the improvement of services. Details on how to provide unit feedback, either electronically or in paper leaflet form should be readily available on the unit.

59.12 Peer Support Services

Many units will have an active parent group. This allows useful discussions about the IC experience to be shared. Additionally, a parent group can function as a source of unit-specific feedback for areas of improvement and development. Parent group members can have representation on Unit Boards and Research Ethics applications supported by the Family liaison service and clinical leads. Other initiatives include Past Patient Party's which can be successful in creating a positive experience for both families and ICU staff.

Beyond the hospital, there are numerous peer-delivered resources available to families. These will be location-specific, and families may wish to approach these groups. Examples include local bereavement groups and condition-specific groups which may have a unique perspective. Additionally, faith-based groups and sibling groups may also be relevant [5]. In the United Kingdom, families who have experienced bereavement can access the Child Death helpline, which is a freephone, confidential service open every day of the year for those affected by the death of a child [16, 52].

59.13 Practical Matters

When considering the care and support of families, it is important that we are doing so in a way that they can understand. The use of formal medical translation services is essential to allow parents to freely communicate with the medical team. This can take the form of telephone translation services in the short term, but, if possible, an in-person translation service can allow for a more natural conversational experience for families.

If required, parents should be able to access breast/chestfeeding rooms, breast pumps and appropriate support to achieve their feeding goals. It is important that these services are highlighted early in the stay, as the stress of an intensive care admission in the initial period of breastfeeding may negatively impact milk supply and, successful breastfeeding.

If children are admitted shortly after birth, parents should be made aware of how to access midwifery services to ensure maternal health is being addressed.

It is important that families have access to facilities to keep themselves well. Orientation of the ward and its facilities should occur as soon as possible. Direct access to food in an ICU is rarely possible. Parents should, however, have access to a small kitchen and comfortable area away from, but relatively near to, their child's bedspace. Provision of information about the neighbourhood around the hospital; places to eat, parks and laundry facilities should be provided. For those travelling to a PIC distant from their homes, access to clean and safe accommodation near their child removes a cause of stress for families.

Take Home Message

The support of families in paediatric intensive care is critical to the long-term morbidity of the patient and families. The care of children is fundamentally intertwined with the care of their families. A multidisciplinary team approach is necessary, and the use of Family liaison nurses is essential to coordinating the care during an admission, following discharge and after death. Providing family-centred care pre- and post-discharge can be a positive experience for staff and patients alike.

We would like to acknowledge and give thanks to the Great Ormond Street Family Liaison Team.

Summary

The support of families in PIC is critical to the long-term morbidity of the patient and families. An MDT approach is required, and the use of FLNs is essential to coordinating the care during an admission, following discharge and after death. Providing family-centred care pre and post-discharge can be a positive experience for staff and patients alike.

References

1. Manning JC, Pinto NP, Rennick JE, Colville G, Curley MAQ. Conceptualizing post intensive care syndrome in children—The PICS-p framework. Pediatr Crit Care Med. 2018;19(4):298–300.
2. Judy E, Rebecca A, Ann C, Davidson J, Aslakson R, Long A, et al. Guidelines for family centered care in the neonatal, pediatric, and adult ICU. Crit Care Med. 2017;45:103–28.
3. Davidson JE, Powers K, Hedayat KM, Tieszen M, Kon A, Shepard E, et al. Clinical practice guidelines for support of the family in the patient-centered intensive care unit. Crit Care Med. 2007;35(2):605–22.
4. Murdock GP. Social structure. 1949.
5. October T, Dryden-Palmer K, Copnell B, Meert KL. Caring for parents after the death of a child. Pediatr Crit Care Med. 2018;19:S61–8.
6. Killien E, Zimmerman J, Di Gennaro JL, Watson R. 507: Association of illness severity with family outcomes following pediatric septic shock. Crit Care Med. 2022;50(1):e0716.
7. Foster JR, AlOthmani FI, Seabrook JA, AlOfisan T, AlGarni YM, Sarpal A. Parental presence at the bedside of critically ill children in a unit with unrestricted visitation. Pediatr Crit Care Med. 2018;19(8):e387–93.
8. Kaplan D, Nkromah T, Eldridge P, Mennella J, Ansari N, Li S, et al. 865: Acute stress in parents and caregivers of patients admitted to the intensive care unit. Crit Care Med. 2018;46(1):11–20.
9. Erçin-Swearinger H, Lindhorst T, Curtis JR, Starks H, Doorenbos AZ. Acute and posttraumatic stress in family members of children with a prolonged stay in a PICU: secondary analysis of a randomized trial. Pediatr Crit Care Med. 2022;23(4):306–14.
10. Alzawad Z, Lewis FM, Walker A. Parents' challenges beyond the pediatric intensive care unit: fraying at the seams while balancing between two worlds, home and hospital. Children (Basel). 2022;9(2):267.
11. Paediatric Clinical Psychology Service. When your child is admitted to the intensive care unit. Great Ormond Street Hospital; 2005.
12. Foster K, Mitchell R, Van C, Young A, McCloughen A, Curtis K. Resilient, recovering, distressed: a longitudinal qualitative study of parent psychosocial trajectories following child critical injury. Injury. 2019;50(10):1605–11.
13. Colville G, Pierce C. Patterns of post-traumatic stress symptoms in families after paediatric intensive care. Intensive Care Med. 2012;38(9):1523–31.
14. Nelson LP, Gold JI. Posttraumatic stress disorder in children and their parents following admission to the pediatric intensive care unit: a review. Pediatr Crit Care Med. 2012;13:338–47.
15. Colville G, Darkins J, Hesketh J, Bennett V, Alcock J, Noyes J. The impact on parents of a child's admission to intensive care: integration of qualitative findings from a cross-sectional study. Intensive Crit Care Nurs. 2009;25(2):72–9.
16. Colville G, Cream P. Post-traumatic growth in parents after a child's admission to intensive care: maybe Nietzsche was right? Intensive Care Med. 2009;35(5):919–23.
17. Rozdilsky JR. Enhancing sibling presence in pediatric ICU. Crit Care Nurs Clin North Am. 2005;17:451–61, xii.
18. O'Meara A, Akande M, Yagiela L, Hummel K, Whyte-Nesfield M, Michelson KN, et al. Family outcomes after the pediatric intensive care unit: a scoping review. J Intensive Care Med. 2022;37(9):1179–98.
19. Colville G. Paediatric intensive care. 2012. https://www.bps.org.uk/psychologist/paediatric-intensive-care.
20. Als LC, Picouto MD, Hau SM, Nadel S, Cooper M, Pierce CM, et al. Mental and physical well-being following admission to pediatric intensive care. Pediatr Crit Care Med. 2015;16(5):e141–9.
21. Colville G, Kerry S, Pierce C. Children's factual and delusional memories of intensive care. Am J Respir Crit Care Med. 2008;177(9):976–82.
22. Miller L, Richard M, Krmpotic K, Kennedy A, Seabrook J, Slumkoski C, et al. Parental presence at the bedside of critically ill children in the pediatric intensive care unit: a scoping review. Eur J Pediatr. 2022;181(2):823–31.
23. Bichard E, Herring D. The psychological burden of restricted parental visiting in paediatric intensive care. Nurs Crit Care. 2020;25:379–81.

24. Yagiela LM, Carlton EF, Meert KL, Odetola FO, Cousino MK. Parent medical traumatic stress and associated family outcomes after pediatric critical illness: a systematic review. Pediatr Crit Care Med. 2019:20, 759–768.
25. Coyne I. Families and health-care professionals' perspectives and expectations of family-centred care: hidden expectations and unclear roles. Health Expect. 2015;18(5):796–808.
26. Landry MA, Lafrenaye S, Roy MC, Cyr C. A randomized, controlled trial of bedside versus conference-room case presentation in a pediatric intensive care unit. Pediatrics. 2007;120(2):275–80.
27. Anand V, Williams E, Elgendi M, Meakins L, Cunningham C, McCrady H, et al. Parental presence at cardiac intensive care unit bedside transfer rounds reduces parental anxiety: results of a randomized controlled trial. Circulation. 2015;132.
28. Phipps LM, Bartke CN, Spear DA, Jones LF, Foerster CP, Killian ME, et al. Assessment of parental presence during bedside pediatric intensive care unit rounds: effect on duration, teaching, and privacy. Pediatr Crit Care Med. 2007;8(3):220–4.
29. Baker SC, Gledhill JA. Systematic review of interventions to reduce psychiatric morbidity in parents and children after PICU admissions*. Pediatr Crit Care Med. 2017;18:343–8.
30. Kentish-Barnes N, Chaize M, Seegers V, Legriel S, Cariou A, Jaber S, et al. Complicated grief after death of a relative in the intensive care unit. Eur Respir J. 2015;45(5):1341–52.
31. Meert KL, Thurston CS, Briller SH. The spiritual needs of parents at the time of their child's death in the pediatric intensive care unit and during bereavement: a qualitative study. Pediatr Crit Care Med. 2005;6(4):420–7.
32. Douglas N, Cooke R, Pearson A. Bereaved parent survey. 2016.
33. Petrinec AB, Daly BJ. Post-traumatic stress symptoms in post-ICU family members. West J Nurs Res. 2016;38(1):57–78.
34. Riley AR, Williams CN, Moyer D, Bradbury K, Leonard S, Turner E, et al. Parental posttraumatic stress symptoms in the context of pediatric post-intensive care syndrome: impact on the family and opportunities for intervention. Clin Pract Pediatr Psychol. 2021;9(2):156–66.
35. Azoulay E, Pochard F, Kentish-Barnes N, Chevret S, Aboab J, Adrie C, et al. Risk of post-traumatic stress symptoms in family members of intensive care unit patients. Am J Respir Crit Care Med. 2005;171(9):987–94.
36. Colville G. The role of a psychologist on the paediatric intensive care unit. Child Psychol Psychiatry Rev. 2001;6(3):102–9.
37. Robinson MR, Thiel MM, Backus MM, Meyer EC. Matters of spirituality at the end of life in the pediatric intensive care unit. Pediatrics. 2006;118(3):e719–29.
38. Gordon BS, Keogh M, Davidson Z, Griffiths S, Sharma V, Marin D, et al. Addressing spirituality during critical illness: a review of current literature. J Crit Care. 2018;45:76–81.
39. Multidisciplinary Working Group. Appendices to the standards for the care of critically ill children. 2010.
40. Meert KL, Briller SH, Schim SM, Thurston C, Kabel A. Examining the needs of bereaved parents in the pediatric intensive care unit: a qualitative study. Death Stud. 2009;33(8):712–40.
41. Curtis JR, Treece PD, Nielsen EL, Gold J, Ciechanowski PS, Shannon SE, et al. Randomized trial of communication facilitators to reduce family distress and intensity of end-of-life care. Am J Respir Crit Care Med. 2016;193(2):154–62.
42. Fulbrook P, Latour J, Albarran J, de Graaf W, Lynch F, Devictor D, et al. The presence of family members during cardiopulmonary resuscitation: European Federation of Critical Care Nursing Associations, European Society of Paediatric and Neonatal Intensive Care and European Society of Cardiology Council on Cardiovascular Nursing and Allied Professions Joint Position Statement. Eur J Cardiovasc Nurs. 2007;6:250–2.
43. Ferreira CAG, Balbino FS, Balieiro MMFG, Mandetta MA. Family presence during cardiopulmonary resuscitation and invasive procedures in children. Rev Paul Pediatr. 2014;32(1):107–13.
44. Tinsley C, Hill JB, Shah J, Zimmerman G, Wilson M, Freier K, et al. Experience of families during cardiopulmonary resuscitation in a pediatric intensive care unit. Pediatrics. 2008;122(4):e799–804.
45. Maxton FJC. Parental presence during resuscitation in the PICU: the parents' experience: sharing and surviving the resuscitation: a phenomenological study. J Clin Nurs. 2008;17(23):3168–76.
46. Meert KL, Briller SH, Schim SM, Thurston CS. Exploring parents' environmental needs at the time of a child's death in the pediatric intensive care unit. Pediatr Crit Care Med. 2008;9(6):623–8.
47. Kessels RPC. Patients' memory for medical information. J R Soc Med. 2003;96:219–22.

48. Eggly S, Meert KL, Berger J, Zimmerman J, Anand KJS, Newth CJL, et al. A framework for conducting follow-up meetings with parents after a child's death in the pediatric intensive care unit. Pediatr Crit Care Med. 2011;12(2):147–52.
49. Colville GA, Cream PR, Kerry SM. Do parents benefit from the offer of a follow-up appointment after their child's admission to intensive care?: An exploratory randomised controlled trial. Intensive Crit Care Nurs. 2010;26(3):146–53.
50. Brooten D, Youngblut JAM. School aged children's experiences 7 and 13 months following a sibling's death. J Child Fam Stud. 2017;26(4):1112–23.
51. Evans D, Booker S, Daykin N, Powell J, Taylor P, Weil S. National evaluation of patient advice and liaison services (PalS), in final report. 2008.
52. Suttle M, Hall MW, Pollack MM, Berg RA, McQuillen PS, Mourani PM, et al. Post-traumatic growth in parents following their child's death in a pediatric intensive care unit. J Palliat Med. 2022;25(2):265–73.

Care of the Critical Care Team

Gillian Colville

Contents

J. Brierley et al. (eds.), *ESPNIC Children's Intensive Care Textbook*,
https://doi.org/10.1007/978-3-031-64762-8_60

Learning Objectives

After reading this chapter, the student will be able to list the main features of three commonly experienced forms of occupational stress associated with working in the emotionally, physically and cognitively demanding setting of a paediatric intensive care unit (PICU): burnout, post-traumatic stress and moral distress. They will also have a better appreciation of the types of extraordinary stress they might encounter in a PICU career and will learn about individual coping strategies and organisational level initiatives which are likely to reduce distress and increase resilience. Furthermore, they will have a better understanding of the type of persisting symptoms that may require professional support and they will learn where to access useful online resources related to enhancing their knowledge in this area. They will also be provided with information about ways to self-monitor their psychological well-being and to maximise the chances of optimising their potential in this challenging, but vital role.

60.1 Introduction

Just as there has been increasing recognition of the psychological impact of admission on intensive care *patients*, awareness has grown of the psychological costs to the *staff* of working in this demanding health setting and of the advantages for patients, family members and staff of moving towards a more trauma-informed working environment [1, 2].

There has been a particular focus on 'burnout' [3] in the literature, but other forms of work-related stress are also coming to light in this population, namely moral distress [4, 5]and post-traumatic stress [6, 7]. These three forms of distress can occur together or independently [8] (See ◘ Fig. 60.1) and need to be distinguished from each other, since they require different remedies.

There is evidence that health professionals experience higher levels of work-related stress than the general population [9] and that these levels are rising [10]. Furthermore, within paediatrics, there are new pressures which specifically apply to intensive care staff. The possibilities offered by modern medical technology present numerous difficult ethical issues [11] and although patient survival rates have increased, so too have their rates of morbidity [12]. In addition, public expectations are high, and the level of scrutiny of clinical decisions to withdraw treatment in situ-

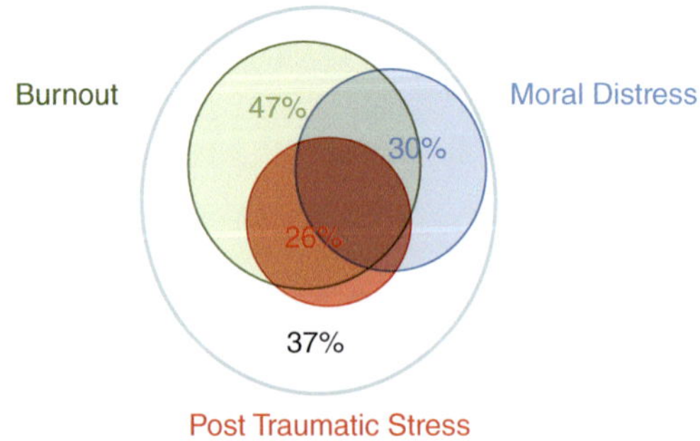

◘ **Fig. 60.1** An illustration of the prevalence and extent of overlap of three types of work-related stress in a sample of $n = 1656$ paediatric intensive care staff [8]

ations of futility is regularly coming under attack, in the full glare of the social media [13]. Also, although there are many advantages of family-centred care [14], increased family presence on PICU can expose staff to greater levels of distress [15].

60.2 Burnout

The term 'burnout' refers to a continuum of symptoms (see ▶ Box 60.1). The three main dimensions measured by the Maslach Burnout Inventory (MBI) [16] are emotional exhaustion, depersonalisation and reduced levels of personal accomplishment. Although 'burnout' is a salient concept for many in the health professions, it is not a formal diagnosis, and even when the best-known scales are used in studies examining its prevalence and associated risks, scores are interpreted differently in different papers [17]. Nevertheless there is compelling evidence across the literature that higher burnout levels are systematically associated with increased risk of suicidality, medical error, depression and alcohol abuse [18, 19]. This has led a group of Critical Care Societies to call for better consensus as to definitions and measurement, and more research into effective interventions [3].

A recent national study of $n = 1656$ healthcare staff working in paediatric intensive care settings, in the UK [8], found an overall prevalence of 47% reporting significant burnout, with those on larger units more likely to report higher scores. The study also found that nurses scored consistently higher than doctors in relation to emotional exhaustion, but that the opposite was true for depersonalisation, with doctors reporting this aspect of burnout more often.

60.3 Post-Traumatic Stress

It is important also to be aware of the risk of developing traumatic stress reactions in relation to working with traumatised populations, such as families in PICU. This type of occupational trauma has been explicitly recognised in the latest international criteria for the diagnosis of post-traumatic stress disorder (PTSD). Caregivers may be traumatised directly by what they witness in the context of their work, or vicariously, in what is known as secondary traumatic stress, as a consequence of being repeatedly exposed to highly distressed people in life-threatening situations.

Symptoms include re-experiencing, avoidance of reminders of the traumatic event(s) and hypervigilance (see ▶ Box 60.2). Although having criteria relating to the number and duration of symptoms are needed for formal diagnosis, having high but sub-threshold levels of these symptoms, sometimes referred to as post-traumatic stress symptoms (PTSS) as opposed to PTSD, is also regarded as clinically significant.

There is evidence that intensive care staff report higher levels of PTSD symptoms than other healthcare workers [6, 7], and some suggest that these symptoms are reported more often in paediatric ICU staff than in adult ICU staff [20], despite the fact that adult units have higher mortality rates. A recent national survey in the UK found that 31% of nurses and 16% of doctors reported clinically significant levels of PTSD symptoms [8].

Meta-analyses have highlighted younger age and previous history of trauma as risk factors associated with a greater chance of developing PTSD symptoms after a traumatic event. In many cases, symptoms naturally abate over time but if they are persistent and affecting functioning, there is a good evidence base for the efficacy of a number of theoretically driven individual treatments, after an initial period of watchful waiting [21].

60.4 Moral Distress

A third form of work-related distress in intensive care settings is moral distress, which refers to the particular psychological strain engendered by not being able to act in alignment with professional or personal values [22] (see ▶ Box 60.3). It is different from having an ethical dilemma, where it is unclear how one should proceed, or other forms of distress, which do not necessarily entail the violation of core values.

Until relatively recently, descriptions of moral distress were confined to qualitative studies only, but a new measure of this phenomenon developed in 2007, and later adapted to include a wider range of potential stressors, is now available. The Measure of Moral Distress in Healthcare Professionals (MMDHP) [4] comprises a list of hypothetical situations which would be expected to produce moral distress, and which are rated both in terms of frequency and intensity.

Moral distress has been found to be more prevalent in intensive care than in other medical settings [23] and there is evidence that it is more common in larger, tertiary paediatric units [8, 24]. The issues most commonly found to be troubling are related to end-of-life care and communication, and over-treatment is more often cited as problematic than under-treatment. It may be that some degree of moral distress is inevitable [25], especially given the speed of technological advancement, which makes so many more treatment options available. And although it may be uncomfortable to experience, it does signify that the person concerned has professional values and is aware of when they are being compromised.

60.5 Special Situations

It is important also to acknowledge that over the course of a career in PICU, staff will occasionally encounter extraordinary stress associated with their work, for which they can never be totally prepared and which will, for a time, overwhelm them. Such situations, which can include terrorist attacks and natural disasters, are sometimes termed ‘Major Incidents’ which, by definition, entail that demands exceed the resources available (e.g. supplies, personnel, beds, ventilators). From a psychological perspective, staff caught up in these situations, whilst able to push themselves to the limit in the immediate crisis for the common good, they may feel seriously depleted and, in some cases, also fearful, angry and guilty, for some time afterwards [26, 27].

There are also examples of unusually stressful situations which affect PICU staff but are not always explicitly conceived of as a single major incident because of their protracted nature. Recent high-profile court cases where PICU staff and families were in dispute as to whether the care of a child was futile, were associated with high levels of distress in staff at follow-up [13] and the recent COVID-19 global pandemic, has left a particular mark psychologically, on healthcare workers in general, as well as more widely on the general population, with specific strains reported by paediatric staff in relation to their redeployment to adult ICU settings [28, 29].

At times such as these, an understanding of the principles of Psychological First Aid (PFA) may be helpful. PFA is based on research demonstrating that people in crisis adapt better psychologically if they are helped to feel safe, calm, efficacious, connected and hopeful at the time of the acute threat to their emotional integrity [30]. Later on, when the emergency has passed, an understanding of the nature of different forms of distress such as those described above is also likely to be useful. Individual coping strategies, and ideally ones which the individual has already identified and tested in calmer times, are likely to be invaluable in relation to the restoration of emotional equilibrium but should also be complemented by the provision of support at the organisational level.

60.6 Self-Care and Organisational Level Interventions

The literature on effective interventions to prevent and reduce staff stress in intensive care settings is still small, but the available data in relation to the prevention of burnout, suggests that interventions are more powerful when they involve strategies at the organisational level, as well as the individual level [31]. There is some evidence that the use of debriefing is associated with a reduction in burnout [20, 32]; that speaking with supervisors, when stressed, is associated with lower rates of post-traumatic stress [20] and that moral distress is lower in units who meet up regularly [5]. Some hospitals have been proactive in launching campaigns to change the prevailing work culture by challenging presenteeism and advocating regular food and rest breaks [33] and others report improvements in burnout and job satisfaction in relation to changes in shift patterns [34]. Organisational interventions associated with lower moral distress include the Nursing Ethics Huddle [35] and the Moral Distress Consultation Service [36].

These findings illustrate the value of prioritising time and space to reflect and recover, emphasised by Highfield (2019) [37] recently. It may be useful to those starting out on careers in this speciality to acknowledge that, whilst it may well be necessary and adaptive at times to suppress emotions acutely in order to focus on the job at hand, they would be wise to schedule downtime later, in order to restore their ability to feel, especially if they notice feeling more numb generally, outside work [38]. Even when it is not possible to share thoughts with colleagues, there is long-standing evidence from psychological research, that the simple acts of labelling feelings [39] and writing thoughts down [40] reduce anxiety and can help with problem-solving. Other individual strategies which have emerged as protective against burnout, and predictive of greater job satisfaction, are 'job crafting' and focusing on finding meaning at work [41].

Finally, the value of self-monitoring has been demonstrated to be an effective strategy for managing well-being, more widely in the literature on physician stress [42], and an evaluation of a new free mobile application, designed to monitor stress levels and promote adaptive coping strategies, such as scheduling regular breaks, has reported significant reductions in distress associated with its use [43]. A number of free self-report tools including 'stresscheckerICU' are also available online, along with other training materials and well-being resources (See ► Box 60.4) (◘ Fig. 60.2).

a b
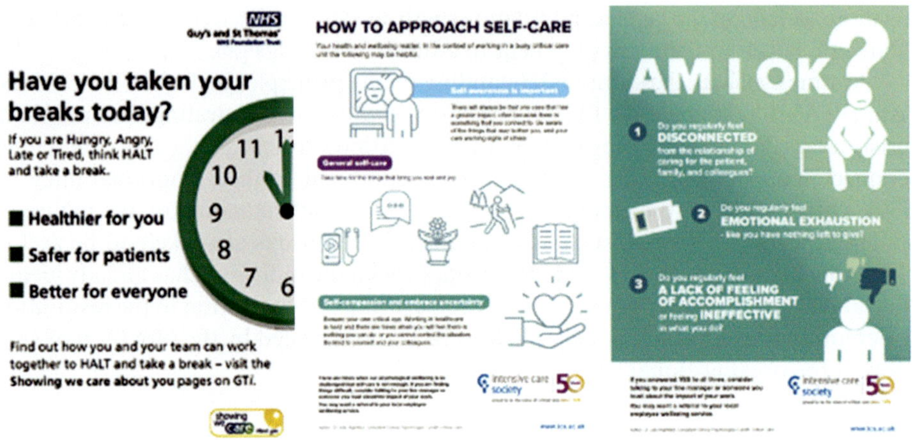

Fig. 60.2 Posters reminding staff to take care of their physical and psychological well-being. (**a**) Guys and St Thomas' Trust, UK [33]. (**b**) UK Intensive Care Society. ▶ https://tinyurl.com/y8ng73wz ▶ https://ics.ac.uk/thriving/online-resources.html

Take-Home Messages

- The causes of stress at work are multifactorial.
- Different types of stress are measured by different instruments and are addressed differently.
- The main dimensions of burnout are emotional exhaustion, depersonalisation and reduced personal achievement.
- High burnout scores are more common than depression or PTSD symptoms in ICU staff.
- The main symptoms of PTSD are re-experiencing, avoidance, hypervigilance and negative mood.
- Moral distress occurs when a person knows the right thing to do in a given situation but is prevented from doing it, often for reasons outside their control.
- Rest, sleep and nutrition all aid psychological well-being.
- Persistent PTSD symptoms indicate that further emotional processing is needed and may require professional input.
- Regular communication in the form of meetings with seniors and unit discussions may facilitate cooing with the more difficult emotional and moral aspects of this work.
- Debriefing initiatives may aid short-term emotional processing after traumatic events.

- In the aftermath of special situations such as major incidents, psychological resources are likely to be temporarily overwhelmed. Staff will benefit from more respite and in some cases, professional support after such events.

Box 60.1. Burnout

Burnout is a continuum of symptoms of work-related stress, made up of three main dimensions:

- Emotional Exhaustion—Reduced energy and enthusiasm in relation to work
- Depersonalisation—Detachment and cynicism
- Reduced Sense of Personal Accomplishment—Diminished sense of efficacy

From Maslach Burnout Inventory [16]

Box 60.2. Post-traumatic Stress Disorder (ICD-11 code 6B40)

- Traumatic experience
- Functional impairment
  - At least one symptom in each of the following three categories, lasting at least 1 month
- Re-experiencing (e.g. nightmares, flashbacks)
- Avoidance (e.g. avoiding talking about it, avoiding reminders)
- Feeling a continuous sense of threat (e.g. hypervigilance, exaggerated startle response)

▶ https://icd.who.int/en

Box 60.3. Moral Distress

Jameton (1984) [22] has defined moral distress as 'when one knows the right thing to do, but institutional constraints make it nearly impossible to pursue the right course of action'.

Examples of items from the questionnaire Measure of Moral Distress for Health Care Professionals (MMDHP) [4] are given below:

- 'Being required to care for more patients than I can safely care for'
- 'Witnessing healthcare providers giving "false hope" to a patient or family'

Box 60.4. Useful Online Resources
Self-Tests

- Compassion Fatigue 7 https://www.aafp.org/fpm/2000/0400/p39.html
- Need for rest ▶ https://renewnow.org/r-o-m/
- StresscheckerICU: Post-traumatic stress symptoms ▶ https://tinyurl.com/y8ng73wz
- StresscheckerICU: Burnout symptoms ▶ https://tinyurl.com/y8ng73wz
- Provider Resilience Mobile App (PRMA), US National Center for Telehealth and Technology

Skills Training

- Slides on Secondary Traumatic Stress ▶ https://www.healthcaretoolbox.org/images/CPTS_-_Secondary_Traumatic_Stress_Healthcare_Staff.pdf
- Resources on Trauma-informed care ▶ https://www.nctsn.org/trauma-informed-care/trauma-informed-systems/healthcare/nctsn-resources

Literature

- Advice on managing sleep and shift work in medical settings: ▶ https://www.guysandstthomaseducation.com/projectsleep-looking-after-your-wellbeing/
- British Medical Journal resources on wellbeing: ▶ https://www.bmj.com/wellbeing
- UK Intensive Care Society wellbeing resources: ▶ https://ics.ac.uk/thrive.html

References

1. Duffee J, Szilagyi M, Forkey H, Kelly ET. Trauma-informed care in child health systems. Pediatrics. 2021;148:e2021052579. https://doi.org/10.1542/peds.2021-052579.
2. Demers LA, Wright NM, Kopstick AJ, et al. Is pediatric intensive care trauma-informed? A review of principles and evidence. Children (Basel). 2022;9:1575. https://doi.org/10.3390/children9101575.
3. Moss M, Good VS, Gozal D, Kleinpell R, Sessler CN. An official critical care societies collaborative statement: burnout syndrome in critical care health care professionals: a call for action. Am J Crit Care. 2016;25(4):368–76. https://doi.org/10.4037/ajcc2016133.
4. Epstein EG, Whitehead PB, Prompahakul C, Thacker LR, Hamric AB. Enhancing understanding of moral distress: the measure of moral distress for health care professionals. AJOB Empir Bioeth. 2019;10(2):113–24. https://doi.org/10.1080/23294515.2019.1586008.

5. Dryden-Palmer K, Moore G, McNeill C, et al. Moral distress of clinicians in Canadian pediatric and neonatal ICUs. Pediatr Crit Care Med. 2020;21(4):314–23. https://doi.org/10.1097/PCC.0000000000002189.
6. Mealer ML, Shelton A, Berg B, et al. Increased prevalence of post- traumatic stress disorder symptoms in critical care nurses. Am J Respir Crit Care Med. 2007;175:693–7.
7. de Boer J, Lok A, Van't Verlaat E, et al. Work-related critical incidents in hospital-based health care providers and the risk of post-traumatic stress symptoms, anxiety, and depression: a meta-analysis. Soc Sci Med. 2011;73:316–26.
8. Jones GAL, Colville GA, Ramnarayan P, et al. Psychological impact of working in paediatric intensive care. A UK-wide prevalence study. Arch Dis Child. 2020;105:470–5. https://doi.org/10.1136/archdischild-2019-317439.
9. Shanafelt TD, Boone S, Tan L, et al. Burnout and satisfaction with work-life balance among US physicians relative to the general US population. Arch Intern Med. 2012;172:1377–85.
10. Shanafelt TD, Hasan O, Dyrbye LN, et al. Changes in burnout and satisfaction with work-life balance in physicians and the general US working population between 2011 and 2014. Mayo Clin Proc. 2015;90:1600–13.
11. Pearson GA. Intensive care: because we can or because we should? Arch Dis Child. 2018;103(6):527–8. https://doi.org/10.1136/archdischild-2017-314731.
12. Heneghan JA, Pollack MM. Morbidity: changing the outcome paradigm for pediatric critical care. Pediatr Clin N Am. 2017;64(5):1147–65.
13. Colville G, Rutt M, Berger Z, Titman P, Brierley J. Moral distress, trauma and burnout in staff in relation to changes in PICU outcomes, challenging cases and media involvement in disagreements about end-of-life care. Arch Dis Child. 2018;103(Suppl 1):A192–3. https://doi.org/10.1136/archdischild-2018-rcpch.459.
14. Davidson JE, Aslakson RA, Long AC, et al. Guidelines for family-centered care in the neonatal, pediatric, and adult ICU. Crit Care Med. 2017;45(1):103–28.
15. Coats H, Bourget E, Starks H, et al. Nurses' reflections on benefits and challenges of implementing family-centered care in Pediatric Intensive Care Units. Am J Crit Care. 2018;27(1):52–8. https://doi.org/10.4037/ajcc2018353.
16. Maslach C, Jackson SE, Leiter MP. The Maslach burnout inventory: manual. Palo Alto: Consulting Psychologists Press; 1996.
17. van Mol MM, Kompanje EJ, Benoit DD, Bakker J, Nijkamp MD. The prevalence of compassion fatigue and burnout among healthcare professionals in intensive care units: a systematic review. PLoS One. 2015;10(8):e0136955. https://doi.org/10.1371/journal.pone.0136955. eCollection.
18. Mion G, Libert N, Journois D. The prevalence of burnout Intensive Care Med. 2018;44(7):1192–4. https://doi.org/10.1007/s00134-018-5200-2.
19. West CP, Dyrbye LN, Sloan JA, et al. Single item measures of emotional exhaustion and depersonalization are useful for assessing burnout in medical professionals. J Gen Intern Med. 2009;24:1318–21.
20. Colville GA, Smith JG, Brierley J, et al. Coping with staff burnout and work-related posttraumatic stress in intensive care. Pediatr Crit Care Med. 2017;18(7):e267–73. https://doi.org/10.1097/PCC.0000000000001179.
21. National Institute for Health and Care Excellence. The management of PTSD in adults and children in primary and secondary care. NICE clinical guideline 116. Manchester: National Institute for Health and Care Excellence; 2018. www.nice.org.uk/guidance/NG116. Accessed 14 Dec 2022.
22. Jameton A. Nursing practice: the ethical issues. Englewood Cliffs: Prentice-Hall; 1984.
23. Whitehead PB, Herbertson RK, Hamric AB, Epstein EG, Fisher JM. Moral distress among healthcare professionals: report of an institution-wide survey. J Nurs Scholarsh. 2015;47:117–25.
24. Larson CP, Dryden-Palmer KD, Gibbons C, et al. Moral distress in PICU and neonatal ICU practitioners: a cross-sectional evaluation. Pediatr Crit Care Med. 2017;18:e318–26.
25. Field D, Deeming J, Smith LK. Moral distress: an inevitable part of neonatal and paediatric intensive care? Arch Dis Child. 2016;101:686–8.
26. De Stefano C, Orri M, Agostinucci JM, et al. Early psychological impact of Paris terrorist attacks on healthcare emergency staff: a cross-sectional study. Depress Anxiety. 2018;35(3):275–82. https://doi.org/10.1002/da.22724.

27. French P, Barrett A, Allsopp K, et al. Psychological screening of adults and young people following the Manchester arena incident. BJPsych Open. 2019;5(5):e85. https://doi.org/10.1192/bjo.2019.61.
28. Ffrench-O'Carroll R, Feeley T, Tan MH, et al. Psychological impact of COVID-19 on staff working in paediatric and adult critical care. Br J Anaesth. 2021;126:e39–41. https://doi.org/10.1016/j.bja.2020.09.040.
29. Mohta S, Alexander J, Colville G. The experience of paediatric staff caring for adults with Covid-19. Arch Dis Childhood. 2021;106(Suppl 1):A344.
30. Hobfoll SE, Watson P, Bell CC, et al. Five essential elements of immediate and mid-term mass trauma intervention: empirical evidence. Psychiatry. 2007;70:283–315. https://doi.org/10.1521/psyc.2007.70.4.283.
31. West CP, Dyrbye LN, Erwin PJ, Shanafelt TD. Interventions to prevent and reduce physician burnout: a systematic review and meta-analysis. Lancet. 2016;388(10057):2272–81. https://doi.org/10.1016/S0140-6736(16)31279-X.
32. Gillen J, Koncicki ML, Hough RF, Palumbo K, Choudhury T, Daube A. The impact of a fellow-driven debriefing program after pediatric cardiac arrests. BMC Med Educ. 2019;19(1):272.
33. Baverstock A, Finlay F. Take a break: HALT—are you hungry, angry, late or tired? Arch Dis Child Educ Pract. 2019;104:200.
34. Mikkelsen ME, Anderson BJ, Bellini L, Schweickert WD, Fuchs BD, Kerlin MP. Burnout, and fulfillment, in the profession of critical care medicine. Am J Respir Crit Care Med. 2019;200:931–3. https://doi.org/10.1164/rccm.201903-0662LE.
35. Chiafery MC, Hopkins P, Norton SA, Shaw MH. Nursing ethics huddles to decrease moral distress among nurses in the intensive care unit. J Clin Ethics. 2018;29(3):217–26.
36. Hamric AB, Epstein EG. A health system-wide moral distress consultation service: development and evaluation. HEC Forum. 2017;29(2):127–43.
37. Highfield JA. The sustainability of the critical care workforce. Nurs Crit Care. 2019;24(1):6–8. https://doi.org/10.1111/nicc.12394.
38. Colville G. To feel or not to feel?—that is the question. Pediatr Crit Care Med. 2020;21(10):912–3. https://doi.org/10.1097/PCC.0000000000002386.
39. Lieberman MD, Eisenberger NI, Crockett MJ, Tom SM, Pfeifer JH, Way BM. Putting feelings into words: affect labeling disrupts amygdala activity in response to affective stimuli. Psychol Sci. 2007;18:421–8. https://doi.org/10.1111/j.1467-9280.2007.01916.x.
40. Pennebaker JW. Writing about emotional experiences as a therapeutic process. Psychol Sci. 1997;8:162–6.
41. Demerouti E. Strategies used by individuals to prevent burnout. Eur J Clin Invest. 2015;45(10):1106–12. https://doi.org/10.1111/eci.12494.
42. Shanafelt TD, Kaups KL, Nelson H, et al. An interactive individualized intervention to promote behavioral change to increase personal well-being in US surgeons. Ann Surg. 2014;259(1):82–8. https://doi.org/10.1097/SLA.0b013e3182a58fa4.
43. Wood AE, Prins A, Bush NE, et al. Reduction of burnout in mental health care providers using the provider resilience mobile application. Community Ment Health J. 2017;53(4):452–9. https://doi.org/10.1007/s10597-016-0076-5.

Management of Older Children in the ICU

Dora Wood and Nwanneka N. Sargant

Contents

J. Brierley et al. (eds.), *ESPNIC Children's Intensive Care Textbook*,
https://doi.org/10.1007/978-3-031-64762-8_61

Learning Objectives

By the end of this chapter, the reader should be able to:

- Understand that the physical, social and emotional changes around adolescence require modifications to usual intensive care practice.
- Use a framework to remember the special considerations needed when caring for young people in the intensive care unit.
- Develop an approach to concepts of consent and confidentiality appropriate for their legal jurisdiction.

61.1 Introduction

The transition from childhood to adulthood is a time of huge physical, social and emotional change [1]. There is increasing recognition of the need to provide 'developmentally appropriate healthcare' to young people undergoing this transition, distinct from the services provided to younger children and older adults. Healthcare settings increasingly meet these needs with dedicated units and services, training and specialists in young people's health.

Many of the principles of caring for critically ill patients apply across the full spectrum of age. Specialised services (including Paediatric and Neonatal Intensive Care Units) allow the delivery of intensive care to be adapted to meet the needs of different patient groups, from premature babies to the elderly. A super-specialised 'Adolescent Intensive Care Unit' is unachievable in most settings, but this chapter describes the ways in which intensive care, whether delivered on a paediatric or adult unit, can be adapted to meet the needs of older children and young adults.

61.2 Definitions

A number of descriptive terms are used to describe young people between the ages of 10 and 25 (▶ Box 61.1). The World Health Organisation defines an adolescent as a young person aged between 10 and 19 years and sub-divides this into early-, mid- and late-adolescence by age. The preferred term for describing this group is 'young people', which includes those up to age 24.

These definitions do not take into account the variability in development between individuals; some 'late adolescents' may be at earlier stages of social and emotional maturity than those who are younger. Prior experience in healthcare, in particular, may affect how well young people can understand and respond to health challenges. If they are one of the growing number of young people with chronic illnesses surviving into adulthood, they may be comfortable interacting with healthcare professionals, whilst previously well young people (possibly used to a greater degree of independence from parents) may require intensive care for the first time after an injury or acute infection.

61.3 Diagnostic Spectrum

Conditions like pneumonia and sepsis cause critical illness across all age groups, but as children approach adolescence, a higher proportion of admissions are due to pathology more commonly seen in young adults.

Some of this difference is a result of increasing independence and risk-taking behaviour. With increasing age, a higher proportion of intensive care unit admissions are related to major trauma, including drowning. Admissions following the use of alcohol or recreational drugs also rise in older age groups, as do the consequences of deliberate self-harm.

As the majority of PICU patients are infants or preschool children, many of these conditions are less common in the PICU than in adult intensive care. Depending on local procedures and expertise, a decision must be made as to whether it is more appropriate to manage some older young people in adult settings or to treat them in the PICU but with specialist input (e.g. from obstetricians).

When managing critically ill young people either in the paediatric or adult intensive care unit, the '6 Ps' (▶ Box 61.2) [2] is a useful aide-memoire.

61.4 Practical Issues

61.4.1 Physical Differences

The most striking difference between young children and those approaching adulthood is size. Manual handling processes that are appropriate for small children must be adapted to allow staff to transfer and reposition larger patients safely. This should include the provision of both appropriate equipment and sufficient staff.

Drug dosing errors are common in this age group when the weight-based dose of a drug exceeds the expected adult dose. For many drugs, this occurs at 40 kg (around age 12 years) but this limit may be considerably lower. Individual prescribers should maintain awareness of these issues, but at an organisational level, processes and alerts may help to reduce errors of this type.

61.4.2 Experiences on ICU

Distressing situations are not uncommon in the intensive care unit. Whilst young children may not notice the death of another patient, resuscitation, or conversations about poor prognoses, many older children will. Even sedated patients may hear and understand nearby conversations. Ward rounds and discussions about other patients should be held well away from the young person's bed space where possible; if this is not possible, music through headphones may provide an auditory shield. Consideration should also be given to what is in the young person's line of sight.

Explanations and reassurance should be given as far as possible whilst maintaining the confidentiality of other patients.

61.5 Privacy

Adolescence is a period of significant physical and social change, which has a direct impact on body image and self-consciousness. Young people are more concerned about physical exposure than any other age group. Same-sex accommodations and wards are often not practical in the PICU, so extra care must be taken to ensure doors and curtains are shut when the young person is uncovered for any reason. Consideration must be given to the adolescent's wishes (or likely wishes, if unable to communicate directly) on the presence of parents during examinations and intimate care. For younger children, involving parents in physical care is desirable, but for many adolescents, this would no longer be acceptable. For similar reasons, when it is possible, adolescents may prefer to have intimate care provided by nursing staff of the same sex.

61.6 Personal Life

Young people value professionals who are approachable, open-minded, trustworthy, and honest, who listen and act on what they hear, explain things in ways young people can understand, take the time to learn how they prefer to communicate and are not patronising. During critical illness, many young people are unable to communicate effectively with caregivers but where this is possible it is important that communication with young people reflects their needs. The validated psychosocial assessment tool, HEADSSS as an interview prompt and vulnerability screening tool provides a useful framework for communication with young people. It follows a simple structure, remembered by the acronym HEADSSS (▶ Box 61.3).

In addition to providing important information about psychosocial functioning, information from a young person directly about their usual alcohol intake or disordered eating, for example, may be different from that given to healthcare providers by their parents. This may change immediate management within the intensive care unit (e.g. prevention of re-feeding syndrome or alcohol withdrawal).

Critical illness often significantly interrupts education. For those young people close to leaving school, these interruptions can have serious consequences, as options for employment and further education can depend on school performance at this stage. Interruption to employment may also be an issue for some young people. Particularly for longer admissions and where possible, consideration should be given to how to enable education to continue, or otherwise mitigate the effects of missing school. This is most effective when done in conjunction with the young person's usual teachers.

Even for those too unwell to undertake education, age-appropriate distraction and entertainment are important. This will vary hugely between individuals, who will by this age have developed distinct interests and preferences. Music, films and other items from home can greatly improve the young person's experience.

Whilst small children primarily relate to the world via their parents, and illness may cause a regression into greater dependence, peer relations become more salient in adolescence. For many young people, peers compete with family as a significant source of emotional well-being. It is thus important that visiting policies reflect the need for peer support, particularly for those requiring prolonged admission. Access to the internet is essential for many young people to maintain relationships with friends and associates; arrangements should be made to enable this.

61.7 Puberty

For post-pubertal females, the possibility of pregnancy must always be considered. This is most often because pregnancy status may alter decisions about treatment or investigations (e.g. avoiding ionising radiation) but occasionally the pregnancy is the cause of critical illness (e.g. ruptured ectopic, eclampsia). Many critically ill patients are unable to provide consent, so indications for proceeding with a pregnancy test in the absence of this consent should be clearly documented.

With the onset of puberty, many young people develop their own skincare and hygiene regimes. Enquiries at or before the point of admission can allow these to be continued, where this is important to the young person.

61.8 Prophylaxis

Deep vein thrombosis and venous thromboembolism (VTE) are much less common in children than in adults but are a significant cause of mortality and morbidity in hospitalised children. VTE prophylaxis in hospitalised adults is widely adopted and well supported by evidence. In contrast, there is no high-quality evidence to guide best practice for DVT prophylaxis in children and young people, either in terms of risk assessment or efficacy of treatments. Existing recommendations are based on data from studies in adults.

The factors that predispose to thrombosis broadly relate to the three categories of Virchow's triad; venous stasis, endothelial injury and hypercoagulability. Critically ill children frequently have multiple risk factors including the presence of an indwelling central venous catheter, infection/inflammation, immobility and a reduced consciousness level. However, overall risk remains low until adolescence, when the coagulation system matures and risk factors, including smoking, obesity and use of hormonal contraceptives, become more common.

Most critically ill young people past the age of puberty should be considered to be at least at moderate risk of VTE, and measures to reduce the risk such as early mobilisation and removal of central venous catheters may not be possible. The benefits of withholding hormonal contraceptives must be balanced against the risk of subsequent unplanned pregnancy. All critically ill young people should be considered for mechanical and/or pharmacological VTE prophylaxis, based on an evaluation of individual risk factors (▶ Box 61.4) [3].

Options for mechanical prophylaxis are anti-embolism stockings (AES) and intermittent pneumatic compression devices. Both are limited by patient size, with limited options for patients below about 40 kg. Anti-embolism stockings provide graduated circumferential pressure that gradually decreases from ankle to thigh. Intermittent compression devices (ICDs) increase venous return from the legs by replicating the 'pumping' action of the calf muscles. Both are safe; in terms of VTE prevention, ICDs are more effective than AES in adults but may be less well tolerated.

Pharmacological prophylaxis (including unfractionated or low molecular weight heparin) should be reserved for those assessed to be at high risk of VTE (generally with more than one risk factor) and where this outweighs the increased risk from bleeding.

61.9 Permission

61.9.1 Communication

Article 12 of the United Nations Convention on the Rights of the Child (UNCRC) outlines the right of young people to participate in matters affecting them, which includes their own healthcare. All healthcare providers should be seeking to include, involve and support the participation of young people in healthcare.

When possible, it is always important to explain treatments and interventions to patients and to take their opinions into account, regardless of their age or legal capacity to consent. However, some important legal differences arise when young people approach adulthood.

61.9.2 Consent

To be capable of consenting for a healthcare intervention, an individual must be able to understand what a proposed procedure involves, and the benefits and risks of undergoing or not undergoing the procedure. They must be able to retain the information for long enough to make a decision, and to communicate it. The capacity to consent depends on how risky or complex the proposed procedure is. For example, a person might be able to consent to treatment with antibiotics, but not for high-risk surgery.

Adults are presumed to have the capacity to consent to their own healthcare decisions unless there is evidence that they are not. Generally, this is not the case for children and young people, but the legal position is not consistent between countries.

In some countries, including Greece, Bulgaria and Italy, the capacity to consent is assumed to start from a fixed age; this may be the age of majority (usually 18 years) or a younger age (often 16 years). For those who have not reached this age, those who have parental responsibility make all decisions about medical care. It is always good practice to take the opinion of the young person into account before making these decisions, and in some countries (e.g. in France) this is legally required.

Several countries, including Belgium, Germany and Austria, have no legal minimum age requirement. In these countries, young people can make their own decisions about medical care as soon as they can demonstrate sufficient intellectual and emotional maturity to do so.

There are also combined approaches. For example, in the UK, which has a predominantly age-based system, young people below the age of majority may be deemed competent to consent to medical treatment. In Spain, dual consent from both parent and young person is required, while in Croatia, the need for parental consent is determined by the risk of the procedure [4, 5].

Of relevance, otherwise competent young people may lose the capacity to consent when they are critically ill, either because of the illness itself or the effects of treatment (e.g. sedative drugs). In this case, decisions about medical treatment may be made by those with parental responsibility or by clinicians, depending on the local legal framework.

61.9.3 Confidentiality

Concerns about confidentiality are heightened during adolescence, and remain one of the critical deterrents to young people accessing and receiving appropriate healthcare. A young person's right to confidentiality is generally assumed when they demonstrate the capacity to consent to treatment. Outside of the intensive care unit, the protection of confidentiality is an important component of adolescent healthcare, promoting the development of maturity and autonomy.

For many critically ill young people, the situation is complicated as they may be too unwell to either understand or share information. In this situation, where decision-making falls to those with parental responsibility, confidentiality is usually compromised in the interest of making sure the decision-makers have all of the medical detail they need.

Take-Home Messages

- Young people requiring intensive care have needs that are distinct both from other critically ill patients and from young people who are not critically ill.
- High-quality responsive care for young people may be most appropriately delivered on either adult or paediatric intensive care units, depending on the clinical situation and physical, social and emotional maturity of the young person.
- The 6 Ps provide an aide-memoire for ways in which intensive care can be optimised for each young person.

Box 61.1 Definitions Pertinent to Adolescent Medicine

WHO definitions:

Adolescent: 10–19 years

Young people: 10–24 years

Youth: 15–24 years

Other:

Teenage: 13–19 years

Young adult: 16–25 years

Adolescent developmental stages:

10–13 years: Early adolescence

14–16 years: Mid adolescence

17–19 years: Late adolescence

19+ years: Emerging adulthood

Box 61.2 The 6 Ps

Practical Issues

- Physical differences (size)
- Experiences on ICU

Privacy

- Physical exposure

Personal life

- HEADSSS
- Education
- Peer support

Puberty

- Pregnancy
- Skincare/hygiene

Prophylaxis

- DVT risk

Permission

- Communication
- Consent
- Confidentiality

Box 61.3 HEADSSS Risk Assessment

H: Home

E: Education/Employment/Eating

A: Activities

D: Drugs

S: Suicidality/depression

S: Sexuality/sexual behavior

S: Safety

Box 61.4 Risk Factors for VTE

Endothelial injury: presence of central venous catheter, trauma

Venous stasis: immobility, reduced conscious level, mechanical ventilation, spinal cord injury

Hypercoagulability: hormonal (pregnancy, exogenous oestrogen use), dehydration, thrombophilia (family or personal history), infection or inflammatory disease, burns, malignancy

References

1. Sargant NN, Hudson L, McDonagh J. Adolescent medicine. In: Lissauer T, Carroll W, editors. The science of paediatrics: MRCPCH mastercourse. 1st ed. Elsevier; 2016. p. 624–639.
2. Tuckwell R, Wood D, Mansfield-Sturgess S, et al. A European Society of Paediatric and Neonatal Intensive Care (ESPNIC) survey of European critical care management of young people. Eur J Pediatr. 2017;176:155–61. https://doi.org/10.1007/s00431-016-2815-6.
3. Faustino EV, Raffini LJ. Prevention of hospital-acquired venous thromboembolism in children: a review of published guidelines. Front Pediatr. 2017;5:9. https://doi.org/10.3389/fped.2017.00009.
4. Sénécal K, Thys K, Vears DF, Van Assche K, Knoppers BM, Borry P. Legal approaches regarding health-care decisions involving minors: implications for next-generation sequencing. Eur J Human Genet. 2016;24(11):1559–64. https://doi.org/10.1038/ejhg.2016.61.
5. European Union Agency for Fundamental Rights. Consenting to medical treatment without parental consent. [Online]. 2020. https://fra.europa.eu/en/publication/2017/mapping-minimum-age-requirements/consent-medical-treatments. Accessed 13 Aug 2020.

Where Do Critically Ill Children Go?

Content

Outcomes in PICU

Karolijn Dulfer, Maayke Hunfeld, Lotte Haverman, and Corinne Buysse

Contents

J. Brierley et al. (eds.), *ESPNIC Children's Intensive Care Textbook*,
https://doi.org/10.1007/978-3-031-64762-8_62

62

Learning Objectives

- Why outcome after critical illness is increasingly important.
- To know the different outcome domains.
- To be aware of the importance and challenges of organizing a follow-up outpatient clinic, both as patient care and research.

62.1 Introduction

In the last decades, mortality in pediatric critical illness in the Western world has decreased to less than 5%, which resulted in increased morbidity. Therefore, the focus on outcomes has shifted from mortality to morbidities after PICU discharge. In adult critical care, these new or worsening morbidities in different domains are well described as post-intensive care syndrome (PICS), which may persist many years after ICU admission [1]. Critically ill children may also experience impairments in different domains in the short-term, e.g., physical, cognitive, emotional, and social health (◘ Fig. 62.1) [2]. Some of these impairments may remain in the long-term. Both the child's preexisting health status and the management of acute pediatric illness might contribute to these impairments. The subjective evaluation of these impairments and their impact on daily life may result in a lower quality of life (QoL). Not only the child but also family members such as caregivers and siblings might be affected by the PICU admission and by experiencing morbidities during the period after PICU discharge.

What makes PICS after critical illness in childhood different than in adults? How do children and parents manage to develop a "new normal" after PICU admission,

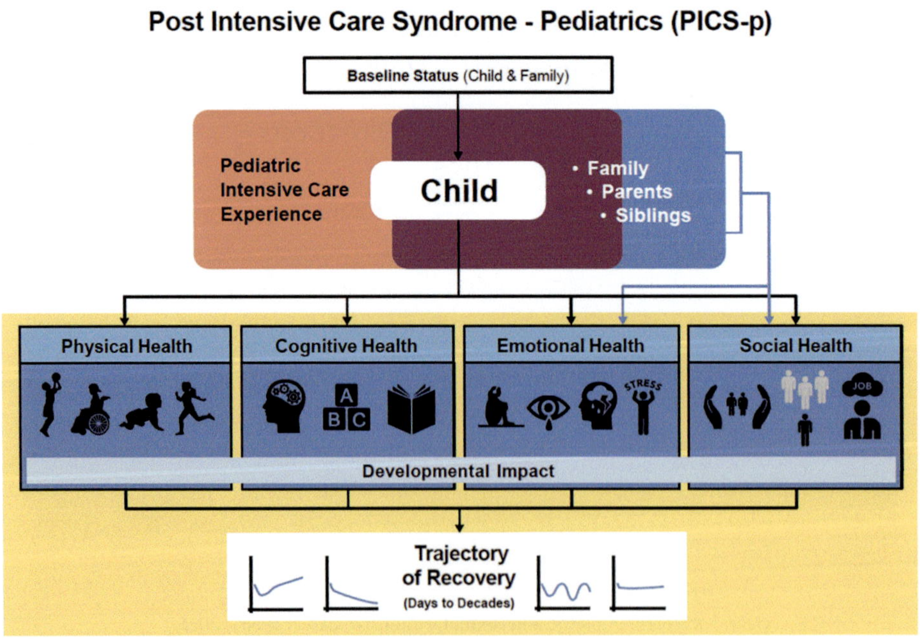

◘ **Fig. 62.1** Post-intensive care syndrome in pediatrics (PICS-p) framework [2]

and what if this does not happen and children grow into deficits? These questions will be addressed in the next chapters.

62.2 Case Reports

Before the physical and psychological outcomes, after pediatric critical illness will be discussed in ▶ Chaps. 68 and 69, respectively; the first two cases are presented below which illustrate how the outcome after a similar event, e.g., near-drowning, may vary.

Patient 1 is a 2-year-old girl, without previous medical history, who experienced a near-drowning event, unwitnessed. After approximately 15 min, Basic Life Support (BLS) was started by laypersons, after which an emergency medical team took over. After 20 min, a return of spontaneous circulation (ROSC) was reached. The girl's first pH was 6.9 and lactate was 16 mmol/L. Her body temperature on arrival at the hospital was 29 °C. She was admitted to the PICU and received post-ROSC care. Unfortunately, she did not regain consciousness and developed severe paroxysmal hyperactivity. An MRI both 5 days and 2 weeks after the event showed minimal hypoxic changes in the basal ganglia and brainstem.

Two years later, the girl is severely disabled; there is no possibility for communication, and she is wheelchair-bound with a spastic quadriplegia.

Patient 2, a previously healthy 5-year-old boy, was the victim of a witnessed near-drowning accident. Bystander BLS was started quickly, 20 min later the medical team arrived, and CPR was continued. Since no ROSC was achieved, ECPR was started on arrival at the emergency department (60 min after the onset of BLS). The boy's first pH was 6.7 and lactate was 24 mmol/L. His body temperature on arrival at the emergency department was 28 °C. Subsequently, he was admitted to the PICU and received post-ROSC care. The day after resuscitation, still on ECMO, he woke up. An MRI 5 days later revealed no ischemic changes.

Two years later, he has only minor neurocognitive deficits, resulting in a lower processing speed than he had before the near-drowning.

62.3 Physical Outcomes After Pediatric Critical Illness

Physical outcomes of critical illness may be organ-specific like cardiorespiratory, neurologically, mobility or more general like the ability to perform daily activities and meet basic needs.

Many studies have found a broad range of adverse physical outcomes like respiratory dysfunctioning, chronic pain, epilepsy, sleep disruption, fatigue, severe muscle weakness, reduced self-care, and feeding disturbance [3–5]. Physical adverse outcomes may be due to the underlying illness (e.g., deafness after meningitis), due to PICU treatment (e.g., subglottic stenosis after endotracheal intubation, postthrombotic syndrome after a central venous catheter) or due to the combination of both (e.g., neurological problems after severe traumatic brain injury).

Unfortunately, lack of uniformity in patient population reported outcome assessment methods and different follow-up intervals after critical illness limits the generalizability of study conclusions, and impedes development of clinical recommendations to improve care.

Commonly used instruments that measure physical outcome (i.e., functional status, neurological functioning, and physical development) after critical illness are summarized in ◘ Table 62.1.

The main limitations of some of these measures are: (1) the lack of precision (e.g., broad category descriptions). For example, the PCPC includes just six categories of cerebral function (normal; mild, moderate, or severe disability; comatose; or dead). (2) The subjective scoring criteria and measurement methods. Some instruments are reported by healthcare providers, others by parents through interviews with healthcare providers or questionnaires. (3) Some important functional problems, including sleep disruption, fatigue, and severe muscle weakness, are not fully captured by the above measures.

◘ **Table 62.1** Physical, psychosocial, neurocognitive, and quality of life outcomes after PICU admission

	Assessment in	**By whom**	**Some examples with administer-time, age range, and translations**
Physical outcomes			
Anthropometrics	Child	Physician	0–18 years; 5 min
Clinical neurological evaluation	Child	Physician	PCPC, GOS-E peds, FSS
Health status, functional status	Child	Physician	FSS: 10 min; 0–18 years; EN
Readmissions	Child	Parent/ physician	
Motor development	Child	Physiotherapist	
Perception/ sensation	Child	Physician	
Psychosocial outcomes			
(Adaptive) behavior	Child	Self and/or parent	VABS: 15–20 min; 0–90 years; EN, SP ABAS: 15–20 min; 0–89 years; EN, SP, DU
Family burden	Parent	Parent	CarerQoL: 5 min; EN, DU, GE, SP, NO, SW, IT, PO OBVL: 10 min; 0–18; EN, SP, DU, FR, AR
Emotions (regulation)	Child Parent	Self and parent Parent	CBCL:15 min; 1.5–18 years; all languages Anxiety: STAI, 10 min; GAD-7, 5 min Depression: BDI, PHQ-9; 5 min

(continued)

Table 62.1 (continued)

	Assessment in	By whom	Some examples with administer-time, age range, and translations
Coping	Child Parent	Self and parent	CCSC: COPE inventory: 5 min, all lang.
Self-esteem	Child	Self and/or parent	CBSK 8–12/CBSA 12–18: 10/15 min RSES: 5 min; 13–90 years
Social functioning	Child	Self	PROMIS-peer: 5 min
Post-traumatic stress	Child Parent	Psychologist Self and parent Parent	CAPS-CA-5: 15 min; 7–18 CRTI: PCL-5: 10 min SRIP: 10 min
Neurocognitive outcomes			
General intelligence	Child	Psychologist	BSID-III: 30–90 min;1–42 m; all languages WPPSI/WISC/WAIS: 30–90 min; 2,5–90 years; all languages
Attention	Child	Psychologist	NEPSY:
Memory (visual/verbal)	Child	Psychologist	CMS: BADS: RCFT:
Visuo-motor integration	Child	Psychologist	Beery VMI:
Executive functioning	Child	Psychologist Parent	ANT: several tasks; 4–90 years; 5–60 min BRIEF: 15 min; DA, DU, EN, FI, FR, NO, DU, SW
Language development	Child	Psychologist	CELF-(preschool): 0–12 years; 20–60 min
Quality of life			
Physical functioning	Child and parent	Self and parent	Children: PedsQL, CHQ, ICHOM-POH, KINDL, KIDSCREEN, PROMIS Parents: SF-36, PROMIS
Emotional functioning	Child and parent	Self and parent	
Social functioning	Child and parent	Self and parent	

PROMIS-Peer PROMIS peer relationships, *CAPS-CA-5* PCL-5: PTSD checklist for DSM-5, *SRIP* self-rating inventory for PTSD, *CRTI* children's responses to trauma inventory, *HRQoL* health-related quality of life, *PedsQL* pediatric quality of life inventory, *OBVL* parenting stress questionnaire, *CCSC* children's coping strategies checklist, *EN* English, *SP* Spanish, *DU* Dutch, *GE* German, *FR* French, *AR* Arabic, *NO* Norwegian, *SW* Swedish, *IT* Italian, *PO* Portuguese, *DA* Danish, *FI* Finnish

62.4 Psychological Outcomes After Pediatric Critical Illness

62.4.1 The "New Normal"

Besides physical impairments, a recently new conceptual framework named Pediatric Post-intensive Care Syndrome-Pediatrics (PICS-p) describes impairments in other domains, such as cognitive, emotional, and social consequences of a PICU admission. In contrast with adult PICS, PICS in children should be seen in the context of growth and development in which parents and/or caregivers are the most important context factors (◘ Fig. 62.1) [6]. Recovery of the critically ill child and caregivers in daily life can best be described through the biopsychosocial model [7] (◘ Fig. 62.2). This model represents the physical, emotional (covering cognitive functioning), and social recoveries which run simultaneously, starting at PICU discharge and concluding in reaching a "new normal."

62.4.2 Quality of Life

This "new normal" for children and their caregivers represents the subjective evaluation of physical, emotional, and social functioning in daily life. This subjective evaluation is captured in an increasingly important outcome in pediatrics, the concept of QoL. Several studies have been done into QoL following pediatric critical illness. Not surprisingly, Aspesberro et al. concluded after their literature review that a significant proportion of children had lower physical and psychosocial QoL [8].

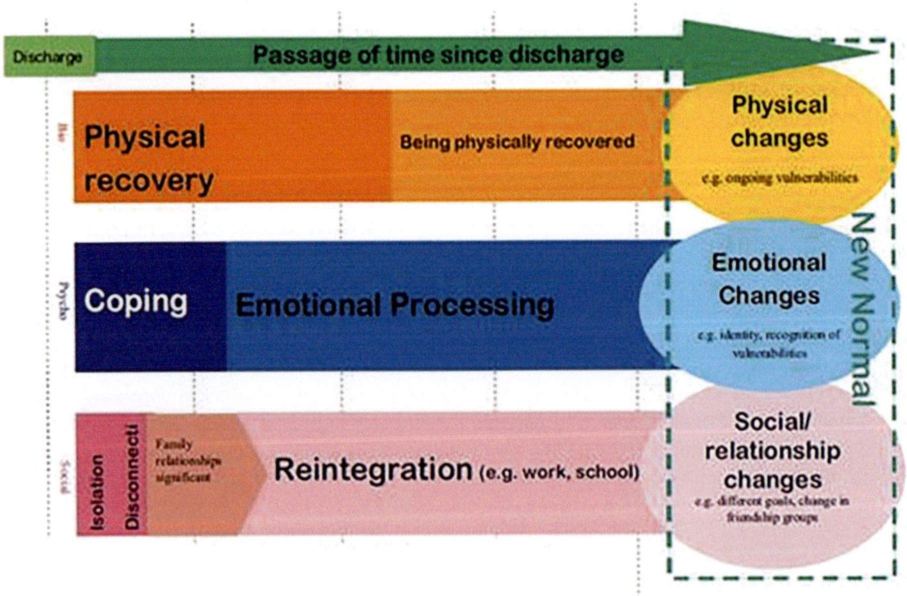

◘ **Fig. 62.2** The biopsychosocial model of recovery in children and families after PICU admission [7]

Several key determinants were related to lower QoL in children surviving a critical illness, including diagnosis at PICU admission, chronic comorbid conditions in which treatment was received, parental anxiety and depression, and social/environmental characteristics.

62.5 Post-traumatic Stress

After PICU discharge, children and parents may experience normal psychological responses such as post-traumatic stress (PTS) as a result of the stressful traumatic event, and treatment and procedures they experienced during the PICU admission. The emotional processing after PICU discharge results in a "new normal"for most of the parents and/or children. Sometimes PTS symptoms fail to decrease and interfere with the recovery to a "new normal." A considerable number of children have persistent PTS. These clinically significant PTS symptoms were reported in 10–28% of children, and rates of subclinical symptoms were even higher [9, 10]. For the children's well-being and future development, it is important to prevent PTS disorder (PTSD) both in children and parents to minimize the intense adverse effects [10]. To be able to develop appropriate interventions and follow-up care, it is important to early identify those children and parents at risk. Over half of parents/caregivers of critically ill children experience significant PTS symptoms 12 months after PICU discharge. These delayed experiences indicate a need for long-term monitoring and supporting families after PICU discharge [11].

In contrast, some parents and children might experience post-traumatic growth after a PICU admission. Post-traumatic growth refers to the positive changes in cognitive and emotional well-being after experiencing a traumatic period in life. It is a result of self-perception ("if I survived this, I can handle anything") and a change in life's priorities (a reevaluation of what is important in life).

62.6 Neurocognitive Outcome

The long-term neurocognitive outcome of critically ill children may theoretically be a result of both the preexisting factors of the child and the acute pediatric critical illness and its management [12]. Neurocognitive outcomes comprise internal mental processes underlying how people perceive stimuli, remember, speak, think, make decisions, and solve problems. The neurocognitive domains are general intellectual functioning, sensation, attention, memory, and executive functioning. Impairment in lower-order functions will affect the development in higher functions. For example, a child has to be able to focus on information (attention) to be able to store this information in their memory. Kachmar et al. (2018) found in a systematic review that younger age at critical illness, lower socioeconomic status, oxygen and mechanical ventilation requirements, and opioids were independently associated with cognitive impairments, whereas severity of illness and corticosteroids were not [13]. In a large 2-years follow-up study of the PEPaNIC trial, a heterogeneous group of critically ill children (0–17 years) admitted to the PICU had worse neurocognitive functioning compared with healthy-matched control children. Benzodiazepines and corticosteroids were independently associated with worse neurocognitive outcomes [14].

62.7 Predictors: What Affects Outcome After a PICU Admission?

As described in the previous paragraphs, there are several factors that determine how and when the child and family successfully adapt to the changes in physical, emotional, social, and cognitive functioning, resulting in a "new normal" for the child and its family. These factors are:

- *Preexisting factors* of the child and family: e.g., medical history, already existing comorbidities, psychological characteristics, socioeconomic status of the family, age of the child.
- *Management during and characteristics of the PICU admission*: e.g., severity of illness, reason for admission (acute, unexpected vs. elective), length of PICU stay, mechanical ventilation, medication usage, nutritional management, coping of parents, subjective evaluation of the traumatic event, PICU-acquired delirium.
- *Recovery phase after PICU discharge*: e.g., anxiety and stress levels of the child and parent, coping strategies, relationship status of parents, readmissions to the hospital, rehabilitation.

62.8 Challenges and Future Directions for Follow-Up

Follow-up assessments should take place in both short-term and long-term, even into adolescence and early adulthood. It is important to understand and monitor the impact of critical illness in childhood on long-term functioning, basic daily skills, and education as children may grow into deficits or develop PTSD.

Therefore, a follow-up in a joint venture of PICU physicians, subspecialists, primary care providers, physiotherapists, and psychologists ideally should be standard of care with standardized follow-up intervals and using well-validated instruments with internationally normative data.

There are some major challenges in developing a follow-up program.

First, the heterogeneity issue of pediatric critical illness: e.g., cause of PICU admission, previously healthy children versus children with severe comorbidities, broad age range (from 1 month to 17 years) with their different developmental stages.

Secondly, to further improve consistency in reporting outcomes after critical illness, there is a need for the development of a core outcome set (COS) [15]. A COS is a standardized minimal set of outcomes to be reported in all effectiveness trials in a specialty, designed to foster consistent reporting of outcomes. To enhance the relevance of outcome assessment for policy and practice, COS development should incorporate the views of all key stakeholders, including providers (e.g., pediatricians, psychologists, physiotherapists) and patients. A COS constitutes the minimum reporting elements but does not limit the reporting of other outcomes. Implementation of standardized assessment and outcome reporting reduces heterogeneity, and outcome reporting bias improves comparability across studies, and enables the pooling of data for meta-analyses. Important in developing a COS is to define a favorable outcome. It could well be that the meaning of quality of life varies among healthcare professionals, caregivers, and patients due to differences in cultural aspects, beliefs, and socioeconomic factors.

Thirdly, as described before, a PICU admission also impacts parents. Therefore, parental outcomes should also be of great interest in follow-up programs. Especially since outcomes such as executive functioning and quality of life in young children are often assessed by one of the parents. Hordijk et al. [2019 Quality of Life Research], found a positive association between parent's own mental QoL and the QoL outcomes they reported in their child. Due to this shared variance, the reported child outcomes might be colored by the subjective well-being of the parent. This indicates the importance of screening for emotional and psychological sequelae of PICU admission in both the child and their parents and focusing on family-centered interventions and care [16].

Finally, from a research point of view, a proper follow-up should be able to identify and prevent/intervene on potentially modifiable factors, already in the PICU, in order to improve short-term and long-term outcomes in critically ill children and their families. This implicates a tight collaboration between research and care. Long-term outcome requires major resources. From a research point of view, this is unfeasible.

Take-Home Messages

- Survivors after critical illness in childhood may experience impairments in different domains, not only short-term but also long-term after PICU discharge. These domains include physical, (neuro)psychological, social, and QoL. Also, family members (caregivers and siblings) can be affected, as a result of the critical illness of a child.

References

1. Needham DM, et al. Improving long-term outcomes after discharge from intensive care unit: report from a stakeholders' conference. Crit Care Med. 2012;40(2):502–9.
2. Manning JC, et al. Conceptualizing post intensive care syndrome in children—The PICS-p framework. Pediatr Crit Care Med. 2018;19(4):298–300.
3. van Zellem L, et al. Cardiac arrest in children: long-term health status and health-related quality of life. Pediatr Crit Care Med. 2015;16(8):693–702.
4. Buysse CM, et al. Long-term skin scarring and orthopaedic sequelae in survivors of meningococcal septic shock. Arch Dis Child. 2009;94(5):381–6.
5. Knoester H, et al. Cardiac function in pediatric septic shock survivors. Arch Pediatr Adolesc Med. 2008;162(12):1164–8.
6. Watson RS, et al. Life after critical illness in children—toward an understanding of pediatric post-intensive care syndrome. J Pediatr. 2018;198:16–24.
7. Atkins E, Colville G, John M. A 'biopsychosocial' model for recovery: a grounded theory study of families' journeys after a Paediatric Intensive Care Admission. Intensive Crit Care Nurs. 2012;28(3):133–40.
8. Aspesberro F, Mangione-Smith R, Zimmerman JJ. Health-related quality of life following pediatric critical illness. Intensive Care Med. 2015;41(7):1235–46.
9. Dow BL, et al. The utility of the Children's Revised Impact of Event Scale in screening for concurrent PTSD following admission to intensive care. J Trauma Stress. 2012;25(5):602–5.
10. Bronner MB, et al. Posttraumatic stress disorder (PTSD) in children after paediatric intensive care treatment compared to children who survived a major fire disaster. Child Adolesc Psychiatry Ment Health. 2008;2(1):9.
11. Colville G, Pierce C. Patterns of post-traumatic stress symptoms in families after paediatric intensive care. Intensive Care Med. 2012;38(9):1523–31.

12. Verstraete S, Van den Berghe G, Vanhorebeek I. What's new in the long-term neurodevelopmental outcome of critically ill children. Intensive Care Med. 2018;44(5):649–51.
13. Kachmar AG, et al. A systematic review of risk factors associated with cognitive impairment after pediatric critical illness*. Pediatr Crit Care Med. 2018;19:e164–71.
14. Verstraete S, et al. Long-term developmental effects of withholding parenteral nutrition for 1 week in the paediatric intensive care unit: a 2-year follow-up of the PEPaNIC international, randomised, controlled trial. Lancet Respir Med. 2019;7(2):141–53.
15. Fink EL, et al. Development of a core outcome set for pediatric critical care outcomes research. Contemp Clin Trials. 2020;91:105968.
16. Williams CN, et al. Postintensive care syndrome in pediatric critical care survivors: therapeutic options to improve outcomes after acquired brain injury. Curr Treat Options Neurol. 2019;21(10):49.

Research Needed in the ICU

Content

What Do We Need to Find Out?

Lyvonne N. Tume

Contents

J. Brierley et al. (eds.), *ESPNIC Children's Intensive Care Textbook*,
https://doi.org/10.1007/978-3-031-64762-8_63

Learning Objectives

At the end of this chapter, the reader will be able to:

- Consider important topics in pediatric critical care for which little or no evidence exists and what we need to know.
- Examine the issues using a clinical case study.
- Discuss why and how we need to do research in pediatric critical care and why existing evidence is not implemented into practice.

63.1 Introduction

Pediatric Critical Care (PCC) is a dynamic, constantly evolving, and complex specialty with a heterogenous patient population, ranging from neonates to 17 years of age or sometimes older. In addition to this, the causes of PCC admission are hugely varied, making this an interesting environment with many important topics, therapies, interventions, treatments, and diseases that we need to understand or understand better. Research is vital to achieving this aim. Historically, paternalistic views around children and their participation in research (or lack of) and strict regulation resulted in little research in this population [1]. This led to a situation where even now, most drugs administered to children in the CCU are prescribed off-label with little pediatric data to support their dosage, safety, and efficacy [2–4]. This is the same for many therapies, leaving PCC is a worse situation than adult critical care.

This has changed though, with the EU law and regulation changes around medicines in 2008 [1], now within Europe and the UK, there are many ongoing clinical studies and trials in critically ill children. These are vital to provide us with evidence of both the safety and effectiveness of the therapies we deliver, but there is still much we need to find out. Recently, what we do know is that hospitals that participate in trials (and are research active) have better patient outcomes, and lower risk-adjusted mortality for acute admissions [5], although exactly why this is, remains unclear. Despite the barriers to conducting clinical trials in PCC, of which lack of time and funding are the two major factors worldwide [6], we must, as a specialty, promote and drive research forward to improve patient, family, and service outcomes.

63.2 So, What Do We Need to Find Out?

Case Study

Consider the common patient case below

A 2-year-old girl (10 kg) is admitted to the PICU after open heart surgery (revision of a right ventricle to pulmonary artery conduit operation). She returns with an arterial and central venous line, both being transduced and receiving continuous flush solutions of heparinized saline at 1 mL/h. She is fluid restricted to 1 mL/kg h (10 mLs h). Prophylactic heparin is running at 10 units/kg/h as per surgical orders. The nurse considers starting enteral feeds after 12 h, but the gastric residual volume is 40 mLs, so she does not. The unit policy is 5 mLs/kg as a threshold for stopping feeds. She is on a fentanyl infusion, a midazolam infusion, and has paravertebral blocks in for pain control. Throughout the whole time, she is ventilated, and her SpO_2 is 100% with her FiO_2 set at 35%. She recovers well and is extubated after 8 h by the physician; the next morning, she is crying and irritable, saying she is thirsty, but with her infusions and drugs, she is allowed virtually no milk/feeds. The parents are by her bedside, but they are asked to leave for the medical ward round.

63.2.1 Consider Now: How Much of the Therapies, Practices, and Policies Above Do We Have Clear Evidence For?

63.2.1.1 Why We Need to Question the Evidence for Our Routine and Historical Practices

Some of the therapies from the case above will now be discussed and challenged. The use of heparinized saline (as opposed to saline solution alone) to maintain arterial line patency in critically ill children remains controversial and variable in practice across PICUs. There are two systematic reviews in adult critical care [7, 8]. Both reviews found insufficient evidence to support the use of heparinized saline to prevent line occlusion in both central or arterial lines in adults. However, children are not just small adults, the diameter of the lines is smaller, and flow rates may be different, so currently we do not know the answer to this. In addition, like this case, many children after heart surgery receive prophylactic heparin infusion for cardiac surgical purposes (no evidence but surgical concerns), thus potentially making this flush solution even more unnecessary.

Extreme fluid restriction (50% of the child's usual maintenance solution or 1 mL/kg/h) after pediatric heart surgery has been used since the beginning of this era [9]. The logical intention of this practice is to avoid fluid overload and worsening heart failure in children with poorly functioning hearts. However, pediatric cardiac surgery, anesthesia, and intensive care management and therapies have dramatically improved over the last 30 years, now including ultrafiltration at the end of cardiopulmonary bypass (CPB) for small children, improved ability to assess cardiac function and tailor inotropic support, improved diuretic therapy, and more effective peritoneal dialysis. Despite these improvements, this extreme "total" fluid restriction still exists in many units, often including enteral fluids/feeds, so that with continuous drug infusions, flush solutions, and bolus drug volumes, there is virtually no "space" allowed for enteral nutrition. This is a problem, as inadequate nutrition is associated with worse outcomes after cardiac surgery [10]. Some units may practice a more "relaxed" approach to enteral feeds, but many still retain this rigid total fluid allowance. Currently do we not know if allowing a more liberal approach to enteral feeds after cardiac surgery improves nutritional and other outcomes without worsening heart failure.

The routine measurement of gastric residual volume (GRV) or the gastric aspirate is another common practice worldwide, with many clinicians worried that a full stomach will lead to vomiting and subsequent pulmonary aspiration [11]. In the UK, all but one of the PICUs measured GRV regularly to guide feeding [12] and used variable thresholds to define how high a GRV was. No evidence exists to support this practice, it is inaccurate (the amount obtained) and does not reflect or predict delayed gastric emptying [13]. Only one small retrospective comparison study [14] showed no difference in outcomes (VAP) but could not demonstrate better energy intake by not measuring. Currently, we do not know whether NOT routinely measuring GRV would improve the energy target achievement in critically ill children. This is currently being investigated in a UK-wide trial and is important to know [15].

The optimal choice of opiate or sedative drug remains an ongoing question for pediatric critical care. Many question the use of benzodiazepines as contributing to iatrogenic withdrawal and delirium, but the ideal drug remains elusive [16]. Other methods to control pain such as the use of paravertebral blocks have also been used, but no evidence exists regarding their effectiveness in reducing opiate doses in children after heart surgery, allowing earlier extubation, and improving patient comfort.

Recent adult research suggests the potential for harm from high levels of arterial oxygenation [16–18] with a recent multicenter UK trial in children [19] showing better outcomes for children with lower saturations (88–92%). Although hypoxia is usually aggressively treated, yet high levels of arterial oxygenation are frequently not acted upon and considered inconsequential.

The composition and education of the pediatric critical care healthcare team are changing, and in many units, advanced nurse practitioners form an important part of the team. Indeed, there is evidence to suggest that protocol-driven (usually delivered by a nurse) weaning of mechanical ventilation, is effective and as safe as that led by a physician. A Cochrane systematic review [20] found a suggestion that protocols shortened the duration of ventilation, but the evidence was inadequate to draw conclusions, and a recent multicenter RCT in the UK found effectively using a team-based approach (involving physicians, nurses, and respiratory physiotherapists) to the weaning of both sedatives and ventilation reduced the duration of ventilation [21].

Finally, asking parents to leave for the medical ward round remains a common practice in PICUs, but this is cultural and country dependent. Healthcare professionals' (HCP) paternalistic arguments for this, are commonly to protect the confidentiality of the other children (in open ICUs) or to avoid upsetting the parents by their misunderstanding of medical terminology [22, 23]. Parents however report they really do not care that other parents hear, as they are all going through the same thing. A prospective study of family-centered ward rounds [23] showed that overall positive feedback from parents and HCPs albeit with some concerns. Despite this, asking parents to leave during rounds persists in many PICUs across the world.

In this situation, and others above, the question remains why are we not using research evidence in our practice, or rather, are we just selecting out the evidence we believe in, to implement? This selective use of research evidence may be even more biased than not using the evidence.

In conclusion, there are many practices and therapies examined in this chapter that we need to find out in pediatric critical care. It is also important to understand and consider what our users, the children, and the parents, think that we need to know to help them. These problems must be examined through a multidisciplinary lens, with studies led by a multidisciplinary (multiprofessional) healthcare team. Finally, and most importantly, we need to ensure we, as clinical staff, know and use the research evidence that exists, effectively implementing this into clinical practice within our units. This is poorly done, with the known lag of implementing research findings into practice of about 10 years [24].

Take-Home Messages

- Hospitals that participate in research studies (are research-active) have better patient outcomes.
- There is still much we need to find out in pediatric critical care.
- This research requires collaboration between disciplines and across multiple centers.
- We need to ensure that robust evidence that does exist is effectively implemented into clinical practice
- Good ethical and research practice is essential to ensure that research carried out in PCC is ethical, clinically relevant, and robust

References

1. Modi N, Vohra J, Preston J, Elliott C, Van't Hoff W, Coad J, et al. Guidance on clinical research involving infants, children and young people: an update for researchers and research ethics committees. Arch Dis Child. 2014;99(10):887–91.
2. Czaja AS, Reiter PD, Schultz ML, Valuck RJ. Patterns of off-label prescribing in the pediatric intensive care unit and prioritizing future research. J Pediatr Pharmacol Ther. 2015;20(3):186.
3. Bavdekar SB, Sadawarte PA, Gogtay NJ, Jain SS, Jadhav S. Off-label drug use in a pediatric intensive care unit. Indian J Pediatr. 2009;76(11):1113–8.
4. de Lima Costa HTM, Costa TX, Martins RR, Oliveira AG. Use of off-label and unlicensed medicines in neonatal intensive care. PLoS One. 2018;13(9):e0204427.
5. Ozdemir BA, Karthikesalingam A, Sinha S, Poloniecki JD, Hinchliffe RJ, Thompson MM, et al. Research activity and the association with mortality. PLoS One. 2015;10(2):e0118253.
6. Duffett M, Choong K, Foster J, Meade M, Menon K, Parker M, Cook DJ, Canadian Critical Care Trials Group. High-quality randomized controlled trials in pediatric critical care: a survey of barriers and facilitators. Pediatr Crit Care Med. 2017;18(5):405–13. https://doi.org/10.1097/PCC.0000000000001144.
7. Zhong L, Wang H-L, Xu B, Yuan Y, Wang X, Zhang Y, et al. Normal saline versus heparin for patency of central venous catheters in adult patients—a systematic review and meta-analysis. Crit Care. 2017;21(1):5.
8. Lee J, Della P. Saline and heparinised flush in maintaining patency of arterial catheters in adult patients—A systematic review. J Health Sci. 2014;2:571–83.
9. Dominiguez T, O'Connor G. Feast and famine: nutrition and fluid restriction after infant cardiac surgery. Pediatr Crit Care Med. 2018;19:168.
10. Larsen B, Goonewardene L, Field K, Joffe A, van Aerde J, Olstad D, Clandinin M. Low energy intakes are associated with adverse outcomes in infants after open heart surgery. JPEN J Parenter Enteral Nutr. 2013;37:254.
11. Tume LN, Latten L, Kenworthy L. Paediatric intensive care nurses' decision-making around gastric residual volume measurement. Nurs Crit Care. 2017;22(5):293–7. https://doi.org/10.1111/nicc.12304.
12. Martinez E, Pereira L, Gura K, Stenquist N, Arigno K, Nurko S, Mehta N. Gastric emptying in critically ill children. JPEN J Parenter Enteral Nutr. 2017;41:1100.
13. Tume LN, Arch B, Woolfall K, Latten L, Deja E, Roper L, Pathan N, Eccleson H, Hickey H, Brown M, Beissel A, Andrzejewska I, Gale C, Valla FV, Dorling J. Gastric residual volume measurement in UK paediatric intensive care units: a survey of practice. Pediatr Crit Care Med. 2019;20(8):707–13.
14. Tume LN, Bickerstaff A, Latten L, Davies S, Lefèvre M, Nicolas G, Valla FV. Routine gastric residual volume measurement and energy target achievement in the PICU: a comparison study. Eur J Pediatr. 2017;176(12):1637–44. https://doi.org/10.1007/s00431-017-3015-8.
15. The GASTRIC-PICU trial. https://fundingawards.nihr.ac.uk/award/NIHR133835.

16. Neubert A, Baarslag M, van Dijk M, van Rosmalen J, Standing J, Sheng Y, et al. The CLOSED trial; CLOnidine compared with midazolam for SEDation of paediatric patients in the intensive care unit: study protocol for a multicentre randomised controlled trial. BMJ Open. 2017;7:e016031.
17. de Jonge E, Peelen L, Keijzers PJ, et al. Association between administered oxygen, arterial partial oxygen pressure and mortality in mechanically ventilated intensive care unit patients. Crit Care. 2008;12:R156. https://doi.org/10.1186/cc715.
18. Elmer J, Scutella M, Pullalarevu R, et al. The association between hyperoxia and patient outcomes after cardiac arrest: analysis of a high-resolution database. Intensive Care Med. 2015;41:49–57. https://doi.org/10.1007/s00134-014-3555-6.
19. Peters M, Gould D, Ray S, et al. Conservative versus liberal oxygenation targets in critically ill children (Oxy-PICU): a UK multicentre, open, parallel-group, randomised clinical trial. Lancet. 2024;403:355–64.
20. Blackwood B, Murray M, Chisakuta A, Cardwell CR, O'Halloran P. Protocolized versus non-protocolized weaning for reducing the duration of invasive mechanical ventilation in critically ill paediatric patients. Cochrane Database Syst Rev. 2013;(7):CD009082. https://doi.org/10.1002/14651858.CD009082.pub2.
21. Blackwood B, Tume L, Morris K. et al.; SANDWICH Investigators. Sedation and ventilator weaning in children: a stepped-wedge cluster trial. JAMA. 2021;326(5):401–410. https://doi.org/10.1001/jama.2021.10296.
22. Tume LN, Latour JM. Invited editorial: family centered rounds in PICU: reality or rhetoric? Pediatr Crit Care Med. 2015;16:875. https://doi.org/10.1097/PCC.0000000000000486.
23. Levin AB, Fisher KR, Cato KD, et al. An evaluation of family-centered rounds in the PICU: room for improvement suggested by families and providers. Pediatr Crit Care Med. 2015;16:801–7.
24. Kristensen N, Nymann C, Konradsen H. Implementing research results in clinical practice—the experiences of healthcare professionals. BMC Health Serv Res. 2016;16:48.

Education

Contents

Online Education

Dennis Daniel and Traci A. Wolbrink

Contents

J. Brierley et al. (eds.), *ESPNIC Children's Intensive Care Textbook*,
https://doi.org/10.1007/978-3-031-64762-8_64

Learning Objectives

- Describe available tools and resources for online medical education
- Develop strategies for implementing online learning experiences targeted at pediatric intensive care clinicians
- Understand the evidence base related to medical educational outcomes associated with different online learning approaches

64.1 Introduction

The explosive growth of the Internet and of the overall volume of medical knowledge have led to fundamental changes in how we learn and teach medicine. Although traditional learning experiences remain prevalent in the ICU [1], including in-person lectures, self-study using texts and manuscripts, and apprenticeship with clinical experts, online (or Web-based or Internet-based) learning is now a standard element in education at all levels and in all professions. The widespread availability of powerful computers and high-speed Internet connectivity has created new opportunities for medical education that did not exist 30 years ago, and even the classic educational approaches mentioned above look and feel different in the Internet era.

Advantages of online learning include [2, 3]:

- A variety of available delivery methods, ranging from static text-based materials to multimedia videos, podcasts, and novel interactive learning experiences
- Easy access to an enormous range of educational materials, many of which are open-access and free to use
- Potential for learners to decide when and where they participate in education
- Options for both synchronous and asynchronous learning
- Greater variety of ways for educators and learners to communicate
- Ability to deliver standardized educational interventions at a large scale, with distribution not limited by physical proximity
- Opportunities to deliver personalized learning experiences

The pediatric intensive care unit is a complex and clinically demanding setting, where learners must maintain a broad, updated fund of knowledge. Frequently, patient care needs also require front-line clinicians to seek answers in a time-sensitive fashion. Online approaches to education and information sharing can offer powerful ways to meet these challenges, but successful utilization of such solutions requires careful consideration of the needs of learners and the unique clinical contexts in which they work.

In this chapter, we will provide pediatric intensive care clinicians with an overview of types of online learning tools, a look into the evidence supporting the use of online approaches to medical education, and some practical suggestions for how to apply the potential benefits of online learning tools to their own clinical and educational circumstances.

64.2 What Qualifies as "Online Education"?

Online education can refer to anything that is delivered via the Internet and that inspires medical learning. Practically speaking, online learning materials and experiences tend to fall into the following categories (◘ Fig. 64.1):

- Individual pieces of content, including text (articles, blog posts, or manuscripts); images, infographics and animations; videos; and podcasts (audio recordings of speakers and interviews)
- Curricula or courses which bring together multiple pieces of content to provide a cohesive overview of a particular domain or topic, and which may also include assessment questions
- Complex, interactive educational experiences, such as screen-based simulations or other "serious games"
- Internet-based collaborative learning and information exchange, which can take place on social media platforms, online discussion boards, or via videoconferencing

Each of the above types of content is provided by a diversity of sources on the Internet in both open-access and restricted forms. In ◘ Table 64.1, we have listed some of the top websites containing high-quality online resources pertinent to pediatric intensive care [7].

Online education can involve either synchronous or asynchronous interactions. Synchronous learning involves real-time interactions among learners and teachers, for example, through videoconferencing or chatrooms. Examples of asynchronous online learning experiences include learners browsing websites or blogs, accessing courses or other pre-developed material when it best suits them, and communicating through media such as email or discussion boards. Hybrid approaches combining both synchronous and asynchronous experiences are also common. In terms of synchronized information sharing via videoconferencing, there are numerous free solutions for videoconferencing on both computers and mobile devices, some of which are proprietary to specific devices (such as Apple FaceTime), and others which are available on multiple platforms (such as Zoom, Skype, and Google Hangouts). Each of these options has different limitations in a number of simultaneous participants, usability on lower-speed Internet connections, and degree of functionality that is provided for free versus requiring payment. Some of these platforms allow videoconferences to be recorded, and these recordings can in turn be shared so that others who are unable to attend at the prescribed time can still benefit.

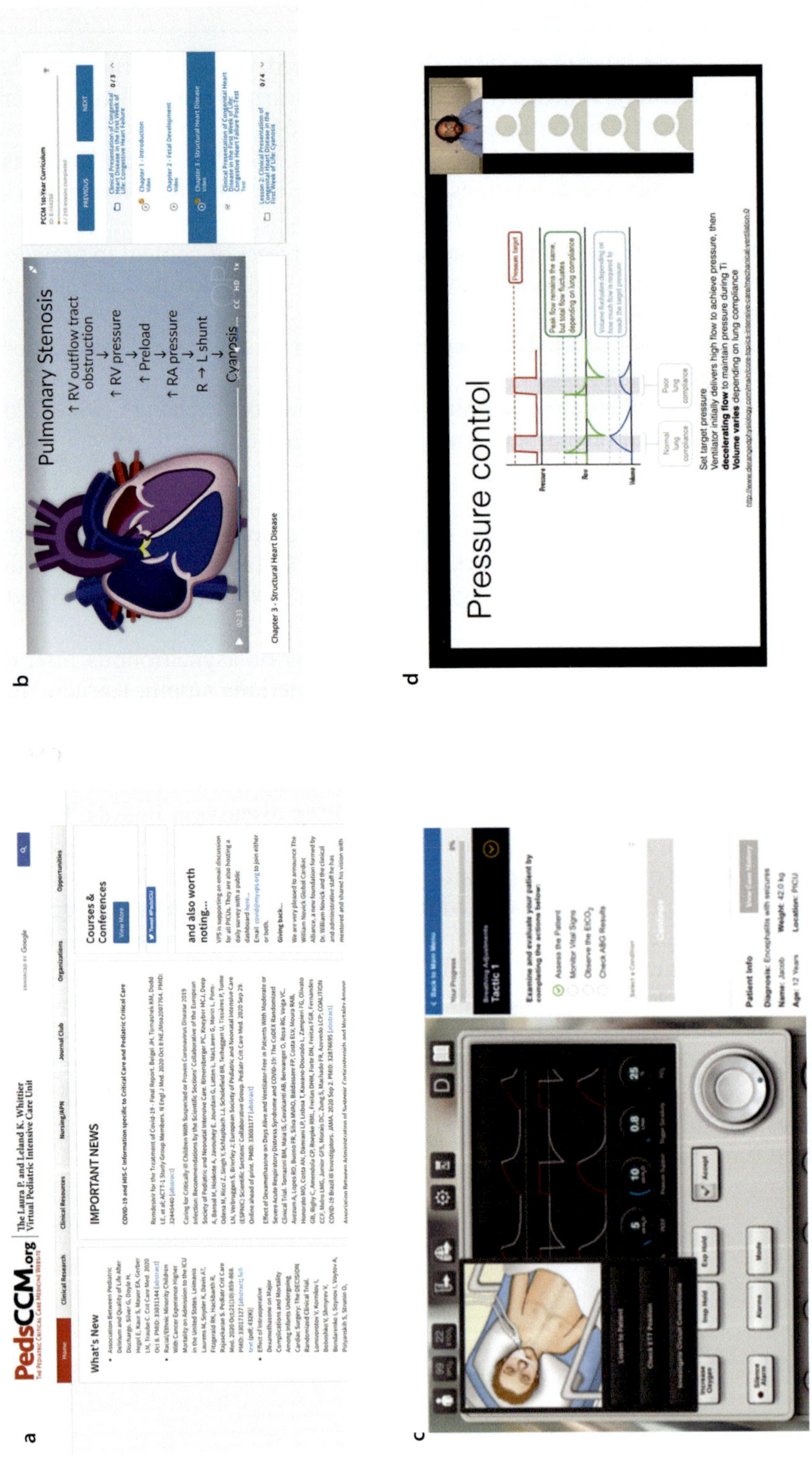

■ **Fig. 64.1** Examples of online learning experiences: **(a)** Individual content (here, text-based) [4]; **(b)** A course bringing together multiple pieces of content in a curated experience [5]; **(c)** A screen-based interactive simulator [6]; and **(d)** Internet-based collaborative learning (here, taking place via videoconferencing)

Table 64.1 List of frequently used online resources for education in pediatric intensive care [7]

Name	Website	Description
American Thoracic Society Critical Care	► https://www.thoracic.org/professionals/clinical-resources/critical-care	Clinical cases, online journal club, podcasts, text-based information, and links to external resources. Website of the American Thoracic Society
Critical Care Project	► http://ccproject.com	Videos, text-based information, and clinical cases with questions. Associated with the University of Maryland, Tulane University, the University of Pennsylvania, and the National Institutes of Health
Intensive Blog	► http://intensiveblog.com	FOAM website with clinical cases, online journal club, and text-based information with videos, graphics, and self-assessment questions. Associated with The Alfred Hospital in Australia
LearnPICU	► http://www.learnpicu.com/home	Text-based information with associated literature summaries and self-assessment questions. Associated with Stanford University
Medscape Critical Care	► https://emedicine.medscape.com/critical_care	Text-based summaries of topics with graphics and videos, interactive CME activities, and updates on news and research in the field
Merck Manual Critical Care Medicine	► http://www.merckmanuals.com/professional/critical-care-medicine	Text-based information with figures, videos, and quizzes
OPENPediatrics	► https://www.openpediatrics.org	Videos, self-paced courses, interactive simulators, congenital heart lesion library, medical calculators, and medical animation and illustration gallery. Associated with Boston Children's Hospital
► PedsCCM.org	► http://pedsccm.org	Online journal club, updates on news and research, and links to external resources
► SurgicalCriticalCare.net	► http://www.surgicalcriticalcare.net	Collection of text-based PDFs, videos, and medical calculators for surgical critical care. Associated with Orlando Regional Medical Center
WikEM	► https://wikem.org/wiki/Category:Critical_Care	Text-based information and reference tables for emergency medicine, with a specific category for critical care

64.3 Implementing Online Education: A Pragmatic Approach

When it comes to meeting the needs of learners, online education is no different from traditional in-person education in the importance of applying a systematic approach to development and implementation. Kern's six-step approach for curriculum development in medical education [8–10] is a popular and generalizable set of best practices that can be applied in all types of educational design. Briefly, Kern's six-step approach involves an orderly approach to curriculum development, starting with problem identification and then progressing through needs assessment, description of goals and objectives, selection of educational strategies, implementation, and finally performing evaluation and gathering feedback.

Similarly, many different conceptual frameworks are potentially relevant in guiding the design of online learning, depending on the context of the learning experience and the goals of the educational intervention. Some examples include Knowles' self-directed learning theory [11, 12], Sweller's cognitive load theory [13], and Kolb's experiential learning cycle [14, 15]. The Technology, Pedagogy, and Content Knowledge (TPCK) framework [16] provides a useful lens for designing and delivering online learning in particular. This framework highlights that the successful development of online learning experiences requires educators to understand the various technologies that can be used for learning, as well as a grasp of educational pedagogy and expertise in the subject matter, in order to successfully develop appropriate, context-specific strategies and experiences.

In this section, we will use Kern's six-step framework as an outline to frame some considerations when deciding to implement online medical education [17].

64.3.1 Problem Identification

As with any educational endeavor, first, it is important to explicitly delineate what problem you hope to address via an online approach. What is the clinical or informational need you are targeting? What do you expect the outcome to be if you successfully address the problem?

64.3.2 Needs Assessment

Once you know what you are targeting, you can systematically evaluate the current situation. The process of needs assessment is essential to make sure the effort you apply in your educational intervention is efficient and worthwhile. Educational needs assessments can be carried out through a variety of mechanisms, including informal discussions, formal interviews or focus groups, surveys, observations in work or learning settings, structured assessments, or tests. Who are the learners you are interested in targeting, and what is their work or learning context? What are their expectations around learning for this given topic or area? What prior experience or preferences do your learners bring? Who are the other stakeholders who should contribute input into understanding the learning needs for this issue? What, if any, solutions currently exist for your problem? What would an ideal solution look like, and what is the gap between the current state and the ideal? What are the potential barriers to enacting your intended solution [18]? How can learners be engaged in creating or delivering your solution?

Also consider whether there are any potential technical supports already in place that can make distribution, user tracking, and evaluation much easier. For example, in some cases, your institution may have a learning management system such as Blackboard or Canvas available, as well as support staff to help with use and administration.

64.3.3 Describing Goals and Objectives

With a clear vision of both the problem you mean to address, as well as a thorough consideration of the stakeholders and their needs and circumstances, you can now develop a concrete plan for intervention. Before you can select content, delivery mechanisms, assessment methods, and approaches to dissemination, it is essential to clearly state the goals and objectives of your intervention. Well-crafted goals and objectives are also of great value to learners, so that they can ensure that a given piece of educational content is relevant for them. Goals are broad and speak to the overall intent of the intervention, whereas objectives should be specific and measurable [8]. When crafting objectives, consider the target audience, the outcome of interest, and the actions your audience members would undertake to achieve the outcome.

64.3.4 Selecting Educational Strategies

When considering the use of online education, one must first establish how and why online approaches are potentially superior to conventional or in-person approaches. As discussed in the Evidence section below, research to date has not demonstrated any inherent superiority of online education when compared to other learning strategies. The most effective use of online education leverages its inherent advantages—such as flexibility, ease of access, and scalability with generally low added cost. Optimal solutions to teaching or learning may consist of blended approaches that integrate both in-person experiences and Web-based self-directed learning. For example, the "flipped classroom" concept [1, 9, 19] promotes learners using self-directed study time to grasp foundational concepts, allowing for in-person time to be spent on higher level content and on more interactive learning experiences. This concept has potential for the intensive care setting but requires striking the right balance between the volume of self-directed learning assigned to or expected of already busy clinicians, versus the limited available time for in-person learning. Overloading the online learning side of the equation with excessive content can lead to learner disengagement.

Remember also that online education will necessarily require learners to interact with educational materials via some sort of Internet-enabled device. Most modern mobile phones are powerful computers in themselves, and most Internet resources are flexible enough to function on a diversity of devices and platforms, but specific resources or tools may not be optimized for the smaller screens and more limited interfaces of mobile devices, and may offer more limited mobile functionality.

(Occasionally, online sites or applications are actually optimized for the mobile environment and limit desktop computer functionality.) Additionally, although cellular data networks are increasingly prevalent, bandwidth (the amount of data that can be sent in a given unit of time) may be limited, which can render some tools or content platforms (especially those heavy on video) more difficult to use.

64.3.5 Implementation of the Intervention

With online education, implementation can range from sharing links via email, posting content to third-party sites such as YouTube, or setting up a dedicated website or other interactive experience for learners. The resources necessary for these different methods will vary, and pre-existing institutional support may or may not be present. Note that more complex methods of distribution, particularly those reliant on proprietary or restricted-access platforms, will increase the complexity for learners looking to access your materials. Open-access platforms and content distribution websites can make it easier for learners to get to content, but may be more limited in their ability to track and support individual users. Whatever distribution methods you choose to employ, it is essential to ensure that both learners and the educators are appropriately trained and supported, as lack of technical familiarity is a common barrier to implementation of online education.

When including any material that you have not created yourself, if that material has not been pre-specified as available for others to use, or you have not obtained permission from the copyright holder, you should ensure that you meet the standard of "fair use" [20]. Fair use refers to the reasonable and limited use of copyrighted materials without first contacting the copyright owner. This doctrine is intended to balance the rights of copyright holders with the public benefits of a wider distribution of creative works. Note that there is not a strict list of criteria for determining what falls under fair use, but generally, four questions are considered.

First, what is the purpose of the use? Nonprofit or educational applications are more likely to be seen as fair use. Second, what is the nature of the work that uses the copyrighted materials? Is the use transformative, or are the copyrighted materials being repurposed for a new audience? Modification, excerption, or application of materials to a different setting than the original will be viewed more favorably. Third, how much of the copyrighted material are you using? Generally, the less material used, the better the chances of qualifying as fair use. Finally, will your use of copyrighted materials cause a loss of money to the owner? If so, this is less likely to be seen as fair use.

64.3.6 Evaluation and Feedback

Evaluation encompasses both assessing whether individuals have met learning goals and objectives, as well as whether the intervention itself is functioning as intended. The former is necessary for providing learners with feedback to drive continued improvement, and the latter is essential for improving the educational experience itself. Such information will also often be necessary to support the continued investment of time and resources needed to maintain and update any meaningful educational effort.

64.4 Evidence for Online Medical Education

There is a large and growing evidence base focused on evaluating the impact of online educational strategies on medical learning outcomes. Multiple meta-analyses have also been conducted. Previous investigations into the efficacy of Internet-based medical education have focused on the following types of comparison, frequently targeting outcomes of learner satisfaction and knowledge gain [21]:

- Online learning interventions versus no intervention
- Online learning versus traditional or non-computer based learning
- Comparison of different online learning approaches

A widely cited meta-analysis of Internet-based learning in the health professions [2] found support for the notion that online educational approaches can have significant positive effects on learners' knowledge, skills, and behaviors, when compared to no educational intervention. However, the same meta-analysis found that the evidence did not support online approaches as consistently superior to conventional educational strategies. Subsequent meta-analyses and other investigations have also not established online approaches as inherently preferable to traditional ones in terms of influencing learning outcomes relating to knowledge, skills, and behaviors [22, 23]. It is important to note the significant heterogeneity among studies in the online medical education evidence base in terms of educational goals, target audiences, structure of online interventions, comparison groups, study methodologies, and outcome measures. Ultimately, we should consider online educational materials and approaches to be tools that may or may not be helpful to achieve our educational and clinical goals, as opposed to pursuing online education as a desirable end in and of itself. This reinforces the importance of a systematic approach to identifying educational goals, determining whether intervention is required, and then developing an appropriate educational strategy.

Take Home Messages

- It is easier than ever to integrate online education into the pediatric critical care context
- Types of online learning materials and experiences can include text documents, images and animations, audio recordings, or videos; complex interactive learning experiences; structured curricula with integrated assessments; and tools for both synchronous and asynchronous communication such as discussion boards and videoconferencing platforms
- As with traditional educational interventions, proper planning and evaluation are necessary for the successful implementation of online learning

64.5 Educational Features (Table 64.2)

Table 64.2 Case examples of applying online learning strategies in the education of pediatric intensive care clinicians

Case 1: Providing an online curriculum for rotating trainees	You are the rotation director for pediatric trainees completing a monthly rotation through your hospital's PICU. Trainees come into the PICU with varying levels of pediatric intensive care knowledge, and while they are in the PICU, the patients and acuity to which they are exposed vary significantly. Thus far, you have mainly provided education through a series of didactics and simulation experiences, but both faculty and trainee availability for in-person teaching is variable, and you want to ensure that the trainees receive consistent exposure to important critical care topics	1. What types of online materials may be most feasible for trainees on a busy clinical rotation to complete? 2. How much material, and what kinds of material, should be delivered through an online curriculum versus in-person? 3. How will you assess the impact of your educational interventions?
Case 2: Supporting communities of practice	In your busy pediatric intensive care division, physicians, nurses, and other clinicians consistently express a desire for more opportunities to share knowledge and to stay abreast of the latest evidence and best practices. The division holds a once-monthly morbidity and mortality conference, as well as a weekly case review conference, both of which are well attended and valued by clinicians. Nonetheless, there is a perception that not all clinicians are promptly made aware of either local institutional changes to practice, or of new knowledge that may lead to changes in care	1. How can Internet-based resources help clinicians stay aware of changes to practice? 2. Who in the institution should be responsible for maintaining and updating online educational resources relating to practice guidelines and policies? 3. What kinds of feedback mechanisms would be helpful for ensuring that newly introduced online resources are meeting the needs of clinicians?

(continued)

Table 64.2 (continued)

Case 3: Promoting collaboration and information-sharing among colleagues remote from each other	You are a member of a pediatric department that includes staff across multiple medical centers and clinics distributed across a wide geographic region. Clinicians are most often only able to meet in-person together in local or regional groupings, and approximately four times per year the entire department is able to convene in the affiliated major academic medical center. You and your colleagues are considering the use of free videoconferencing software to promote more regular engagement with each other	1. What kinds of collaborative experiences can be best facilitated by videoconferencing? What about discussion boards? 2. Should third-party social media platforms be utilized for conversations and collaboration with potential clinical content? 3. What kinds of institutional support would be most useful for ensuring the success of this initiative?

References

1. Tainter CR, Wong NL, Cudemus-Deseda GA, Bittner EA. The “flipped classroom” model for teaching in the intensive care unit: rationale, practical considerations, and an example of successful implementation. J Intensive Care Med. 2017;32(3):187–96.
2. Cook DA, Levinson AJ, Garside S, Dupras DM, Erwin PJ, Montori VM. Internet-based learning in the health professions: a meta-analysis. JAMA. 2008;300(10):1181–96.
3. Cook DA, Levinson AJ, Garside S, Dupras DM, Erwin PJ, Montori VM. Instructional design variations in internet-based learning for health professions education: a systematic review and meta-analysis. Acad Med. 2010;85(5):909–22.
4. Markovitz B, editor. PedsCCM.org. http://www.pedsccm.org. Accessed 13 Oct 2020.
5. Delsignore L, Daniel D, van der Velden M, Wolbrink T (course directors). PCCM 1st-year curriculum. OPENPediatrics https://learn.openpediatrics.org/learn/course/3717/pccm-1st-year-curriculum. Accessed 13 Oct 2020.
6. Wolbrink TA, Lehmann S, Brecher R, Daniel D, Marques B, Perez J, Tegtmeyer K, Craig N, Olszewski A, Smallwood, C. Ventilator simulator: HTML5 release. 04/2020. Online simulator. OPENPediatrics. https://learn.openpediatrics.org/learn/course/2965/ventilator-simulator. Accessed 13 Oct 2020.
7. Wolbrink TA, Rubin L, Burns JP, Markovitz B. The top ten websites in critical care medicine education today. J Intensive Care Med. 2019;34(1):3–16.
8. Thomas PA, Kern DE, Hughes MT, Chen BY, editors. Curriculum development for medical education: a six-step approach. JHU Press; 2016.
9. Chen BY, Kern DE, Kearns RM, Thomas PA, Hughes MT, Tackett S. From modules to MOOCs: application of the six-step approach to online curriculum development for medical education. Acad Med. 2019;94(5):678–85.
10. Zackoff MW, Real FJ, Abramson EL, Li ST, Klein MD, Gusic ME. Enhancing educational scholarship through conceptual frameworks: a challenge and roadmap for medical educators. Acad Pediatr. 2019;19(2):135–41.
11. Knowles MS. Self-directed learning: a guide for learners and teachers. Association Press; 1975
12. Loeng S. Self-directed learning: a core concept in adult education. Educ Res Int. 2020;2020.

13. Van Merriënboer JJ, Sweller J. Cognitive load theory in health professional education: design principles and strategies. Med Educ. 2010;44(1):85–93.
14. Kolb DA. Experience as the source of learning and development. Hoboken: Prentice Hall; 1984.
15. Kolb A, Kolb D. Eight important things to know about the experiential learning cycle. Aust Educ Leader. 2018;40(3):8.
16. Mishra P, Koehler MJ. Technological pedagogical content knowledge: a framework for teacher knowledge. Teachers College Record. 2006;108(6):1017–54.
17. Cook DA, Dupras DM. A practical guide to developing effective web-based learning. J Gen Intern Med. 2004;19(6):698–707.
18. O'Doherty D, Dromey M, Lougheed J, Hannigan A, Last J, McGrath D. Barriers and solutions to online learning in medical education—an integrative review. BMC Med Educ. 2018;18(1):130.
19. Wittich CM, Agrawal A, Wang AT, Halvorsen AJ, Mandrekar JN, Chaudhry S, Dupras DM, Oxentenko AS, Beckman TJ. Flipped classrooms in graduate medical education: a national survey of residency program directors. Acad Med. 2018;93(3):471–7.
20. Lyons MG. Open access is almost here: navigating through copyright, fair use, and the TEACH Act. J Contin Educ Nurs. 2010;41(2):57–64.
21. Moreau KA. Has the new Kirkpatrick generation built a better hammer for our evaluation toolbox? Med Teach. 2017;39(9):999–1001.
22. Richmond H, Copsey B, Hall AM, Davies D, Lamb SE. A systematic review and meta-analysis of online versus alternative methods for training licensed health care professionals to deliver clinical interventions. BMC Med Educ. 2017;17(1):227.
23. Pei L, Wu H. Does online learning work better than offline learning in undergraduate medical education? A systematic review and meta-analysis. Med Educ Online. 2019;24(1):1666538.

Simulation in Pediatric Critical Care

Anna Zanin

Contents

J. Brierley et al. (eds.), *ESPNIC Children's Intensive Care Textbook*,
https://doi.org/10.1007/978-3-031-64762-8_65

Learning Objectives

- Definition and understanding of experiential learning as a teaching strategy
- Advantages of simulation-based education in pediatric settings compared to standard education training
- Structure of the role-play simulated scenario session and the key role of the debriefing phase
- Role and definition of Crisis Resource Management principles in pediatric critical care education

65.1 Introduction

The evolution of medical education in recent years has been impressive and pointed out the importance of "experiential learning". John Dewey [1] was an early promoter of the idea of learning by action and reflection and defines it as "a process that allows the individual to build their own knowledge, develop skills and reinforce their values directly from experience" [1]. Based on Dewey's work, David Kolb conceptualized the process of experiential learning describing the different steps known as Kolb's cycle (◘ Fig. 65.1) [2]. This process is the basis of education through simulation and simulators that, before being applied in the medical environment, were initially used for the training and formation of aviation pilots and in a military context [3].

In medical education, we can recognise three distinct areas of learning: (a) patient-centered skills, (b) process-centered skills, and (c) environment-centered skills [4]. Patient-centered skills are those related to the direct care of patients, including communication skills and technical skills. Process-centered and environment-centered skills are fundamental to interact successfully with colleagues and the environment (management skills, situational awareness, teamwork skills,

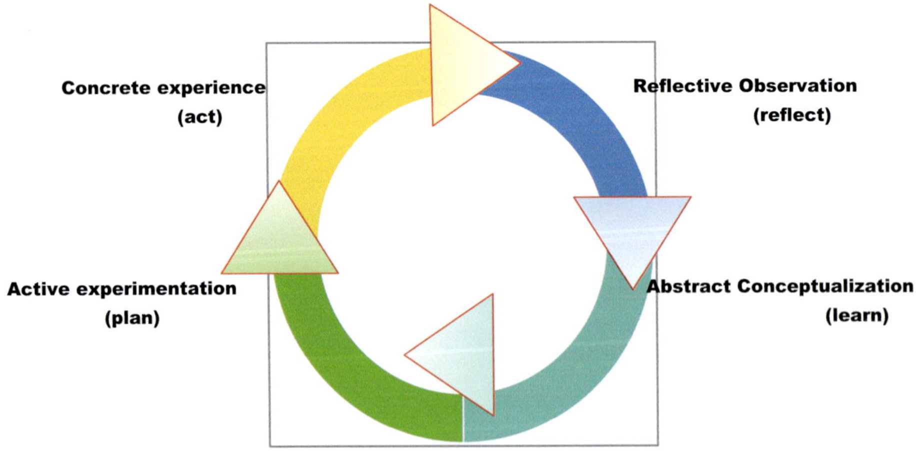

◘ **Fig. 65.1** Different component of experiential learning accordingly to Kolb's cycle: students have an experience (Concrete Experience), reflect on observations about that (Reflective Observation), analyze responses and formulate new ideas (Abstract Conceptualization), then actively test these new ideas in new situations (Active Experimentation)

Table 65.1 List of different simulation modalities

Simulation modalities
Standardized patient (actor)
Task trainer
Computerized case management scenarios (Virtual avatar/virtual environment)
Manikin
Role play (with or without simulators)

patient advocacy skills and self-directed learning skills, leadership). These are essential cognitive and behavioural skills required by all competent practitioners, especially in acute care settings, that can be collected in the concept of crisis resource management (CRM). This concept originates from the "crew resource management" applied in aviation [3], and it has been extended into different domains and specialties, also in medical settings.

In the late 1980s, David Gaba for the first time shifted the focus of traditional learning from technical aspects of patient management towards behavioural aspects of team performance. He developed a simulation training course, defining this tool "as a technique, not a technology, to replace or expand real experiences through guided experiences, which evoke or replicate substantial aspects of the real world, in a fully interactive way" [5] (Table 65.1). Simulation-based CRM training programs were rapidly developed in other high-risk, medical specialties, including pediatric critical care settings [6].

65.1.1 Challenges in Pediatric Critical Care Education

Medical education had been based for decades on internships where students with theoretical knowledge, experienced the "see one, do one, teach one" model, being directly in contact with patients. This model has shown its failures, especially in connection with a marked increase in the number of students, higher attention to prevention and clinical risk and, especially in intensive care units, a change in working practice with a higher service pressure and progressively a decreasing training time with a consequent reduction of exposure of young people to more complicated cases. This situation is even more marked in pediatric intensive care units (PICUs) where the resident or medical student is faced with rare and critical conditions that need specialized techniques and very high expertise. In PICUs most complex interventions and the most critical cases are infrequent, so, the interval between initial training and the concrete practice can be very long. Moreover, any senior clinician has to maintain his competencies and pursue lifelong training even when once formal training is completed. For all these peculiar characteristics, in this particular pediatric context, simulation has been very well accepted as an effective training tool, moving to a new concept: "See One, Sim One, Do One" [7].

65.2 Evolution of Paediatric Resuscitation Training

One of the main applications of simulation-based training (SBT) is advanced life support teaching. Over the years simulation has been used both as a teaching and evaluation methodology in pediatric resuscitation: from low-fidelity task trainers used for basic cardiopulmonary resuscitation (CPR) training to the more sophisticated technology supporting high-fidelity simulators with real-time feedback or even virtual reality.

65.2.1 History of CPR Training

It is interesting how the history of CPR has been tied since the beginning to the need for its teaching. In the 1940s Peter Safar and James Elam described the cardiopulmonary resuscitation techniques used up to that time, especially "mouth-to-mouth" ventilation [8, 9]. Dr. Safar immediately realized the need to train as many people as possible in CPR, even if they were not healthcare professionals (HCPs). He also commissioned Asmund Laerdal—a Norwegian toymaker—to design a life-size doll for him to model and teach CPR sessions. He was very sensitive to this issue because a few months before his drowned son was resuscitated with the same technique, so he enthusiastically took part in Safar's project. Dr. Safar has pioneered not only the establishment of CPR techniques and the need for its teaching but also the creation of out-of-hospital assistance services. These two points still remain fundamental pillars for the management and diffusion of medical and social awareness of cardiac arrest. In this context, the use of low-fidelity simulators has given the possibility of implementing the training of residents and senior doctors with standardized courses in addition to improving performance during CPR.

65.2.2 Quality CPR Training in Pediatrics

Historically, residents during their training in intensive care learned CPR and medical procedures directly in contact with the patient in the emergency department or the intensive care. These situations are much less frequent in children than in adult patients, so generally result in a lower degree of exposure to pediatricians. A study by Hunt et al. reported that the largest number of residents in the third year of residency had never participated in a real CPR code [10]. Knowing that the patient's outcome depends on the quality of resuscitation (Neumar et al. 2015), all CPR training programs such as Advance Pediatric Life Support (APLS), Pediatric Advanced Life Support (PALS), Neonatal Resuscitation Program (NRP) and equivalents over time have been implemented regularly and any pediatrician involved in acute care needs a re-certification every two to three years (Atkins et al. 2015; Machonochie et al. 2015).

Despite this ongoing training effort, several studies showed that trained health professionals do not perform high-quality resuscitation [11] and that standard education models do not guarantee the maintenance of competencies over time [12, 13].

In the same way, the teaching of CPR in recent years has been implemented, thanks to a greater focus on the quality of CPR [14–17]. Quality CPR (qCPR) improves the survival rate after sudden cardiac arrest, and rescuers should apply compressions with the correct depth (5–6 cm or 2–2.4 inches) of the correct frequency (100–120 compressions/min), ensuring not staying on the chest and keeping interruptions to an absolute minimum (compression fraction of the chest >60%) and finally avoiding excessive ventilation, following the 2015 guidelines (Atkins et al. 2015, 2017).

At this level, qCPR monitoring is necessary and SBT is giving concrete support: thanks to technological resources, it is quite accessible to have simulators or defibrillators with the use of feedback systems for the frequency, depth and interruption of live chest compressions, to generate a form of control over the quantitative part of the CPR. In addition, resuscitation teams must coordinate their efforts to ensure CPR also with qualitative values during cardiac arrest: this may be based on the assessment of the performance of the resuscitation teams or the physiological responses of patients to resuscitation manoeuvres, all of which must be continuously adjusted according to the response obtained. Despite these changes and interventions, Sutton et al. in their data on the qCPR underline that we have to take into account not only the quantitative and qualitative aspects but that the "CPR quality improves when feedback is combined with a structured training effort" [18].

65.2.3 Basic Concept of Role-Play Simulated Scenarios

Thanks to task trainers and mannequins it is possible to focus on the learning objectives for students and trainees towards quantitative aspects of CPR. This is a very important aspect of patient-centred skills that enable the learner to improve CPR psychomotor skill performance. In order to empower also the qualitative aspect of team behaviour, another aspect of SBT is required.

Role-play simulation is based on experiential learning: a specific scenario, designed according to the learning objectives, allows the learners "to react to problems or conditions as they would under genuine circumstances" [19]. This is a powerful technique that permits anyone participating in the scenario to have first-person experiences in a safe and supportive environment. In healthcare simulation, three phases are identified in each role-play session [20] (◘ Fig. 65.2):

- the briefing
- the simulated scenario
- the debriefing

The *briefing* is the very first part of the educational activity, essential to present the simulation session to the learners by the facilitators, to set the stage and familiarization with the equipment. This phase is very important because if not well planned, it can negatively affect also the debriefing [21]. At this point it is also important to set a sort of a fictional contract between the participants and the facilitators, inviting them to "suspend disbelief" regarding potential limitations of the simulation and reassuring them about the confidentiality in order to guarantee a real safe learning environment [22]. In general, the group of learners is divided into *participants* and *observers* in the *scenario* phase. Participants are acting first while the observers are watching the simulation with a live audio and video stream in a classroom, and then they switch. The scenario can be run in a dedicated simulation laboratory and in situ,

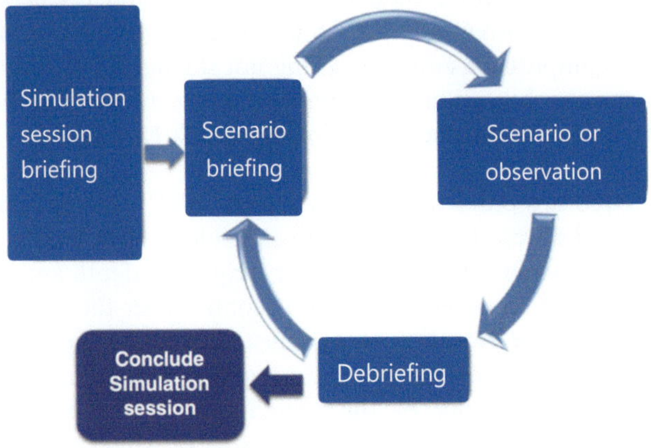

Fig. 65.2 General simulation session process diagram (modified from Oriot D, Alinier G (2018) Pocket Book for Simulation Debriefing in Healthcare. Springer International Publishing)

directly in the ward. The last and most important component of the SBT session is the *debriefing* [23]. It has been defined as a facilitated "post-event analysis" encounter or as a "learner-centred technique, non-offensive, in order to help a professional or a team to improve one's performance by a reflective practice" conversation [24]. The debriefing phase is a valuable moment for the learners where they can reflect on their actions in the scenario and discuss within the team and the facilitators. They can analyse their reactions starting from their feelings, explore and understand their actions, review the best evidence guidelines and recommendations through an abstraction process, and finally identify which learning points they can transfer into their future practice. The debriefing allows the facilitators to discuss not only technical skills but also human factors [25] and CRM principles [26]. The introduction of this kind of analysis in addition to standard education has shown how the learning and maintenance of knowledge and skills are much greater than standard education [27, 28]. This phase is also the most challenging one for the facilitators who need adequate training in conducting the debriefing and in the technical aspects of simulation.

65.2.4 Importance of Simulation and Debriefing in CPR Training

The introduction of SBT and retrospective debriefing systems have been developed widely and radically changed the structure of the education program related to resuscitation [14, 16]. This process has led to a deeper analysis of the information that emerged during simulated scenarios and also boosted clinicians to start debriefing real resuscitation codes, applying "debriefing rules" as a part of the implementation of local quality systems. Systematic use of debriefing, the presence of supervisors (or "coach") monitoring the performance of resuscitators [27] and broader involvement in multicenter registries are the concrete signs of a revolution that is impacting not only education but also patients' outcomes [27, 29]. A simulation, regardless if it involves standardized patients (SPs), computerized case management scenarios, mannequins, simulators or a combination of these methods, guarantees the safety of the patient and also the psychological safety of the student and the environment, keeping in mind that the ultimate aim is to improve patient outcome [30].

These results confirm that the ability to perform complex procedures requires a balance of psychomotor skills, knowledge, clinical judgment, communicative ability, decision-making capacity, and not only technical performance. Many different forms of education programs in pediatric critical care settings are integrated with simulation because to improve the quality of CPR or any other technique, it is mandatory to develop CRM principles and teamwork.

65.3 Crisis Resource Management in Pediatric Resuscitation Teams

CRM principles have been described widely [31, 32] covering some key behaviours such as leadership and followership, communication, teamwork, material resource use, and situational awareness (◘ Table 65.2).

65.3.1 Leadership and Followership

Effective resuscitation teams require effective leadership [33] and effective followership. A team should include a team leader and additional team members with clearly assigned roles. The team leader is responsible for monitoring other members' actions, maintaining an overall view of the patient, and synthesizing key information from the team and adapting to the changes in the situation. Team members should have a clear and common view of the team's goals, to perceive their individual roles within the team, to support each other, and feel free to ask for help if needed or share information with the rest of the team [34]. This process of continuing fruitful interactions between the team leader and the team members is a concept defined as "flattening hierarchy" [35]. Extending this training to a multidisciplinary staff and including junior doctors in the management of acute response can potentially produce a change in the culture of the participants. It is possible to empower and point out the advantages of this flattened hierarchy with a safe environment that allows anyone to speak up with the common ultimate aim of achieving a safer intervention.

65.3.2 Communication

Most of the medical errors reported are caused primarily by a failure in communication [36]. Effective communication is crucial for a successful team and important to establish a collaborative environment. Communication should be complete, clear, brief, and timely [33]. There are some strategies to enhance this including: (1) assertive communication, (2) closed-loop communication, and (3) information sharing and inquiry [6].

- *Assertive communication* is the ability to express positive and negative ideas and feelings in a respectful, honest and direct way to any member of the team. It recognises our rights while respecting the rights and the roles of others,

Table 65.2 Tips for incorporating crisis resource management elements into simulated paediatric scenarios (from Oriot D, Alinier G (2018) Pocket Book for Simulation Debriefing in Healthcare. Springer International Publishing)

Crisis resource management principles	Strategy to incorporate crisis resource management principle into the scenario
Leadership	Wave effect[a]—introduce team members in a sequential fashion (e.g., nurses → residents → fellows) Introduce a new team member Introduce a potential new team leader (e.g., critical care physician, anesthesiologist) Introduce a parent or caregiver as a potential distractor
Communication	Take people out of their comfort zone (e.g., start scenario without nurses/without doctors) Introduce "handover," e.g., paramedic handing over to emergency team; nursing handover at shift change Introduce a scripted medication error Withhold information (e.g., relevant medical history) Give critical information to a team member (e.g., blood glucose) during crisis point in scenario (e.g., cardiac arrest) Introduce a parent or caregiver as a potential distractor Use phone calls
Teamwork (human resources)	Challenge team with multiple tasks/problems (e.g., hypoglycemia, seizure, hypotension, respiratory arrest) Wave effect[a]—introduce team members in a sequential fashion (e.g., nurses → residents → fellows) Introduce a junior team member (e.g., medical student) Introduce parents or team members who are distractors Introduce a team member who makes some mistakes Use phone calls Provide fewer team members
Resource use	Withhold critical equipment (e.g., defibrillator) Provide broken or improperly sized equipment (e.g., rupture endotracheal tube cuff) Provide an abundance of resources (e.g., scatter multiple endotracheal tubes on top of crash cart) Use a phone call to introduce the case and allow time for team to prepare for resuscitation (e.g., trauma arriving to emergency department)
Situational awareness	Design challenging scenario with more frequent physiological changes Design scenario history, physical or case progression to promote fixation error (e.g., cardiogenic shock from myocarditis presenting as vomiting and diarrhea) Challenge team leader to prioritize by providing laboratory and radiology results or introducing team members during critical points in scenario (e.g., during intubation) Introduce a team member who makes mistakes

helping again to "flatten the hierarchy". This can represent a constructive communication strategy to compare different positions and find a mutually satisfying solution.

- *Closed-loop* communication: once the team leader has requested information or asked for a procedure to be performed by a named person, the members of the team should acknowledge the request explicitly and confirm when it is done.
- *Information-sharing and inquiry* refers to an ongoing process of knowledge-sharing and corrective action when necessary. This can help to prevent inappropriate actions and the development of fixation errors [6].

65.3.3 Use of Resources

Optimal resource use includes appropriate management of *human* resources and also *equipment* and *cognitive aids.*

It is very important to ensure the presence and participation of the appropriate team in terms of the number of HCPs, in order to avoid that individual team members can rapidly become overwhelmed if asked to perform too many tasks. Furthermore, an appropriate allocation of roles to qualified team members is mandatory. During medical emergencies, teams have sometimes to perform a multitude of tasks simultaneously and often beyond their skill set. If possible, teams should distribute roles and tasks paying attention to the overall workload and trying to preplan as much as possible at the beginning of a critical situation.

The management of material resources will depend on the specific needs of the team and the complexity of the situation. In general, teams should be aware of the equipment available and eventually be able to call for help early and activate additional resources if needed. Critical situations are also a stress test to identify if the correct equipment is used properly by designated personnel.

65.3.4 Situational Awareness

Situational awareness has been defined as an individual's ability to perceive relevant data from their surroundings, process the information, and determine its impact on current goals and utilise this understanding to predict future events [37]. The capacity of the team to continually reassess a patient, updating each member of the team on the current situation is defined as "shared cognition" or "shared mental model". This overall collective thought process [38] is very important to find out the right decision or approach for the patient.

In pediatric acute care medicine as in all acute care settings, the coordination of resuscitation teams is crucial to deliver a safe and effective treatment. Team members function in a dynamic fashion and great attention has to be paid to each member's behaviour. CRM will help teams to deliver coordinated and effective care to critically ill children and represent an effective tool in emergency training [39, 40]. The staff trained in this way has the possibility to experience the meaning of changing roles when appropriate, how to choose priorities and completing tasks, and moreover how to communicate to minimize errors and optimize safety.

65.4 Future Perspectives

In the following section some new simulation-based education models, applied to pediatric critical care settings, are briefly presented.

65.4.1 Rapid Cycle Deliberate Practice and Repeated Encounters

Shorter and more repeated educational encounters over time have been shown to be more efficient than longer and punctual standard training formats, increasing significantly the retention of learning [41, 42]. This strategy has been used as an effective implementation program, increasing the confidence of HCPs in managing the critical child [43]. Rapid-Cycle Deliberate Practice (RCDP) is a simulation-based instructional strategy that focuses on the rapid acquisition of defined skills where students have multiple opportunities to perform the procedure, receiving live feedback correcting their gaps [44]. In this way the students are exposed to micro-debriefing during the activity and have the possibility to reflect during the action, eventually stopping to discuss, and then trying the procedure again. Some recent studies have taught how this technique can be applied effectively in the teaching of skills training such as intubation [45]. Compared with traditional debriefing, this strategy provides the opportunity for an immediate repetitive practice [46], with immediate and direct feedback and assessment of the learner.

65.4.2 Gaming

"Simulation gaming" or "serious game" (as computer-based video games) identify games with a special focus on education. These terms generally are used when a game structure is applied in a context where traditionally it is not present. In medical education, it is integrated with other training strategies to increase the degree of involvement of the attendees, regardless they are new millennial students or more senior learners. Ghoman et al. reviewing the games available for neonatology training, show how these games have the potential to improve health professionals' knowledge, technical skills, and adherence to resuscitation algorithms [47]. The authors analyzed 12 games dedicated to learning neonatology topics (4 board games, 5 video games and 3 virtual reality games) capable of enhancing knowledge in professionals as a valid alternative or resource to complement traditional SBT courses. Games can increase working memory, improve decision-making capacity and also positively influence teamwork [48].

The added value of these games is the possibility of using them without time or space limits, together with the freedom of choosing the topic without following a compulsory scheme, according to the learner's need [15, 17, 49]. In addition, games can be exported in areas with limited resources and in low- or middle-income countries, although accessibility to computers, networks, and smartphones as the initial costs for software development and updating represent some clear limitations [47].

As virtual games guarantee immediate feedback, they can be used easily as assessment tools [50], for example as pre- or post-evaluation of a frontal course.

Another form of gaming is represented by direct competitions of residents, on role-play simulated scenarios with national or international diffusion in multiple specialties (SIMCUP, SimWars, Pediatric simulation games, etc.) [51, 52]. The residents or fellows are divided into teams in a real competition where knowledge and skills related to a defined topic are tested.

The success of serious games is associated with self-determination theory: this has two basic aspects related to the intrinsic motivation of the student (the amusement related to the activity) and the extrinsic motivation (the evaluation of the activity only as an external reward or penalty). Both are related to the wish to play and improve knowledge [53].

Whether the application of gaming in medical training really improves the learning process and the acquisition of long-term knowledge is still an open question. Further investigations are also needed to understand if there are some conditions that can enhance or reduce the learning process (gamification in action).

65.4.3 Boot Camp

Over the last 10 years in the United States, it is common practice to organise educational meetings called "boot camps", right before the beginning of the residency or fellowship. They consist of an intensive curriculum (from 5 days to 10 weeks) characterized by a training plan of simulations and activities aimed at a specific subspecialty, in order to help future residents to recognize their gaps. This model has been exported worldwide not only for residences but also as a transition plan from medical school to residency [54–56].

Between 2004 and 2011, in Israel, 85 workshops including 4172 trainees participated in a national annual boot camp: 85% of the participants considered this project essential for professional development and 87% recommended it as mandatory [7].

In the United States, since 2009, a common orientation boot camp for pediatric intensive care fellows has been organized by nine institutions (two days and a half). High-fidelity simulation topics cover airway management, vascular access, resuscitation, sepsis, trauma, cranial trauma, and how to deliver bad news to parents. In the first report of 2009, each fellow had 15.5 h of training distributed as 2.75 h in a group for didactic sessions (17.7%), 1.08 h for interaction in small groups (7.0%), 4.67 h for task training (30.1%), and 7 h for training (45.2%) with high fidelity simulators and CRM. A questionnaire revealed that this type of training has been highly appreciated by students and has been very effective in improving clinical performance and increasing confidence [57].

65.4.4 Coaching, Codes and Mock Codes

Dr. Betsy Hunt and her team at Johns Hopkins Children's Center have recently introduced the concept of CPR Coach. They have developed a prospective observational study on the quality of compressions during in-hospital cardiac arrest associated with an implementation and development program (bundle) [27]. The objectives were (1) implementing the debriefing program, (2) identifing the obstacles to performing effective compressions, (3) developing a resuscitation quality bundle, and (4) evaluating the impact of these measures. The resuscitation quality bundle called CODE ACES2 includes: CPR Coaching, evaluation of objective states, phrases chanted to actions, choreography, ergonomics, structured debriefing and simulation. During the simulations, as in real life, there is a dedicated person called "CPR coach" who stays by the defibrillator, focused on the quality of the CPR performed by the team, giving positive reinforcements and following corrections [28]. The coach provides corrective information, and ensures coordination between ventilations, compressions and breaks that may suggest a team change if fatigue in rescuers overlaps.

In Cheng's prospective and observational multicenter study, it has been shown how the teams exposed to the coach's presence have performed more effective compressions and ventilations than the group that only had technological feedback. The authors point out how all the monitoring technologies are not able to replace the need for human supervision which is much more effective during cardiopulmonary resuscitation. Hunt et al.'s data confirm that updating the CPR coach added to all other CODE ACES2 measures has led to progressive implementation during the years of adherence to the AHA CPR guidelines 44.3% in 2015 (35.3–53.3) versus 19.9% (6.9–32.9) in 2013; (odds ratio 3.2 [95% confidence interval: 1.3–8.1], $P = 0.01$). Another comment that comes out of these studies is the need for a dedicated team for the emergency of cardiopulmonary resuscitation. In the different countries and also in the different university hospitals, these teams have an extremely varied composition. The application of the model proposed for Dr. Hunt offers a clear and effective line of application, surely the dedicated repeated practice of these teams also with the introduction of a "mock code" for training is the key to success and improvement of outcomes.

Andreatta et al. present the experience of a false emergency call (mock code) every month for 4 years. After one year there was a 17% increase in survival after cardiac arrest [39] in their institution. More studies are necessary to define the clinical impact of learning in the simulation environment. There are still very few studies in the literature highlighting how increased patient safety and patient outcomes are associated with SBT.

65.4.5 Telesimulation

Telesimulation is an innovative educational model that has been developed in recent decades. In 2016 a new definition was approved by the Society for Simulation in Healthcare (SSH) defining telesimulation as "a process in which telecommunication of simulation courses is used to give teaching education to evaluate students who are in another place" [58]. Through internet connection distances are abolished and it is possible to spread knowledge very quickly and effectively, for example, to countries with fewer resources [59] or rural areas [60, 61]. A specific application in pediatric and neonatal intensive care units (NICUs) is the Managing Emergencies in Pediatric Anesthesia (MEPA) course that allows the participation of students who are very far from the place where the training takes place [62]. Donohue et al. report their experience at UC Davis Children's Hospital where, for 8 years, they offered training in neonatal resuscitation and urgent consultation via telemedicine to rural communities lacking a NICU consultant. In this case, thanks to the combination of telesimulation and telemedicine, it has been possible to increase the quality of care and reduce the difference in care between neonates born in a third-level center and those in first- and second-level centres [63]. The problem of centralization of neonatal care affects several countries. Another recent contribution by Dr. Gross [64] evidences in a prospective monocentric randomized neonatal simulation study, the superiority of having a neonatal team leader ("teleleader") versus a remote "consultant" ("teleconsultant"). The possibility of having technical resources to conduct a remote simulation also offers the possibility of teledebriefing on scenarios that take place at a distance. In the medical education community, since February 2020, due to the SARS-COV-2 outbreak, social distancing transformed classrooms and universities into online remote learning platforms [65]. Some reports of interactive telesimulation programs or hybrid approaches have been successfully reported in providing timely education during a coronavirus pandemic [66]. The current market offers almost unlimited connection options and many free or low-cost applications to potentially connect teachers and students. Once educators are familiar with these resources, the learning objectives and educational contents are identified, and it will be easily possible to start programming [67].

Take Home Messages

- Simulation-based training (SBT) is founded on experiential learning, the learner can build his own knowledge, and develop technical and non-technical skills directly from experience.
- The development of SBT has been driven by the dual aspect of the patient's and the learner's safety.
- Simulation is a "technique" with several modalities that can be differently applied according to the learning objective: there is no "one size fits all".
- The principles of crisis resource management (CRM) can help prevent and manage difficulties during medical care from both an individual and team-oriented point of view.
- There is growing evidence in the literature that procedural and teamwork skills are enhanced by SBT.
- There is a need for more studies to elucidate if the use of SBT and debriefing improves patient outcomes.

? Questions

1. Describe Kolb's cycle and the experiential learning.
2. How is crisis resource management defined?
3. List and define some effective communication strategies.
4. What is the debriefing phase in a role-play simulation?

✓ Answers

1. Kolb's learning theory is a ► learning theory based on experiential learning, a process that allows the individual to build his knowledge and develop skills directly from experience. It is a four-stage cycle. It starts from concrete learning, passing through reflective observation, abstract conceptualization and finally active experimentation. Effective learning can be seen when the learner progresses through the cycle.

2. The concept of Crisis Resource Management (CRM) collects a set of principles dealing with interpersonal interactions and behaviours that HCPs experience in their daily practice: leadership and followership, communication, teamwork and resource use, and situational awareness. They can contribute to optimal team functioning during crises.
3. *Assertive communication* is the ability to express positive and negative ideas and feelings in a respectful, direct way to any member of the team. *Closed-loop* communication is based on the integration of the answer by any member of the team to the team leader, with an acknowledgement of the request and a confirmation when the action is done. *Information-sharing and inquiry* refer to an ongoing process of knowledge-sharing and corrective action when necessary during a crisis.
4. The debriefing phase is the last and most important part of the role-play simulation session, after performing the scenario. In this phase, the students can reflect on their actions and discuss with the team and the facilitators. They can analyse their reactions starting from their feelings, explore and understand their actions, review the best evidence guidelines and recommendations through an abstraction process, and finally identify which learning points they can transfer into their future practice.

▪▪ Guidelines

1. Meaney PA, Bobrow BJ, Mancini ME, Christenson J, de Caen A, Bhanji F, et al. Cardiopulmonary resuscitation quality: [corrected] improving cardiac resuscitation outcomes both inside and outside the hospital: a consensus statement from the American Heart Association. Circulation. 2013;128(4):417–35.
2. Neumar RW, Shuster M, Callaway CW, Gent LM, Atkins DL, Bhanji F, et al. 2015 American Heart Association guidelines update for cardiopulmonary resuscitation and emergency cardiovascular care. Circulation. 2015;132 Suppl 2:S315–S367.
3. Atkins DL, Berger S, Duff JP, Gonzales JC, Hunt EA, Joyner BL, et al. Part 11: Pediatric basic life support and cardiopulmonary resuscitation quality 2015 American Heart Association guidelines update for cardiopulmonary resuscitation and emergency cardiovascular care. Circulation. 2015;132:S519–S525.
4. Atkins DL, de Caen AR, Berger S, Samson RA, Schexnayder SM, Joyner BL Jr, et al. 2017 American Heart Association focused update on pediatric basic life support and cardiopulmonary resuscitation quality: an update to the American Heart Association guidelines for cardiopulmonary resuscitation and emergency cardiovascular care. Circulation. 2018;137(1):e1–e6.
5. Maconochie IK, Bingham R, Eich C, López-Herce J, Rodríguez- Núñez A, Rajka T, et al. European resuscitation council guidelines for resuscitation 2015 section 6. Paediatric life support. Resuscitation. 2015; 95:223–248.

References

1. Dewey J. Experience and education. New York: MacMillan; 1938.
2. Kolb D. Experiential learning: Experience as the source of learning and development. Hoboken: Prentice-Hall; 1984.
3. Rosen KR. The history of medical simulation. J Crit Care. 2008;23:157–66.
4. Lane JL, Slavin L, Ziv A. Simulation in medical education: a review. Simul Gaming. 2001;32(3):297–314.
5. Gaba DM. The future vision of simulation in health care. Qual Saf Health Care. 2004;13(Suppl 1):i2–i10.
6. Cheng A, Donoghue A, Gilfoyle E, Eppich W. Simulation-based crisis resource management training for pediatric critical care medicine: a review for instructors. Pediatr Crit Care Med. 2012;13(2):226–7.
7. Minha S, Shefet D, Sagi D, Berkenstadt H, Ziv A. "See One, Sim One, Do One"—A national pre-internship boot-camp to ensure a safer "Student to Doctor" transition. PLoS One. 2016;11(3):e0150122. https://doi.org/10.1371/journal.pone.0150122.
8. Elam JO. Rediscovery of expired air methods for emergency ventilation. In: Safar P, editor. Advances in cardiopulmonary resuscitation. New York: Springer Verlag; 1977. p. 263–5.
9. Safar P. History of cardiopulmonary-cerebral resuscitation. In: Kay W, Bircher N, editors. Cardiopulmonary resuscitation. New York: Churchill Livingston; 1989. p. 1–53.
10. Hunt EA, Patel S, Vera K, Shaffner DH, Pronovost PJ. Survey of paediatric resident experiences with resuscitation training and attendance at actual cardiopulmonary arrests. Pediatr Crit Care Med. 2009;10(1):96–105.
11. Sutton RM, Niles D, French B, et al. First quantitative analysis of cardiopulmonary resuscitation quality during in-hospital cardiac arrests of young children. Resuscitation. 2014;85(1):70–4.
12. Grant EC, Marczinski CA, Menon K. Using paediatric advanced life support in paediatric residency training: does the curriculum need resuscitation? Pediatr Crit Care Med. 2007;8(5):433–9.
13. Hunt EA, Hohenhaus SM, Luo X, Frush KS. Simulation of paediatric trauma stabilization in 35 North Carolina emergency departments: identification of targets for performance improvement. Paediatrics. 2006;117(3):641–8.
14. Cheng A, Brown LL, Duff JP, et al. Improving cardiopulmonary resuscitation with a CPR feedback device and refresher simulations (CPR CARES study). JAMA Pediatr. 2015a;169(2):137.
15. Rutledge C, Walsh C, Swinger N, Auerbach M, Castro D, Dewan M, et al.; for the Quality Cardiopulmonary Resuscitation (QCPR) leaderboard investigators of the International Network for Simulation-based Pediatric Innovation, Research, and Education (INSPIRE). Gamification in action: theoretical and practical considerations for medical educators. Acad Med. 2018a;93(7):1014–1020.
16. Cheng A, Donoghue A, Bhanji F. Time to incorporate real-time CPR feedback and CPR debriefings into advanced life support courses. Resuscitation. 2015b;5(90):e3–4. https://doi.org/10.1016/j.resuscitation.2015.02.012.
17. Rutledge C, Walsh C, Swinger N, Auerbach M, Castro D, Dewan M, Khattab M, Rake A, Harwayne-Gidansky I, Raymond TT, Maa T, et al.; Quality Cardiopulmonary Resuscitation (QCPR) Leaderboard Investigators of the International Network for Simulation-based Pediatric Innovation, Research, and Education (INSPIRE). Gamification in action: theoretical and practical considerations for medical educators. Acad Med. 2018b;93(7):1014-1020.
18. Sutton M, et al. "Putting it all together" to improve resuscitation quality. Emerg Med Clin North Am. 2012;30(1):105–22.
19. Tekian A, McGuire C, McGaghie W. Innovative simulations for assessing professional competence: from paper-and-pencil to virtual reality. Illinois: University of Illinois Chicago; 1999.

20. Oriot D, Alinier G. Pocket book for simulation debriefing in healthcare. Springer International Publishing; 2018.
21. Lioce L, Meakim CH, Fey MK, Chmil JV, Mariani B, Alinier G. Standards of best practice: simulation standard IX: simulation design. Clin Simul Nurs. 2015;11(6):309–15.
22. Dieckmann P, Gaba D, Rall M. Deepening the theoretical foundations of patient simulation as social practice. Simul Healthc. 2007;2(3):183–93.
23. Fanning RM, Gaba DM. The role of debriefing in simulation-based learning. Simul Healthc. 2007;2(2):115–25.
24. O'Donnell J, Rodgers D, Lee W, Edelson D, Haag J, Hamilton M, et al. Structured and supported debriefing. Dallas: American Heart Association; 2009.
25. Carayon P. Handbook of human factors and ergonomics in health care and patient safety. Boca Raton: CRC Press; 2011.
26. Gaba D, Howard SK, Fish KJ, Smith BE, Sowb Y. Simulation-based training in anesthesia crisis resource management (ACRM): a decade of experience. Simul Gaming. 2001;32(2):175–93.
27. Hunt E, Jeffers J, McNamara L, Newton H, Ford K, Bernier M. Improved CPR performance with CODE-ACES2, a resuscitation quality bundle. J Am Heart Assoc. 2018;7(24):e009860. https://doi.org/10.1161/JAHA.118.009860.
28. Cheng A, Kessler D, Lin Y, et al. Influence of cardiopulmonary resuscitation coaching and provider role on perception of cardiopulmonary resuscitation quality during simulated pediatric cardiac arrest. Pediatr Crit Care Med. 2019;20(4):e191–8.
29. Reeder RW, Girling A, Wolfe H, Holubkov R, Berg RA, et al.; on behalf of Eunice Kennedy Shriver National Institute of Child Health and Human Development Collaborative Pediatric Critical Care Research Network (CPCCRN). Improving outcomes after pediatric cardiac arrest—the ICU-resuscitation project: study protocol for a randomized controlled trial. Trials. 2018;19(1):213. https://doi.org/10.1186/s13063-018-2590-y.
30. Aggarwal R, Mytton OT, Derbrew M, Hananel D, Heydenburg M, Issenberg B, et al. Training and simulation for patient safety. Qual Saf Health Care. 2010;19(Suppl 2):i34–43.
31. Risser DT, Rice MM, Salisbury ML, et al.; The MedTeams Research Consortium. The potential for improved teamwork to reduce medical errors in the emergency department. Ann Emerg Med. 1999;34:373–383.
32. Brindley P, Cardinal P. Optimizing crisis resource management to improve patient safety and team performance—A handbook for acute care health professionals: ©Royal College of Physicians and Surgeons of Canada; 2017. Endorsed by the Canadian Critical Care Society and Canadian Association of Critical Care Nurses. isbn:978-1-926588-41-4. Accessed 31 May 2020.
33. Clancy CM, Tornberg DN. TeamSTEPPS: assuring optimal teamwork in clinical settings. Am J Med Qual. 2007;22(3):214–7.
34. Burtscher MJ, Manser T. Team mental models and their potential to improve teamwork and safety: a review and implications for future research in healthcare. Saf Sci. 2012;50:1344–54.
35. Clapper TC. TeamSTEPPS® is an effective tool to level the hierarchy in healthcare communication by empowering all stakeholders. J Commun Healthc. 2018;11(4):241–4.
36. Joint Commission International Center for Patient Safety. Communication: a critical component in delivering quality care. Oak-brook Terrace: Joint Commission on Accreditation of Healthcare Organizations; 2009.
37. Schulz CM, Endsley MR, Kochs EF, Gelb AW, Wagner KJ. Situation awareness in anesthesia: concept and research. Anesthesiology. 2013;118(3):729–42.
38. Eppich WJ, Brannen M, Hunt EA. Team training: implications for emergency and critical care pediatrics. Curr Opin Pediatr. 2008;20:255–60.
39. Andreatta P, Saxton E, Thompson M, Annich G. Simulation-based mock codes significantly correlate with improved paediatric patient cardiopulmonary arrest survival rates. Pediatr Crit Care Med. 2011;12(1):33–8.
40. Shapiro MJ, Morey JC, Small SD, et al. Simulation based teamwork training for emergency department staff: does it improve clinical team performance when added to an existing didactic teamwork curriculum? Qual Saf Health Care. 2004;13:417–21.
41. Kerfoot BP. Adaptive spaced education improves learning efficiency: a randomized controlled trial. J Urol. 2010;183(2):678–81.

42. Toppino TC, Fearnow-Kenney MD, Kiepert MH, Teremula AC. The spacing effect in intentional and incidental free recall by children and adults: limits on the automaticity hypothesis. Mem Cognit. 2009;37(3):316–25.
43. Ojha R, Liu A, Rai D, Nanan R. Review of simulation in pediatrics: the evolution of a revolution. Front Pediatr. 2015;3:106.
44. Hunt EA, Duval-Arnould JM, Nelson-McMillan KL, Bradshaw JH, Diener-West M, Perretta JS, Shilkofski NA. Pediatric resident resuscitation skills improve after "rapid cycle deliberate practice" training. Resuscitation. 2014;85:945–51.
45. Gross IT, Abrahan DG, Kumar A, et al. Rapid cycle deliberate practice (RCDP) as a method to improve airway management skills—A randomized controlled simulation study. Cureus. 2019;11(9):e5546.
46. Doughty C, Welch-Horan T, Hsu D, Fielder E, Pereira F, Little-Wienert K, Kaziny B, McManemy J, Lemke D. Rapid cycle deliberate practice pediatric simulation scenarios. MedEdPORTAL Publications; 2015. Accessed 31 May 2020.
47. Ghoman SK, et al. Serious games, a game changer in teaching neonatal resuscitation? A review. Arch Dis Child Fetal Neonatal Ed. 2020;105(1):98–107.
48. Langhan TS, Rigby IJ, Walker IW, et al. Simulation-based training in critical resuscitation procedures improves residents' competence. CJEM. 2009;11:535–9.
49. Williams J, Jones D, Walker R. Consideration of using virtual reality for teaching neonatal resuscitation to midwifery students. Nurse Educ Pract. 2018;31:126–9.
50. Cutumisu M, Patel SD, Brown MRG, et al. RETAIN: a board game that improves neonatal resuscitation knowledge retention. Front Pediatr. 2019;7(1):13. https://doi.org/10.3389/fped.2019.00013. eCollection 2019.
51. Ingrassia PL, Franc JM, Carenzo L. A novel simulation competition format as an effective instructional tool in post-graduate medical education. Adv Simul (Lond). 2018;3(17):2–8.
52. Okuda Y, Godwin SA, Jacobson L, Wang E, Weingart S. SimWars. J Emerg Med. 2014;47(5):586–93.
53. Young J. Using a role-play simulation game to promote systems thinking. J Contin Educ Nurs. 2018;49:10–1.
54. Dversdal RK, Gold JA, Richards MH, Chiovaro MH, Iossi KA, Mansoor AM, et al. A 5-day intensive curriculum for interns utilizing simulation and active-learning techniques: addressing domains important across internal medicine practice. BMC Res Notes. 2018;11(1):916. https://doi.org/10.1186/s13104-018-4011-4.
55. Lerner V, Higgins EE, Winkel A. Re-boot: simulation elective for medical students as preparation bootcamp for obstetrics and gynecology residency. Cureus. 2018;10(6):e2811. https://doi.org/10.7759/cureus.2811.
56. Karmali RJ, Sim JM, You DZ, Spano S, Winthrop AL, Rudan JF, et al. The Surgical Skills and Technology Elective Program (SSTEP): a comprehensive simulation-based surgical skills initiative for preclerkship medical students. Am J Surg. 2018;216(2):375–81. https://doi.org/10.1016/j.amjsurg.2017.09.012.
57. Nishisaki A, Hales R, Biagas K, Cheifetz I, Corriveau C, Garber N, et al. A multi-institutional high-fidelity simulation "boot camp" orientation and training program for first year pediatric critical care fellows. Pediatr Crit Care Med. 2009;10(2):157–62.
58. Official IMSH. Onsite program guide. 2016. http://www.ssih.org/Portals/48/IMSH%202016/IMSH2016-Onsite-web.pdf. Accessed 31 May 2020.
59. Mikrogianakis A, Kam A, Silver S, et al. Telesimulation: an innovative and effective tool for teaching novel intraosseous insertion techniques in developing countries. Acad Emerg Med. 2011;18:420–7.
60. Okrainec A, Smith L, Azzie G. Surgical simulation in Africa: the feasibility and impact of a 3-day fundamentals of laparoscopic surgery course. Surg Endosc. 2009;23:2493–8.
61. Reznick R, MacRae H. Teaching surgical skills—changes in the wind. N Engl J Med. 2006;355:2664–9.
62. Everett T, Ng E, Power D, et al. The managing emergencies in paediatric anaesthesia global rating scale is a reliable tool for simulation-based assessment in pediatric anaesthesia crisis management. Paediatr Anaesth. 2013;23:1117–23.
63. Donohue L, Hoffmann K, Marcin J. Use of telemedicine to improve neonatal resuscitation. Children (Basel). 2019;6(4):50. https://doi.org/10.3390/children6040050.

64. Gross IT, Whitfill T, Redmond B, Couturier K, Bhatnagar A, Joseph M, et al. Comparison of two telemedicine delivery modes for neonatal resuscitation support: a simulation-based randomized trial. Neonatology. 2020;117(2):159–66. https://doi.org/10.1159/000504853. Epub ahead of print.
65. Association of American Medical Colleges. Updated interim guidance for medical students' participation in patient care during the Coronavirus (COVID-19) outbreak. 2020. https://www.aamc.org/news-insights/press-releases/updated-interim-guidance-medical-students-participation-patient-care-during-coronavirus-covid-19. Accessed 31 May 2020.
66. Naik N, Finkelstein RA, Howell J, Rajwani K, Ching K. Telesimulation for COVID-19 ventilator management training with social-distancing restrictions during the coronavirus pandemic. Simul Gaming. 2020;51(4):571–7. https://doi.org/10.1177/1046878120926561.
67. McCoy CE, Sayegh J, Alrabah R, Yarris MK. Telesimulation: an innovative tool for health professions education. AEM Educ Train. 2017;1:132–6.

MIX
Papier aus verantwortungsvollen Quellen
Paper from responsible sources
FSC® C105338

If you have any concerns about our products,
you can contact us on
ProductSafety@springernature.com

In case Publisher is established outside the EU,
the EU authorized representative is:
Springer Nature Customer Service Center GmbH
Europaplatz 3, 69115 Heidelberg, Germany

Printed by Libri Plureos GmbH
in Hamburg, Germany